Anesthesiologist's Manual of Surgical Procedures

Second Edition

Editors

Richard A. Jaffe, M.D., Ph.D.
Associate Professor of Anesthesia

and

Stanley I. Samuels, M.B., B.Ch., F.F.A.R.C.S.
Professor of Anesthesia

Stanford University School of Medicine
Stanford, California

LIPPINCOTT WILLIAMS & WILKINS
A **Wolters Kluwer** Company
Philadelphia • Baltimore • New York • London
Buenos Aires • Hong Kong • Sydney • Tokyo

Acquisitions Editor: R. Craig Percy
Developmental Editor: Dee Mosteller
Production Editor: Tim Reynolds
Manufacturing Manager: Robert Pancotti
Cover Designer: David Levy
Indexer: Dee Mosteller
Compositor: QualiType, Inc.
Printer: Courier Westford

Illustrations new to this edition were rendered by Laura Pardi Duprey.

Printed in the United States of America

9 8 7 6 5 4

Library of Congress Cataloging-in-Publication Data

Anesthesiologist's manual of surgical procedures / editors, Richard A. Jaffe and Stanley I. Samuels, with 115 contributors. —2nd ed.
p. cm.
Includes bibliographical references and index.
ISBN 0-7817-1471-0
1. Anesthesiology—Handbooks, manuals, etc. 2. Surgery, Operative—Handbooks, manuals, etc. 3. Operations, Surgical—Handbooks, manuals, etc. I. Jaffe, Richard A. II. Samuels, Stanley I.
[DNLM: 1. Anesthesia—methods. 2. Surgical Procedures, Operative. WO 235A5795 1999]
RD82.2.A54 1999
617.9′6—dc21
DNLM/DLC
For Library of Congress 98-34027
CIP

Anesthesiologist's Manual of Surgical Procedures

Second Edition

This book is respectfully dedicated to
our friend, mentor, teacher, and colleague,

C. Philip Larson, Jr, MD, MS

TABLE OF CONTENTS

Appendices

Authors: *Sandra Leigh Bardas, Stephen P. Fischer, Alvin Hackel, Gregory B. Hammer, Richard A. Jaffe, Cathy R. Lammers, C. Philip Larson, Jr., Yuan-Chi Lin, Cathy M. Russo, Stanley I. Samuels*

Subject Index

CONTRIBUTORS

John R. Adler, MD
Professor of Neurosurgery
Stanford University School of Medicine
(*Stereotactic Neurosurgery*)

Edward J. Alfrey, MD
Assistant Professor of Transplant Surgery
Department of Surgery
Stanford University School of Medicine
(*Kidney Transplantation*)

Edward R. Baer, MD
Clinical Assistant Professor of Anesthesia
Associated Anesthesiologists
Stanford University Medical Center
(*Skull Base Surgery*)

Sandra Leigh Bardas, RPh, BS
Clinical Pharmacist
Stanford University Medical Center
(*Drug Interactions*)

J. Augusto Bastidas, MD
Associate Professor of Surgery
Stanford University School of Medicine
(*Trauma Surgery*)

M. Gail Boltz, MD
Assistant Professor of Anesthesia
Division of Pediatric Anesthesia
Stanford University School of Medicine
Pediatric Anesthesiologist
Lucile Salter Packard Children's Hospital at Stanford
(*Pediatric Interventional Cardiology*)

John G. Brock-Utne, MD, PhD, FFA(SA)
Professor of Anesthesia
Stanford University School of Medicine
(*Otolaryngology*)

Jay B. Brodsky, MD
Professor of Anesthesia
Stanford University School of Medicine
(*Thoracic Surgery*)

Gordon A. Brody, MD
Clinical Associate Professor of Orthopedics
Stanford University School of Medicine
Sports, Orthopedics and Rehabilitation
Medicine Associates, Menlo Park, CA
(*Hand Surgery*)

Sally R. Byrd, MD
Clinical Assistant Professor of Ophthalmic Surgery
Stanford University School of Medicine
Chief, Department of Ophthalmology
Veterans Affairs Palo Alto Health Care System
(*Ophthalmic Surgery*)

Walter B. Cannon, MD
Clinical Professor
Department of Cardiothoracic Surgery,
Division of Thoracic Surgery
Stanford University School of Medicine
(*Thoracic Surgery*)

Eugene J. Carragee, MD
Assistant Professor of Orthopedic Surgery
Director, Orthopedic Spine Service
Stanford University School of Medicine
(*Spine Surgery*)

Michael W. Champeau, MD
Clinical Associate Professor of Anesthesia
Associated Anesthesiologists
Stanford University Medical Center
(*Surgery for Sleep-Disordered Breathing*)

Annette C. Cholon, MD
Resident, Division of Plastic Surgery
Department of Functional Restoration
Stanford University School of Medicine
(*Aesthetic Surgery*)

Sheila E. Cohen, MB, ChB, FRCA
Professor of Anesthesia
Director, Obstetrical Anesthesia
Stanford University School of Medicine
(*Obstetric Surgery*)

George W. Commons, MD
Clinical Assistant Professor
Department of Functional Restoration
Stanford University School of Medicine
(*Liposuction*)

John J. Csongradi, MD
Director, Department of Pediatric Orthopedic Surgery
Santa Clara Valley Medical Center, San Jose CA
Clinical Professor of Orthopedics
Stanford University School of Medicine
(*Orthopedic Surgery of Lower Extremities*)

Donald C. Dafoe, MD
Associate Professor of Surgery
Chief, Division of Transplantation
Director, Multi-Organ Transplant Center
Stanford University School of Medicine
(*Kidney Transplantation*)

Michael D. Dake, MD
Associate Professor of Radiology
Division of Cardiovascular and Interventional Radiology
Stanford University School of Medicine
(*Endovascular Stent-Grafting; TIPS*)

Charles DeBattista, MD
Assistant Professor of Psychiatry
Stanford University School of Medicine
(*Electroconvulsive Therapy*)

Steven A. Deem, MD
Assistant Professor of Anesthesia
University of Washington, Seattle WA
(*Urology*)

Jayshree B. Desai, MD
Anesthesiologist
Alta Bates Medical Center, Berkeley, CA
(*Ophthalmic Surgery*)

Sarah S. Donaldson, MD, FACR
Professor of Radiation Oncology
Stanford University School of Medicine
Director of Radiation Oncology
Lucile Salter Packard Children's Hospital at Stanford
(*Pediatric Radiation Therapy*)

Babak Edraki, MD
Clinical Assistant Professor of Gynecology and Obstetrics
Stanford University School of Medicine
(*Gynecologic Oncology; Obstetric Surgery*)

Talmage D. Egan, MD
Assistant Professor of Anesthesia
University Hospital, Salt Lake City, UT
(*Hand, Shoulder Surgery*)

Peter R. Egbert, MD
Professor of Ophthalmology
Stanford University School of Medicine
(*Ophthalmic Surgery*)

Yasser El-Sayed, MD
Clinical Assistant Instructor of Maternal-Fetal Medicine
Department of Gynecology and Obstetrics
Stanford University School of Medicine
(*Obstetric Surgery*)

Carlos O. Esquivel, MD, PhD
Professor of Surgery
Director, Liver Transplant Program
Stanford University School of Medicine
(*Liver Transplantation*)

James I. Fann, MD
Clinical Assistant Professor of Cardiothoracic Surgery
Stanford University School of Medicine
Staff Physician, Department of Cardiovascular Surgery
Veterans Affairs Palo Alto Health Care System
(*Vascular Surgery; Heart/Lung Transplantation*)

Willard E. Fee, Jr, MD
Professor and Chairman
Department of Otolaryngology
Stanford University School of Medicine
(*Otolaryngology*)

Stephen P. Fischer, MD
Assistant Professor of Anesthesia
Medical Director, Anesthesia
Preoperative Evaluation Clinic
Stanford University School of Medicine
(*Preoperative Laboratory Testing/Diagnostics*)

Brett G. Fitzmaurice, MD, FRCP
Clinical Associate Professor of Anesthesia
Vancouver General Hospital, Vancouver, Canada
(*Thoracic Surgery*)

Linda E. Foppiano, MD
Clinical Assistant Professor of Anesthesia
Stanford University School of Medicine
(*Trauma Surgery*)

Fuad S. Freiha, MD, FACS
Chief, Urologic Oncology
Professor of Urology
Stanford University School of Medicine
(*Urology*)

Edward C. Gabalski, MD
Clinical Instructor of Otolaryngology/Head and Neck Surgery, Department of Surgery
Stanford University School of Medicine
(*Otolaryngology*)

Raymond R. Gaeta, MD
Assistant Professor of Anesthesia
Director, Pain Management Services
Stanford University School of Medicine
(*Otolaryngology*)

Michael W. Gaynon, MD
Clinical Associate Professor of Ophthalmology
Stanford University School of Medicine
(*Retinal Surgery*)

Ronald N. Gibson, MD
Obstetrician and Gynecologist
Maui Medical Clinic
Maui, HI
(*Obstetric Surgery*)

Rona G. Giffard, PhD, MD
Associate Professor of Anesthesia
Stanford University School of Medicine
(*Aesthetic, Burn Surgery*)

Harcharan S. Gill, MD
Assistant Professor of Urology
Stanford University School of Medicine
(*Urology*)

Alexandra J. Golby, MD
Resident, Department of Neurosurgery
Stanford University School of Medicine
(*Stereotactic Neurosurgery*)

Stuart B. Goodman, MD, MSC, FRCSC, FACS
Professor of Orthopedic Surgery
Stanford University School of Medicine
(*Orthopedic Surgery of Lower Extremities*)

Alvin Hackel, MD
Professor of Anesthesia and Pediatrics
Stanford University School of Medicine
Pediatric Anesthesiologist
Lucile Salter Packard Children's Hospital at Stanford
(*Pediatric General Surgery*)

Gordon R. Haddow, MB, ChB, FFA(SA)
Associate Professor of Anesthesia
Stanford University School of Medicine
(*Cardiac, Vascular Surgery; Liver/Kidney Transplantation*)

Bruce D. Halperin, MD
Clinical Associate Professor of Anesthesia
Associated Anesthesiologists
Stanford University Medical Center
(*Aesthetic Surgery*)

Gregory B. Hammer, MD
Associate Professor
Division of Pediatric Anesthesia
Stanford University School of Medicine
Associate Director, Pediatric Intensive Care Unit
Lucile Salter Packard Children's Hospital at Stanford
(*Pediatric Otolaryngology, Urology, Oncology, Endoscopy, Imaging, Anesthetic Protocols, Pain Management*)

Gary E. Hartman, MD
Professor of Surgery and Pediatrics
Chairman, Department of Pediatric Surgery
Children's National Medical Center, Washington, DC
(*Pediatric General Surgery; ECMO*)

W. LeRoy Heinrichs, MD, PhD
Professor Emeritus of Gynecology and Obstetrics
Stanford University School of Medicine
(*Gynecology/Infertility Surgery*)

Gary Heit, MD, PhD
Assistant Professor of Neurosurgery
Stanford University School of Medicine
(*Surgery for Movement Disorders*)

R. Harold Holbrook, Jr, MD
Associate Professor of Maternal-Fetal Medicine
Department of Gynecology and Obstetrics
Stanford University School of Medicine
(*Obstetric Surgery*)

Terri D. Homer, MD
Clinical Assistant Professor of Anesthesia
Associated Anesthesiologists
Stanford University Medical Center
(*Aesthetic Surgery*)

Steven K. Howard, MD
Staff Anesthesiologist
Veterans Affairs Palo Alto Health Care System
Assistant Professor of Anesthesia
Stanford University School of Medicine
(*General Surgery*)

Stephen L. Huhn, MD
Assistant Professor of Neurosurgery
Stanford University School of Medicine
Chief, Pediatric Neurosurgery
Lucile Salter Packard Children's Hospital at Stanford
(*Pediatric Neurosurgery*)

Kenneth C. W. Hui, MD, FACS
Assistant Professor of Plastic Surgery
Stanford University School of Medicine
(*Functional Restoration, Microsurgery*)

Richard A. Jaffe, MD, PhD
Associate Professor of Anesthesia
Stanford University School of Medicine
(*Stereotactic Neurosurgery; Ophthalmic, Dental, Spine Surgery; Functional Restoration; Out-of-OR Procedures; Anesthetic Protocols*)

Stefanie S. Jeffrey, MD, FACS
Chief of Breast Surgery
Assistant Professor, Division of Surgical Oncology
Stanford University School of Medicine
(*Breast Surgery*)

Daniel S. Kapp, MD
Professor of Radiation Oncology
Stanford University School of Medicine
(*Gynecological Oncology*)

Stephen T. Kee, MD
Assistant Professor of Radiology
Division of Cardiovascular and Interventional Radiology
Stanford University School of Medicine
(*Endovascular Stent-Grafting; TIPS Procedure*)

Alexsander R. Komar, MD
Research Fellow, Department of Surgery
Stanford University Medical Center
(*Trauma Surgery*)

Amy L. Ladd, MD
Assistant Professor of Functional Restoration
Stanford University School of Medicine
Chief, Hand Clinic
Veterans Affairs Palo Alto Health Care System
Chief, Hand Clinic
Lucile Salter Packard Children's Hospital at Stanford
(*Hand, Shoulder Surgery*)

Cathy R. Lammers, MD
Assistant Professor of Anesthesia
University of California–Davis Medical Center
(*Pediatric Otolaryngology, Urology, Interventional Cardiology*)

Steven P. LaPointe, MD
Post Doctoral Fellow, Department of Urology
Stanford University School of Medicine
(*Pediatric Urology*)

C. Philip Larson, Jr, MD, MS
Professor of Anesthesia and Neurosurgery
University of California at Los Angeles
(*Intracranial, Spinal, Pediatric Neurosurgery; Fiber Optic Intubation*)

Kasey K. Li, DDS, MD
Clinical Instructor
Sleep Disorders Clinic and Research Center
Stanford University School of Medicine
(*Surgery for Sleep-Disordered Breathing*)

I. Bing Liem, DO
Associate Director, Cardiac Electrophysiology
Assistant Professor of Cardiology
Stanford University School of Medicine
(*DC Cardioversion*)

Yuan-Chi Lin, MD
Associate Professor of Anesthesia
Stanford University School of Medicine
Director, Pediatric Pain Management Services
Lucile Salter Packard Children's Hospital at Stanford
(*Repair of Congenital Malformations; Hand Surgery; Pediatric Orthopedic Surgery, Pain Management*)

William C. Lineaweaver, MD, FACS
Associate Professor of Plastic Surgery
Department of Functional Restoration
Stanford University School of Medicine
(*Functional Restoration, Microsurgery*)

M. Thomas Margolis, MD
Director, Center for Pelvic Reconstructive Surgery
Women's Cancer Center, Palo Alto, CA
Clinical Assistant Professor of Gynecology and Obstetrics
Stanford University School of Medicine
(*Gynecology/Infertility Surgery*)

James B. D. Mark, MD
Johnson and Johnson Professor
Department of Cardiothoracic Surgery
Professor Emeritus, Division of Thoracic Surgery
Stanford University School of Medicine
(*Thoracic Surgery*)

Anna H. Messner, MD
Assistant Professor of Surgery/Head and Neck Surgery
Division of Otolaryngology, Department of Surgery
Stanford University School of Medicine
(*Pediatric Otolaryngology*)

Frederick G. Mihm, MD
Professor of Anesthesia
Stanford University School of Medicine
(*Orthopedic Surgery of Lower Extremities*)

R. Scott Mitchell, MD
Associate Professor of Cardiovascular Surgery
Stanford University School of Medicine
Chief, Division of Cardiac Surgery
Veterans Affairs Palo Alto Health Care System
(*Cardiac, Vascular Surgery*)

Camran R. Nezhat, MD
Director, Endoscopy Training Center
Clinical Professor of Gynecology and Obstetrics and Surgery
Stanford University School of Medicine
(*Laparoscopic Procedures for Gynecologic Surgery*)

Alexander M. Norbash, MD
Assistant Professor of Radiology
Department of Diagnostic Radiology and Nuclear Medicine Services
Stanford University School of Medicine
(*Interventional Neuroradiology*)

Harry A. Oberhelman, MD, FACS
Professor Emeritus, Division of Gastrointestinal Surgery
Stanford University School of Medicine
(*Esophageal, Intestinal, Hepatic, Pancreatic, Peritoneal, Endocrine Surgery*)

B. Hannah Ortiz, MD
Administrative Chief Resident
Department of Gynecology and Obstetrics
Stanford University School of Medicine
(*Laparascopic Procedures for Gynecologic Surgery*)

Ronald G. Pearl, MD, PhD
Associate Professor of Anesthesia
Stanford University School of Medicine
(*Urology*)

Kristi L. Peterson, MD
Assistant Professor of Anesthesia
Stanford University School of Medicine
Pediatric Anesthesiologist
Lucile Salter Packard Children's Hospital at Stanford
(*Vascular Surgery; Pediatric Cardiovascular Surgery*)

Paul T. Pitlick, MD
Associate Professor of Pediatrics
Department of Pediatric Cardiology
Stanford University School of Medicine
Pediatric Cardiologist
Lucile Salter Packard Children's Hospital at Stanford
(*Pediatric Interventional Cardiology*)

Nelson B. Powell, MD
Associate Clinical Professor
Co-Director, Sleep Disorders Clinic and Research Center
Stanford University Medical Center
(*Surgery for Sleep-Disordered Breathing*)

Barry H. J. Press, MD, FACS
Clinical Associate Professor of Plastic Surgery
Stanford University School of Medicine
(*Burn Surgery*)

Jon W. Propst, MD, PhD
Attending Anesthesiologist
Marian Medical Center, Santa Maria CA
(*Gynecologic Oncology*)

Emily F. Ratner, MD
Assistant Professor of Anesthesia
Stanford University School of Medicine
(*Gynecology/Infertility Surgery*)

Bruce A. Reitz, MD
Professor and Chairman
Department of Cardiothoracic Surgery
Stanford University School of Medicine
Chief, Pediatric Cardiac Surgical Service
Lucile Salter Packard Children's Hospital at Stanford
(*Heart/Lung Transplantation; Pediatric Cardiovascular Surgery*)

Edward T. Riley, MD
Assistant Professor of Anesthesia
Stanford University School of Medicine
(*Laparoscopic Procedures for Gynecologic Surgery*)

Robert W. Riley, DDS, MD
Associate Clinical Professor
Sleep Disorders Clinic and Research Center
Stanford University Medical Center
(*Surgery for Sleep-Disordered Breathing*)

Lawrence A. Rinsky, MD
Professor of Orthopedic Surgery
Stanford University School of Medicine
Chief, Pediatric Orthopedics
Lucile Salter Packard Children's Hospital at Stanford
(*Pediatric Orthopedic Surgery*)

Joseph B. Roberson, MD
Assistant Professor of Otolaryngology
Division of Otolaryngology/Head and Neck Surgery
Stanford University School of Medicine
(*Skull Base Surgery*)

Myer H. Rosenthal, MD, FACCP
Professor of Anesthesia, Medicine and Surgery
Stanford University School of Medicine
(*Gynecologic Oncology*)

Cathy M. Russo, MD
Clinical Assistant Professor of Anesthesia
Pain Management Services
Stanford University School of Medicine
(*Adult Postoperative Pain Management*)

Stanley I. Samuels, MB, BCh, FFARCS
Professor of Anesthesia
Stanford University School of Medicine
(*Stereotactic Neurosurgery; Ophthalmic, Dental, Spine Surgery; Functional Restoration; Out-of-OR Procedures; Anesthetic Protocols*)

Stephen A. Schendel, MD, DDS
Professor and Head
Division of Plastic and Reconstructive Surgery
Department of Functional Restoration
Stanford University Medical Center
Director, Craniofacial Anomalies Center
Lucile Salter Packard Children's Hospital at Stanford
(*Dental Surgery; Functional Restoration; Repair of Congenital Malformations*)

Charles P. Semba, MD
Assistant Professor of Radiology
Division of Cardiovascular and Interventional Radiology
Stanford University Medical Center
(*TIPS Procedure*)

Linda D. Shortliffe, MD
Professor and Chair
Department of Urology
Stanford University School of Medicine
(*Pediatric Urology*)

Carol A. Shostak, RN, RTT, CMD
Chief Medical Dosimetrist
Department of Radiation Oncology
Stanford University School of Medicine
(*Pediatric Radiation Therapy*)

Lawrence M. Shuer, MD
Associate Professor of Neurosurgery
Stanford University School of Medicine
(*Intracranial, Spinal, Pediatric Neurosurgery*)

Norman E. Shumway, MD, PhD
Professor Emeritus
Department of Cardiovascular and Cardiothoracic Surgery
Stanford University School of Medicine
(*Cardiac Surgery*)

Lawrence C. Siegel, MD
Clinical Associate Professor of Anesthesia
Stanford University Medical Center
(*Port-Access Surgery; Heart/Lung Transplantation*)

Gerald D. Silverberg, MD
Professor of Neurosurgery
Stanford University School of Medicine
(*Surgery for Movement Disorders*)

Robert J. Singer, MD
Chief Resident, Department of Neurosurgery
Vanderbilt University Medical Center, Nashville, TN
(*Interventional Neuroradiology*)

Lynn D. Solem, MD
Associate Professor of Surgery
University of Minnesota Medical Center
Director, Burn Center of Regions Hospital, St. Paul, MN
(*Burn Surgery*)

Gary K. Steinberg, MD, PhD
Professor and Chair
Department of Neurosurgery
Stanford University School of Medicine
(*Neurovascular Surgery, Pediatric Neurosurgery*)

James M. Stone, MD
Northern California Surgical Group, Redding, CA
(*Colorectal Surgery*)

E. Price Stover, MD
Assistant Professor of Anesthesia
Stanford University School of Medicine
(*Multi-Organ Procurement for Transplantation*)

Jeffrey D. Swenson, MD
Assistant Professor of Anesthesiology
University Hospital, Salt Lake City, UT
(*Hand, Shoulder Surgery*)

Daniel Y. Sze, MD, PhD
Acting Assistant Professor of Radiology
Division of Cardiovascular and Interventional Radiology
Stanford University School of Medicine
(*Imaging, Image-Guided Procedures*)

Nelson N. Teng, MD, PhD
Associate Professor of Gynecology and Obstetrics
Director, Gynecological Oncology
Department of Gynecology and Obstetrics
Stanford University School of Medicine
(*Gynecologic Oncology*)

David J. Terris, MD
Assistant Professor of Otolaryngology
Stanford University School of Medicine
(*Otolaryngology*)

Robert J. Troell, MD
Clinical Instructor, Department of Surgery and Sleep Disorders Clinic and Research Center
Stanford University Medical Center
(*Surgery for Sleep-Disordered Breathing*)

Andrew E. Turk, MD
Assistant Professor of Functional Restoration and
Plastic Reconstructive Surgery
Stanford University School of Medicine
(*Aesthetic Surgery*)

George F. Van Hare, MD
Assistant Professor of Pediatrics
Division of Pediatric Cardiology
Stanford University School of Medicine
(*Electrophysiologic Study*)

Mark A. Vierra, MD
Assistant Professor of Surgery, Division of
Gastrointestinal Surgery
Stanford University School of Medicine
(*Stomach, Biliary Tract, General Laparascopic Surgery*)

Lars M. Vistnes, MD, FRCS(C)
Professor Emeritus of Plastic and Reconstructive Surgery
Department of Functional Restoration
Stanford University School of Medicine
(*Aesthetic Surgery*)

Ronald J. Weigel, MD, PhD
Associate Professor of Surgery
Stanford University School of Medicine
(*Endocrine Surgery*)

David D. Yuh, MD
Chief Resident, Department of Surgery
Stanford University School of Medicine
(*Pediatric Cardiovascular Surgery*)

FOREWORD

A New Surgeon Is in Town: An Anesthesiologist's Dilemma

Imagine that you have recently moved to a new private practice location or a new academic department and have been assigned to provide anesthesia for a patient undergoing a surgical procedure with which you are either unfamiliar or have had no practical experience following residency. Your case may involve, for example, a patient with moyamoya disease undergoing extracranial-to-intracranial vascular anastomosis; or a patient with morbid obesity needing laparoscopic gastric bypass; or a patient requiring minimally invasive coronary artery surgery; or, perhaps, a patient with sleep apnea undergoing palatal surgery. What do you do? More importantly, what do you do quickly?

Certainly one option is to ask a colleague who, depending on his or her experience, may or may not be able to help. Alternatively, you can search the literature for relevant articles that describe the special anesthesia-related requirements for the particular procedure. In all likelihood, this will be time-consuming and often unsuccessful in terms of obtaining the most current information, especially for recently developed surgical procedures. Of course, there is the option of querying the surgeon; however, surgeons, as familiar as they may be with the surgery and their surgical needs, are not as likely to be of help in defining the anesthesia requirements.

There is another solution—the one I turned to when, shortly after moving to my new department, I was asked to provide care to a patient undergoing a procedure with which I had no previous experience. That is, to use a copy of this textbook, *Anesthesiologist's Manual of Surgical Procedures*, to obtain a description of the procedure and its anesthetic needs. Edited by my colleagues, Drs. Richard Jaffe and Stanley Samuels, it contains, in a concise yet complete manner, a description of the surgical considerations and anesthetic requirements for virtually every surgical procedure—from the most common to the most exotic.

This volume is the second edition—the first was published in 1994—and represents a substantial revision of the first. For example, in addition to updating and revising each of the original procedures, there are six new chapters (including laparoscopic general surgery and laparoscopic obstetric/gynecologic surgery and a host of out-of-OR procedures), more than 70 new surgical procedures (including minimally invasive cardiac surgery and surgery for sleep disorders), and five new appendices (including protocols for adult and pediatric pain management as well as preoperative evaluation and testing). Just think how useful it is for the anesthesiologist to be able to anticipate what is needed when asked to provide anesthesia for a patient of the newly recruited surgeon, interventional radiologist, or endoscopist specializing in procedures heretofore not performed at the institution.

The format used for this textbook is, to my knowledge, unique in our specialty. Surgical subspecialties comprise the major sections, which, in turn, are subdivided into surgical procedures. Each procedure is described by a surgical expert, who includes a description of the procedure and all of the factors that should be of interest to the anesthesiologist, including patient position, expected duration of the surgery, common complications, and special needs, such as the use of a nerve stimulator that mitigates against neuromuscular blocking drugs. The surgeon's contribution is followed by the anesthetic considerations, written by an anesthesiologist with special expertise in providing anesthesia to patients undergoing the particular surgery being described. Rather than rigidly prescribing specific agents, which can vary among anesthesiologists, a technique that "works for that anesthesiologist" is provided, along with suggested monitoring modalities, most common intra- and postoperative complications, and suggestions for postoperative pain management.

This presentation provides information that can be used by the reader as a suggestion for devising an anesthetic plan best suited for the individual patient, as well as for the surgery planned. Although most of the contributors are Stanford University anesthesiologists and surgeons, the approach is not provincial, and I am impressed that the advice advocated by these authors represents the most advanced and current information available as of the date of publication. This textbook is a wonderful aid for the harried anesthesiologist (and surgeon, for that matter) who is confronted increasingly by new surgeons and unfamiliar surgical procedures.

Lawrence J. Saidman, M.D.
Professor of Anesthesiology
Stanford University School of Medicine
September, 1998

PREFACE

It was with mixed feelings that we received the news from our publishers that they wanted a second edition of the *Anesthesiologist's Manual of Surgical Procedures*. The response to the first edition had been most gratifying, and we were, indeed, flattered by both our readers' and publisher's interest in having a new version. Pragmatists that we are (or were), however, we viewed the Herculean task of preparing another *Manual* with some trepidation. Unlike the lyrics of the old Sinatra song, we realized that editing is not necessarily easier "the second time around."

The goals of the second edition are unchanged from those of the first—that is, to provide an easily accessible source of clinically specific information about a wide variety of surgical procedures. As with the first edition, this one does not pretend to be either a textbook of anesthesia or a textbook of surgery. Indeed, in the formulation of an anesthetic plan, there is no substitute for experience and sound clinical judgment.

Those familiar with the first edition will notice that the format and organization of this edition remain unchanged. Procedure codes have been eliminated to protect the innocent, and page thickness was reduced to help disguise the significantly increased page count, the result of adding five new chapters and dozens of new procedures. Every existing procedure was reviewed and revised as necessary to reflect current practices.

In the interval between the first and second editions, we have seen a dramatic increase in endoscopic or minimally invasive surgical procedures and in the demand for out-of-OR anesthetic services. Accordingly, we have greatly expanded our coverage in these areas with entirely new sections devoted to laparoscopic general surgery, laparoscopic gynecologic surgery, and minimally invasive cardiac surgery. Within each of the other surgical specialties, individual descriptions of endoscopic procedures have been added. The section on out-of-OR procedures has been completely rewritten and expanded to include electroconvulsive therapy, interventional radiology, transjugular intrahepatic portosystemic shunts (TIPS), and image-guided procedures. The coverage of pediatric surgery has been increased to include separate sections on otolaryngology, urology, and a greatly expanded section on cardiovascular surgery. Information in the appendices has been revised and expanded with entirely new sections for preoperative testing, pediatric anesthesia, and both adult and pediatric pain management. The section on drug interactions now includes a table on herbal remedies, an increasing and potentially unrecognized problem for the anesthesiologist.

Once again we have made extensive use of abbreviations, medical symbols, and telegraphic sentence structure to present a large quantity of information in a condensed format. While we realize that it may be aesthetically more pleasing to read, "Hypoxia or hypercapnia can lead to the development of tachycardia and hypertension," it takes up a lot less space to write, "$\uparrow PaCO_2$ or $\downarrow PaO_2 \rightarrow \uparrow$HR + $\uparrow$BP."

Finally, we have attempted to incorporate the many constructive comments we received from our readers and reviewers of the first edition. However, it must be left up to you, the reader, to decide if we have created an improved and more balanced edition the second time around.

Richard A. Jaffe and Stanley I. Samuels
Stanford University School of Medicine
September, 1998

ACKNOWLEDGMENTS

Immediately upon completion of the first edition of this book, our developmental editor, Dee Mosteller, fled to the East Coast, "forgetting" to provide us with a forwarding address. When the publisher asked us to edit a second edition, a search of the usual sources failed to reveal her whereabouts, so we were forced to begin work without her assistance. It quickly became apparent that her unique organizational ability and insights were not to be easily replaced. In desperation, we engaged the services of San Francisco's Rat Dog Dick Detective Agency to locate her (which took about 15 minutes and the best $85 we ever spent). Incredibly, she agreed to help us with the second edition. We have no doubt that without her help we might still be working on this project. The logistics involved in dealing with 600+ procedures, 115 authors, and two very heavy-handed editors present challenges that can be known only to those few brave enough or foolish enough to be involved in such a project. We remain eternally grateful for her extraordinary act of bravery.

We would also like to thank our Contributors; the editorial staff at Lippincott Williams & Wilkins—most particularly our executive editor, Craig Percy, his assistant, Andrea Allison-Williams, and our perfect word processor, Eileen Jackson—for their patient and enthusiastic support of this project; and our typesetters at QualiType, Inc., for service above and beyond. Finally, we thankfully acknowledge the generous forbearance of our families, friends, and Stanford colleagues. Their continuing support is greatly appreciated.

1.0 NEUROSURGERY

Surgeons

Gary K. Steinberg, MD, PhD (*Neurovascular surgery*)
Lawrence M. Shuer, MD (*General neurosurgery*)
Alexandra J. Golby, MD (*Stereotactic neurosurgery*)
John R. Adler, MD (*Stereotactic neurosurgery*)
Gary Heit, MD, PhD (*Surgery for movement disorders*)
Gerald D. Silverberg, MD (*Surgery for movement disorders*)

1.1 INTRACRANIAL NEUROSURGERY

Anesthesiologists

C. Philip Larson, Jr, MD, MS (*General neurosurgery*)
Richard A. Jaffe, MD, PhD (*Stereotactic neurosurgery*)
Stanley I. Samuels, MB, BCh, FFARCS (*Stereotactic neurosurgery*)

CRANIOTOMY FOR INTRACRANIAL ANEURYSMS

SURGICAL CONSIDERATIONS

Gary K. Steinberg

Description: Clipping of intracranial aneurysms is the treatment of choice for preventing aneurysmal rupture (with subarachnoid or intraparenchymal hemorrhage), aneurysmal enlargement or distal embolization from the aneurysm. **Hunt** and **Hess** described a clinical grading system for patients with ruptured intracranial aneurysms[13] that has prognostic value in terms of ultimate clinical outcome and is also used to determine the timing of surgery. Grading is based on the neurological examination and ranges from Grade I (minimal headache, no neurologic deficit) to Grade V (moribund). Common sites of aneurysms are shown in Fig 1.1-1.

Through a **craniotomy** or **craniectomy**, using microscopic techniques, the parent vessel giving rise to the aneurysm is identified. The aneurysm neck is isolated, and a small, nonferromagnetic alloy spring clip is placed across the aneurysm neck, excluding it from the circulation. A **frontotemporal (pterional) craniotomy** normally is used to approach anterior circulation aneurysms. This requires extensive drilling of the medial sphenoid wing (pterion) and allows access to most aneurysms on the anterior and lateral Circle of Willis vessels: internal carotid-paraclinoid/superior hypophyseal artery; internal carotid-ophthalmic artery; posterior communicating artery; anterior choroidal artery; internal carotid artery bifurcation; middle cerebral artery; and anterior communicating artery. Posterior circulation aneurysms are approached via a pterional or subtemporal exposure (upper basilar artery, posterior cerebral artery, superior cerebellar artery), a suboccipital exposure (vertebral artery, posterior inferior cerebellar artery), or a combined subtemporal and suboccipital exposure (basilar trunk, vertebrobasilar junction). Circulatory arrest under CPB with deep hypothermia (16-20°C) is used for repairing some giant (> 2.5 cm) aneurysms.

Usual preop diagnosis: Cerebral aneurysm; subarachnoid hemorrhage; intracerebral hemorrhage; progressive neurological deficits (mass effect on cranial nerves or CNS structures); TIAs; cerebral infarct

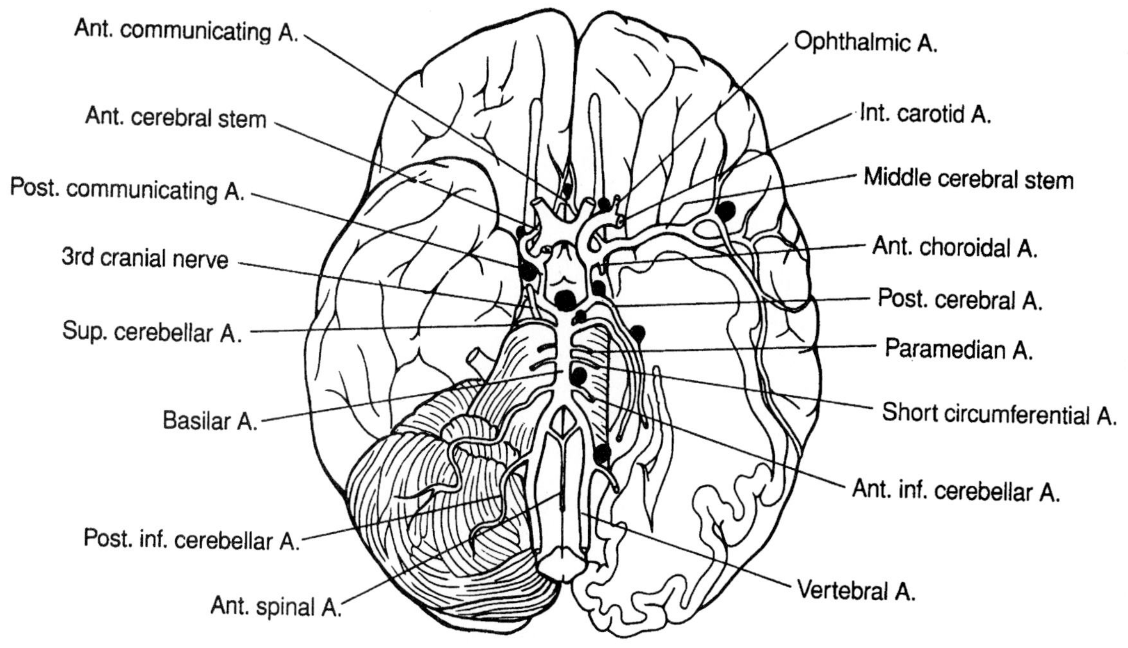

Figure 1.1-1. Cross-section of the Circle of Willis, showing sites of aneurysms; the majority (~90%) are located in the anterior half of the circle. (Reproduced with permission from Adams RD: *Principles of Neurology*, 4th edition. McGraw-Hill: 1989.)

SUMMARY OF PROCEDURE

	Anterior Circulation Aneurysms	Posterior Circulation Aneurysms	Circulatory Arrest (CPB) W/Deep Hypothermia
Position	Supine, head in Mayfield headrest, turned 30-45° to side away from aneurysm, vertex dropped (Fig 1.1-4)	⇐ Or lateral decubitus, head lateral in Mayfield headrest	⇐ + Both groins must be accessible for arterial + venous cannulation; access to chest for defibrillation.
Incision	Frontotemporal	⇐ Or temporal, temporosub-occipital or suboccipital	⇐
Special instrumentation	Operating microscope; aneurysm clips; radiolucent table and headrest for intraop angiography	⇐ + Aperture clips to accommodate cranial nerves and critical vessels.	⇐ + CPB pump; femoral cannulae; defibrillator; CUSA for partially thrombosed aneurysms
Unique considerations	Temporary arterial clipping; mild hypothermia (33°C); intraop angiography with access to femoral artery; electrophysiological monitoring (SEPs, BAERs); brain relaxation; ± lumbar subarachnoid CSF drainage; dexamethasone 8-12 mg iv	⇐	⇐ + No manipulation of brain retractors after systemic heparinization; meticulous attention to hemostasis
Antibiotics	Nafcillin (1-2 g iv q 6 h) + cefotaxime (1 g iv q 6 h)	⇐	⇐
Surgical time	3-5 h	3-6 h	6-8 h
Closing considerations	Rewarming	⇐	⇐
EBL	250-1000 ml	⇐	2000-4000 ml
Postop care	ICU × 1-7 d; postop CBF monitoring. TCD monitor	⇐	⇐ + ICP monitoring
Mortality	Unruptured: 0.5%	1.5%	5-10% (giant aneurysms)
	Ruptured:		
	Hunt and Hess grades I-III: < 10%	< 15%	5-15%
	Hunt and Hess grades IV-V: 20-40%	20-50%	15-50%
Morbidity	Neurological: 5-20%	10-30%	10-50%
	Cranial nerve injury	⇐	⇐
	Stroke	⇐	⇐
	Hydrocephalus	⇐	⇐
	Hyponatremia	⇐	⇐
	Respiratory failure: Rare	⇐	⇐
	Thromboembolism: Rare	⇐	⇐
	CSF leak: Rare	⇐	⇐
	Infection: Rare	⇐	⇐
	Massive blood loss: Rare	⇐	⇐
Pain score	3-4	3-4	4-5

PATIENT POPULATION CHARACTERISTICS

Age range	30-70 yr
Male:Female	44:56
Incidence	12/100,000/yr for ruptured aneurysms with subarachnoid hemorrhage
Etiology	Idiopathic (probably acquired and related to hemodynamic stress at arterial branch points, although may have congenital predisposition to loss of internal elastic lamina); traumatic; infectious; familial
Associated conditions	Polycystic kidney disease; coarctation of the aorta; Marfan syndrome; Ehlers-Danlos syndrome; intracranial arteriovenous malformations (AVMs); aortic aneurysm; fibromuscular dysplasia; pseudoxanthoma elastica; Rendu-Osler-Weber syndrome

ANESTHETIC CONSIDERATIONS

C. Philip Larson, Jr.

PREOPERATIVE

Aneurysms may occur in any age group, although they generally become symptomatic and are diagnosed in young or middle-aged adults who are usually in otherwise good health. Most patients have warning Sx before the first major bleed, but these tend to be mild and nonspecific (e.g., headache, dizziness, orbital pain, slight motor or sensory disturbances). The symptoms are generally disregarded by both patients and physicians.

Respiratory Usually not significant unless the patient has Hx of smoking, or has pulmonary aspiration as a result of a neurological deficit from an intracranial hemorrhage.
Tests: As indicated from H&P.

Cardiovascular Generally, these patients do not have other cardiovascular diseases, although intracerebral aneurysms occur more commonly in patients with certain congenital disorders, such as polycystic disease of the kidneys, coarctation of the aorta, fibromuscular hyperplasia, Marfan and Ehlers-Danlos syndromes. Patients who have had a recent intracranial hemorrhage from leaking or rupture of a cerebral aneurysm are prone to develop systemic HTN, hypovolemia[2] and electrocardiographic abnormalities.[1] The HTN is thought to be due to autonomic hyperactivity, and is generally treated with antihypertensive medication, which should be continued up to the time of anesthesia and surgery. Why hypovolemia occurs following subarachnoid hemorrhage is not clear, but may be due in part to cerebral vasospasm, and to sustained bed rest. ECG abnormalities occur in 50-80% of patients who sustain an intracranial hemorrhage. Appropriate preop preparation includes ECG characterization of the abnormality. If patient has Hx of ischemic heart disease, then ECHO and cardiac enzyme studies may be helpful in determining whether ECG changes are due to heart disease or intracranial hemorrhage.
Tests: ECG; others as indicated from H&P.

Neurological Seldom do aneurysms produce neurological Sx by enlarging to the point that they compress adjacent neural tissue or cause ↑ICP. If an intracranial hemorrhage occurs, the neurological dysfunction will vary, depending on the site and extent of the hemorrhage. These patients may complain of severe headache, be confused and disoriented, have a motor deficit of one or more extremities, or be comatose. A major complication of an intracerebral hemorrhage is the development of cerebral vasospasm or vasoconstriction of cerebral vessels. The vasospasm may be local or diffuse, and may be mild or severe. If severe, it causes worsening of the neurological deficits. It usually occurs in the first wk after the bleed, peaks at ~10 d, and is usually resolved within 2-3 wk. The exact mechanism for the vasospasm is not known; but it is believed that the precipitating agent is free oxyhemoglobin which, in turn, may cause release of vasospastic substances such as serotonin, prostaglandin or potassium from brain tissue. If the neurosurgeon suspects that the patient may have focal cerebral edema or vasospasm from an intracranial hemorrhage, surgery will generally be delayed until neurologic Sx have stabilized or resolved, and the CT scan is normal. Treatment during this waiting period usually involves support of BP and vigorous hydration to induce hypervolemic hemodilution, thereby increasing CBF and improving the rheological characteristics of the blood.
If a patient is evaluated by a neurosurgeon within 6-8 h of sustaining an intracranial hemorrhage, and if the severity of the neurological injury or deficit is minimal, the neurosurgeon may decide to ligate the aneurysm immediately. The rationale behind this approach is that failure to ligate promptly may result in an acute rebleed and death. Although control of BP is important in all patients with aneurysms, it is particularly critical in this subset of patients. Any substantial increase in BP may cause a serious rebleed, permanent neurological deficits or death; and any substantial decrease in BP may cause cerebral ischemia and infarction in the area of the original bleed. Arterial catheterization and continuous beat-to-beat monitoring of BP prior to induction of anesthesia is essential in these patients.
Tests: CT; MRI; cerebral angiogram, which the anesthesiologist should examine preop to identify the nature and site of the aneurysm.

Hematologic **Tests:** Hct; PT; PTT

Laboratory CT or MRI scan; cerebral angiogram; others as indicated from H&P.

Premedication Seldom necessary; detailed discussion with the patient about the anesthetic plan, with appropriate reassurance, is usually enough. Should an intracranial aneurysm leak or rupture in the immediate preop period, its signs may be difficult to distinguish from those associated with excessive responses to premedication. If medication is desirable, small doses of sedative/hypnotics (e.g., midazolam 2-5 mg iv) are preferable to opiates.

INTRAOPERATIVE

Anesthetic technique: GETA. The goals of anesthesia for this operation are to: (1) maintain optimum CPP (cerebral arterial pressure minus cerebral venous or intracranial pressure, whichever is greater), but be prepared to increase or decrease CPP rapidly and profoundly if intracranial hemorrhage occurs during surgical clipping; (2) decrease intracranial volume (blood and tissue) to optimize working space for surgeons within the cranial compartment, thereby minimizing the need for surgical retraction of brain tissue; and (3) minimize metabolic rate and $CMRO_2$, with the expectation that the brain will tolerate severe hypotension and ischemia if sudden decreases in MAP and, hence, CPP become necessary.

Induction STP 5-10 mg/kg or propofol 2-3 mg/kg iv to provide amnesia and ↓ cerebral blood volume by inducing cerebral vasoconstriction. Fentanyl 7-10 μg/kg iv to provide analgesia for the first hours of surgery. Vecuronium 0.15 mg/kg or rocuronium 0.7-1 mg/kg to provide muscle relaxation for tracheal intubation and positioning of the patient.

Maintenance Isoflurane ≤ 1% (≤ 0.6% if evoked potential monitoring is used), inspired with O_2. N_2O > 50% is not used because of its potential for reversing the protective effects of STP.[5,15] Propofol (75-100 μg/kg/min) may be used to further ↓ cerebral blood volume, ↓ cerebral metabolism and ↓ $CMRO_2$. Generally, no additional neuromuscular blocking drugs are needed, but if movement is of concern, rocuronium 0.15-0.3 mg/kg/h will provide adequate neuromuscular blockade.

Emergence With this technique, patients will be sufficiently responsive within 30 min of conclusion of operation to permit gross neurological evaluation, and will not have any recall of the operative period. As recovery from anesthesia occurs, the patient's BP will generally increase in response to the emergence stimuli. Titration of β-adrenergic blocking drugs such as esmolol and/or vasodilators such as SNP may be needed; if so, the dose should be stabilized prior to transport to ICU. (See Control of BP, below.) If the brain has not been injured by the surgical procedure, patient should awaken from anesthetic within 30 min after cessation of isoflurane administration. As the patient is awakening, it is important to assure full reversal from neuromuscular blockade and close regulation of BP. If the patient begins to cough on ETT, either it should be removed or cough reflex suppressed with lidocaine sprayed down ETT (LTA kit) while patient is still anesthetized. Patient is placed in bed in a 30° head-up position and transported to ICU for monitoring overnight. Supplemental O_2 should be administered and close regulation of BP maintained. Prophylactic antiemetic (e.g., metoclopramide 10 mg or ondansetron 4 mg) should be given 30-60 min before extubation.

Blood and fluid requirements	IV: 18 ga × 2 NS/LR @ < 10 ml/kg + UO Expand blood volume with albumin 5% if Hct > 30%. Albumin + PRBC if Hct < 30% Hetastarch may → coagulopathy.[3]	What fluid and how much to give depends on patient's condition. If blood volume is normal, crystalloid fluid should not exceed 10 ml/kg beyond that required to replace UO. If blood volume is low because of vasospasm or prolonged bed rest, albumin 5% is given if Hct > 30%; combinations of albumin and blood, if Hct is < 30%. Hetastarch 6% may be used in place of albumin, but do not exceed 20 ml/kg because of its potential for inducing a coagulopathy.
Control of brain volume (ICP)	Hyperventilate to $PaCO_2$ = 25-30 mmHg ($PetCO_2$ = 20-25 mmHg). PaO_2 >100 mmHg ↓fluids < 10 ml/kg + UO STP or propofol infusion ↓isoflurane < 1% Mannitol 1 g/kg ± Furosemide 0.3 mg/kg Control BP & CVP: low normal. ± Steroids	↓$PaCO_2$ → ↓cerebral vascular volume (better surgical access) + ↑CBF to ischemic areas ("Robin Hood" effect) + ↓anesthetic requirements + ↑lactic acid buffering. Mannitol/furosemide → ↓K^+; monitor level and replace as necessary. If mannitol is administered too rapidly, hypotension may occur, probably from peripheral vasodilation.

ICP, cont.	± Lumbar CSF drain Head up 20-30°	CSF drain often placed after induction of anesthesia, and may be opened as required.
Monitoring	Standard monitors (see p. B-1). ± Bladder temperature Arterial line (before induction)	Direct monitoring of arterial pressure is essential because of the marked fluctuations in BP that may occur, necessitating hypertensive or hypotensive drug therapy, as well as need for ABGs. Recording transducer should always be at the level of the head rather than the heart.
	CVP line UO (Foley catheter) ± Evoked potentials[6]	Monitoring CVP via a right atrial catheter is desirable in virtually all patients to assess adequacy of fluid therapy intraop and postop. The catheter also is essential for infusion of vasoactive drugs commonly used during and/or after this operation. The ideal site for insertion of the catheter, in order of preference, is: right IJ, right subclavian, and right EJ vein. Localization of the catheter can be determined by CXR, ECG tracing (noting P-wave changes), or pressure-wave contour and value as the catheter is withdrawn from the RV into the right atrium.
Hypothermia	Ice packs Thermal blanket Cool air blower Cold OR	Mild hypothermia (33°C) is used in some centers during this operation for two purposes: 1) to ↓ $CMRO_2$ and 2) to ↓ brain size.[6] ↓ $CMRO_2$ decreases about 7% for every degree C decrease in brain temperature; so, at 33°C, cerebral metabolism is decreased about 30% below normal. From studies in animals, it is generally believed that this level of hypothermia is beneficial, although there are no studies in patients documenting decreased morbidity or mortality from its use. This level of hypothermia does not interfere appreciably with coagulation, nor it is generally associated with cardiac dysrhythmias. Warming is begun several h before the conclusion of the operation by using thermal blanket, Bair Hugger, and warming lights, by warming inspired gases, and by increasing the ambient temperature in the OR. Usually by the time the operation is completed, patient temperature is near normal.
Control of BP	During application of head fixation device (Mayfield) Prior to clipping: ↓ MAP to 80-100% of baseline. Temporary clipping of aneurysm: ↑ MAP to 90-110 mmHg. In event of aneurysmal rupture: ↓ MAP to 40-50 mmHg, if necessary. Postclipping: MAP usually kept @ 80-100 mmHg. If HR > 80 bpm, esmolol 50-300 μg/kg/min to ↓ HR to 50-60 bpm. If HR already slow, or if esmolol alone does not produce satisfactory control of BP, administer SNP 0.1-2 μg/kg/min to desired effect. Generally try to maintain postop BP at 80% of preop range.	Control of BP is critical to the successful outcome of both anesthetic and operation. Substantial increases in BP will increase transmural pressure across the aneurysmal wall, and increase likelihood of rupture of the aneurysm. Many neurosurgeons apply a temporary clip on the major feeding vessel(s) in advance of clipping the aneurysm.[11] This technique collapses the aneurysm and makes the clipping easier, more complete and less likely to cause inadvertent rupture. Temporary clipping of feeding vessel(s) is also performed if an aneurysm ruptures during surgical dissection and exposure. If this technique is used, it is essential for the anesthesiologist to ↑ BP 20-30% above baseline pressure to maximize collateral flow while the feeding vessel(s) is occluded. Phenylephrine is preferred because it has minimal dysrhythmogenic potential. If necessary, BP may be reduced with isoflurane alone or in combination with a short-acting β-adrenergic blocking drug such as esmolol. Responses to vasoactive drugs are much easier to regulate if a normal blood volume has been established and maintained throughout the anesthetic period.
Positioning	For most aneurysms: Supine, head turned	Anesthetic gas hoses and all monitoring and vascular catheter lines are directed to patient's side or feet, where the

Positioning, cont.	Three-point fixation (beware of marked ↑BP with use of pins). Use shoulder roll. ✓ and pad pressure points. ✓ eyes.	anesthesiologist is positioned during surgery. Antiembolism stockings and SCDs used to minimize DVT. Shoulder roll to ↓ brachial plexus stretch. Remifentanil (4-5 μg/kg) to minimize ↑BP during skull pinning.
Complications	Hypothermia (mild)	

POSTOPERATIVE

Complications	Intracranial hemorrhage Stroke Cerebral vasospasm	If any of these complications occur, it is likely that the patient's trachea will have to be reintubated and the patient transported to CT scanner for further neurological evaluation or possible reoperation.
Pain management	Meperidine (10-20 mg iv prn) Codeine (30-60 mg im q 4 h prn)	Meperidine will ↓ postop shivering.
Tests	CT scan, if any change in neurological status	

References

1. Andreoli A, dePasquale G, Pinelli G, et al: Subarachnoid hemorrhage: frequency and severity of cardiac arrhythmias. A survey of 70 cases studied in the acute phase. *Stroke* 1987; 18(3):558-64.
2. Brazenor GA, Chamberlain MJ, Gelb AW: Systemic hypovolemia after subarachnoid hemorrhage. *J Neurosurg Anesthesiol* 1990; 2:42-9.
3. Cully MD, Larson CP Jr, Silverberg GD: Hetastarch coagulopathy in a neurosurgical patient. *Anesthesiology* 1987; 66(5):706-7.
4. Drake CG, Peerless SJ, Ferguson GG: Hunterian proximal arterial occlusion for giant aneurysms of the carotid circulation. *J Neurosurg* 1994; 81:656-65.
5. Hartung J, Cottrell JE: Nitrous oxide reduces STP-induced prolongation of survival in hypoxic and anoxic mice. *Anesth Analg* 1987; 66(1):47-52.
6. Mooij JJ, Buchthal A, Belopavlovic M: Somatosensory evoked potential monitoring of temporary middle cerebral artery occlusion during aneurysm operation. *Neurosurgery* 1987; 21(4):492-96.
7. Ojemann RG, Ogilvy CS, Heros RC, Crowell RM: *Surgical Management of Cerebrovascular Disease*. Williams & Wilkins, Baltimore: 1995.
8. Peerless SJ, Drake CG: Surgical management of posterior cerebral aneurysms. In *Operative Neurosurgical Techniques: Indications, Methods, and Results*, Vols I-II. Schmidek HH, Sweet WH, eds. WB Saunders Co, Philadelphia: 1995.
9. Samson DS, Batjer HH: *Intracranial Aneurysm Surgery: Techniques*. Futura Publishing Co, Mount Kisco: 1990.
10. Schmidek HH, Sweet WH, eds: *Operative Neurosurgical Techniques: Indications, Methods, and Results*, Vols I-II. WB Saunders Co, Philadelphia: 1995.
11. Steinberg GK, Drake CG, Peerless SJ: Deliberate basilar or vertebral artery occlusion in the treatment of intracranial aneurysms. Immediate results and long-term outcome in 201 patients. *J Neurosurg* 1993; 79:161-73.
12. Sundt TM Jr: *Surgical Techniques for Saccular and Giant Intracranial Aneurysms*. Williams & Wilkins, Baltimore: 1990.
13. Weir B: *Aneurysms Affecting the Nervous System*. Williams & Wilkins, Baltimore: 1987.
14. Wilkins RH, Rengachary SS, eds: *Neurosurgery*, Vols 1-3. McGraw-Hill, New York: 1996.
15. Warner DS, Zhou JG, Ramani R, Todd MM, McAllister A: Nitrous oxide does not alter infarct volume in rats undergoing reversible middle cerebral artery occlusion. *Anesthesiology* 1990; 73(4):686-93.
16. Youmans JR, ed: *Neurological Surgery*, Vols 1-6. WB Saunders Co, Philadelphia: 1990.

ANESTHETIC CONSIDERATIONS FOR CRANIOTOMY FOR GIANT INTRACRANIAL ANEURYSMS

(Requiring deep hypothermic circulatory arrest)

PREOPERATIVE

Aneurysms are classified as "giant" when they are > 2.5 cm in diameter. These giant aneurysms represent ~5% of all aneurysms. They occur twice as often in women, usually become symptomatic in the 4th or 5th decade of life, and present particularly difficult surgical challenges:[3,6] (1) their large size makes direct visualization of the vascular anatomy difficult; (2) vascular branches essential to maintaining flow to normal brain may be an integral part of the giant aneurysm, and cannot be included in the clipping without causing permanent neurological injury; (3) standard aneurysm clips may not occlude a large, turgid aneurysm, or may slip or move, once applied; and (4) giant aneurysms may rupture during dissection or clip application, resulting in severe neurological morbidity or mortality. A special anesthetic and surgical management, using deep hypothermia to 18°C, achieved with fem-fem CPB and temporary circulatory arrest, has evolved.[2,3] These techniques decompress the aneurysm, making it easier to clip, and protect the brain during circulatory arrest. The duration of cardiac arrest may be as long as 45 min.

Respiratory None unless patient has Hx of smoking, or has sustained pulmonary aspiration as a result of a neurological deficit from an intracranial hemorrhage.
Tests: As indicated from H&P.

Cardiovascular Generally, these patients do not have other cardiovascular diseases. (See Anesthetic Considerations for Intracranial Aneurysms, p. 7.)
Tests: ECG; others as indicated from H&P.

Neurological These patients usually present with complaints of intermittent or persistent headaches or visual disturbances that are probably due to aneurysmal compression of adjacent neural tissue or ↑ICP. If an intracranial hemorrhage occurs, neurological dysfunction varies, depending on site and extent of the hemorrhage. Cerebral vasospasm is a major complication of intracranial hemorrhage (see discussion in Anesthetic Considerations for Intracranial Aneurysms, p. 7).
Tests: CT; MRI; angiogram. The anesthesiologist should examine the cerebral angiogram preop to visualize the size and site of aneurysm.

Hematologic T&C for 6 U PRBCs.
Tests: Hct; PT; PTT; hemogram; others as indicated from H&P.

Laboratory Other tests as indicated from H&P.

Premedication Premedication is seldom necessary in this procedure. Detailed discussion with patient about the anesthetic plan, with appropriate reassurance, is usually sufficient. Should an intracranial aneurysm leak or rupture in the immediate preop period, it may be difficult to distinguish this event from changes associated with excessive responses to premedication. If premedication is desirable, however, small doses of sedative/hypnotics (e.g., midazolam 2-5 mg) are preferable to opiates.

INTRAOPERATIVE

Anesthetic technique: GETA. The goals of anesthesia for this procedure are to: (1) provide adequate surgical anesthesia; (2) decrease intracranial volume (blood and tissue) and optimize working space within the cranial compartment, thereby minimizing the need for surgical retraction of brain tissue; and (3) increase tolerance of the brain to ischemia by decreasing $CMRO_2$, which occurs with the use of deep hypothermia, barbiturate therapy and isovolemic hemodilution.

Induction STP 10-20 mg/kg or propofol 2-3 mg/kg iv to provide amnesia and decrease cerebral blood volume by inducing cerebral vasoconstriction. Fentanyl 7-10 μg/kg iv to provide analgesia for the first hours. Vecuronium 0.15 mg/kg or rocuronium 0.7-1 mg/kg to provide relaxation for intubation and positioning.

Maintenance STP 20 mg/kg by continuous infusion, to be completed within 2 h of induction, for a total dose of 30-40 mg/kg, or propofol 100-200 μg/kg/min administered by constant-infusion pump. These doses provide additional amnesia and decrease cerebral blood volume and $CMRO_2$. Isoflurane ≤ 1%. N_2O not used because of its potential for reversing the protective effects of STP.[1,2] An additional dose of neuromuscular blocking drug is administered just prior to the start of CPB.

Emergence Because of the length and nature of the operation, and the potential for temporary neurological injury, it is advisable to leave the ETT in place immediately postop, and send patient to the ICU on controlled ventilation. If patient begins to cough, the reflex should be suppressed with opiates, neuromuscular blocking drugs, and/or LTA sprayed down the ETT. The patient is placed in bed in a 30° head-up position and transported to ICU for overnight monitoring. Supplemental O_2 should be administered and close regulation of BP maintained. Prophylactic antiemetic (e.g., metoclopramide 10 mg or ondansetron 4 mg) should be given 30-60 min before extubation.

Blood and fluid requirements
IV: 16 ga × 2
NS/LR @ 1-2 ml/kg/h — Cold NS up to 10 ml/kg, + a volume equal to UO, is administered during surgery.
PRBC 4-6 U

Isovolemic hemodilution	5% albumin 8 × 250 ml NS 4 × 1000 ml	Albumin and NS are placed in a refrigerator at 4°C the night before surgery to be used for cooling during isovolemic hemodilution.
	CPD bags	After induction of anesthesia, a 2nd arterial cannula is placed for removal of blood into CPD bags. Generally, about 1000 ml of blood are removed and replaced with 1 L of cold albumin 5%. This usually results in a decrease in Hct to 22-26%. Frequent intraop Hct checks are appropriate. The withdrawn blood is held at room temperature for reinfusion at the conclusion of operation. In addition, the perfusate from the CPB unit is spun down and packed cells returned to patient.
Control of brain volume (ICP)	Hyperventilate to $PaCO_2$ = 25-30 mmHg. Limit crystalloid < 10 ml/kg + UO. Limit isoflurane ≤ 1%. High-dose STP Mannitol 1 g/kg ± Furosemide 0.3 mg/kg ± Lumbar CSF drainage Dexamethasone 8-12 mg	Ventilation is controlled and TV and RR adjusted such that $PaCO_2$ ranges from 25-30 mmHg. There are several advantages to hypocarbia, including: decreasing cerebral vascular volume to provide more surgical working space, thereby lessening need for vigorous retraction of brain tissue; improving regional distribution of CBF by preferentially diverting blood to potentially ischemic areas of the brain; better buffering of brain lactic acid that may form as a result of focal ischemia; and decreasing anesthetic requirement.
Monitoring	Standard monitors (see p. B-1). Temperature = esophageal, bladder and brain surface Arterial line × 2	
	CVP (triple-lumen) line	CVP (triple-lumen) with multiple stopcocks is used for infusions of esmolol, SNP and phenylephrine. Frequent checks are made of Hct, electrolytes, ACT values, before, during and after CPB.
	UO	Keep UO > 0.5 cc/kg/hr.
Control of BP	Maintain BP normal-to-20% below normal with esmolol infusion, SNP or propofol. Phenylephrine	BP control is critical to successful surgery. ↑BP during induction or prior to CPB will ↑ transmural pressure across the aneurysmal wall and ↑ likelihood of rupture. Prior to CPB, BP is generally kept to normal-to-20% below normal for patient, using anesthetic agents alone or with an esmolol infusion to ↓ HR to a range of 50-60 bpm. If desired level of BP is not achieved with this combination, SNP or propofol infusion may be added. SNP also facilitates both cooling and rewarming because of its vasodilatory effect. If a vasoconstrictor is needed, particularly during CPB while patient is still cold, a pure α-adrenergic stimulant such as phenylephrine is preferred because of its minimal dysrhythmogenic potential. Responses to vasoactive drugs are much easier to regulate if normal blood volume has been established and maintained throughout the anesthetic period.
Positioning	Shoulder roll 180° table rotation ✓ and pad pressure points. ✓ eyes. Circuit extension tubes Antiembolism stockings and SCD	Anesthetic gas hoses and all monitoring and vascular catheter lines are directed to patient's feet, where the anesthesiologist is positioned during operation. In planning anesthetic equipment to be used, the anesthesiologist must make sure that all will reach the foot of operating table. Antiembolism stockings and SCDs used to minimize DVT.
Deep hypothermia and CPB	Surface cooling: Thermal blanket Ice packs	Surface cooling is begun as soon as induction is complete, using thermal blankets above and below patient, ice packs and infusion of cold fluids during establish-

Hypothermia, cont.	SNP infusion Heparinization Rewarming	ment of isovolemic hemodilution, and infusion of SNP, as tolerated, to induce cutaneous vasodilatation. Once the neurosurgeons have exposed the giant aneurysm and determined that it cannot be clipped without resorting to CPB, systemic **heparinization** (load: 300 U/kg; maintenance: 100 U/kg/h) is established and patient is put on CPB using fem-fem bypass and cooled to ~18°C. During CPB cooling, the heart will usually fibrillate between 22-26°C. Once 18°C is reached, the CPB unit is shut off to deflate the aneurysm; it may be activated and shut off several times during clipping to evaluate adequacy of the surgical occlusion of the aneurysm and to apply additional clips. ★ **Total circulatory arrest time should not exceed 45 min.** When clipping is complete, CPB is resumed and warming instituted. Partial CPB is continued until normal cardiac rhythm is established, and body temperature reaches ~36°C. Once partial CPB is D/C, patient will tend to cool unless vigorous efforts at warming are continued. Warming the OR and iv fluids, and use of warming lights and Bair Hugger will facilitate the warming process. ACT analysis is performed to establish that heparin reversal is complete 5-10 min after protamine (1 mg/100 U heparin activity). If coagulation seems inadequate following heparin reversal, blood is sent for clotting studies, and Plts, FFP and calcium gluconate are administered as needed. Hetastarch 6% is not used in these patients because of its potential for inducing a coagulopathy.[1]
Complications	↓↓BP 2° failure to maintain circulating volume Dysrhythmias 2° ↓K^+ from diuresis and cold	

POSTOPERATIVE

Complications	HTN Vasospasm Intracranial hemorrhage, stroke Hypothermia Hypervolemia Coagulopathy DVT Seizures PE	HTN Rx: esmolol + SNP titrated to effect Vasospasm Rx: fluid-loading Patient should be rewarmed to 36-37°C before terminating CPB. ✓ coagulation status. Seizure Rx: Phenytoin (1 g iv slowly to avoid ↓BP) ★ **NB:** Incompatible with dextrose-containing solutions.
Pain management	Meperidine (10-20 mg iv prn) Codeine (30-60 mg im q 4 h prn)	Meperidine minimizes postop shivering.
Tests	CT scan Coagulation panel	If any question about neurological status arises, a CT scan is performed postop. Coagulation studies are needed early postop to assure normal coagulation.

References

1. Cully MD, Larson CP Jr, Silverberg GD: Hetastarch coagulopathy in a neurosurgical patient. *Anesthesiology* 1987; 66(5): 706-7.
2. Silverberg GD: Giant aneurysms: surgical treatment. *Neurol Res* 1984; 6(1-2):57-63.
3. Silverberg GD, Reitz BA, Ream AK: Hypothermia and cardiac arrest in the treatment of giant aneurysms of the cerebral circulation and hemangioblastoma of the medulla. *J Neurosurg* 1981; 55(3):337-46.
4. Steinberg GK, Chung M: Giant cerebral aneurysms: Morphology and structural pathology. In: Olwad IA, Barrow DL, eds: *Giant Cerebral Aneurysms.* American Association of Neurological Surgeons. Park Ridge: 1995, 1-11.

5. Steinberg GK, Drake CG, Peerless SJ: Deliberate basilar or vertebral artery occlusion in the treatment of intracranial aneurysms: Immediate results and long-term outcome in 201 patients. *J Neurosurg* 1993; 79:161-73.
6. Whittle IR, Dorsch NW, Besser M: Giant intracranial aneurysms: diagnosis, management, and outcome. *Surg Neurol* 1984; 21(3):218-30.

CRANIOTOMY FOR CEREBRAL EMBOLECTOMY

SURGICAL CONSIDERATIONS

Gary K. Steinberg

Description: This procedure is performed within 6 h following the onset of a neurological deficit 2° a documented thrombotic or embolic occlusion of a major intracranial vessel. A craniotomy is fashioned and the occluded intracranial artery is exposed using microscopic techniques. The involved arterial segment is isolated, temporarily occluded with miniature clips, and an **arteriotomy** is performed to remove the thrombus or embolus. Then the arteriotomy is closed. With the advent of intraarterial or iv tissue plasminogen activator delivered by endovascular techniques, this procedure may become less frequently performed.

Usual preop diagnosis: Stroke; transient ischemic attack (TIA); intracranial arterial occlusion; catheter embolization to intracranial artery

SUMMARY OF PROCEDURE

Position	Supine or lateral decubitus
Incision	Frontal, temporal or occipital
Special instrumentation	Microscopic instruments (fine forceps, miniature vascular clips, operating microscope)
Unique considerations	Neuroprotective agents during arterial segment occlusion (barbiturates, mannitol), mild hypothermia (33°C)
Antibiotics	Nafcillin (1-2 g iv q 6 h) + cefotaxime (1 g iv q 6 h)
Surgical time	3-4 h
Closing considerations	Avoid hypotension (MAP 80-100); induced mild HTN (MAP 90-110) during temporary arterial occlusion.
EBL	100-250 ml
Postop care	Control BP (MAP 80-100 mmHg); start aspirin postop d 1; ICU: 1-2 d.
Mortality	5-10%
Morbidity	Intracerebral hemorrhage Stroke MI: Rare Thromboembolism: Rare Respiratory failure: Rare Infection: Rare
Pain score	3-4

PATIENT POPULATION CHARACTERISTICS

Age range	50-80 yr
Male:Female	1:1
Incidence	Rare
Etiology	Atherosclerosis; carotid artery disease; atrial fibrillation; iatrogenic endovascular catheter complication
Associated conditions	HTN; CAD; PVD; carotid artery disease; hyperlipidemia; smoking; alcohol abuse; obesity; atrial fibrillation

ANESTHETIC CONSIDERATIONS

See Anesthetic Considerations for Craniotomy for Intracranial Aneurysms, p. 7.

References

1. Ojemann RG, Ogilvy CS, Heros RC, Crowell RM: *Surgical Management of Cerebrovascular Disease.* Williams & Wilkins, Baltimore: 1995.
2. Schmidek HH, Sweet WH, eds: *Operative Neurosurgical Techniques: Indications, Methods, and Results*, Vols I-II. WB Saunders Co, Philadelphia: 1995.
3. Sundt TM Jr: *Surgical Techniques for Saccular and Giant Intracranial Aneurysms.* Williams & Wilkins, Baltimore: 1990, 467-76.
4. Wilkins RH, Rengachary SS, eds: *Neurosurgery*, Vols 1-3. McGraw-Hill, New York: 1996.
5. Youmans JR, ed: *Neurological Surgery*, Vols 1-6. WB Saunders Co, Philadelphia: 1990.

CRANIOTOMY FOR INTRACRANIAL VASCULAR MALFORMATIONS

SURGICAL CONSIDERATIONS

Gary K. Steinberg

Description: Intracranial vascular malformations are congenital abnormalities that cause intracranial hemorrhage, seizures, headaches, progressive neurological deficits or audible bruits. Intracranial vascular malformations comprise high-flow, arteriovenous malformations (AVMs); low-flow, angiographically occult vascular malformations (AOVMs), including cavernous malformations, "cryptic" AVMs, capillary telangiectasias and transitional malformations; and low-flow, venous angiomas (developmental venous anomalies). **Microsurgical resection** is the optimal treatment for these lesions, although preop endovascular embolization, and preop or postop focused **stereotactic radiosurgery** (heavy particle or photon) may be useful adjuncts.

Most moderate-sized and large AVMs (> 3 cm diameter) are resected using a standard scalp flap and with craniotomy centered over the area of the AVM. The patient is positioned appropriately to place the craniotomy site uppermost in the field and parallel to the floor. For instance, a patient with a left frontal AVM would be positioned supine, head turned to the right, a left frontal or bicranial scalp flap raised and a left frontal craniotomy bone flap removed. A patient with a right medial occipital AVM would be positioned in the left lateral decubitus position with head turned semiprone and a right occipital scalp flap and craniotomy performed. Smaller AVMs (< 3 cm diameter), many low-flow AOVMs, and many deep-seated vascular malformations (AVMs and AOVMs) require a small, stereotactic craniotomy. This is performed by attaching a stereotactic base frame to the patient's skull (using local anesthetic and sedation). Next, a CT or MRI scan is obtained, using a radio-opaque localizer fixed to the base frame. The location of the AVM in relation to the frame is calculated, using a computer and stereotactic geometric principles. The patient is then taken to the OR, intubated fiber optically (because of the frame position) and positioned for surgery. A three-dimensional arc frame is fixed to the base frame and coordinates appropriately set to localize the vascular malformation within the brain.

In many centers, this traditional approach has been replaced with a frameless OR surgical navigation system (e.g., Radionics Optical Tracking System). With this frameless system, small radioopaque localizers are glued to the scalp, a CT or MRI scan is obtained, and the patient is taken to the OR, anesthetized and positioned for surgery. The surgical navigation system reference is attached to the headrest or microscope and calibrated. The location of the AVM is calculated, using a computer and stereotactic geometric principles. A small scalp flap and a small craniotomy (a few cm in diameter) can be fashioned precisely for microscopic exposure of the malformation. Microsurgical resection of brain stem and thalamic vascular malformations often necessitate special positioning.

Usual preop diagnosis: Cerebral AVM; dural AVM; cavernous malformation; angiographically occult vascular malformation; intracerebral hemorrhage; subarachnoid hemorrhage; seizures; epilepsy; progressive neurological deficit; migraine or vascular headaches

SUMMARY OF PROCEDURE

	Standard Craniotomy (High-Flow AVM)	Stereotactic Craniotomy (Low-Flow AOVM)	Brain Stem/Thalamic Vascular Malformations
Position	Supine, lateral, Concorde (modified prone) (Fig 1.1-2)	⇐	Lateral, Concorde, semisitting (Fig 1.1-3)
Incision	Frontal, temporal, parietal, occipital, suboccipital, or combination	⇐	Suboccipital (midline), paramedian or occipital
Special instrumentation	Operating microscope; irrigating bipolar coagulation; radiolucent table and headrest. Sundt mini aneurysm and micro AVM clips. Access to femoral artery for intraop angiography.	⇐ + Surgical navigation system	⇐
Unique considerations	Induced hypotension (MAP 60-65 mmHg) during resection, use of neuroprotective agents (see Craniotomy for Aneurysms, p. 6). Relaxed brain. Mild hypothermia (33°C); ± lumbar CSF drain.	Use of neuroprotective agents and relaxed brain (see Craniotomy for Aneurysms, p. 6). ⇐	⇐
Antibiotics	Nafcillin (1-2 g iv q 6 h) + cefotaxime (1 g iv q 6 h)	⇐	⇐
Surgical time	4-10 h	2-5 h	3-6 h
Closing considerations	Maintain MAP 60-65 mmHg. Avoid ↑venous pressure. For supratentorial vascular malformations, administer additional anticonvulsants; give loading dose of phenytoin (1 g iv for adults) if not previously on anticonvulsants.	Keep MAP 70-90 mmHg. ⇐	⇐ No anticonvulsants necessary
EBL	500-3000 ml	< 250 ml	⇐
Postop care	ICU × 1-2 d. Maintain MAP 60-65 mmHg for 2-4 d. ICP monitoring, ventricular drain; normovolemic in ICU.	ICU × 1 d; normovolemic in ICU	⇐
Mortality	1-10%, depending on AVM size, location, and venous drainage pattern	< 0.5%	< 2%
Morbidity	Overall: 5-30%	< 5%	10-50% (transient)
	Neurological	⇐	⇐
	Intracranial hemorrhage	⇐	⇐
	Cerebral edema	⇐	⇐
	Stroke	⇐	⇐
	Hydrocephalus	⇐	⇐
	Massive blood loss: Occasional	⇐	⇐
	Thromboembolism: Rare	⇐	⇐
	Infection: Rare	⇐	⇐
Pain score	3-4	3-4	3-4

PATIENT POPULATION CHARACTERISTICS

Age range	15-40 yr (most common), 41-60 yr (less frequent)
Male:Female	1:1
Incidence	0.5-1% of U.S. population
Etiology	Congenital; traumatic for dural AVM
Associated conditions	Von Hippel-Lindau disease; Rendu-Osler-Weber syndrome; familial cavernous malformation syndrome

ANESTHETIC CONSIDERATIONS

C. Philip Larson, Jr.

PREOPERATIVE

Arteriovenous malformations (AVMs) are direct arterial-to-venous communications without intervening capillary circulation.[8] With the gross and radiologic appearance of "a bag of worms," they can occur anywhere in the brain or spinal cord, varying in size from small lesions called "cryptic malformations" to very large lesions occupying a major portion of a cerebral hemisphere. Thought to be congenital, AVMs usually do not manifest themselves clinically until patients are in their late teens or 20's. Typically, these patients are otherwise healthy. On histological exam, the vessel walls are thin and lack a muscular layer; consequently, the vessels exhibit loss of normal vasomotor control or responsiveness to changes in $PaCO_2$. Treatment consists of surgical excision, radiologic embolization or stereotactic radiosurgery, alone or in combination.[12] **Stereotactic localization** is essential for safe excision of deep-seated AVMs (e.g., those located in the corona radiata, basal ganglia, visual center, cerebellar white matter or corpus callosum).

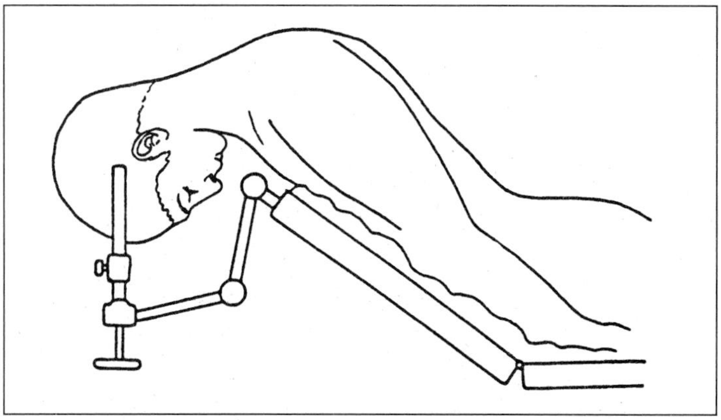

Figure 1.1-2. Concorde (modified prone) position for resection of posterior fossa vascular malformations. (Reproduced with permission from Sugita K: *Microsurgical Atlas*. Springer-Verlag Berlin Heidelberg: 1985.)

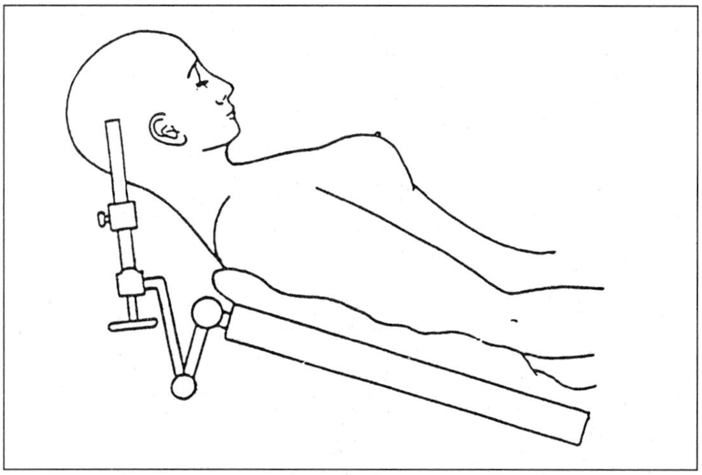

Figure 1.1-3. Semisitting position for resection of deep posterior corpus callosum or thalamic vascular malformations. (Reproduced with permission from Sugita K: *Microsurgical Atlas*. Springer-Verlag Berlin Heidelberg: 1985.)

Respiratory Not usually significant unless patient has Hx of smoking, or has pulmonary aspiration as a result of a neurological deficit from an intracranial hemorrhage.

Tests: As indicated from H&P.

Cardiovascular Generally, these patients do not have other cardiovascular diseases. Occasionally, ECG changes are noted following intracranial hemorrhage, and may simply reflect the extent of brain injury.

Tests: ECG; others as indicated from H&P.

Neurological Presenting Sx depend on location and size of AVM, and whether it is a low- or high-flow lesion. Hemorrhage with resultant neurological deficits is the most common Sx, although patients also may present with intractable seizure disorder, recurrent headaches or Sx of cerebral ischemia, including seizures 2° high-flow arteriovenous shunts, causing an intracerebral steal. Surgical treatment is vital not only to eliminate recurrent headaches or seizures but, more importantly, to prevent future hemorrhage (incidence of 3-4%/yr) and substantial mortality (6-30%) or severe morbidity (15-80%).[14] Hemorrhages from AVMs located deep in the brain (thalamus, caudate nucleus) or in the brain stem are particularly devastating. Unlike hemorrhages from an intracerebral aneurysm (generally intraventricular), hemorrhages from an AVM are usually intraparenchymal; hence, they are seldom associated with cerebral vasospasm.

Tests: CT; MRI; cerebral angiogram. Preop cerebral angiogram indicates size and location of the AVM, and whether it is likely to be a low- or high-flow lesion.

Hematologic After 7-8 h of surgery for AVM, it is fairly common for surrounding brain tissue to swell and vascular surgery sites to bleed. The cause of this is unknown, but it may be related to the fact that the brain is rich in thromboplastin, which, in turn, may cause a local coagulopathy. Thus, it is advisable to obtain coagulation studies preop and stage excision over more than one sitting when AVM is large.
Tests: Hct; PT; PTT; Plt count

Laboratory CBC; other tests as indicated from H&P.

Premedication Seldom necessary; detailed discussion with patient about the anesthetic plan, with appropriate reassurance, is usually enough. If medication is desirable, small doses of sedative/hypnotic (e.g., midazolam 2-5 mg iv) are useful.

INTRAOPERATIVE

Anesthetic technique: GETA. The goals of anesthesia for this operation are to: (1) maintain a somewhat decreased (10-20% below normal) CPP to lessen blood loss during excision of the AVM (CPP = cerebral arterial pressure minus cerebral venous or ICP, whichever is greater); (2) decrease intracranial volume (blood and tissue) to optimize surgical working space within the cranial compartment and minimize the need for surgical retraction of brain tissue; (3) decrease cerebral oxygen consumption ($CMRO_2$) to lessen the dependence, at least acutely, of normal brain on vessels feeding the AVM. For stereotactic surgery, either a frame is placed on the patient's head under local anesthesia or scalp localizing markers are attached. The patient is then sent to CT or MR where the exact coordinates defining the AVM and critical adjacent structures are established. The patient is brought to OR and anesthesia is induced.

Induction STP 5 mg/kg or propofol 2-3 mg/kg iv provides amnesia and decreases cerebral blood volume by inducing cerebral vasoconstriction. Fentanyl 9-10 μg/kg iv provides analgesia for the first hours. High-dose opiates used as a primary anesthetic technique do not alter CBF or $CMRO_2$ enough to provide any special benefits beyond their GA effects. Vecuronium (0.15 mg/kg) or rocuronium (0.7-1 mg/kg) provide muscle relaxation for intubation and patient positioning.
If patient is in a stereotactic frame, ET intubation must be accomplished before anesthesia is induced, because the frame partially occludes the mouth, making conventional laryngoscopy impossible. Oral fiber optic intubation of the trachea is the easiest method for accomplishing this (see p. B-6).

Maintenance Isoflurane 1% or less (0.6% maximum if evoked potential monitoring is used) with 1:1 O_2/N_2O. Propofol 75-150 μg/kg/min by continuous infusion may be administered to provide ↓cerebral blood volume and ↓$CMRO_2$. Mild hypothermia (33°C) provides additional cerebral protection (see below). Additional neuromuscular blocking drugs are not necessary, but can be administered if patient movement is of concern.

Emergence If the brain has not been injured by the surgical procedure and patient is adequately rewarmed, awakening from the anesthetic should occur within 30 min after cessation of isoflurane administration. As patient is awakening, it is important to assure full reversal from neuromuscular blockade, and closely regulate BP. If the intubated patient begins to cough, either the ETT should be removed or the cough suppressed with lidocaine sprayed down the tube (LTA) while patient is still anesthetized. Patient is placed in bed in a 30° head-up position and transported to ICU for overnight monitoring. Supplemental O_2 should be administered, and close regulation of BP maintained to prevent breakthrough bleeding from the raw surface areas left behind. Prophylactic antiemetic (e.g., metoclopramide 10 mg or ondansetron 4 mg) should be given 30-60 min before extubation.

Blood and fluid requirements

IV: 16 ga × 2
NS/LR @ < 10 ml/kg + UO

If blood volume is normal, NS/LR – not to exceed 10 ml/kg beyond that required to replace UO – is given. If hypovolemic, albumin 5% is given if Hct > 30%; combinations of albumin and blood, if Hct < 30%. Hetastarch may be used but should not exceed 20 ml/kg because of its potential for inducing a coagulopathy.[2]

Hypothermia

Ice packs
Thermal blanket
Cool air blower (or Polar Bair)
Cold OR

Mild hypothermia (33°-34°C) is used in some centers during this operation to decrease $CMRO_2$ and brain size.[13] $CMRO_2$ decreases about 7% for every degree C decrease in brain temperature; so at 33°C, cerebral metabolism is

Hypothermia, cont.		decreased about 30% below normal. From studies in animals, it is generally believed that this level of hypothermia is beneficial,[1,4] although there are no studies in patients documenting decreased morbidity or mortality from its use. This level of hypothermia does not interfere appreciably with coagulation, nor is it generally associated with cardiac dysrhythmias. Warming is begun several h before the conclusion of surgery by using thermal blanket, Bair Hugger and warming lights, by warming inspired gases, and by increasing the ambient temperature in OR. Usually by the time the operation is completed, patient temperature is near normal.
Control of brain volume (ICP)	Hyperventilate to $PaCO_2$ = 25-30 mmHg or $PetCO_2$ = 20-25 mmHg. Limit isoflurane ≤ 1%. Limit fluids. High-dose STP Mannitol 1 g/kg Furosemide 0.3 mg/kg Lumbar CSF drainage	↓$PaCO_2$ has several advantages, including ↓cerebral vascular volume, which provides surgeons more working space and lessens need for vigorous retraction of brain tissue. ↓$PaCO_2$ also improves the regional distribution of CBF by: preferentially diverting blood to potentially ischemic areas of the brain; better buffering of the brain lactic acid that may form as a result of focal ischemia; and decreasing anesthetic requirement. If AVM is superficial, decreasing brain volume is less important, and the first 4 techniques listed (at left) are usually sufficient. If AVM is deep, the additional listed therapies may be needed.
Monitoring	Standard monitors (see p. B-1). + Bladder temperature Arterial line CVP line UO	Direct monitoring of arterial pressure prior to induction is essential for rapid control of BP. Transducer should always be placed at the level of the head rather than the heart, since CPP is arterial pressure at the brain level minus cerebral venous or ICP, whichever is higher. Monitoring CVP via a right atrial catheter is desirable in virtually all patients to assess adequacy of fluid therapy and for infusion of vasoactive drugs. The ideal site for insertion of the catheter, in order of preference, is: right IJ, right subclavian, and right EJ vein. Localization of the catheter can be determined by CXR, ECG tracing, noting P-wave changes, or pressure-wave contour and value as the catheter is withdrawn from the right ventricle into the right atrium. If patient has a high-flow AVM causing a large arteriovenous shunt, venous blood may appear arterialized (or bright red) during central venous catheterization, suggesting that the operator has punctured an artery rather than a central vein.
Control of BP	Isoflurane/sevoflurane Esmolol infusion SNP infusion Maintain normovolemia.	Close regulation of BP during induction and prior to excision of AVMs may be less critical than for aneurysmal surgery.[13] Once surgical excision is underway, however, modest decreases in MAP (≤ 20% below normal) using isoflurane, alone or in combination with esmolol and/or SNP, should be used to prevent excessive bleeding. Responses to vasoactive drugs are much easier to regulate if normal blood volume has been established and maintained throughout the anesthetic period.
Positioning	Shoulder roll 3-point fixation ✓ and pad pressure points. ✓ eyes. 180° rotation	For most AVMs, patient is positioned supine, head turned laterally in 3-point fixation and a roll under shoulder on the side of operation (Fig 1.1-4). Anesthetic hoses and all monitoring and vascular catheter lines are directed toward patient's feet or side where the anesthesiologist is

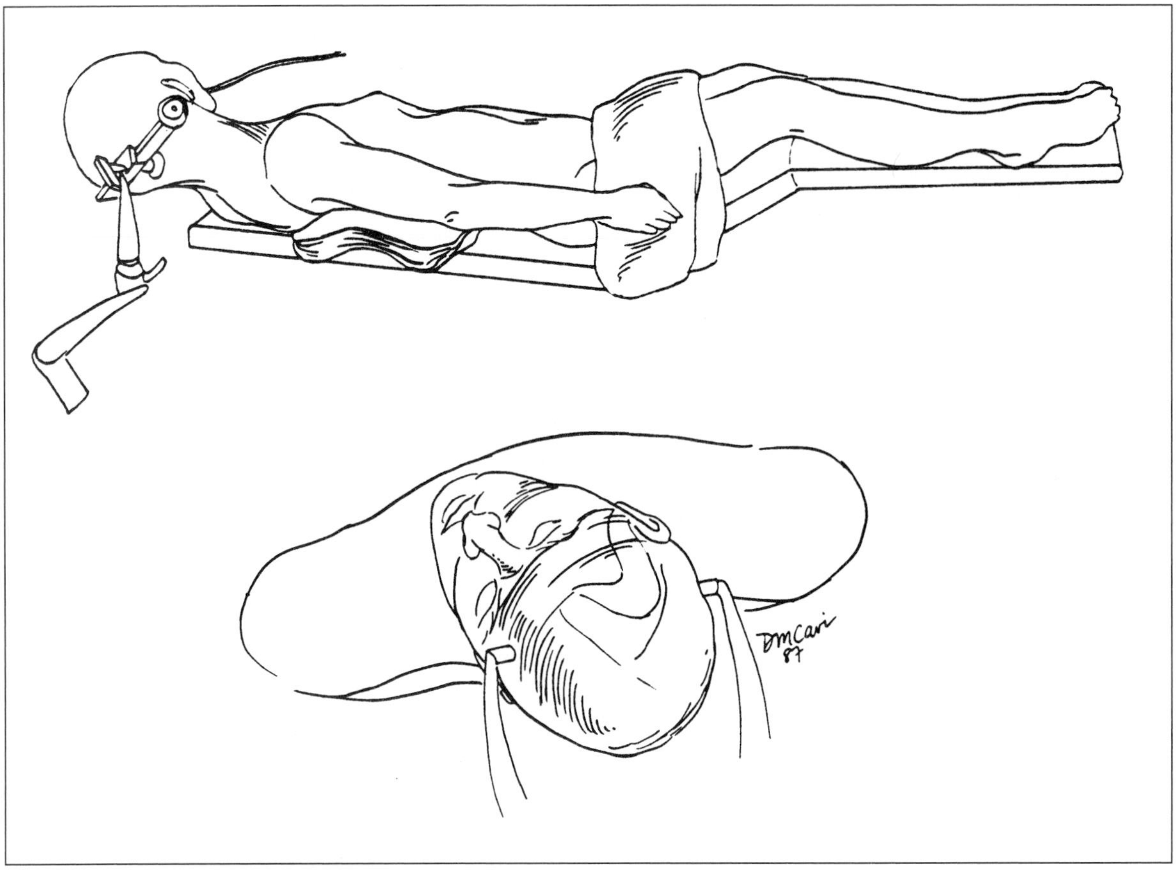

Figure 1.1-4. Supine position, head elevated above heart, turned 30-45° to side, vertex dropped for approach to anterior circulation aneurysms and frontal vascular malformations. (Reproduced with permission from Long DM: *Atlas of Operative Neurosurgical Technique*, Vol 1. Williams & Wilkins: 1989.)

Positioning, cont.

positioned. In planning anesthetic equipment, make sure that all will reach the foot of operating table. Antiembolism stockings and SCDs used to minimize DVT. Remifentanil (4-5 μg/kg) to minimize ↑BP during skull pinning.

POSTOPERATIVE

Complications	Neurological deficits Cerebral edema and ↑ICP Intracerebral hemorrhage	If any of these complications occur, it is likely that patient will have to be reintubated and transported to the CT scanner for further neurological evaluation or possible reoperation. Careful regulation of BP is essential to avoid postop hemorrhage.
	Seizures	★ Seizure Rx: Phenytoin (1 g loading dose). **NB:** Incompatible with dextrose-containing solutions.
Pain management	Meperidine 10-20 mg iv Codeine (30-60 mg im q 4 h prn)	Meperidine minimizes postop shivering.
Tests	CT scan if neurological status changes.	

References

1. Berntman L, Welsh FA, Harp JR: Cerebral protective effect of low-grade hypothermia. *Anesthesiology* 1981; 55(5):495-98.
2. Cully MD, Larson CP Jr, Silverberg GD: Hetastarch coagulopathy in a neurosurgical patient. [Letter] *Anesthesiology* 1987; 66(5):706-7.
3. Ojemann RG, Ogilvy CS, Heros RC, Crowell RM: *Surgical Management of Cerebrovascular Disease*. Williams & Wilkins, Baltimore: 1995.

4. Sano T, Drummond JC, Patel PM, Grafe MR, Watson JC, Cole DJ: A comparison of the cerebral protective effects of isoflurane and mild hypothermia in a model of incomplete forebrain ischemia in the rat. *Anesthesiology* 1992; 76(2):221-28.
5. Schmidek HH, Sweet WH, eds: *Operative Neurosurgical Techniques: Indications, Methods, and Results*, Vols I-II. WB Saunders Co, Philadelphia: 1995.
6. Smith RM, Stetson JB: Therapeutic hypothermia. *N Engl J Med* 1961; 265:1097-1103, 1147-51.
7. Stein B, Soloman R: Arteriovenous malformations of the brain. In: *Neurological Surgery*, Vols 1-6. Youmans JR, ed. WB Saunders Co, Philadelphia: 1990, 1831-63.
8. Stein BM, Wolpert SM: Arteriovenous malformations of the brain. I: Current concepts and treatment. *Arch Neurol* 1980; 37(1):1-5.
9. Steinberg GK, Chang SD: Surgical management of angiographically occult vascular malformations of the brainstem, thalamus and basal ganglia. In: *Neurosurgical Atlas*. Rengachary SS, ed. American Association of Neurological Surgeons, Park Ridge: 1998 (in press).
10. Steinberg GK, Chang SD, Levy RP, Marks MP, Frankel K, Marcellus M: Surgical resection of intracranial arteriovenous malformations following stereotactic radiosurgery. *J Neurosurg* 1966; 84:920-28.
11. Steinberg GK, Marks MP: Intracranial arteriovenous malformations: Therapeutic options. In: *Cerebrovascular Disease*, Batjer HH, ed. Lippincott-Raven Publishers, Philadelphia: 1997; 727-42.
12. Steinberg GK, Vanefsky MA: Management of the patient with an angiographically occult vascular malformation. In: *Perspectives in Neurological Surgery,* Hadley MN, ed. Quality Medical Publishing, Inc., St. Louis: 1994; 5:18-39.
13. Szabo MD, Crosby G, Sundaram P, Dodson BA, Kjellberg RN: Hypertension does not cause spontaneous hemorrhage of intracranial arteriovenous malformations. *Anesthesiology* 1989; 70(5):761-3.
14. Wilkins RH: Natural history of intracranial vascular malformations: a review. *Neurosurgery* 1985; 16(3):421-30.
15. Wilkins RH, Rengachary SS, eds: *Neurosurgery*, Vols 1-3. McGraw-Hill, New York: 1996.
16. Yasargil MG: *Microneurosurgery*. Thieme Medical Publishers Inc, New York: 1988.
17. Youmans JR, ed: *Neurological Surgery*, Vols 1-6. WB Saunders Co, Philadelphia: 1990.

CRANIOTOMY FOR EXTRACRANIAL-INTRACRANIAL REVASCULARIZATION (EC-IC BYPASS)

SURGICAL CONSIDERATIONS

Gary K. Steinberg

Description: Extracranial-intracranial (EC-IC) revascularization procedures are performed when: (1) deliberate occlusion of a major cervical artery (carotid or vertebral) is necessary and inadequate collateral CBF is available; or (2) stenosis or occlusion of major cervical or intracranial arteries causes transient ischemic attacks (TIAs) or stroke, despite the use of maximum medical therapy (aspirin, heparin or Coumadin). A donor extracranial scalp artery or interposition vein segment is sutured to a cervical artery and anastomosed to an intracranial artery, using microscopic techniques, through a **craniotomy**. The most common EC-IC procedure is a **superficial temporal artery (STA)-to-middle cerebral artery (MCA) branch anastomosis**. Other grafts include STA-to-posterior cerebral artery, STA-to- superior cerebellar artery, occipital artery-to-posterior inferior cerebral artery or interposition saphenous vein segment graft from the cervical external carotid artery to the middle cerebral artery, posterior cerebral artery or superior cerebellar artery.

Variant procedure or approaches: Encephalo-duro-arterio-synangiosis (EDAS) is a variant procedure wherein the STA is dissected circumferentially with its adventitia in the scalp, left in continuity and laid on the surface of the brain after opening the dura. **Omentum-to-brain transposition** is another variant wherein the omentum, with its luxuriant blood supply, is lengthened, left attached to the right gastroepiploic artery, tunneled subcutaneously in the chest and neck, and laid over a large area of poorly vascularized cerebral cortex after opening the dura. Sometimes a free omental graft is transposed to the brain by anastomosing the omental gastroepiploic artery and vein to the superficial temporal artery and vein. Revascularization is induced by angiogenesis factors and growth substances secreted by the omentum.

Usual preop diagnosis: Stroke; TIA; carotid artery stenosis (inaccessible to carotid endarterectomy); carotid artery occlusion; middle cerebral artery stenosis or occlusion; vertebral artery stenosis or occlusion; basilar artery stenosis or occlusion; moyamoya disease (cerebral ischemia due to occlusion of vessels at base of the brain)

SUMMARY OF PROCEDURE

	EC-IC Bypass	EC-IC Bypass With Vein Graft	Omentum-to-Brain Transposition
Position	Supine or lateral decubitus	⇐	⇐
Incision	Frontal, parietal, temporal or occipital, or a combination of these, depending on area to be vascularized.	⇐ + Medial aspect of leg and thigh for harvesting greater saphenous vein	⇐ + Vertical abdominal incision for harvesting omentum; chest/neck incision for tunneling
Special instrumentation	Microscopic instruments; microvascular Doppler to identify scalp donor artery course and confirm graft patency.	⇐ + Tunneling instruments	⇐
Unique considerations	Neuroprotective agents (barbiturates, mannitol) and induced mild HTN (MAP 90-110) during cross-clamp of recipient intracranial artery. Avoid excessive brain relaxation. Mild hypothermia (33°C). Dexamethasone 8-12 mg iv.	⇐ + Attention to proper alignment of vein when tunneled, to avoid kinking; heparinization if major cervical artery (carotid, vertebral) is temporarily occluded.	⇐ + Avoid devascularizing omentum during dissection and compromise to omental blood supply during tunneling and skin closure.
Antibiotics	Nafcillin (1-2 g iv q 6 h) + cefotaxime (1 g iv q 6 h)	⇐	⇐
Surgical time	3-5 h	⇐	⇐
Closing considerations	Careful attention to hemostasis. Avoid compromise of graft with dural closure, bone replacement or scalp closure.	⇐	⇐
EBL	< 100 ml	⇐	100-500 ml
Postop care	Start aspirin on postop d 1; monitor for subdural hygroma (CSF fluid collection in subdural space); ICU × 1 d.	⇐	⇐
Mortality	< 0.5%	⇐	⇐
Morbidity	Subdural hygroma: Rare	⇐	Abdominal hernia: Rare
	Wound infection: Rare	⇐	⇐
	Stroke: Rare	⇐	⇐
Pain score	3	3	3

PATIENT POPULATION CHARACTERISTICS

Age range	40-80 yr; 2-20 yr for moyamoya disease
Male:Female	1:1 for atherosclerotic disease; 1:1.4 for moyamoya disease
Incidence	Thromboembolic stroke common, but indications for EC-IC bypass rare; 1/million/yr for moyamoya disease
Etiology	Atherosclerosis; embolism from heart or carotid artery
Associated conditions	HTN; CAD; PVD; hyperlipidemia; smoking; alcohol abuse; obesity; moyamoya disease

ANESTHETIC CONSIDERATIONS

C. Philip Larson, Jr.

PREOPERATIVE

EC-IC bypass is used to make an anastomosis between external (usually superficial temporal artery) and internal carotid circulation. Patients with symptomatic moyamoya disease or bilateral carotid stenosis or occlusion also seem to be good candidates for EC-IC bypass, especially since there are no other forms of therapy which have proven to be effective.

Respiratory None unless patient has Hx of smoking or has sustained pulmonary aspiration as a result of a neurological deficit.
Tests: As indicated from H&P.

Cardiovascular These patients may have generalized vascular disease, including CAD, so a careful cardiac Hx, physical exam and ECG analysis should be done. If findings are positive, consider a more complete evaluation, including ECHO and coronary angiography. Be aware that cardiac insufficiency is the cause of about half of the deaths in patients with cerebrovascular disease.[5]
Tests: Consider ECG, others as indicated from H&P.

Neurological Patients present with Sx of focal ischemic lesions. Cerebral angiography to rule out other causes of transient ischemic attacks and characterize collateral circulation. Regional CBF studies generally not helpful because measurement does not distinguish between low flow due to cerebrovascular obstruction from low flow due to low metabolic demands 2° prolonged cerebral ischemia.
Tests: CT; MRI; angiogram

Hematologic Anticoagulants or platelet-suppressive drugs such as NSAIDs should be D/C 2 wk before surgery to avoid excessive bleeding.
Tests: Hct; PT; PTT; hemogram

Laboratory Tests as indicated from H&P.

Premedication Seldom necessary; detailed discussion with patient about the anesthetic plan, with appropriate reassurance, is usually enough. If premedication is desirable, small doses of sedative/hypnotics (e.g., midazolam 2-5 mg) are preferable to opiates.

INTRAOPERATIVE

Anesthetic technique: GETA. The goals of anesthesia for this procedure are to: (1) provide adequate surgical anesthesia; (2) decrease intracranial volume (blood and tissue) to optimize working space within the cranial compartment, thereby minimizing the need for surgical retraction of brain tissue; and (3) increase tolerance of the brain to ischemia by decreasing $CMRO_2$ with the use of mild hypothermia (33°-34°C) and barbiturate or propofol therapy, and maximizing flow to the ischemic area through collateral channels by maintaining BP at normal or somewhat elevated values.

Induction STP (5 mg/kg iv) or propofol (2-3 mg/kg) provides amnesia and decreases cerebral blood volume by inducing cerebral vasoconstriction in the normally reactive vessels. Ischemic vessels will not contract in response to these drugs. Fentanyl (7-10 μg/kg iv) provides analgesia for first hours of case). Vecuronium (0.15 mg/kg) or rocuronium (0.7-1 mg/kg) for intubation and positioning of patient.

Maintenance Isoflurane ≤ 1% inspired with O_2/N_2O (≤ 50% N_20 because of its potential for reversing the protective effects of STP for focal ischemia). STP (5 mg/kg) or propofol (2-3 mg/kg) is given just prior to surgical occlusion of the cerebral vessel in preparation for anastomosis. This dose is given over 5-10 min to avoid sudden ↓BP. The concentration of isoflurane is decreased during STP or propofol administration.

Emergence Generally, ETT can be removed at the conclusion of anesthetic, unless the operation has been particularly long or complex. Prophylactic antiemetic (e.g., metoclopramide 10 mg or ondansetron 4 mg) should be given 30-60 min before extubation.

Blood and fluid requirements
IV: 18 ga × 2
NS/LR @ < 10 ml/kg + UO
CVP (triple-lumen)

Triple-lumen CVP with multiple stopcocks for connection of esmolol, SNP, phenylephrine infusions. One lumen is used for monitoring CVP.

Control of brain volume (ICP)
Hyperventilate to $PaCO_2$ = 25-30 mmHg.
↓fluids < 10 ml/kg + UO
STP or propofol infusion
↓isoflurane < 1%, or sevoflurane < 2%
Mannitol 1 g/kg
± Furosemide 0.3 mg/kg
± Lumbar CSF drain
Dexamethasone 8-12 mg

Generally, vigorous control of brain volume is not necessary since surgeon is working with cerebral vessels on the surface of the brain. If an omental graft is to be placed on the brain, however, additional brain shrinkage is useful. Ventilation is controlled and TV and RR are adjusted such that $PaCO_2$ ranges from 25-30 mmHg. Hypocarbia has several advantages, including decreasing cerebral vascular volume, providing more surgical working space and lessening need for vigorous retraction of brain tis-

Brain volume, cont.		sue; improving the regional distribution of CBF by: preferentially diverting blood to potentially ischemic areas of the brain; better buffering of brain lactic acid that may form as a result of focal ischemia; and decreasing anesthetic requirement.
Monitoring	Standard monitors (see p. B-1). ± Bladder temperature Arterial line CVP (triple-lumen IJ catheter) UO	
Control of BP	Maintain normal BP.	Maintenance of normal BP is important because of the dependence of flow on collateral circulation, particularly during temporary occlusion of the surgical vessel being anastomosed. If a vasoconstrictor is needed, a pure α-adrenergic stimulant such as phenylephrine is preferred because it has minimal dysrhythmogenic potential. Responses to vasoactive drugs are much easier to regulate if a normal blood volume has been maintained throughout the anesthetic period.
Positioning	✓ and pad pressure points. ✓ eyes. Shoulder roll	If omental graft is used, chest and abdomen must be clear of anesthetic apparatus. Anesthetic hoses and monitoring and vascular lines directed to patient's feet where anesthesiologist is positioned during surgery.
	Antiembolism stockings, SCDs	Antiembolism stockings and SCDs used to minimize DVT.
Deliberate hypothermia	Cold-water circulating blanket, ice packs or cold air blanket Maintain body temperature of ~33-34°C Warm OR and iv fluids.	Surface cooling is begun as soon as induction of anesthesia is complete, using a cold-water circulating blanket underneath patient, ice packs or a cold air blanket (e.g., Polar Bair) above the patient. When anastomosis is nearly complete, vigorous efforts at warming, including warming OR and iv fluids, are initiated.
Complications	Seizures Stroke Hemorrhage at anastomosis	★ Seizure Rx: Phenytoin (1 g loading dose). **NB:** Incompatible with dextrose-containing solutions)

POSTOPERATIVE

Complications	Localized scalp necrosis	Major complications uncommon; localized scalp necrosis unique to this procedure.
Pain management	Meperidine (10 mg iv prn) Codeine (30-60 mg im q 4 h prn)	
Tests	Cerebral angiogram	Cerebral angiography documents patency of graft and collateral flow.
	Regional blood flow studies	Some centers have the capability of performing regional blood flow studies.
	CT scan	If any question about neurological status, a CT scan is performed.

References

1. Ausman JI, Diaz FG: Critique of the extracranial-intracranial bypass study. *Surg Neurol* 1986; 26(3):218-21.
2. Chang SD, Steinberg GK: Other surgical options for stroke prevention. In: *Cerebrovascular Disease: Pathophysiology, Diagnosis and Management.* Ginsberg M, Bougosslavsky J, eds. Blackwell Science, Cambridge: 1998, 1945–63.
3. Cockcroft KM, Steinberg GK: Cerebral revascularization. In *Principles of Neurosurgery,* 2nd edition. Grossman RG, Loftus CM, eds. Lippincott-Raven Publishers, Philadelphia: 1999, 367-84.
4. Day AL, Rhoton AL, Little JR: The extracranial-intracranial bypass study. *Surg Neurol* 1986; 26(3):222-26.

5. EC/IC Bypass Study Group: Failure of extracranial-intracranial arterial bypass to reduce the risk of ischemic stroke. Results of an international randomized trial. *N Engl J Med* 1985; 313(19):1191-1200.
6. Fox JL, et al: Microsurgical treatment of neurovascular disease. *Neurosurgery* 1978; 3:285-337.
7. Ojemann RG, Ogilvy CS, Heros RC, Crowell RM: *Surgical Management of Cerebrovascular Disease.* Williams & Wilkins, Baltimore: 1995.
8. Samson DS, Boone S: Extracranial-intracranial (EC-IC) arterial bypass: past performances and current concepts. *Neurosurgery* 1978; 3(1):79-86.
9. Schmidek HH, Sweet WH, eds: *Operative Neurosurgical Techniques: Indications, Methods, and Results*, Vols I-II. WB Saunders Co, Philadelphia: 1995.
10. Sundt TM Jr: *Surgical Techniques for Saccular and Giant Intracranial Aneurysms.* Williams & Wilkins, Baltimore: 1990.
11. Wilkins RH, Rengachary SS, eds: *Neurosurgery*, Vols 1-3. McGraw-Hill, New York: 1996.
12. Yonekawa Y, Gots Y, Ogata N: Moyamoya disease: diagnosis, treatment and recent achievement. In *Stroke: Pathophysiology, Diagnosis and Management*, 2nd edition. Barnett HJM, Mohr JP, Stein BM, Yabu F, eds. Churchill Livingstone, New York: 1992, 721-47.
13. Youmans JR, ed: *Neurological Surgery*, Vols 1-6. WB Saunders Co, Philadelphia: 1990.

CRANIOTOMY FOR TUMOR

SURGICAL CONSIDERATIONS

Lawrence M. Shuer

Description: Tumors of the brain fall into various categories, which can be classified as: supratentorial and infratentorial, intraaxial (e.g., astrocytoma, oligodendroglioma, glioblastoma) and extraaxial (e.g., meningioma, acoustic neuroma). The surgical approach depends on the location of the lesion, whether there is a need for brain relaxation or whether exposure will require brain resection or incision. The positioning of the patient also depends on the location of tumor; e.g., the sitting position is often utilized for pineal tumors and for some other posterior fossa tumors (cerebellar tumors and acoustic neuromas) and the supine position is used for craniopharyngiomas and subfrontal tumors. Surgeons may prefer the lateral position for temporal lobe or parietal lobe lesions and the prone position for occipital lobe lesions and some cerebellar lesions. The prone or lateral position may be used for acoustic neuromas and the semisitting position may be used for occipital lesions. The patient's head is placed in a head holder (suction cup, horseshoe or Shea headrest or pin fixation (Mayfield). There are several common types of incisions, and the type used is customized to the lesion. The bone normally is removed by creating burr holes and then cutting a flap with the neuro bone saw. Some surgeons routinely use a "free-bone flap," in which the bone is completely removed and stored for the duration of the case. Other surgeons turn an osteoplastic flap, where the bone is left attached to muscle and/or pericranium to keep it partially vascularized. In the **suboccipital**, or **posterior fossa craniotomy**, the bone is often removed piecemeal, with either a drill or a series of rongeurs. Once the bone is removed, the dura is opened and, depending on tumor location and type, the surgeon either proceeds with tumor removal or obtains exposure within the brain in order to remove the tumor. Brain relaxation is requested if it is needed to expose and remove the lesion. When operating around the brain stem, vasomotor instability (bradycardia or HTN) may occur. The surgeon will need to know when these events occur, as they may signal injury to vital areas. Once the tumor is removed, the surgeon establishes hemostasis prior to dural closure. Occasionally, it is necessary to use a dural graft to close the dura. In supratentorial cases, the bone is usually replaced; however, the bone can be stored up to 6 months for subsequent replacement if swelling is anticipated. Patients undergoing this type of procedure usually require intensive postop care.

Variant procedure or approaches: Patient positioning varies from supine to prone to lateral to sitting, depending on surgeon's preference, as well as tumor location. Tumors on the convexity or close to the surface may not require much brain relaxation or exposure; however, tumors at the base of the brain may require extensive relaxation and exposure in order to be reached. Tumors at the base of the brain or deep within the ventricular system are usually removed with the aid of the operating microscope. Some are easily removed (e.g., convexity meningioma), while others are tedious and involve lengthy surgical time (e.g., craniopharyngioma and acoustic neuroma). Surgeons may use evoked potential monitoring techniques to aid in the removal of the tumors at the base of the brain in and about the cranial nerves.

Usual preop diagnosis: Brain tumor; glioma; glioblastoma; astrocytoma; oligodendroglioma; ependymoma; primitive neuroectodermal tumor; meningioma; craniopharyngioma; choroid plexus papilloma; hemangioblastoma; medulloblastoma; acoustic neuroma; pituitary adenoma

SUMMARY OF PROCEDURE

Position	Supine, lateral, prone or sitting
Incision	Dependent on location of tumor
Special instrumentation	Operating microscope; laser; CUSA; neuro drill (craniotome); ± evoked potential monitoring equipment
Unique considerations	ETT must be taped securely in a location satisfactory to the surgeon; anode or RAE tube is helpful in certain situations. Brain relaxation techniques may be required. The patient with ↑ICP may require special consideration for induction of anesthesia.
Antibiotics	Nafcillin 1-2 g; cefotaxime 1 g iv
Surgical time	2.5-12 h
Closing considerations	Possible requirement for fascia lata graft or lyophilized (cadaveric) dura. Drain often left in epidural space. The surgeon often requests control of BP to avoid hemorrhage into bed of tumor.
EBL	25-500 ml
Postop care	ICU or close observation unit x 1-3 d. Fluid and electrolytes require frequent monitoring, as the patient may develop SIADH following this procedure. BP may need to be controlled with hypotensive agents or ß-blockers.
Mortality	0-5% (higher for tumors in critical locations)
Morbidity	Infection Neurological: neurologic disability, nerve injury Endocrine disorder: panhypopituitarism, diabetes insipidus (DI) CSF leak Massive blood loss: venous sinus injury
Pain score	2-6

PATIENT POPULATION CHARACTERISTICS

Age range	Infant–85 yr (usually 20-60 yr)
Male:Female	~1:1
Incidence	Common neurosurgical procedure
Etiology	Neoplastic; traumatic

ANESTHETIC CONSIDERATIONS

C. Philip Larson, Jr.

PREOPERATIVE

Typically this is a healthy patient population, apart from Sx attributable to intracranial pathology (↑ ICP, seizures, headache, N/V, visual disturbances, etc.).

Respiratory	No special considerations, unless indicated from H&P.
Cardiovascular	Benign or malignant brain tumors cause edema formation in adjacent normal brain tissue, which may lead to ↑ICP. If ICP increases sufficiently to cause herniation of the brain stem, patients develop the "Cushing triad" of HTN, bradycardia and ↓RR. These changes will resolve when ICP is reduced, so vigorous attempts to regulate BP and HR prior to craniotomy are not warranted. Once the diagnosis of brain tumor is made, most patients are placed on high-dose steroid therapy to lessen edema in surrounding normal brain. Steroids are extremely effective in this setting, and Sx of ↑ICP will often abate. **Tests:** Consider ECG, others as indicated from H&P.
Neurological	Patients may present with complaints of headache, N/V, recent onset of seizures, visual changes or neurological deficits from compression of motor area, or as a result of hemorrhage from the tumor or edema in surrounding normal brain. Document preop physical findings.

Neurological, cont. **Tests:** A CT scan or MRI will delineate the site and size of the tumor, especially if iv contrast material, such as gadolinium, is administered to enhance the margins of the tumor.

Laboratory Other tests as indicated from H&P.

Premedication Standard premedication (except for patients with the possibility of ↑ICP → no sedation).

INTRAOPERATIVE

Anesthetic technique: Small tumors, particularly those located in deeper brain structures, may be localized and resected using stereotactic and microsurgical techniques. Generally, the stereotactic frame is placed on patient's head under local anesthesia; then patient is taken to CT for determination of the coordinates to be used for stereotactic guidance to tumor site. In children, GETA may be needed both for placing the stereotactic frame and for completion of CT scan. GETA is almost invariably used for tumor removal, although MAC is used on rare occasions when the surgeon needs to assess motor or sensory function during resection of tumor adjacent to critical motor or sensory areas.

Induction If patient is in a stereotactic frame, or a difficult intubation is anticipated, orotracheal intubation will need to be accomplished before induction of GA. Awake fiber optic intubation is the best choice, since fitting a mask on the face with the stereotactic frame in place is impossible (see p. B-6). Once the airway is secured, anesthesia is usually induced with STP (3-5 mg/kg) or propofol (2-3 mg/kg) and an opiate (e.g., meperidine 1.5-2 mg/kg), in combination with a nondepolarizing muscle relaxant (e.g., vecuronium 10 mg or rocuronium 0.7-1 mg/kg). To minimize ↑↑BP and ↑↑ICP with ET intubation, it is important that the patient be well anesthetized (and paralyzed, if appropriate) before undertaking laryngoscopy. Induction doses of STP (8 mg/kg), propofol (3 mg/kg) or midazolam (0.5 mg/kg) may not be sufficient to abolish increases in MAP, CPP and, hence, ↑ICP associated with laryngoscopy and tracheal intubation.[8] Consideration should be given to using fentanyl (5-10 μg/kg) or lidocaine (1.5-2 mg/kg iv) as part of the induction technique. Once anesthesia is induced, a nondepolarizing neuromuscular blocking drug (vecuronium 10 mg or rocuronium 50-70 mg) is administered for ET intubation and subsequent positioning of the patient. Both of these nondepolarizing neuromuscular blocking drugs have been shown not to increase ICP in patients with brain tumors.[21] In contrast, both d-tubocurarine and succinylcholine increase ICP in patients with brain tumors. The succinylcholine effect, however, can be abolished by a "defasciculating" dose of metocurine (0.03 mg/kg) or other nondepolarizing drugs.[17]

Maintenance The ideal drug for maintenance of anesthesia is one that decreases ICP and $CMRO_2$, maintains cerebral autoregulation, redistributes flow to the potentially ischemic areas and provides protection of the brain from focal ischemia. STP and propofol meet all of these criteria, and are excellent anesthetics for this operation. An effective, safe and reliable method of delivery is a continuous infusion of STP, 0.5-1% solution administered at a rate of 0.2-0.3 mg/kg/min, to a total dose of 20-25 mg/kg or propofol 70-150 μg/kg/min. If using STP, the administration should be complete by the time the dura is ready for opening. At these doses, CBF will be decreased by 50%, thereby decreasing cerebral blood volume and ICP and lessening need for brain retraction during operation. These agents also may provide cerebral protection from focal ischemia by decreasing $CMRO_2$ (by ~50%), and by redistributing flow to potentially ischemic areas where surgical retraction is occurring. It is generally believed that cerebral reactivity to changes in $PaCO_2$ is preserved during STP or propofol anesthesia.

High-dose narcotic (e.g., fentanyl 10 μg/kg load + 2 μg/kg/h infusion) has become an attractive technique for maintenance of anesthesia in patients undergoing craniotomy for tumor because of the circulatory stability these agents confer. Fentanyl does not have any direct effect on cerebral vasculature and, hence, does not increase ICP; but both alfentanil and sufentanil may cause mild cerebral vasodilatation and ↑ICP in patients with brain tumors, unless hypocarbia is instituted.[12] What evidence exists suggests that the opioids have minimal protective effect in the presence of focal cerebral ischemia.[18]

Isoflurane is regarded as the best volatile agent for patients undergoing neurosurgical procedures. Although isoflurane causes dose-dependent increases in CBF and volume and ↑ICP, these effects tend to be mitigated by the prior administration of STP or propofol, institution of hyperventilation, and limitation of the inspired isoflurane concentration to ≤ 1%. If STP induction dose is low (5-6 mg/kg), however, and the inspired isoflurane concentration is ≥ 1%, some patients with supratentorial tumors will evidence ↑↑ICP, even if $PaCO_2$ is maintained at < 30 mmHg.[18] At inspired isoflurane concentrations of ≤ 1%, CBF responses to changes in $PaCO_2$ are maintained, and cerebral autoregulation remains

Maintenance, cont.

intact.[11,14] Finally, isoflurane (and possibly sevoflurane) appears to provide protection from incomplete focal ischemia,[2,15] but whether it is as effective as STP in this regard remains controversial. N_2O, a modest cerebrovascular dilator which increases ICP, does not appear to provide any cerebral protection in the presence of incomplete focal ischemia,[23] and, in fact, may attenuate the protective effects of STP or isoflurane.[10] Also, it has been suggested that N_2O may increase likelihood of postop tension pneumocephalus, but this has recently been challenged.[5] Because the evidence relating to N_2O is controversial and its risks and benefits are unclear, its use is best left to the discretion of the anesthesiologist.

Generally, no further neuromuscular blocking drugs are administered beyond that used for tracheal intubation. With adequate anesthesia, and the head in Mayfield-Kees skeletal fixation, patient movement of any consequence is highly unlikely. Furthermore, it is useful to see movement of an extremity as an indicator of inadequate depth of anesthesia.

Emergence

Using sevoflurane (< 2%) for the last hour of surgery allows for rapid emergence and early evaluation of neurological function. It has been suggested that use of N_2O during closure of a craniotomy may worsen a tension pneumocephalus; however, a recent study suggested that N_2O did not increase ICP during closure.[5] With normal emergence, ETT should be removed before vigorous coughing ensues. If surgeon suspects that patient may have a slow recovery or a neurological injury from tumor removal, or if the anesthesiologist believes that recovery from anesthesia may be delayed, it is advisable to leave ETT in place at least overnight. Prophylactic antiemetic (e.g., metoclopramide 10 mg or ondansetron 4 mg) should be given 30-60 min before extubation.

Blood and fluid requirements

IV: 16-18 ga × 2
NS/LR @ 2-3 ml/kg/h

Brain tumors can be highly vascular, so it is prudent to plan accordingly. To minimize postop cerebral edema, limit NS/LR to ≤ 10 ml/kg plus replacement of UO. If volume is needed, administer albumin 5% as required or hetastarch 6% ≤ 20 ml/kg. Transfuse for Hct < 25%. Controlled hypotension is generally not used in this operation unless bleeding becomes profuse, diffuse and difficult for the neurosurgeon to control.

Monitoring

Standard monitors (see p. B-1).
Arterial line
CVP line
UO
± Doppler
± BAE, SSEP

If the tumor is in the posterior fossa and patient is in the seated position, a Doppler precordial chest stethoscope is necessary. If the tumor is an acoustic neuroma, the surgeon will request evoked potential monitoring, in which case the dose of barbiturate should be limited to ≤ 10 mg/kg to avoid interference with this monitoring.

Positioning

✓ and pad pressure points.
✓ eyes.

For brain tumors in the frontal, parietal or temporal lobes, patient will be supine with head in Mayfield-Kees skeletal fixation, turned to the side and a roll under the shoulder on the operative side (Fig 1.1-4). For occipital or posterior fossa tumors, patient may be prone or, preferably, sitting (see Anesthetic Considerations for Cervical Neurosurgical Procedures, p. 73). Acoustic neuromas are generally most easily removed with patient in the lateral ("park-bench") position with a roll under the axilla. Patient generally lies on a bean bag which, when aspirated, holds her/him firmly in the lateral position.

Control of ICP

Control BP & CVP = low normal.
PaO_2 > 100 mmHg
↓fluids < 10 ml/kg + UO
Propofol or STP infusion
↓isoflurane < 1%, or sevoflurane < 2%
± Steroids
Hyperventilate to $PaCO_2$ = 25-30 mmHg ($PetCO_2$ = 20-25 mmHg).

Patients with intracranial tumors may be on the steep portion of the intracranial compliance curve such that any increase in intracranial volume may cause ↑↑ICP. Transient increases in ICP—even up to 50-60 mmHg—are tolerated, provided they are promptly terminated. Sustained increases in ICP > 25-30 mmHg are associated with severe neurologic injury and poor outcome.

↓$PaCO_2$ → ↓cerebral vascular volume (providing better surgical access) + ↑CBF to ischemic areas ("Robin Hood" effect) + ↓anesthetic requirements + ↑lactic acid buffering.

ICP, cont.	Mannitol 1 g/kg ± Furosemide 0.3 mg/kg	Mannitol/furosemide → ↓K^+; monitor level and replace as necessary. If mannitol is administered too rapidly, profound hypotension will occur, probably from peripheral vasodilation.
	± Lumbar CSF drain Head up 20-30°	CSF drain often placed after induction of anesthesia, and may be opened as required to ↓ CSF volume.

POSTOPERATIVE

Complications	Seizures Neurologic deficits Hemorrhage requiring re-exploration Edema and ↑ICP Tension pneumocephalus	★ Seizure Rx: Phenytoin (1 g loading dose). **NB:** Incompatible with dextrose-containing solutions. In seated position, additional rare, but possible complications include quadriplegia from excessive flexion of head or tension pneumocephalus from air in cerebral cavities. Severe tension pneumocephalus may delay emergence from anesthesia, or cause postop neurologic deficits.
Pain management	Meperidine (10-20 mg iv prn) Codeine (30-60 mg im q 4 h)	Meperidine minimizes postop shivering.
Tests	CT scan	If patient exhibits any delay in emergence from anesthesia and surgery, or any new neurologic deficits emerge postop, a CT scan is invariably obtained.

References

1. Apuzzo MLJ: *Brain Surgery: Complication, Avoidance and Management.* Churchill Livingstone, New York: 1993, 175-688.
2. Baughman VL, Hoffman WE, Thomas C, Miletich DJ, Albrecht RF: Comparison of methohexital and isoflurane on neurologic outcome and histopathology following incomplete ischemia in rats. *Anesthesiology* 1990; 72(1):85-94.
3. Black PM: Brain tumors. *N Engl J Med* 1991; 324(21):1471-76, 1555-64.
4. Domaingue CM, Nye DH: Hypotensive effect of mannitol administered rapidly. *Anaesth Intensive Care* 1985; 13(2):134-36.
5. Domino KB, Hemstad JR, Lam AM, Laohaprasit V, Hamberg TA, Harrison SD, Grady MS, Winn HR: Effect of nitrous oxide on intracranial pressure after cranial-dural closure in patients undergoing craniotomy. *Anesthesiology* 1992; 77(3):421-25.
6. Eng C, Lam AM, Mayberg TS, Lee C, Mathisen T: The influence of propofol with and without nitrous oxide on cerebral blood flow velocity and CO_2 reactivity in humans. *Anesthesiology* 1992; 77(5):872-79.
7. From RP, Warner DS, Todd MM, Sokoll MD: Anesthesia for craniotomy: a double-blind comparison of alfentanil, fentanyl, and sufentanil. *Anesthesiology* 1990; 73(5):896-904.
8. Giffin JP, Cottrell JE, Shwiry B, Hartung J, Epstein J, Lim K: Intracranial pressure, mean arterial pressure, and heart rate following midazolam or STP in humans with brain tumors. *Anesthesiology* 1984; 60(5):491-94.
9. Grosslight KR, Foster R, Colohan AR, Bedford RF: Isoflurane for neuroanesthesia: risk factors for increases in intracranial pressure. *Anesthesiology* 1985; 63(5):533-36.
10. Hartung J, Cottrell JE: Nitrous oxide reduces STP-induced prolongation of survival in hypoxic and anoxic mice. *Anesth Analg* 1987; 66(1):47-52.
11. Hoffman WE, Edelman G, Kochs E, Werner C, Segil L, Albrecht RF: Cerebral autoregulation in awake versus isoflurane-anesthetized rats. *Anesth Analg* 1991; 73(6):753-57.
12. Jung R, Shah N, Reinsel R, Marx W, Marshall W, Galicich J, Bedford R: Cerebrospinal fluid pressure in patients with brain tumors: impact of fentanyl versus alfentanil during nitrous oxide-oxygen anesthesia. *Anesth Analg* 1990; 71(4):419-22.
13. Kochs E, Hoffman WE, Werner C, Thomas C, Albrecht RF, Schulte am Esch J: The effects of propofol on brain electrical activity, neurologic outcome, and neuronal damage following incomplete ischemia in rats. *Anesthesiology* 1992; 76(2):245-52.
14. McPherson RW, Traystman RJ: Effects of isoflurane on cerebral autoregulation in dogs. *Anesthesiology* 1988; 69(4): 493-99.
15. Michenfelder JD, Sundt TM Jr, Fode N, Sharbrough FW: Isoflurane when compared to enflurane and halothane decreases the frequency of cerebral ischemia during carotid endarterectomy. *Anesthesiology* 1987; 67(3):336-40.
16. Milde LN, Milde JH, Lanier WL, Michenfelder JD: Comparison of the effects of isoflurane and STP on neurologic outcome and neuropathology after temporary focal cerebral ischemia in primates. *Anesthesiology* 1988; 69(6):905-13.
17. Minton MD, Grosslight KR, Stirt JA, Bedford RF: Increases in intracranial pressure from succinylcholine: prevention by prior nondepolarizing blockade. *Anesthesiology* 1986; 65(2):165-69.
18. Nehls DG, Todd MM, Spetzler RF, Drummond JC, Thompson RA, Johnson PC: A comparison of the cerebral protective effects of isoflurane and barbiturates during temporary focal ischemia in primates. *Anesthesiology* 1987; 66(4):453-64.
19. Pinaud M, Lelausque JN, Chetanneau A, Fauchoux N, Menegalli D, Souron R: Effects of propofol on cerebral hemodynamics and metabolism in patients with brain trauma. *Anesthesiology* 1990; 73(3):404-09.
20. Ridenour TR, Warner DS, Todd MM, Gionet TX: Comparative effects of propofol and halothane on outcome from temporary middle cerebral artery occlusion in the rat. *Anesthesiology* 1992; 76(5):807-12.

21. Stirt JA, Maggio W, Haworth C, Minton MD, Bedford RF: Vecuronium: effect on intracranial pressure and hemodynamics in neurosurgical patients. *Anesthesiology* 1987; 67(4):570-73.
22. Van Hemelrijck J, Fitch W, Mattheussen M, Van Aken H, Plets C, Lauwers T: Effect of propofol on cerebral circulation and autoregulation in the baboon. *Anesth Analg* 1990; 71(1):49-54.
23. Warner DS, Zhou J, Ramani R, Todd MM, McAllister A: Nitrous oxide does not alter infarct volume in rats undergoing reversible middle cerebral artery occlusion. *Anesthesiology* 1990; 73(4):686-93.

CRANIOTOMY FOR SKULL TUMOR

SURGICAL CONSIDERATIONS

Lawrence M. Shuer

Description: Tumors of the skull fall into the classification of other bony tumors. Examples of types of skull tumors often requiring surgery include eosinophilic granuloma, histiocytosis, hemangioma, osteoma, epidermoid, dermoid tumor, metastatic tumors, osteosarcoma, fibrous dysplasia and meningioma. They may occur anywhere on the skull. The exact positioning of the patient depends on the location of tumor. For example, the sitting position is often used for tumors in the occipital or suboccipital regions and the supine position is used for frontal, temporal or parietal tumors. Some surgeons prefer the lateral position for temporal or parietal bone lesions and the prone position for occipital and some suboccipital bone lesions. The patient's head is placed in a head holder (either pins, suction cup, horseshoe or Shea headrest). The bone is usually removed by creating burr hole(s) and then cutting a flap with the neuro bone saw. In the suboccipital or posterior fossa craniotomy, the bone is often removed piecemeal with either a drill or a series of rongeurs. The dura usually is not opened unless it is involved with the tumor. The surgeon may elect to perform a **cranioplasty** to cover the defect, depending on size and location of the bone defect. The defect can be repaired using methylmethacrylate at the time of surgery, or bone may be harvested from either another location on the skull or another site (hip or rib) for reconstruction. Once the reconstruction is completed, the skin incision is closed. Occasionally, the tumor of the skull will be approached intracranially, if its location favors that approach. Examples include tumors of the petrous portion of the temporal bone or fibrous dysplasia involving the optic canal.

Usual preop diagnosis: Eosinophilic granuloma; histiocytosis; hemangioma; osteoma; epidermoid; dermoid tumor; metastatic tumors; osteosarcoma; fibrous dysplasia; meningioma

SUMMARY OF PROCEDURE

Position	Supine, lateral, prone or sitting
Incision	Dependent on location of tumor
Special instrumentation	Neuro drill
Unique considerations	ETT must be taped securely in a location satisfactory to the surgeon. Anode or RAE tube may be helpful in certain situations.
Antibiotics	Cefazolin 1 g iv
Surgical time	1-4 h
Closing considerations	Drain often left in epidural space. Surgeon often requests control of BP to avoid hemorrhage into the bed of tumor.
EBL	25-500 ml
Postop care	ICU or close observation unit
Mortality	0-2% (higher for tumors in critical locations)
Morbidity	Usually < 5%: Infection Neurological disability CSF leak Massive blood loss—venous sinus injury
Pain score	2-5

PATIENT POPULATION CHARACTERISTICS

Age range	Infant–85 yr (usually 20-60 yr)
Male:Female	~1:1
Incidence	Unknown
Etiology	Neoplastic; traumatic

ANESTHETIC CONSIDERATIONS

See Anesthetic Considerations for Craniotomy for Tumor, p. 26. Note, however, that patients with skull tumors rarely have problems with ICP.

Reference

1. Voorhies RM, Sundaresan N: Tumors of the skull. In *Neurosurgery*. Wilkins RH, Rengachary SS, eds. McGraw-Hill, New York: 1985, 984-1001.

CRANIOTOMY FOR TRAUMA

SURGICAL CONSIDERATIONS

Lawrence M. Shuer

Description: Head injuries occasionally require emergent surgical procedures to evacuate mass lesions or debride contused or contaminated brain. The majority of these injuries are supratentorial. The surgical procedure depends on the exact type and location of the injury (e.g., epidural, subdural, intracerebral hematomas or depressed skull fracture). Often the entire head is shaved and placed in a headrest (pins, suction cups or horseshoe). An incision is made according to the location and extent of the injury. The skin is incised and reflected and the skull is perforated with a cranial drill. If the abnormality is a chronic, subdural hematoma, it may be drained via burr holes. If there is a clot or depressed fracture or penetrating wound, a formal bone flap is elevated. Mass lesions are identified or removed, and the dura is repaired if lacerated. Depending on the injury and the presence of brain swelling, the dura may be patched and the bone flap replaced. An ICP monitor may be placed at the end of the procedure.

Usual preop diagnosis: Epidural hematoma; subdural hematoma; intracerebral hematoma; depressed skull fracture; cerebral contusions; gunshot wound of the brain

SUMMARY OF PROCEDURE

Position	Supine, lateral, prone or sitting, depending on site of injury
Incision	Varies with location of injury
Unique considerations	The patient may have ↑↑ICP. Because incipient herniation and/or associated injuries may be a concern, timing is critical.
Antibiotics	Nafcillin 1-2 g iv + cefotaxime 1 g iv
Surgical time	1.5-6 h
Closing considerations	Application of head dressing may jostle ETT at end of case → ↑BP. Patient may stay intubated postop. ICP monitor may be placed. Phenytoin may be given for seizure prophylaxis.
EBL	25-500 ml
Postop care	ICU or close observation unit until stable. Fluid and electrolytes require frequent monitoring, as the patient may develop SIADH following this procedure. BP may need to be controlled with vasodilators and β-blockers.
Mortality	10-50%, depending on lesion; higher for acute subdural hematomas, lower for epidural hematomas.

Morbidity	Infection Neurologic disability Nerve injury CSF leak Endocrine disorders: SIADH Panhypopituitarism Diabetes insipidus (DI) Massive blood loss: venous sinus injury
Pain score	2-4

PATIENT POPULATION CHARACTERISTICS

Age range	Infant–85 yr (usually 15-40 yr)
Male:Female	2:1
Incidence	Relatively common
Etiology	Trauma
Associated conditions	Abdominal injuries; cervical spine fractures

ANESTHETIC CONSIDERATIONS

C. Philip Larson, Jr.

PREOPERATIVE

Head injury is the leading cause of death of persons under 24 years of age.[3] A penetrating injury of the skull will usually cause major damage to the brain as a result of diffuse neuronal injury and hemorrhage into brain tissue. Surgery is necessary to control intracranial bleeding, to debride the wound, and to remove bone fragments, foreign material and damaged brain so that the cranial vault can better accommodate the brain swelling that inevitably occurs. Head injury also can be focal in nature, most commonly in the form of an epidural, subdural or intracranial hematoma. Epidural hematomas form between the skull and dura, and are usually due to bleeding from an artery (e.g., anterior cerebral or middle meningeal). Hence, time is of the essence and rapid evacuation and control of the bleeding is essential if permanent neurological injury is to be avoided. Subdural bleeding occurs between the dura and the leptomeninges lining the brain surface. This bleeding is usually venous in origin, and usually occurs more gradually. Focal intracranial hemorrhages may be either arterial or venous, and, as with subdural hematomas, must be evacuated if they are enlarging.

Respiratory

Localized injuries to the frontal or parietal lobes may not cause any respiratory changes. If ↑ICP, respirations may become slow (< 10/min) and deep, and result in substantial hypocapnia. Many patients with head injuries demonstrate partial airway obstruction from the tongue falling back into the posterior pharyngeal space. If this occurs, or if the patient is comatose and unable to protect the airway and prevent aspiration of gastric contents, immediate tracheal intubation should be performed. Head injuries in the region of the occipital lobes may → apnea.
Tests: As indicated from H&P and as time allows.

Cardiovascular

Most patients with head injuries evidence ↑BP and ↑HR. If ICP increases sufficiently to cause herniation of brain stem, patients develop the "Cushing triad" of ↑BP, ↓HR and ↓RR. These changes resolve when ↑ICP is relieved, so vigorous attempts to regulate BP and prior to craniotomy are not warranted. Patient, however, should be taken to OR as quickly as possible.
Tests: As indicated from H&P, and as time allows.

Neurological

Neurological evaluation of the head-injured patient is based on the Glasgow Coma Scale (Table 1.1-1). The scale involves evaluation of three functions: eye opening, verbal response and motor response. Using this scoring system, the severity of brain injury may be classified as mild (13-15 points), moderate (9-12 points), or severe (8 points or less). By definition, any patient having 8 points or less is in coma. Additional useful neurological examinations include assessment of pupillary size and reactivity to the light, reflex responses, and evidence of asymmetry or flaccidity of the extremities or decerebrate or decorticate posturing. Head-injured patients whose neurological function is deteriorating rapidly, and in whom an epidural or subdural hemorrhage is suspected, should be taken to OR immediately without CT scan.

Neurological, cont. **Tests:** CT scan

Hematologic Severe head injury may be associated with a progressively worsening coagulopathy, resulting in a clinical picture similar to that of DIC. The reason for this is not known, but the brain is rich in thromboplastin and other coagulation factors.
Tests: Hct; PT; PTT; others as indicated from H&P.

Laboratory Other tests as indicated from H&P, and as time permits.

Premedication Usually none

INTRAOPERATIVE

Anesthetic technique: GETA

Induction ↑ICP is likely in most patients with head injury requiring operation, and induction of anesthesia is best accomplished with drugs that ↓ ICP. If patient is hemodynamically stable and not hypovolemic, induction with STP (≤ 10 mg/kg), propofol (1.5-3 mg/kg), ± opiate supplementation (meperidine 1.5-2 mg/kg, fentanyl 5 μg/kg) is satisfactory. If hemodynamically unstable, etomidate (0.1-0.4 mg/kg) is suitable for induction. Ketamine is not used because of its ability to ↑ ICP. If patient is comatose, anesthetic requirement is less, needing only O_2 and muscle relaxant, or N_2O 60% or low-dose isoflurane (≤ 0.5%) or sevoflurane (< 2%). A nondepolarizing muscle relaxant (vecuronium [0.1 mg/kg] or rocuronium [1 mg/kg]) is administered for ET intubation.[17] Succinylcholine can be used if a "defasciculating" dose of a nondepolarizing neuromuscular blocking drug is administered first.[14] Nasotracheal intubation is not recommended for patients with maxillary and/or basilar skull fractures because of the potential for inserting the tube through the fracture site into the brain stem.
To minimize ↑↑BP and ↑↑ICP with ET intubation, it is important that the patient be anesthetized and paralyzed before undertaking laryngoscopy. Induction doses of STP or propofol may not be sufficient to abolish increases in MAP, CPP and, hence, ICP associated with laryngoscopy and tracheal intubation.[13] In addition, consideration should be given to using lidocaine 2 mg/kg iv and fentanyl 5 μg/kg as part of the induction technique. Lidocaine has the amnesic effects of STP without the myocardial depressant effects. In hypovolemic patients, hydration with a mixture of crystalloid and colloid should be initiated prior to induction.

Maintenance The ideal drug for maintenance of anesthesia decreases ICP and $CMRO_2$, maintains cerebral autoregulation, redistributes flow to potentially ischemic areas and provides protection of the brain from focal ischemia. STP meets these criteria, and is an excellent anesthetic for the head-trauma patient, provided the circulation tolerates the drug. A total dose of 15-20 mg/kg given by intermittent bolus injection or continuous infusion is sufficient. A continuous infusion of propofol 150 mg/kg/min to a total dose of 10 mg/kg can be used for the same purpose because it also decreases cerebral blood volume and ICP while maintaining cerebral autoregulation.[5,15]
Isoflurane is regarded as the best volatile agent for patients undergoing neurosurgical procedures. Although isoflurane causes dose-dependent increases in CBF and volume and, hence, ↑ICP, these effects tend to be mitigated by the prior administration of STP, hyperventilation, and by limiting the inspired isoflurane concentration to ≤ 1%. At

Table 1.1-1. Glasgow Coma Scale (GCS)

Category	Score
I. Eyes open:	
Never	1
To pain	2
To verbal stimuli	3
Spontaneously	4
II. Best verbal response:	
None	1
Incomprehensible sounds	2
Inappropriate words	3
Patient disoriented and converses	4
Patient oriented and converses	5
III. Best motor response:	
None	1
Extension (decerebrate rigidity)	2
Flexion abnormal (decorticate rigidity)	3
Flexion withdrawal	4
Patient localizes pain	5
Patient obeys	6
I + II + III Total = 3-15	

Maintenance, cont.

< 1% isoflurane, CBF responses to changes in $PaCO_2$ are maintained, and cerebral autoregulation remains intact.[1,10] Finally, isoflurane appears to provide protection from incomplete focal ischemia.[7,11] Sevoflurane (≤ 2%) is also a good choice for maintenance because of its low solubility and, hence, rapid emergence. Its CNS properties appear to be similar to those of isoflurane.

N_2O may be administered, recognizing that it is a modest cerebrovascular dilator, thereby increasing ICP, an effect that would not be desirable in patients with a space-occupying lesion. Also, N_2O does not appear to provide any cerebral protection in the presence of incomplete focal ischemia,[12] and, in fact, may attenuate the protective effects of STP or isoflurane.[16]

Generally, no further neuromuscular blocking drugs are administered beyond that used for tracheal intubation. With adequate anesthesia, and head in Mayfield-Kees skeletal fixation, patient movement of any consequence is highly unlikely. Furthermore, it is useful to see movement of an extremity as an indicator of inadequate depth of anesthesia.

Emergence

Because recovery from head injury is so unpredictable, it is generally advisable to leave the ETT in place and maintain controlled hyperventilation until there is sufficient clinical evidence that normal neurological recovery is occurring. Prophylactic antiemetic (e.g., metoclopramide 10 mg or ondansetron 4 mg) should be given 30-60 min before extubation.

Blood and fluid requirements	Possible marked blood loss IV: 16-18 ga × 1 NS @ 2-4 ml/kg/h	Blood transfusion is often necessary. To minimize postop cerebral edema, total crystalloid volume should be limited to < 10 ml/kg plus replacement of UO. Glucose-containing solutions should be avoided; blood glucose levels should be maintained between 80-200 mg%. If volume is needed, albumin 5% (or hetastarch 6% up to 20 ml/kg) should be administered.
Control of blood loss	Low normal BP HR = 50-70	Blood loss is best minimized by maintaining MAP at low normal for that patient. Controlled hypotension generally is not used unless bleeding becomes profuse and difficult to control. HR is easily controlled with an esmolol infusion, and if additional ↓MAP is needed, SNP is begun. Hypotension is better treated with volume replacement than vasopressors.
Monitoring	Standard monitors (see p. B-1). ± Arterial line ± CVP line ± UO	For minor head injuries, no special monitoring is needed. If the injury is extensive or unknown, or if the patient is unstable, invasive monitoring is mandatory.
Positioning	✓ and pad pressure points. ✓ eyes.	For occipital or posterior fossa injuries, patient may be prone or sitting (see Anesthetic Considerations for Cervical Neurosurgical Procedures, p. 73). Otherwise, patient will be supine with head in Mayfield-Kees skeletal fixation and turned to the side, and a roll placed under the shoulder on the operative side.
Control of ICP	Adequate anesthesia Head up 20-30° STP or propofol infusion	Patients with skull fractures or intracranial bleeding may be on the steep portion of intracranial compliance curve such that any increase in intracranial volume may cause ↑↑ICP. Transient increases in ICP—even up to 50-60 mmHg—are tolerated, provided they are promptly terminated. Sustained increases in ICP > 25-30 mmHg are associated with severe neurologic injury and poor outcome.
	Hyperventilation to $PaCO_2$ = 25-30 mmHg PaO_2 >100 mmHg	Hypocarbia is a potent cerebral vasoconstrictor, thereby decreasing cerebral blood volume and ICP. It should be recognized that some patients with diffuse brain injury will have lost cerebrovascular sensitivity to $PaCO_2$, such that hyperventilation will have little or no effect on vascular volume (or brain size). Maintaining PaO_2 will prevent cerebral vasodilatation from hypoxemia. Despite maintaining adequate ventilation, oxygenation and BP,

ICP, cont.		patients with diffuse head injury often exhibit arterial and CSF lactic acidosis, a further indication of the metabolic derangement that exists in the brain from the injury.[14]
	Keep MAP low normal.	Control MAP and cerebral venous pressure so that CPP is maintained in the low normal range for that patient. Because most patients with head injury of any consequence lose cerebral autoregulation, ↑CPP → ↑cerebral blood volume and ↑ICP. Also, with loss of autoregulation, hypotension should be avoided to avoid cerebral ischemia. In severe, diffuse head injury with loss of autoregulation, some parts of the brain may exhibit "luxury perfusion," while other areas exhibit severe ischemia.[8]
	Mannitol 1 g/kg	With mannitol at a dose of 1 g/kg, vigorous diuresis will commence in about 30 min (if blood volume is adequate), and brain shrinkage will follow. It is often necessary to provide supplemental potassium (20-30 mEq iv slowly).
	Furosemide 10-20 mg	Simultaneous administration of furosemide (10-20 mg) is recommended to avoid the transient increases in cerebral blood volume and ICP that accompany mannitol administration. If mannitol is administered too rapidly, profound hypotension will occur, probably from peripheral vasodilatation.

POSTOPERATIVE

Complications	Seizures Neurologic deficits Hemorrhage Edema ↑ICP	★ Seizure Rx: phenytoin (1 g loading dose). **NB:** Incompatible with dextrose-containing solutions. Some patients with severe head injury remain unconscious for weeks or months, without evidencing any substantial neurological recovery. A late complication of head injury is hydrocephalus requiring a shunt procedure.
Pain management	Codeine (30-60 mg im q 4 h)	
Tests	CT scan ICP monitor	Unless neurological recovery is rapid, periodic CT scans are obtained postop to follow the intracranial changes. In addition, in many institutions, a device for monitoring ICP postop is placed at the time of operation.

References

1. Adams RW, Cucchiara RF, Gronert GA, Messick JM, Michenfelder JD: Isoflurane and cerebrospinal fluid pressure in neurosurgical patients. *Anesthesiology* 1981; 54(2):97-99.
2. Baughman VL, Hoffman WE, Thomas C, Miletich DJ, Albrecht RF: Comparison of methohexital and isoflurane on neurologic outcome and histopathology following incomplete ischemia in rats. *Anesthesiology* 1990; 72(1):85-94.
3. Cooper PR: Traumatic intracranial hematomas. In *Neurosurgery*. Wilkins RH, Rengachary SS, eds. McGraw-Hill, New York: 1985, 1657-69.
4. Domaingue CM, Nye DH: Hypotensive effect of mannitol administered rapidly. *Anaesth Intensive Care* 1985; 13(2):134-36.
5. Giffin JP, Cottrell JE, Shwiry B, Hartung J, Epstein J, Lim K: Intracranial pressure, mean arterial pressure, and heart rate following midazolam or STP in humans with brain tumors. *Anesthesiology* 1984; 60(5):491-94.
6. Hartung J, Cottrell JE: Nitrous oxide reduces STP-induced prolongation of survival in hypoxic and anoxic mice. *Anesth Analg* 1987; 66(1):47-52.
7. Hoffman WE, Edelman G, Kochs E, Werner C, Segil L, Albrecht RF: Cerebral autoregulation in awake versus isoflurane-anesthetized rats. *Anesth Analg* 1991; 73(6):753-57.
8. King LR, McLaurin RL, Knowles HC Jr: Acid-base balance and arterial and CSF lactate levels following human head injury. *J Neurosurg* 1974; 40(5):617-25.
9. Kochs E, Hoffman WE, Werner C, Thomas C, Albrecht RF, Schulte am Esch J: The effects of propofol on brain electrical activity, neurologic outcome, and neuronal damage following incomplete ischemia in rats. *Anesthesiology* 1992; 76(2):245-52.
10. McPherson RW, Traystman RJ: Effects of isoflurane on cerebral autoregulation in dogs. *Anesthesiology* 1988; 69(4):493-99.
11. Michenfelder JD, Sundt TM Jr, Fode N, Sharbrough FW: Isoflurane when compared to enflurane and halothane decreases the frequency of cerebral ischemia during carotid endarterectomy. *Anesthesiology* 1987; 67(3):336-40.

12. Overgaard J, Tweed WA: Cerebral circulation after head injury. Part 1: Cerebral blood flow and its regulation after closed head injury with emphasis on clinical correlations. *J Neurosurg* 1974; 41(5):531-41.
13. Stirt JA, Grosslight KR, Bedford RF, Vollmer D: "Defasciculation" with metocurine prevents succinylcholine-induced increases in intracranial pressure. *Anesthesiology* 1987; 67(1):50-53.
14. Stirt JA, Maggio W, Haworth C, Minton MD, Bedford RF: Vecuronium: effect on intracranial pressure and hemodynamics in neurosurgical patients. *Anesthesiology* 1987; 67(4):570-73.
15. Van Hemelrijck J, Fitch W, Mattheussen M, Van Aken H, Plets C, Lauwers T: Effect of propofol on cerebral circulation and autoregulation in the baboon. *Anesth Analg* 1990; 71(1):49-54.
16. Warner DS, Zhou J, Ramani R, Todd MM, McAllister A: Nitrous oxide does not alter infarct volume in rats undergoing reversible middle cerebral artery occlusion. *Anesthesiology* 1990; 73(4):686-93.
17. White RJ, Likavec MG: The diagnosis and initial management of head injury. *N Engl J Med* 1992; 327(21):1507-11.

MICROVASCULAR DECOMPRESSION OF CRANIAL NERVE

SURGICAL CONSIDERATIONS

Lawrence M. Shuer

Description: Microvascular decompression is used to treat various disorders of the cranial nerves. The conditions in which this procedure is utilized most frequently include trigeminal neuralgia, hemifacial spasm and, more rarely, glossopharyngeal neuralgia. These conditions are thought to be caused by cross-compression of a cranial nerve by a vascular structure (usually an artery). A **craniectomy** is performed just behind the ear on the affected side. The dura at the junction of the transverse and sigmoid sinus is exposed. At this point, there is a risk of venous sinus bleeding. With brain relaxation, the cerebellum is retracted, exposing the cerebellopontine angle. The operating microscope allows the surgeon to explore the involved cranial nerve. If an offending vessel is identified, it is carefully dissected off the nerve and a pad (Teflon sponge or muscle) is placed to keep the vessel from returning to its original position. In the case of trigeminal or glossopharyngeal neuralgia, occasionally a partial section of the nerve is performed, if no offending vessel is identified. With glossopharyngeal neuralgia, partial section of the 9th or 10th cranial nerve may cause some vasomotor instability. The main variations in this procedure are in patient positioning and surgeon's preference for various adjuncts. Patient positioning may be lateral, prone, supine or sitting. Intraop, mannitol (1 g/kg) and a spinal drain (for CSF removal) may be needed for brain relaxation.

Usual preop diagnosis: Trigeminal neuralgia; tic douloureux; hemifacial spasm; tinnitus; glossopharyngeal neuralgia

SUMMARY OF PROCEDURE

Position	Normally, lateral ("park-bench"), head elevated 30°; less frequently, sitting, prone or supine
Incision	Retroauricular (mastoid)
Special instrumentation	Operating microscope; cranial perforator; ± facial nerve monitoring; ± EMG; ± brain stem auditory evoked response (BAER)
Unique considerations	Risk of air embolus
Antibiotics	Cefotaxime 1 g + nafcillin 1-2 g iv slowly
Surgical time	2-3 h
EBL	25-250 ml
Postop care	ICU or close observation unit. Observe for change in neurologic status (e.g., level of alertness, response to commands), usually for 12-24 h.
Mortality	0-3%
Morbidity	Usually < 5%: Infection Deafness Facial weakness Facial sensory deficit CSF leak Massive blood loss 2° vertebral artery injury
Pain score	4-6

PATIENT POPULATION CHARACTERISTICS

Age range	40-85 yr (usually 60-70 yr)
Male:Female	~2:3
Incidence	Common
Etiology	Vascular compression of cranial nerve; multiple sclerosis plaque
Associated conditions	HTN; multiple sclerosis

ANESTHETIC CONSIDERATIONS

C. Philip Larson, Jr.

PREOPERATIVE

Microvascular decompression involves a full craniotomy for decompression of a nerve which is causing facial pain and/or spasm of facial muscles. Generally, these patients have trigeminal neuralgia or tic douloureux which has not been responsive to medical management (carbamazepine [Tegretol] therapy) and percutaneous rhizotomy or glycerol injection has failed.

Respiratory None unless the patient has a long-standing Hx of smoking and has COPD.

Cardiovascular Many patients will have Hx of idiopathic HTN and take any one of a variety of antihypertensive medications. Good control of BP preop is important because it will make intraop and postop management of BP easier.

Neurological The presenting symptom is pain ± muscle spasm in the maxillary and/or mandibular division of the trigeminal nerve, unaccompanied by any motor or sensory deficits.

Laboratory None, except for routine preop studies.

Premedication Generally, patients for these procedures are elderly and do not require any special premedication. Midazolam 2-4 mg im will provide amnesia for the preop events, if that is desired by patient or surgeons.

INTRAOPERATIVE

Anesthetic technique: GA is necessary because a full craniotomy is performed. ICP is not increased in these patients, so special precautions in that regard are not necessary. Brain shrinkage, however, is important to provide the surgeon with sufficient space to identify and relieve the pressure on the offending nerve without requiring excessive brain retraction in the process.

Induction Induction is best accomplished with drugs that cause brain shrinkage, including STP (10 mg/kg) or propofol (1-2 mg/kg), followed by neuromuscular blockade and ET intubation.

Maintenance STP ≤ 20 mg/kg, or an equivalent dose of propofol, associated with an opiate such as fentanyl 2-3 μg/kg or meperidine 1.5 mg/kg, and isoflurane (≤ 1%) or sevoflurane (< 2%) with N_2O 60-70%, is satisfactory. BP is maintained in the normal range during the operation. Hyperventilation to achieve a $PaCO_2$ of 25-30 mmHg is helpful in decreasing brain size and providing adequate space for the surgeon to work. Once the nerve has been stented or transected, hyperventilation can be terminated and brain size can be allowed to return to normal. Sometimes the surgeon will also insert a spinal drain to remove CSF during the operation and improve exposure. The drain is usually opened at the time of dural opening and closed as soon as surgery on the nerve is complete.

Emergence The ETT is removed at the conclusion of operation. Postop HTN may need to be controlled with esmolol and/or SNP by continuous pump infusion. Prophylactic antiemetic (e.g., metoclopramide 10 mg or ondansetron 4 mg) should be given 30-60 min before extubation.

Blood and fluid requirements	Minimal blood loss IV: 18 ga × 1 NS @ 2-4 ml/kg/h	Mannitol 1-1.5 mg/kg is sometimes necessary to provide sufficient brain shrinkage to permit adequate surgical exposure.
Monitoring	Standard monitors (see p. B-1). Arterial line CVP line ± EMG and/or SSEP	Sometimes EMG and/or SSEP monitoring of the facial nerve is performed.

Positioning	✓ and pad pressure points. ✓ eyes. Pillow between legs	Patients usually will be positioned laterally in the "park-bench" position. Padding of the axillae and elbows and placing a pillow between the legs are necessary. A bean bag is often used to hold patient stable in the lateral position.

POSTOPERATIVE

Complications	Bleeding Brain edema	Major complications from this operation are uncommon, and postop recovery is usually uneventful. On rare occasion, significant brain edema or bleeding may be experienced.
Pain management	Codeine (30-60 mg im q 4 h)	
Tests	CT scan, if neurological recovery is delayed.	

Reference

1. Jannetta PJ: Supralateral exposure of the trigeminal nerve in the cerebellopontine angle for microvascular decompression. In *Brain Surgery: Complication, Avoidance and Management*. Apuzzo MLJ, ed. Churchill Livingstone, New York: 1993, 2085-96.

BIFRONTAL CRANIOTOMY FOR CSF LEAK

SURGICAL CONSIDERATIONS

Lawrence M. Shuer

Description: CSF leaks may develop 2° trauma and, occasionally, to tumors or congenital malformations. Most of these leaks involve the floor of the anterior cranial fossa. The surgical repair for this type of problem is fairly standard: **bifrontal craniotomy** is performed with a bicoronal skin flap. The patient's head is stabilized with either suction cups or pins, and a bifrontal free-bone flap is used. Brain relaxation (minimum volume) is usually necessary for the procedure and may require placement of a spinal lumbar subarachnoid drain to remove CSF. The dura is opened across the sagittal sinus and an intradural exploration is undertaken to determine the site of the leak. The frontal lobes are elevated, and the olfactory tracts are often sacrificed. If the site of leak can be determined, the repair can be performed by use of some dura or graft material (either fascia lata, pericranium or cadaveric dura). It usually is necessary to strip the dura off the anterior cranial fossa to complete the repair. Defects in the bone can be plugged with some material (e.g., fat, muscle, bone or wax). Once the repair is complete, the dura can be closed and the bone flap replaced, often with a drain left in the epidural space. At this point, relaxation is no longer required; thus, if hyperventilation has been used, it can be reversed. The wound is closed with glial stitches and skin closure.

Another approach is used for dealing with CSF leaks 2° tumor at the base of the anterior cranial fossa which may invade dura and the cribriform plate region. In these cases, the procedure is often performed with an otorhinolaryngologist. This procedure is identical to bifrontal craniotomy, except that bone and tumor are removed at the floor of the anterior cranial fossa and the otorhinolaryngologist makes an incision on the face and performs surgery in the nasal cavity. A common space is created between the two operative fields. Closure involves isolating the two cavities once again. The dural repair is as above. The mucosa of the nasal cavity is recreated with use of a skin graft.

Usual preop diagnosis: CSF leak or rhinorrhea; fracture of the anterior cranial fossa; intranasal encephalocele; cribriform plate tumor; esthesioneurocytoma

SUMMARY OF PROCEDURE

Position	Supine
Incision	Bicoronal
Special instrumentation	Operating microscope (optional)
Unique considerations	Brain relaxation desired; lumbar subarachnoid catheter; fascia lata graft
Antibiotics	Nafcillin 1-2 g + cefotaxime 1 g iv
Surgical time	2-3.5 h, depending on extent of leak or lesion
Closing considerations	Drain often left in epidural space. Application of head dressing will jostle patient and ETT → ↑BP.
EBL	75-500 ml
Postop care	ICU or close observation unit
Mortality	≤ 5%
Morbidity	Infection CSF leak Neurologic disability Nerve injury Massive blood loss: venous sinus injury
Pain score	3-5

PATIENT POPULATION CHARACTERISTICS

Age range	15-65 yr
Male:Female	~3:2
Incidence	Relatively rare neurosurgical procedure
Etiology	Traumatic; congenital; neoplastic

ANESTHETIC CONSIDERATIONS

See Anesthetic Considerations for Transsphenoidal Resection of Pituitary Tumor, p. 42.

Reference

1. Couldwell WT, Weiss MH: Cerebrospinal fluid fistulas. In *Brain Surgery: Complication, Avoidance and Management.* Apuzzo MLJ, ed. Churchill Livingstone, New York: 1993, 2329-42.

TRANSORAL RESECTION OF THE ODONTOID

SURGICAL CONSIDERATIONS

Lawrence M. Shuer

Description: The transoral approach often provides excellent access to the odontoid process of the C2 vertebral body, as well as the skull base just anterior to the brain stem. This is important for conditions where there is pressure on the brain stem (such as in cases of basilar impression) or spinal cord (odontoid fractures or rheumatoid arthritis with pannus behind the odontoid). In these cases, the operation is performed through the oral cavity with an incision at the back of the mouth. Special retractors hold the mouth open and keep the tongue out of the way. Fluoroscopic guidance helps the surgeon maintain proper trajectory. Normally, drills are used to remove the bone of the basisphenoid or first and second vertebral bodies. Upon completion of the decompression, the mucosa is closed. It may be necessary to fuse the occiput to the upper cervical spine if the patient is made unstable by this procedure. This may take place at the same time, or at a later date. Cervical spine precautions normally are used during and after the case. The patient may be in traction with tongs or a halter and, thus, a fiber optic intubation may be required.

Usual preop diagnosis: Basilar impression (platybasia); odontoid fracture; rheumatoid arthritis with atlantoaxial instability and anterior impingement of the cord

SUMMARY OF PROCEDURE

Position	Supine; head in traction or pins
Incision	Back of oropharynx
Special instrumentation	Operating microscope; image intensifier; micro drill; intraoral retractors for exposure
Unique considerations	ETT must be taped securely in a location satisfactory to surgeon. Anode or RAE tube may be helpful. Occasionally, a **tracheostomy** is performed in advance.
Antibiotics	Ampicillin (or vancomycin) 1 g iv + cefotaxime 1 g
Surgical time	2.5-3 h
Closing considerations	Patient may remain intubated postop.
EBL	25-250 ml
Postop care	ICU or close observation unit; monitor airway for swelling (✓ for stridor).
Mortality	0-3%
Morbidity	All < 20%: Infection CSF leak Neurological Massive blood loss
Pain score	2-4

PATIENT POPULATION CHARACTERISTICS

Age range	18-85 yr (usually 20-60 yr)
Male:Female	~1:2
Incidence	Rare
Etiology	Neoplastic; traumatic; congenital; degenerative
Associated conditions	Rheumatoid arthritis; traumatic injury

ANESTHETIC CONSIDERATIONS

See Anesthetic Considerations for Transsphenoidal Resection of Pituitary Tumor, p. 42.

References

1. Crockard AH: Transoral approach to intra/extradural tumors. In *Surgery of Cranial Base Tumors*. Sekhar LN, Janecka ID, eds. Raven Press, New York: 1993, 225-34.
2. Menezes AH: Transoral approach to the clivus and upper cervical spine. In *Neurosurgery Update*, Vol I. Wilkins RH, Rengachary SS, eds. McGraw-Hill, New York: 1990, 306-313.

TRANSSPHENOIDAL RESECTION OF PITUITARY TUMOR

SURGICAL CONSIDERATIONS

Lawrence M. Shuer

Description: The transsphenoidal approach to the sella turcica is a direct procedure used to gain access to the pituitary gland and sella region and is associated with relatively fewer complications than a craniotomy. The procedure usually is performed through a sublabial incision in the maxillary gingiva or via an incision in or alongside the nose. An otorhinolaryngologist may participate in obtaining the exposure, which involves creating a tunnel to the sphenoid sinus through a plane between the septum of the nose and nasal mucosa. Once the sphenoid sinus is reached, it is entered by removing a portion of the vomer. The mucosa of the sphenoid sinus is stripped and the sella is entered by removing a portion of the sella floor. Under fluoroscopic guidance and with the aid of the operating microscope, the surgeon can operate safely within the region of the pituitary gland. The tumor is removed with a series of microdissectors and suctioned out with curettage. Following tumor removal, the surgeon may harvest fat from the thigh or abdomen to place in the sella to serve as a graft to seal the dura if CSF is found. The surgeon also may reconstruct the floor of the sella with bone salvaged from the exposure.

Usual preop diagnosis: Pituitary tumor; prolactin-secreting tumor; growth hormone-secreting tumor (acromegaly); ACTH-secreting tumor (Cushing's disease); visual compromise 2° intrasellar tumor; craniopharyngioma; occasionally, diabetes or prostate cancer; Forbes-Albright syndrome

SUMMARY OF PROCEDURE

Position	Supine, head elevated 30°
Incision	Sublabial, maxillary gingiva; abdomen or thigh for fat graft
Special instrumentation	Operating microscope; image intensifier; micro drill; laser (occasionally)
Unique considerations	ETT must be taped securely in a location satisfactory to surgeon. Anode or RAE tube may be helpful. Dissection in the nasal cavity can be noxious stimulus, thus elevating BP and ICP and risking air embolus.
Antibiotics	Ampicillin (or vancomycin) 1 g iv + cefotaxime 1 g iv
Surgical time	2.5-3 h
Closing considerations	Possible abdominal or thigh-fat graft. Closure quite fast, requiring only gingival suture and nasal packs.
EBL	25-250 ml
Postop care	ICU or close observation unit; fluid and electrolytes require frequent monitoring as the patient may develop diabetes insipidus (DI) transiently following this procedure.
Mortality	0-3%
Morbidity	All < 5%: Infection CSF leak Endocrine disorder: panhypopituitarism, DI Cavernous sinus syndrome Optic nerve injury Massive blood loss: carotid injury
Pain score	2-4

PATIENT POPULATION CHARACTERISTICS

Age range	18-85 yr (usually 20-60 yr)
Male:Female	~1:2
Incidence	Relatively uncommon
Etiology	Neoplastic; traumatic
Associated conditions	Cushing's disease; acromegaly; amenorrhea/galactorrhea

ANESTHETIC CONSIDERATIONS

(Procedures covered: bifrontal craniotomy for CSF leak; transoral resection of odontoid; transsphenoidal resection of pituitary tumor)

C. Philip Larson, Jr.

PREOPERATIVE

Endocrine — Tumors of the pituitary gland are either nonfunctional or secretory. If nonfunctional, they will produce Sx either by their mass effect on adjacent pituitary tissue, or because of extension outside of the sella turcica. Rarely, the mass effect may cause the clinical picture of panhypopituitarism requiring preop treatment with thyroxine, glucocorticoid and vasopressin. Functional tumors secrete varying quantities of prolactin (→ lactation), growth hormone (→ acromegaly) and ACTH (→ adrenal hyperplasia).
Tests: Preop endocrine studies, including serum and urinary levels of pituitary, thyroid and adrenal hormones; appropriate replacement therapy established before proceeding with surgery.[3]

Respiratory — No special requirements, unless patient has acromegaly,[1] in which case large facial features, long neck, large tongue and redundant soft tissue in the oropharynx may make mask fit and ET intubation difficult. If these patients evidence hoarseness or inspiratory stridor, they should have a full clinical and radiological evaluation of the upper airway.
Tests: As indicated from H&P.

Cardiovascular — No special requirements unless patient has acromegaly, in which case they may have HTN, ischemic heart disease or diabetes.
Tests: As indicated from H&P.

Neurological — Secretory tumors of the pituitary are usually small, confined to the sella, rarely cause ↑ICP, and produce Sx of endocrine dysfunction early in their growth. In contrast, nonfunctional pituitary tumors may not produce Sx until they extend beyond the boundaries of the sella, causing headaches or pressure effects on the optic chiasm, producing visual field defects.
Tests: A CT or MRI will delineate the site and size of the tumor, especially if iv contrast material, such as gadolinium, is administered to enhance the margins of the tumor.

Musculoskeletal — If growth hormone is the primary secretant, patient will exhibit Sx of acromegaly, including large hands, feet, head and tongue.
Tests: As indicated from H&P.

Laboratory — Hct and others as indicated from H&P.

INTRAOPERATIVE

Anesthetic technique: GETA is required for this operation, since the surgical approach is through the mouth above the maxillary gum line and behind the nose.

Induction — If a difficult intubation is anticipated, orotracheal intubation will need to be accomplished before induction of GA. Awake FOL is the best choice (see p. B-6). Since these tumors are generally confined to the sella turcica and, hence, ICP usually is not increased, a standard induction technique is appropriate (see p. B-2). If ↑ICP is of concern, induction should be similar to that used for patients with other kinds of brain tumors (see Anesthetic Considerations for Craniotomy for Tumor, p. 26). To minimize the cardiovascular responses to ET intubation, it may be helpful to administer lidocaine 1-1.5 mg/kg, and then wait a few minutes before proceeding with ET intubation. Since the surgeon will be working from the patient's right side, the ETT and esophageal stethoscope must be positioned at the far left side of the mouth. An oral airway should not be used.

Maintenance — Standard maintenance (see p. B-3). Generally, no further neuromuscular-blocking drugs are administered beyond that used for ET intubation. With adequate anesthesia, and the head in Mayfield-Kees skeletal fixation, patient movement of any consequence is highly unlikely. Furthermore, it is useful to see movement of an extremity as an indicator of inadequate depth of anesthesia. Ventilation is controlled with $PaCO_2$ maintained in the normal range. Hyperventilation is not desired because it makes it more difficult for the neurosurgeon to locate the tumor in the sella, and establish that it has been removed in its entirety.

Emergence At the conclusion of operation, a decision must be made regarding extubation of the trachea. If the patient evidences normal emergence from anesthesia, the ETT should be removed before vigorous coughing ensues. Before removing the ETT, however, the anesthesiologist must make certain that all blood accumulated in the back of the throat is suctioned out, and that oropharyngeal packs placed in the back of the throat by the surgeon have been removed. The surgeon will have packed the nose at the end of operation, forcing the patient to be an obligatory mouth breather until the nasal packs are removed. If there is any question about airway patency because of a large tongue, small mouth or soft-tissue redundancy in the oropharynx, the ETT should be left in place until patient is fully awake from anesthesia. Prophylactic antiemetic (e.g., metoclopramide 10 mg or ondansetron 4 mg) should be given 30-60 min before extubation.

Blood and fluid requirements	Minimal blood loss usual Potential large blood loss IV: 16-18 ga × 1 NS/LR @ 4-8 ml/kg/h	Blood loss is minimal, unless the surgeon inadvertently enters the internal carotid artery or cavernous sinus during the course of dissection and drilling into the sella.
Control of blood loss	Deliberate hypotension	Controlled hypotension not used in this operation unless bleeding becomes profuse, diffuse or hard to control.
Monitoring	Standard monitors (see p. B-1). Arterial line CVP line UO Doppler	Monitor for VAE in semisitting position.
Positioning	✓ and pad pressure points. ✓ eyes. Shoulder roll Table turned 180°	The surgeon will use an operating microscope, which means that the anesthesiologist will be positioned near patient's feet. Anesthetic hoses and intravascular lines must be long enough to be accessible at patient's feet.

POSTOPERATIVE

Complications	Hypopituitarism Diabetes insipidus (DI)	Replacement therapy with steroids is necessary until normal pituitary function returns. Occasionally, patients will develop DI postop, as evidenced by polyuria and decreased urine-specific gravity. Rarely, this may occur near the conclusion of anesthetic, necessitating vigorous fluid replacement and vasopressin therapy (5-10 U sc or im bid).
Pain management	Codeine (30-60 mg im q 4 h)	
Tests	CT scan	If a patient exhibits any delay in emergence from anesthesia and surgery, or any new neurologic deficits emerge postop, a CT scan is invariably obtained.

References

1. Chan VWS, Tindal S: Anesthesia for transsphenoidal surgery in a patient with extreme giantism. *Br J Anaesth* 1988; 60:464-68.
2. Hardy J: Transsphenoidal approach to the pituitary gland. In *Neurosurgery*. Wilkins RH, Rengachary SS, eds. McGraw-Hill, New York: 1985, 889-98.
3. Matjasko J: Perioperative management of patients with pituitary tumors. *Semin Anesth* 1984; 111:155-67.

VENTRICULAR SHUNT PROCEDURES

SURGICAL CONSIDERATIONS

Lawrence M. Shuer

Description: Many conditions exist whereby it is necessary to divert CSF from the ventricles to another body cavity for absorption. Most commonly, the patient has developed hydrocephalus where there is dilation of the ventricular system due to some blockage in the spinal fluid pathways or absorption of the fluid at the level of the arachnoid villi. The procedure involves shaving the scalp over either the parietal or the coronal region of the skull. A continuous surgical field is created from the cranium to the peritoneum in the case of a **VP shunt**. An incision is made over the intended region of cannulation of the ventricle. A burr hole is placed in the cranium, and a ventricular catheter is placed into the ventricle. A separate incision is made over the peritoneum and dissection is carried down to the level of the posterior rectus sheath or peritoneum. A length of catheter is then passed from the abdominal incision to the cranial incision in a subcutaneous tunnel created by a special tunneling instrument. It may be necessary to use one or more jump incisions between the head and abdominal incision. A pocket is created beneath the skin, usually behind the ear, for the valve. Connections are made between the ventricular catheter, valve and the peritoneal tubing. Once the system is found to be functioning satisfactorily, the peritoneal end is placed into the peritoneum and all wounds are closed. Any component of a shunt may malfunction; thus, it may be necessary to test each component at the time of the revision in order to identify the problem. Usually, the malfunctioning part is replaced. Valves usually are passive and have a preset pressure setting (e.g., low, medium, high).

Variant procedure or approaches: The ventricular catheter can be placed in either lateral ventricle; occasionally, both lateral ventricles are cannulated. This procedure is also used to shunt the fourth ventricle and, sometimes, subarachnoid cysts. The terminal end may alternatively be the right atrium (**VA shunt**) or the pleural cavity. To place the distal end into the atrium, a vein is cannulated in the neck (usually IJ or EJ), and the catheter is fed into the atrium under fluoroscopic guidance. It may be necessary to inject radiopaque contrast in order to verify proper placement. The pleural cavity is a less common site. The catheter is threaded into the pleural cavity, and a Valsalva maneuver is performed upon closure to reinflate the lung.

Usual preop diagnosis: Hydrocephalus; obstructive or communicating hydrocephalus; aqueductal stenosis; Dandy-Walker malformation; occult hydrocephalus; normal pressure hydrocephalus; subarachnoid cyst

SUMMARY OF PROCEDURE

	VP Shunt	VA Shunt
Position	Supine, with head turned	⇐
Incision	Scalp, either coronal and retroauricular, or parietal; + neck and abdomen	Scalp, either coronal and retroauricular or parietal; + neck
Special instrumentation	Ventricular endoscope (optional)	⇐ + Image intensifier
Unique considerations	Patient to be treated as if there is ↑ICP.	⇐
Antibiotics	Cefotaxime 1 g iv and nafcillin 1-2 g iv	⇐
Surgical time	1 h	⇐
EBL	5-25 ml	⇐
Postop care	PACU → room; usually kept flat for 24 h.	⇐
Mortality	< 1%	⇐
Morbidity	Infection: < 15% Neurological: Intracranial bleed: < 1% Subdural hematoma: < 1% Hardware failure: < 1%	⇐
Pain score	4-6	2-4

PATIENT POPULATION CHARACTERISTICS

Age range	Newborn-elderly
Male:Female	1:1
Incidence	Common
Etiology	Congenital; acquired; neoplastic; infectious; posthemorrhagic
Associated conditions	Myelodysplasia; spina bifida; intraventricular hemorrhage; intraventricular tumor

ANESTHETIC CONSIDERATIONS

C. Philip Larson, Jr.

PREOPERATIVE

Ventricular shunts are inserted to ameliorate hydrocephalus or cyst formations, which are either congenital or acquired.

Cardiovascular ↑ICP → ↑BP & ↓↓HR (Cushing's response)
Tests: As indicated from H&P.

Neurological The most common presenting Sx is headache. If hydrocephalus is severe, Sx of ↑ICP (>15 mmHg) (e.g., N/V, drowsiness, papilledema, seizures and focal neurological defects) develop.

Laboratory Tests as indicated by H&P.

Premedication Usually not required; should be avoided in patients with ↑ICP.

INTRAOPERATIVE

Anesthetic technique: GETA

Induction If ↑ICP, iv induction with STP (3-5 mg/kg) or propofol (0.15-0.3 mg/kg) is preferred, because of their ability to decrease cerebral blood volume and, hence, ICP. ET intubation is accomplished with the use of a nondepolarizing neuromuscular blocking drug (e.g., vecuronium [0.1 mg/kg] or rocuronium [0.7-1 mg/kg]).

Maintenance Isoflurane 1.5% or less or sevoflurane < 2% inspired with N_2O/O_2 mixture to maintain O_2 sat ~99%. Depending on duration of operation, additional doses of vecuronium (0.1 mg/kg) or rocuronium (0.2 mg/kg) may be needed. Maintain normal temperature in children by keeping OR warm (78°F) and using warming lights as needed. Ventilation is controlled mechanically (ventilator) or manually from the start of anesthesia until the surgical wound is closed. TV and frequency are adjusted such that the $PetCO_2$ = 35-40 mmHg. Hyperventilation and hypocarbia are undesirable because they make cannulation of the ventricle(s) more difficult for the surgeon. Maintain normotension.

Emergence ETT is removed at the conclusion of the anesthetic. Prophylactic antiemetic (e.g., metoclopramide 10 mg or ondansetron 4 mg) should be given 30-60 min before extubation.

Blood and fluid requirements	IV: 18-20 ga × 1 NS/LR @ 4-6 ml/kg/h	Administer crystalloid, usually NS (via measured volume system in a child). Blood is rarely, if ever, necessary.
Monitoring	Standard monitors (see p. B-1).	
Positioning	Table turned 180° ✓ and pad pressure points. ✓ eyes.	Supine with a bolster under the shoulder on the operative side. The head, chest and abdomen are prepped, so all anesthesia equipment and lines must be at the sides of the patient.
Complications	Infection Valve malfunction	Major complications from this operation are uncommon, but include infection at the valve site or in the tubing, and malfunction of the valve, either draining too little or too much CSF.

POSTOPERATIVE

Pain management Children < 2 yr: Tylenol suppositories (10-15 mg/kg q 4 h)
Adults: meperidine 10-20 mg iv prn

Reference

1. Ruge JR, McLone DG: Cerebrospinal fluid diversion procedures. In *Brain Surgery: Complication, Avoidance and Management*. Apuzzo MLJ, ed. Churchill Livingstone, New York: 1993, 1463-94.

CRANIOCERVICAL DECOMPRESSION (CHIARI MALFORMATION)

SURGICAL CONSIDERATIONS

Lawrence M. Shuer

Description: Certain congenital malformations known as **Chiari malformations** cause crowding of structures at the craniocervical junction. These are anomalies in which portions of the cerebellum protrude through the foramen magnum such that there is little room for the brain stem and upper cervical spinal cord at this level. Frequently, the malformation is accompanied by syringomyelia, a condition in which CSF is abnormally located within the spinal cord. The craniocervical decompression is designed to make room for the structures at this level. The foramen magnum is opened by removing bone from the suboccipital skull. The posterior arch of C1 is removed and as many upper cervical lamina as are needed to fully decompress the malformation are removed. Next, the dura is opened; and, under microscopic guidance, the tonsils are dissected apart to gain an opening into the fourth ventricle. To make a patulous cisterna magna, the dura is patched with pericranium, fascia lata or tissue-bank dura. This procedure may be performed in either the prone or seated position. Some surgeons plug the foramen cecum with muscle or prosthetic material, which may lead to cardiorespiratory instability. A stent may be placed in the fourth ventricle and brought out to the subarachnoid space to ensure adequate drainage. At the same time, a shunt or stent may be placed into the syrinx cavity (see Thoracic Laminectomy, p. 63).

Usual preop diagnosis: Chiari Malformation I or II, Arnold-Chiari malformation; syringomyelia. (Chiari I malformations usually are not associated with conditions other than syringomyelia. Chiari II is commonly associated with spina bifida or myelodysplasia [Arnold-Chiari malformation]).

SUMMARY OF PROCEDURE

Position	Prone or sitting
Incision	Midline posterior, posterolateral thigh for fascia lata graft (optional)
Special instrumentation	Operating microscope
Unique considerations	Risk of air embolus; brain stem manipulation can cause BP and pulse instability.
Antibiotics	Cefotaxime 1 g and nafcillin 1 g iv
Surgical time	2.5-3.5 h
Closing considerations	Application of head dressing with consequent head movement → ↑BP and need for BP control.
EBL	25-250 ml
Postop care	ICU or constant observation unit; neurological function monitored.
Mortality	0-3%
Morbidity	All < 5%: Infection Neurological Aseptic meningitis CSF leak Postop instability Massive blood loss; vertebral artery injury
Pain score	5-7

PATIENT POPULATION CHARACTERISTICS

Age range	Infant-70 yr (usually 9-40 yr)
Male:Female	~1:1
Incidence	Relatively rare neurosurgical procedure
Etiology	Congenital; acquired, S/P lumboperitoneal shunting
Associated conditions	Hydrocephalus; syringomyelia; scoliosis; myelodysplasia

ANESTHETIC CONSIDERATIONS

See Anesthetic Considerations for Cervical Neurosurgical Procedures, p. 73.

References

1. Batzdorf U: Chiari malformation and syringomyelia. In *Brain Surgery: Complication, Avoidance and Management.* Apuzzo MLJ, ed. Churchill Livingstone, New York: 1993, 1985-2001.
2. Batzdorf U: *Syringomyelia: Current Concepts in Diagnosis and Treatment.* Williams & Wilkins, Baltimore: 1991.

STEREOTACTIC NEUROSURGERY

SURGICAL CONSIDERATIONS

Alexandra J. Golby and John R. Adler

Description: Stereotaxis applies simple rules of geometry to radiologic images to allow precise localization within the brain. Such techniques can be applied to a variety of neurosurgical procedures, providing up to 1-mm accuracy. This precision makes it possible to perform certain intracranial procedures less invasively. Methods include both frame-based and frameless systems as well as specific stereotactic applications for functional neurosurgery and radiosurgery.

Frame-based stereotaxy: Stereotactic localization was developed using frames, and these continue to be the most commonly performed stereotactic surgeries. These procedures begin with the attachment of a frame to the patient's head using four pins or screws that anchor to the skull. This is typically done outside the OR, using local anesthetic and sometimes light sedation. In the cooperative adult, frame application takes only 5-10 min; however, GA is typically used for children. Once the frame is in place, access to the patient's airway is restricted. A key for emergency removal of the frame is kept with the patient at all times. With the stereotactic frame in place, CT, MRI and/or cerebral angiography are used for target identification and localization. During imaging, a set of fiducials (radiographically visible markers) is attached to the frame. These markers provide the geometric reference points needed for localization. Data from imaging studies are used to calculate, by hand or computer, the spatial coordinates of the target(s). In nearly all cooperative patients, there is no need for sedation or analgesia during this stage of the procedure.

Frame-based stereotaxy is most frequently used for biopsy of intracranial lesions; however, drainage of cystic lesions or placement of a catheter or depth electrodes also can be performed. These common procedures involve relatively minor surgery, usually requiring only light sedation and local anesthesia. After prepping and draping, specialized operating tools are attached to the stereotactic frame. These instruments provide spatial guidance throughout the surgical procedure. A burr or twist drill hole is the usual form of intracranial access. Maximal sedation is needed during drilling and dural opening. Anesthetic considerations include ensuring adequate oxygenation and ventilation which may be compromised by the sterile drapes. At the completion of the case the frame is removed and the patient is brought to the recovery room.

Image-guided "frameless" stereotaxy: Over the last several years, techniques have been developed to provide neurosurgeons with a real-time computer display of position and trajectory. Spatial information is displayed as two-dimensional images and 3-D renderings obtained from CT and/or MRI. These devices have the added advantage of being frameless; instead of a frame providing a system of reference, small markers (fiducials) are affixed to the scalp and forehead with adhesive.

Image-guided surgery begins with an imaging study performed with fiducials in place. The remainder of the case is performed in the OR, usually under GA. Once the patient's head is appropriately positioned, the locations of the fiducials are entered into a computer, using any one of several different commercially available digitizing techniques. The most common system uses triangulation of infrared light from LEDs to determine the position of a pointer in space. The computer calculates the position of the pointer with respect to the patient and displays on the monitor the images from the scan with a representation of the pointer superimposed. Since the process of localization assumes a constant frame of reference, it is important that fiducials do not move between the time of imaging and registration in the OR. A further refinement—the dynamic reference frame—may be affixed to the craniotomy headrest to allow intraop repositioning of the patient. The OR must be set up to accommodate the computer and monitor as well as to allow a direct line-of-sight between the operative site and an array of infrared sensors. (See Fig 1.1-5.)

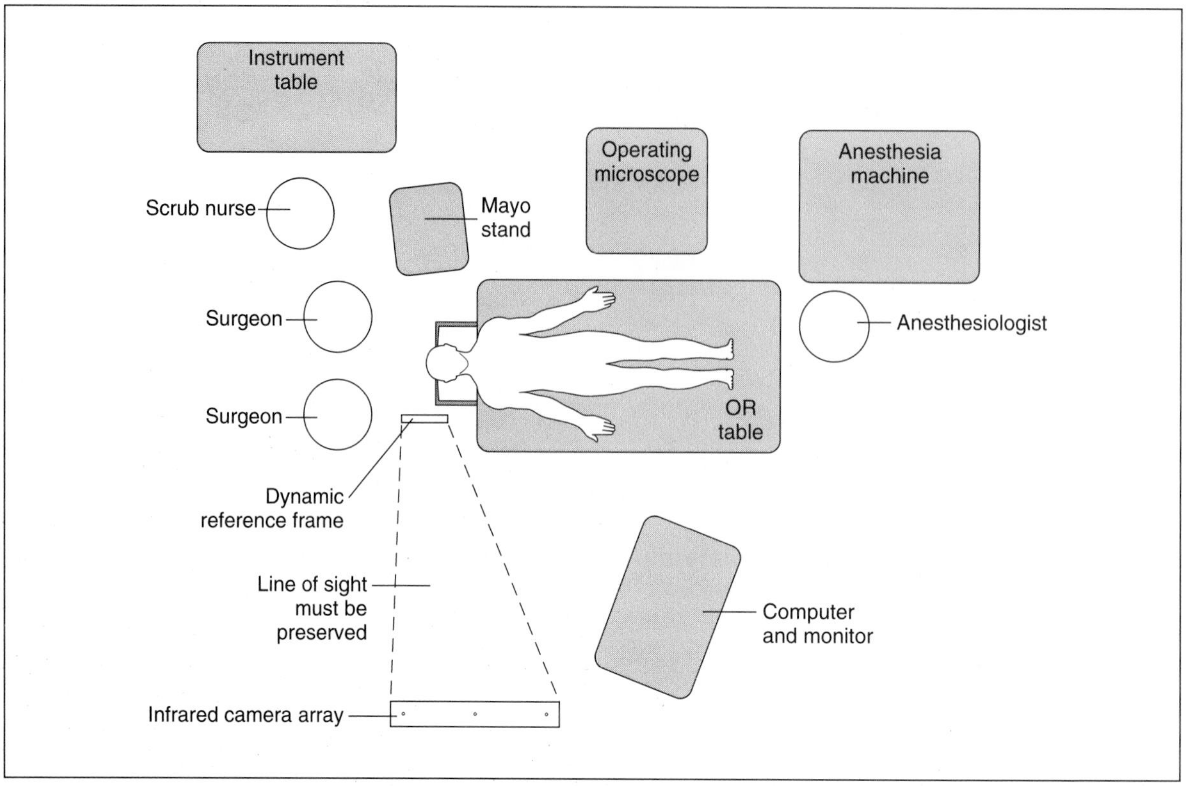

Figure 1.1-5. OR layout for frameless stereotactic surgery.

The spatial information provided to neurosurgeons by image guidance can be used to access deep or critically located lesions through the most direct trajectory and a smaller craniotomy. These techniques have been used primarily during craniotomy for tumor or vascular malformation; however, image guidance can also be used for biopsy or other smaller procedures. As with most craniotomies, GA is used. Maneuvers that alter the spatial relationship of the intracranial contents, such as hyperventilation or diuresis, will result in brain shift relative to the presurgical images and should be avoided if possible, particularly during the early stages of surgery.

Radiosurgery: This technique allows the ablation of small tumors and malformations through the closed cranium with focused doses of radiation. In contrast to other stereotactic operations, radiosurgery is performed outside the OR, using a linear accelerator or other specialized irradiation device. Cooperative adults need little or no sedation during the procedure. Children, however, almost always require GA from the beginning of frame placement through the actual treatment, which may last from 5-8 h. Consequently, anesthesia must be administered at several locations in the hospital, as well as during transport between these sites. Ideally GA is initiated in the imaging suite just prior to frame placement. After transport to the recovery unit, the child is maintained under anesthesia while radiosurgical treatment is being planned, which takes from 1-3 h. The patient is then transported to the radiosurgery suite, still anesthetized, and treatment is performed. Depending on complexity, radiosurgery itself may last from 1-2 h. At the completion of treatment, the stereotaxic frame is removed and the child is awakened.

Functional Neurosurgery: Surgery using precisely placed lesions (e.g., **pallidotomy**, **thalamotomy**) or stimulators for the treatment of movement disorders, pain, and certain psychiatric syndromes is encompassed by the term "functional stereotaxy." These techniques depend on absolutely precise localization and are usually frame-based. Concurrent neuroanatomic localization using electrophysiologic techniques is often employed. In order to preserve neural potentials and allow the patient to cooperate with neurologic testing, no general anesthesia is used. These procedures begin, as do other frame-based cases, with placement of the frame and imaging. In the OR, a burr hole is made with the patient under local anesthesia. The patient must remain awake and cooperative with his or her head immobilized throughout a several-hour procedure, which may require patient participation in various neurologic tests. Production of the lesion itself is brief and painless. After closure, the frame is removed and the patient monitored in a postop observation unit.

Usual preop diagnosis: Brain disease requiring biopsy; brain tumor; vascular malformation; Parkinson's disease; pain syndromes; psychiatric syndromes

SUMMARY OF PROCEDURE

	Frame-Based Biopsy	Frameless Craniotomy	Pediatric Radiosurgery	Functional Neurosurgery
Position	Supine or prone	Sitting, supine, prone or lateral	Supine or prone	Supine, head fixed to floor stand
Incision	0.5-2 cm, scalp	1-12 cm, scalp	None	1-3 cm, scalp
Special instrumentation	Stereotactic treatment arc	Sensor array, pointer, computer, monitor, dynamic reference frame	LINAC	Electrophysiologic monitoring equipment, lesion generator, stimulator
Unique considerations	Key for emergency: removal of frame	Minimize brain shift	Extended anesthesia in several different locations	Patient must be awake, able to cooperate with testing.
Antibiotics	Cefazolin 1 g	Nafcillin 1-2 g + cefotaxime 1 g	None	Cefazolin 1 g
Surgical time	0.5-1.5 h	2-6 h	5-8 h	2-6 h
EBL	< 10 ml	20-1000 ml	None	< 100 ml
Postop care	PACU	ICU	PACU	Neuroobservation unit
Mortality	< 0.5%	1%	None	< 1%
Morbidity	Overall: < 1% Symptomatic intracerebral hemorrhage	Infection Hemorrhage Seizures Worsening edema	N/V: 10%	N/V: 1-10% Intracerebral hemorrhage New neurologic deficits
Pain score	2	4	2	2

PATIENT POPULATION CHARACTERISTICS

Age range	All ages	⇐	0-12 yr	18-90 yr
Male:Female	1:1	⇐	⇐	⇐
Incidence	Uncommon	Unusual	⇐	Rare
Etiology	Tumor; infection; AIDS	Tumor; vascular malformations	⇐	Parkinson's disease; pain syndromes; psychiatric syndromes

ANESTHETIC CONSIDERATIONS

Richard A. Jaffe and Stanley I. Samuels

PREOPERATIVE

Neurosurgical procedures are performed using stereotactic control when the lesion is small and/or is located deep within brain tissue, or as a means of obtaining a biopsy of a lesion for diagnosis. For example, focal, deep-seated arteriovenous malformations (AVMs) may be resected under stereotactic control. These patients are often otherwise healthy.

Neurological Neurological Sx vary (depending on site and size of the lesion) and they should be carefully documented. In addition to the usual tests, a CT or MRI scan is obtained preop with the frame in place to determine stereotactic coordinates. Once the coordinates are established, the frame or fiducial markers must not be moved until the operation is complete.

Laboratory Tests as indicated from H&P.

INTRAOPERATIVE

Anesthetic technique: GETA or MAC. In adults, fiducial markers or a stereotactic frame is placed before surgery and the patient is taken to the radiological suite for CT/MRI scan to determine stereotactic coordinates. The patient is then brought to OR with the frame or fiducial markers in place. The "key" for removing the stereotactic frame must be readily available in the event of an airway emergency. Biopsies generally are done under local anesthesia with MAC. If a complete resection is planned (e.g., AVM resection), GETA is used. In children, it is usually necessary to induce GA before placing the frame, thus necessitating the maintenance of GA during the CT/MRI scan. The child is then moved to the OR, still anesthetized, and the operation is completed.

Induction If MAC is planned, O_2 by nasal prongs is administered, and the patient is lightly sedated with combinations of droperidol 0.01 mg/kg to prevent N/V; midazolam 0.07 mg/kg in divided doses to provide amnesia; and meperidine 1.5 mg/kg or fentanyl 3.5 μg/kg in divided doses to provide analgesia. It is important that the patient be able to communicate with the surgeon as needed throughout the operation. For functional neurosurgery (e.g., pallidotomy), sedation should be minimized to preserve normal electrophysiological activity. If GETA is needed, FOL is necessary before inducing anesthesia because the frame precludes intubation by direct laryngoscopy (see p. B-6). Once ET intubation is established, anesthesia may be induced with STP 5-10 mg/kg or propofol 1.5-2 mg/kg, followed by a nondepolarizing neuromuscular blocking drug to facilitate positioning of patient.

Maintenance If GA is used, maintenance is the same as for a tumor (see Anesthetic Considerations for Craniotomy for Tumor, p. 26) or AVM (see Anesthetic Considerations for Craniotomy for Intracranial Vascular Malformations, p. 17). If children are to be transported from the site of placement of the stereotactic frame to the radiological suite and then to the OR, it is best to use inhalation anesthesia with isoflurane 1-1.5% or sevoflurane 2-3% in O_2 with spontaneous ventilation to assure adequate ventilation and oxygenation during transport and study. Opiates and nondepolarizing neuromuscular-blocking drugs should not be administered until the child is in the operating suite.

Emergence ETT is generally removed at the conclusion of the operation. Prophylactic antiemetic (e.g., metoclopramide 10 mg or ondansetron 4 mg) should be given 30-60 min before extubation.

Blood and fluid requirements	IV: 16-18 ga × 2 (adults); 20-22 ga (children) NS/LR @ 4-6 ml/kg/h	Blood loss is minimal since the volume of tissue removed is small.
Monitoring	If local anesthesia: standard monitors (see p. B-1). If GA: Arterial line CVP line UO	
Positioning	✓ and pad pressure points. ✓ eyes.	

POSTOPERATIVE

Complications	Bleeding	Focal bleeding may occur postop, causing onset of a neurological deficit.
Pain management	Vicodin (1-2 mg po q 4 h prn)	
Tests	CT or MRI scan, if a new neurological deficit occurs.	

Reference

1. Heilbrun MP, ed: *Stereotactic Neurosurgery*. Williams & Wilkins, Baltimore: 1988.

STEREOTACTIC NEUROSURGERY FOR MOVEMENT DISORDERS

SURGICAL CONSIDERATIONS

Gary Heit and Gerald D. Silverberg

Description: The surgical treatment of movement disorders—mainly Parkinson's disease—is now focused on the globus pallidus interna (posteroventral pallidotomy [PVP]) and the ventral intermedialis nucleus of the thalamus (VIM) thalamotomy or stimulation.[2]

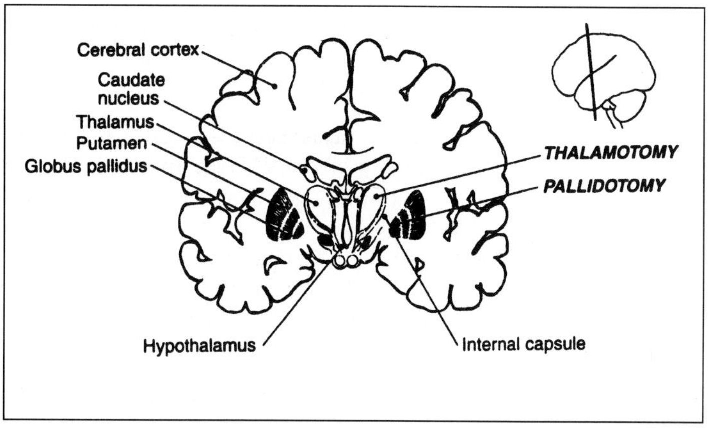

Figure 1.1-6. Anatomical locations for therapeutic lesions (thalamotomy and pallidotomy) for the surgical treatment of Parkinson's disease. Inset shows the plane of the coronal section through the diencephalon, identifying the lesions. (Reproduced with permission from Mason LJ, Cojocaru TT, Cole DJ: Surgical Intervention and Anesthetic Management of the Patient with Parkinson's Disease. In *International Anesthesiology Clinics: Topics in Neuroanesthesia.* Jaffe RA, Giffard RG, eds. Little, Brown, Boston: 1996 4(34):141.)

For Parkinson's disease, **PVP** produces nearly complete resolution of dyskinesia in over 89% of patients. Approximately 70% of patients receive moderate-to-marked relief of bradykinesia, fluctuations in medication response and rigidity. PVP for dystonia can produce nearly complete resolution of symptoms. PVP for tremor is problematic, and tremor is not considered to be a major indication for PVP.

In contrast, **thalamotomy** is highly efficacious for the control of tremor; for example, for unilateral essential tremor, 85-92% of patients gain excellent control of the tremor. Parkinsonian tremor responds, to a similar degree. Unilateral thalamotomy has a complication rate of 5-8%; however, there is a significant rise in morbidity (9-20% across series) with bilateral thalamotomies and the procedure is not widely used.

Deep-brain stimulation, which recently has emerged as a viable alternative to either ablative procedure for movement disorders, has been used to treat bilateral tremor. The current indications for VIM thalamic deep brain stimulation in the United States are essential tremor or Parkinsonian tremor. Marked-to-moderate improvement in essential tremor and Parkinsonian tremor was seen in 62% and 89% of patients, respectively.

All procedures are currently performed with frame-based stereotactic techniques with intracranial access via a burr hole or twist drill. As in most stereotactic procedures, MAP should be ≤ 90 mmHg. There are two approaches to target identification following initial stereotactic CT or MRI radiographic localization; both require patient cooperation. In one approach, the target is confirmed by assessing symptomatic resolution during high-frequency macrostimulation, and by identifying surrounding structures using their characteristic stimulation-evoked responses. In the other system, prior to stimulation testing, single-neuron recordings are performed to localize the appropriate target through somatotopic kinesthetic and/or somatosensory responses. This technique utilizes specialized high-impedance microelectrodes and amplifiers susceptible to interference from monitoring equipment, which may necessitate manual measurements of BP and clinical assessment of oxygenation. Anesthesia or sedation can significantly modify neuronal activity and, thus, interfere with functional mapping. For example, propofol has been shown to inhibit globus pallidus neurons for several minutes beyond its behavioral effects.[3] Additionally, many of these agents have been shown to change evoked potential responses, raising the possibility that they could alter stimulation thresholds for either the internal capsule or optic tract. Thermal ablation typically is performed with a radiofrequency lesion generator operating at 500 kHz, which may interfere with some types of monitoring equipment; however, the ablation process only lasts approximately 10 minutes.

For deep-brain stimulation, implantation of the intracranial electrode is performed under local anesthesia to permit monitoring of behavioral and physiological responses. The implantable pulse generator may be placed in an infraclavicular, subcutaneous pocket at the time of the intracranial electrode implantation. Implantation of the pulse generator and subcutaneous tunneling of the electrode lead can be done under MAC, but is best tolerated under GETA. To facilitate induction and intubation, the calvarial wound is closed temporally and the stereotactic frame is removed.

Usual preop diagnosis: **PVP**—medically intractable idiopathic Parkinson's disease with disabling L-Dopa-induced dyskinesia, bradykinesia or rigidity; severe fluctuations in medication responses; dystonia musculorum deformans; post-CVA dystonia; and, occasionally, severe torticollis. **VIM thalamotomy**—essential tremor, severe Parkinson's disease tremor and, occasionally, cerebellar tremor disorders. **Deep-brain stimulation**—movement disorders

SUMMARY OF PROCEDURE

Position	Supine or semirecumbent
Incision	2-3 cm linear (burr hole access) or stab wound (twist-drill access), 30-40 mm from midline and 1 cm anterior to coronal suture
Special instrumentation	Stereotactic frame; radiofrequency lesion generator; single-neuron recording system; deep-brain stimulation hardware; external trial stimulator
Unique considerations	Minimal or no sedation. Patient cooperation necessary. If single-neuron recordings are used, then avoid propofol; use low-dose remifentanil infusion. Local anesthetic should contain no epinephrine. Sedation with meperidine in patients taking selegiline is contraindicated. No dopaminergic agonist or antagonist (e.g., metoclopramide, droperidol) should be given. To enhance single-cell responses, withhold medications prescribed for target symptoms for 8-24 h. May need manual monitoring techniques to avoid interference with single-cell recordings.
Antibiotics	Cefazolin 1 g and dexamethasone 6-8 mg iv
Surgical time	2-5 h
Closing considerations	Single, interrupted suture for stab wounds or two-layer suture/staple closure for burr hole
EBL	< 25 ml
Postop care	Overnight observation in neurosurgical unit (risk of intracranial hemorrhage). Ambulate only with assistance 2° risk of falls after PVP.
Mortality	< 0.3%
Morbidity	Visual field defect (pallidotomy): ≤ 14% Intracranial hematoma or hemorrhage: 2-8% Inadvertent ablation of nontarget structures: 1-5% Infection: 1-5%
Pain score	2-3

PATIENT POPULATION CHARACTERISTICS

	Parkinson's Disease	Dystonia*	Essential Tremor
Age range	40-80 yr	10-70 yr	50-80 yr
Male:Female	50:50	Varies by type	50:50
Incidence	40-50/100,000	Varies by type	100-120/100,000
Etiology	Idiopathic	Varies by type*	Idiopathic
Associated conditions	Depression; autonomic dysfunction	Multiple*	Multiple

*Dystonia is a symptomatic description for a variety of disorders (e.g., facial tics versus dystonia musculorum deformans).

ANESTHETIC CONSIDERATIONS

Stanley I. Samuels and Richard A. Jaffe

PREOPERATIVE

Parkinson's disease is the most common movement disorder, affecting ~1% of the population > 60 yr. It is caused by the loss of dopaminergic neurons in the substantia nigra → ↓dopamine (dopamine/acetocholine imbalance) in basal ganglia → movement disorder. Medical treatment is directed primarily to restoring dopamine levels by increasing the availability of the dopamine precursor (L-dopa), inhibiting liver dopa decarboxylase (carbidopa, usually given in combination with L-dopa as Sinemet), by releasing endogenous dopamine (amantadine [Symmetrel]) and by blocking MAO-B (selegiline [Eldepryl]). Medical treatment also may include dopamine agonists (pergolide [Permax]; bromocriptine [Parlodel]), and acetylcholine antagonists (amantadine [Symmetrel], benztropine [Cogentin]) to correct the dopamine/acetylcholine imbalance. Patients presenting for surgery have failed medical therapy, and will have been taken off their antiparkinsonian medications 8-24 h before surgery. This will maximize their symptoms to help assess treatment effects intraop; thus, preop assessment on the day of surgery will be difficult.

Respiratory	Autonomic dysfunction → esophageal dysfunction → ↑risk of aspiration. Patients typically have ↓vital capacity 2° rigidity, dyskinesia → ↓respiratory function and ↓cough. Laryngospasm and respiratory failure may occur following withdrawal of antiparkinsonian medications. **Tests:** CXR; consider ABG; PFTs may be difficult to obtain.

Cardiovascular	Autonomic dysfunction → orthostatic hypotension. Dopamine replacement therapy → cardiac dysrhythmias, ↓BP and hypovolemia. In patients taking selegiline (MAO inhibitor): meperidine → ↑↑BP, rigidity, agitation; sympathomimetics → exaggerated ↑BP.	
Neurological	The primary Sx of Parkinson's disease include rigidity, tremor, bradykinesia, muscle weakness. Secondary symptoms include dementia, depression and speech difficulty. Patients may alternate between a state of immobility and one of exaggerated tremor (which may interfere with intraop monitoring).	
Renal	Urinary retention is common.	
Gastrointestinal	Autonomic dysfunction → gastroparesis, ↑incidence of reflux. Poor nutrition. Pharyngeal muscle dysfunction → dysphagia.	
Laboratory	As indicated from H&P.	
Premedication	None. These patients often will have received small doses of fentanyl and/or midazolam to facilitate placement of the stereotactic frame.	

INTRAOPERATIVE

Anesthetic technique: MAC, with minimal or no sedation, as patient cooperation is essential for the success of the procedure.

Induction	Low-dose remifentanil (0.01-0.05 μg/kg/min) may be used for sedation.	
Maintenance	BP control is important to minimize the risk of intracranial hemorrhage. MAP should be kept at or, preferably, somewhat below normal for that patient. This usually can be accomplished without an arterial line by using small doses of labetalol (2.5-5 mg increments) and/or an infusion of NTG titrated to effect. Postop BP control can be continued by using NTG paste applied 30-60 min before the end of the procedure. In the event of an airway emergency, a means of releasing the patient from the stereotactic frame must be readily available.	
Emergence	Antiparkinsonian medication should be given when the procedure is complete. The patient is usually transported directly to the neurology ward for postop monitoring.	
Blood and fluid requirements	Minimal blood loss IV: 18-20 ga × 1 NS/LR @ 1-2 ml/kg/h	IV should be placed in the ipsilateral arm (relative to side of surgery).
Monitoring	Standard monitors (see p. B-1).	Exaggerated tremors in these patients may interfere with monitoring. It may be helpful to place the BP cuff on a leg (less tremor). No monitor should be placed on contralateral arm, which must be kept free for testing. Monitors (oximeter, BP, gas analyzer) may interfere with intraop electrophysiology and may need to be replaced with manual techniques during this period.
Positioning	✓ and pad pressure points. ✓ stereotactic frame clearance.	Patient comfort may be improved by placing pillows under the knees to relieve lower back strain.
Complications	Intracerebral hemorrhage	Dx: ↓mental status and hemiparesis. CT scan usually required to confirm Dx. Emergency craniotomy may be necessary.
	Loss of airway	Rx: remove stereotactic frame and secure airway.

POSTOPERATIVE

Complications	Intracranial hemorrhage Motor deficit Visual field deficit Aphasia	Intracranial hemorrhage may require emergency craniotomy.
Tests	None	
Pain management	Usually not necessary	

References

1. Benabid A, Pollak P, Gao D, Hoffman D, Limousin P, Gay E, Payen I, Benazzouz A: Chronic electrical stimulation of the ventralis intermedius nucleus of the thalamus as a treatment of movement disorders. *J Neurosurg* 1996; 84:203-14.
2. Guridi J, Lozano A: A brief history of pallidotomy. *Neurosurgery* 1997; 41(5):1169-83.
3. Heit G, Murphy G, Jaffe R, Golby A, Silverberg GS: The effects of propofol on human globus pallidus neurons. *Stereotact Funct Neurosurg* 1997; 67(1-2):74.
4. Mason LJ, Cojocaru TT, Cole DJ: Surgical intervention and anesthetic management of the patient with Parkinson's disease. In *Topics in Neuroanesthesia.* Jaffe RA, Giffard RG, eds. Little, Brown, Boston: 1996; 34(4):133-150.

EPILEPSY SURGERY

SURGICAL CONSIDERATIONS

Lawrence M. Shuer

Description: In the U.S., the prevalence of epilepsy is approximately 5-20/1,000 (0.5-2%), meaning that at least 1.5 million people have epilepsy.[2,3] In childhood, the incidence and prevalence is higher, with 90% of all new cases occurring before the age of 20. Intractable epilepsy is defined as persistent seizure activity of such frequency or severity that prevents normal function and/or development. This diagnosis is made only after an adequate trial of anticonvulsant medication(s), with therapeutic levels, has been documented.[4] Of all those with epilepsy, 10-20% prove to be intractable; and it is estimated that approximately 20-30% of patients with intractable epilepsy may benefit from a surgical procedure.[5]

The causes of epilepsy are varied, ranging from idiopathic to neoplastic. Epilepsy surgery is most beneficial in patients with partial epilepsy 2° a structural lesion. Most commonly, this lesion is located in the temporal lobe; and, therefore, the most common operation is a **temporal lobectomy** in both children and adults. Cerebral dominance and, hence, the location of speech, must be determined using a preop Wada test (intracarotid amobarbital injection to localize language function).[1] Temporal lobe surgery may involve removal of only the structural lesion and associated epileptogenic cortex, cortical resection alone, excision of the amygdala and hippocampus or removal of the entire anterior temporal lobe, with the extent of posterior resection dependent on dominance. Depending on the center, intraop electrocorticography may be employed, requiring neuroleptic anesthesia. In addition, the speech center may need to be identified intraop, necessitating an awake procedure. These differing options will significantly alter the choice of anesthesia and must be established prior to surgery.

A standard **temporal lobectomy** is detailed as follows: The patient is placed supine on the operating table with the head turned 90° and held with pin fixation. A "question mark" temporal incision is often used, and hemostasis is achieved with skin clips. A flap—either a free temporal bone flap or an osteoplastic flap, based on the temporalis muscle—is elevated with a high-speed craniotome. A **subtemporal craniectomy** allows visualization of the entire anterior temporal lobe. The dura is opened, widely exposing the anterior 6-6.5 cm of the temporal lobe. Labbe's vein must be preserved. At this point, surface and/or depth electrocorticography may be employed and **inhalation anesthetics must not be used**. After mapping the lesion, amygdala and hippocampus or anterior temporal lobe is removed. Temporal lobectomy involves resection of both the lateral and medial temporal structures, and is commonly performed in two steps. Often an operating microscope will be used to completely resect medial structures, including the uncus and hippocampal formation. Injury to the brain stem, 3rd and 4th cranial nerves, and either the middle cerebral or posterior cerebral arteries, can occur; these are known complications of this surgery. Closure of the dura, bone flap and scalp is routine.

Variant procedure or approaches: There are three common alternate procedures. The first is sectioning of the corpus callosum, known as a **corpus callosotomy**. This is commonly used for patients with atonic seizures or partial seizures with secondary generalization. Either the anterior two-thirds or the entire corpus callosum is divided in the midline. The approach is the same as any transcallosal, intraventricular procedure, and uses a bifrontal, paramedian scalp incision and elevation of free-bone flap adjacent to the midline in the region of the coronal suture. Injury to the sagittal sinus is possible and must be avoided. In addition, numerous bridging veins across the interhemispheric fissure must be preserved to avoid venous congestion and possible infarction. The right cerebral hemisphere is gently retracted from the falx, exposing the paired anterior cerebral arteries and underlying corpus callosum. If an anterior two-thirds transection is performed, an intraop x-ray is required to determine the posterior border.

The second alternate procedure is either a **frontal**, **temporal** or **occipital craniotomy** for resection of a structural, epileptogenic focus such as a tumor or AVM. This procedure may employ **stereotaxic localization** and the resultant craniotomy may be performed in the stereotaxic head frame, which alters the method of intubation. The subsequent craniotomy is similar to the excision of any structural lesion, with the exception of intraop electrocorticography of surrounding cortex, if used. Such monitoring alters the choice of anesthetic.

The third alternate procedure is diagnostic and involves placement of **surface and/or depth electrodes**. This may be performed with or without stereotaxic localization. Often only burr holes, outlining the future craniotomy flap, are used.

Usual preop diagnosis: Temporal lobe epilepsy; partial epilepsy; intractable epilepsy

SUMMARY OF PROCEDURE

Position	Supine, rarely prone for occipital lesions; or table 180°
Incision	Temporal question mark, reverse question mark, paramedian, frontal or occipital
Special instrumentation	Operating microscope; Cavitron; bipolar cautery; surface electrode grids and strips; depth electrode
Unique considerations	Electrocorticography requiring neuroleptic anesthesia; awake procedures for mapping of temporal and/or frontal speech areas; stereotaxic craniotomy and lesionectomy
Antibiotics	Nafcillin 1-2 g + cefotaxime 1 g iv
Surgical time	3 h
EBL	Minimal for diagnostic procedures; 250-500 ml with craniotomy (adults)
Postop care	After craniotomy, ICU for 12-24 h
Mortality	< 1%
Morbidity	Hemiplegia Dysphasia Ophthalmoplegia Brain stem surgery
Pain score	1-3

PATIENT POPULATION CHARACTERISTICS

Age range	2-50 yr
Male:Female	1:1
Incidence	150,000/yr (new cases of epilepsy): ~10% eventually present for surgery/yr (1500)
Etiology	Idiopathic (mesial temporal sclerosis); infectious (brain abscess, encephalitis); traumatic (glial scar); vascular (AVM, infarct); neoplastic (glioma, hamartoma, ganglioglioma); congenital (cortical dysplasia)
Associated conditions	Tuberous sclerosis; Sturge-Weber syndrome; infantile hemiplegia; encephalitis; hemimegalencephaly

ANESTHETIC CONSIDERATIONS

C. Philip Larson, Jr.

PREOPERATIVE

Epilepsy is a common disorder among young adults. Antiepileptic medication, such as phenytoin, will abolish seizure disorders in most patients, but some develop intolerable side effects to such medications; others are refractory to medical therapy. Surgical ablation of the seizure focus may be the only effective therapy for some patients if they are to become self-sufficient and be able to operate a motor vehicle. Several operations may be done, the most common being placement of surface or depth electrodes to determine the focus of the seizure, with subsequent temporal lobectomy for removal of the focus. In some cases, the lesion may be very focal and amenable to stereotactic localization and removal.

Neurological Usually the only neurological findings are a Hx of uncontrollable seizures, either focal or generalized. Obtain a description of seizure and prodromal Sx.

Tests: A Wada test (intracarotid injection of a barbiturate) is usually performed to determine whether the area of proposed surgery has any cerebral dominance or speech function.

Gastrointestinal Abnormal liver function may be associated with valproate and carbamazepine use.
Tests: LFT and others as indicated from H&P.

Hematologic Phenytoin/phenobarbital → ↓Hct; carbamazepine/valproate/ethosuximide/primidone → ↓Plt; Carbamazepine/primidone → ↓WBC

Tests: CBC and others as indicated from H&P.

Laboratory Tests as indicated from H&P.

Premedication Standard premedication (see p. B-2) is usually appropriate.

INTRAOPERATIVE

Anesthetic technique: Local anesthesia and GETA. The placement of surface or depth electrodes is done under GETA, as is a temporal lobectomy in the nondominant hemisphere. If the seizure focus is in the dominant hemisphere and/or if there is any question about possible neurological injury by temporal lobectomy, the procedure is performed under local anesthesia, with intraop localization of the seizure focus. In this case, the patient should be told that the operation will be performed under local anesthesia, that every effort will be made to control discomfort, and that he/she will be expected to respond to some pictures and questions once the head is opened and the seizure area is identified. The patient should also be told that he/she probably will be amnesic for the operative events.

Induction Standard induction (see p. B-2). If a difficult intubation is anticipated (e.g., stereotactic frame), orotracheal intubation is best accomplished before induction of GA. An awake fiber optic intubation is the best technique (see p. B-2). Once anesthesia is induced, a nondepolarizing neuromuscular relaxant is administered.

Maintenance Standard maintenance (see p. B-3). Generally, no further neuromuscular-blocking drugs are administered beyond that used for tracheal intubation. With adequate anesthesia, and the head fixed in the Mayfield-Kees skeletal fixation, patient movement of any consequence is highly unlikely. Furthermore, it is useful to see movement of an extremity as an indicator of inadequate depth of anesthesia.

Emergence No special considerations. Prophylactic antiemetic (e.g., metoclopramide 10 mg or ondansetron 4 mg) should be given 30-60 min before extubation.

Wake-up testing: At some institutions an asleep-awake-asleep technique is used in which the patient is placed under general-endotracheal anesthesia for positioning and craniotomy. After surgical exposure of the seizure area, the patient is allowed to awaken to assess neurologic function while areas of the brain are stimulated. When the seizure focus has been adequately delineated, GA is reinstituted for the remainder of the operation. An excellent anesthetic technique under these circumstances includes the use of N_2O and sevoflurane for amnesia, and remifentanil (0.05-2 μg/kg/min) by continuous infusion for analgesia. The advantage of these drugs is that they are quickly eliminated, allowing for rapid emergence for the awake component of the procedure, followed by rapid reinduction of anesthesia when the testing period is over. To allow the patient to talk during the awake portion of the procedure, the ETT must be removed. This is best accomplished by inserting a small or medium-sized tube changer through the ETT before it is removed. The tube changer can then be used as a guide for reinsertion of the ETT, and it will not prevent normal vocalization by the patient during the awake phase.

Local anesthesia: Initial sedation may be achieved with a combination of midazolam (0.07 mg/kg) and meperidine (1-1.5 mg/kg) or fentanyl (2-3 μg/kg). Nasal prongs should be placed on the patient and supplemental O_2 administered. If local anesthesia is used, continuous pump infusions of propofol (50-150 μg/kg/min) and an opiate (e.g., remifentanil 0.05-2 μg/kg/min) are extremely effective in providing amnesia and analgesia, while allowing the anesthesiologist to awaken the patient for about 30-60 min of testing, once the temporal lobe has been exposed surgically.

Blood and fluid requirements	Moderate blood loss IV: 18 ga × 2 NS/LR @ 4-6 ml/kg/h	If local anesthesia used, 2 iv cannulae are useful–one for fluid administration, another for infusion of anesthetic and other drugs. If GA used, 1 peripheral iv and a CVP cannula are inserted. Blood transfusions seldom are needed for this operation since blood loss is usually < 500 ml.
Monitoring	Standard monitors (see p. B-1). Arterial line CVP line (if GA) UO	O_2 sat and $ETCO_2$ monitoring will indicate the adequacy of ventilation and oxygenation.

Positioning	Table rotated 180° ✓ and pad pressure points ✓ eyes	Semisitting position with head held in Mayfield-Kees skeletal fixation and rotated laterally with a roll under the shoulder on the operative side. Anesthetic hoses and intravascular lines must be long enough to be accessible.
Complications	Anxiety Agitation Seizure	Local anesthetic toxicity may produce agitation and seizures.

POSTOPERATIVE

Complications	Seizure Bleeding Cerebral edema	Monitor carefully for altered mental status.
Pain management	Codeine 30-60 mg im q 4 h	Avoid oversedation.
Tests	CT scan	If a patient exhibits any delay in emergence from anesthesia and surgery, or any new neurologic deficits appear, a CT scan is invariably obtained.

References

1. Blume WT, Grabow JD, Darley FL, Aronson AE: Intracarotid amobarbital test of language and memory before temporal lobectomy for seizure control. *Neurology* 1973, 23(8):812-19.
2. Hauser WA: *Epilepsy: frequency, causes, and consequences*. Demos, New York: 1990, 21-48.
3. Hauser WA, Kurland LT: The epidemiology of epilepsy in Rochester, Minnesota, 1935 through 1967. *Epilepsia* 1975; 16(1):1-66.
4. Morrison G, Duchowny M, Resnick T, Alvarez L, Jayakan P, Prats AR, Dean P, Penate M: Epilepsy surgery in childhood. A report of 79 patients. *Pediatr Neurosurg* 1992, 18(5-6):291-7.
5. NIH Consensus Development Conference. Consensus Statement: *Surgery for Epilepsy*. 1990, Mar 19-21; 8(2) 2, and *JAMA* 1990; 264:729-33.
6. O'Donohoe NV: *Epilepsies of Childhood*. Butterworths, Boston: 1985, 4.

Surgeon

Lawrence M. Shuer, MD

1.2 SPINAL NEUROSURGERY

Anesthesiologist

C. Philip Larson, Jr., MD, MS

LUMBAR FUSION

SURGICAL CONSIDERATIONS

Description: The goal of a **lumbar spinal fusion** is to have two or more spinal segments unite as one over time. The procedure is often performed when there is instability of the spine, such as spondylolisthesis, or cases where the patient may have a known instability due to damage of the normal support structures (e.g., facets). Through a midline vertical incision, the paraspinal muscles are exposed and dissected off of the spinous processes, lamina and facets. Next, dissection is carried down to the transverse processes and/or sacral alae of the segments to be fused. Blood loss can be significant during this stage of surgery.

A **discectomy** or **nerve-root decompression** may be incorporated (see Lumbar Laminotomy, Laminectomy, p. 62). The bone surfaces are decorticated and bone graft material (usually harvested from the ilium) is placed in contact with them. Instrumentation may be used to achieve internal fixation. These types of hardware may include Knodt distraction rods, Harrington rods, various types of pedicle screw and rod/plate combinations, or interspace cages. Intraop x-rays may be taken to verify proper placement of the pedicle screws. The wound is closed in layers; and a drain is left in the wound at the end of the procedure.

Variant procedure or approaches: Some surgeons perform an **interbody lumbar fusion** following a **complete bilateral discectomy**. This procedure begins as a **lumbar laminectomy** and involves preparation of the vertebral body end plates for graft placement by the surgeon. This is achieved by removing the cartilaginous surface of the vertebral body. Rectangular bone grafts are shaped appropriately and countersunk into the disc space with retraction of the dural sack. The bone grafts may be taken from the patient's ilium or the tissue bank. This type of fusion also may be supplemented with some form of internal fixation as described above.

Usual preop diagnosis: Lumbar instability; spondylolisthesis; pseudospondylolisthesis; spondylolysis; mechanical back syndrome

SUMMARY OF PROCEDURE

	Lateral Transverse Process	Posterior Lumbar Interbody
Position	Prone	⇐
Incision	Posterior midline	⇐
Special instrumentation	Drill for decortication; internal hardware, optional (see description of types of hardware, above)	⇐
Unique considerations	Localizing intraop spine x-ray is used to assess level for operation (optional); fluoroscopy or films for pedicle screw placement.	⇐
Antibiotics	Cefazolin 1 g iv	⇐
Surgical time	2-4 h for single level; additional levels, add 1-2 h each.	2-3 h for single level; additional levels, add 0.5 h each.
Closing considerations	No cast or brace	⇐
EBL	250-500 ml	50-300 ml
Postop care	PACU → room	⇐
Mortality	0-5%	⇐
Morbidity	Infection CSF leak Nerve root injury Postop instability Massive blood loss: injury to retroperitoneal vessels	⇐
Pain score	6-10	6-10

PATIENT POPULATION CHARACTERISTICS

Age range	15-85 yr (usually 30-60 yr)
Male:Female	~3:2
Incidence	Common
Etiology	Degenerative; congenital; neoplastic; traumatic; infectious

ANESTHETIC CONSIDERATIONS

See Anesthetic Considerations for Thoracolumbar Neurosurgical Procedures, p. 64.

References

1. Dunsker SB: Lumbar spine stabilization: indications. *Clin Neurosurg* 1990; 36:147-58.
2. Egnatchik JG: Lumbar spine stabilization: techniques. *Clin Neurosurg* 1990; 36:159-67.

LUMBAR LAMINOTOMY, LAMINECTOMY

SURGICAL CONSIDERATIONS

Description: Lumbar laminotomy (partial removal of lamina) and **laminectomy** (complete removal of lamina) are procedures for decompressing the neural elements of the lumbar spine via a posterior approach. They can be used to treat lumbar radiculopathy 2° degenerative disc disease (e.g., herniated discs or osteophytes). **Decompressive laminectomy** can be used to treat compression of the cauda equina, usually 2° degenerative disease, congenital stenosis, neoplasm and, occasionally, trauma. Lumbar laminectomy is also used to gain access to the spinal canal for dealing with intradural tumors, arteriovenous malformations (AVMs) and other spinal cord lesions.

Through a vertical midline incision, the lumbodorsal fascia is exposed and then the paraspinal muscles are dissected off of the spinous process and lamina of the segments intended for decompression. The level may need to be checked by intraop x-ray if the surgeon is not able to identify location based on visual confirmation of anatomic level. The bone landmarks are identified and ligamentous attachments are cut. The bone is removed piecemeal with either rongeurs, gouges or power drills. Care is taken not to injure the underlying dura. If a dural tear is made, it must be repaired. The surgeon may want a Valsalva-like maneuver (sustained inspiration at 30-40 cmH_2O) performed to test the integrity of the repair. If disc is to be removed, the dura is retracted and the annulus incised. The disc is removed piecemeal with a series of curettes and disc-biting rongeurs. There is a risk of damage to retroperitoneal structures (e.g., great vessels or intestines) during this portion of the procedure. More commonly, there may be troublesome epidural bleeding which may be difficult to control and will necessitate transfusion. Hemostasis is obtained prior to closure. The wound is closed in layers; a drain may be left in the epidural space. The patient is rolled onto his/her back on a hospital bed at the completion of the procedure.

Variant procedure or approaches: The extent of the procedure depends on the indications for treatment. When the patient has single nerve-root-compression syndrome, the laminotomy consists of decompressing that one root. When there is diffuse narrowing of the spinal canal, an extensive lumbar decompression over several segments may be indicated. The amount of bone removal varies from case to case. Occasionally, the procedure includes a fusion of some type (e.g., plate and screws), if it is felt that the patient has some instability.

Usual preop diagnosis: Lumbar radiculopathy (nerve-root compression); lumbar disc disease (herniation or degeneration of one or more lumbar discs); lateral recess stenosis; herniated disc, lumbar stenosis; neurogenic claudication; metastatic carcinoma or tumor to spine; lumbar spine tumor; spondylosis (arthritic degeneration); spondylolysis (structural defect in the pars interarticularis of the vertebra); spondylolisthesis (misalignment or slip of vertebra)

SUMMARY OF PROCEDURE

	Lumbar Laminotomy	Laminectomy
Position	Prone	⇐
Incision	Posterior midline	⇐
Special instrumentation	Operating microscope (optional)	⇐
Unique considerations	Localizing intraop spine x-ray taken to assess correct level for operation (optional)	⇐

	Lumbar Laminotomy	Laminectomy
Antibiotics	Cefazolin 1 g iv	⇐
Surgical time	1-2 h for single level; additional levels, add 0.5-1 h each.	2 h for single level; additional levels, add 0.5 h each.
EBL	25-500 ml	50-1500 ml
Postop care	PACU → room	⇐
Mortality	0.5%	⇐
Morbidity	The following usually occur in < 5% of cases:	⇐
	Infection	⇐
	CSF leak	⇐
	Nerve-root injury	⇐
	Postop instability	⇐
	Massive blood loss: injury to retroperitoneal vessels	⇐
Pain score	4-10	4-10

PATIENT POPULATION CHARACTERISTICS

Age range	15-85 yr (usually 30-60 yr)
Male:Female	~3:2
Incidence	Common
Etiology	Degenerative; neoplastic; traumatic; infectious

ANESTHETIC CONSIDERATIONS

See Anesthetic Considerations for Thoracolumbar Neurosurgical Procedures p. 64.

Reference

1. Rothman RH, Simeone FA: The operative treatment of lumbar disc disease. In *The Spine*, 4th edition. WB Saunders Co, Philadelphia: 1998.

THORACIC LAMINECTOMY, COSTOTRANSVERSECTOMY

SURGICAL CONSIDERATIONS

Description: Thoracic laminectomy (midline removal of the lamina) and costotransversectomy (off midline removal of the rib head and transverse process) are procedures for decompressing the neural elements of the thoracic spine via a posterior approach. **Costotransversectomy** is used to treat thoracic radiculopathy 2° degenerative disc disease (e.g., herniated discs or osteophytes). **Decompressive thoracic laminectomy** is used to treat thoracic spinal cord compression usually 2° neoplasm and, occasionally, trauma. It is also used to gain access to the spinal canal or spinal cord for dealing with intradural or intramedullary tumors, etc. For the **laminectomy**, a midline incision is used to expose the thoracodorsal fascia. The paraspinal muscles are dissected off the spinous processes and lamina. The bone is then removed piecemeal with rongeurs or drills. The extent of the procedure depends on the indications for treatment. When there is diffuse narrowing of the spinal canal, an extensive thoracic decompression over several segments may be indicated. Hemostasis is achieved with bipolar cautery. The raw bone surfaces are sealed with bone wax. Topical hemostatic agents are used to aid in hemostasis in the epidural gutters. If the patient has an intradural tumor or process such as syringomyelia, the dura is opened and the operating microscope is used for this portion of the procedure. Once the intradural portion of the procedure is completed, the dura is closed. The surgeon may wish to test the integrity of the closure with a Valsalva-like maneuver (sustained inspiration at 30-40 cmH_2O). The wound is closed in layers; a drain may be left in the epidural space.

Variant procedure or approaches: When the patient has only a single nerve-root compression syndrome, the costotransversectomy consists of decompressing that one root. The spinal cord cannot be retracted, thus necessitating a lateral approach to the disc rather than the standard laminectomy. A paramedian approach is made to the junction of the rib head with the vertebral body. The paraspinal muscles are split on that side. Intraop x-rays are required to assess appropriate level. The rib head is dissected out and removed piecemeal with rongeurs. The transverse process is removed. This gives access to the lateral opening of the neural foramen. A thoracic disc can be removed with disc-biting rongeurs. Hemostasis is obtained and the wound is closed in layers.

Usual preop diagnosis: Thoracic radiculopathy (nerve-root compression); thoracic disc disease (herniation or degeneration of one or more thoracic discs); thoracic myelopathy (spinal-cord compression); metastatic carcinoma or tumor to spine; thoracic spine tumor; syringomyelia; intractable pain

SUMMARY OF PROCEDURE

	Thoracic Laminectomy	Costotransversectomy
Position	Prone; pin fixation or horseshoe headrest may be used.	⇐
Incision	Posterior midline	⇐ + Paramedian
Special instrumentation	Operating microscope (optional); evoked potential monitoring equipment (optional)	⇐
Unique considerations	Localizing intraop spine x-ray taken to assess correct level for operation.	⇐
Antibiotics	Cefazolin 1 g iv	⇐
Surgical time	1.5-2 h for single level; additional levels, add 0.5-1 h each.	2 h for single level; additional levels, add 0.5 h each.
EBL	25-1500 ml	50-500 ml
Postop care	PACU → room; neurologic monitoring to check for change	⇐
Mortality	0-5%	⇐
Morbidity	All < 5%: Infection CSF leak Neurological: myelopathy; root injury Massive blood loss Postop instability	⇐
Pain score	6-10	6-10

PATIENT POPULATION CHARACTERISTICS

Age range	7-85 yr (usually 30-60 yr)
Male:Female	~1:1
Incidence	Relatively uncommon neurosurgical procedure
Etiology	Degenerative; neoplastic; traumatic; infectious
Associated conditions	Paraplegia

ANESTHETIC CONSIDERATIONS FOR THORACOLUMBAR NEUROSURGICAL PROCEDURES

(Procedures covered: lumbar fusion; laminotomy; laminectomy; thoracic laminectomy; costotransversectomy)

PREOPERATIVE

Surgery of the lumbar or thoracic spine is common, primarily because of the frequency of herniation of a lumbar or thoracic intervertebral disk causing compression of the adjacent spinal cord or nerve roots. In general, these patients are fit and healthy. Other, less frequent indications for thoracolumbar neurosurgery include: chronic instability of the back, either of congenital or acquired origin, requiring Knodt rod fusion, removal of a tumor of the spinal cord, or placement of a shunt from a spinal cord cyst into the subarachnoid or peritoneal spaces.

Neurological Patients with herniation of a thoracic or lumbar disc generally complain first of pain, usually radiating into the pelvis or down one or both legs. Temporary relief may be obtained by standing or lying down, in combination with the use of a back brace, local heat, and nonsteroidal anti-inflammatory drugs. As nerve compression continues, patients begin to develop weakness and atrophy of specific leg muscle groups. These Sx, however, are not specific to herniation of a disc, and may be caused by a spinal cord tumor or cyst. Although myelography has been the standard method in the past for evaluating the presence of a herniated intervertebral disc, MRI of the spinal cord has virtually replaced it as the diagnostic test, because it will distinguish disc from tumor from cyst. The image may be enhanced by the use of gadolinium or other contrast material.
Tests: MRI

Hematologic None, unless antiplatelet agents have been used.

Laboratory Other tests as indicated from H&P.

Premedication Premedication is very useful in this patient population for purposes of relieving pain and lessening anxiety related to forthcoming surgery. Many of these patients have had prior back operations, and dread further surgery on their backs. Midazolam 2-4 mg iv and meperidine 20-40 mg iv in divided doses prior to entering the OR will make these patients amnestic and tractable.

INTRAOPERATIVE

Anesthetic technique: GA is almost invariably used for these operations because it maximizes patient comfort, provides airway control and permits use of controlled hypotension. Spinal and epidural anesthesia are, in principle, excellent techniques for lumbar surgery, particularly for removal of a lumbar intervertebral disc, but they are seldom used because of the medicolegal concern that the regional anesthetic may be blamed for a new neurological deficit, if one should occur as a result of the surgery. Regional anesthesia is generally not suitable for lumbar fusion or removal of a spinal cord tumor or cyst because the duration of operation is usually unpredictable, and may be prolonged.

Induction Because the operation is performed with the patient in the prone position, it may be desirable to place ETT under local anesthesia and have patient position him/herself prone before induction of GA. This technique eliminates the need for others to lift and position patient, and allows the anesthesiologist opportunity to confirm patient comfort and that no pressure points exist before inducing GA. (See technique for fiber optic intubation, p. B-6.) Once the intubated patient has moved into the prone position, and monitors have been reattached, anesthesia is induced with STP 3-5 mg/kg or propofol 2-3 mg/kg iv. Recently, neurosurgeons and orthopedic surgeons have elected to approach isolated disease of the anterior thoracic spine through the chest using thoracoscopy. Three or four entry ports are made in the anterolateral chest wall, and disc excision, fusion or tumor removal is performed thorascopically. For this surgical approach it is mandatory that a DLT be inserted and the lung fully deflated on the side of operation.

Maintenance Standard maintenance (see p. B-3). It is helpful to surgeons if a single dose of neuromuscular-blocking drug (vecuronium 10 mg or rocuronium 50-70 mg) is administered to relax the strap muscles of the back.

Emergence If an opiate-based anesthetic is used, the orotracheal tube often can be removed at the end of surgery while the patient is still in the prone position. This is not advisable if the original intubation was difficult, or if the operation was prolonged and airway edema or respiratory depression are likely.

Blood and fluid requirements	IV: 16-18 ga × 1-2 NS/LR @ 4-6 ml/kg/h	Blood transfusion is rarely necessary for simple disc surgery. Autologous blood obtained preop and/or from a Cell Saver generally will be needed if an extensive laminectomy and fusion are performed.
Control of blood loss	Deliberate hypotension	Deliberate hypotension helps minimize blood loss when extensive laminectomy and fusion are performed. This is most easily achieved with a combination of esmolol and SNP administered by means of continuous infusion to achieve a HR of 50-70 bpm and MAP = 70-80 mmHg.

Monitoring	Standard monitors (see p. B-1). ± Arterial line ± CVP line ± Urinary catheter	For simple back surgery, standard monitors are sufficient. If deliberate hypotension is planned, an arterial catheter is necessary to monitor BP, and a CVP catheter is recommended for infusion of vasoactive drugs and monitoring of CVP. A urinary drainage catheter is also desirable if surgery is expected to last several h or substantial fluid shifts are anticipated.
Positioning	✓ and pad pressure points. ✓ eyes and ears frequently. ✓ breasts and genitals. ✓ free abdominal movement. Neutral C-spine	Except for syringoperitoneal shunts, which are performed with patient in lateral position, patients are positioned prone on a Wilson frame or on bolsters. Generally, the head is turned to one side on a pillow or towels or a Shea headrest. If patient has limited lateral movement of the head, or has cervical disk disease, placement of the head in the midline, using a horseshoe headrest or Gardner-Wells tongs, should be considered. Elbows and knees should be padded to avoid pressure sores. It is very useful to have patient position him/herself prior to induction of anesthesia to assure that all body parts are properly positioned and comfortable.
Complications	↓BP Bowel or ureteral injury Hemorrhage	↓BP may be 2° abdominal compression and ↓venous return. ↑blood loss may occur 2° epidural vein engorgement, abdominal compression or vascular injury.

POSTOPERATIVE

Complications	Hemorrhage ↓BP Nerve-root injury	If hypotension persists despite vigorous blood and fluid administration, the anesthesiologist should suspect bleeding into the retroperitoneal space or abdomen. Alert the surgeon of this possibility and prepare for immediate exploration of the abdomen.
Pain management	Epidural opiate	Some surgeons may place a mixture consisting of Duramorph, steroid, bupivacaine and Avitene hemostat into the epidural space before closing.
Tests	Hct; document neurological status.	If postop bleeding is suspected, serial Hct determinations are useful.

Reference

1. Sonntag VRH, Hadley MN: Surgical approaches to the thoracolumbar spine. In *Clinical Neurosurgery*, Vol 36. Williams & Wilkins, Baltimore: 1990, 168-85.

CERVICAL LAMINECTOMY FOR TUMOR

SURGICAL CONSIDERATIONS

Description: A **decompressive laminectomy** is used to expose a cervical tumor, which may be extradural, intradural, extramedullary or intramedullary. Depending on the location of the tumor, the surgeon may need to open the dura and/or spinal cord. Obviously, the intradural intramedullary tumors involve more risk and are more delicate to remove. Many lamina may be removed in order to expose and excise the tumor. Surgical adjunctive tools (e.g., CUSA, laser, surgical microscope, etc.) may be used to aid in removal of the tumor. Intraop evoked potential monitoring may be used during these procedures to test the integrity of the dorsal columns. Once the tumor has been removed, the wound is closed in layers, as in a simple laminectomy. These procedures may be performed in the prone or seated position.

Usual preop diagnosis: Cervical myelopathy (spinal-cord compression) 2° tumor; spinal tumor; spinal cord tumor; meningioma; schwannoma; ependymoma; astrocytoma; neurofibromatosis; von Hippel-Lindau disease; hemangioblastoma; metastatic tumor (carcinoma)

SUMMARY OF PROCEDURE

Position	Prone or seated, head in pin fixation
Incision	Posterior midline
Special instrumentation	Operating microscope; evoked potential monitoring (optional); laser; CUSA
Unique considerations	Fiber optic intubation occasionally indicated. Localizing intraop lateral cervical spine x-ray taken to assess correct level for operation.
Antibiotics	Nafcillin 1 g iv slowly + cefotaxime 1 g iv
Surgical time	2.5-8 h
Closing considerations	Cervical orthosis (collar or halo vest)
EBL	50-1000 ml
Postop care	PACU → room; occasionally patients may require ICU or constant observation.
Mortality	0-5%
Morbidity	Infection CSF leak Myelopathy Nerve injury Postop instability
Pain score	5-7

PATIENT POPULATION CHARACTERISTICS

Age range	5-85 yr (usually 30-60 yr)
Male:Female	1:1
Incidence	3-10/100,000
Etiology	Degenerative; traumatic; neoplastic – metastatic, primary CNS, known syndrome (e.g., neurofibromatosis); infectious
Associated conditions	Von Recklinghausen's disease; neurofibromatosis; Von Hippel-Lindau disease

ANESTHETIC CONSIDERATIONS

See Anesthetic Considerations for Cervical Neurosurgical Procedures, p. 73.

Reference

1. Wilkins RH, Rengachary SS, eds: Spinal tumors. In *Neurosurgery*. McGraw-Hill, New York: 1985, 1039-83.

ANTERIOR CERVICAL DISCECTOMY, WITH OR WITHOUT FUSION

SURGICAL CONSIDERATIONS

Description: Anterior cervical discectomy is a common procedure for excising herniated or degenerated discs and osteophytes which may be causing radiculopathy or myelopathy. Occasionally, the procedure is used for unstable conditions in which there is ligamentous laxity on either a degenerative or traumatic basis.

An incision is made in the anterolateral neck and dissection is carried down between the carotid sheath (carotid and jugular vessels) and the trachea and esophagus to the prevertebral fascia (Fig 1.2-1). At this point, the surgeon has

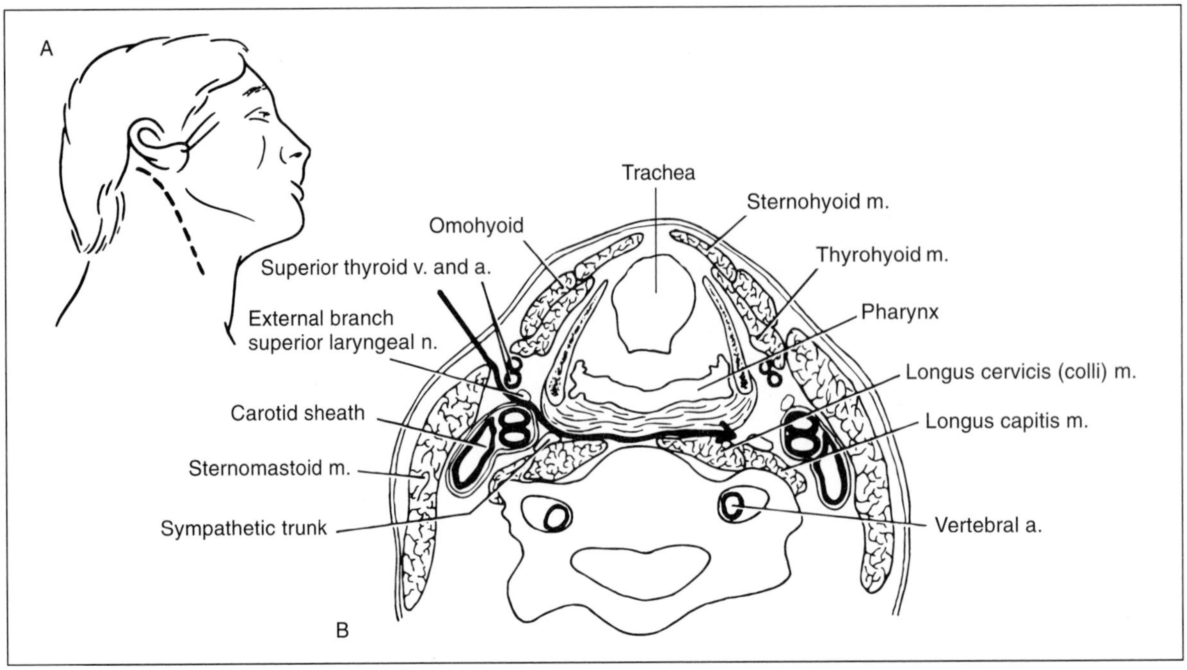

Figure 1.2-1. (A) Longitudinal incision along anterior border of sternomastoid muscle. (B) Cross-section of the neck at the level of the thyroid cartilage. Plane of dissection anterior to the carotid sheath and sympathetic trunk is shown. (Reproduced with permission from Rothman RH, Simeone FA, eds: *The Spine*, 2nd edition. WB Saunders Co: 1982.)

exposed the anterior aspect of the vertebral bodies and discs. A lateral x-ray usually is taken to identify the appropriate levels. The disk is then removed via curettage. The posterior longitudinal ligament is often removed, along with any spurs compressing the spinal canal or nerve roots.

Variant procedure or approaches: This procedure can be performed with or without an **interbody fusion**, depending on surgeon's preference. Approximately 70% of patients who undergo an anterior discectomy without fusion will go on to fuse spontaneously (over 2-4 months) following the procedure. There are several variant approaches to surgical fusion. The fusion is usually performed by placing a bone graft into the disc space, after removal of the disc and osteophytes and after preparation of the graft recipient site. The bone grafts may be autologous (removed from the patient's iliac crest through a separate incision) or from a bone bank. Occasionally, the bone fusion may be supplemented by incorporating internal stabilizing hardware; for example, AO or Caspar stainless steel plates and screws.

Usual preop diagnosis: Cervical radiculopathy (nerve-root compression); cervical myelopathy (spinal cord compression); cervical instability (ligamentous laxity or disruption); cervical disc disease (herniation or degeneration of one or more cervical discs)

SUMMARY OF PROCEDURE

	Simple Discectomy	Discectomy with Fusion
Position	Supine	⇐
Incision	Anterolateral neck	⇐ + Anterolateral ilium, if autologous bone graft)
Special instrumentation	Operating microscope (optional)	⇐ + Titanium plates and screws (optional)
Unique considerations	FOL occasionally indicated. Patient may be in cervical traction during procedure. Localizing intraop lateral cervical spine x-ray taken to assess correct level of operation.	⇐ + Intraop x-rays may be taken to assess graft placement or instrumentation, if used.
Antibiotics	Cefazolin 1 g iv	⇐
Surgical time	1.5-2.5 h for single level; additional levels, add 0.5-1 h for each.	1.5-2.5 h for single level; add 0.5 h for autologous graft; 0.5-1 h for instrumentation.
Closing considerations	Cervical collar (optional)	Cervical orthosis collar; occasionally, halo vest
EBL	25-250 ml	50-500 ml

	Simple Discectomy	Discectomy with Fusion
Postop care	PACU → room	⇐
Mortality	< 1%	⇐
Morbidity	Esophageal perforation: < 1%	⇐
	Infection: < 1%	⇐
	Massive blood loss – carotid or jugular injury, epidural ooze: < 1%	⇐
	Neurological myelopathy: < 1%	⇐
	Neurological nerve injury:	
	Root: < 1%	⇐
	Recurrent laryngeal nerve: 5%	⇐
	Sympathetic chain: < 1%	⇐
	Postop instability: < 1%	⇐
		Instrument failure: <1%
		Slipped graft: < 1%
Pain score	3-4	3-4 (6 if bone graft harvested from patient)

PATIENT POPULATION CHARACTERISTICS

Age range	18-85 yr (usually 30-60 yr)
Male:Female	1:1
Incidence	Common
Etiology	Degenerative; traumatic; infectious

ANESTHETIC CONSIDERATIONS

See Anesthetic Considerations for Cervical Neurosurgical Procedures, p. 73.

Reference

1. Rothman RH, Simeone FA, eds: Surgical approaches to the cervical spine. In *The Spine*, 4th edition. WB Saunders Co, Philadelphia: 1998.

CERVICAL LAMINOTOMY, FORAMINOTOMY AND LAMINECTOMY

SURGICAL CONSIDERATIONS

Description: Cervical laminotomy (removal of a portion of the lamina), foraminotomy (opening of the neural foramina), and laminectomy (removal of the lamina) are procedures for decompressing the neural elements of the cervical spine via a posterior approach. These procedures can be used to treat cervical radiculopathy 2° degenerative disc disease (i.e., herniated discs or osteophytes). **Decompressive laminectomy** can be used to treat cervical spine stenosis, which is present either on a congenital or degenerative basis, or to gain access to the spinal canal or spinal cord. The extent of the procedure depends on the indications for treatment. When the patient has only a single nerve-root-compression syndrome, the procedure may consist of decompressing that one root. When there is diffuse stenosis of the cervical canal, an extensive cervical decompression over several cervical vertebral segments may be indicated. The cervical dorsal fascia is exposed via a midline posterior incision. The paraspinal muscles are dissected off the spinous processes and lamina, and the bone is removed piecemeal with rongeurs or drills. The extent of the procedure depends on the indications for treatment. Hemostasis is achieved with bipolar cautery, and raw bone surfaces are sealed with bone wax. Topical hemostatic agents are used to aid in hemostasis in the epidural gutters. If the patient has an intradural tumor or process such as syringomyelia, the dura is opened and the operating microscope is used for this portion of the procedure. Once the intradural procedure is complete, the dura is closed, and the surgeon may wish to test the integrity of the closure with a Valsalva-like maneuver (sustained inspiration to 30-40 cmH_2O). The wound is closed in layers, and a drain may be left in the epidural space.

Variant procedure or approaches: The major variation in these procedures is patient position. Either prone or sitting position (using a pin fixation device with an overhead bar) may be used, depending on surgeon's preference.

Usual preop diagnosis: Cervical radiculopathy (nerve-root compression); cervical myelopathy (spinal cord compression); cervical disc disease (herniation or degeneration of one or more cervical discs)

SUMMARY OF PROCEDURE

	Cervical Laminotomy or Foraminotomy	Cervical Laminectomy
Position	Prone or sitting; pin fixation or horseshoe headrest	⇐
Incision	Posterior midline neck	⇐
Special instrumentation	Operating microscope (optional)	⇐
Unique considerations	Fiber optic intubation occasionally is indicated; a localizing intraop lateral cervical spine x-ray is taken to assess correct level for the operation.	⇐
Antibiotics	Cefazolin 1 g (optional)	⇐
Surgical time	1.5-2 h for single level; additional levels, add 0.5-1 h for each.	2 h for single level; additional levels, add 0.5 h for each.
EBL	25-250 ml	50-500 ml
Postop care	PACU → room	⇐
Mortality	0-3%	⇐
Morbidity	All < 5%:	⇐
	Infection	⇐
	Neurological: myelopathy; root injury	⇐
	CSF leak	⇐
	Postop instability	⇐
	Air embolism	⇐
	Massive blood loss	⇐
Pain score	7-10	7-10

PATIENT POPULATION CHARACTERISTICS

Age range	18-85 yr (usually 30-60 yr)
Male:Female	~1:1
Incidence	Common
Etiology	Degenerative; traumatic; infectious

ANESTHETIC CONSIDERATIONS

See Anesthetic Considerations for Cervical Neurosurgical Procedures, p. 73.

Reference

1. Tarlov EC: Extradural spinal cord and nerve root compression from benign lesions of the cervical area and their management by the posterior approach. In *Neurological Surgery*, 4th edition. Youmans JR, ed. WB Saunders Co, Philadelphia: 1996, 2241.

VERTEBRAL CORPECTOMY WITH STRUT FUSION

SURGICAL CONSIDERATIONS

Description: **Vertebral corpectomy** (removal of vertebral body) with fusion is used to treat conditions in which there is anterior impingement of the spinal cord or narrowing of the spinal canal at the level of the vertebral body (not just the disc). This is utilized for pathologic fractures of the spine (e.g., metastatic carcinoma) or certain infections of the vertebral body. Conditions such as ossification of the posterior longitudinal ligament (OPLL) are best treated in this manner. This procedure is also used to treat some fractures of the cervical spine. Occasionally, this approach may be used to remove intradural lesions anterior to the spinal cord. The vertebral body or bodies can be removed, allowing for decompression of the anterior spinal canal. The spine must be stabilized following corpectomy, usually with a bone graft (autologous ilium, fibula or bone-bank bone). This procedure is performed using the same exposure as described in the section on **anterior cervical discectomy**. In this case, however, the exposure is more generous. More bone is removed and a fusion is performed at the completion of bone removal. Some patients with limited life expectancy may be candidates for use of a prosthesis instead of bone graft. This may involve use of a polymerizing acrylic to replace bone. Occasionally, the bone fusion may be supplemented by incorporating internal stabilizing hardware (e.g., AO or Caspar stainless steel plates and screws).

Usual preop diagnosis: Cervical myelopathy (spinal cord compression) 2° fracture of the cervical spine (traumatic or pathologic); narrowing of the spinal canal due to congenital conditions; degenerative conditions such as severe disc disease with osteophyte formation; OPLL; cervical instability (ligamentous laxity or disruption or destruction of bone due to tumor or infection); failed previous spinal fusion

SUMMARY OF PROCEDURE

Position	Supine
Incision	Anterolateral neck; anterolateral ilium, or possibly lateral lower leg for bone graft
Special instrumentation	Operating microscope (optional); stainless steel plates and screws (optional)
Unique considerations	Fiber optic intubation occasionally indicated. Patient may be in cervical traction during the procedure. Localizing intraop lateral cervical spine x-ray taken to assess correct level for operation. Intraop x-rays may be taken to assess graft placement or instrumentation.
Antibiotics	Cefazolin 1 g
Surgical time	2.5-3 h for single level; additional levels, add 0.5-1 h for each; add 0.5-1 h for instrumentation; add 0.5 h for harvesting autologous bone.
Closing considerations	Cervical orthosis (collar or halo vest)
EBL	50-1000 ml
Postop care	PACU → room
Mortality	0-5%
Morbidity	Infection
	Neurological: myelopathy; nerve-root injury
	Recurrent laryngeal nerve injury
	Sympathetic chain
	Esophageal perforation
	Postop instability
	Slipped graft
	Instrument failure
	CSF leak
	Massive blood loss: carotid or jugular injury, epidural ooze
Pain score	4-7

PATIENT POPULATION CHARACTERISTICS

Age range	18-85 yr (usually 30-60 yr)
Male:Female	1:1
Incidence	Relatively common
Etiology	Degenerative; traumatic; OPLL; neoplastic; infectious

ANESTHETIC CONSIDERATIONS

See Anesthetic Considerations for Cervical Neurosurgical Procedures, p. 73.

Reference

1. Rengachary SS, Redford JB: Partial median corpectomy for cervical spondylotic myelopathy. In *Neurosurgery Update*, Vol II. Wilkins RH, Rengachary SS, eds. McGraw-Hill, New York: 1991, 356-59.

CERVICAL OR CRANIOCERVICAL FUSION

SURGICAL CONSIDERATIONS

Description: Certain conditions, including those where there is instability of the spine due to traumatic, degenerative and/or certain neoplastic conditions, require posterior fusion of the cervical spine. The fusion usually involves two or possibly three vertebral segments. Occasionally, it is necessary to fuse the occiput to the upper cervical spine.

The operation involves exposing the spinous processes, lamina and facets of the levels to be fused. A bone graft will be harvested from the posterior iliac crest and fashioned appropriately. The bone graft is secured with wire to the decorticated segments to be fused. The wire will be either sublaminar, through the base of the spinous process or lamina, or through the facet. X-rays may be taken to verify alignment. The wound is closed in layers, possibly with a drain in place. Some of the fusions will be supplemented with instrumentation. Luque rectangles with sublaminar wires or lateral mass plate and screws may be incorporated to internally fixate a fusion. An orthopedic surgeon may be cosurgeon on some of these procedures.

Usual preop diagnosis: Spinal fracture; cervical instability; atlantoaxial instability; odontoid fracture; pseudarthrosis

SUMMARY OF PROCEDURE

Position	Prone, head in tong traction or pins
Incision	Midline posterior, posterior ilium for graft
Special instrumentation	Luque rectangles and other hardware for fixation
Unique considerations	Unstable cervical spine preop may require fiber optic intubation.
Antibiotics	Cefazolin 1-2 g iv
Surgical time	2.5-3.5+ h (longer for complicated cases)
Closing considerations	Possible need for halo vest placement or other cervical brace upon closure
EBL	100-500 ml
Postop care	Patient to PACU; then close observation unit or routine floor; neurological function monitoring during observation
Mortality	0.3%
Morbidity	Infection Neurological impairment CSF leak Massive blood loss
Pain score	5-9

PATIENT POPULATION CHARACTERISTICS

Age range	3-70 yr (usually 9-40 yr)
Male:Female	~2:1
Incidence	Relatively common
Etiology	Congenital; traumatic; degenerative; inflammatory; rheumatic; neoplastic
Associated conditions	Spinal cord injury; rheumatoid arthritis

ANESTHETIC CONSIDERATIONS FOR CERVICAL NEUROSURGICAL PROCEDURES

(Procedures covered: cervical laminectomy for tumor; anterior cervical discectomy; cervical laminotomy, foraminotomy, laminectomy; vertebral corpectomy; cervical or craniocervical fusion; craniocervical decompression)

PREOPERATIVE

Surgery of the cervical spine is common, primarily because of the frequency of herniation of a cervical intervertebral disc causing compression of the adjacent spinal nerve roots. Other, less frequent indications for cervical surgery include: acute or chronic instability of the neck, of either congenital or acquired origin, requiring fusion; removal of a tumor of the spinal cord; or craniocervical decompression for Arnold-Chiari malformation (see p. 46).

Respiratory Acute fractures of the cervical spine may be associated with sufficient trauma to the spinal cord to cause acute respiratory insufficiency and inability to handle oropharyngeal secretions. If this occurs, immediate tracheal intubation is necessary. Before initiating intubation, the neck must be stabilized, preferably in Gardner-Wells tongs or a body jacket; lacking those, a tight neck collar with sandbags on each side of the head will suffice. The objective is to **not flex or extend the head or move it laterally** during the course of tracheal intubation.
Tests: Consider ABG to substantiate degree of respiratory impairment, if present.

Cardiovascular Acute fractures of the cervical spine and associated spinal cord trauma may result in loss of sympathetic tone, which, in turn, may cause peripheral vasodilation and bradycardia. Generally, this condition can be treated effectively with crystalloid and/or colloid infusion, and atropine to ↑ HR. Rarely is it necessary to use vasopressors to maintain BP or HR.
Tests: As indicated from H&P.

Neurological Patients with herniation of a cervical disc generally complain first of pain in the neck, particularly with lateral rotation of the head. The pain may radiate down one or, rarely, both arms. As nerve compression continues, patients begin to develop weakness and atrophy of specific muscle groups in the arm. These Sx, however, are not specific to herniation of a disc, and may be caused by a spinal cord tumor or cyst. Patients with acute fractures of the neck and attendant spinal cord trauma at T1 level will be paraplegic, while fractures above C5 may result in quadriplegia and loss of phrenic nerve function. Injuries between these two levels result in variable loss of motor and sensory functions in the upper extremities. A careful documentation of preop sensory and motor deficits is important.
Tests: MRI has replaced myelography as the primary diagnostic test, because it distinguishes disc from tumor from cyst. Emergency CT is invaluable in the assessment of patients with acute neck injuries and suspected cervical fracture; if not available, A-P and lateral x-rays of the neck generally will reveal the site and extent of bony injury.

Hematologic Antiplatelet agents should be stopped 10 d before surgery.
Tests: Hct; others as indicated from H&P.

Laboratory Other tests as indicated from H&P.

Premedication Premedication is very useful in this patient population. Midazolam 2-4 mg iv and meperidine 20-40 mg iv in divided doses prior to entering the OR makes patients amnestic and tractable.

INTRAOPERATIVE

Anesthetic technique: GETA

Induction For patient with stable neck, orotracheal intubation using standard laryngoscopy, if possible, is acceptable. If patient's neck is unstable, with head in tongs, a halo device or a body jacket, or if findings on H&P suggest that tracheal intubation may be difficult, it is preferable to place ETT with FOL under local anesthesia before induction of GA. In skilled hands, **orotracheal fiber optic intubation** is the easiest, quickest and most pleasant method for placing the ETT. Nasotracheal intubation is rarely, if ever, needed for this type of surgery. (For details of fiber optic intubation, see p. B-6.) Once ETT is in place, anesthesia is induced with STP 3-5 mg/kg or propofol 1.5-2.5 mg/kg iv.

Maintenance Standard maintenance (see p. B-3). It is helpful to surgeons if a neuromuscular blocking drug—

Maintenance, cont.

vecuronium 10 mg or rocuronium 50-70 mg—is administered to facilitate positioning and relax neck muscles. Additional doses of relaxants are usually not necessary.

Emergence

If a cervical fusion has been performed, and the patient is returned to a halo device or body jacket, it is desirable to leave ETT in place until patient is fully awake and able to manage his/her own airway. To permit tolerance of the ETT and minimize coughing during emergence, it is useful to spray lidocaine (4 ml 4%) down the orotracheal tube, or inject the same dose of lidocaine through ★ the secondary port of a cuff system designed for this purpose. **NB:** Immediate airway obstruction 2° soft-tissue occlusion or superior laryngeal nerve damage may occur on extubation. A useful way to test for airway patency is to deflate the cuff of the tracheal tube and determine that patient is able to breathe around the tube as well as through it. If there is any concern about ability of the patient to maintain an airway following removal of the ETT, a tube changer should be inserted into the trachea prior to removal of the ETT. The tube changer can be left in the trachea for a time and will facilitate reintubation if that should become necessary. The patient can vocalize with the tube changer in place.

Blood and fluid requirements

IV: 16-18 ga × 1
NS/LR @ 4-6 ml/kg/h

Blood transfusion is rarely needed for operations on the cervical spine.

Monitoring

Standard monitors (see p. B-1).
± Arterial line
± CVP line
± Doppler
± Urinary catheter

If a posterior surgical approach with patient in seated position is planned, an arterial catheter is useful for monitoring BP, and a CVP catheter is necessary for monitoring CVP and aspiration of air, should an air embolism occur. If patient is seated, an ultrasonic Doppler flow probe also should be placed on the anterior chest wall with confirmation of its performance by injecting 1 ml of agitated NS into CVP line and listening for the change in Doppler sound.

SSEP

If SSEP monitoring is planned, the combination of sevoflurane, O_2, opiates (fentanyl or meperidine), and neuromuscular blockage (rocuronium) is the ideal anesthetic regimen for optimizing the potentials. N_2O and isoflurane make SSEP monitoring less satisfactory.

Positioning

Supine:
✓ and pad pressure points.
✓ eyes.
Shoulder roll
Cervical traction

For **anterior cervical discectomy** and/or fusion, patient is positioned supine with a roll under the shoulders and head is moderately hyperextended. A cervical strap is placed below the chin and behind the occiput, and attached to a weight of 5-10 lbs hung over the head of the bed. If patient is in a halo or tongs, 5-10 lbs of weight are attached to the device. Alternatively, the surgeon may request measured traction of 20-50 lbs intermittently during insertion of bone plugs for fusion. The surgical incision is made in the right side of the neck.

Prone:
- ✓ and pad pressure points.
- ✓ eyes.
- ✓ genitalia.

Sitting:
- ✓ and pad pressure points.
- ✓ eyes.

VAE monitoring:
- ✓ ETT position.

A **posterior approach** is used if the operation is for spinal stenosis or craniocervical decompression. With this approach, patient is positioned either prone (on a Wilson frame or on bolsters), or sitting, with the head in 3-point fixation. There are advantages to both neurosurgeon and anesthesiologist, as well as the patient, for using a seated position. For the neurosurgeon: (1) easier access to the lesion; (2) less blood loss, since both arterial and venous pressures are lower than if patient were prone;[2] (3) less interference from CSF, since it readily drains away from the operative site; and (4) lower incidence of postop neurological injury.[2] Advantages to the anesthesiologist are: (1) less chance that ETT and other arterial and venous catheters will become dislodged than with patient prone; (2) less chance for inadvertent pressure injury; (3) easier assessment and management of ventilation; and (4) easier access to patient for insertion of additional catheters, if necessary.

Complications	VAE	The major disadvantage of the sitting position is the risk of VAE, particularly paradoxical air embolism to the left side of the heart through a PFO (or, rarely, through the pulmonary circulation) → CNS or coronary emboli. Incidence of VAE is 25-45% in patients operated on in the seated position.[2,3] VAE is easily detected using a combination of Doppler, $ETCO_2$ and ETN_2 analysis; and complications are rare.[1,2] If VAE is suspected (Sx = ↓$ETCO_2$, ↑ETN_2, ↓BP, dysrhythmias), notify the surgeon and aspirate the right atrial catheter using a 10 ml syringe. This generally will confirm the diagnosis as well as provide treatment. If VAE continues, and the surgeon has difficulty identifying the site of air entrainment, consider using PEEP ≤ 10 cmH_2O or bilateral jugular compression to increase CVP and cerebral venous pressure. Low levels of PEEP applied and released gradually will not promote paradoxical air embolism.[4,6]
	↓BP	Hypotension caused by venous pooling, inadequate venous return to the heart, and decreased CO can be treated by wrapping lower extremities while patient is supine, infusing adequate fluid volume to maintain right heart filling pressure, and avoiding excessive depth of anesthesia.

POSTOPERATIVE

Complications	Airway obstruction Hematoma Neurologic deficit	The cause of the airway obstruction is usually from soft tissue falling back against the posterior pharyngeal wall which cannot be corrected by forward displacement of the mandible because of the neck fusion or postop traction/stabilization device (halo or body jacket). May require oral or nasal airway.
	Tension pneumothorax	Delayed respiratory insufficiency is usually caused by either development of a tension pneumothorax from entrainment of air via the surgical wound or an unsuspected oropharyngeal laceration during tracheal intubation, or from bleeding into the neck at the surgical site, with progressive compression and occlusion of the airway. If a tension pneumothorax is suspected and circulatory signs are stable, immediate CXR should confirm the diagnosis. If circulation is failing, an 18- or 20-ga needle catheter should be inserted immediately anteriorly at the 2nd intercostal space on the suspected side to relieve the pneumothorax. If the diagnosis is airway obstruction from bleeding into the neck, the wound should be opened immediately and clots and blood removed. This should be done **before attempting tracheal intubation**. Intubation of the airway is futile and wastes valuable time if the cause is airway compression by blood in the wound. It is sometimes difficult to distinguish airway obstruction from tension pneumothorax by physical signs. One useful way is to check for the "puff sign." With airway obstruction from any cause, what gas moves in and out of the airway does so very slowly because of the obstruction. In contrast, with tension pneumothorax, gas moves in and out of airway with great speed because of high intrapleural pressure. By applying positive pressure to airway and listening at patient's mouth for the sound of gas escaping as airway pressure is released, one hears either a puff or jet of air escaping (tension pneumothorax) or slow, gradual exit of air (airway obstruction).

Pain management	Meperidine (10 mg iv prn) Codeine (20 mg iv or po prn)	
Tests	CXR Hct	Repeat neurological exam prior to discharge from PACU.

References

1. Black S, Cucchiara RF, Nishimura RA, Michenfelder JD: Parameters affecting occurrence of paradoxical air embolism. *Anesthesiology* 1989; 71(2):235-41.
2. Black S, Ockert DB, Oliver WC Jr, Cucchiara RF: Outcome following posterior fossa craniectomy in patients in the sitting or horizontal positions. *Anesthesiology* 1988; 69(1):49-56.
3. Cucchiara RF, Nugent M, Seward JB, Messick JM: Air embolism in upright neurosurgical patients: Detection and localization by two-dimensional transesophageal echocardiography. *Anesthesiology* 1984; 60(4):353-55.
4. Pearl RG, Larson CP Jr: Hemodynamic effects of positive end-expiratory pressure during continuous venous air embolism in the dog. *Anesthesiology* 1986; 64(6):724-29.
5. Sonntag VKH, Hadley MN: Management of upper cervical spinal instability. In *Neurosurgery Update*, Vol II. Wilkins RH, Rengachary SS, eds. McGraw-Hill, New York: 1991, 222-33.
6. Zasslow MA, Pearl RG, Larson CP Jr, Silverberg G, Shuer LF: PEEP does not affect left atrial-right atrial pressure difference in neurosurgical patients. *Anesthesiology* 1988; 68(5):760-63.

SURGERY FOR SPASTICITY

SURGICAL CONSIDERATIONS

Description: Neurologic conditions associated with spasticity of the extremities include spinal cord injury, multiple sclerosis, stroke, etc. The spasticity is often managed with oral medications. An alternative approach is to infuse baclofen (GABA-agonist that decreases frequency and amplitude of tonic impulses to the muscle spindles) into the subarachnoid space via an implanted pump. When these therapeutic modalities fail, it may be necessary to perform surgery. Some of the procedures are destructive in that a lesion is placed in certain nerves or the spinal cord to destroy the reflex arc which is contributing to the spasticity. There are both percutaneous and open techniques for placing the lesion. In the **open procedures**, a **laminectomy** is performed (see Lumbar Laminotomy, Laminectomy, p. 62). In a case where a **myelotomy** is to be performed, the lower spinal cord is exposed and incised at the appropriate location to interrupt the reflex arc. In certain cases, selective electrical stimulation can be performed on isolated dorsal rootlets from the involved extremity. Abnormal responses in the extremities are monitored via EMG and direct observation. When abnormal responses are detected, that particular rootlet is divided (dorsal rhizotomy). This procedure is somewhat tedious and requires that stable anesthetic conditions be maintained so that appropriate monitoring can be carried out during the procedure. The surgeon usually must sacrifice 40-60% of the dorsal rootlets in cases of spastic diplegia found in cerebral palsy.

Variant procedure or approaches: Percutaneous **radiofrequency rhizotomy** is another procedure used for spasticity. A thermal lesion is placed in the appropriate dorsal roots with a radiofrequency generator. Needles are passed into the neural foramen via a posterolateral trajectory for levels L1-L5, and then from a midline approach to the S1 root. The needle position is determined by A-P and lateral fluoroscopy and by stimulus mapping. Stimulating current is delivered via an electrode passed through the needle. A low-level stimulating current causes muscle twitching in the appropriate leg if the needle is in the proper location. Once placed and verified, the radiofrequency generator is used to produce the lesion. At the termination of this procedure, the patient's legs should be flaccid. Patients with spinal cord injury-producing anesthesia below T10 may not require additional anesthetic for the procedure.

Usual preop diagnosis: Spasticity; multiple sclerosis; spinal cord injury

SUMMARY OF PROCEDURE

	Open Rhizotomy or Myelotomy	Radiofrequency Rhizotomy
Position	Prone	⇐
Incision	Midline	Needles placed in lumbar region
Special instrumentation	EMG monitor; nerve stimulator	Radiofrequency generator; fluoroscope
Unique considerations	Anesthetic which allows EMG recordings	May not require anesthesia if anesthetic below waist (spinal cord surgery).
Antibiotics	Nafcillin 1 g iv + cefotaxime 1 g iv	None
Surgical time	4 h	2 h
Closing considerations	Surgeon may wish to test dural closure with Valsalva maneuver.	
EBL	50-250 ml	Negligible
Postop care	Head flat; PACU → room	⇐
Mortality	< 1%	⇐
Morbidity	All < 5%: CSF leak Infection Hemorrhage Neurological impairment	⇐
Pain score	4	2

PATIENT POPULATION CHARACTERISTICS

Age range	3-55 yr
Male:Female	~3:2
Incidence	Relatively uncommon neurosurgical procedure
Etiology	Hyperactivity of gamma stretch reflex
Associated conditions	Multiple sclerosis; cerebral palsy; spinal cord injury

ANESTHETIC CONSIDERATIONS

See Anesthetic Considerations for Surgical Correction of Spinal Dysraphism, Pediatric Neurosurgery, p. 858.

References

1. Kennemore DE: Percutaneous electrocoagulation of spinal nerves for the relief of pain and spasticity. In *Radionics Procedure Technique Series*. Radionics, Burlington MA: 1978.
2. Peacock WJ, Staudt LA, Nuwer MR: A neurosurgical approach to spasticity: selective posterior rhizotomy. In *Neurosurgery Update*, Vol II. Wilkins RH, Rengachary SS, eds. McGraw-Hill, New York: 1991, 403-7.

Surgeons

Lawrence M. Shuer, MD (*Percutaneous procedures*)
Gary K. Steinberg, MD, PhD (*Carotid endarterectomy*)

1.3 OTHER NEUROSURGERY

Anesthesiologist

C. Philip Larson, Jr, MD, MS

CAROTID ENDARTERECTOMY

SURGICAL CONSIDERATIONS

Gary K. Steinberg

Description: Carotid endarterectomy (CEA) is frequently used to treat severe atherosclerotic occlusive disease involving internal carotid arteries at the common carotid artery bifurcation. Atherosclerotic carotid artery disease commonly causes thromboembolic or hemodynamic stroke and transient ischemic attacks (TIAs). Recent studies[35] proved the efficacy of this operation, compared with medical treatment for symptomatic high-grade stenoses (> 70%), and asymptomatic high-grade stenosis (≥ 60%). Ongoing studies are evaluating its benefit for symptomatic lesions of moderate stenoses (50-70%).

The operation involves opening the common carotid arteries and the proximal internal carotid arteries in the neck (Fig 1.3-1), removing atherosclerotic plaque from the inside of the artery, and resuturing the wall of the arteries (media and adventitia). Opening the carotid artery (**arteriotomy**) requires temporary occlusion of the proximal common carotid artery, distal internal carotid artery, external carotid artery and usually its first branch, the superior thyroid artery. The entire procedure can be achieved under continued occlusion of these vessels, if the collateral blood flow to the territory supplied by the occluded internal carotid is deemed adequate (on the basis of intraop EEG monitoring, internal carotid artery back-bleeding, stump pressures, CBF studies or angiography). Alternatively, an internal shunt between the proximal common carotid artery and distal internal carotid artery can be placed after the arteriotomy for use during the endarterectomy. Sometimes a vein graft or synthetic graft (Gortex, Dacron) is used to reconstruct ("patch") the arteriotomy site.

Usual preop diagnosis: Stroke; TIAs; carotid artery stenosis; carotid artery dissection

SUMMARY OF PROCEDURE

Position	Supine
Incision	Anterolateral neck; occasionally if "patching" arteriotomy, may have to harvest portion of greater saphenous vein from leg.
Special instrumentation	Magnification loupes; vascular instruments ± shunt (Bard, Javid, Pruitt-Inahara)
Unique considerations	Techniques for monitoring collateral blood flow: EEG-spectral analysis or raw EEG, back-bleeding or internal carotid artery stump pressure (> 50 mmHg), CBF measurements using Xenon, transcranial Doppler; full anticoagulation with heparin (5,000-7,500 U iv) during arterial occlusion ± reversal with protamine (25-75 mg iv) at end of arteriotomy repair and 10 min after reopening of carotid arteries; maintaining mild HTN during internal carotid artery occlusion (MAP 90-110); use of intraop neuroprotective agents during internal carotid artery occlusion (e.g., iv STP 4-5 mg/kg).
Antibiotics	Cefazolin (1 g iv q 6 h)
Surgical time	2-2.5 h
Closing considerations	Avoid HTN or hypotension (MAP 80-110); meticulous hemostasis.
EBL	50-150 ml
Postop care	Control of BP (MAP 80-100 mmHg); start aspirin on postop d 1; ICU × 1 d.
Mortality	0.5-1%
Morbidity	Cranial nerve injury: Up to 39% Stroke: 1-2% MI: ≤ 1% Wound infection: Rare
Pain score	3

PATIENT POPULATION CHARACTERISTICS

Age range	50-80 yr
Male:Female	1:1
Incidence	100,000 CEAs/yr in U.S.
Etiology	Atherosclerosis; occasionally, traumatic (dissection)
Associated conditions	HTN; CAD; PVD; smoking; obesity; alcohol abuse; hyperlipidemia

ANESTHETIC CONSIDERATIONS

(Procedure covered: carotid endarterectomy—neurosurgery, vascular)

PREOPERATIVE

The incidence of occlusive or ulcerative lesions of the extracranial or intracranial vasculature increases with advancing years. Generally, these lesions are asymptomatic until the cross-sectional area of the vessel is decreased by at least 50%.[39] This is because the cerebral vasculature has excellent collateral circulation, most importantly the Circle of Willis, but also the carotid-basilar anastomosis via the trigeminal artery and the extra- to intracranial collateral flow via the ophthalmic artery or branches of the vertebral artery. Systemic hypotension such as that arising from a cardiac dysrhythmia may be a cause of cerebral ischemia in some patients with carotid stenosis. Patients presenting for CEA generally fall into one of three categories: (1) Those with TIAs, presenting with symptoms that may be focal or generalized. Clinical trials[9,28,38] document that CEA is superior to medical management in preventing the development of strokes in patients who are either asymptomatic (stenosis ≥ 60%) or symptomatic (stenosis ≥ 70%). (2) Patients with completed stroke. If the stroke is recent (< 2-4 wk), most surgeons will not operate on the patient for fear of converting an ischemic infarct into a hemorrhagic infarct. Angiographic evaluation following recovery from an acute stroke usually demonstrates a stenotic and/or ulcerative lesion at the carotid bifurcation. (3) Patients with asymptomatic bruit, which usually is found during a routine physical examination of the neck. These are of concern because they may signal the development of carotid stenosis[37] and may benefit from surgical intervention.[38]

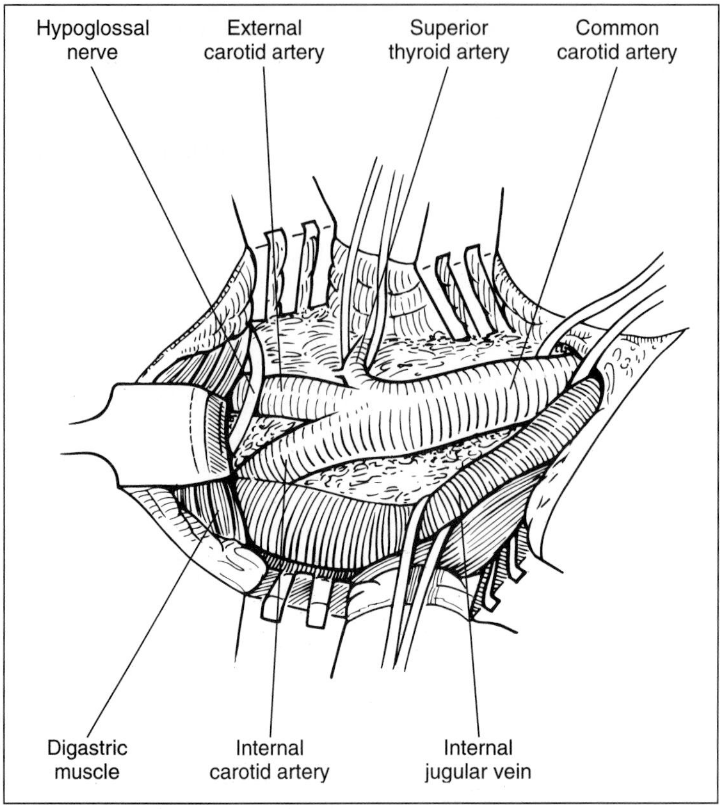

Figure 1.3-1. Exposure and control of carotid artery. (Reproduced with permission from Calne R, Pollard SG: *Operative Surgery*. Gower Medical Pub: 1992.)

Respiratory If there is evidence of pulmonary infection, appropriate antibiotic therapy should be instituted. If secretions are excessive, preop pulmonary physiotherapy, including bronchodilator therapy, may be indicated. Patients should be asked to stop smoking prior to anesthesia, even if only the night before. While cessation of smoking for such a short time will not lessen the volume of secretions appreciably, or make the airways less irritable to a foreign body such as an ETT, it will provide sufficient time for the carbon monoxide levels in the blood to decrease, thereby enhancing O_2 carrying capacity. Any Hx of pulmonary disease should be evaluated with spirometry, ABGs and CXR.
Tests: ABGs; spirometry; CXR, if indicated from H&P.

Cardiovascular In addition to the usual measures taken in preop evaluation of any patient undergoing anesthesia, there are special considerations that relate to patients who are to undergo a CEA. Most important is a careful evaluation of cardiovascular status, including a detailed Hx of cardiovascular function and serial determinations of BP in both arms to establish the range of pressures that normally occur, and whether there are regional differences. If BP is different in the two arms, it should be measured intraop and postop in the arm with the higher values. Also, a preop ECG is mandatory. The reason for concern about cardiovascular function is twofold: (1) It is often necessary to administer vasoactive drugs to artificially regulate BP during CEA, either to maintain it at a normal value, or sometimes to increase it as much as 20% above the highest resting pressure to maintain optimal collateral circulation during surgical carotid occlusion. (2) The incidence of perioperative

MI in this surgical population is at least 1%, and represents the most common major postop complication in this operation. Except in the case of emergencies, anesthesia and operation should not proceed in the face of severe, uncontrolled HTN, diabetes or a MI within the last 3 mo. Antihypertensive medications should be continued up to the time of anesthesia.
Tests: ECG; others as indicated from H&P.

Neurological The Sx of cerebrovascular insufficiency are due to either critical stenosis or occlusion of cerebral vessels, combined with inadequate collateral circulation, or the development of ulcerative lesions at arterial branch points. The degenerative plaques or mural thrombi readily break off from the vessel wall and cause focal ischemic lesions. Manual occlusion of the carotid arteries is not an appropriate test of tolerance to temporary circulatory occlusion, as it may endanger the patient by precipitating embolization from an ulcerative lesion or by inducing bradycardia and hypotension from activation of the carotid sinus reflex. It is desirable, however, to position the patient's head in the operative position as a test of the effect of that position on CBF. It is well documented that hyperextension and lateral rotation of the head may occlude vertebral-basilar flow between the scalenus anticus and longus coli muscles and, if sustained, contribute to postop cerebral ischemia. Sx of dizziness or diplopia will emerge with this maneuver if CBF is compromised.
Tests: Cerebral angiography will identify type of lesion (ulcerative or stenotic), its location, and extent of collateral circulation. Other commonly used techniques include MR angiography, CT rapid spiral angiography, duplex ultrasonography and digital subtraction angiography (DSA). DSA involves iv injection of a contrast agent, and through the use of computer reconstruction, an arterial image is formed. This circumvents the need for arterial catheterization,[24] but does not give as clear or detailed an image as conventional angiography. As part of the preop evaluation, the anesthesiologist should examine the angiograms of the patient to become familiarized with the type, location and extent of the lesion.

Hematologic If a patient is on long-term aspirin therapy to minimize platelet aggregation and thrombus formation, it should be stopped at least 2 wk prior to surgery.
Tests: PT; PTT

Laboratory Tests as indicated from H&P.

Premedication Use of premedication in patients undergoing CEA is controversial. Should a new TIA or stroke occur in the immediate preop period, its Sx may be difficult to distinguish from those associated with excessive responses to premedication. In this population, detailed discussion about the anesthetic and surgical plan, with appropriate reassurance, is usually enough. If medication is desired, midazolam 1-3 mg is preferable to opiates.

INTRAOPERATIVE

Anesthetic technique (regional): In the developmental stage of CEA, regional anesthesia—in the form of a superficial and deep cervical plexus block, supplemented as needed by a local field block—was used by most anesthesiologists and surgeons. It provided the opportunity to evaluate cerebral function during a trial occlusion of 2-3 min. If the patient showed no adverse effects, the operation was completed under regional anesthesia. If the patient developed neurological changes, a shunt was inserted or GA was induced and ET intubation performed, following which the operation was completed. However, regional anesthesia has several disadvantages: absence of cerebral protection; patients may tolerate occlusion for 10 min or more before suddenly losing consciousness or developing a seizure; and conversion to GETA may be technically difficult. Nevertheless, the technique has an increasing number of advocates among anesthesiologists and surgeons.[1,2,5,6,7,8,12,29,33] It is claimed that: it decreases the need for a surgical shunt and thereby avoids the complications of shunt insertion;[2,5,7] it decreases the length of stay in the ICU;[12] and as an anesthetic technique it is well accepted by some patients.[8]

Anesthetic technique (GETA): GETA offers both direct and indirect advantages for patients undergoing CEA: cerebral protection by decreasing $CMRO_2$ and redistributing flow toward the potentially ischemic area; greater patient comfort; and the ability to regulate PO_2, PCO_2 and MAP. Despite these arguments favoring GA, recent studies comparing regional and GA suggest that there is no clear outcome advantage of one technique over the other.[1,2,29]

Induction Both STP (3-5 mg/kg) and propofol (1-2 mg/kg), when slowly administered, are suitable for induction agents as arterial blood pressure will generally remain at acceptable levels (± 20% of baseline) in normovolemic patients. These agents will ↓ $CMRO_2$, constrict normally reactive cerebral vessels, and lead to a redistribution of CBF toward potentially ischemic areas. Propofol has the additional advantages of antiemesis and prompt recovery. Etomidate (0.1-0.4 mg/kg) may be useful for induction of anesthesia in hemodynamically unstable patients. A muscle relaxant, such as vecuronium (0.15 mg/kg), cisatracurium (0.1-0.2 mg/kg) or rocuronium (0.5-0.6 mg/kg) is administered for tracheal intubation. An analgesic such as meperidine (2-3 mg/kg), fentanyl (2-5 μg/kg) or remifentanil (0.05-2 μg/kg/min) may be given to minimize the cardiovascular responses to ET intubation. These opiates have minimal effects on CBF or $CMRO_2$.[37]

Maintenance Isoflurane up to 0.6% inspired either alone or in combination with N_2O 60% and/or remifentanil (0.05-0.2 μg/kg/min) is satisfactory. Just prior to surgical cross-clamping of the carotid artery, an additional dose of STP sufficient to produce burst suppression on the EEG (usually 3-5 mg/kg) may be administered for its cerebral protective effects. Frawley, et al, have suggested that STP adequately protects the brain during CEA, and that a surgical shunt is obsolete and never needed.[11]

Emergence Upon removal of the carotid cross-clamps, total carotid occlusion time should be noted on the anesthetic record. Once bleeding from the arteriotomy site has been controlled, protamine (typically 0.5 mg/100 U heparin) is administered iv slowly over at least 10 min. If ↓BP occurs, rate of protamine administration is slowed. If vasopressors were used during operation, patient should be weaned from them during emergence, because HTN is likely as patient awakens from anesthesia. The need to control BP with a combination of esmolol and SNP is likely in the emergence phase.

Blood and fluid requirements	IV: 18 ga × 2 NS/LR @ 5-10 ml/kg/h	Blood replacement is seldom an issue. Studies indicate that glucose may worsen the tolerance of brain to ischemia; thus, it is prudent to avoid glucose-containing solutions.
	Hetastarch 6% < 20 ml/kg	Hetastarch stays in the intravascular compartment longer (2-3 d) than crystalloid solutions (1-3 h).
Monitoring	Standard monitors (see p. B-1). Arterial line UO	Marked fluctuations in BP may occur, necessitating hypertensive or hypotensive drug therapy. The arterial pressure transducer should be placed at the level of the head to accurately assess CPP. A CVP catheter is seldom necessary. Vasoactive drugs usually can be given quickly and safely through a cannula placed in the arm.
Cerebral perfusion monitoring	rCBF	Regional CBF (rCBF) >24 ml/min/100 g brain is satisfactory, and < 18 ml/min/100 g indicates potential for cerebral ischemia; however, capability for making rCBF measurements is not generally available in OR.
	EEG	A variety of spectral compression EEG techniques permit computerized EEG analysis in OR. The major disadvantages of this analysis are: the EEG usually does not change until severe cerebral ischemia occurs, so it is not a good prodromal indicator of ischemia; the EEG may not identify small focal areas of ischemia; the depth of anesthesia and level of ventilation must be held stable or the EEG will not be interpretable; and there is a high incidence of false positives and negatives.
	Stump pressure	Stump pressure (pressure distal to the carotid clamp – also called "back pressure") – is used to evaluate the adequacy of cerebral perfusion. Cerebral ischemia rarely occurs at stump pressures > 60 mmHg. The major criticism of stump pressure is the large number of false positives; that is, a stump pressure < 60 mmHg and a rCBF > 24 ml/min/100 g brain. This occurs in about a third of patients[21] and results in a shunt being placed when none is needed. The simplicity of the measurement and its validity when pressure > 60 mmHg still make it a useful clinical method for assuring adequate perfusion.
	Cerebral oximetry	Cerebral oximetry has been used to evaluate cerebral perfusion during CEA.[32] Cerebral oximeters are placed on

Cerebral perfusion, cont.		the forehead, where it is presumed they measure O_2 saturation in the superficial distal cortex. With carotid occlusion, ipsilateral oximetric values may decrease. Oximetry values have been extremely variable among patients both before and during carotid occlusion, and no correlation with cerebral ischemia has been made.
	SSEP	Monitoring of SSEPs has been advocated as a means of determining the adequacy of cerebral perfusion during temporary occlusion of a major cerebral artery,[25] although its reliability as an indicator of cerebral ischemia has been questioned.
	Transcranial Doppler (TCD)	TCD scanning alone[13] or combined with EEG monitoring[10] is a useful method for detecting microemboli (air or particulate matter) during CEA. It also has been suggested that TCD can be used as a guide for regulating BP postop to minimize the occurrence of post endarterectomy cerebral hyperperfusion states.[10]
Control of BP	Keep MAP ≥ awake levels. Autoregulation Vasopressors	It is highly desirable to maintain MAP at or slightly above the patient's highest recorded resting pressure while awake. Surgical occlusion of the carotid artery will often decrease distal perfusion pressure (stump pressure) < 60 mmHg. Volatile anesthetics impair autoregulation; therefore, the higher the pressure, the more likely it is that cerebral perfusion will be adequate during surgical occlusion. A pure α-adrenergic agonist (e.g., phenylephrine) is ideal to support BP because it has minimal dysrhythmogenic potential. The modified V-5 lead will usually indicate if the ↓BP is causing myocardial ischemia. If hypertensive episodes occur during surgery, infusions of esmolol ± SNP work well.
Positioning	✓ and pad pressure points. ✓ eyes.	

POSTOPERATIVE

Complications	Circulatory instability	Circulatory instability is common.[36] Hypotension may be due to hypovolemia, depression of circulation by anesthetic or other drugs, dysrhythmias or exposure of the baroreceptor mechanism to a new higher pressure, causing an exaggerated reflex response. Rx by volume expansion and pressors.
	HTN MI	HTN may be due to loss of the normal carotid baroreceptor mechanism. It may → excessive bleeding, increased myocardial O_2 consumption or dysrhythmias and MI, intracerebral hemorrhage and increased ICP from cerebral edema.
	Loss of carotid body function	Chemoreceptor function is lost in most patients after CEA, as evidenced by a loss of ventilatory and circulatory responses to hypoxia and a modest increase in resting arterial $PaCO_2$.[36] These patients should be given supplemental O_2 postop. Special attention must be directed toward preventing atelectasis or other pulmonary or circulatory abnormalities that might cause hypoxemia, and to which the patient could only respond by further respiratory and circulatory depression and loss of consciousness.
	Respiratory insufficiency	Acute respiratory insufficiency may occur 2° hematoma formation with tracheal deviation, vocal cord paralysis from surgical traction on laryngeal nerves, or tension

Complications, cont.		pneumothorax from dissection of air through the wound into the mediastinum and pleural space. Unexpected respiratory distress should immediately bring these 3 possibilities to mind with appropriate diagnosis and therapy. A hematoma which causes respiratory distress always should be evacuated before reintubation is attempted.
	Tension pneumothorax	Likewise, if there is evidence of circulatory insufficiency, a tension pneumothorax should be relieved immediately by needle evacuation.
	Intimal flap → stroke	Should a patient emerge from anesthesia with a new neurological deficit, immediate cerebral angiography should be performed to determine if an intimal flap has formed at the site of operation. This is a surgically correctable lesion and, if corrected immediately, may lessen the severity of the subsequent neurological deficit.
Pain management	Meperidine (10 mg iv prn) Codeine (30-60 mg im q 4 h)	Emerging stroke → suspect intimal flap → emergency cerebral angiography or immediate surgical exploration of operative site.
Tests	Cerebral angiography	

References

1. Allen BT, Anderson CB, Rubin BG, Thompson RW, Flye MW, Young-Beyer P: The influence of anesthetic technique on perioperative complications after carotid endarterectomy. *J Vasc Surg* 1994; 19:834-42.
2. Anthony T, Johansen K: Optimal outcome for "high-risk" carotid endarterectomy. *Am J Surg* 1994; 167:469-71.
3. Archer DP, Tang TKK: The choice of anaesthetic for carotid endarterectomy: does it matter? *Can J Anaesth* 1995; 42:566-70.
4. Bandyk DF, Thiele BL: Noninvasive assessment of carotid artery disease. *West J Med* 1983; 139:486-501.
5. Benjamin ME, Silva MB Jr, Watt C, McCaffrey MT, Burford-Foggs A, Flinn WR: Awake patient monitoring to determine the need for shunting during carotid endarterectomy. *Surgery* 1993; 114:673-79.
6. Chang BB, Darling RC, Shah DM, Paty PS, Leather RP: Carotid endarterectomy can be safely performed with acceptable mortality and morbidity in patients requiring coronary artery bypass grafts. *Am J Surg* 1994; 168:94-6.
7. Davies MJ, Mooney PH, Scott DA, Silbert BS, Cook RJ: Neurologic changes during carotid endarterectomy under cervical block predict a high risk of postoperative stroke. *Anesthesiology* 1993; 78:829-33.
8. Davies MJ, Murrell GC, Cronin KC, Meads A, Dawson AR: Carotid endarterectomy under cervical plexus block: a prospective clinical audit. *Anaesth Intensive Care* 1990; 18:219-23.
9. European Carotid Surgery Trialists' Collaborative Group: MCR European carotid surgery trial: interim results for symptomatic patients with severe (70-99%) or with mild (0-29%) carotid stenosis. *Lancet* 1991; 337:1235-43.
10. Fiori L, Parenti G, Marconi F: Combined transcranial Doppler and electrophysiologic monitoring for carotid endarterectomy. *J Neurosurg Anesthesiol* 1997; 9:11-16.
11. Frawley JE, Hicks RG, Gray LJ, Niesche JW: Carotid endarterectomy without a shunt for symptomatic lesions associated with contralateral severe stenosis or occlusion. *J Vasc Surg* 1996; 23:421-27.
12. Gabelman CG, Gann DS, Ashworth CJ, Carney WI: One hundred consecutive carotid reconstructions: local versus general anesthesia. *Am J Surg* 1983; 145:477-82.
13. Gaunt ME, Ratliff DA, Martin PJ, Smith JL, Bell PR, Naylor AR: On-table diagnosis of incipient carotid artery thrombosis during carotid endarterectomy by transcranial Doppler scanning. *J Vasc Surg* 1994; 20:104-7.
14. Hobson RW II, Weiss DG, Fields WS, Goldstone J, Moore WS, Towne JB, Wright CB: Efficacy of carotid endarterectomy for asymptomatic carotid stenosis. The Veterans Affairs Cooperative Study Group. *N Engl J Med* 1993; 328(4):221-27.
15. Kearse LA Jr, Brown EN, McPeck K: Somatosensory evoked potentials sensitivity relative to electroencephalography for cerebral ischemia during carotid endarterectomy. *Stroke* 1992; 23:498-505.
16. Kearse LA Jr, Lopez-Bresnahan M, McPeck K, Zaslavsky A: Preoperative cerebrovascular symptoms and electroencephalographic abnormalities do not predict cerebral ischemia during carotid endarterectomy. *Stroke* 1995; 26:1210-14.
17. Kearse LA Jr, Martin D, McPeck K, Lopez-Bresnahan M: Computer-derived density spectral array in detection of mild analog electroencephalographic ischemic pattern changes during carotid endarterectomy. *J Neurosurg* 1993; 78:884-90.
18. Kraft SA, Larson CP Jr, Shuer LM, Steinberg GK, Benson GV, Pearl RG: Effect of hyperglycemia on neuronal changes in a rabbit model of focal cerebral ischemia. *Stroke* 199; 21(3):447-50.
19. Kresowik TF, Khoury MD: Limitations of EEG monitoring in the detection of cerebral ischemia accompanying carotid endarterectomy. *J Vasc Surg* 1991; 13:439-43.
20. Lanier WL, Stangland KJ, Scheithauer BW, Milde JH, Michenfelder JD: The effects of dextrose infusion and head position on neurologic outcome after complete cerebral ischemia in primates: examination of a model. *Anesthesiology* 1987; 66(1):39-48.

21. McKay RD, Sundt TM, Michenfelder JD, et al: Internal carotid artery stump pressure and cerebral blood flow during carotid endarterectomy: modification by halothane, enflurane, and Innovar®. *Anesthesiology* 1976; 45(4):390-99.
22. Michenfelder JD, Milde JH, Sundt TM Jr: Cerebral protection by barbiturate anesthesia. Use after middle cerebral artery occlusion in Java monkeys. *Arch Neurol* 1976; 33(5):345-50.
23. Michenfelder JD, Sundt TM, Fode N, Sharbrough FW: Isoflurane when compared to enflurane and halothane decreases the frequency of cerebral ischemia during carotid endarterectomy. *Anesthesiology* 1987; 67(3):336-40.
24. Mirko MK, Morasch MD, Burke K, Greisler HP, Littooy FN, Baker WH: The changing face of carotid endarterectomy. *J Vasc Surg* 1996; 23:622-27.
25. Mooij JJ, Buchthal A, Belopavlovic M: Somatosensory evoked potential monitoring of temporary middle cerebral artery occlusion during aneurysm operation. *Neurosurgery* 1987; 21:492-96.
26. Moore WS: Carotid endarterectomy for prevention of stroke. *West J Med* 1993; 159:37-43.
27. Mutch WAC, White IWC, Donin N, Thomson IR, Rosenbloom M, Cheang M, West M: Haemodynamic instability and myocardial ischaemia during carotid endarterectomy: a comparison of propofol and isoflurane. *Can J Anaesth* 1995; 42:577-87.
28. North American Symptomatic Carotid Endarterectomy Trial Collaborators: Beneficial effect of carotid endarterectomy in symptomatic patients with high-grade carotid stenosis. *N Engl J Med* 1991; 325(7):445-53.
29. Ombrellaro MP, Freeman MB, Stevens SL, Goldman MH: Effect of anesthetic technique on cardiac morbidity following carotid artery surgery. *Am J Surg* 1996; 171:387-90.
30. Pulsinelli WA, et al: Moderate hyperglycemia augments ischemic brain damage: a neuropathologic study in the rat. *Neurology* 1982; 32(11):1239-46.
31. Ropper AH, Wechsler LR, Wilson LS: Carotid bruit and the risk of stroke in elective surgery. *N Engl J Med* 1982; 307(22):1388-90.
32. Samra SK, Dorje P, Zelenock GB, Stanley JC: Cerebral oximetry in patients undergoing carotid endarterectomy under regional anesthesia. *Stroke* 1996; 27:49-55.
33. Shah DM, Darling RC, Chang BB, Bock DE, Paty PS, Leather RP: Carotid endarterectomy in awake patients: its safety, acceptability, and outcome. *J Vasc Surg* 1994; 19:1015-19.
34. Smith A, Hoff JT, Nielsen SL, Larson CP Jr: Barbiturate protection in acute focal cerebral ischemia. *Stroke* 1974; 5(1):1-7.
35. Steinberg GK, Anson JA: Carotid endarterectomy: update. *West J Med* 1992; 158:64-65.
36. Wade, JG, Larson CP Jr, Hickey RF, Ehrenfeld WK, Severinghaus JW: Effect of carotid endarterectomy on carotid chemoreceptor and baroreceptor function in man. *N Engl J Med* 1970; 282(15):823-29.
37. Warner DS, Hindman BJ, Todd MM, Sawin PD, Kirchner J, Roland CL, Jamerson BD: Intracranial pressure and hemodynamic effects of remifentanil versus alfentanil in patients undergoing supratentorial craniotomy. *Anesth Analg* 1996; 83:348353.
38. Wolf PA, Kannel WB, Sorlie P, McNamara P: Asymptomatic carotid bruit and risk of stroke. The Framingham Study. *JAMA* 1981; 245(14):1442-45.
39. Wylie EJ, Ehrenfeld WK, eds. *Extracranial Occlusive Cerebrovascular Disease; Diagnosis and Management.* WB Saunders Co, Philadelphia: 1970.
40. Zasslow MA, Pearl RG, Shuer LM, Steinberg GK, Lieberson RE, Larson CP Jr: Hyperglycemia decreases acute neuronal ischemic changes after middle cerebral artery occlusion in cats. *Stroke* 1989; 20(4):519-23.

PERCUTANEOUS PROCEDURES FOR TRIGEMINAL NEURALGIA

SURGICAL CONSIDERATIONS

Lawrence M. Shuer

Description: Two percutaneous procedures are commonly used to treat trigeminal neuralgia (a well defined pain disorder of the face). Each involves placing a needle percutaneously from the cheek into the foramen ovale at the base of the skull under a light iv anesthetic. For the **glycerol injection**, it is necessary for the surgeon to verify that the needle is placed in the cistern of the trigeminal nerve or gasserian ganglion. This is usually done via image intensification or x-ray films. There should be free flow of CSF through the needle. The patient is placed in the seated position, with head flexed, and sterile glycerol is injected into the cistern. The patient is taken to the recovery room, with the head still flexed, for an hour. The glycerol damages neurons in the ganglion, which usually causes mild sensory loss and relieves the tic pain in most cases. Injection of the glycerol is often very painful.

Radiofrequency rhizotomy is the other percutaneous procedure used for trigeminal neuralgia. This procedure differs from glycerol injection in that a radiofrequency generator is used to place a thermal lesion in the appropriate portion of the gasserian ganglion. The needle is actually an insulated electrode with a portion of the tip exposed. The proper needle position is determined by applying stimulating current, with the patient awake, while assessing patient's responses. Multiple brief periods of anesthesia may be required to adjust needle position or to lesion the nerve. It is important for the patient to awaken quickly and be able to cooperate with the stimulus localization throughout this procedure.

Usual preop diagnosis: Trigeminal neuralgia; tic douloureux

SUMMARY OF PROCEDURE

	Glycerol Injection	Radiofrequency Rhizotomy
Position	Supine	⇐
Incision	Needle placed lateral to mouth on cheek	⇐
Special instrumentation	Image intensifier	⇐ + Radiofrequency generator
Unique considerations	Hypertensive response to needle placement	⇐ + Requirement for periodic deep sedation with rapid awakening for radiofrequency lesioning.
Antibiotics	Usually none	⇐
Surgical time	0.5 h	1-1.5 h
EBL	None	⇐
Postop care	Seated position with head flexed for 1 h	None
Mortality	< 1%	⇐
Morbidity	Usually < 5%: Infection Complete facial numbness (anesthesia dolorosa) Extraocular muscle paresis CSF leak Carotid puncture Facial hematoma	⇐
Pain score	2-4	2-4

PATIENT POPULATION CHARACTERISTICS

Age range	40-85 yr (usually 60-70 yr)
Male:Female	~2:3
Incidence	Relatively common neurosurgical procedure
Etiology	Vascular compression of a cranial nerve; multiple sclerosis plaque
Associated conditions	HTN; multiple sclerosis

ANESTHETIC CONSIDERATIONS

PREOPERATIVE

Trigeminal neuralgia, or tic douloureux, is a condition that develops in adults usually over the age of 60 yr. It is more common in women in whom an intermittent, severe, lancinating pain arises over the maxillary and/or mandibular divisions of the trigeminal nerve. The ophthalmic division of the trigeminal nerve is rarely involved. The pain is unilateral and often can be precipitated by stimulating a trigger point, such as by rubbing the cheek, mastication or brushing the teeth. The cause of this condition is not known. Medical management consists of therapy with carbamazepine (Tegretol), an anticonvulsant and analgesic specific for this condition. Surgery is considered when medical management fails to control pain, or complications of drug therapy develop (anemia, bleeding disorders, dizziness, etc.). One of two types of percutaneous procedures is performed: either **glycerol injection** or **radiofrequency rhizotomy** of the symptomatic branches of the trigeminal ganglion. If these treatments fail, surgical exploration of the trigeminal ganglion is considered.

Respiratory	No special considerations, unless patient has a longstanding Hx of smoking and has COPD. **Tests:** As indicated from H&P.
Cardiovascular	Most patients have Hx of idiopathic HTN and take any one of a variety of antihypertensive medications. Good control of BP preop is important because most patients become hypertensive

during the operative procedure. Intraop HTN is unavoidable because of the surgical need to have the patient awake during much of the procedure.
Tests: As indicated by H&P.

Neurological The presenting symptom is pain in the maxillary and/or mandibular division of the trigeminal nerve, unaccompanied by motor or sensory deficits.

Laboratory As indicated from H&P.

Premedication None, except for atropine 0.5 mg or glycopyrrolate 0.2 mg iv shortly before induction of anesthesia to minimize oral secretions while the surgeon is working in the mouth positioning the needle.

INTRAOPERATIVE

Anesthetic technique: GA, regardless of which percutaneous technique is to be used. O_2 by nasal cannula should be administered before induction of anesthesia. To keep the cannula out of the surgeon's field, it must be taped above the eye on the side of operation.

Induction Because the surgeon will want the patient awake as soon as the needle is in place to check for symptoms of pain, the induction drug must be potent, but short-acting. Either methohexital 1-1.5 mg/kg or propofol (1-2 mg/kg) alone or at a reduced dose in combination with remifentanil (0.5 μg/kg) are suitable for this purpose. The drug should be injected by bolus into a rapidly flowing iv to achieve a high concentration of drug in the brain quickly. Continuous infusion of the drug is not satisfactory, because it either fails to achieve a high brain concentration quickly, or its continuous administration prolongs the time before the patient is sufficiently arousable to communicate with the surgeon. In experienced hands, the needle is placed within a matter of 2-3 min. If difficulty is encountered in placing the needle, additional doses of induction drug may be needed. Patients invariably develop apnea for 1-2 min, followed by partial or total airway obstruction, while the surgeon has his hand in the mouth positioning the needle. Prior to induction of anesthesia, therefore, it is essential that the anesthesiologist optimize ventilation and oxygenation by asking patient to take a series of deep breaths through the nose with the mouth closed. This will increase the O_2 level and decrease the CO_2 level in the lungs prior to induction. To maintain adequate spontaneous ventilation and oxygenation, it is usually necessary to institute forward displacement of the mandible while the surgeon inserts the needle. Another alternative is to insert a nasal airway.
If **glycerol injection** is used, needle position is verified by radiological imaging, using a radio-opaque dye. Patient is awakened and placed in a seated position with head flexed. The glycerol is injected, causing severe pain. Patient is then moved to recovery room still in seated position with the head forward to keep the glycerol localized to the region of the trigeminal ganglion.
If **radiofrequency rhizotomy** is performed, the patient is awakened and the position of the needle is verified by stimulating the ganglion with heat and determining the site of pain. The patient is then reanesthetized with a smaller bolus of the same drug to permit high-intensity heat stimulation for ~1 min. This procedure may be repeated several times. Each time, the patient needs less anesthetic, because of both the cumulative effects of the drug, and the fact that the trigeminal ganglion is becoming permanently damaged by the heat.

Emergence In the recovery room, patients are maintained in a seated position with an ice pack on the cheek at the site of needle insertion to minimize postop bleeding and swelling. Following glycerol injection, patients often complain of pain in the face, requiring opiate analgesics. Following radiofrequency rhizotomy, the face is usually numb, which is the end point for concluding the operation.

Blood and fluid requirements IV: 18 ga × 1
NS/LR @ 4-6 ml/kg/h

Monitoring Standard monitors (see p. B-1).

Control of BP Clonidine patch
Labetalol

Patients almost invariably become hypertensive during this therapy. Attempts to lessen these episodes with a clonidine patch preop or use of intermittent doses of labetalol prophylactically or therapeutically are only partially successful.

Positioning Table turned 180°
✓ and pad pressure points.
✓ eyes.

Patient supine with head in the midline.

Complications	Failure of needle placement Bleeding Respiratory arrest	Major complications from this operation are uncommon, but include: (1) Failure to identify the foramen ovale, through which the needle must be inserted to reach the trigeminal ganglion. If the needle cannot be placed within 30-40 min, the procedure is usually aborted until another day. (2) Bleeding into cheek from puncture of a branch of the facial artery. (3) Apnea from spillover of the neurolytic solution into circulating CSF, presumably affecting the respiratory center in the 4th ventricle.

POSTOPERATIVE

Pain management Parenteral opiates (see p. C-1).

Reference

1. Young RF: Stereotactic procedures for facial pain. In *Brain Surgery: Complication, Avoidance and Management*. Apuzzo MLJ, ed. Churchill Livingstone, New York: 1993, 2097-113.

Surgeons

Sally R. Byrd, MD (*Ophthalmic surgery*)
Peter R. Egbert, MD (*Ophthalmic surgery*)
Michael W. Gaynon, MD (*Retinal surgery*)

2.0 OPHTHALMIC SURGERY

Anesthesiologists

Stanley I. Samuels, MB, BCh, FFARCS
Richard A. Jaffe, MD, PhD
Jayshree B. Desai, MD

CATARACT EXTRACTION WITH INTRAOCULAR LENS INSERTION

SURGICAL CONSIDERATIONS

Description: The **extracapsular cataract technique** involves removing the lens in pieces. A small (3-10 mm) incision is made at the superior corneal scleral junction. The anterior capsule of the lens is removed, and the nucleus is then either expressed intact or is emulsified and sucked out by the **phacoemulsification technique** (**ultrasonic fragmentation**). Finally, the cortex is aspirated using a manual irrigation aspirating needle or the automatic aspiration device attached to the phacoemulsification machine. A plastic intraocular lens is placed behind the iris and supported by the remaining intact posterior capsule of the natural lens or placed directly into the capsular bag (Fig 2-1). The wound is closed with multiple 10-0 nylon sutures or left unsutured if small and watertight.

Variant procedure or approaches: **Intracapsular cataract extraction** is rarely done anymore given the superior results of extracapsular surgery. In intracapsular extraction, the entire lens is removed intact by application of a cryoprobe. It is most commonly done when the lens has lost its zonular support 2° trauma or a genetic condition.

Usual preop diagnosis: Cataract

SUMMARY OF PROCEDURE

Position	Supine
Incision	3-10 mm at periphery of cornea
Special instrumentation	Surgical microscope; automated irrigation/aspiration machine; sometimes phacoemulsification machine
Antibiotics	Subconjunctival cefazolin (50-100 mg) or gentamicin (20-40 mg)
Surgical time	30-60 min
EBL	None
Mortality	Minimal
Morbidity	Corneal edema: 1% Retinal detachment: < 1% Wound rupture: < 1% Infection: < 0.1%
Pain score	1-3

PATIENT POPULATION CHARACTERISTICS

Age range	50-90+ yr
Male:Female	1:1
Incidence	> 1,000,000/yr in U.S.
Etiology	Formation may be accelerated by poor nutrition, UV light exposure or steroids.
Associated conditions	Associated systemic diseases of the elderly (common); HTN; diabetes; heart disease

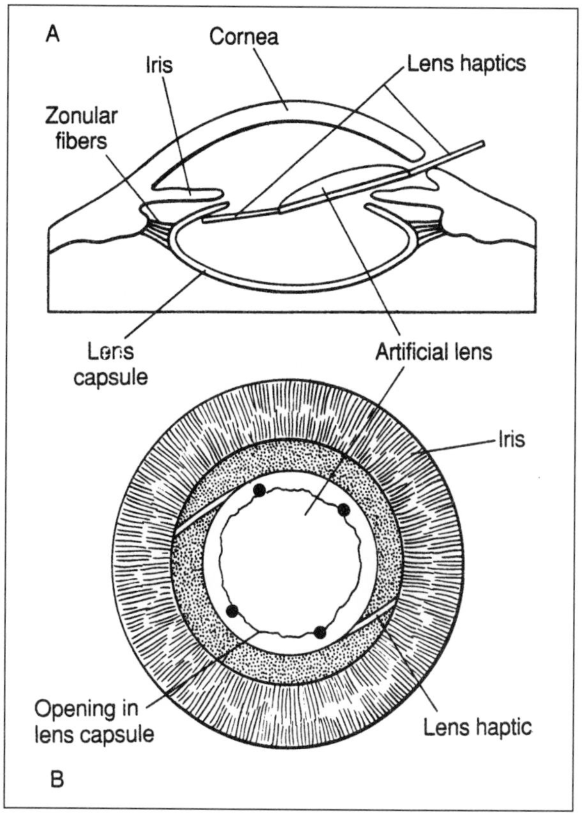

Figure 2-1. (A) Placement of intraocular lens into remaining capsular bay. (B) "In-the-bag" insertion. (Reproduced with permission from Spaeth GL, ed: *Ophthalmic Surgery: Principles & Practice*, 2nd edition. WB Saunders: 1990.)

ANESTHETIC CONSIDERATIONS

See Anesthetic Considerations for Ophthalmic Surgical Procedures under MAC, p. 100.

References

See General References following Ophthalmic Surgery section, p. 116.

CORNEAL TRANSPLANT

SURGICAL CONSIDERATIONS

Description: The eye may be removed from a suitable donor up to a maximum of 24 h before transplantation; the cornea is removed from the donor eye in the OR just before transplantation. The central portion of the recipient's cornea (generally an 8 mm button) is removed, using a round trephine followed by corneal scissors. At this time, there is a large hole in the patient's eye and pressure on the eye must be avoided. If the patient needs a cataract extraction, a plastic **intraocular lens insertion** or **anterior vitrectomy** may be done concurrently. The donor cornea is sutured into place with multiple 10-0 nylon sutures in order to achieve a watertight closure (Fig 2-2).

Usual preop diagnosis: Corneal scar; corneal dystrophy; keratoconus

SUMMARY OF PROCEDURE

Position	Supine
Incision	Corneal
Special instrumentation	Surgical microscope
Unique considerations	Open-globe precautions
Antibiotics	Subconjunctival gentamicin (20-40 mg) or cefazolin (50-100 mg)
Surgical time	60-90 min
EBL	Minimal
Postop care	Patients must be followed closely for evidence of tissue rejection in immediate postop period.
Mortality	Minimal
Morbidity	Graft rejection: 5% Infection: < 1% Wound dehiscence
Pain score	2

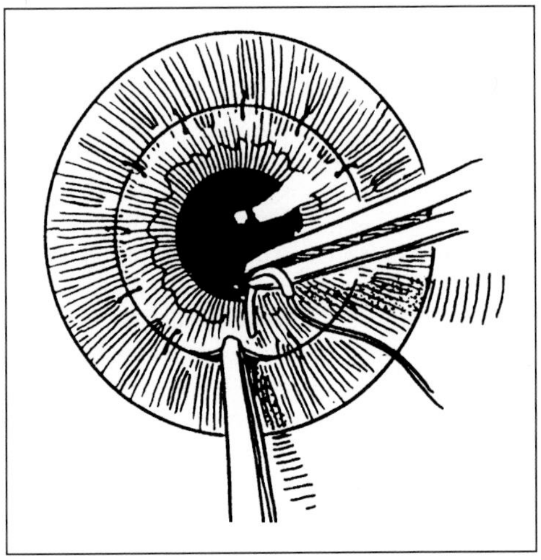

Figure 2-2. Suturing donor cornea on recipient eye. (Reproduced with permission from Phelps CD, ed: *Manual of Common Ophthalmic Surgical Procedures*. Churchill Livingstone: 1986.)

PATIENT POPULATION CHARACTERISTICS

Age range	Any age
Male:Female	1:1
Incidence	1,000/yr in U.S.
Etiology	Scarring, infection or trauma; various inheritable conditions; damage to the cornea (decompensation) 2° cataract surgery (rare)
Associated conditions	Trauma; infection; corneal dystrophies; congenital malformations which may involve cornea (rare)

ANESTHETIC CONSIDERATIONS

See Anesthetic Considerations for Ophthalmic Surgical Procedures under MAC, p. 100.

References

See General References following Ophthalmic Surgery section, p. 116.

TRABECULECTOMY

SURGICAL CONSIDERATIONS

Description: Trabeculectomy is the most commonly performed surgery to lower intraocular pressure (IOP) in patients with glaucoma. The goal is to create a fistula from the anterior chamber to the subconjunctival space, thus giving the intraocular fluid an alternate exit route and lowering eye pressure. The conjunctiva near the cornea is reflected back from the sclera. Antimetabolites such as mitomycin or 5-fluorouracil are often applied briefly to lessen subsequent scarring. An opening approximately 2 × 2 mm is made into the anterior chamber under a partial-thickness scleral flap (Fig 2-3), and an **iridectomy** is performed. The scleral flap partially retards leakage of aqueous from the anterior chamber through the subconjunctival space and decreases the amount of postop hypotony. The sclera is closed and the conjunctiva sutured. A full-thickness procedure varies only in the absence of a scleral flap.

Variant procedure or approaches: In certain patients for whom glaucoma surgery has failed, or who have particularly refractive glaucoma, a **glaucoma seton implant** (e.g., **Molteno** or **Baerveldt**) may be used to maintain drainage fistulas. This involves dissecting the conjunctiva away from sclera and inserting a small tube (usually Silastic) directly into the anterior chamber from the corneal limbus. The tube is connected to one or two small plates which are sewn to the sclera. Exposed tube is covered by sclera, usually from a donor eye, and then the conjunctiva is brought back down and sewn into place. The plates prevent conjunctiva from scarring back down to sclera, thus allowing the fluid draining from the anterior chamber to collect and then reabsorb.

In infants and children with congenital glaucoma, the procedures of choice involve making a long opening directly into the drainage angle of the anterior chamber, either as a goniotomy or trabeculotomy. A **goniotomy** is performed by passing a small knife across the anterior chamber into the angle and then, under direct visualization with a goniotomy lens, making an incision over trabecular meshwork extending 1-2 quadrants. In a **trabeculotomy,** a cutdown is made at the limbus and Schlemm's canal is identified. A special instrument is passed into Schlemm's canal and rotated into the anterior chamber, opening the canal directly to the anterior chamber.

Usual preop diagnosis: Glaucoma

SUMMARY OF PROCEDURE

Position	Supine
Incision	Superior portion of eye
Special instrumentation	Surgical microscope
Antibiotics	Subconjunctival cefazolin (50-100 mg), gentamicin (20-40 mg), and dexamethasone (2-4 mg)
Surgical time	30-60 min
EBL	Minimal
Postop care	May involve additional treatment with antimetabolite drugs (e.g., fluorouracil) to retard scarring; also may involve cutting scleral flap sutures with laser to control postop pressure.
Mortality	Minimal
Morbidity	Excessive drainage with low IOP: 5%
Pain score	1

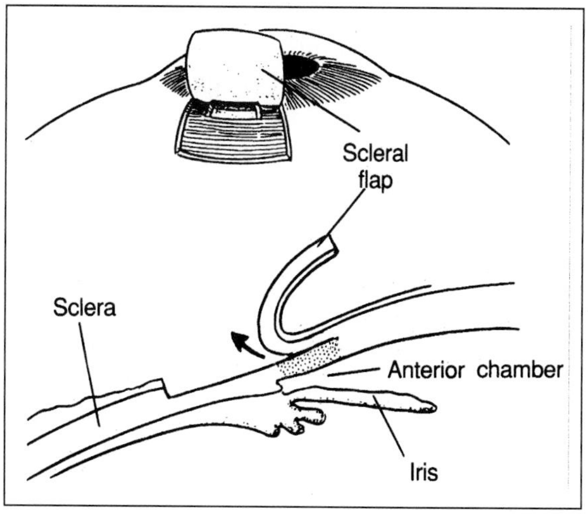

Figure 2-3. Small opening made in anterior chamber under a scleral flap. Opening corresponds to shaded area in lower diagram. (Reproduced with permission from Phelps CD, ed: *Manual of Common Ophthalmic Surgical Procedures.* Churchill Livingstone: 1986.)

PATIENT POPULATION CHARACTERISTICS

Age range	Infants–adults; more common in elderly
Male:Female	1:1
Incidence	10,000/yr in U.S.
Etiology	Unknown for most part; occasionally results from eye trauma, inflammation, abnormal vascular growth or certain congenital anomalies with abnormal eye development.

Associated conditions	Congenital glaucoma may be associated with other congenital syndromes: Rieger's syndrome—hypoplastic maxilla Neurofibromatosis—possible ↑ICP, spinal cord involvement, airway involvement Sturge-Weber syndrome—CNS Sx may be present.

ANESTHETIC CONSIDERATIONS

See Anesthetic Considerations for Ophthalmic Surgical Procedures under MAC, p. 100.

References

See General References following Ophthalmic Surgery section, p. 116.

ECTROPION REPAIR

SURGICAL CONSIDERATIONS

Description: Ectropion is a malposition of either the upper or lower eyelid in which the lid margin is everted away from the globe. Surgical repair can be approached in a variety of ways, depending on the underlying pathology. Generally speaking, ectropion involves either loose or excess lid tissue which causes the lid to fall away from the eye, or scarring (cicatrix) of the skin of the lid which pulls it away from the globe. In the first case, a lid-tightening procedure is performed, either by simply removing a full-thickness wedge of lid and reapproximating the cut edges, or with the "lateral canthal strip" procedure. In this operation, the inferior cruz of the lateral canthal tendon is disinserted (Fig 2-4) and a strip of lateral tarsus is isolated by dissecting it free from overlying skin and orbicularis muscle and then by removing conjunctiva from the posterior surface. This strip of tarsus is then shortened to a length necessary to restore proper lid tension and sutured in place to the periosteum of the lateral orbital rim. Excess skin is excised and the defect closed.

Variant procedure or approaches: In the case of cicatricial ectropion, the contracted scar can sometimes be released by using a z-plasty technique to release vertical tension. Alternatively, a full-thickness skin graft taken from upper lid or the postauricular or supraclavicular regions is used to fill in any defects after all scar bands have been lysed.

Usual preop diagnosis: Ectropion of the eyelid

SUMMARY OF PROCEDURE

Position	Supine
Incision	Generally at lateral canthus for involutional ectropion; in area of scarring
Antibiotics	Postop topical antibiotics
Surgical time	0.5-1 h
EBL	Minimal
Mortality	Minimal
Morbidity	Infection: < 1%
Pain score	2

PATIENT POPULATION CHARACTERISTICS

Age range	Elderly; cicatricial ectropion may occur in younger patients 2° trauma or burns.
Male:Female	1:1
Incidence	Common
Etiology	Aging

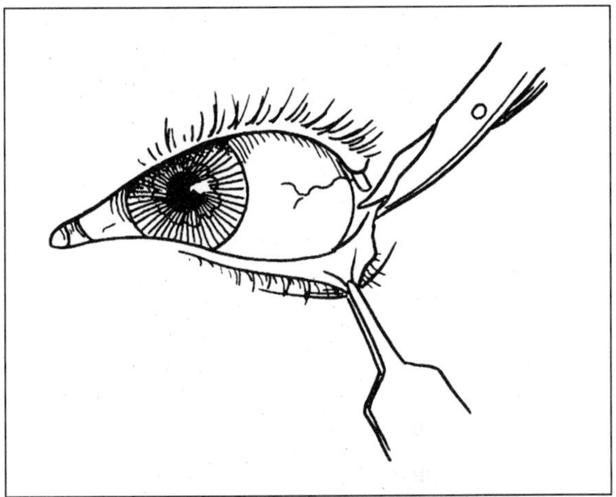

Figure 2-4. Disinsertion of the inferior cruz of the lateral canthal tendon. (Reproduced with permission from Phelps CD, ed: *Manual of Common Ophthalmic Surgery*. Churchill Livingstone: 1986.)

ANESTHETIC CONSIDERATIONS

See Anesthetic Considerations for Ophthalmic Surgical Procedures Under MAC, p. 100.

References

See General References following Ophthalmic Surgery section, p. 116.

ENTROPION REPAIR

SURGICAL CONSIDERATIONS

Description: Entropion involves the inward rotation of the eyelid toward the globe. As with ectropion repair, multiple procedures have been described, their use depending on concomitant lid findings and surgeon's preference. In senile or involutional entropion, which involves primarily the lower lids, the most common underlying pathology is dehiscence or weakening of the lower lid retractor muscles, often in combination with horizontal lid laxity. One approach is to make a horizontal lid incision through skin and orbicularis muscle approximately 2 mm from the lashes. Orbital septum is then incised and the lower lid retractor muscles identified and sewn back onto the inferior tarsal border. Skin is closed after excising redundant tissue. If horizontal lid laxity also exists, a lateral tarsal strip procedure, similar to that described for ectropion repair, can also be done.

Variant procedure or approaches: In the case of cicatricial entropion, involving either the upper or lower lids, there is scarring or shrinkage of the conjunctival tarsal surface. This pulls the lid margin inward toward the globe. In mild cases, a **Weis procedure** may be performed. This involves making a full-thickness horizontal lid incision, fracturing the tarsus and everting it with carefully placed sutures and reclosing the skin. For more severe cicatricial entropion, a full-thickness mucosal graft may be needed on the inner lid surface. This is commonly taken from the lower lip.

Usual preop diagnosis: Entropion of eyelid

SUMMARY OF PROCEDURE

Position	Supine
Antibiotics	Topical antibiotics postop
Surgical time	0.5-1.5 h
EBL	Minimal
Mortality	Minimal
Morbidity	Infection: < 1%
Pain score	2

PATIENT POPULATION CHARACTERISTICS

Age range	Involutional entropion, primarily in elderly; cicatricial entropion, any age
Male:Female	1:1
Incidence	Common
Etiology	Cicatricial entropion associated with trauma, chemical injury or chronic infection or inflammation
Associated conditions	Stevens-Johnson syndrome—may require epidermolysis bullosa-type precautions; cicatricial pemphigoid; trachoma

ANESTHETIC CONSIDERATIONS

See Anesthetic Considerations for Ophthalmic Surgical Procedures under MAC, p. 100.

References

See General References following Ophthalmic Surgery section, p. 116.

PTOSIS SURGERY

SURGICAL CONSIDERATIONS

Description: The most frequently performed procedure for ptosis correction involves shortening, or simply reattaching, the levator palpebrae aponeurosis at its site of insertion on the superior tarsus. **Levator aponeurosis surgery** in adults is performed preferably under local anesthesia so that lid position with eyes open can be adequately assessed and adjusted. An incision is made through the skin along the upper eyelid crease, and the dissection is carried down through the orbicularis muscle and orbital septum until the levator aponeurosis is isolated and sewn to the superior tarsus. The exact position is adjusted according to lid height and contour. The skin incision is closed, with any excess being excised.

Variant procedure or approaches: Patients with little or no levator function, as assessed by their preop eyelid excursion, may require a **frontalis suspension** operation. This involves suspending the upper lid from the brow so that the lid is opened by raising the brow and closed by contracting the orbicularis muscle. For this purpose, autogenous, or cadaver fascia lata or an alloplastic material (e.g., silicone rod) is tunneled beneath the skin and muscle from the brow to the upper lid margin and then tied at a length appropriate for the desired lid height. Frontalis suspension in both children and adults is done under GA.

Usual preop diagnosis: Congenital or acquired ptosis

SUMMARY OF PROCEDURE

	Ptosis Corrections	Frontalis Suspension
Position	Supine. When levator surgery is performed under local anesthesia, patient may be required to sit upright for more accurate assessment of lid position.	Supine
Incision	Generally through upper lid crease	Small incisions above lid margin and brow
Antibiotics	Topical antibiotics postop	⇐
Surgical time	1-1.5 h	1 h
EBL	Minimal	⇐
Mortality	Minimal	⇐
Morbidity	Infection: < 1%	⇐
	Corneal exposure from overcorrection	⇐
Pain score	3	3

PATIENT POPULATION CHARACTERISTICS

Age range	Generally elderly unless congenital
Male:Female	1:1
Incidence	Common
Etiology	Stretching or dehiscence of the levator aponeurosis associated with aging (common); neurogenic (e.g., 3rd nerve palsy) or congenital ptosis
Associated conditions	Systemic disorders such as myasthenia gravis, myotonic dystrophy or progressive external ophthalmoplegia

ANESTHETIC CONSIDERATIONS

See Anesthetic Considerations for Ophthalmic Surgical Procedures under MAC, p. 100.

References

See General References following Ophthalmic Surgery section, p. 116.

EYELID RECONSTRUCTION

SURGICAL CONSIDERATIONS

Description: Tumors of the lids, both benign and malignant, frequently need to be excised, making it necessary to reconstruct the lid to protect and maintain eye function and give the best cosmetic results. When a tumor is known to be malignant, resection is usually carried out under frozen-section control. In some instances, however, particularly with tumors involving the medial canthal area, resection is first done by a Mohs surgeon (a dermatologist trained in this technique) with reconstruction being undertaken during a separate operation. Mohs surgery involves horizontal sectioning of tumor under microscopic control, allowing the tumor to be completely removed with the least sacrifice of normal tissue. If the remaining defect is 25% or less of the total lid length, closure can be accomplished often by simply closing the defect. Deep bites are taken through tarsus before closing the skin, and special care is taken in reapproximating the lid margin so as not to leave a notch or step.

Variant procedure or approaches: If the lid defect cannot be pulled together, but is lacking only a few millimeters, a **lateral canthotomy** may be performed with lysis of the corresponding branch of the lateral canthal tendon. For larger defects affecting up to 40-50% of the medial or central lids, a **semicircular flap** is often utilized. This is made laterally, extensively undermined and used in conjunction with lateral canthal lysis. For larger lid defects, a variety of full- and partial-thickness flaps and grafts can be used, depending on the location of the defect and surgeon's preference. Some procedures involve using a tunnel flap, which advances tissue from one lid to another, and closing the eye for 3-12 weeks, at which time the flap can be separated from its pedicle.

Usual preop diagnosis: Basal-cell carcinoma; malignant tumor; squamous-cell carcinoma; sebaceous-cell carcinoma; malignant melanoma; nevi

SUMMARY OF PROCEDURE

Position	Supine
Incision	Variable, depending on tumor location
Antibiotics	Topical, following surgery
Surgical time	0.5-2 h
EBL	Minimal
Mortality	Minimal
Morbidity	Infection: < 1%
	Dry eye
	Secondary lid deformity
Pain score	3

PATIENT POPULATION CHARACTERISTICS

Age range	More common in elderly, but young adults included
Male:Female	1:1
Incidence	Common
Etiology	Skin cancers related to sun exposure

ANESTHETIC CONSIDERATIONS

See Anesthetic Considerations for Ophthalmic Surgical Procedures under MAC, below.

References

See General References following Ophthalmic Surgery section, p. 116.

PTERYGIUM EXCISION

SURGICAL CONSIDERATIONS

Description: Pterygia are vascular fleshy growths arising from the conjunctiva and extending onto the cornea. Pterygium removal is often performed under local anesthetic with a subconjunctival, rather than a retrobulbar injection. It is frequently done in the clinic setting, with an operating microscope, if the planned dissection is not too extensive. They are removed by carefully dissecting the head from the cornea, undermining and excising a portion of the body, and leaving an area of bare sclera or relaxing the adjacent conjunctiva and pulling it closed. The defect also may be covered with a conjunctival graft taken from the same or opposite eye.

Variant procedure or approaches: Due to the general high recurrence rate, many minor variations in the approach have been attempted, including folding part of the pterygium under itself and applying β-radiation or mitomycin at the limbus to prevent it from growing back.

Preop diagnosis or indications: Pterygium causing decreased vision or motility, excessive irritation or cosmetic disfigurement

SUMMARY OF PROCEDURE

Position	Supine
Incision	In area of pterygium—most commonly medial interpalpebral region
Antibiotics	Topical antibiotics postop
Surgical time	15-45 min
EBL	None
Mortality	Minimal
Morbidity	High recurrence rate, often in more aggressive form
Pain score	2-3

PATIENT POPULATION CHARACTERISTICS

Age range	Young-to-middle-age adults
Male:Female	1:1
Incidence	Common in tropical regions; unusual in temperate climates
Etiology	Related to solar exposure

ANESTHETIC CONSIDERATIONS FOR OPHTHALMIC SURGICAL PROCEDURES UNDER MAC

(Procedures covered: cataract extraction and other procedures; corneal transplant; trabeculectomy; ectropion-entropion repair; ptosis surgery; eyelid reconstruction; pterygium excision)

PREOPERATIVE

Ophthalmic procedures that are of relatively short duration and those that result in minimal blood loss are being performed increasingly more often on an outpatient basis, usually with local anesthesia (e.g., retrobulbar or peribulbar blocks)

under MAC (see p. B-4). Ophthalmologists also have made use of topical anesthetic administered repeatedly and, often, in combination with intracameral lidocaine. This eliminates the risk of injection as well as the need for iv sedation at the time of the block. Since eye movements are not blocked, however, one needs cooperative patients who can tolerate seeing their surgery in progress. The majority of these ocular procedures are performed on elderly patients who usually have multiple medical problems; thus, anesthesiologists are faced with monitoring and managing these potentially challenging patients. A thorough preop H&P, along with appropriate lab workup, are mandatory, even if local anesthesia/MAC is to be used. Contraindications to use of local anesthesia for ocular surgery include: coagulation abnormalities; open-eye injuries; patients with chronic cough, claustrophobia, or inability to lie flat; and patients who refuse local anesthesia.

Respiratory Elderly patients have increased incidence of hiatal hernia and, therefore, are at increased risk for pulmonary aspiration. Assess the patient's ability to lie flat for the duration of the procedure.
Tests: As indicated from H&P.

Cardiovascular Hx of HTN, CAD, CHF or poor exercise tolerance should prompt a thorough investigation into the patient's cardiac status, including efficacy of current medications and recent ECG (compared with previous ECGs). Consultation with a cardiologist may be appropriate to optimize the patient's condition before surgery.
Tests: ECG; others (e.g., ECHO) as indicated from H&P.

Diabetes Diabetic patients are at increased risk for silent myocardial ischemia. Pulmonary aspiration 2° diabetic gastroparesis is also a risk in this population. Patients usually take 1/2 or 1/3 of their normal NPH insulin dose (on the morning of surgery); fasting blood sugar is checked; and an iv infusion of D5 LR is started if glucose < 90 mg/dl, or treated with regular insulin if glucose > 200 mg/dl. Blood sugar is checked intraop and postop.

Musculoskeletal Arthritic changes make lying flat difficult for some patients.

Hematologic ✓ for recent aspirin/NSAID use, particularly in patients undergoing lid or orbital procedures.
Tests: As indicated from H&P.

Laboratory Creatinine usual in patients > 64 yr; in other patients, as indicated from H&P.

Premedication For patients with increased risk of aspiration (e.g., with hiatal hernia or diabetic gastroparesis) and for the obese and very anxious patients, metoclopramide 10 mg iv may enhance gastric emptying. Patients will benefit from a detailed explanation of events prior to surgery (including iv placement, application of monitors, performance of local block, ocular pressure, prepping eye and draping of the whole face, provision of supplemental O_2 and the assurance that the anesthesiologist will always be nearby, monitoring the patient. Midazolam (0.5-1 mg iv) is often beneficial.

INTRAOPERATIVE

Anesthetic technique: MAC (see p. B-4). Placement of the retrobulbar or peribulbar blocks may be painful and very short-acting agents (e.g., remifentanil, 0.5-1 μg/kg, alfentanil 5-7 μg/kg or propofol 30-50 mg) should be administered to minimize patient discomfort. Dose requirements vary significantly among patients, and the anesthesiologist should be prepared to treat ↓BP and apnea. Usually further sedation is unnecessary and may interfere with patient cooperation during the surgery. Coughing should be avoided during the procedure, and the anesthesiologist must always be prepared to administer GA if necessary.

Retrobulbar block: Using a 25- or 27-ga needle (1.5"), the retrobulbar space is approached from the infratemporal quadrant of the orbit. The eye should be in a neutral or downward and medial position. Once the needle is positioned and there is no return of blood or CSF on aspiration, 3-5 ml of anesthetic solution is injected slowly. A facial nerve block is necessary to prevent eyelid movement. This can be accomplished by injecting 4-8 ml of anesthetic solution above and below the lateral aspect of the orbit. Typically, the anesthetic solution consists of a 50:50 mixture of 0.5% bupivacaine and 2% lidocaine with hyaluronidase.

Peribulbar block: Using a 25- or 27-ga 5/8"-1" needle, 5-6 ml of anesthetic solution is injected into the peribulbar space, entering just superior to the inferior rim of the orbit at the junction of the lateral and middle thirds of the lower lid. While perforation of the globe and hemorrhage are still possible, direct injury to the optic nerve and subdural injection are unlikely due to the length and position of the needle. Peribulbar blocks generally take longer to take effect than retrobulbars and are more likely to cause conjunctival swelling, which may interfere with surgery.

Blood and fluid requirements	IV: 18 ga × 1 NS/LR @ 1.5-3 ml/kg/h	Excessive fluids → bladder distention → ↑BP

Monitoring	Standard monitors (see P. B-1). Verbal response	It is important to remain in communication with the patient throughout the procedure. (Take care to avoid evoking head movement.)
Positioning	✓ and pad pressure points. ✓ nonoperated eye.	Pillows under knees to relieve back strain.
Complications	Dysrhythmias, especially ↓HR	Usually 2° traction on ocular/periocular strabismus (see OCR, p. 107).
	↑BP	2° anxiety, pain, etc. Rx: labetalol 5 mg or hydralazine 4-mg increments, as appropriate.
	Retrobulbar hemorrhage	Rx: pressure bandage; usually cancel surgery.
	Globe perforation	If needle perforation, no repair usually necessary.
	Convulsions 2° iv local anesthetic	Supportive treatment with IPPV
	Respiratory arrest	2° subarachnoid injection. Rx: CPR.
	Oculocardiac reflex (OCR)→ ↓↓HR, ↓↓BP	Rx: Stop stimulation; use atropine (see OCR discussion: p. 107).

POSTOPERATIVE

Complications	Myocardial ischemia	Rx: Provide O_2; ✓ BP; sublingual NTG; ✓ ECG; cardiology consultation.
	Corneal abrasion	
	Photophobia	
	N/V	Rx: Metoclopramide 10 mg iv, droperidol 0.625 mg iv, or ondansetron 4 mg iv.
	Diplopia	
Pain management	Acetaminophen 325-1000 mg po	

Table 2-1. Commonly Used Ophthalmic Drugs and Their Systemic Effects

Phenylephrine	An α-adrenergic agonist which causes mydriasis (pupillary dilation) and vasoconstriction to aid ocular surgery; however, it also can precipitate significant HTN and dysrhythmias.
Echothiophate	An irreversible cholinesterase inhibitor used in glaucoma treatment to cause miosis and ↓IOP. Its systemic absorption can reduce plasma cholinesterase activity and thereby prolong paralysis 2° to succinylcholine (usually not more than 20-30 min).
Timolol	A nonselective β-adrenergic antagonist which decreases production of aqueous humor → ↓IOP. Rarely it may be associated with atropine-resistant bradycardia, asthma, CHF and hypotension.
Acetazolamide	A carbonic anhydrase inhibitor used to ↓ IOP. It also can cause diuresis and a hypokalemic metabolic acidosis.
Atropine	An anticholinergic which produces mydriasis to aid with ocular examination and surgery. It also can precipitate central anticholinergic syndrome. (Sx range from dry mouth, tachycardia, agitation, delirium and hallucinations to unconsciousness.) Physostigmine 0.01-0.03 mg/kg will increase central acetylcholine and reverse the symptoms. (It may be repeated after 15-30 min.)

References

1. Barash PG, Cullen BF, Stoelting RK, eds: *Clinical Anesthesia, 3rd edition.* JB Lippincott, Philadelphia: 1997.
2. McGoldrick KE, ed: *Anesthesia for Ophthalmic and Otolaryngologic Surgery.* WB Saunders Co, Philadelphia: 1992.
3. McGoldrick KE, Mardirossian J: Ophthalmic Surgery. In *Ambulatory Anesthesiology: A Problem Oriented Approach.* Williams & Wilkins, Baltimore:, 1995, 507-35.

REPAIR OF RUPTURED OR LACERATED GLOBE

SURGICAL CONSIDERATIONS

Description: The goal of this surgery is to repair the cornea and sclera sufficiently to create a watertight wound. The laceration often contains a prolapsed iris, which must be removed or reposited. The cornea is then carefully closed with 10-0 nylon suture. An associated cataract may need to be removed and the associated scleral laceration may need to be closed. Lacerations extending beyond the equator of the globe, however, are generally inaccessible to closure. At times, a laceration may involve one of the extraocular muscle tendons, necessitating reattachment to the globe.

Usual preop diagnosis: Ruptured or lacerated globe

SUMMARY OF PROCEDURE

Position	Supine
Incision	A conjunctival incision may be indicated to improve exposure, if the laceration extends past the corneal limbus onto the sclera
Special instrumentation	Surgical microscope
Antibiotics	Subconjunctival cefazolin 100 mg or gentamicin 20-40 mg; iv broad spectrum antibiotics (cephalosporin or vancomycin) and an aminoglycoside
Closing considerations	Until wound is closed, avoid coughing, bucking, etc.
Surgical time	0.5-2 h
EBL	Minimal
Postop care	IV antibiotics are usually continued 5 d.
Mortality	Minimal
Morbidity	Infection-variable, depending on type of injury Wound leak: 5% Sympathetic ophthalmia: < 1%
Pain score	4

PATIENT POPULATION CHARACTERISTICS

Age range	Any age
Male:Female	2:1
Incidence	Fairly common, but depends on patient population.
Etiology	Trauma
Associated conditions	May be associated with orbital or facial trauma.

ANESTHETIC CONSIDERATIONS

PREOPERATIVE

This is a generally healthy patient population; however, patients with penetrating eye injuries present the anesthesiologist with two special challenges: (1) They invariably have full stomachs, resulting in risk of aspiration. (2) They are at risk of blindness 2° increased intraocular pressure (IOP) and loss of ocular contents, which may be a result of coughing, crying and/or struggling during induction. Normal IOP ranges from 10-22 mmHg, depending on the rate of formation and drainage of aqueous humor, choroidal blood volume, scleral rigidity, extraocular muscle tone, as well as extrinsic pressure on the eye (e.g., a poorly fitting mask or retrobulbar hematoma). Patient movement, coughing, straining, vomiting, hypercarbia, HTN and ET intubation may also increase IOP as much as 40 mmHg or more.

Full-stomach precautions: Consider patient to have a full stomach if the injury occurred within 8 h of the last meal. Pain and anxiety due to trauma will delay gastric emptying. Goal is to minimize risk of aspiration pneumonitis by decreasing gastric volume and acidity. Consider premedication with metoclopramide (10-20 mg iv), antacids such as Na citrate (15-30 ml orally immediately prior to induction) and H_2-histamine receptor antagonists (ranitidine [50 mg iv]). H_2-histamine receptor antagonists, however, have no effect on the pH of gastric secretions present in the stomach prior to administration, and are, therefore, of limited value in patients presenting for emergency surgery. If patient has Hx of smoking or is an asthmatic, consider preop use of inhalers such as albuterol (2-4 puffs).

Laboratory Tests as indicated from H&P.

Premedication Patients often are very anxious and may benefit from benzodiazepines (e.g., for pediatric population, midazolam 0.5-0.75 mg/kg po in cola or apple juice, 15-30 ml). Avoid narcotic premedication, which may increase nausea and possibility of emesis.

INTRAOPERATIVE

Anesthetic technique: GETA. Regional anesthesia (e.g., retrobulbar block) is contraindicated in patients with open-eye injury because of ↑IOP, which may accompany injection of local anesthetic behind the globe. Thus, in spite of the increased risk of aspiration from a full stomach, GETA is recommended.

Induction To protect the airway and prevent ↑IOP, a rapid-sequence induction with cricoid pressure and a smooth intubation are required. While the choice of induction agent is relatively straightforward—propofol 1-2 mg/kg or STP 3-5 mg/kg—the choice of neuromuscular blocking agents for facilitating intubation is controversial. Succinylcholine provides a rapid onset, short duration of action and excellent intubating conditions, but it also transiently increases IOP. This ↑IOP is not always attenuated by pretreatment with a nondepolarizing agent (e.g., d-tubocurarine). Rocuronium (1 mg/kg) produces muscle relaxation in 1-2 min and may be a satisfactory alternative to succinylcholine; however, a premature attempt at intubation may significantly ↑ IOP as a result of coughing and straining. Of interest, there are no reports in the literature documenting exacerbation of eye injuries with the use of succinylcholine following pretreatment with a nondepolarizing muscle relaxant. Given that the anesthesiologist's main concern is safe airway management, the following is a suggested induction plan:

(1) Preoxygenation, avoiding external pressure on the eye from face mask.

(2) Pretreatment with a nondepolarizing relaxant (e.g., d-tubocurarine 0.06 mg/kg), followed by iv lidocaine (1 mg/kg) and fentanyl (2-3 μg/kg) to blunt the cardiovascular response to laryngoscopy and intubation.

(3) Consider 5-10 mg labetalol, also to blunt cardiovascular response to laryngoscopy and intubation (if patient does not have reactive airway disease).

(4) 4 min later, with cricoid pressure, induce with propofol (1.5-2.5 mg/kg) and succinylcholine (1.5 mg/kg). Intubate with oral RAE tube. Note: for pediatric patients, it might be appropriate to induce with sevoflurane while maintaining cricoid pressure and intubating when the patient is deeply anesthetized. Trying to start an iv prior to induction may precipitate struggling and crying, leading to further eye injury.

Maintenance Standard maintenance (see p. B-3). Avoid hypercapnia, which → ↑IOP. Muscle relaxation is mandatory until the eye is surgically closed. Humidify gasses for pediatric patients.

Emergence Decompress the stomach with OG tube. Goal is smooth emergence and extubation with patient awake with intact airway reflexes. IV lidocaine (1.5 mg/kg) 5 min before extubation; posterior pharyngeal suctioning with patient deeply anesthetized, combined with a small amount of narcotic (remifentanil 1-2 μg/kg), may blunt cough reflex prior to extubation. The common occurrence of postop N/V requires administration of intraop antiemetics (e.g., metoclopramide 10 mg iv, droperidol 0.625 mg iv or ondansetron 4 mg iv 30 min before end of surgery).

Blood and fluid requirements IV: 18 ga × 1 (adult)
20 ga × 1 (child)
NS/LR @ 5-10 ml/kg/h
Warm fluids.

Monitoring Standard monitors (see p. B-1). Neuromuscular blockade must be monitored closely and additional relaxant given as necessary to prevent patient movement during surgery.

Positioning ✓ and pad pressure points.
✓ nonoperated eye.

Complications ↑IOP with extrusion of intraocular contents
Aspiration of gastric contents

IOP (normal = ~10-22 mmHg) increased by: blink = 10-15 mmHg; forced closure = > 70 mmHg

POSTOPERATIVE

Complications	N/V Corneal abrasion Aspiration pneumonitis Photophobia Diplopia Hemorrhagic retinopathy	Rx: Metoclopramide 10 mg iv, droperidol 0.625, ondansetron 4 mg iv. Provide O_2 by face mask, if not intubated. Follow O_2 saturation. ✓ CXR.
Pain management	Acetaminophen	Occasionally, parenteral opiates (see p. C-1).

References

1. Barash PG, Cullen BF, Stoelting RK, eds: *Clinical Anesthesia, 3rd edition.* JB Lippincott, Philadelphia: 1997.
2. McGoldrick KE, ed: *Anesthesia for Ophthalmic and Otolaryngologic Surgery*. WB Saunders Co, Philadelphia: 1992.
Also see General References following Ophthalmic Surgery section.

STRABISMUS SURGERY

SURGICAL CONSIDERATIONS

Description: Strabismus surgery is performed on patients with ocular malalignment, and involves lengthening or shortening individual muscles or pairs of muscles with an eventual goal of straightening the eyes cosmetically and allowing binocular vision. An incision is made transconjunctivally in the proximity of the muscle being worked on (Fig 2-5A). The muscle is then isolated and either recessed by disinserting it and sewing it further back on the globe, which effectively decreases the muscle tension, or resected (Fig 2-5B) by removing a segment of muscle, which increases its tension. Depending on the pattern of strabismus, oblique muscles are sometimes totally disinserted or partially transected to weaken their action.

Variant procedure or approaches: In adults and very cooperative older children, an **adjustable suture approach** is sometimes used. The muscle is tied in such a way that it can be either lengthened or shortened postop before being tied securely in place.

Usual preop diagnosis: Strabismus

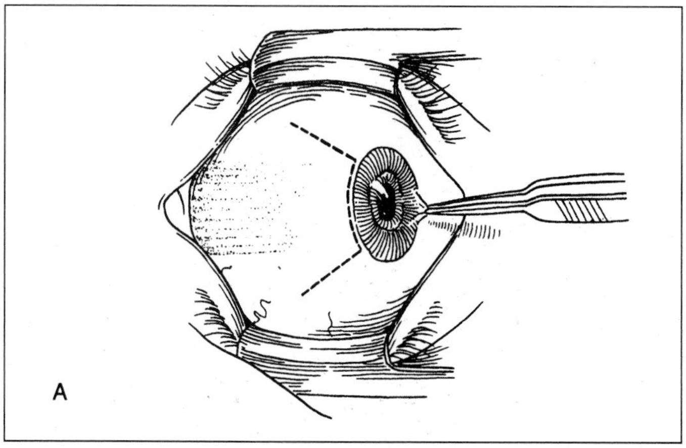

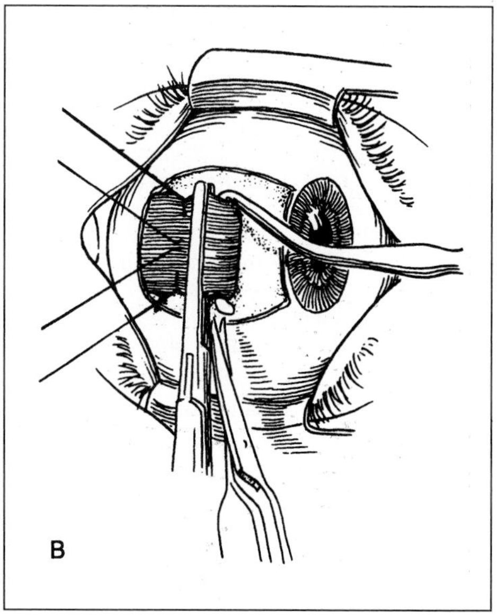

Figure 2-5. (A) Conjunctival incision in region of horizontal rectus muscle. (B) Resection of horizontal rectus muscle – sutures have been passed through muscle prior to its disinsertion from the globe. (Reproduced with permission from Phelps CD: *Manual of Common Ophthalmic Surgical Procedures*. Churchill Livingstone: 1986.)

SUMMARY OF PROCEDURE

Position	Supine
Incision	Transconjunctival (Fig 2-5A)
Antibiotics	Topical antibiotics at end of surgery
Surgical time	0.5-1 h
EBL	Minimal
Mortality	Minimal
Morbidity	Continued malalignment: 30% Infection: < 1%
Pain score	3-4

PATIENT POPULATION CHARACTERISTICS

Age range	Children (most common)
Male:Female	1:1
Incidence	Relatively common (~ 5% of population)
Etiology	Generally idiopathic; ocular muscle palsies may be associated with trauma, inflammation, tumors and local ischemia
Associated conditions	Higher incidence in premature infants and certain congenital syndromes (e.g., Apert and Down syndromes and Crouzon's disease); myopathy; CNS disease (e.g., meningomyelocele, cerebral palsy)

ANESTHETIC CONSIDERATIONS

PREOPERATIVE

In children, strabismus is the most frequent ophthalmic condition requiring surgical repair. Although most patients with this condition are otherwise healthy, there is an increased incidence of strabismus in children with cerebral palsy or meningomyelocele with hydrocephalus. Unlike many adult eye surgeries, which can be performed under regional anesthesia (retrobulbar or peribulbar block), in children, GA is almost always required to ensure good surgical conditions. The anesthesiologist should be aware of the potential problems that are associated with strabismus surgery, including: increased risk of malignant hyperthermia (MH); occurrence of the oculocardiac reflex (OCR); and increased incidence of postop N/V. It has been noted that individuals at risk for MH often have musculoskeletal abnormalities, such as strabismus or ptosis. It is, therefore, important to obtain a thorough family history of anesthetic problems. Avoid the use of succinylcholine since it can induce a tonic contracture of the extraocular muscles, which can interfere with the forced duction test (FDT). The surgeon performs the FDT by grasping the sclera of the operative eye and moving it into each field of gaze in order to determine if the strabismus is a result of paretic or restrictive extraocular muscles. This helps in forming the surgical plan.

Respiratory Surgery should be postponed for patients presenting with Sx of acute URI, and recent fever or chills. These patients may be predisposed to bronchospasm and laryngospasm → difficulty with ventilation and oxygenation. A thorough H&P should be performed.
Tests: As indicated from H&P.

Cardiovascular Patients with associated myopathies may have abnormal cardiac function.
Tests: ECG and ECHO, if indicated from H&P.

Malignant hyperthermia ✓ for personal or family Hx of MH. If patient is MH-susceptible (had previous episodes of MH or had developed masseter spasm [trismus] with succinylcholine), avoid succinylcholine and potent inhalational agents. N_2O also may be a weak triggering agent. "Safe" agents include STP, propofol, pancuronium, droperidol, opiates and benzodiazepines. A "clean" anesthetic machine without vaporizers or one that was flushed overnight with O_2 and has fresh CO_2 absorbent should be used. Dantrolene and ice should be readily available.
Tests: Halothane and caffeine contracture test of skeletal muscle Bx if indicated from H&P.

Laboratory Other tests as indicated from H&P.

Premedication Use midazolam 0.5-0.7 mg/kg po in apple juice or cola (15-30 ml). The child should be made

Premedication, cont.	aware that one or both eyes may have patches on them after the surgery and that blurred or diminished vision may be present during emergence.	

INTRAOPERATIVE

Anesthetic technique: GETA

Induction	Standard mask induction (see p. B-2). Following induction, give atropine 0.02 mg/kg or glycopyrrolate 0.01 mg/kg iv to attenuate the OCR. Surgeons perform a FDT; then the patient is given a nondepolarizing neuromuscular blocker and intubated (oral RAE).	
Maintenance	Standard maintenance (see p. B-3).	
Emergence	To decrease incidence of postop emesis, administer metoclopramide 0.1 mg/kg iv about 30 min prior to end of surgery; suction stomach while patient is deeply anesthetized. The common occurrence of postop N/V requires the administration of intraop antiemetics.	
Blood and fluid requirements	IV: 20 or 22 ga × 1 NS/LR @ 5-10 ml/kg/h Warm fluids, humidify gasses.	
Monitoring	Standard monitors (see p. B-1).	
Positioning	✓ and pad pressure points. ✓ eyes.	
Complications	OCR → ↓↓HR, ↓↓BP	OCR is triggered by pressure, pain and/or traction on ocular or periocular structures. The most common cardiac dysrhythmia is bradycardia. Others that are seen include junctional rhythm, multifocal PVCs, AV block, VT and asystole. Rx: D/C stimulus, provide adequate depth of anesthesia and consider atropine (7 μg/kg iv) for refractory bradycardia. Lidocaine infiltration near the eye muscles may be helpful. With repeated manipulation, the OCR often fatigues.
	Malignant hyperthermia (MH)	Consider MH if the following are noted: unexplained tachycardia; ↑$ETCO_2$; muscular rigidity, masseter spasm; ↑temperature (a late sign). To evaluate, obtain ABGs. MH produces ↓PaO_2, ↑$PaCO_2$, ↑K^+ and acidosis. If MH is suspected, stop anesthetics and change anesthetic tubing and CO_2 absorbent. Stop surgery as soon as possible, hyperventilate patient with 100% O_2, treat acidosis with bicarbonate, and treat hyperkalemia (e.g., 15 U regular insulin/50 g glucose). Give dantrolene 2.5 mg/kg iv as soon as possible. Also cool the patient and maintain UO. Further doses of dantrolene may be necessary (can give up to 10 mg/kg).

POSTOPERATIVE

Complications	N/V	Rx: Metoclopramide 10 mg iv, droperidol 0.625 mg iv, ondansetron 4 mg iv.
	MH	See discussion above.
Pain management	Acetaminophen suppositories 15-20 mg/kg q 4-6 h	

References

1. Barash PG, Cullen BF, Stoelting RK, eds: *Clinical Anesthesia, 3rd edition.* JB Lippincott, Philadelphia: 1997.
2. McGoldrick KE, ed: *Anesthesia for Ophthalmic and Otolaryngologic Surgery.* WB Saunders Co, Philadelphia: 1992.
3. McGoldrick KE, Mardirossian J: Ophthalmic Surgery. In *Ambulatory Anesthesiology: A Problem Oriented Approach.* Williams & Wilkins, Baltimore: 1995, 507-35.

DACRYOCYSTORHINOSTOMY (DCR)

SURGICAL CONSIDERATIONS

Description: Dacryocystorhinostomy (DCR) is performed in patients who have chronic epiphora or dacryocystitis 2° obstruction at the level of the nasolacrimal duct. The goal is to create a new drainage path for tears from the lids to the nose. A 15 mm incision is made on the side of the nose near the medial canthus (Fig 2-6). A subperiosteal dissection is made to the lacrimal sac and the lacrimal sac is identified. The thin bone separating the lacrimal fossa from the middle fossa of the nose is broken and rongeured to make a 10-15 mm-diameter opening. The mucosa of the lacrimal sac is then anastomosed to the mucosa of the nose. Sometimes a silicone tube is placed through the lacrimal canaliculi through the anastomosis and tied in the nose to prevent closure by scarring. The wound closure is a simple skin closure.

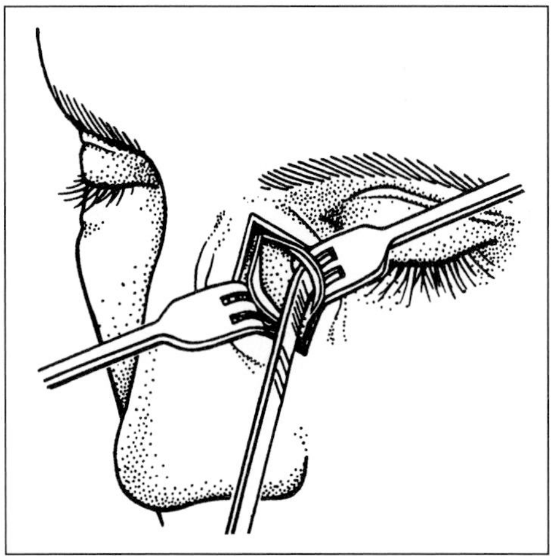

↑**Figure 2-6.** Incision site. (Reproduced with permission from Levine MR, ed: *Manual of Oculoplastic Surgery*. Churchill Livingstone: 1988.)

Variant procedure or approaches: In certain older patients with recurrent dacryocystitis 2° nasolacrimal duct (NLD) blockage, epiphora may not be a problem because of concomitant low-tear production. In these cases, it may be possible to do a **dacryocystectomy** or **tear-sack resection** without making a new passage into the nose. When blockage to tear drainage is at the level of the canaliculi, it may be necessary to do a **conjunctivorhinostomy** with insertion of a Jone's tube (Fig 2-7). The initial steps for this procedure are essentially the same as those for the DCR; however, the canaliculi are bypassed by inserting a small Pyrex tube through the conjunctiva in the region of the caruncle (which is excised) so that it passes through the bony opening, with the nasal-to-lacrimal-sac anastomosis and into the nose. There is a congenital form of NLD obstruction which generally occurs at the level of the nose. Often the obstruction will decrease with time; however, if it persists, a **NLD probing** may be done. This involves passing a bent wire from the upper and lower puncti through the canaliculi, tear sac, nasolacrimal duct and then into the nose. At times, a Silastic stent is also passed through the lacrimal drainage tract and left in place for several months.

Usual preop diagnosis: Occlusion of the nasal lacrimal duct

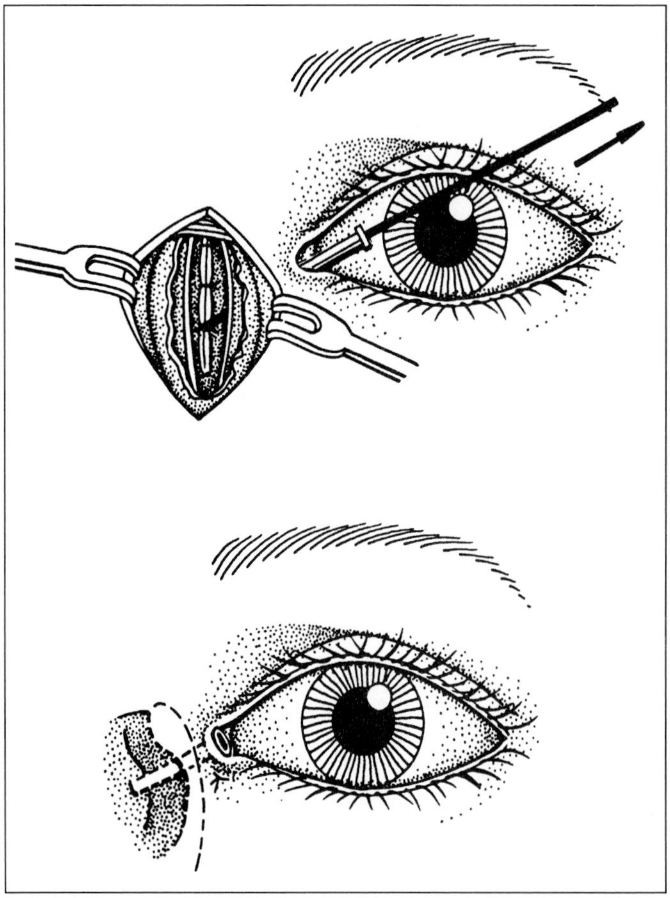

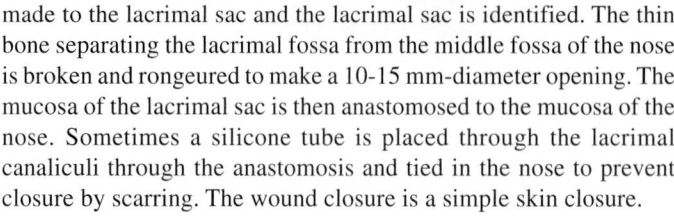

←**Figure 2-7**. Insertion of a Pyrex Jone's tube into the region of the caruncle for **conjunctivorhinostomy** procedure. (Reproduced with permission from Levine MR: *Manual of Oculoplastic Surgery*. Churchill Livingstone: 1988.)

SUMMARY OF PROCEDURE

Position	Supine
Incision	2 cm at side of nose (Fig 2-6)
Special instrumentation	Headlight; bone equipment
Unique considerations	Nasal pack with vasoconstrictor used at start of procedure. Blood often drains into throat during surgery.
Antibiotics	IV antibiotics at time of surgery, followed by a short course of oral antibiotics, used by some surgeons.
Surgical time	1-1.5 h
EBL	100 ml; may be considerably larger from unusual nasal or ethmoid bleeding that is difficult to stop.
Postop care	Usually outpatient; may have bleeding from nose, especially in children.
Mortality	Minimal
Morbidity	Bleeding from nose: 5% Infection: < 1%
Pain score	2

PATIENT POPULATION CHARACTERISTICS

Age range	30-70 yr
Male:Female	1:1
Incidence	Fairly common
Etiology	Infection in nasolacrimal duct

ANESTHETIC CONSIDERATIONS

See Anesthetic Considerations following Orbitotomy – Anterior and Lateral, p. 112.

References

See General References following Ophthalmic Surgery section, p. 116.

ENUCLEATION

SURGICAL CONSIDERATIONS

Description: Enucleation involves removal of the entire globe and a portion of the optic nerve. The overlying conjunctiva, Tenon's fascia and extraocular muscles are left behind and then sewn over the orbital implant to keep it in position and give it motility. The procedure starts with a 360° conjunctival incision adjacent to the cornea. The conjunctiva and Tenon's fascia are dissected from the sclera and the four rectus muscles are cut from the globe, passing suture through the cut ends so that the muscles may be sewn over or onto the implant later. With outward traction on the eye, the oblique muscles are cut, the optic nerve is sectioned and the globe is removed. The empty socket is tamponaded for 2-5 minutes or until all bleeding has stopped. An implant, commonly a polyethylene sphere, is selected and Tenon's fascia and conjunctiva, along with the recti muscles, are sewn securely closed over it. An alternative implant is a hydroxyapatite (coral) sphere which, because of its roughness, is frequently covered with eye bank sclera or temporalis fascia harvested at the time of enucleation.

Variant procedure or approaches: Evisceration involves removing the intraocular contents and leaving behind the scleral shell with the attached extraocular muscles. It affords better motility but there is increased risk of sympathetic ophthalmia (an autoimmune condition which may affect the remaining eye, causing severe inflammation) and it should not be performed for tumor removal because of the increased chances of incomplete removal.

Usual preop diagnosis: Blind eye 2° to trauma or end-stage glaucoma; to decrease risk of sympathetic ophthalmia or for pain relief; intraocular tumors such as melanoma or retinoblastoma; endophthalmitis with total loss of vision

SUMMARY OF PROCEDURE

Position	Supine
Incision	360° conjunctival incision
Antibiotics	Topical antibiotics at end of case
Surgical time	1-1.5 h
EBL	Approx 20 ml
Mortality	Minimal
Morbidity	Infection: < 1%
Pain score	6

PATIENT POPULATION CHARACTERISTICS

Age range	Any age, although trauma requiring enucleation is more frequent in young males
Male:Female	Male > Female
Incidence	Relatively common
Etiology	Trauma; ocular tumors; phthisis
Associated conditions	In the past, rubeotic glaucoma in patients with diabetes mellitus was a common cause for enucleation; fortunately, this complication is less frequently found.

ANESTHETIC CONSIDERATIONS

See Anesthetic Considerations following Orbitotomy – Anterior and Lateral, p. 112.

References

See General References following Ophthalmic Surgery section, p. 116.

ORBITOTOMY—ANTERIOR AND LATERAL

SURGICAL CONSIDERATIONS

Description: Surgical access to the orbit may be necessary to biopsy or remove an orbital tumor, repair orbital fractures, drain an orbital abscess or remove a foreign body. For the purpose of surgery, the orbit may be divided into several compartments (Fig 2-8), including the peripheral surgical space, subperiosteal space, sub-Tenon's space and central surgical space. The particular approach to the orbit depends on the lesion's location, size and suspected pathology. In general, anterior orbitotomy is used to biopsy lesions throughout the orbit or remove small tumors from the anterior orbit. A lateral orbitotomy is generally required for larger, more posteriorly located tumors, and when complete exposure of the lacrimal gland is required. Occasionally, a combined anterior and lateral approach is used for very extensive lesions.

Anterior orbitotomies are generally approached in three basic ways. The **transconjunctival approach** is used for lesions in the sub-Tenon's space. The area within the muscle cone also can be reached by disinserting the lateral or medial rectus muscles. This, for example, would be a common approach for biopsy or decompression of the optic nerve.

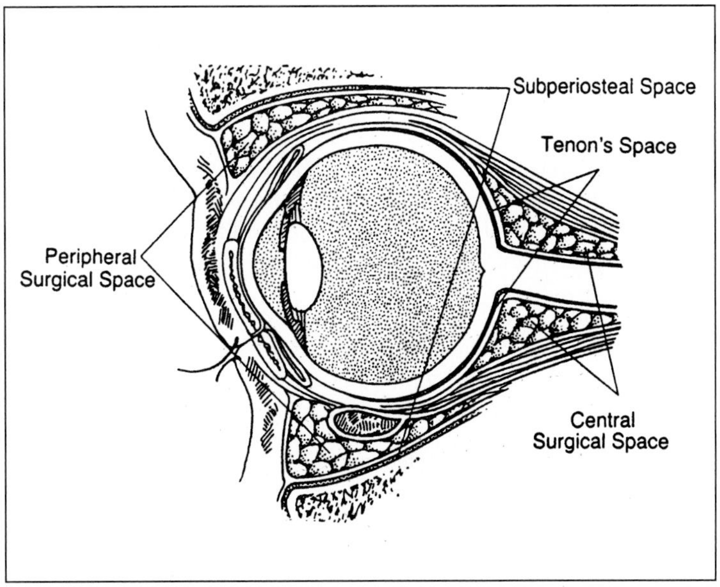

Figure 2-8. Orbital compartments. (Reproduced with permission from Levine MR: *Manual of Oculoplastic Surgery*. Churchill Livingstone, 1988.)

The **transseptal approach** is particularly useful for anteriorly located tumors palpable through the eyelids. The incision is made through the skin and orbital septum directly into the peripheral orbital space. It is often used for lesions such as hemangiomas, lymphomas and dermoids. Finally, the **transperiosteal** or **extraperiosteal approach** is used primarily for lesions along the superior, medial or inferior orbital walls or within the frontal or ethmoid sinuses. A skin incision is made just outside the orbital rim in the desired quadrant. Periosteum is identified and incised and then reflected from the orbital margin and wall. It is the common approach for orbital wall fractures, and mucoceles of the frontal or ethmoid sinuses. It is also used for drainage of subperiosteal hematomas or abscesses and for orbital decompression in thyroid disease.

Variant procedure or approaches: Lateral orbitotomies involve removing a portion of the bone from the lateral wall to give access to the retrobulbar space. It is also the only approach which gives complete exposure of the lacrimal gland, a necessity in removing certain tumors. A skin incision is made over the lateral brow and extended to the zygomatic arch. Dissection is carried out down to the periosteum, which is then incised along the lateral orbital rim and reflected. The lateral bony wall is removed using a saw and rongeurs, and the inner periosteum (periorbital) is opened to expose the orbit. After removal or biopsy of the lesion, the bone is wired back into place and the wound closed in layers.

Usual preop diagnosis: Tumors such as hemangiomas, inflammatory pseudotumors, lymphomas, lacrimal gland tumors, rhabdomyosarcoma; trauma resulting in orbital wall fractures or retained foreign body; infection with abscess formation

SUMMARY OF PROCEDURE

Position	Generally supine. May have head slightly elevated to reduce venous pressure and rotate face away from the operative site when using the lateral approach.
Incision	Variable (see above).
Special instrumentation	Operating microscope sometimes used for deep orbitotomies, especially when working around optic nerve.
Antibiotics	Variable; some surgeons use iv antibiotics both prophylactically and following surgery.
Surgical time	1-3 h
EBL	Usually minimal; may be considerable if vascular tumor and extensive dissection are involved.
Mortality	Minimal
Morbidity	Decreased ocular motility Secondary infection Loss of vision
Pain score	3-6

PATIENT POPULATION CHARACTERISTICS

Age range	Any age
Male:Female	1:1
Incidence	Rare
Etiology	Tumor; trauma; infection

ANESTHETIC CONSIDERATIONS

(Procedures covered: dacryocystorhinostomy (DCR); enucleation; anterior and lateral orbitotomy.)

PREOPERATIVE

Patients presenting for DCR, enucleation and orbitotomy represent a diverse population. These patients are generally healthy, aside from the infection, tumor or trauma underlying their ocular or periocular pathology. Preop evaluation should focus on possible coexisting disease and the systemic manifestations of previous therapeutic intervention (e.g., chemotherapy and drugs used to treat glaucoma).

Laboratory	Tests as indicated from H&P.	
Premedication	Standard premedication (see p. B-2).	

INTRAOPERATIVE

Anesthetic technique: GETA.

Induction	Standard induction (see p. B-2). An oral RAE ETT may be preferred.	
Maintenance	Standard maintenance (see, p. B-3). Muscle relaxation is not required.	
Emergence	No special considerations. The common occurrence of postop N/V requires the administration of intraop antiemetics (e.g., metoclopramide 10 mg iv, droperidol 0.625 mg iv or ondansetron 4 mg iv).	
Blood and fluid requirements	Blood loss variable IV: 18 ga × 1 NS/LR @ 4-6 ml/kg/h	
Monitoring	Standard monitors (see p. B-1).	
Positioning	Table rotated 90° ✓ and pad pressure points. ✓ nonoperated eye.	
Complications	Oculocardiac reflex (OCR) → ↓↓HR	See discussion in Anesthetic Considerations for Strabismus Surgery, p. 107.

POSTOPERATIVE

Complications	N/V	Rx: Metoclopramide 10 mg iv, droperidol 0.625 mg iv, ondansetron 4 mg iv.
Pain management	Acetaminophen	Occasionally parenteral opiates (see p. C-1).

RETINAL SURGERY

SURGICAL CONSIDERATIONS

Michael W. Gaynon

Description: Retinal surgery is performed for: retinal detachment; vitreous hemorrhage or opacification; macular epiretinal membranes or other surgically correctable macular conditions; dislocated intraocular lenses; endophthalmitis; and posterior segment trauma, including repair of ruptured globes and removal of intraocular foreign bodies. Most retinal detachments are due to one or more small tears in the retina caused by traction following a vitreous separation. Less commonly, retinal detachments are induced by vitreoretinal traction or by trauma, which may involve an open globe. Care must be taken to avoid any increase in intraocular pressure (IOP) in an eye which may harbor a rupture. On rare occasion, a retinal detachment is due to the formation of a giant retinal tear. Just as rarely, retinal surgery is done on premature infants in an effort to prevent or repair retinal detachments. The ultimate aim of retinal surgery is the preservation or recovery of vision through the restoration of normal posterior segment anatomy. (Anatomy of the eye shown in Fig 2-9.)

Retinal surgery may involve various procedures alone or in combination, including scleral buckling, vitrectomy, gas-fluid exchange, and injection of vitreous substitutes. **Scleral buckles** are silicone rubber appliances sutured to the sclera to indent the eye wall, thereby relieving vitreous traction and functionally closing retinal tears. This is an external procedure in which the eye may either not be entered at all or entered with a small needle puncture through the sclera for drainage of subretinal fluid.

Vitrectomy is an intraocular procedure in which three 20-ga openings are made into the vitreous cavity with a myringotomy blade 3-4 mm posterior to the limbus (junction of the cornea and sclera.) One of these openings in the inferotemporal quadrant is used for infusion of balanced salt solution via a sutured cannula. The remaining openings are at the 9:30 and 2:30 o'clock positions. One is used for a hand-held fiber optic light; the other, for insertion of a variety of manual and automated instruments, including suction cutters, scissors and forceps used to remove and section abnormal tissue within the vitreous cavity.

Visualization of the retina during vitrectomy is made possible by a contact lens, which is either sutured to the eye or held in position by the assistant. Balanced salt solution replaces the vitreous and other tissues removed during the operation. A bubble of gas is sometimes introduced into the vitreous cavity during a scleral buckle or a vitrectomy when the surgeon wants an internal tamponade of retinal tears which cannot be adequately closed by a scleral buckle alone.

In the case of a giant retinal tear, a **gas-fluid exchange** formerly was performed with the patient in the prone position toward the end of the operation. This required that the patient be on a Stryker frame, so that he or she could be moved from the supine to the prone position for the gas-fluid exchange. Perfluorocarbon liquids now obviate the need for a Stryker frame.

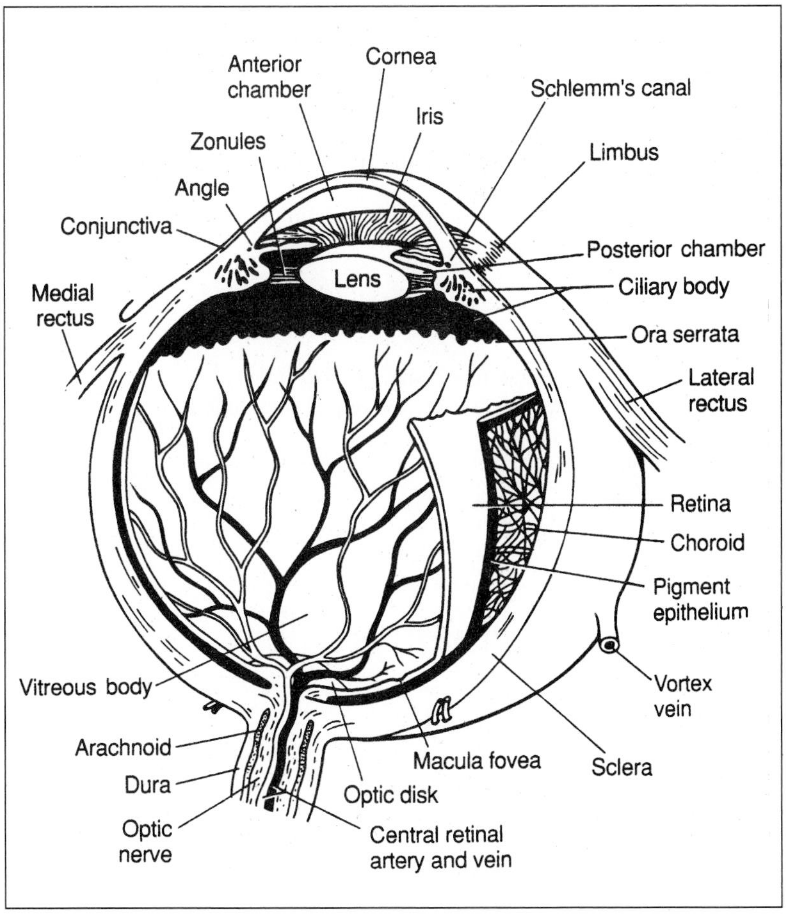

Figure 2-9. Eye anatomy. (Reproduced with permission from Langstom D, ed: *Manual of Ocular Diagnosis and Therapy*. Little, Brown, New York: 1985. Adapted from Peck P: *Anatomy of the Eye*. Lederle Laboratories, Pearl River, NY.)

Liquid vitreous substitutes, such as perfluorocarbon liquids or silicone oil, are sometimes introduced into the vitreous cavity during a vitrectomy. Perfluorocarbon liquids are heavier than water and are used as an intraop tool to unfold the detached retina; they are then removed at the end of the procedure. Perfluorocarbon liquids make possible repair of giant retinal tears in the supine position, thus eliminating the need for a Stryker frame. Silicone oil is used for complex detachments in which a long-term, internal tamponade of retinal tears is deemed necessary to prevent redetachment. It sometimes is removed a few months postop with a second operation. Cryotherapy or lasers are used frequently to establish chorioretinal adhesions around retinal tears. Cryotherapy is applied to the sclera; a laser is applied with a fiber optic cable introduced into the vitreous cavity during vitrectomy surgery. It also can be administered with an indirect ophthalmoscope delivery system for those eyes not undergoing vitrectomy.

Simple detachments frequently can be repaired by a **pneumatic retinopexy**, in which retinal tears are treated with cryotherapy or laser and an expanding gas is injected into the vitreous cavity. This technique is usually done in phakic eyes (which have not undergone cataract extraction) with tears in the superior 8 clock hours (clockwise from 8-4 o'clock). Pneumatic retinopexy usually is done as an outpatient office procedure, with local anesthesia or MAC. The other procedures discussed are done with MAC or GA, according to surgeon's preference and patient's systemic condition. Some surgeons inject retrobulbar or subconjunctival bupivacaine at the end of a procedure done under GA to decrease postop pain.

Usual preop diagnosis: Retinal detachment; diabetic retinopathy; vitreous hemorrhage or opacification; epiretinal membrane; ruptured globe; retinopathy of prematurity (ROP)

SUMMARY OF PROCEDURE

Position	Supine
Incision	Transconjunctival
Special instrumentation	Vitrectomy machine; cryoprobe; laser; indirect ophthalmoscope; microscope
Unique considerations	Ruptured globe—avoid increased IOP. Stop N_2O 5-10 min before a gas-fluid exchange.
Antibiotics	May use iv antibiotics at the start of surgery, in addition to subconjunctival antibiotics at conclusion of surgery.
Surgical time	Pneumatic retinopexy: 1 h Scleral buckle: 1-3 h Vitrectomy: 1-4+ h Giant tear: 2-4+ h
Closing considerations	Try to avoid postop bucking or vomiting.
EBL	None
Postop care	Prone positioning, if gas was injected.
Mortality	Extremely rare
Morbidity	Hemorrhage: < 5% Retinal detachment: < 5% Infection: < 1%
Pain score	6

PATIENT POPULATION CHARACTERISTICS

Age range	Usually adults; occasionally premature infants (ROP) and children (retinal detachment or trauma)
Male:Female	1:1
Incidence	1/20,000 phakic; 1/250 pseudophakic (postcataract extraction with placement of intraocular lens)
Etiology	Majority idiopathic; some induced by trauma
Associated conditions	Idiopathic: retinal detachment, epiretinal membrane, macular hole Diabetic retinopathy: vitreous hemorrhage or traction retinal detachment Prior eye surgery: retinal detachment Trauma: vitreous hemorrhage, retinal detachment, ruptured globe HTN: vitreous hemorrhage Extreme prematurity: ROP, retinal detachment

ANESTHETIC CONSIDERATIONS

PREOPERATIVE

Retinal detachments are classified as traction, exudative (not usually treated with surgery) or rhegmatogenous (rupture, tear). Children, especially those with ROP or trauma, may develop retinal detachments. In adults, retinal detachments are most frequently associated with diabetes, myopia, trauma and previous cataract surgery. Rhegmatogenous retinal detachments (more common in adults) start off with a small retinal tear, which allows the vitreous to seep in between the retina and pigment epithelium, forcing retinal separation. Symptoms range from floaters and flashes to showers of black specks and, ultimately, to a dark shadow that impinges on the field of vision. Surgeons prefer a normotensive eye during retinal reattachment surgery and, therefore, patients may be given acetazolamide or mannitol to decrease IOP.

Cardiovascular Mannitol decreases IOP by increasing plasma oncotic pressure relative to aqueous humor pressure.

Cardiovascular, cont.	It is usually given just prior to or during surgery. Total dosage should not exceed 1.5-2 g/kg iv over a 30-60 min period. Rapid infusion of large doses of mannitol may precipitate CHF, pulmonary edema, electrolyte abnormalities, HTN and, possibly, myocardial ischemia; hence, the importance of a thorough evaluation of the patient's renal and cardiovascular status prior to administering mannitol. **Tests:** As indicated from H&P.
Diabetes	Diabetic patients are at increased risk for silent myocardial ischemia. Pulmonary aspiration 2° diabetic gastroparesis is also a risk in this population. Patients usually take 1/2 or 1/3 of their normal NPH insulin dose (on the morning of surgery); fasting blood sugar is checked; and an iv infusion of D5 LR is started if glucose < 90 mg/dl, or treated with regular insulin if glucose > 200 mg/dl. Blood sugar is checked intraop and postop.
Renal	Acetazolamide, a carbonic anhydrase inhibitor, decreases secretion of aqueous humor. It also inhibits renal carbonic anhydrase, thereby facilitating the loss of HCO_3, Na^+, K^+ and water. Thus, patients on chronic therapy may be acidotic, hypokalemic and hyponatremic. **Tests:** Electrolytes; others as indicated from H&P.
Hematologic	✓ for sickle-cell disease. Sickle-cell trait is not commonly associated with perioperative complications. Patients with sickle-cell anemia should be well hydrated and transfused preop, as necessary to increase HbA concentration > 40%.
Laboratory	Tests as indicated from H&P.
Premedication	Midazolam 0.5 mg po for pediatric patients, and midazolam 1-2 mg iv incrementally for adults, to alleviate anxiety. Avoid excessive sedation (respiratory depression) in sickle-cell patients.

INTRAOPERATIVE

Anesthetic technique: Retinal detachment surgery may be performed under regional anesthesia, but some anesthesiologists prefer GETA, especially if the surgery is expected to be > 2 h.

Induction	Standard induction (see p. B-2) is appropriate for these patients, with care being taken not to put pressure on the affected eye with the face mask.
Maintenance	Standard maintenance (see p. B-3). Ophthalmologists, however, may use expanding gases such as sulfur hexafluoride (SF_6) or perfluoropropane (C_3F_8) for internal tamponade of the retinal breaks; and if N_2O is used, the injected bubble may expand rapidly, causing a dramatic rise in IOP. This can impair retinal blood flow. N_2O should be discontinued at least 15 min before gas injection. If patient needs a second surgery and GA after the first gas injection, N_2O should be avoided for 5 d for air injection, 10 d for SF_6 injection, 15-30 d for C_3F_8. Nondepolarizing muscle relaxants may be advantageous, especially if N_2O is discontinued.
Emergence	Use narcotics for pain control and iv lidocaine 1.0-1.5 mg/kg 5 min prior to extubation to provide smooth emergence. The common occurrence of postop N/V requires the administration of intraop antiemetics (e.g., metoclopramide 10 mg iv, droperidol 0.625 mg iv, or ondansetron 4 mg iv 30 min before the end of surgery).

Blood and fluid requirements	IV: 18 ga × 1 (adult) 20 ga × 1 (child) NS/LR @ 4-6 ml/kg/h	Keep sickle-cell patients well hydrated, oxygenated and warm to avoid sickle-cell crisis.
Monitoring	Standard monitors (see p. B-1).	
Positioning	✓ and pad pressure points. ✓ and pad nonsurgical eye.	Careful padding and frequent repositioning will help avoid circulatory stasis in sickle-cell patients.
Complications	Oculocardiac reflex (OCR)	See Intraoperative Complications under Anesthetic Considerations for Strabismus Surgery, p. 107.

POSTOPERATIVE

Complications	N/V Corneal abrasion Vitreous hemorrhage Glaucoma	Rx: Metoclopramide 10 mg iv, droperidol 0.625 iv, or ondansetron 4 mg iv; however, eye pain (e.g., 2° to corneal abrasion) may also cause N/V. If this is the case, treat pain also (ophthalmology consult).

Complications, cont.	Ptosis Diplopia Loss of vision Infection	
Pain management	Meperidine 0.5-1 mg/kg/h iv Retrobulbar anesthesia	Avoid excessive sedation in sickle-cell patients.
Tests	None routinely required.	

References

1. Barash PG, Cullen BF, Stoelting RK, eds: *Clinical Anesthesia*, 3rd edition. Lippincott-Raven, Philadelphia: 1997.
2. McGoldrick KE, ed: *Anesthesia for Ophthalmic and Otolaryngologic Surgery*. WB Saunders Co, Philadelphia: 1992.
3. Ryan SJ, ed: *Retina, 2nd edition.* CV Mosby Co, St. Louis: 1994.

General Ophthalmology References

1. Levine MR, ed: *Manual of Oculoplastic Surgery*, 2nd edition. Butterworth-Heinmann, New York: 1996.
2. Phelps CD, Hansjoerg EJ, eds: *Manual of Common Ophthalmic Surgical Procedures.* Churchill Livingstone, New York: 1986.
3. Spaeth GL, ed: *Ophthalmic Surgery: Principles and Practice*, 2nd edition. WB Saunders Co, Philadelphia: 1990.
4. Nesi FA, Smith BC, eds: *Ophthalmic Plastic and Reconstructive Surgery*, 2nd edition. Mosby-Year Book. St. Louis: 1997.
5. Waltman SR, Keates RH, Hoyt CS, Frueh BR, Herschler J, Carroll DM, eds: *Surgery of the Eye.* Churchill Livingstone, New York: 1988.

Surgeons

Willard E. Fee, Jr., MD
David J. Terris, MD
Edward C. Gabalski, MD
Robert J. Troell, MD (*Sleep-disordered breathing*)
Robert W. Riley, DDS, MD (*Sleep-disordered breathing*)
Nelson B. Powell, MD (*Sleep-disordered breathing*)
Kasey K. Li, DDS, MD (*Sleep-disordered breathing*)
Joseph B. Roberson, MD (*Skull base surgery*)

3.0 OTOLARYNGOLOGY—HEAD AND NECK SURGERY

Anesthesiologists

John G. Brock-Utne, MD, PhD, FFA(SA)
Raymond R. Gaeta, MD
Edward R. Baer, MD (*Skull base surgery*)
Michael W. Champeau, MD (*Sleep-disordered breathing*)

OTOLARYNGOLOGY—HEAD AND NECK SURGERY

INTRODUCTION—SURGEON'S PERSPECTIVE

AIRWAY COMPETITION

Induction and maintenance of anesthesia for surgery of the head and neck requires interdisciplinary cooperation. Thorough communication both preop and intraop is required for a satisfactory outcome. Of necessity, anesthesiologists cannot have control of the head for many of the cases and competition for the airway produces some anxiety on the part of both physicians. For many procedures, head movement is the norm and unless the tube is properly secured, extubation can occur. Inflammatory or neoplastic lesions of the upper aerodigestive tract produce some degree of airway obstruction and may make intubation extremely difficult—in some cases impossible—necessitating tracheostomy under local anesthesia before induction of GA. Airway obstruction upon induction of anesthesia can occur even with seemingly simple procedures such as tonsillectomy. Communication between the surgeon and anesthesiologist is crucial to assure success.

PREMEDICATION

There are few areas in surgery that have as many functional and/or cosmetic consequences as surgery of the head and neck. The properly informed patient understands the consequences and comes to the OR with a certain degree of anxiety. For oral cavity procedures or endoscopy, a drying agent facilitates performance of the procedure, making a combination of morphine or meperidine and scopolamine the agents of choice for people < 70 years. A small percentage of patients > 70 years of age will have a postscopolamine psychosis that will be unpleasant for all concerned. For that reason, atropine or glycopyrrolate is substituted. Anxiolytics must be used with great caution to avoid airway compromise.

TUBES AND TUBE SIZE

Seldom is there a need for anything larger than a size 6.0 mm ETT. The surgeon may need to lift the tube to examine the larynx adequately, and having to move a larger tube around can be difficult. For procedures on the oral cavity and pharynx, or for endoscopy, a cuffed tube is required to prevent anesthesia blow-by or aspiration of blood into the tracheobronchial tree. If a mouth gag is utilized, an anode or armored tube should be used to prevent compression of the tube by the gag. Although rare, anode tube obstruction does occur, and constant vigilance is required. If intraoral or laryngeal surgery is performed with the laser, compatible ETTs must be used to prevent ignition of the tubes, resulting in intratracheal or laryngeal fires. Maintenance of anesthesia for laser cases should be performed without N_2O and with $FiO_2 < 0.3$. If FiO_2 must be raised beyond that for any reason, the laser should not be used until the $FiO_2 < 0.3$.

MUSCLE RELAXATION

In some cases, muscle relaxation is mandatory; in others, it is contraindicated. In the case of parotidectomy, visual or monitored facial muscle movements are required; thus, no muscle relaxant is indicated. In the case of rigid esophagoscopy, muscle relaxation is often helpful in passing through the cricopharyngeal muscle. As a matter of habit, it is best to ask, as there is nothing more frustrating than having to wait for muscle relaxation to wear off before proceeding.

PATIENT POSITIONING

It is rare that anything other than the supine position is used. Prior to induction, the shoulders should always be at the break in the table so that head and neck can be flexed and/or extended as required intraop. This is especially true for endoscopy. A reverse Trendelenburg position is utilized for esophagoscopy to prevent gastric contents from seeping into the esophagus and slowing down the performance of the procedure. For most major head and neck procedures, elevating the head to ~30° increases venous return, decreases blood loss and expedites the procedure.

HYPOTENSIVE ANESTHESIA

Anything that can be done to reduce blood loss results in faster surgery and less morbidity to the patient. One-third of the anatomy of the entire body is concentrated in the head and neck, and most surgical procedures are designed to preserve function, making some dissections quite tedious. Anything that can be done to maintain relative hypotension is very much appreciated by the surgeon (SBP = 80-100 mmHg is desirable). True hypotensive anesthesia is usually only required for excisions of angiofibromas, AV malformations, hemangiomas or glomus tumors.

TONSILLECTOMY AND/OR ADENOIDECTOMY

SURGICAL CONSIDERATIONS

Description: The dissection for **tonsillectomy** is carried out with the patient supine, shoulders elevated on a small pillow (Fig 3-1). A mouth gag is inserted; and, if an **adenoidectomy** is being done concurrently, adenoids are removed first, with a curette, and the nasopharynx packed. The tonsillectomy is then accomplished by firmly grasping the upper pole of the tonsil and drawing it medially, allowing a mucosal incision to be made over the anterior faucial pillar. The tonsil is dissected from its bed and removed. A snare may be used to snip the dissected tonsil off at the lower pole. Hemostasis is secured with gauze packs and the use of electrocautery. Packs are removed from the nasopharynx and tonsillar beds before extubation. Tonsillectomy may be combined with **palatopharyngoplasty** in cases of obstructive sleep apnea or stertorous breathing (see p. 157).

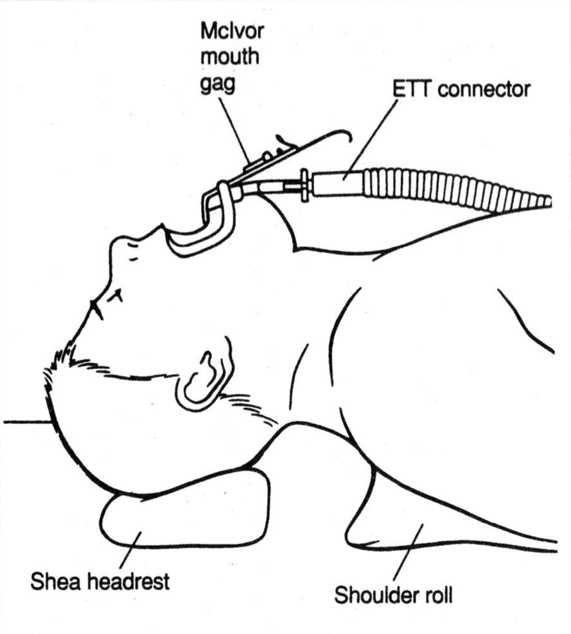

Figure 3-1. The "Rose" position for tonsillectomy.

Variant procedure or approaches: Guillotine technique (rarely used)

Usual preop diagnosis: Chronic tonsillitis and/or adenoiditis (most common); sleep apnea; asymmetric enlargement of tonsils (to rule out cancer); nasal airway obstruction; snoring; peritonsillar abscess

SUMMARY OF PROCEDURE

Position	"Rose" (supine, shoulder roll, head extended); surgeon at head of table (turned 90°-180°)
Incision	Intraoral mucosal
Special instrumentation	Mouth gag (McIvor)
Unique considerations	Use of armored ETT prevents compression of tube by mouth gag. Tube should be secured to lower lip in midline.
Antibiotics	Not used routinely.
Surgical time	30 min-1 h
Closing considerations	If patient has sleep apnea, heightened sensitivity to narcotics and sedatives may make emergence difficult. Avoid hypercapnia on emergence to prevent vasodilation and resultant bleeding. Awake extubation provides maximum airway protection.
EBL	25-200 ml. Monitor suction bottle contents and irrigation as an indication of blood loss.
Postop care	Lateral position; head down; gentle suctioning
Mortality	Rare
Morbidity	Bleeding: 4%[1] Infection: 4% Delayed bleeding: 3.2% Aspiration: Rare Tooth damage: Rare
Pain score	4-6

PATIENT POPULATION CHARACTERISTICS

Age range	2+ yr
Male:Female	1:1
Incidence	750,000 cases/yr in U.S.
Etiology	Chronic infection; sleep apnea; peritonsillar abscess; snoring; cancer
Associated conditions	Nonspecific

ANESTHETIC CONSIDERATIONS

PREOPERATIVE

Most T/A patients are young and otherwise healthy; however, a subset of both pediatric and adult patients may present with Sx of obstructive sleep apnea (OSA) or URI. It is important to distinguish between a child with chronic sniffles and one who presents with an acute URI, which may necessitate postponing an elective surgical procedure. For many children, this is their first anesthetic; therefore, it is imperative to check family Hx for anesthetic problems.

Respiratory Large tonsils and lymphoid hypertrophy may make intubation difficult. In patients presenting with Sx of acute URI (purulent sputum or nasal secretions, fever, etc.), the general recommendation is to postpone any elective procedure until symptoms have abated, usually within 7-14 d. The rationale for postponing surgery includes: the possibility of progression from a URI to a lower respiratory tract infection; presence of secretions which may obstruct the ETT and plug small airways; predisposition to laryngospasm, and ↓respiratory reserve. The patient with OSA is often obese, with a potentially difficult airway, consequent to a short, thick neck, large tongue and redundant pharyngeal tissue. These patients may require an awake FOL.
Tests: As indicated from H&P.

Dental Parents should be informed that loose teeth in pediatric patients may be dislodged/damaged. Physical exam should include a careful dental assessment.

Cardiovascular Rarely, chronic airway obstruction (e.g., OSA) may lead to pulmonary HTN and right heart failure.
Tests: As indicated from H&P.

Musculoskeletal For patients with Down syndrome, neck extension should be avoided to prevent atlantoaxial subluxation. In children with short stature syndrome, including achondroplastic dwarfs and selected cases of Down syndrome, a C1-C2 subluxation and stenosis of the spinal canal may be present. SSEP monitoring may be necessary during intubation and positioning.

Hematologic ✓ for recent aspirin use and Hx of excessive bleeding following minor trauma or tooth extraction.

Laboratory Other tests as indicated from H&P.

Premedication Sedative premedication should be avoided in OSA patients because of their sensitivity to sedative drugs. Otherwise, midazolam iv 0.5 mg/kg po may provide satisfactory preop sedation.

INTRAOPERATIVE

Anesthetic technique: GETA

Induction A standard induction (p. B-2) is suitable for many of these patients; however, in patients with chronic upper airway obstruction, the airway may obstruct following inhalation induction and anesthesia. Use of an oral airway or nasal airway frequently resolves the problem (especially if the mouth is sprayed with local anesthetic prior to induction). In adults with OSA, an awake FOL may be indicated. In patients with peritonsillar abscess, great care must be exercised to prevent rupture of the abscess. Patients with peritonsillar abscess may have trismus. Typically, an oral RAE tube should be used, held in place by means of a mouth gag (Boyle-Davis). Following placement of the gag, the ETT may be dislodged, kinked or inadvertently advanced into a mainstem bronchus. Thus, it is essential to verify tube placement (e.g., chest movement, bilateral and equal breath sounds and normal PIP).

Maintenance Standard maintenance (p. B-3). Muscle relaxation not required.

Emergence At the end of the procedure, the patient should be turned onto the side in the tonsillar position (semiprone, with head down). Patient can be prevented from rolling onto his/her face by using a large pillow beneath the chest, and from rolling supine by extending the lower arm behind the body. Patients are usually extubated awake when protective airway reflexes have returned. Remember to verify removal of throat pack before extubation. Use care when suctioning pharynx.

Blood and fluid requirements
IV: 18 ga × 1 (adult)
20 ga × 1 (child)
NS/LR @ 5-10 ml/kg/h

Blood loss typically averages 4 ml/kg, although it may be difficult to assess 2° drainage into stomach.

Monitoring	Standard monitors (p. B-1).	Careful monitoring of blood loss is important in the pediatric population.
Positioning	✓ and pad pressure points. ✓ eyes.	
Complications	ETT damage/obstruction ETT dislodgement	ETTs (with stylet) of different sizes should be readily available. Readjust Boyle-Davis gag as necessary.

POSTOPERATIVE

Complications	Retention of throat pack	Manifested by severe postop respiratory distress. Under direct laryngoscopy, remove pack with Magill forceps.
	Laryngospasm and/or bronchospasm	A relatively common complication. Rx: 100% O_2 via mask ventilation with jaw thrust and CPAP is generally sufficient. Rapid-sequence induction and direct laryngoscopy/intubation for persistent spasm.
	Bleeding tonsil	This is a serious complication and common cause of mortality following tonsillectomy in children. Sx include ↑HR, ↑RR, ↓BP and pallor. The patient may swallow most of the blood being lost and should be treated as a high risk for aspiration. Blood loss (Hct < 25%) should be replaced, if possible, before reinduction of anesthesia. Following volume resuscitation, anesthesia (etomidate 0.2-0.3 ml/kg or ketamine 1-2 mg/kg) should be induced by rapid-sequence technique with cricoid pressure. Suction must always be available. Before extubation, NG tube should be passed and stomach contents aspirated.
	Postobstructive pulmonary edema	Negative-pressure pulmonary edema is a rare complication; however, it may require reintubation and postop ventilatory support.
Pain management	Meperidine 0.5-1 mg/kg/h iv Acetaminophen suppositories q 4-6 h, 240 mg (4-5 yr), 325-650 mg (10-11 yr)	
Tests	Hct (if blood loss suspected).	Frequent swallowing, especially in children, may be a sign of ongoing hemorrhage.

References

1. Breson K, Diepeveen J: Dissection tonsillectomy—complications and follow-up. *J Laryngol Otol* 1969; 83(6):601-8.
2. Brown BR Jr: *Anesthesia and ENT Surgery*. FA Davis Co, Philadelphia: 1987.
3. Morrison JD: *Anesthesia for Eye, Ear, Nose and Throat Surgery*, 2nd edition. Morrison JD, Mirakhur RK, Craig HJL, eds. Churchill Livingstone, New York: 1985.
4. Randall DA, Hoffer ME: Complications of tonsillectomy and adenoidectomy. *Otolaryngol Head Neck Surg* 1998; 118(1), 61-8.

LARYNGOSCOPY/BRONCHOSCOPY/ESOPHAGOSCOPY

SURGICAL CONSIDERATIONS

Description: **Laryngoscopy** is used for visualization of the pharynx, hypopharynx or larynx for diagnostic and/or therapeutic benefit. The patient is supine with cervical spine flexed and atlantoaxial joint extended (this position is best achieved with a headrest); and the teeth are protected with a mouth guard. The laryngoscope is introduced (Fig 3-2); then, with a lifting motion, a thorough examination of the oropharynx, hypopharynx, laryngopharynx and larynx is carried out and biopsies can be taken. Any bleeding encountered normally can be controlled easily with pressure. Laryngoscopy is often combined with esophagoscopy, bronchoscopy or direct nasopharyngoscopy to survey the aerodigestive tract for malignancy. If the procedure is diagnostic, the surgeon may need to visualize the airway prior to intubation and/or muscle relaxation. If a laser is to be utilized, use of a special laser ETT, < 30% O_2 concentration, and avoidance of N_2O are required.

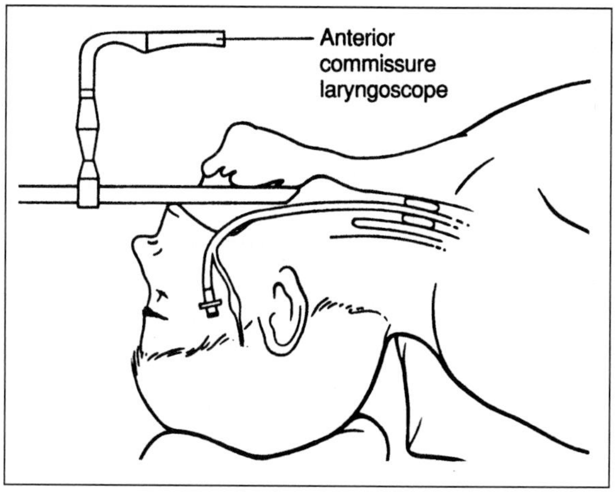

Figure 3-2. Placement of anterior commissure laryngoscope for laryngoscopy.

Usual preop diagnosis: Oropharyngeal, hypopharyngeal or laryngeal tumors

Bronchoscopy is used for visualization of the tracheobronchial tree for both diagnostic and therapeutic purposes. The patient is supine with head elevated and neck extended at the upper cervical level. The bronchoscope is directed along the right side of the tongue forward toward the midline to visualize the epiglottis. Next, the bronchoscope tip is used to lift the epiglottis and advance the bronchoscope through the vocal cords, into the trachea and bronchus (Fig 3-3). The scope can be directed for inspection of the carina, main bronchi and, with the aid of telescopes, the segmental bronchi. This is often performed with direct laryngoscopy, esophagoscopy or as part of **panendoscopy**.

Usual preop diagnosis: Head and neck squamous-cell carcinoma; foreign body in bronchus

Esophagoscopy is used for visualization of the esophagus for either diagnostic or thera-

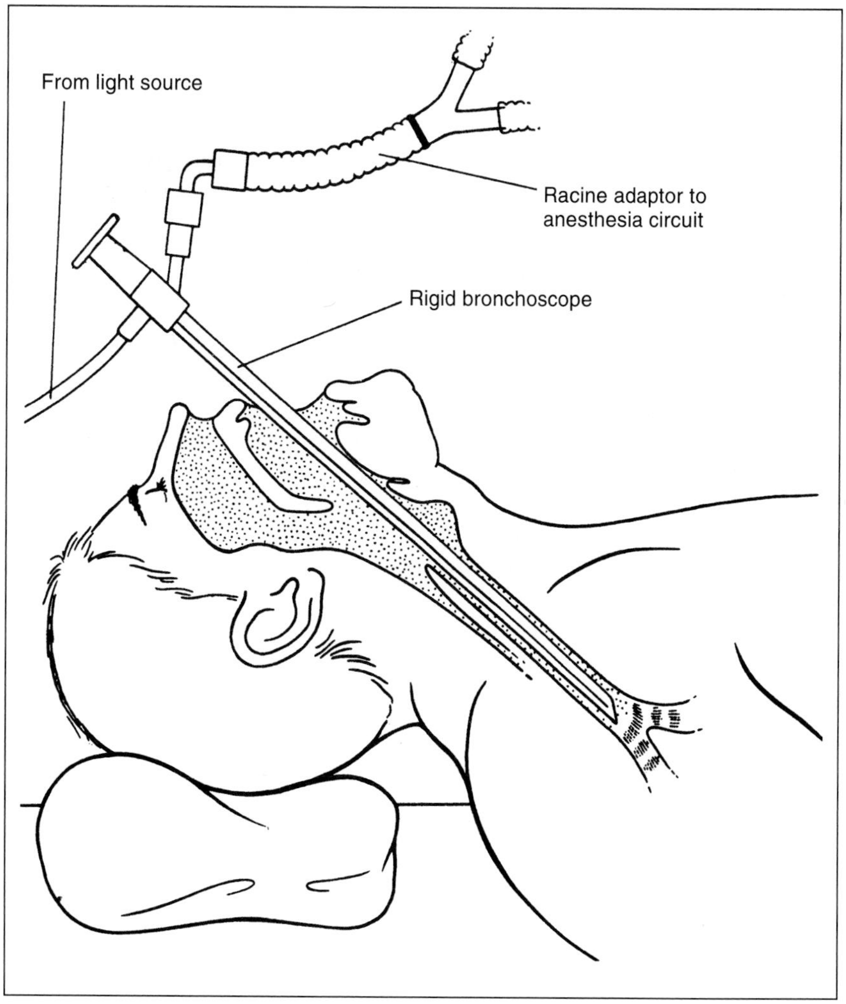

Figure 3-3. Rigid bronchoscopy showing adaptor (Racine) for anesthesia machine. Note neck flexion and head extension to align oropharyngeal and tracheal axes.

peutic benefit. The patient is supine with head elevated and neck extended at the upper cervical level. The esophagoscope (held in the right hand) is advanced through the mouth behind the arytenoids, gently using the left thumb. The bevel of the scope is then used to advance through the cricopharyngeal muscle (upper esophageal sphincter) with an upward lifting movement, entering the cervical esophagus. As the scope advances, the head may have to be lowered or the neck extended and the scope directed slightly toward the left. It should be advanced only when a visible lumen is seen all the way down to the cardia. A biopsy may be taken through the scope. Esophagoscopy also is often performed as part of **panendoscopy**.

Usual preop diagnosis: Head and neck squamous-cell carcinoma; foreign body ingestion

SUMMARY OF PROCEDURE

	Laryngoscopy	Bronchoscopy	Esophagoscopy
Position	Supine; table 90°	⇐	⇐ + Reverse Trendelenburg or head up 30° to prevent gastric reflux
Special instrumentation	Laser ETT; microscope (both used occasionally)	Rigid or flexible bronchoscopes of various sizes. If rigid scope used, an adaptor connects it to anesthesia tubing. If flexible scope used, accessory port adaptor should be connected to the ETT.	Rigid esophagoscope or flexible gastroscope
Unique considerations	Steroids (dexamethasone 4-12 mg) may be helpful if airway is compromised and extensive manipulation or therapeutic procedure required.	With laser ablation, keep O_2 < 30%, avoid N_2O. Bleeding following biopsy or removal of tumors is rare, but may require re-bronchoscopy and suctioning to adequately ventilate the patient.	May need to deflate ETT cuff to introduce scope or retrieve foreign body.
Antibiotics	None	Usually none	None
Surgical time	10 min-1.5 h (diagnostic vs therapeutic)	10-60 min	⇐
EBL	Minimal	⇐	⇐
Postop care	Rarely may require overnight ICU monitoring if airway compromised and no tracheostomy performed.	Usually PACU. If surgery 2° airway obstruction, it may worsen immediately postop, requiring ICU observation.	PACU; may require overnight observation to rule out perforation.
Mortality	< 1%	⇐	< 0.1%
Morbidity	Laryngospasm: < 5%	–	⇐
	Airway obstruction upon induction: 1%	⇐	< 1%
	Damaged teeth: < 1%	1%	⇐
	Laryngeal edema requiring tracheostomy or reintubation: < 1%	Pneumonia: 1%	Perforation of esophagus: 1%
Pain score	1-2	1-2	1-2

PATIENT POPULATION CHARACTERISTICS

Age range	Newborn–old age	⇐	⇐
Male:Female	1:1	⇐	⇐
Incidence	Common	⇐	⇐
Etiology	Neoplasia; foreign bodies; congenital webs/cysts	⇐	⇐

ANESTHETIC CONSIDERATIONS

(Procedures covered: direct laryngoscopy, bronchoscopy, esophagoscopy)

PREOPERATIVE

Attention to airway management is paramount in these procedures. Surgeons and anesthesiologists must share the airway; hence, close communication is essential.

Airway Occult airway compromise may be present in these patients. Airway assessment may require indirect laryngoscopy with topical anesthetic (usually performed by surgeons preop; ✓ surgeon's notes for findings). Patients with lesions in the mediastinum may have involvement of the recurrent laryngeal nerve, with hoarseness, and potential airway management problems (e.g., difficult mask ventilation, difficult intubation, ↑aspiration risk). (See Anesthetic Considerations for Mediastinoscopy, p. 194.)

Respiratory In laryngoscopy/bronchoscopy patients, respiratory function may be impaired. COPD and tobacco use are common. PFTs may show ↓FEV_1, ↓FVC, or ↓FEV_1/FVC ratio. ABGs may demonstrate ↓PaO_2 and/or ↑$PaCO_2$. Lesions of the upper airway may impede intubation and ventilation. For esophagoscopy patients, obstructing lesions of the esophagus can be associated with regurgitation of fluid or particulate matter on induction. Patients requiring urgent endoscopy for GI bleeds or foreign bodies should be considered at risk for aspiration.
Tests: CXR; consider ABG, PFTs, as indicated from H&P.

Dental Patients (or parents, as appropriate) should be informed that loose teeth may be dislodged/ damaged. Physical exam should include a careful dental assessment and documentation.

Cardiovascular Tobacco use (> 40 pack-years) increases the incidence of heart disease. Carefully assess patient, including exercise tolerance. Look for Sx of CAD (e.g., angina) and CHF (e.g., orthopnea, PND, peripheral edema) in patients with cardiac risk factors (including age > 40 yrs, male, HTN, hypercholesteremia, long Hx of smoking, obesity and family Hx). The volume status of debilitated patients who are unable to eat because of obstructing lesions of the esophagus should be assessed.
Tests: Consider ECG, if indicated from H&P. Orthostatic BP and HR changes >10 mmHg, ↓SBP, and/or 15 bpm ↑HR suggest significant (> 20%) hypovolemia.

Neurologic Some patients may have Hx of alcohol abuse which may result in increased anesthetic requirements because of hepatic enzyme induction.

Hematologic Patients with malignancy or chronic disease may have evidence of anemia or coagulopathy.
Tests: Consider CBC, PT, PTT, Plt, as indicated from H&P.

Gastrointestinal In obstructing lesions, a CXR should be obtained for evidence of esophageal dilatation and retained fluids, which may be regurgitated during induction. Hypokalemia and hypomagnesemia should be corrected preop. Patients with malignant tumors may be malnourished.
Tests: CXR; electrolytes

Laboratory LFTs, and others, if indicated from H&P.

Premedication A drying agent (e.g., glycopyrrolate 0.2 mg iv) given preinduction, facilitates panendoscopy; however, ↑HR may be detrimental in those with CAD. Benzodiazepines and/or opiates may be appropriate ★ (see Standard Premedication, p. B- 2). **NB:** Care must be taken not to oversedate these patients.

INTRAOPERATIVE

Anesthetic technique: GETA. The challenge of airway management in these cases requires careful planning and continuous communication with the surgeon. Fiber optic esophagoscopy can be performed under MAC (p. B-4) with appropriate sedation, using short-acting agents, including midazolam, fentanyl or propofol. Rigid esophagoscopy requires GA to provide adequate anesthesia and muscle relaxation.

Induction With a normal airway, standard induction (p. B-2) is appropriate. Any patient at risk for aspiration, however, requires rapid-sequence induction with cricoid pressure. A cuffed ETT should be placed and cricoid pressure released only after the airway is secured. In cases where there is the potential for airway obstruction, an awake fiber optic intubation under topical and transtracheal anesthesia should be performed. Generally, small ETTs (5-6 mm) are used to facilitate visualization of the larynx by the surgical team. For laser cases, a shielded tube, manufactured specifically for laser surgery, is required. The cuff should be filled with NS, rather than air.

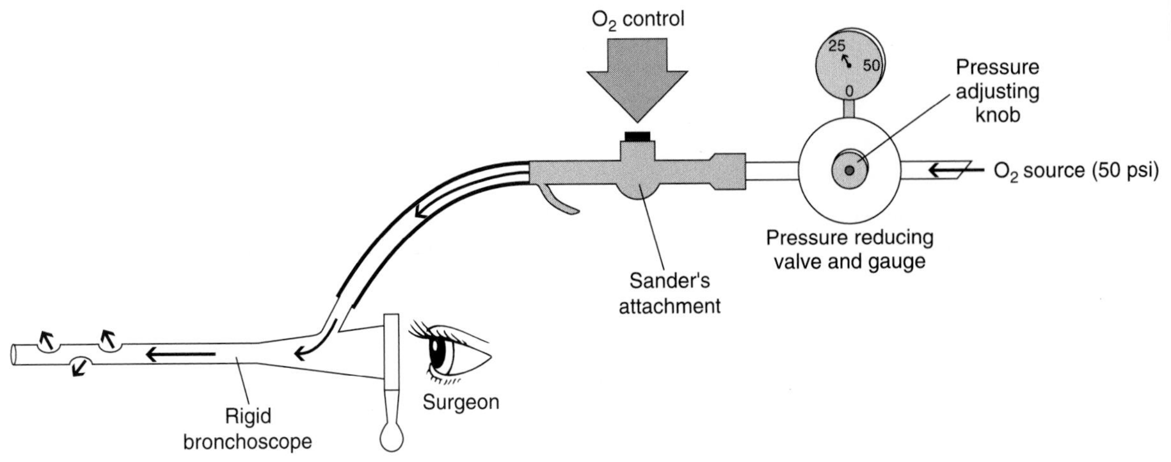

Figure 3-4. Rigid bronchoscope with modified Sanders jet ventilation technique. The wall oxygen supply at 50 psi is connected to a reducing valve that allows the pressure to be adjusted from 0 to 50 psi. The side port of the bronchoscope is used as the Venturi injector site, and the open end can be used for continuous viewing by the endoscopist. (Redrawn with permission from Ehrenwerth J, Burll S: Anesthesia for thoracic diagnostic procedures. In: *Anesthesia*, 2nd edition. Kaplan JA, ed. Churchill Livingstone, New York: 1991, 331.)

Maintenance Standard maintenance (p. B-3) with muscle relaxation and 100% O_2. Anesthesia may be supplemented with iv agent (e.g., fentanyl or meperidine titrated to effect). Ventilation can be achieved by a variety of methods (see discussion below). For laser cases, dilute O_2 (FiO_2 = 0.3) with air, N_2 or helium. High FiO_2 and FiN_2O support combustion. Cover patient's eyes with protective glasses. Complete muscle relaxation is essential during rigid esophagoscopy to prevent esophageal perforation. ETT should be firmly secured and held manually throughout the procedure, as movement of the esophagoscope may dislodge the ETT. Hand ventilation will allow detection of disconnects and/or airway occlusion related to procedure.

Emergence Patient should have full return of protective airway reflexes prior to extubation.

Blood and fluid requirements	IV: GI bleeder: 14-16 ga × 2 Others: 18 ga × 1 NS/LR @ 3-5 ml/kg/h For esophagoscopy: NS/LR @ 4-6 ml/kg/h	Blood loss is usually minimal; however, in case of GI bleed, blood loss may be massive. T&C patient for 2 U PRBC, with blood immediately available in OR.
Monitoring	Standard monitors (p. B-1). ± Arterial line	+ other monitors as indicated by patient condition. In cases of potential hemorrhage, an arterial line is desirable.
Positioning	Table rotated 90° ✓ and pad pressure points. ✓ eyes.	Patient should have a shoulder roll with neck extension to facilitate endoscopy. For flexible fiber optic endoscopy, patients will generally be in the lateral decubitus position.
Ventilation	Small cuffed ETT	The use of a small, cuffed ETT offers the usual advantages of airway protection, controlled ventilation and ease of respiratory gas monitoring. The potential for interfering with surgical visualization, however, may preclude its use.
	Jet ventilation (Sanders attachment) (Fig 3-4)	Jet ventilation in patients with adequate pulmonary compliance will provide good surgical visibility, but it requires iv anesthesia, special equipment, and can cause barotrauma.
	Racine adapter (rigid bronchoscopy) (Fig 3-3)	
	Apneic oxygenation	Apneic oxygenation is limited by ↑$PaCO_2$ (1-2 mmHg/min) producing acidosis and dysrhythmias. Apnea periods should be < 5 min.

Complications	Inadequate ventilation Loss of airway Perforation of airway Pneumothorax Dysrhythmias	Inadequate ventilation → ↑$PaCO_2$, ↓PaO_2 → dysrhythmias. Mechanical or laser perforation of the airway may lead to bronchospasm or uncontrollable hemorrhage.
	Eye trauma Bleeding post biopsy	Eye trauma from surgical instruments used during endoscopy may require ophthalmology consult.
Airway fire	Stop ventilation/clamp ETT. Extinguish fire with NS. Remove ETT. Reestablish airway. Resume ventilation with air until all burning is stopped. Resume 100% FiO_2. ✓ airway for extent of damage. Save tube for later examination.	This is an acute, life-threatening emergency requiring prompt treatment. O_2 and N_2O both support combustion; hence, these need to be turned off while the fire is extinguished. Once the fire is out, ventilation should be resumed with 100% O_2. Replace ETT over tube exchanger. Bronchoscopy is required to ✓ extent of damage and airway edema.

POSTOPERATIVE

Complications	Dental trauma Massive bleeding Eye trauma Esophageal rupture	Dental trauma may result from surgical manipulation of the airway.
	Pneumothorax Pneumomediastinum Hemothorax Coughing Aspiration	Pneumothorax, mediastinal air or hemothorax from esophageal rupture may present as hypotension, cardiovascular collapse or increased airway pressures.
Pain management	Acetaminophen ± opiates	Generally, mild analgesics may be required after a simple endoscopy.
Tests	CXR Hct	For evidence of pneumothorax, hemothorax, mediastinal air.

References

1. Brown BR Jr: *Anesthesia and ENT Surgery.* FA Davis Co, Philadelphia: 1987.
2. Loré JM: *An Atlas of Head and Neck Surgery*, 3rd edition. WB Saunders Co, Philadelphia: 1988.
3. Lyon ST, Holinger LD: Endoscopic evaluation of the patient with head and neck cancer. *Clin Plast Surg* 1985; 12(3): 331-41.
4. Morrison JD: *Anesthesia for Eye, Ear, Nose and Throat Surgery*, 2nd edition. Morrison JD, Mirakhur RK, Craig HJL, eds. Churchill Livingstone, New York: 1985.

NASAL SURGERY

(RHINOPLASTY, SEPTOPLASTY, SEPTORHINOPLASTY)

SURGICAL CONSIDERATIONS

Description: Nasal surgery is performed for either cosmetic or functional restoration of the airway, or both. Functional restoration is usually performed for either congenital or posttraumatic deviations of the septum. The procedure varies in each case, although in all nasal surgery, the nasal cavity is first cocainized with 4% cocaine-soaked pledgets placed in each nostril for 5-10 min. **Septoplasty** (reconstruction of the nasal septum) usually can be carried out under sedation with local anesthesia, using 1% lidocaine with 1:100,000 epinephrine. **Rhinoplasty-septorhinoplasty** is usually carried out under local anesthesia, but if GA is used, a mouth pack is inserted. Local infiltration with 1% lidocaine with 1:100,000 epinephrine is used to ensure vasoconstriction and to minimize bleeding. Intranasal incisions are made and septal problems corrected. Generally, an anterior hemitransfixion incision is made down to the cartilage, and a submucoperichondrial flap is elevated the length of the septum. A similar flap may be elevated on the contralateral side. Bony deformities are resected with an osteotome, while cartilaginous deformities are either resected or weakened by morselizing, either *in situ* or after removal, and then replaced. The incision is closed with interrupted absorbable sutures. In **rhinoplasty**, tip remodelling, hump reduction and bony osteotomies are done to remodel the nasal contour. Surgery on the inferior turbinates in the form of intramural cautery, resection of turbinate bone, resection of turbinate mucosa or, in some cases, complete turbinectomy may be required to produce a satisfactory airway. After the surgery is complete, both nasal cavities are packed and external splints may be used for rhinoplasty and septorhinoplasty cases.

Usual preop diagnosis: Nasal deformity or deviation; deviated septum

SUMMARY OF PROCEDURE

Position	Head up 30° to decrease bleeding. Table may be turned 90°-180°.
Incision	Intranasal, usually; extended only in open septorhinoplasty
Unique considerations	Nose initially cocainized; use of 1% lidocaine with 1:100,000 epinephrine to decrease bleeding.
Antibiotics	Cefazolin 1 g iv; routinely used as long as nasal packs are in place.
Surgical time	1-2.5 h
Closing considerations	Nose often packed postop, necessitating oral airway after extubation.
EBL	50-100 ml (excessive blood loss rare)
Postop care	PACU
Mortality	Minimal
Morbidity	Septal perforation: 5% Bleeding: 4% Infection: 4%
Pain score	4-6

PATIENT POPULATION CHARACTERISTICS

Age range	Young teens–young adults
Male:Female	1:1
Incidence	Common
Etiology	Congenital/traumatic septal and/or nasal deviation

ANESTHETIC CONSIDERATIONS

See Anesthetic Considerations for Nasal and Sinus Surgery, p. 130.

References

1. Niechajev I, Haraldsson PO: Two methods of anesthesia for rhinoplasty in outpatient setting. *Aesthetic Plast Surg* 1996; 20(2):159-63.
2. Sheen JH: *Aesthetic Rhinoplasty*, 2nd edition. Sheen JH, Sheen AD, eds. CV Mosby, St. Louis: 1987.
3. Toriumi DM: Surgical correction of the aging nose. *Facial Plast Surg* 1996; 12(2):205-14.

SINUS SURGERY

(EXTERNAL OR ENDOSCOPIC)

SURGICAL CONSIDERATIONS

Description: Sinus surgery is performed to eliminate infection, polyps or neoplastic conditions that result in obstruction of the sinuses → secondary infection. Providing aeration of the sinuses so that mucous secretion can adequately drain into the nose and nasopharynx is the goal. The patient should be intubated orally and pharynx packed. Nasal mucosa is cocainized with 4% cocaine, and a local injection of 1% lidocaine with 1:100,000 epinephrine is used before making incisions. **Endoscopic sinus surgery** is carried out intranasally using endoscopes with a video monitor. Biting forceps are used to remove polyps, diseased mucosa or biopsy material.

External approaches include: **Caldwell-Luc** (a sublabial approach to the maxillary sinus), **transantral ethmoidectomy**, **external ethmoidectomy**, **transseptal sphenoidectomy**, and **frontal osteoplastic flap** via coronal or brow incision. These procedures accomplish the same end as endoscopic sinus surgery. They involve external incisions and tend to be done for persistent diseases that recur despite intranasal surgery. The **Caldwell-Luc** is performed through an intraoral incision placed in the gingival-buccal sulcus just posterior to the canine fossa. A submucoperiosteal flap is elevated superiorly, exposing the infraorbital nerve. The sinus is entered just inferior to this nerve using a small osteotome. The opening is widened with biting forceps, and the mucosal lining of the diseased sinus is usually exenterated. Typically, a nasoantral window is placed through the inferior meatus to allow additional drainage. The gingival-buccal incision is then closed with interrupted absorbable sutures. The external methods are also the preferred approaches to deal with neoplastic conditions. A craniofacial **combined neurosurgical-external sinus approach** is occasionally required to clear neoplastic nasal and sinus disease. After endoscopic or external sinus surgery, the nose/sinus is usually packed; thus, an oral airway will aid postop mouth breathing on extubation until patient is fully awake.

Usual preop diagnosis: Infection; nasal polyps; neoplasia (benign or malignant)

SUMMARY OF PROCEDURE

Position	Head up 30° (minimizes bleeding). Table may be turned 90°-180°.
Incision	Endoscopic: intranasal. External: sublabial, medial orbital or bicoronal.
Special instrumentation	Nasal endoscopes; video monitor setup; microscope (may be used for external approaches).
Unique considerations	Nose may be packed bilaterally, necessitating use of oral airway on emergence. 1% lidocaine with 1:100,000 epinephrine normally used to decrease bleeding.
Antibiotics	Cefazolin 1 g iv
Surgical time	1-3 h
EBL	50-300 ml (excessive blood loss rarely anticipated). Watch suction bottle and measure irrigation.
Postop care	PACU
Mortality	Minimal
Morbidity	Bleeding: 4%
	Infection: 4%
Pain score	2-4 (4-6 for external approaches)

PATIENT POPULATION CHARACTERISTICS

Age range	Children–adults
Male:Female	1:1
Incidence	Common
Etiology	Infectious; allergic; neoplastic
Associated conditions	Asthma patients most often will benefit from sinus surgery, with reduction in the incidence and/or severity of asthmatic attacks. Rarely, surgery itself may precipitate an asthmatic attack upon emergence or in the immediate postop period. Cystic fibrosis patients may be assisted by postop bronchoscopy at the termination of procedure to facilitate pulmonary toilet in the immediate postop period.

ANESTHETIC CONSIDERATIONS FOR NASAL AND SINUS SURGERY

PREOPERATIVE

These cases are typically elective and can be performed on an outpatient basis.

Respiratory Patients with nasal polyps and asthma often have a hypersensitivity to aspirin, which can precipitate bronchospasm; hence, NSAIDs, including ketorolac, should be avoided. Some patients undergoing nasal surgery may have obstructive sleep apnea (OSA), which can be associated with redundant pharyngeal tissues and/or chronic airway obstruction. (See Anesthetic Considerations for Tonsillectomy and/or Adenoidectomy, p. 121.)

Tests: CXR (to assess for pulmonary HTN); ABGs, PFTs with flow-volume loops in patients with sleep apnea

Cardiovascular The intraop use of topical vasoconstrictors, including cocaine, to control bleeding may result in ↑BP, dysrhythmias, coronary artery spasm and seizures; therefore, a careful evaluation of the cardiovascular system is essential. Patients with OSA may have evidence of cor pulmonale.

Tests: ECG; Consider ECHO, if indicated from H&P.

Premedication Standard premedication (p. B-2). Sedation should be avoided in patients with Hx of OSA.

INTRAOPERATIVE

Anesthetic technique: Rhinoplasty or repair of septal defects is commonly performed under local anesthesia with MAC (p. B-4) and sedation. Other types of nasal and sinus surgery may require GA.

Induction For those procedures done under GA, standard induction (p. B-2) is appropriate. ETT may be taped to one side; if a RAE tube is used, it should be taped in the midline.

Maintenance Standard maintenance (p. B-3).

Emergence The oropharynx should be suctioned under direct vision to avoid aspiration. These patients may have a nasal or pharyngeal pack, which must be removed prior to emergence. Also, patients may have surgical packs placed in the nares, which makes them obligate mouth breathers. Patients should have return of full airway reflexes before extubation.

Blood and fluid requirements	Blood loss generally minimal IV: 18 ga × 1 NS/LR @ 4-6 ml/kg/h	Blood loss controlled with surgical hemostasis and topical applications of vasoconstrictors, including cocaine or epinephrine.
Monitoring	Standard monitors (p. B-1).	
Positioning	Head elevated 30° Table turned 90°-180° ✓ and pad pressure points. ✓ eyes.	Extension tubing for the anesthesia circuit should be available.
Complications	Dysrhythmias	Dysrhythmias related to vasoconstrictor agents may be a problem, particularly in patients with CAD. Halothane should be avoided, if possible, as dysrhythmias may occur with low doses of epinephrine.

POSTOPERATIVE

Complications	Occult postop bleeding	Occult postop bleeding may cause the patient to swallow large quantities of blood, which may be aspirated if a second anesthetic induction is required.
Pain management	Acetaminophen ± codeine or hydrocodone	

References

1. Brown BR Jr: *Anesthesia and ENT Surgery*. FA Davis Co, Philadelphia: 1987.
2. Kennedy DA, Senior BA: Endoscopic sinus surgery: a review. *Otolaryngol Clin North Am* 1997; 30(3):313-30.

3. Morrison JD: *Anesthesia for Eye, Ear, Nose and Throat Surgery*, 2nd edition. Morrison JD, Mirakhur RK, Craig HJL, eds. Churchill Livingstone, New York: 1985.
4. Rice DH: *Endoscopic Paranasal Surgery*. Rice DH, Schaefer SD, eds. Raven Press, New York: 1988.
5. Rontal M, Rontal E, Anon JB: An anatomic approach to local anesthesia for surgery of the nose and paranasal sinuses. *Otolaryngol Clin North Am* 1997; 30(3): 403-20.

EAR SURGERY

SURGICAL CONSIDERATIONS

Description: Surgery on the external ear is performed for reconstruction of a congenitally deformed ear or following trauma, and may therefore involve multiple cosmetic procedures. More commonly, surgery is performed to restore hearing, eliminate infections, remove cholesteatoma or for neoplastic conditions. The surgical approaches, techniques, and instrumentation are highly variable and individualized according to the surgeon; however, anesthesia for ear surgery is relatively generic. Since the facial nerve travels in the temporal bone, most surgeons do not want the patient paralyzed, so that they can either observe or monitor facial nerve function intraop. If **tympanoplasty** (repair of the ear drum) or a **tympanomeatal flap** is being created (as in the case of **stapedotomy** or **stapedectomy**), N_2O is not used. This is to prevent pressurization of the middle ear space, which leads to displacement of either the tympanic membrane or the graft. There are many approaches to the middle ear, but, basically, the procedures are performed via a **transcanal approach**, using the microscope, or from a **postauricular approach**, through the mastoid. A **myringotomy** typically is made in radial fashion in the anterior/ inferior quadrant of the tympanic membrane and fluid liberated with a suction. If long-term ventilation is indicated, a tympanostomy tube is placed with the flange on the medial and lateral surface of the tympanic membrane. In most cases, these procedures can be performed using mask GA. **Exploratory tympanotomy** begins with injection of 2% lidocaine, **1:20,000** of epinephrine, followed by a curved incision along the posterior external

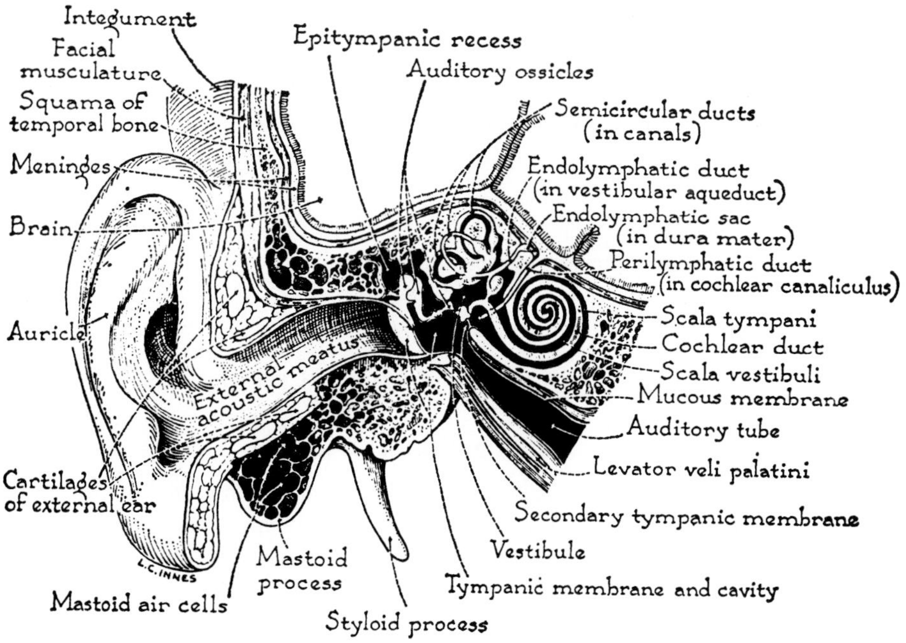

Figure 3-5. Middle ear anatomy. (Reproduced with permission from Anson BJ, McVay CB: *Surgical Anatomy*, 5th edition. WB Saunders Co: 1981.)

auditory canal. The canal skin and the tympanic membrane are elevated forward to expose the middle ear contents, which can be approached either through the canal, or by a postauricular approach. A tympanic membrane perforation can be repaired by placing a temporalis fascia graft, while abnormalities in the ossicular chain can be repaired with prosthesis. Gelfoam is frequently placed in the middle ear, and the tympanic membrane is returned to its anatomic position. The external canal is likewise packed with Gelfoam. A postauricular approach is usually employed for a **simple mastoidectomy**. After gaining exposure of the mastoid cortex, a large burr is used to drill away the diseased mastoid air cells, exposing the facial nerve, the semicircular canals and the middle ear space. The incision is then closed and a mastoid dressing applied. A **modified radical mastoidectomy** is similar to a simple mastoidectomy, except that the posterior wall of the external auditory canal is removed, so that the mastoid can be visualized through the external canal during postop visits. Finally, a **radical mastoidectomy** includes not only removal of the posterior external canal, but of the tympanic membrane, malleus and incus as well. This surgery is rarely performed. Glomus tumors may extend into the neck and require both a transmastoid and a transcervical approach. Removal of large glomus tumors may result in rapid and profound blood loss (> 1000 ml) and require intraarterial monitoring and the ability to provide rapid transfusion. (Middle ear anatomy is shown in Fig 3-5.)

Usual preop diagnosis: Congenitally deformed ear; conductive hearing loss; chronic otitis media ± perforation of the tympanic membrane; cholesteatoma; neoplasia; trauma

SUMMARY OF PROCEDURE

Position	Supine
Incision	Postauricular, endaural or transcanal
Special instrumentation	Ear instruments; microscope; occasionally laser; microdrill
Unique considerations	Facial nerve monitoring or observation; therefore, no muscle relaxation. D/C N_2O 30 min before laying down tympanic membrane graft.
Antibiotics	Varies with situation and type of surgery.
Surgical time	1.5-4 h
EBL	Negligible for most; the rare exception is excision of glomus tumors (mentioned above).
Mortality	Minimal
Morbidity	The incidence of these complications varies according to type of surgery and primary pathology: Infection Vertigo Sensorineural hearing loss Facial nerve paralysis Perilymph fistula
Pain score	2–6, depending on extent of surgery

PATIENT POPULATION CHARACTERISTICS

Age range	Infants–adults
Male:Female	1:1
Incidence	Common
Etiology	Infectious; traumatic; congenital; neoplastic

ANESTHETIC CONSIDERATIONS

PREOPERATIVE

This patient population is generally young and healthy. Myringotomy and pressure equalization (PE) tube insertion are generally very short procedures. In contrast, ossicular reconstruction and tympanic membrane reconstruction are much longer. External ear reconstructions may be associated with other congenital abnormalities, which should be considered preop.

Respiratory Many pediatric patients present with concurrent Sx of URI. These patients may have a predisposition to laryngospasm intraop and postop. In patients presenting with Sx of acute URI (purulent sputum or nasal secretions, fever, etc.), the general recommendation is to postpone any elective procedure until symptoms have abated, usually within 7-14 d. The rationale for postponing surgery includes:

the possibility of progression to a lower URI; secretions which may obstruct the ETT and plug small airways; a predisposition to laryngospasm; and ↓respiratory reserve.
Tests: As indicated from H&P.

Dental Any loose teeth in young children should be identified preop.

Premedication Standard premedication (p. B-2).

INTRAOPERATIVE

Anesthetic technique: GETA, or mask GA (for uncomplicated PE tube placement or myringotomy).

Induction In children, inhalation induction with N_2O, O_2, and sevoflurane/halothane is appropriate. In adults or pediatric patients with an established iv line, standard induction (p. B-2) may be used. A RAE tube is helpful in avoiding intrusion onto the surgical field.

Maintenance For short cases where an adequate airway can be maintained, use of face mask (or LMA) anesthesia with volatile agents is desirable; otherwise, standard maintenance (p. B-3) is appropriate. In longer cases, opiates may be administered, provided an antiemetic is used to avoid postop nausea. N_2O should be D/C at least 1/2 h before placement of a tympanic membrane graft, as the diffusion of N_2O into closed spaces may unseat the graft. Muscle relaxants should be used to eliminate patient movement during microscopic surgery. In cases in which the facial nerve is exposed, however, the surgeon may wish to use a nerve stimulator and muscle relaxants should be avoided.

Emergence Extubation should be smooth to avoid straining, which may unseat the tympanic membrane graft or disrupt other repairs; hence, deep extubation should be considered in this patient population. This consists of giving a spontaneously breathing patient 3-4% sevoflurane or 2-3% isoflurane in 100% O_2 for 3-5 min; then the airway is inspected using a laryngoscope. If clear, the trachea is extubated with the patient in the tonsillar (lateral) position; and 100% O_2 is administered by mask. The anesthesiologist maintains the airway until patient is fully awake. Antiemetics (e.g., metoclopramide 0.15 mg/kg iv) should be used in cases of middle-ear surgery.

Blood and fluid requirements	IV: 18 ga × 1 (adult) 20-22 ga × 1 (child) NS/LR @ 2-4 ml/kg/h	In small children, initial fluid deficit should be replaced with a dextrose-containing solution (e.g., D5 ¼ NS). Blood loss is minimal in these cases.
Control of bleeding	Head-up position Injection of epinephrine-containing solutions by surgeon Deliberate hypotension	These special considerations are applicable to microscopic surgical procedures, where even the smallest quantity of blood may interfere with visualization.
Monitoring	Standard monitors (p. B-1).	
Positioning	✓ and pad pressure points. ✓ eyes. ✓ opposite ear.	Surgeon may request unobstructed access to the head. Under those circumstances, a RAE or anode tube should be used to secure airway.

POSTOPERATIVE

Complications	N/V Facial nerve injury	Liberal prophylactic use of antiemetics is indicated.
Pain management	Pediatric: acetaminophen 15 mg/kg pr Adult: acetaminophen + codeine po	If patient is npo, the use of iv PCA is appropriate in older children and adults.

References

1. Brown BR Jr: *Anesthesia and ENT Surgery*. FA Davis Co, Philadelphia: 1987.
2. Glasscock ME: *Surgery of the Ear*, 4th edition. Glasscock ME, Shambaugh GE, eds. WB Saunders Co, Philadelphia: 1990.
3. Gonzales RM, et al: Prevention of endotracheal tube-induced coughing during emergence from general anesthesia. *Anesth Analg* 1994; 79:792-95.
4. Goycoolea MV, Paparella MM, Nissen RL, eds: *Atlas of Otologic Surgery*. WB Saunders Co, Philadelphia: 1989.
5. Morrison JD: *Anesthesia for Eye, Ear, Nose and Throat Surgery*, 2nd edition. Morrison JD, Mirakhur RK, Craig HJL, eds. Churchill Livingstone, New York: 1985.

PAROTIDECTOMY: SUPERFICIAL, TOTAL, RADICAL

SURGICAL CONSIDERATIONS

Description: A **superficial parotidectomy** (better called a **supraneural parotidectomy**) removes all of the parotid gland lateral to the facial nerve, dissecting and protecting the facial nerve (Fig 3-6). It is usually performed for a tumor, but occasionally is performed for infectious disorders or to enable the surgeon to approach tumors of the deep lobe. A **total parotidectomy** is performed for either infectious disorders or for tumors that arise in the parotid gland medial to the facial nerve. The integrity of the facial nerve is preserved during total parotidectomy, as long as it is not involved with malignancy. It may be combined with neck dissection (radical or functional) or with modified temporal bone resections when the tumor extends into the ear canal or middle ear or invades the facial nerve at the base of the skull.

A **radical parotidectomy** removes the total parotid gland, together with the facial nerve, which usually is reconstructed with a facial-nerve graft. The mastoid may have to be drilled to get a healthy proximal end of the facial nerve. **Microsurgical techniques** are then used to graft the resected nerve. The graft may be harvested from the opposite greater auricular nerve or the sural nerve may be used.

Usual preop diagnosis: Superficial parotidectomy: benign or malignant tumor of the superficial lobe of the parotid gland; infectious disorders. Total parotidectomy: malignant tumors or benign tumors of the deep lobe of the parotid gland. Radical parotidectomy: invasive malignant parotid tumors.

SUMMARY OF PROCEDURE

	Superficial	Total	Radical
Position	Supine; head turned slightly to opposite side	⇐	⇐
Incision	Preauricular, extending into neck; has many variations, including modified face-lift incision.	⇐	May require postaural extension for mastoid access.
Special instrumentation	Facial nerve stimulator, facial nerve monitor	⇐	⇐ + Drill for mastoidectomy; microscope/microsurgical instruments and 9-0 nylon for nerve reanastomosis
Unique considerations	Muscle relaxation is not indicated 2° facial nerve identification. Tape oral ETT to the opposite side of the mandible.	Nasal intubation may be necessary to dislocate mandible anteriorly. Be certain that the ETT is well below vocal cords to allow for anterior dislocation → 1-2 cm of superior ascent of ETT.	⇐
Antibiotics	None or cefazolin 1 g	Cefazolin 1 g	⇐
Surgical time	1.5-2 h	2-4 h	4-6 h
EBL	25-200 ml	200-300 ml	500-700 ml for total parotidectomy, neck dissection and modified temporal bone resection. Sudden, large blood losses do not occur; transfusion usually not necessary.
Mortality	Very rare	⇐	⇐
Morbidity	Dysesthesia or anesthesia of the greater auricular nerve: 100% (almost all will recover within 1 yr). Facial nerve weakness (temporary): 20-50% Frey's syndrome: 35% will have measurable gustatory sweating, but only 5% will have clinical symptoms.	⇐	Facial nerve loss: With graft, function returns slowly over 1 yr.

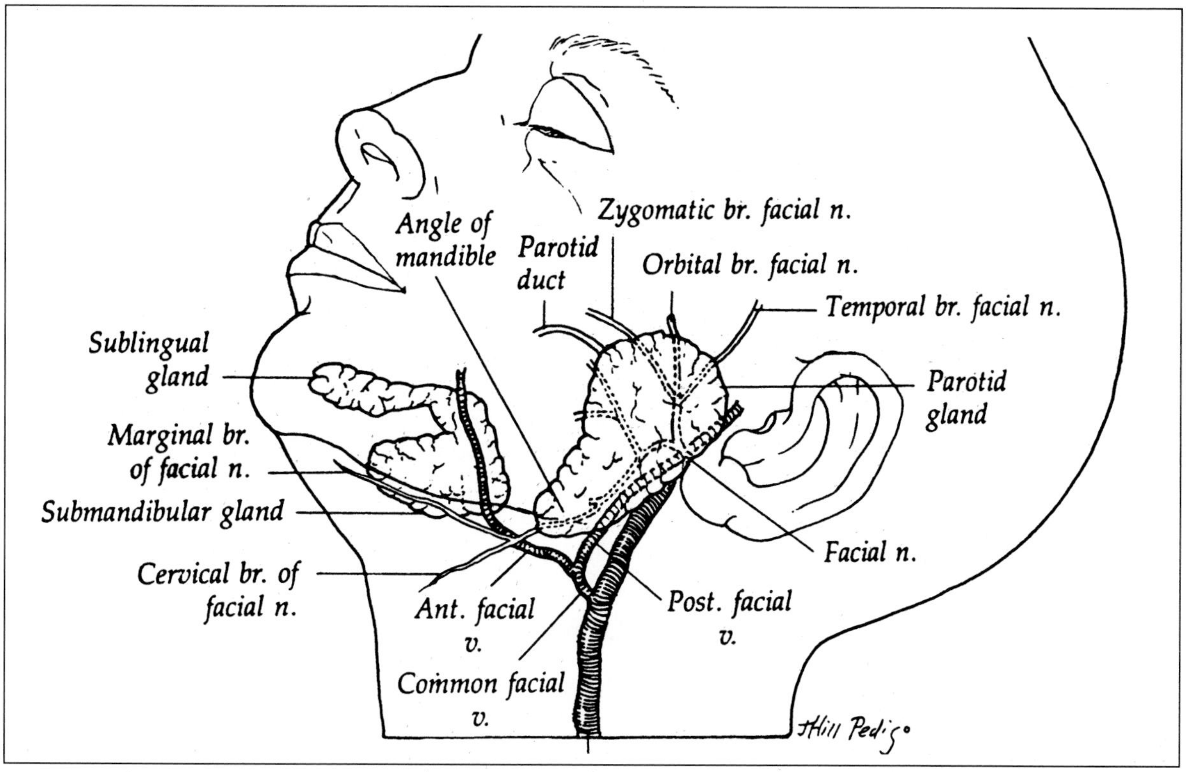

Figure 3-6. Relationship of parotid gland and neurovascular structures. (Reproduced with permission from Ballenger JJ: *Diseases of the Nose, Throat, Ear, Head & Neck.* Lea & Febiger: 1991.)

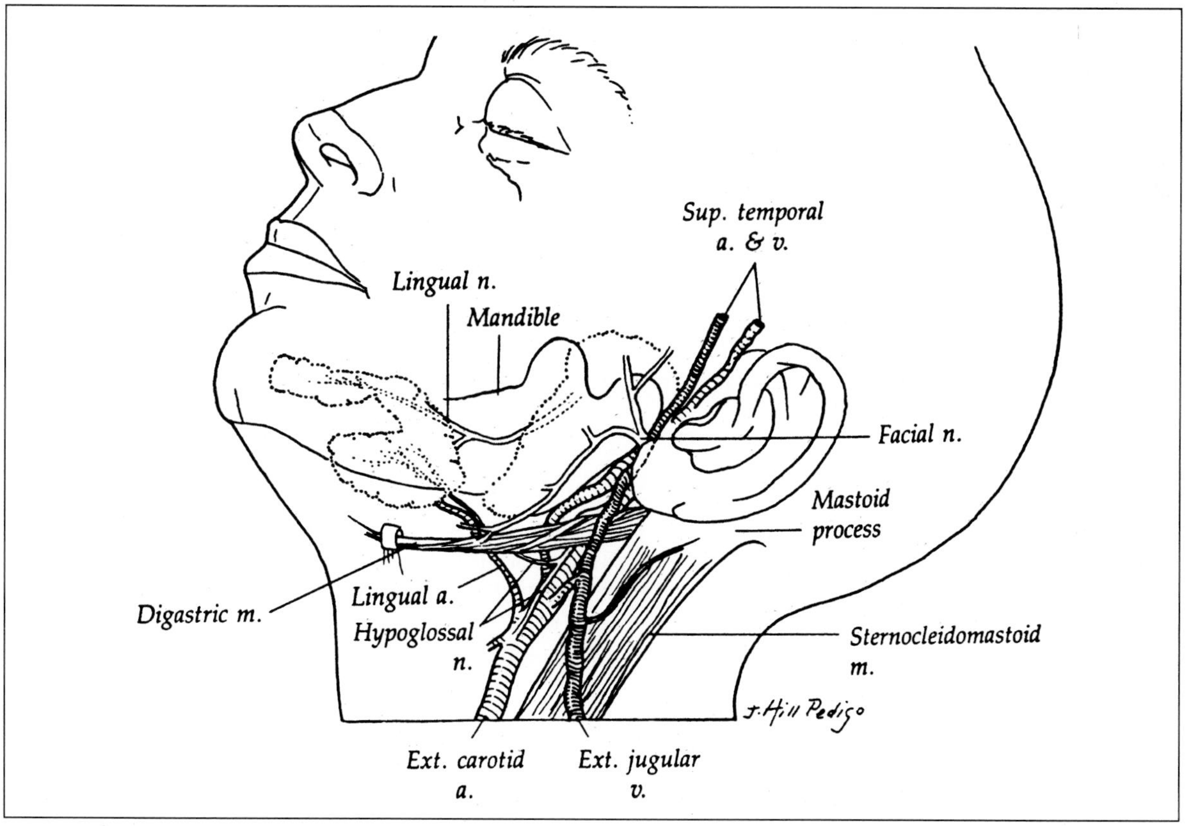

Figure 3-7. Relationship of submandibular gland and adjunct structures. (Reproduced with permission from Ballenger JJ: *Diseases of the Nose, Throat, Ear, Head & Neck.* Lea & Febiger: 1991.)

	Superficial	Total	Radical
Morbidity, cont.	Bleeding: 4% Infection: 4% Permanent facial nerve paralysis: < 1%		
Pain score	2-3	3-4	4-6

PATIENT POPULATION CHARACTERISTICS

Age range	Infants–old age
Male:Female	1:1
Incidence	Common
Etiology	Benign mixed tumor (pleomorphic adenoma) (75%); variety of low- to high-grade malignant cancers (25%); chronic sialoadenitis (results from ductal strictures and/or stones) (rare)
Associated conditions	Nonspecific

ANESTHETIC CONSIDERATIONS

See Anesthetic Considerations following Submandibular Gland Excision, p. 137.

References

1. Terris DJ, Fee WE: Current issues in nerve repair. *Arch Otolaryngol. Head Neck Surg* 1993; 119(7):725-31.
2. Thawley SE, Panje WR, eds: *Comprehensive Management of Head and Neck Tumors.* WB Saunders Co, Philadelphia: 1987.

SUBMANDIBULAR GLAND EXCISION

SURGICAL CONSIDERATIONS

Description: Removal of the submandibular gland is performed for either chronic sialoadenitis due to ductal strictures and/or stones or benign or malignant tumors of the submandibular gland. (General anatomy of the area is shown in Fig 3-7.) The patient lies supine with a pillow under the shoulder and head turned slightly to the opposite side. A skin crease incision is made below the mandible and skin flaps elevated. The marginal mandibular nerve usually is carefully identified or can be avoided by identifying the facial vein and dissecting deep to its plane, employing the **Hayes-Martin maneuver**. Dissection is carried out within the capsule of the submandibular gland, which is then excised and removed. Frozen section usually is performed; and, if necessary, further excision, including a neck dissection for high-grade malignancies, is done.

Variant procedure or approaches: Occasionally, it may be necessary to perform a **neck dissection** (radical or functional) in the case of high-grade malignancy.

Usual preop diagnosis: Chronic sialoadenitis; stones; benign or malignant tumors

SUMMARY OF PROCEDURE

Position	Supine
Incision	Upper neck skin crease
Special instrumentation	Occasionally, facial nerve stimulator
Unique considerations	If surgeon plans to use facial nerve stimulator, muscle relaxation is contraindicated.
Antibiotics	Usually not indicated
Surgical time	0.5-1 h
EBL	25 ml (400 ml if neck dissection is done)
Postop care	PACU → room or home
Mortality	Minimal
Morbidity	Marginal mandibular nerve paresis or paralysis: 20% Bleeding: 4% Infection: 4% Lingual dysesthesia: 1% XIIth nerve paresis or paralysis: < 1%
Pain score	2-4

PATIENT POPULATION CHARACTERISTICS

Age range	Unlimited
Male:Female	1:1
Incidence	Rare
Etiology	Chronic infection Neoplasia: ~60% of tumors are benign, with the remaining being low- and high-grade malignancies.
Associated conditions	Nonspecific

ANESTHETIC CONSIDERATIONS

(Procedures covered: parotidectomy, submandibular gland excision)

PREOPERATIVE

Diseases of the parotid gland have been associated with the use of alcohol and autoimmune disease; therefore, Sx of alcohol abuse and alcohol-related diseases should be sought.

Respiratory Rarely, the submandibular gland may be enlarged enough to cause upper respiratory tract obstruction. Evaluate airway carefully and consider FOL.
Tests: As indicated from H&P.

Neurological Surgical approach to the parotid gland will place the facial nerve at jeopardy; thus, all preop facial nerve deficits should be documented. Note Sx of alcohol abuse, since chronic alcohol intake may cause hepatic enzyme induction with increased anesthetic requirement. Sx of alcohol withdrawal should be controlled prior to surgery in consultation with the patient's primary physician.

Hematologic Submandibular and parotid malignancies may be associated with chronic debilitation and anemia.
Tests: Hb

Laboratory Other tests as indicated from H&P.

Premedication Standard premedication (p. B-2).

INTRAOPERATIVE

Anesthetic technique: GETA

Induction Standard induction (p. B-2). Should tumor extend into upper respiratory tract, however, a tracheostomy under local anesthesia or fiber optic intubation should be considered. ETT should be secured on the nonoperative side. An oral or nasal RAE tube may be indicated, depending on surgical requirements.

Maintenance	Standard maintenance (p. B-3). Muscle relaxants should be avoided if nerve stimulation is done for facial nerve preservation. If muscle relaxants are used, very short-acting agents, such as mivacurium (0.15 mg/kg), should be used and coordinated with the surgeons so that adequate nerve-stimulation tests can be performed.	
Emergence	✓ that throat pack (if used) has been removed before extubation.	
Blood and fluid requirements	IV: 18 ga × 1 NS/LR @ 3-6 ml/kg/h	
Monitoring	Standard monitors (p. B-1).	Invasive monitoring may be indicated, depending on patient's general health.
Positioning	Table may be rotated 90°-180°. ✓ & pad pressure points. ✓ eyes.	Extension tubes for the anesthesia circuit should be available.

POSTOPERATIVE

Complications	Facial paralysis 2° surgical trauma	Notify surgeons.
Pain management	PCA (p. C-3) Parenteral opiates (p. C-1)	

References

1. Brown BR Jr: *Anesthesia and ENT Surgery*. FA Davis Co, Philadelphia: 1987.
2. Johns ME, Price JC, Mattox DE: *Atlas of Head and Neck Surgery*. BC Decker, Philadelphia: 1990.
3. Morrison JD: *Anesthesia for Eye, Ear, Nose and Throat Surgery*, 2nd edition. Morrison JD, Mirakhur RK, Craig HJL, eds. Churchill Livingstone, New York: 1985.

NECK DISSECTION: FUNCTIONAL, MODIFIED RADICAL, RADICAL

SURGICAL CONSIDERATIONS

Description: A **radical neck dissection** consists of a complete **cervical lymphadenectomy**, together with the resection of the sternocleidomastoid muscle, IJ vein and cranial nerve XI. A **modified neck dissection** is a variation between a functional neck dissection and a radical neck dissection, and includes supraomohyoid neck dissection, posterior neck dissection, anterior neck dissection, etc. A **functional neck dissection** is a complete cervical lymphadenectomy, preserving the sternocleidomastoid muscle, IJ vein and cranial nerve XI. Neck dissections are seldom performed as isolated surgical procedures; usually they are combined with resection of the primary lesion, which may involve the tongue, pharynx, larynx, etc.

Typically, the neck dissection is performed through 1 or 2 horizontal neck incisions—occasionally extending vertically to expose the neck from the mandible down to the clavicle. The procedure usually begins with transection of the sternocleidomastoid muscle at its sternal attachment, if this muscle is to be removed. The IJ vein is isolated, cut and tied (again, if it is to be removed). The inferior portion of the dissection includes identification and preservation of the brachial plexus, the phrenic nerve, the vagus nerve and the carotid artery. As the dissection specimen is swept superiorly, cervical sensory branches are divided. The accessory nerve (XI) is identified and carefully preserved (Fig 3-8). When the digastric muscle is encountered, the submandibular portion of the dissection is complete. The hypoglossal nerve (XII) and lingual nerve are identified and preserved. The submental triangle may or may not be resected. The specimen is attached at the skull base and after retraction of the digastric muscle, the IJ vein is ligated and cut at the skull base. The sternocleidomastoid muscle is divided at the mastoid and the specimen is removed. Drains are placed posteriorly, and the wound is closed in layers.

Variant procedure or approaches: In a **composite resection** (**"commando,"** a radical neck dissection + partial mandibulectomy ± partial glossectomy), the neck dissection normally is done first, and an attempt is made to keep the neck specimen in continuity with the primary resection.

Although the upper limb of the neck incision is commonly extended through the chin and lip to gain exposure to the oral cavity and oropharynx, this is not necessary. A combination of intraoral exposure and external approach through the neck incision is sufficient to visualize the primary lesion, and resect it, usually with a segment of mandible. The resultant defect is closed either primarily, with a split-thickness skin graft, or with a chest flap (pectoralis major or deltopectoral). More recently, free flaps may be brought in for closure and revascularized using the facial artery or superior thyroid artery. A **tracheostomy** is almost always performed as part of a composite resection.

Usual preop diagnosis: Cancer of the mouth, oropharynx or tonsil, with documented or suspected spread from a primary source to the cervical lymph nodes

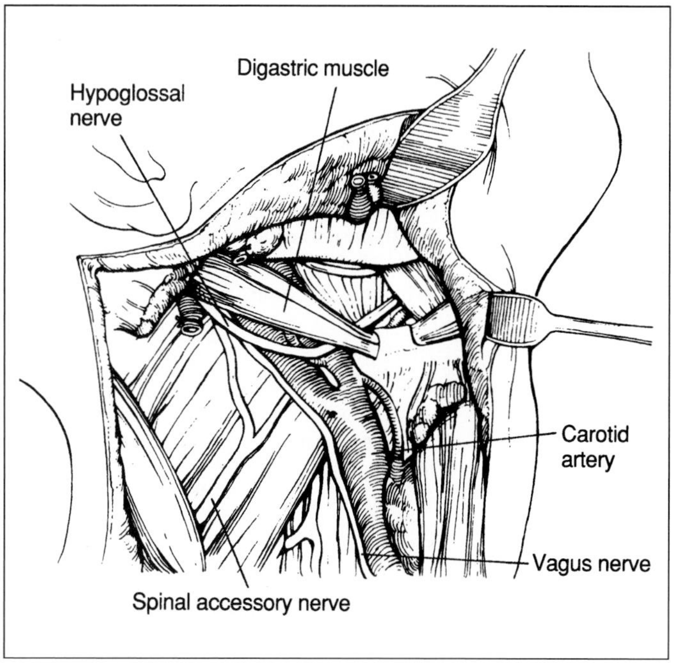

Figure 3-8. Surgical field after completion of accessory nerve-sparing neck dissection. (Reproduced with permission from Thawley SE, Panje WR, et al, eds: *Comprehensive Management of Head and Neck Tumors.* WB Saunders Co: 1987.)

SUMMARY OF PROCEDURE

	Functional	Modified Radical	Radical
Position	Supine; head turned to opposite side; pillow below shoulders	⇐	⇐
Incision	Various neck incisions (e.g., utility, McFee, lip split, etc.), depending on site of primary.	⇐	⇐
Unique considerations	If neck dissection performed on opposite side, significant laryngeal edema may ensue, necessitating tracheostomy.	If cranial nerve XI is dissected/preserved, nerve stimulator may be needed, so muscle relaxation is undesirable.	Rarely, carotid artery needs to be resected or resected/reconstructed, making vascular instruments desirable.
	Dissection around the carotid bulb may result in profound bradycardia, responsive to local anesthetic injection of the bulb and/or iv atropine.	⇐	⇐
Antibiotics	Cefazolin 1 g iv (+ metronidazole 500 mg if aerodigestive mucosa is involved).	⇐	⇐
Surgical time	Neck dissection: 1.5-3 h With resection of primary and reconstruction: 3-6 h	⇐	⇐
EBL	Neck dissection: 150-200 ml	⇐	⇐
	Postradiated patients: 200-400 ml	⇐	⇐
	If primary is also resected: 400-700 ml	⇐	⇐
	If flap reconstructions are required: 700-1200 ml	⇐	⇐ Uncontrolled bleeding of IJ vein at skull base (rare) can result in sudden large blood loss. Usually can be controlled by

	Functional	Modified Radical	Radical
EBL, cont.			surgeon with digital pressure, allowing anesthesiologist to prepare for increasing fluid volume or transfusion.
Postop care	Routine ward care for neck dissection; tracheostomy care if opposite neck also dissected. ICU overnight if 6-8 h operating time.	⇐	⇐
Mortality	Rare	⇐	⇐
Morbidity	Bleeding	⇐	⇐
	Infection	⇐	Painful shoulder syndrome: 20%
	Cranial nerve injury	⇐	
	Chyle leak	⇐	
Pain score	4-6 (Depending on 1° site, pain score may be 6-8.)	6-8	6-8

PATIENT POPULATION CHARACTERISTICS

Age range	Adults
Male:Female	3:1
Incidence	Common
Etiology	Head and neck tumors
Associated conditions	COPD; atherosclerosis

ANESTHETIC CONSIDERATIONS

See Anesthetic Considerations following Glossectomy, p. 143.

References

1. Loré JM Jr: *An Atlas of Head and Neck Surgery*, 3rd edition. WB Saunders Co, Philadelphia: 1988, 650-65.
2. Reed GF, Rabuzzi DD: Neck dissection. *Otolaryngol Clin North Am* 1969; 2:547-63.

LARYNGECTOMY: TOTAL, SUPRAGLOTTIC, HEMI

SURGICAL CONSIDERATIONS

Description: A **total laryngectomy** involves removal of the vallecula (or, if necessary, the posterior third of the tongue) to the first or second tracheal rings. An apron flap incision allows exposure in a subplatysmal plane from the hyoid bone to the clavicle. A **tracheostomy** is performed and an anode tube placed. The strap muscles are divided inferiorly and the hyoid bone is skeletonized. The thyroid gland is resected away from the trachea, unless it is to be included in the specimen. Typically, the larynx is transected just above the hyoid bone, and the specimen is removed. The pharynx is closed in a T-shape and the trachea is brought out to the skin as an end-tracheostomy. No ET or tracheostomy tube is required.

A **supraglottic laryngectomy** involves resection of the larynx from the ventricle to the base of tongue, leaving the true cords. The exposure is similar to that for a total laryngectomy; however, the strap muscles are preserved intact. Once the thyroid cartilage is exposed, subperichondrial flaps are elevated off of the thyroid lamina, and used later for reconstruction. Cuts are made either with a knife or saw through the midthyroid cartilage at a level just above the true vocal cords and completed at the base of tongue. The specimen includes the false vocal cords and supraglottic larynx, the epiglottis and a portion of the base of tongue. Closure is obtained by approximating the thyroid perichondrium to the base of tongue and then the strap muscles also to the base of tongue. A temporary tracheostomy is required.

A **hemilaryngectomy** (also called a **vertical partial laryngectomy**) involves removal of a unilateral true and false cord, retaining the epiglottis and opposite side true and false cord, with various methods of reconstruction. The exposure required for a hemilaryngectomy is similar to that for a supraglottic laryngectomy. A perichondrial flap is similarly raised; however, it is limited to the ipsilateral thyroid lamina. Cuts on the ipsilateral thyroid cartilage are made with either a knife or saw and the anterior commissure is divided with Pott's scissors. After the tumor is resected, closure is obtained utilizing the thyroid perichondrium. Typically, the sternohyoid muscle is used to reconstruct the vocal cord. The wound is then closed in layers and drains are placed. Again, a tracheostomy is required.

A **near-total laryngectomy** involves removal of all of the larynx except for one arytenoid in constructing a phonatory shunt for speaking. All of the techniques involve creation of a temporary or permanent **tracheostomy**, and may be combined with **neck dissection** (radical or functional) and with partial or total **pharyngectomy**, which necessitates flap reconstruction.

Usual preop diagnosis: Cancer of larynx; intractable aspiration, with resultant pneumonia unresponsive to other techniques

SUMMARY OF PROCEDURE

	Total	Supraglottic	Hemi
Position	Supine	⇐	⇐
Incision	Various neck incisions, depending on whether or not reconstruction is anticipated, and requirements of neck dissection.	Horizontal	⇐
Special instrumentation	Major head/neck set; headlights; sterile anesthesia connecting tubes; 6 Fr anode tube; No. 8 and No. 10 cuffed laryngectomy tubes	⇐	Newborn Finochetto rib retractor
Unique considerations	Tumors of the larynx necessarily produce distortion of the airway and, occasionally, a compromised airway prior to onset of anesthesia. A patient with compromised airway is probably best treated by tracheostomy under local anesthesia prior to the start of GA. Intubation can be exceedingly difficult.	⇐	⇐
Antibiotics	Cefazolin 1 g; metronidazole 500 mg	⇐	⇐
Surgical time	2-6 h	⇐	⇐ Rarely is neck dissection necessary.
EBL	Total laryngectomy: 200-300 ml Total laryngectomy with neck dissection: 500-700 ml Total laryngectomy, pharyngectomy and flap reconstruction: 700-1200 ml.	⇐	25-100 ml

	Total	Supraglottic	Hemi
EBL, cont.	Sudden large blood losses do not occur; transfusion usually is not necessary.		
Postop care	Suctioning of tracheal secretions as in tracheostomy.	⇐	⇐
Mortality	< 1%	⇐	⇐
Morbidity	Fistula (radiation salvage): 20%	1%	⇐
	Fistula formation (unirradiated): 5%	–	–
	Bleeding: 4%	⇐	–
	Infection: 4%	⇐	–
Pain score	4-6	4-6	4-6

PATIENT POPULATION CHARACTERISTICS

Age range	40-80 yr
Male:Female	3:1
Incidence	Common
Etiology	Smoking; alcohol
Associated conditions	COPD; atherosclerosis

ANESTHETIC CONSIDERATIONS

See Anesthetic Considerations following Glossectomy, p. 143.

References

1. Friedman M, ed: Laryngeal Surgery. *Operative Techniques in Otolaryngology/Head and Neck Surgery* 1990; 1(1):1-82.
2. Roberson JB Jr, Fee WE Jr: Conservation surgery for laryngeal carcinoma. *Ann Acad Med Singapore* 1991; 20(5):656-64.

GLOSSECTOMY

SURGICAL CONSIDERATIONS

Description: Glossectomy, either **partial** or **total**, is performed for neoplastic lesions of the tongue. During this procedure, nasal intubation is helpful, but not mandatory. On the other hand, complete relaxation is necessary. Additionally, a drying agent, such as scopolamine or glycopyrrolate, helps reduce oral secretions and facilitates surgery. A side-biting or Dingman mouth gag is used to gain adequate surgical exposure. The lesion is resected with electrocautery and can usually be closed primarily. Depending on the extent of resection, and location on the tongue, a **tracheostomy** may be indicated; or oral intubation alone may suffice, for a period of 24-48 h. If neither is done, a short course of steroids helps reduce the lingual edema. A NG tube is placed for postop feeding. A **total glossectomy** is performed in similar fashion, but is frequently combined with a **laryngectomy** because of the aspiration that ensues.

Variant procedure or approaches: Glossectomy can be done with a **neck dissection** or **mandibulectomy** and, on occasion, also can be combined with a **total laryngectomy**.

Usual preop diagnosis: Neoplastic disease of the tongue or adjacent structures (e.g., alveolus, floor of mouth) with involvement of the tongue

SUMMARY OF PROCEDURE

	Partial	Total
Position	Supine	⇐
Incision	Intraoral	⇐ + Suprahyoid approach/neck approach
Special instrumentation	Dingman mouth gag	⇐
Unique considerations	Hypotensive anesthesia Nasal intubation Postop tracheostomy Steroids, if a tracheostomy will not be performed.	⇐
Antibiotics	Cefazolin 1 g, metronidazole 500 mg	⇐
Surgical time	30 min-1 h	2-4 h
Closing considerations	Usually primary closure. May keep patient intubated 24-48 h if minimal tongue edema expected.	Flap repair required; laryngeal suspension usually required. Tracheostomy mandatory postop.
EBL	50-100 ml	200-400 ml
Postop care	Intubated 24-48 h	Tracheostomy care
Mortality	< 1%	⇐
Morbidity	Bleeding Infection Aspiration	Aspiration Bleeding Infection
Pain score	1-2	2-4

PATIENT POPULATION CHARACTERISTICS

Age range	Adults
Male:Female	3:1
Incidence	Uncommon
Etiology	Neoplasia
Associated conditions	Nonspecific

ANESTHETIC CONSIDERATIONS

(Procedures covered: neck dissection; laryngectomy; glossectomy)

PREOPERATIVE

A radical neck dissection generally is done for carcinomas of the head and neck. Since ENT malignancies are commonly associated with the chronic use of tobacco and alcohol, which may lead to significant cardiopulmonary disorders, evidence of physiologic alterations related to this abuse should be sought. In addition, these patients may be malnourished, suffer from Sx of alcohol withdrawal, and present problems in airway management. A laryngectomy is frequently preceded by panendoscopy (see p. 123) and tracheostomy (see p. 148).

Airway Tumor or edema may distort normal anatomy and compromise the airway. These changes may become more pronounced with the induction of anesthesia. A CXR may show tracheal deviation. Flow volume loops can show characteristic patterns of obstruction. Lesions of the upper airway, previous surgery and prior XRT may impede intubation and ventilation. Review of preop indirect and direct laryngoscopies and/or CT scan may be helpful in planning intubation. Preliminary tracheostomy may be required in cases of significant compromise.

Respiratory Smoking (> 40 pack-years) may cause impaired respiratory function, and COPD is common, with ↓FEV_1, ↓FVC or FEV_1/FVC ratio; and ABGs may demonstrate hypoxemia and/or CO_2 retention.
Tests: Consider CXR; as indicated from H&P.

Cardiovascular Since tobacco use raises incidence of heart disease, assess exercise tolerance. Note Sx of CAD (e.g., angina) and CHF (e.g., orthopnea, PND, peripheral edema) in patients with cardiac risk factors (e.g., age > 40 yr, male gender, HTN, hypercholesteremia, smoking, obesity, family Hx).
Tests: Consider ECG, CXR, treadmill stress test, ECHO, if indicated from H&P.

Neurologic Look for Sx of alcohol abuse. Patients may have increased anesthetic requirements because of hepatic enzyme induction. Alcohol withdrawal seizures may occur. Signs of alcohol withdrawal (e.g., tremulousness, increased sympathetic activity and altered mental status) should be sought.
Tests: Consider hepatic function tests, if indicated from H&P.

Hematologic In cases of malignancy or chronic disease, anemia or coagulopathies may be present.
Tests: Hb; consider Plt, PT; PTT

Laboratory Other tests as indicated from H&P.

Premedication Standard premedication (p. B-2). A preinduction drying agent (e.g., glycopyrrolate 0.2 mg iv) facilitates panendoscopy prior to a laryngectomy. Consider contraindications such as ↑HR in patients with CAD.

INTRAOPERATIVE

Anesthetic technique: GETA

Induction With a normal airway, standard induction (p. B-2) is appropriate. In cases with the potential for airway obstruction, an awake FOL under topical and transtracheal anesthesia should be performed. Efforts to maintain spontaneous ventilation prior to intubation are paramount. Occasionally, a tracheostomy under local anesthesia may be necessary to manage a severely compromised airway. A reinforced (anode) tube is desirable.

Maintenance Standard maintenance (p. B-3). Muscle relaxants should be avoided if nerve stimulation is done for facial nerve localization. If muscle relaxants are used, short-acting agents, such as atracurium or mivacurium, are indicated and coordinated with the surgeons so that adequate nerve stimulation tests can be performed. If the procedure includes a tracheostomy or laryngectomy, it is prudent to give the patient 100% O_2 before removing the oral ETT. Following tracheostomy, a sterile anode tube with breathing circuit is inserted and connected by the surgeon. The anode tube is frequently sutured to the chest wall to ensure stability. ✓ bilateral breath sounds, airway compliance and $ETCO_2$ waveform to ensure correct placement of tube.

Emergence Typically no special considerations. Many patients will have a tracheostomy. Gradual emergence allows maintenance of baseline hemodynamic parameters, very important in patients with CAD. In patients without a tracheostomy, extubation over a tube changer may be advisable.[4]

Blood and fluid requirements	Moderate blood loss 1° iv: 16 ga or larger 2° iv: 18 ga or larger NS/LR @ 3-5 ml/kg/h Fluid warmer and humidifier	Blood loss may be massive if the jugular vein or carotid artery are damaged. T&C patient so blood will be immediately available in OR. Initial blood loss may be replaced with NS/LR.
Control of blood loss	Surgical hemostasis Topical vasoconstrictors Deliberate hypotension Head-up tilt 30°	Hemostasis is the primary means of blood-loss control. Vasoconstrictive agents (e.g., phenylephrine or epinephrine) used topically, can be helpful. Deliberate hypotension utilizing a volatile anesthetic or SNP may be useful.
Monitoring	Standard monitors (p. B-1) ± Arterial line Foley catheter CVP line	An arterial line is useful in the course of a neck dissection (serial Hct, ABG, electrolytes, etc.); it is required for the use of deliberate hypotension. CVP, if indicated by coexisting disease (basilic/cephalic vein approach preferred).
Positioning	Usually supine, head elevated 30° Table turned 180° ✓ and pad pressure points. ✓ and pad eyes.	Extension tubes should be available.
Complications	Vagal reflexes → ↓HR and ↓BP	Rx: stop surgery; iv atropine; lidocaine infiltration by surgeons. Prepare for CPR.
	Dysrhythmias	When dysrhythmias are detected, surgeon should stop manipulation of the carotid sinus region. Atropine may be used for marked bradycardia. Infiltration of the surgical field with local anesthetic may blunt or ablate further episodes.

Complications, cont.	↑Q-T interval	Interruption of cervical sympathetic outflow to heart (with right radical neck dissection) → ECG changes.
VAE	↓$ETCO_2$ ↓BP ↓ST segment "Mill wheel" murmur Dysrhythmias	With large veins open in the neck, VAE is possible, and may account for unexplained hypotension and/or dysrhythmia. Rx: notify surgeon, flood field with NS, head down, aspirate CVP, 100% O_2 circulatory support (fluid, pressors, as required).
	POSTOPERATIVE	
Complications	Nerve injury	Facial nerve injury can cause facial droop. Recurrent laryngeal nerve injury can result in vocal cord dysfunction. The phrenic nerve also may pass in the surgical field and respiratory problems may develop if diaphragmatic paralysis occurs.
	Diaphragmatic paralysis	
	Pneumothorax	Pneumothorax may occur with low neck dissection. Dx: ↑RR, ↓BP, ↑CVP, wheezing, ↓O_2 saturation, SOB, chest pain, ↓breath sounds, ↓ECG amplitude, dullness on percussion CXR. Rx: chest tube or needle aspiration, 100% O_2, ventilation and volume expansion.
	Agitation	Agitation → ↑$PaCO_2$, ↓PaO_2, ↑HR. Rx: ✓ restrictive neck dressings; evacuate hematoma; reestablish airway with ETT; 100% O_2; ventilate patient as required.
	Laryngospasm	Coating the ETT with lidocaine ointment or using a Sheridan LITA tube[5] can reduce the incidence of coughing/bucking → bronchospasm/laryngospasm.
Pain management	PCA (p. C-3) Parenteral opiates (p. C-1)	
Tests	CXR ECG	CXR for position of tracheostomy tube and evidence of pneumothorax; ECG for diagnosis of rhythm disturbances.

References

1. Brown BR Jr: *Anesthesia and ENT Surgery*. FA Davis Co, Philadelphia: 1987.
2. Loré JM Jr: *An Atlas of Head and Neck Surgery*, 3rd edition. WB Saunders Co, Philadelphia: 1988, 626-29.
3. Morrison JD: *Anesthesia for Eye, Ear, Nose and Throat Surgery*, 2nd edition. Morrison JD, Mirakhur RK, Craig HJL, eds. Churchill Livingstone, New York: 1985.
4. Robles B, Hester J, Brock-Utne JG: Remember the gum-elastic bougie at extubation. *J Clin Anesth* 1993; 5:329-31.
5. Tunink B, Brock-Utne JG: Bucking is suppressed during emergency from general anesthesia: laryngotracheal lidocaine through a modified endotracheal tube. *Anesthesiology* 1994; 81:A489.

MAXILLECTOMY

SURGICAL CONSIDERATIONS

Description: Maxillectomy is performed for benign or malignant neoplastic lesions of the maxillary sinuses. There are two basic types of this procedure: (1) **partial maxillectomy** and (2) **total maxillectomy**, with or without orbital exenteration, depending on tumor extent. Dental obturator is usually fitted immediately after the surgical resection. A Weber-Ferguson incision is made along the nasofacial groove and ala, exposing the face of the maxilla. An intraoral Caldwell-Luc incision is made and connected with the Weber-Ferguson incision. An **external ethmoidectomy** is usually performed at this time. The proposed osteotomy sites are then outlined with electrocautery and the bone is exposed. A sagittal saw or osteotome is used to make the bony cuts through the palate, maxillary tuberosity, and maxilla at a point dictated by the tumor. Frequently, the specimen must be dissected away from the pterygoid musculature and the internal maxillary artery. After bleeding is controlled, the defect is lined with a split-thickness skin graft and packed with gauze, which is held in place by a dental obturator. For a partial or medial maxillectomy, the palate and lateral maxilla are preserved intact, so that a split-thickness skin graft and dental obturator are not necessary.

Variant procedure or approaches: Maxillectomy may be included in a **craniofacial *en-bloc* resection**.

Usual preop diagnosis: Neoplastic disease of maxillary sinus or lateral wall of nose

SUMMARY OF PROCEDURE

	Partial Maxillectomy	Total Maxillectomy
Position	Supine, with head elevated 30°	⇐
Incision	Oral approach for partial palatal resections. Weber-Ferguson incision for medial maxillectomy.	Weber-Ferguson, with extension around eyelids if orbital exenteration involved.
Special instrumentation	Power saw, drill; dermatome; nasal osteotomes; curved Lambottes osteotomes; dental instruments for tooth extraction	⇐
Unique considerations	Hypotensive anesthesia during procedure to reduce blood loss	⇐
Antibiotics	Cefazolin 1 g + metronidazole 500 mg	⇐
Surgical time	1-2 h	2-4 h
Closing considerations	Nose may be packed, mandating oral airway upon extubation.	⇐
EBL	100-200 ml. Sudden brisk bleeding due to transection of internal maxillary artery occurs when posterior maxillary cut is made with curved osteotome. Control of this bleeding often cannot be achieved until maxillectomy specimen is removed. A 200-300 ml blood loss within 5 min is not unusual. Although not often needed, T&C for 1-2 U PRBCs is wise. Watch suction bottle and measure irrigation.	200-700 ml
Postop care	Mist via face mask is helpful (especially if the nose is packed) to prevent drying of oral mucous membranes immediately postop.	⇐
Mortality	< 1%	⇐
Morbidity	Bleeding: 5% Diplopia (if eye saved): 5% Infection: 4%	⇐
Pain score	2-3	3-6

PATIENT POPULATION CHARACTERISTICS

Age range	Usually 6th-7th decade
Male:Female	3:1
Incidence	Common
Etiology	Benign and malignant paranasal sinus and nasal neoplasia; inverting papilloma

ANESTHETIC CONSIDERATIONS

PREOPERATIVE

Typically, these patients are in relatively good health, apart from some symptoms referable to nose and sinuses.

Airway A careful inspection is warranted, although it is unlikely that the disease process will result in airway compromise. XRT is typically done postop.

Cardiovascular Preop evaluation should focus on suitability for controlled hypotension.
Tests: As indicated from H&P.

Laboratory	Tests as indicated from H&P.	
Premedication	Standard premedication (p. B-2)	

INTRAOPERATIVE

Anesthetic technique: GETA

Induction	Standard induction (see p. B-2).	
Maintenance	Standard maintenance (p. B-3). Deliberate hypotension may be beneficial during a maxillectomy (if patient's medical condition permits), to minimize blood loss and improve visibility within the surgical field.	
Emergence	The oropharynx should be suctioned carefully to avoid aspiration of pharyngeal contents. The patient may have a pharyngeal pack in place which must be removed prior to emergence. They may also have surgical packs, sutured to the nose at the conclusion of surgery. Patients should have return of airway reflexes before extubation.	
Blood and fluid requirements	Blood loss moderate-to-severe IV: 16 ga × 1-2	Blood loss controlled with surgical hemostasis, topical applications of vasoconstrictors (cocaine or epinephrine) and perhaps deliberate hypotension.
Monitoring	Standard monitors (p. B-1) ± Arterial line ± CVP line	Invasive monitoring may be necessary for deliberate hypotension; otherwise, as indicated from patient's medical condition.
Positioning	Head elevated 30° Table turned 90°-180° ✓ and pad pressure points. ✓ eyes.	Have extension tubes for anesthetic circuit available.
Complications	Dysrhythmias	Dysrhythmias 2° to vasoconstrictor agents may be a problem, particularly in those patients with CAD.

POSTOPERATIVE

Complications	Occult postop bleeding	Postop bleeding may cause the patient to swallow large quantities of blood, which may be aspirated, especially if patient needs to be reanesthetized to obtain hemostasis.
Pain management	PCA (p. C-3) Other analgesia	

References

1. Brown BR Jr: *Anesthesia and ENT Surgery*. FA Davis Co, Philadelphia: 1987.
2. Loré JM: *An Atlas of Head and Neck Surgery*. WB Saunders Co, Philadelphia: 1988.
3. Maniglia AJ, Phillips DA: Midfacial degloving for the management of nasal, sinus, and skull base neoplasms. *Otolaryngol Clin North Am* 1995; 28(6):1127-43.
4. Morrison JD: *Anesthesia for Eye, Ear, Nose and Throat Surgery*, 2nd edition. Morrison JD, Mirakhur RK, Craig HJL, eds. Churchill Livingstone, New York: 1985.

TRACHEOSTOMY

SURGICAL CONSIDERATIONS

Description: Tracheostomy is performed either prophylactically in anticipation of upper airway obstruction due to major head and neck surgery, or to establish an airway in acute infectious processes of the head and neck associated with airway obstruction. Other indications are: laryngeal fractures, sleep apnea, inability to intubate for various reasons, requirements for prolonged ventilatory assistance, etc. A tracheostomy tube is placed, or a permanent tracheostomy can be fashioned by using interdigitating neck skin flaps and tracheal flaps. Rarely, an ETT may serve as a tracheostomy securing an airway. Tracheostomy under local anesthesia is the preferred technique for anyone with upper airway obstruction. After infiltrating the operative site with 1% lidocaine, with 1:100,000 epinephrine, a horizontal incision is made 1 cm below the cricoid, exposing the strap muscles, which are separated in the midline. The thyroid isthmus is encountered and divided with electrocautery. The pretracheal fascia is removed (Fig 3-9), and the cricoid cartilage identified. The trachea is entered, usually at the 2nd or 3rd ring, with either a horizontal or cruciate incision, or a segment of tracheal wall may be removed. In infants, a vertical incision is used with stay sutures attached to each flap. The tracheotomy tube is introduced and secured with trach ties and/or sutures.

Variant procedure or approaches: Cricothyroidotomy (incision placed just over the cricothyroid membrane into the subglottic larynx) is the preferred technique to obtain a rapid airway in an emergency. Conversion to a conventional tracheostomy should be performed either immediately or within the first 24 h to prevent development of cricoid cartilage chondritis with resultant subglottic stenosis.

Usual preop diagnosis: Acute upper airway obstruction; respiratory failure with ventilator dependence

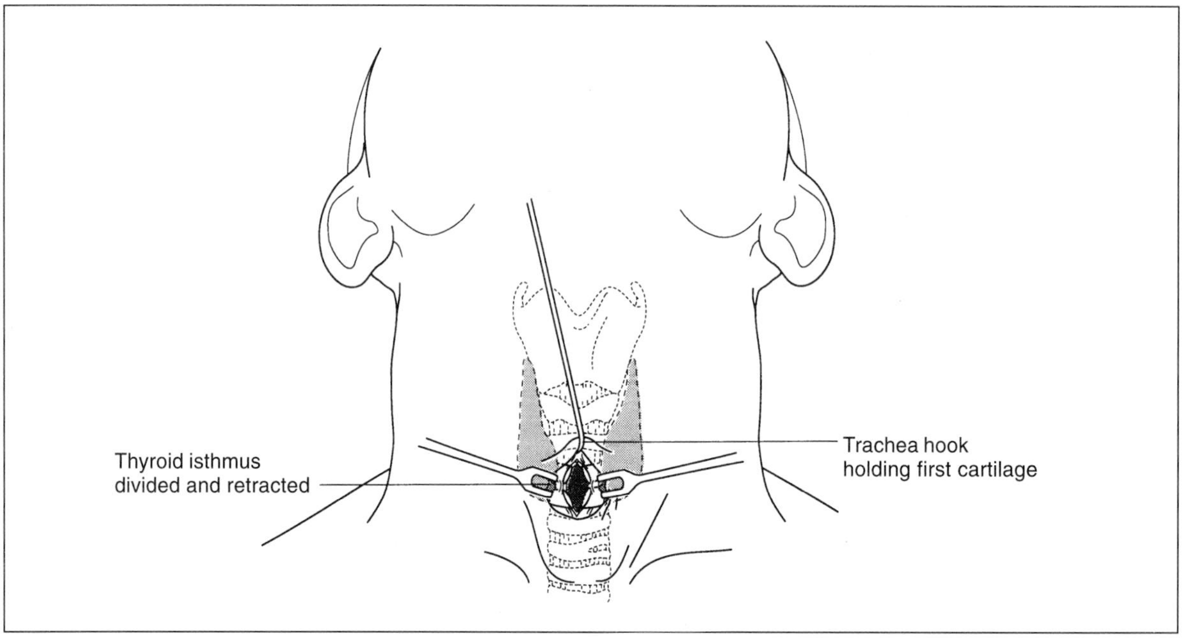

Figure 3-9. Standard tracheostomy using a vertical incision through the second and third tracheal rings. (Reproduced with permission from Greenfield LJ, et al, eds: *Surgery: Scientific principles and Practice*, 2nd edition. Lippincott-Raven, Philadelphia: 1997, 143.)

SUMMARY OF PROCEDURE

	Tracheostomy	Cricothyrotomy
Position	Supine; head extended; sandbag under shoulder, if tolerated.	⇐
Incision	Transverse skin crease, midway between thyroid notch and suprasternal notch	Transverse skin crease between thyroid and cricoid cartilage
Special instrumentation	None	Cricothyrotome or minitracheostomy set

	Tracheostomy	Cricothyrotomy
Unique considerations	Most often performed under controlled conditions, if possible with patient intubated. Can be performed under local anesthesia.	Usually performed in acute emergency situations and converted to standard tracheostomy when patient stabilized.
Antibiotics	None	⇐
Surgical time	3-20 min	3-5 min
EBL	5-25 ml	Minimal
Postop care	Warm mist to replace humidification, warm inhaled air. Hospitals should have full protocol for tracheostomy suctioning and cleaning.	⇐
Mortality	< 1%	⇐
Morbidity	Bleeding: < 5%	⇐
	Infection: < 5%	Subglottic stenosis
	Tracheomalacia: 1%	
	Tracheostenosis: 1%	
Pain score	1-2	2-3

PATIENT POPULATION CHARACTERISTICS

Age range	Adults
Male:Female	2:1
Incidence	Common
Etiology	Upper airway obstruction; prolonged intubation; airway toilet

ANESTHETIC CONSIDERATIONS

PREOPERATIVE

Typically, there are 3 patient populations presenting for tracheostomy: (1) intubated patients in chronic respiratory failure or following major trauma; (2) patients for whom tracheostomy is part of a scheduled procedure (e.g., radical neck dissection); and (3) the rare patient who, having failed intubation, presents in acute respiratory distress and may require immediate transtracheal jet ventilation and subsequent tracheostomy. An example of this group is the patient presenting with **Ludwig's angina,** a severe indurated cellulitis resembling an abscess of the sublingual and submaxillary spaces of the floor of the mouth. The tongue may be elevated against the roof of the mouth and the airway may become obstructed rapidly. An emergency tracheostomy under local anesthetic may be necessary. Primary treatment of Ludwig's angina includes antibiotics and, if necessary, incision and drainage under local anesthesia. The following preop considerations apply only to patients in groups 1 and 2. Of these, the first group presents little or no airway challenge to the anesthesiologist; however, the second group does. Thus, the focus of the preop evaluation in group 2 is to identify those patients who may prove to be difficult or impossible to ventilate or intubate.

Features of the H&P which may be associated with a difficult airway include: (1) specific anatomic characteristics (e.g., bull neck, large tongue, receding jaw, limited mouth opening, difficulty visualizing posterior pharynx, ↓C-spine ROM and obesity); (2) stridor (inspiratory = obstruction at or above larynx; expiratory = subglottic or intrathoracic obstruction). (3) Hoarseness (vocal cord lesion or dysfunction); (4) tachypnea; (5) marked respiratory effort; (6) dyspnea; (7) previous Hx of thyroid gland and neck surgery, trauma or XRT; (8) Hx of previous difficult intubation, vocal cord paralysis; and (9) infections such as epiglottitis or Ludwig's angina.

Respiratory Patients in group 1 may have respiratory insufficiency, requiring mechanical ventilation with PEEP to maintain adequate oxygenation. The continued application of PEEP may be an important consideration during transport from ICU to OR. Patients in group 2 require a careful airway evaluation as outlined above. Based on the assessment, the anesthesiologist must decide whether to choose a direct laryngoscopy, an awake FOL or a tracheostomy under local anesthesia to secure the airway. These patients often have a long Hx of smoking, with consequent COPD.
Tests: CXR; PFT (if Sx of pulmonary dysfunction); ABG

Cardiovascular Patients in group 2 may have significant cardiac risk factors, including smoking (> 40-pack-years Hx), alcohol abuse, male gender, ↑cholesterol, family Hx and HTN). Assess exercise tolerance. Look for Sx of CAD (e.g., angina) and CHF (e.g., orthopnea, PND, edema, DOE).
Tests: ECG in patient with cardiac risk factors

Neurological Look for Sx of ETOH abuse. These patients may require more anesthetic because of hepatic enzyme induction. The perioperative period may be complicated by Sx of ETOH withdrawal.

Hematologic In cases of malignancy or chronic disease, coagulopathies or anemia may be present.
Tests: Hb; PT; PTT; Plt

Laboratory Other tests as indicated from H&P.

Premedication Standard premedication (p. B-2) in elective cases. Premedication is best avoided if airway is compromised, or in emergencies.

INTRAOPERATIVE

Anesthetic technique: GETA (intubated or intubatable patients) or local anesthesia (in the presence of airway compromise or anticipated difficult intubation).

Induction If already intubated, convert preexisting sedation to GA using carefully titrated induction agents (e.g., etomidate 0.3 mg/kg iv). If not intubated and no airway problems are anticipated, a standard induction (p. B-2) may be appropriate. If airway problems are anticipated, an awake fiber optic intubation is the method of choice. In any event, the anesthesiologist should be prepared to deal with a failed intubation and have a surgeon immediately available to perform a tracheostomy if ventilation proves impossible.

Maintenance Standard maintenance (see p. B-3).

Emergence No special considerations

Blood and fluid requirements	IV: 18 ga × 1 NS/LR @ 1-2 ml/kg/h	Generally, little blood loss when done as an isolated procedure.
Monitoring	Standard monitors (p. B-1)	Avoid monitor placement in prepped area. Invasive monitoring may be appropriate, depending on patient condition.
Positioning	Shoulder roll ✓ and pad pressure points. ✓ eyes.	Generally, patient will have a shoulder roll with neck extension to optimize surgical field.
Airway management	100% O_2 prior to tracheostomy Sterile ventilation hoses	Frequently, when tracheostomy is a prelude to a more major procedure, an anode tube is inserted through the tracheostomy by surgeons and sutured in place. It is replaced at the end of surgery by a cuffed tracheostomy tube.
Complications	Pneumothorax Hemorrhage Aspiration of blood Difficult ETT insertion/reinsertion Pneumomediastinum	Pneumothorax may occur with low neck dissection. Dx: ↑RR, ↓BP, ↑CVP, wheezing, ↓O_2 saturation, SOB, chest pain, ↓breath sounds, ↓ECG amplitude, dullness on percussion CXR. RX: chest tube or needle aspiration, 100% O_2, ventilation and volume expansion.

POSTOPERATIVE

Complications	Pneumothorax	(See pneumothorax Dx/Rx in Intraoperative Complications, above.)
	Recurrent laryngeal nerve damage Blood loss	Bilateral recurrent laryngeal nerve injury → airway obstruction, necessitating reintubation.
	Airway compromise	Airway compromise may also be the result of a hematoma, requiring emergent evacuation and reintubation.
Pain management	PCA (p. C-3)	IV opiates, as patient will remain npo postop.
Tests	CXR	For position of tracheostomy tube, evidence of pneumothorax, pneumomediastinum

References

1. Brown BR Jr: *Anesthesia and ENT Surgery*. FA Davis Co, Philadelphia: 1987.
2. Peterson JL: Odontogenic Infections. In *Otolaryngology–Head & Neck Surgery*, Vol. 2, 2nd edition. Cummings CW, Schuller DE, eds. Mosby-Year Book, St Louis: 1993, 1199-1215.

INTUBATION FOR EPIGLOTTITIS

ANESTHETIC CONSIDERATIONS

PREOPERATIVE

Epiglottitis is an acute inflammation and swelling of the epiglottis associated with a generalized systemic toxicity, usually due to hemophilus influenza Type B. It also can be caused by ß-hemolytic streptococci, staphylococci or pneumococci. It occasionally results in total laryngeal obstruction and death due to asphyxia. Formerly, the typical patient was a previously healthy child between 1-4 years of age; however, since the advent of the H-flu vaccine, epiglottitis is more common in adults than in children. In both, the treatment of choice is ET intubation and antibiotics. About 80% of hemophilus influenza infections are sensitive to ampicillin. Steroids also have been recommended, but no difference in outcome has been reported.

Respiratory — Symptoms may be sore throat, fever, muffled voice, dysphagia and rapidly increasing stridor. The child sits upright, leaning forward and drools saliva. It is imperative to realize that total airway ★ obstruction can occur suddenly and without warning. **NB:** Rapid treatment should be instituted instead of performing time-consuming investigations. The sudden development of respiratory obstruction in the x-ray suite could have a disastrous outcome.

Hematologic — A high leukocyte count is usually found in these patients.
Tests: Blood drawing before the airway is secured may be inadvisable.

Premedication — None

INTRAOPERATIVE

Anesthetic technique: GETA. It is essential that an experienced anesthesiologist be present for this procedure. It is important that no exam of the throat be made (as this may precipitate complete airway obstruction) except under an anesthetic. In adults, it has been suggested that indirect laryngoscopy or FOB may be performed without the risk of precipitating complete laryngeal obstruction, although this is controversial.

Induction — While the patient is breathing spontaneously, atropine 0.02 mg/kg is given to prevent vagal reflexes and bradycardia from manipulation of the inflamed epiglottis. An experienced ENT surgeon with an emergency tracheostomy set must be available. Inhalation induction, with sevoflurane and 100% O_2, is used, with patient sitting. Induction may be prolonged and intubation extremely difficult. Smaller than usual oral ETT is used initially, then may be changed to a nasal tube at the end of the procedure; however, this may prove hazardous.

Maintenance — Standard maintenance (see p. B-3).

Emergence — The patient will remain intubated for 24-48 h and should be kept sedated and restrained to prevent accidental extubation. (The mean duration of intubation in one series was 36 h.) It is believed that direct observation of the epiglottis is the only reliable way to determine the stage at which the ETT is no longer necessary.

Blood and fluid requirements	Minimal blood loss IV: 18 ga (adult) 22-26 ga (child) NS/LR @ 4-7 ml/kg/h (adult) @ 2-3 ml/kg/h (child)	If possible, iv should be placed following induction of anesthesia because subsequent crying and struggling may → acute respiratory obstruction.
Monitoring	Standard monitors (p. B-1)	
Positioning	✓ and pad pressure points. ✓ eyes.	
Complications	Pulmonary edema	A short-lived pulmonary edema occasionally occurs after relief of the obstruction and must be treated with IPPV.

POSTOPERATIVE

Complications	Accidental extubation ETT blockage	Accidental extubation and ETT blockage are serious complications that can prove fatal. The blockages are some-

Complications, cont.		times due to crusting of the ETT because of insufficient humidification. The tube should be changed after 24 h.
Pain management	PCA (see p. C-3).	Postop sedation and manual restraints

References

1. Brown BR Jr: *Anesthesia and ENT Surgery*. FA Davis Co, Philadelphia: 1987.
2. Crockett DM, Healy GB, McGill TJ, Friedman EM: Airway management of acute supraglottitis at the Children's Hospital, Boston: 1980-1985. *Ann Otol Rhinol Laryngol* 1988; 97(2Pt1):114-19.
3. Dort JC, Frohlich AM, Tate RB: Acute epiglottis in adults: diagnosis and treatment in 43 patients. *J Otolaryngol* 1994; 23(4):281-85.
4. Morrison JD: *Anesthesia for Eye, Ear, Nose and Throat Surgery*, 2nd edition. Morrison JD, Mirakhur RK, Craig HJL, eds. Churchill Livingstone, New York: 1985.
5. Senior BA, Radkowski D, MacArthur C, Spredner RC, Jones D: Changing patterns in pediatric supraglottitis: a multi-institutional review, 1980 to 1992. *Otolaryngol Head Neck Surg* 1994; 110(2):203-10.

SKULL BASE SURGERY

SURGICAL CONSIDERATIONS

Description: **Posterior fossa craniotomy** (translabyrinthine, transcochlear, far lateral or infratemporal fossa craniotomy) is carried out with the patient supine, rotated 180° from the anesthesiologist. The patient's head is rotated to the side to allow access to the cranium posterior and inferior to the ear. An incision is made from the supraauricular area into skin overlying the mastoid and, in some cases, into the neck. Bone is removed around, and sometimes including, the inner ear structures to allow access to the posterior cranial fossa and internal auditory canal. Continuous intraop monitoring of cranial nerves 5-12, SSEPs and auditory evoked potentials may be used. The patient should be placed on the table and secured with two seat belts, as lateral rotation is frequently necessary during the procedure. A CSF leak is produced, and then repaired with tissue (fat) taken from the abdomen during closure.

In contrast to the standard neurosurgical approach, the **translabyrinthine approach** to the posterior fossa remains extradural, avoiding direct retraction of the cerebellum or other brain structures. We believe the advantages include a decreased incidence of seizures, prolonged headaches, CSF leaks and aseptic meningitis. Most importantly, however, is the advantage of finding the facial nerve in a normal position and tracing it over the tumor. From the suboccipital approach, the facial nerve is on the opposite side of the tumor from the surgeon and may be difficult to locate. This can slow down the surgery and has been associated with abnormal facial nerve function. In the translabyrinthine approach, however, the facial nerve is identified in the mastoid and then followed (after removal of bone) back to the internal auditory canal. The nerve is then traced over the top of the tumor, permitting removal of the tumor without damaging the nerve.

Usual preop diagnosis: Vestibular schwannoma (acoustic neuroma); vestibular neuritis; Meniere's disease; cholesterol granuloma; meningioma; cholesteatoma; facial nerve paralysis; aneurysms; primary intracranial tumor; glomus tumors of the skull base

Middle fossa craniotomy also is carried out with the patient supine, rotated 180° from the anesthesiologist. The head is turned to the side to allow access to the cranium superior to the ear. An incision is made from the pretragal area in a curved fashion onto the side of the head. A craniotomy of approximately 3" × 3" is performed superior to the ear (Fig 3-10). Elevation of the dura and placement of retractors allows exposure of the bone at the base of the skull. Bone is removed over the areas of interest to allow access to pathologic tissues for resection (Fig 3-11). Continuous intraop monitoring of cranial nerves 5-12, SSEPs and auditory evoked potentials may be used. The patient should be placed on the table and secured with two seat belts, since lateral rotation is frequently necessary during this procedure. Trendelenburg and reverse Trendelenburg changes also are necessary during the procedure to allow for exposure of critical structures. As in posterior fossa craniotomy, a CSF leak is produced, and then repaired with tissue (fat) taken from the abdomen during closure.

Usual preop diagnosis: Vestibular schwannoma (acoustic neuroma); vestibular neuritis; Meniere's disease; cholesterol granuloma; cholesteatoma; facial nerve paralysis; aneurysms in the cerebellar pontine angle and prepontine space

→ **Figure 3-10.** Right middle fossa approach: surgeon is looking down at patient's head, which is turned to the left. The temporalis has been reflected inferiorly and a square craniotomy has been performed. The dura is visible, with the middle meningeal artery visible on it.

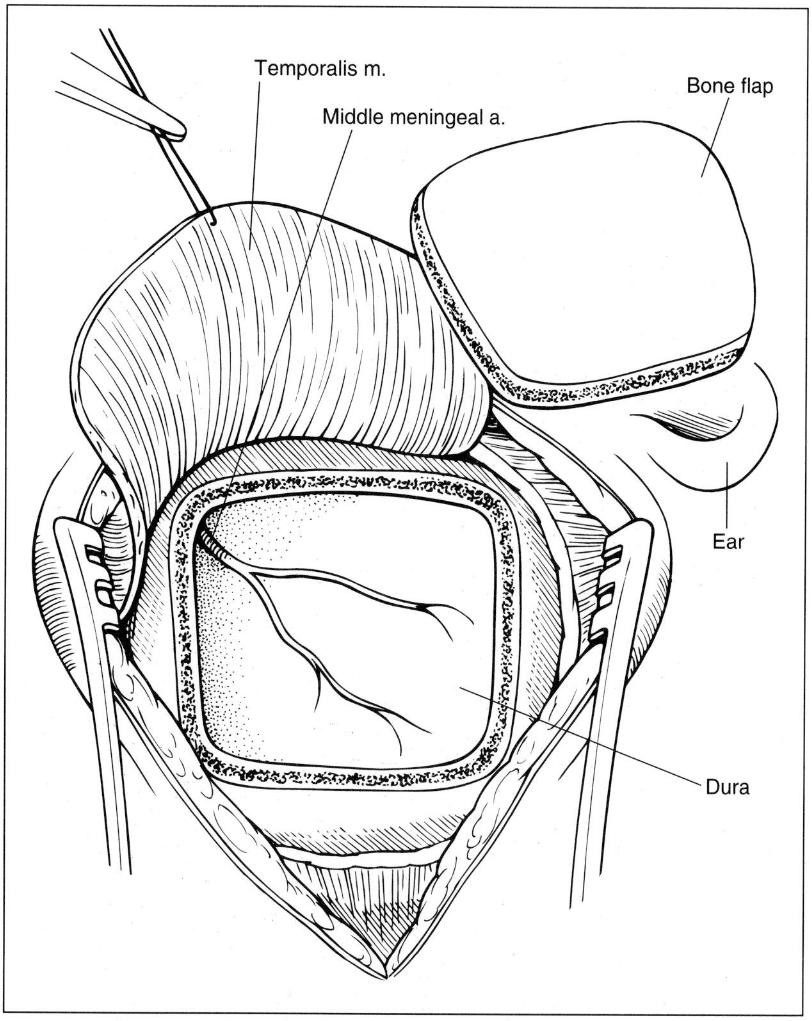

↓ **Figure 3-11**. Right middle fossa approach with House-Urban retractor holding dura off the middle cranial fossa floor. The anatomic structures shown are under the floor and not visible except for the greater superficial petrosal nerve and a prominent bony outcropping over the superior semicircular canal, which allows the location of the other structures to be calculated.

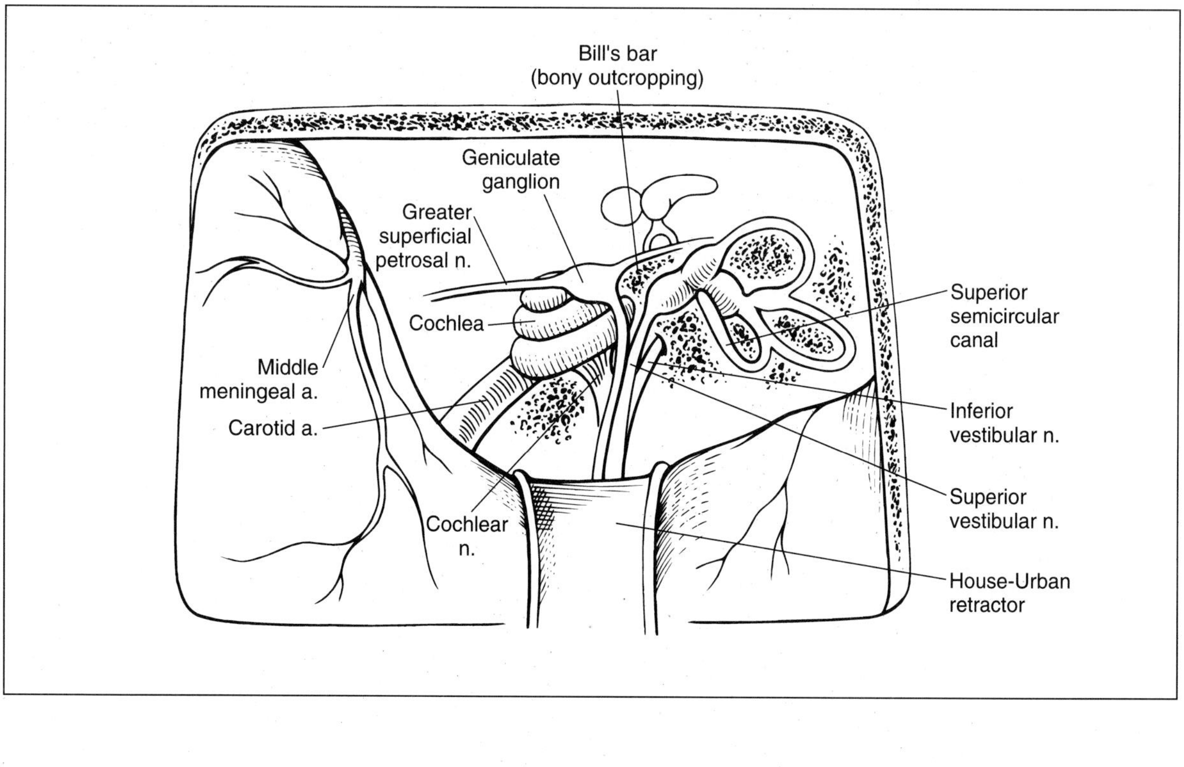

SUMMARY OF PROCEDURE

	Posterior Fossa Craniotomy	Middle Fossa Craniotomy
Position	Supine, table turned 180°, surgeon sitting to the side of the patient's head, with scrub nurse directly across and microscope in between (Fig. 3-12)	Supine, surgeon at head of table, table turned 180°, patient secured with 2 seat belts (Fig. 3-13).
Incision	Temporal/mastoid ± neck extension	Pretragal to lateral temporal
Special instrumentation	Microscope, cranial nerve monitor, bipolar cautery, US aspirator, BAER computer	⇐
Unique considerations	TED hose, SCDs, Foley catheter, arterial line ± CVP monitoring, at the discretion of the anesthesiologist. Lumbar drainage with some patients.	TED hose, SCDs, Foley catheter, arterial line ± CVP monitoring
Special medications	Dexamethasone 8 mg iv. (Note: hyperventilation and osmotic diuretic agents are usually not necessary with posterior fossa craniotomy.)	Mannitol 0.5-1.0 g/kg infusion, started after induction of anesthesia. Furosemide (10 mg iv); dexamethasone (8 mg iv).
Antibiotics	Vancomycin 1 g iv + ceftazidime 1 g iv q 8 h	Vancomycin 1 g iv, ceftazidime 1 g iv
Procedure time	3-12 h	3-6 h
Closing considerations	Sterile dressing placed after all drapes are removed (3-5 min application time). Attempt to minimize coughing and Valsalva to reduce risk of intracranial bleeding. It is acceptable to use muscle relaxants after dural closure.	Minimize coughing and Valsalva to reduce risk of intracranial bleeding.
EBL	150-1000 ml (Have 1 U autologous blood available.)	150-500 ml (Have 1 U autologous blood available.)
Postop care	Direct transfer to ICU after extubation. Transport with ECG/O_2 sat/BP monitor. Establish level of consciousness and hemodynamic stability in ICU.	ICU
Mortality	Rare	⇐
Morbidity	Hearing loss: 5-100% (depending on approach)	30%
	Transient facial weakness: 20-30%	10-30%
	Permanent facial nerve weakness: ≤ 10%	⇐
	CSF leak: ≤ 2%	–
	Infection: ≤ 2%	⇐
	Delayed bleeding 1-2%	⇐
	Meningitis: 1-2%	⇐
	Stroke: ≤ 1%	–
	Aspiration: Rare	⇐
Pain score	6	6

PATIENT POPULATION CHARACTERISTICS

Age range	Usually adults (occasional approaches of this type are used in children).	10+ yr
Male:Female	1:1	1:1
Incidence	1/20,000 population/yr in U.S.	1/40,000 population/yr in U.S.
Etiology	Neoplasm; chronic infection; recurrent dizziness; congenital lesions	Neoplasm; chronic infection; recurrent dizziness
Associated conditions	Hearing impairment in some patients (look for a hearing device, which should be removed after patient is asleep); balance disturbance	Hearing impairment

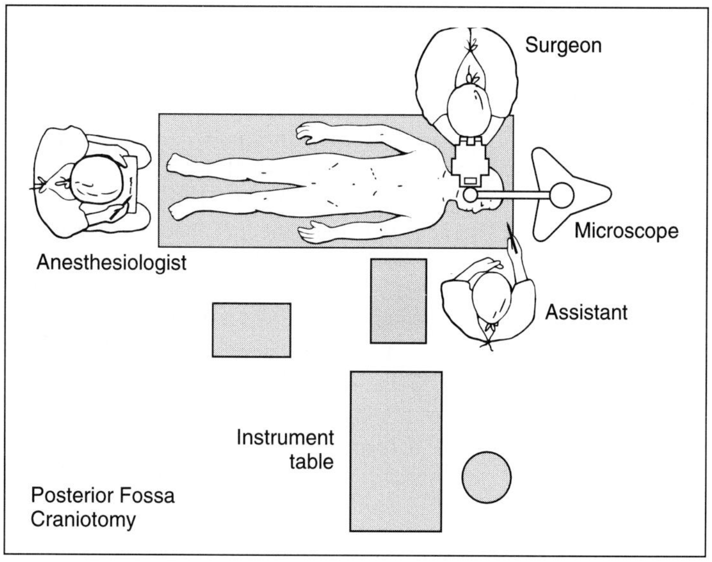

Figure 3-12. OR configuration for posterior fossa craniotomy.

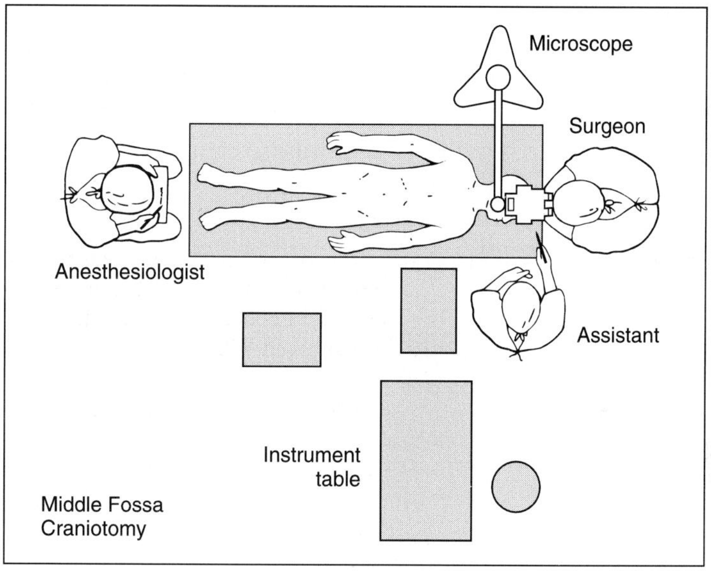

Figure 3-13. OR configuration for middle fossa craniotomy.

ANESTHETIC CONSIDERATIONS

PREOPERATIVE

Typically, these patients are otherwise healthy, and ↑ICP occurs only infrequently.

Respiratory Elective surgery is contraindicated in patients with active upper or lower respiratory infections.

Cardiovascular HTN is a risk for perioperative bleeding and should be controlled before surgery.
Tests: ECG and others, if indicated from H&P

Neurological Any Sx of ↑ICP (e.g., headache, N/V, papilledema) warrant further evaluation. Some patients may have hearing aids, which may be removed after induction of anesthesia.

Hematologic Recent use of an NSAID may force delay of elective surgery. ✓ family Hx for bleeding disorder.
Tests: As indicated from H&P.

Laboratory **Tests:** HCT and others, if indicated from H&P.

Premedication In the absence of ↑ICP, midazolam 1-3 mg commonly is used.

INTRAOPERATIVE

Anesthetic technique: GETA, controlled ventilation. Use of cranial nerve monitors precludes use of muscle relaxants during most of the procedure.

Induction Defasciculate with nondepolarizing muscle relaxant (e.g., dTC 3 mg). Induce anesthesia with STP (3-5 mg/kg) or propofol (1.5-2.5 mg/kg), an opiate (e.g., fentanyl 5 μg/kg) and succinylcholine (1.5 mg/kg). The airway will be inaccessible during surgery, so the ETT must be well secured. An alternative to taping the ETT is to secure the tube with a suture or dental floss. First tie the suture around the base of an incisor at the gingiva; then wrap and tie the suture around the ETT. A Flexibend ETT is especially well suited for this. The ETT is cut so that the flexible, corrugated connector begins at the teeth. The suture is wrapped and tied to the corrugated plastic. This ensures that the ETT remains in place when the patient's head is turned or extended during surgery. A small dose of mivacurium (e.g.) may be used, if necessary, to facilitate placement of the CVP line and positioning of patient. Occasionally, a modified ETT and vocal cord electrode are required for cranial nerve monitoring (Xomed NIM-2 EMG ETT). After the table is turned 180°, the surgeon performs direct laryngoscopy and inserts the vocal cord electrodes. Intramuscular needle electrodes are placed before prep and drape for monitoring: CN7 (face), CN8 (hearing), CN9 (pharynx), CN10 (vocal cord), CN11 (trapezius) and CN12 (tongue).

Maintenance Standard maintenance (p. B-3). Usually, a balanced technique combining low doses of an opiate, propofol and a volatile agent ± N_2O. Dexamethasone 8 mg is given. Commonly, only mild hyperventilation for posterior fossa craniotomies. Middle fossa craniotomies, at surgeon's request, may require hyperventilation and mannitol (0.5-1 g/kg). Vasodilators (e.g., SNP) or β-blockers (e.g., labetalol or esmolol) may be necessary to prevent HTN.

Emergence As the surgeon begins to close, the cranial nerve monitoring is D/C, and it is possible to add an intermediate-acting muscle relaxant (e.g., mivacurium 0.1 mg/kg) to the technique. Application of the surgical dressings takes several minutes and involves much manipulation of the head and neck. It is important to prevent coughing or Valsalva, which will ↑ ICP and ↑ BP. The use of a muscle relaxant prevents coughing, while allowing the patient to be rapidly awakened after the dressings are applied. If a vocal cord electrode has been used, it may be pulled out gently (without direct visualization) before the ETT is removed. The ETT is removed in the OR and the patient taken to ICU. (If any significant neurologic injury is suspected, the ETT should not be removed.) A rapid-acting agent (e.g., SNP) should be available to treat HTN.

Blood and fluid requirements	IV: 18 ga × 1 NS/LR @ 5-10 ml/h UO ≥ 0.5 ml/h	NS to maintain UO ≥ 0.5 ml/h. Avoid hypotonic fluids and glucose. Colloid may be used for volume. Maximum blood loss occurs with opening. Blood loss with glomus tumors can be brisk (100-300 ml over 5 min) during tumor resection. Transfusions usually not required, but patients with cardiovascular disease may fare better with an Hct ≥ 30.
Monitoring	Standard monitors (p. B-1) Arterial line CVP catheter UO	Cranial nerve monitoring typically performed by surgical team. Controlled hypotension may be required.
Positioning	✓ & pad pressure points. ✓ eyes.	Consider covering the eyes with rigid shields. ✓ & pad pressure points with careful attention to arms. As the table is frequently tilted from side-to-side, the patient is secured with two belts.
Complications	Labile BP Pneumothorax (2° CVP)	Occasional BP lability during tumor resection for large lesions impacting the brain stem or involving the 9th and 10th nerve complex.

POSTOPERATIVE

Complications	Neurologic deficits Intracranial bleeding	Uncontrolled HTN → intracranial bleeding. Occasional 9th or 10th nerve damage → smaller than usual glottic

Complications, cont.	Pneumothorax Peripheral nerve injury N/V	opening. (Fully awake patients can be extubated safely.) Stroke frequently predicted with intraop monitoring techniques. Sx of depressed consciousness (2° intracranial bleeding or acute obstructive hydrocephalus) can occur several h following surgery. Follow level of consciousness closely in the immediate postop period. Patients who have resection of either the cochlear vestibular nerve or removal of the inner ear are expected to be vertiginous with strong nystagmus after awakening. This is also manifested as N/V in the immediate postop period. IV ondansetron (4 mg iv), prochlorperazine (Compazine) (5-10 mg iv), and promethazine (Phenergan) (12.5-50 mg iv) used most frequently. Minimization of antiemetic medications allows more rapid patient recovery.
Pain management	Fentanyl or morphine iv	
Tests	Neurological exam	If intracranial bleeding is suspected, a CT or MRI.
	Hct	
	CXR	To rule out pneumothorax and confirm that tip of the central venous line is outside the heart.

References

1. Brackmann DE: Middle cranial fossa approach. In *Acoustic Tumors*, Vol. 2. House WF, Leutje C, eds. University Park Press, Baltimore: 1979, 15-41.
2. Brackmann DE, Green JD: Translabyrinthine approach. *Otolaryngol Clin North Am* 1992; 24:311-30.
3. Gantz BJ, Parnes LS, Harker LA, McCabe BF: Middle cranial fossa acoustic neuroma excision: results and complications. *Ann Otol Rhinol Laryngol* 1986; 95:454-59.
4. House WF, Hitselberger WE: The transcochlear approach to the skull base. *Arch Otolaryngol* 1976; 102:334-42.
5. House WF, Shelton C: Middle fossa approach for acoustic tumor removal. *Otolaryngol Clin North Am* 1992; 25:347-60.
6. Kawaguchi M, Sakamoto T, Ohnishi H, Karasawa J, Furuya H: Do recently developed techniques for skull base surgery increase the risk of difficult airway management? Assessment of pseudoankylosis of the mandible following surgical manipulation of the temporalis muscle. *J Neurosurg Anesthesiol* 1995;7(3):183-6.
7. Morrison AW: Translabyrinthine surgical approach to the internal acoustic meatus. *JR Soc Med* 1978; 71:269-73.
8. Sekhar LN, Estonillo R: Transtemporal approach to the skull base: an anatomical study. *Neurosurgery* 1986; 19:799-808.
9. Shelton C, Brackmann DE, House WF, Hitselberger WE: Middle fossa acoustic tumor surgery: results in 106 cases. *Laryngoscope* 1989; 99:405-8.
10. Stetchison MT: Neurophysiologic monitoring during cranial base surgery. *J Neurooncol* 1994; 20(3):313-25.
11. Tos M, Hashimoto S: Anatomy of the cerebellopontine angle visualized through the translabyrinthine approach. *Acta Otolaryngol* 1989; 108:238-45.

RECONSTRUCTIVE SURGERY FOR SLEEP-DISORDERED BREATHING

SURGICAL CONSIDERATIONS

Description: There are a number of surgical approaches available to treat sleep-related upper airway obstruction. These fall into three categories: 1) classic procedures that directly enlarge the upper airway; 2) specialized procedures that directly enlarge the upper airway; and 3) tracheotomy to bypass the pharyngeal portion of the upper airway.

Uvulopalatopharyngoplasty (UPPP) is a procedure designed to enlarge the retropalatal airway by excision of tonsils, if present, excision of the uvula and posterior soft palate, and trimming and reorienting the anterior and posterior tonsillar pillars (Fig 3-14).

Uvulopalatal flap (UPF) is a reversible procedure to enlarge the retropalatal area by reflecting the uvula up toward the hard palate. The mucosa of the oral surface of the uvula and midline soft palate are removed, the distal aspect of the uvula is amputated and the soft palate is sutured into this new position (Fig 3-15).

Uvulopalatopharyngoglossoplasty (UPPGP) is an intraoral procedure incorporating a modified UPPP with limited resection of the base of tongue for both retropalatal and retrolingual collapse.

Laser midline glossectomy (LMG) is designed to enlarge the retrolingual airway by excision of approximately 2.5 cm × 5 cm of midline tongue tissue through an intraoral approach. This also may require lingual tonsillectomy, reduction of the aryepiglottic folds and partial epiglottectomy (Fig 3-16A). LMG is usually combined with a tracheotomy for airway protection.

Lingualplasty (LP) is the same procedure as LMG except that additional tongue tissue is extirpated posteriorly and laterally to that portion removed by LMG (Fig 3-16B). It is usually combined with a tracheotomy (see below) for airway protection.

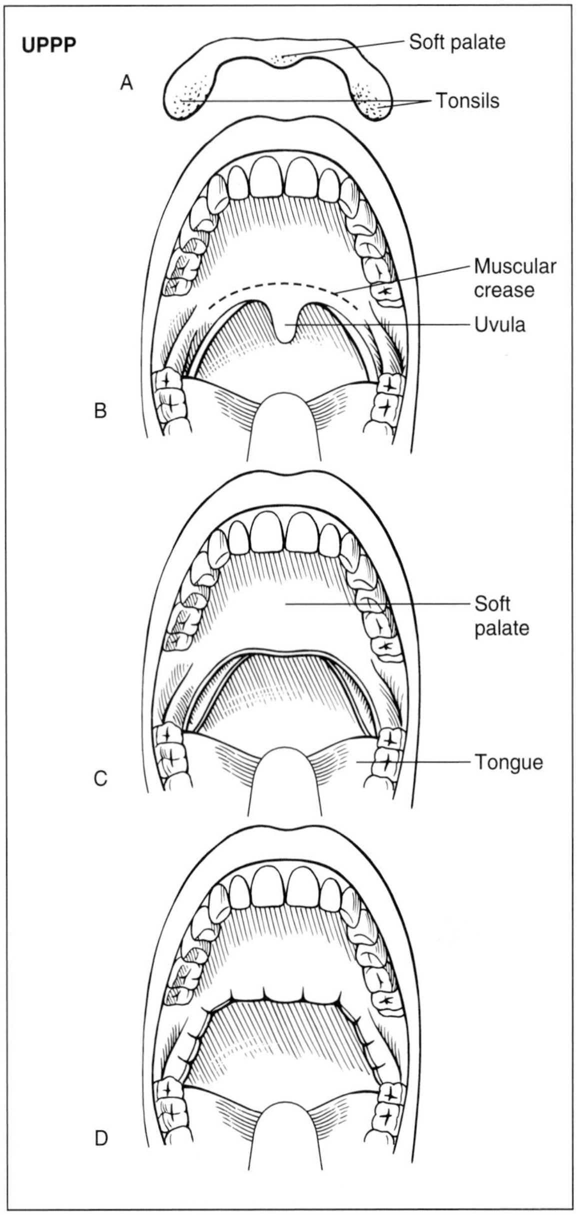

Figure 3-14. The uvulopalatopharyngoplasty (UPPP) technique: (A&B) tonsils and redundant soft palate are excised.; (C) mucosal flaps are prepared for closure; (D) the soft palate is closed to itself and the anterior and posterior tonsillar pillars are sutured to each other.

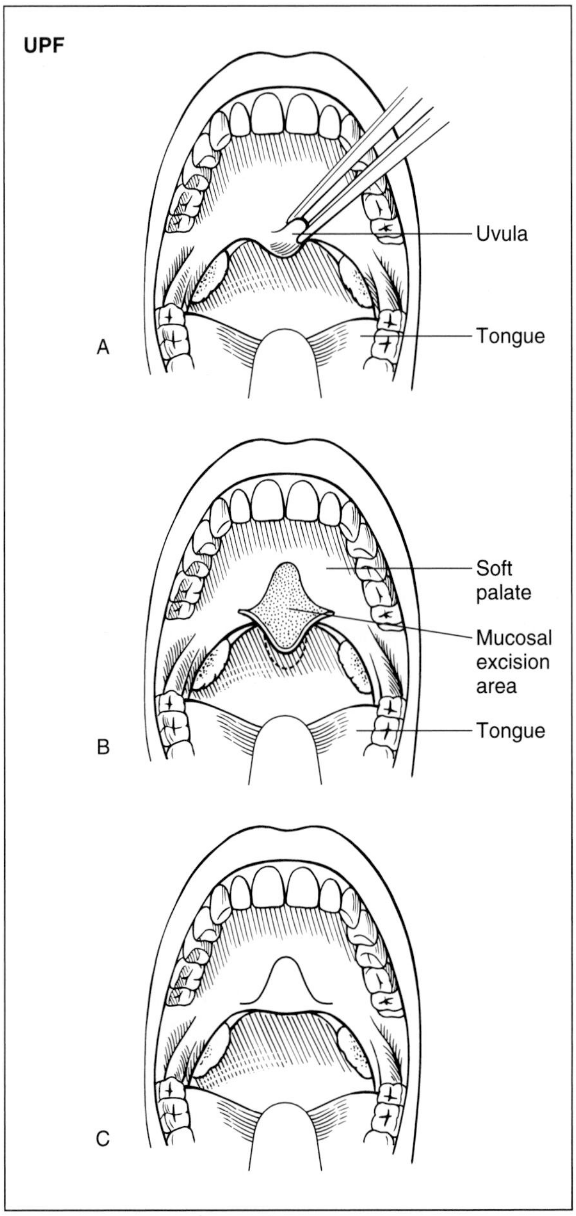

Figure 3-15. The uvulopalatal flap (UPF): (A) The uvula is reflected back to the hard palate to identify the muscular crease. (B) Mucosa on the oral side of the uvula and soft palate are removed, and part of the uvula is amputated. (C) The mucosal incisions are closed with absorbable suture.

Inferior sagittal mandibular osteotomy and genioglossal advancement (MOGA) is an intraoral approach designed to enlarge the retrolingual area. The genial tubercle—the anterior attachment of the genioglossus muscle—is mobilized by osteotomies. The segment is advanced and rotated to allow bony overlap to lock the inner (lingual) surface of the mandible and the geniotubercle at the outer (labial) surface. The fragment is fixed at the inferior aspect of the osteotomy with a titanium screw (Fig 3-17).

Hyoid myotomy and suspension (HM) is a retrolingual procedure that alleviates obstruction by redundant lateral pharyngeal tissue or a retrodisplaced epiglottis. A horizontal cervical incision above the hyoid bone is performed, and the dissection is carried down to the suprahyoid musculature. The midline hyoid bone is isolated and then advanced over the thyroid ala. It is then immobilized with two medial and two lateral permanent sutures (Fig 3-18). The wound is closed, a drain placed and a pressure dressing applied.

Maxillomandibular osteotomy and advancement (MMO) prevents retropalatal collapse through stenting of the superior pharyngeal muscles and widening of the nasopharyngeal inlet. It also minimizes retrolingual obstruction by placing the genioglossus muscle under tension, providing more room in the oral cavity for soft tissues, and stenting the lateral pharyngeal wall. An outer-table cranial bone graft usually is performed, along with archbar placement (or orthodontic banding in an outpatient setting) prior to the osteotomies. A LeFort I maxillary osteotomy and bilateral sagittal-split mandibular osteotomy are performed. The skeletal

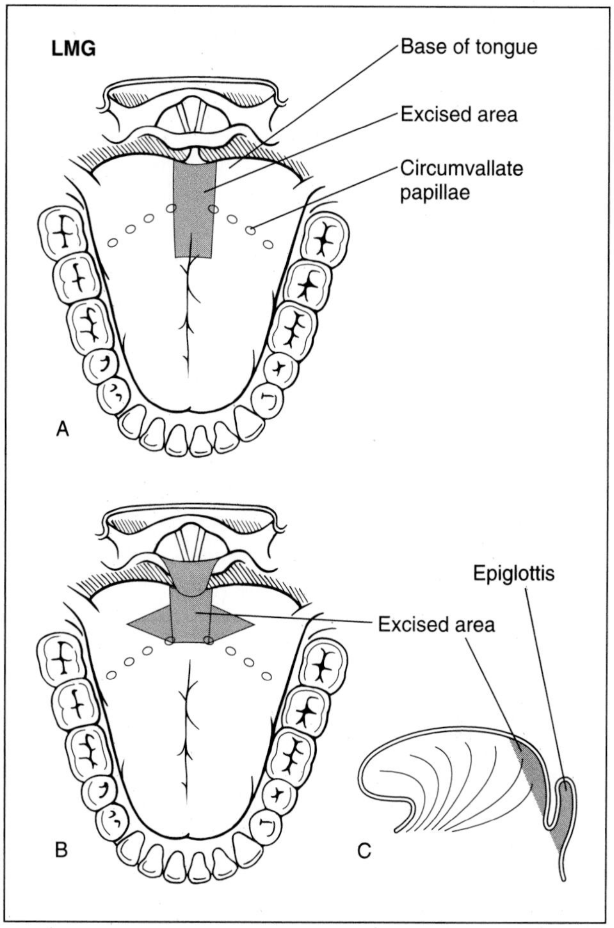

Figure 3-16. LMG/lingualplasty technique: (A) Excision of a midline segment of the base of the tongue is performed with a laser or electrocautery; this excision occasionally is carried lateral. (B) The remaining tongue muscle edges are reapproximated with absorbable suture. (C) Lateral view of tongue.

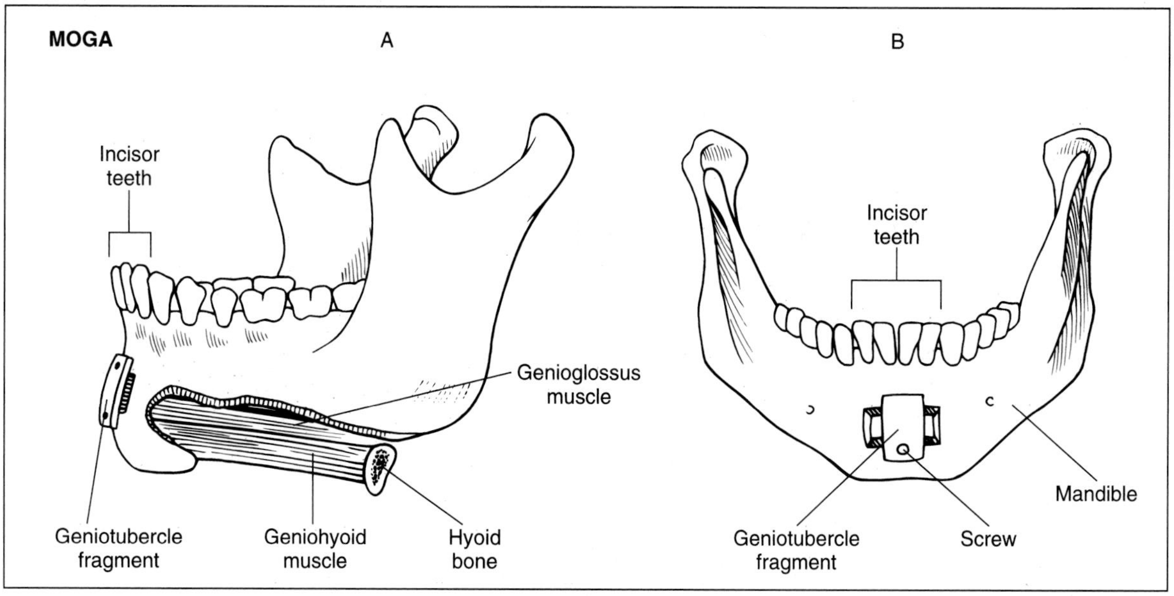

Figure 3-17. The mandibular osteotomy and genioglossus advancement (MOGA) technique: (A) Lateral view. (B) Anterior view. A rectangular anterior mandibular osteotomy below the incisor teeth is advanced, rotated and immobilized.

arches are advanced forward approximately 10 mm and secured with the aid of a methylmethacrylate dental splint (Fig 3-19). Immobilization with wires, plates and screws follows, then wound closure, intermaxillary fixation and pressure dressing application. This procedure usually is performed if previous upper airway procedures have not completely relieved the sleep-related obstruction.

Tracheotomy is a procedure in which a horizontal or vertical cervical incision is performed midway between the manubrium and the cricoid cartilage. Dissection is carried out in the midline down to the trachea, frequently transecting the thyroid gland; then, an opening in the superior trachea allows placement of a tracheotomy tube (Fig 3-9).

Usual preop diagnosis: Sleep disordered breathing, including upper airway resistance syndrome and obstructive sleep apnea (OSA) syndrome

SUMMARY OF PROCEDURES

Position	Supine
Incision	Intraoral (except HM–horizontal cervical above hyoid bone)
Special instrumentation	For osteotomy cases (MOGA, MMO), sagittal and reciprocating saws, drills
Unique considerations	When using a CO_2 laser (LMG, LP), a laser-safe ETT or, more commonly, tracheotomy tube is required. MMO requires a nasal intubation. Tracheotomy may be performed with patient sitting with iv sedation and/or local infiltration. Dexamethasone 8 mg iv.
Antibiotics	Cefazolin 1 g iv
Surgical time	UPPP, UPF: 20-60 min UPPGP, LMG, LP: 1-3 h MOGA, HM: 30-60 min MMO: 3-5 h
EBL	UPPP, UPF, MOGA, HM: 0-100 ml UPPGP, LMG, LP: 50-250 ml MMO: 100-500 ml
Postop care	UPPP, UPF: PACU → ward Multiple procedures, MMO, labile HTN: ICU → ward
Mortality	Rare
Morbidity	Bleeding Infection Wound dehiscence Hematoma/seroma formation Parasthesias HTN Upper airway obstruction
Pain score	UPPP, UPPGP, LMG, LP: 8-10 UPF, MOGA, HM, MMO: 6-8

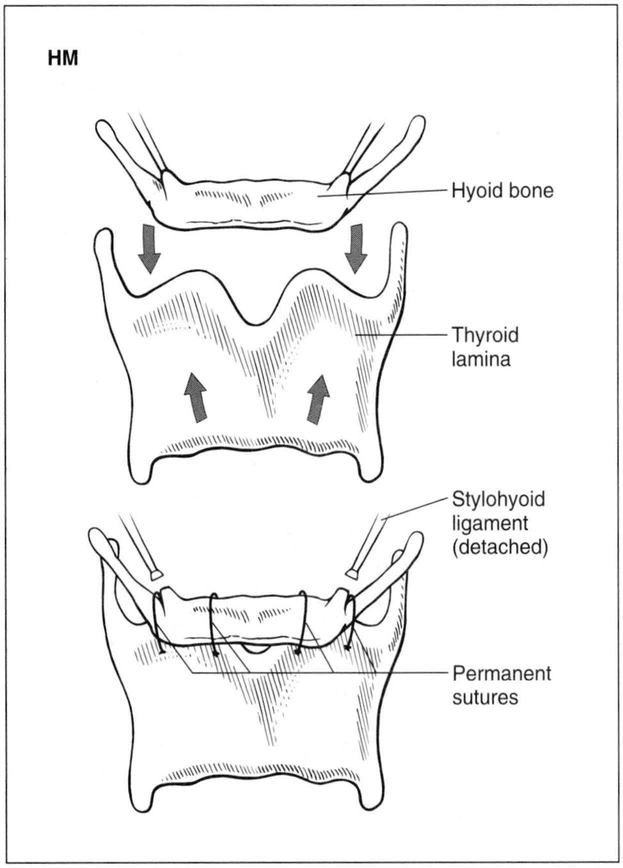

Figure 3-18. The hyoid myotomy (HM) and suspension technique: the hyoid is advanced over the thyroid lamina and immobilized.

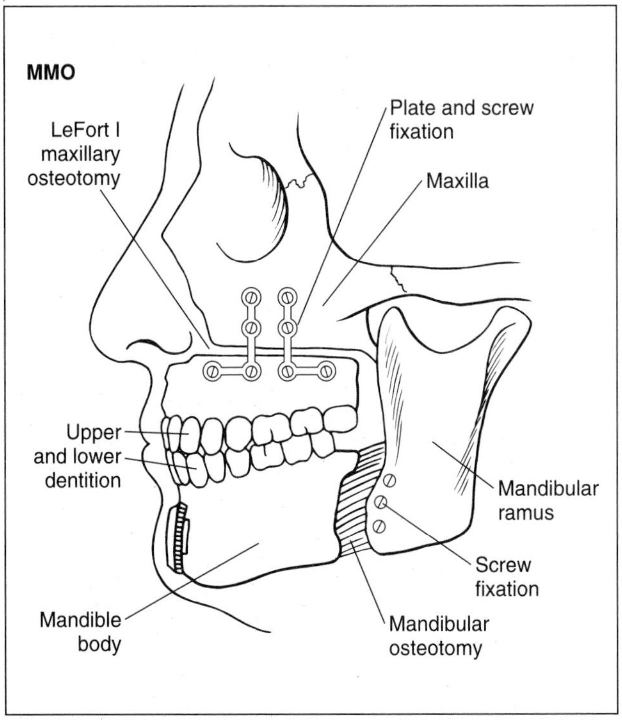

Figure 3-19. Maxillomandibular osteotomy (MMO) and advancement surgery technique.

PATIENT POPULATION CHARACTERISTICS

Age range	Children, adolescents, adults
Male:Female	3-10: 1
Incidence	4-10% of adult males; 2-4% of adult females
Etiology	Upper airway collapse by frank obstruction or muscular relaxation
Associated conditions	Systemic and pulmonary HTN; CAD; cardiac arrhythmias; GERD; depression; obesity; polycythemia

ANESTHETIC CONSIDERATIONS

PREOPERATIVE

Patients with OSA often present with a variety of related medical conditions. These may range from chronic fatigue to an increased risk of sudden death. Some patients may have OSA associated with morbid obesity (see p. 354). Typically, these patients are exquisitely sensitive to sedative drugs. Preop evaluation should include their ability to tolerate the supine position without obstructing.

Respiratory Chronic OSA → hypoxia/hypercarbia → pulmonary HTN → right heart failure. Careful assessment of the airway is essential (suitability for mask ventilation vs need for awake FOL or tracheostomy). Typically, 25% of the patients will present with airway management problems that may require awake FOL (4%) or tracheostomy (3%). Preop evaluation should include a discussion with the surgeon of the results of preop fiber optic nasopharyngoscopy.
Tests: CXR; PFT; ABG, if indicated from H&P.

Cardiovascular Patients are at ↑risk for systemic and pulmonary HTN (Sx: loud P_2, clubbing, ↑JVD, cyanosis, RVH, right-axis deviation), cardiac arrhythmias, cerebrovascular disease and CAD. These patients may have dyspnea on exertion and at rest, making difficult the routine assessment of cardiovascular function and reserve.
Tests: ECG; ECHO; others as indicated from H&P.

Neurologic These patients may be chronically fatigued and irritable due to disrupted sleep patterns. Daytime sleepiness also may be associated with hypothyroidism or anemia, which should have been ruled out.
Tests: As indicated by H&P.

Hematologic Chronic hypoxia → polycythemia (Sx: clubbing, cyanosis) → ↑risk of CVA.
Test: Hct

Gastrointestinal This patient population has a higher incidence of GERD and hiatal hernia; thus, full-stomach precautions (see p. B-5) may be required.

Laboratory **Tests:** As indicated from H&P.

Premedication Typically, all sedative medication should be avoided in this patient population; however, if sedative premedication is to be given, the anesthesiologist must remain with the patient and be prepared to manage the airway.

INTRAOPERATIVE

Anesthetic technique: Typically GETA; however, patients undergoing UPF, MOGA and HM may only require MAC.

Induction Consideration must be given to securing the airway before induction of anesthesia if a difficult intubation is anticipated. Fiber optic intubation with minimal sedation is recommended for these patients (see Awake FOL, p. B-7). Otherwise, standard induction with no muscle relaxant until ability to mask ventilate is assured. A short-acting (e.g., mivacurium 0.15 mg/kg) or intermediate-acting (e.g., vecuronium 0.1 mg/kg) muscle relaxant may be administered after mask ventilation is established. MMO requires nasal intubation.

Maintenance Maintenance with N_2O, propofol and narcotics, in conjunction with low-dose inhalational agents, will facilitate smooth emergence compared to maintenance with higher doses of inhalational agents. Anticipate ↑BP in response to surgical procedure, especially in patients with preexisting HTN, during UPPP, and with fracture of pterygoid plate in MMO. Resist temptation to treat ↑BP with ↑inhalational anesthetics alone, as emergence will be compromised. Labetalol (5-10 mg increments)

	and hydralazine (5 mg increments) frequently are required, while esmolol and SNP infusions are occasionally needed.	
Emergence	The patient should remain intubated until sufficiently awake to respond to a series of commands. Premature extubation can cause complete loss of airway or laryngospasm. Airway is likely to be worse upon emergence than preop because of surgically induced edema. Extubation over a tube changer may be appropriate in some cases. Anticipate ↑BP during emergence, which will continue into first postop day. Antihypertensive agents frequently required as postop HTN can cause bleeding, particularly from osteotomy sites.	
Blood and fluid requirements	IV: 16-18 ga × 1 NS/LR @ 1-3 ml/kg/h	Minimal-to-little blood loss with all except MMO. EBL with MMO is 100-500 ml. Attempt to minimize fluids to reduce severity of postop airway edema (< 1000 ml of NS/LR for all except MMO; < 2000 ml for MMO).
Monitoring	Standard monitors (p. B-1) Arterial line (MMO)	Arterial line also suggested for postop BP control in all patients with preexisting HTN and in any patient who displays labile BP intraop. Control of BP in the postop period is a high priority.
Positioning	✓ and pad pressure points. ✓ eyes.	Occasional requests for minimal Trendelenburg or sitting maneuvers.
Complications	ETT damage Hemorrhage	ETT may be cut during MMO, necessitating rapid reintubation.

POSTOPERATIVE

Complications	Airway compromise Airway obstruction	Airway compromise 2° hematoma, edema, excessive sedation or underlying disease. Consider observation in ICU for patients having multiple procedures, MMO or labile HTN.
	HTN Aspiration	Postop HTN is extremely common, and can contribute significantly to likelihood of postop airway obstruction 2° hematoma.
Pain management	Minimize iv narcotics.	Avoid excessive postop sedation. UPPP patients, in particular, should be warned preop of anticipated significant postop discomfort.

References

1. Burgess L, Derderian S, Morin G, et al: Postoperative risk following uvulopalatopharyngoplasty for obstructive sleep apnea. *Otolaryngol Head Neck Surg* 1992; 106:81-6.
2. Conway W, Fujita S, Zorick F, et al: Uvulopalatopharyngoplasty. One-year followup. *Chest* 1985; 88:385-87.
3. Escalamado RM, Glenn MG, McCulloch TM, Cummings CW: Perioperative complications and risk factors in the surgical treatment of obstructive sleep apnea. *Laryngoscope* 1989; 99:1125-29.
4. Fairbanks, DN: Snoring: Surgical vs nonsurgical management. *Laryngoscope* 1984; 94:1188-92.
5. Fujita S, Conway W, Zorick F, et al: Surgical correction of anatomic abnormalities in obstructive sleep apnea syndrome: Uvulopalatopharyngoplasty. *Otolaryngol Head Neck Surg* 1981; 89:923-34.
6. Mickleson SA, Rosenthal L: Midline glossectomy and epiglottidectomy for obstructive sleep apnea syndrome. *Laryngoscope* 1997; 107:614-19.
7. Powell N, Riley R, Guilleminault C, Troell R: A reversible uvulopalatal flap for snoring and sleep apnea syndrome. *Sleep* 1996; 19(7):593-99.
8. Riley R, Powell N, Guilleminault C: Obstructive sleep apnea and the hyoid: a revised surgical procedure. *Otolaryngol Head Neck Surg* 1994; 111:717-21.
9. Riley RW, Powell NP, Guilleminault C, Pelayo R, Troell RJ: Obstructive sleep apnea surgery: Risk management and complications. *Otolaryngol Head Neck Surg* 1997; (6):648-52.
10. Riley R. Powell N, Guilleminault C: Obstructive sleep apnea syndrome: a review of 306 consecutively treated surgical patients. *Otolaryngol Head Neck Surg* 1993; 108:117-25.
11. Sher A, Schechtman K, Piccirillo J: The efficacy of surgical modifications of the upper airway in adults with obstructive sleep apnea syndrome. *Sleep* 1996; 19(2):156-77.
12. Woodson BT, Fujita S: Clinical experience with lingualplasty as part of the treatment of severe obstructive sleep apnea. *Otolaryngol Head Neck Surg* 1992; 107:40-8.

Surgeon

Stephen A. Schendel, MD, DDS

4.0 DENTAL SURGERY

Anesthesiologists

Richard A. Jaffe, MD, PhD
Stanley I. Samuels, MB, BCh, FFARCS

TEMPOROMANDIBULAR JOINT ARTHROSCOPY/ARTHROPLASTY

SURGICAL CONSIDERATIONS

Description: Temporomandibular joint (TMJ) arthroplasty is a common procedure that usually is performed bilaterally. This involves a preauricular incision with opening of the joint compartment and, normally, a repositioning of the disc. Severely damaged discs require removal and replacement. When a disc removal is required, a substitute material, consisting chiefly of temporalis fascia flaps, free dermagrafts or auricular cartilage grafts, is usually placed. Associated with this may be procedures to smooth and reshape the condylar head and eminence of the glenoid fossa. **TMJ arthroscopy** may be performed prior to the actual arthroplasty, or as a separate procedure. This involves placing a scope into the joint from a preauricular approach and visualizing the internal structures of the superior compartment for the purpose of irrigation and debridement.

Usual preop diagnosis: Internal derangement, subluxation and ankylosis of TMJ

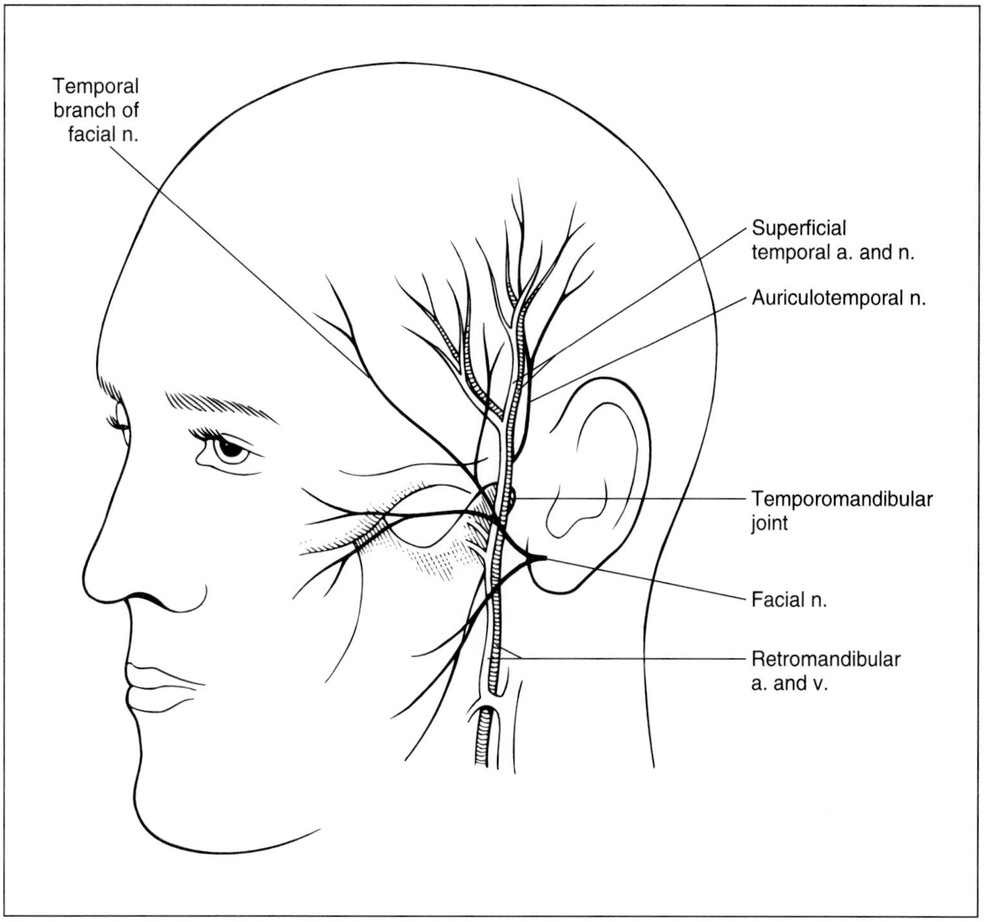

Figure 4-1. Anatomy for TMJ procedure.

SUMMARY OF PROCEDURE

	Arthroscopy	Arthroplasty
Position	Supine	⇐
Incision	Preauricular	⇐
Special instrumentation	Arthroscope; laser	Air power tools
Antibiotics	Penicillin 2 million U q 6 h	⇐
Surgical time	0.5 h	1.5 h/side
EBL	Minimal	⇐

	Arthroscopy	Arthroplasty
Postop care	May be an outpatient procedure; PACU → room.	⇐
Mortality	Minimal	⇐
Morbidity	VII nerve damage: 7-32%[2,4]	⇐
	Hemorrhage	
	V nerve damage	
Pain score	5	6

PATIENT POPULATION CHARACTERISTICS

Age range	20-40 yr
Male:Female	1:9
Incidence	Up to 17% of the population suffers from TMJ dysfunction (TMJD).
Etiology	TMJD possibly 2° muscle spasm, bruxism, osteoarthritis; idiopathic; trauma
Associated conditions	Psychiatric problems—typically depression; trismus; pain on opening mouth

ANESTHETIC CONSIDERATIONS

See Anesthetic Considerations for Dental/Oral Surgery, p. 168.

ORAL SURGERY

SURGICAL CONSIDERATIONS

Description: Surgery of the oral cavity, frequently performed under GA, includes the removal of impacted teeth, multiple dental extractions, preprosthetic surgery (e.g., vestibuloplasties [surgical modifications of the gingival mucous membrane relationships]) and the insertion of osteointegrated implants.

SUMMARY OF PROCEDURE

	Surgical Removal of Teeth	Preprosthetic Surgery	Dental Implants
Position	Supine	⇐	⇐
Incision	Intraoral	⇐	⇐
Special instrumentation	None	⇐	Specific dental implant insertion kit and implants
Unique considerations	Nasotracheal intubation; throat pack used.	⇐	⇐
Antibiotics	Penicillin × 5 d po	⇐	⇐
Surgical time	0.5-1 h	1-2 h	0.5-2 h
EBL	Minimal	⇐	⇐
Postop care	PACU → home	⇐	⇐
Mortality	Minimal	⇐	⇐
Morbidity	Pain	⇐	⇐
	Aspiration of dental debris	–	–
	Swelling	–	–
	Infection	–	Loss of implant
Pain score	3	3	2

PATIENT POPULATION CHARACTERISTICS

	Surgical Removal of Teeth	Preprosthetic Surgery	Dental Implants
Age range	15-20 yr	> 40 yr	⇐
Male:Female	1:1	⇐	⇐
Incidence	Unknown	⇐	⇐
Etiology	Congenital; idiopathic	⇐	⇐
Associated conditions	Loose teeth	⇐	

ANESTHETIC CONSIDERATIONS

See Anesthetic Considerations for Dental/Oral Surgery, p 168.

RESTORATIVE DENTISTRY

SURGICAL CONSIDERATIONS

Description: Multiple dental restorative procedures are performed under GA when there is rampant caries, and an extensive amount of dental work must be performed at one time. The second most common indication for GA is for procedures that need to be performed on mentally retarded patients who are not candidates for a local anesthetic. The actual amount of restorative dentistry is quite variable, depending on the individual case; thus, surgical time can be quite variable. Generally, blood loss is not a problem.

SUMMARY OF PROCEDURE

Position	Supine
Incision	Intraoral
Special instrumentation	Dental armamentarium
Unique considerations	Nasal intubation; throat pack
Antibiotics	Penicillin × 5 d po
Surgical time	0.5-3 h
EBL	Minimal
Postop care	PACU → home
Mortality	Minimal
Morbidity	Pain Aspiration of dental debris Swelling
Pain score	1-3

PATIENT POPULATION CHARACTERISTICS

Age range	2 yr - adult
Male:Female	1:1
Incidence	Unknown
Etiology	Idiopathic or congenital anomalies
Associated conditions	Mental retardation (majority); Down syndrome, seizures

ANESTHETIC CONSIDERATIONS FOR DENTAL/ORAL SURGERY

PREOPERATIVE

Most patients presenting for dental or oral surgery usually will require only local anesthesia provided by the dentist/oral surgeon. GA may be required, however, for several unique patient groups: (1) young children (some with systemic diseases such as CHD, hemophilia); (2) the mentally retarded; (3) those with poorly controlled seizure disorders; (4) those presenting for TMJ procedures; and (5) those with an oral septic focus, who may be quite ill. If the patient does not fall into one of these readily identifiable categories, the reasons for GA should be ascertained.

Airway Patients presenting for TMJ procedures may have problems with mouth opening (2° pain, trismus and arthritis), making airway examination difficult. Mouth opening may not improve with GA and muscle relaxation. Nasotracheal intubation using FOL (done awake in patients with difficult airways) should be planned. Examine nares for patency; check for loose teeth.

Respiratory Surgery should be postponed (2 wk) in patients presenting with Sx of acute RTI (fever, coughing, purulent sputum, etc.). Sx of chronic respiratory disease should be sought and treated before surgery.
Tests: As indicated from H&P.

Cardiovascular Patients with dysrhythmias may be sensitive to the epinephrine used in local anesthetic solutions administered intraop. As with other types of elective surgery, preexisting cardiovascular problems should be treated before inducing anesthesia. Prophylactic antibiotics for endocarditis may be required in some patients.
Tests: As indicated from H&P.

Neurological Patients with seizure disorders should be on optimal medical therapy before surgery. Discuss precipitating factors and prodromal Sx with the patient.
Tests: ✓ therapeutic levels of anticonvulsant (e.g., phenytoin = 10-20 μg/ml; carbamazepine = 3-12 μg/ml; phenobarbital = 10-40 μg/ml).

Musculoskeletal In addition to TMJ problems, rheumatoid arthritis is associated with cricoarytenoid joint immobility and cervical spine immobility/instability that may complicate intubation.

Laboratory Other tests as indicated from H&P.

Premedication Standard premedication (see p. B-2) usually is appropriate, although in patients with limited airway access, sedation may be inappropriate. If FOL is planned, pretreatment with an antisialagogue (e.g., glycopyrrolate 4 μg/kg) is useful.

INTRAOPERATIVE

Anesthetic technique: GETA. Typically a nasotracheal intubation is required, using an ET tube 0.5-1 mm smaller than for oral intubation. In patients with difficult airways, an awake nasal FOL is indicated. (See general discussion of Awake FOL, p. B-6.)

Induction In patients with normal airways, a standard induction (see p. B-2) is appropriate. Following loss of consciousness, topical intranasal cocaine is applied (4% on pledgets, 4 ml maximum) to shrink the nasal mucosa and for vasoconstriction. The well lubricated ETT is passed through the nose into the trachea, either blindly or assisted by McGill's forceps under direct laryngoscopy. ETT is often sewn to nasal septum.

Maintenance Standard maintenance (see p. B-3).

Emergence No special considerations except that throat packs must be removed prior to extubation.

Blood and fluid requirements IV: 18 ga × 1
NS/LR @ 4-6 ml/kg/h

Monitoring Standard monitors (see p. B-1).

Positioning ✓ and pad pressure points.
✓ eyes.

POSTOPERATIVE

Complications Airway obstruction 2° retained throat pack

Complications, cont.	N&V	These patients may swallow blood, with consequent N&V. Rx: metoclopramide 10 mg iv.
Pain management	Oral analgesics (see p. C-1).	

References for Dental/Oral Surgery

1. Coplans MP, Green RA: *Anesthesia and Sedation in Dentistry*. Elsevier Science Pub Co, New York: 1983.
2. Dolwick MF, Kretzschmar DP: Morbidity associated with the preauricular and perimeatal approaches to the temporomandibular joint. *J Oral Maxillofac Surg* 1982; 40(11):699-700.
3. Gotta AW, Sullivan CA, Rocanelli L: Oral surgery and temporomandibular joint arthroscopy. In *Ambulatory Anesthesiology: A Problem-Oriented Approach*. McGoldrick KE, ed. Williams & Wilkins, New York: 1995, 572-79.
4. Zide BM: The temporomandibular joint. In *Plastic Surgery*, Vol 2. McCarthy JG, ed. WB Saunders Co, Philadelphia: 1990, 1475-1513.

Surgeons

Walter B. Cannon, MD
James B.D. Mark, MD

5.0 THORACIC SURGERY

Anesthesiologists

Brett G. Fitzmaurice, MD
Jay B. Brodsky, MD

THORACIC SURGERY

INTRODUCTION—SURGEON'S PERSPECTIVE

AIRWAY AND LUNG ACCESS CONFLICTS

As in Head and Neck Surgery, induction and maintenance of anesthesia for thoracic surgery requires interdisciplinary cooperation. Perioperative communication between the surgeon and anesthesiologist is required for a satisfactory outcome. For example, during periods of OLV, significant hypoxia and hypotension may occur. Surgery may need to be stopped temporarily while the hypoxia is corrected by reinflation of the unventilated lung. Hypotension in the absence of bleeding can be corrected by less vigorous retraction of the lung and heart by the surgeon. Quick and timely communication between the anesthesiologist and the surgeon can be life-saving. Occasionally, during critical parts of the dissection, cessation of all respiration for short periods of time can make the surgeon's job much easier.

TUBES AND TUBE SIZES

Although the size of the ET tubes may not be particularly critical for most anesthetics, thoracic surgical procedures may be different. Fiber optic bronchoscopy through the ETT is a common event. The standard fiber optic bronchoscope just fits through the 8.0 ET tube. The fiber optic laryngoscope used for difficult intubations will fit smaller ETTs and DLTs. Proper lubrication of the bronchoscope with a Carbowax ointment (rather than an aqueous jelly that will dry out quickly) makes manipulation quite easy. The fiber optic laryngoscope can be used for correct positioning of the DLT. If the bronchial portion of the DLT cannot be advanced into the left main bronchus, the bronchoscope can be advanced through the bronchial side of the DLT into the left main bronchus. Then, through use of the bronchoscope as a stent, the DLT can be advanced over the bronchoscope into the left bronchus. The depth of the tube can be determined by bronchoscopic observation of the right main bronchus through the tracheal side of the DLT. If a laser is to be involved, have a laser-compatible ETT available, keep FiO_2 to less than 0.3 and do not use N_2O.

PATIENT POSITIONING

The standard thoracotomy requires either a left or a right lateral decubitus position. After the patient is anesthetized and intubated, he/she is placed on the left or right side. (Note: reviewing a recent CXR in the OR will help ensure that the thoracotomy is performed on the correct side). An axillary roll and pads under the down knee and between the knees will prevent damage to nerves (brachial plexus and peroneal). A bean bag under the chest, abdomen and hip helps to stabilize the patient. Adhesive tape can be strapped across the patient at the hip level for safety. The arm can be supported by pillows or a standard airplane arm support. The down knee should be bent about 90 degrees and the upper leg should be straight and supported by pillows. Breaking (flexing) the operating table to increase the separation between the hip and stomach will improve surgical access. Prior to wound closure, the operating table should be returned to the flat position. If requested by the surgeon, downward pressure on the upper shoulder by the anesthesiologist or assistant helps with wound closure.

LOBECTOMY, PNEUMONECTOMY

SURGICAL CONSIDERATIONS

Description: It is generally agreed that appropriate **pulmonary resection**, including lymph node dissection, is the mainstay of treatment for a curable carcinoma of the lung. The operations most often carried out are **lobectomy** (or **bilobectomy** on the right) or **pneumonectomy**, depending on the extent of the disease. (Fig 5-1 shows segmental anatomy of the lung.) If the cancer is encompassable and entirely removable by lobectomy, then pneumonectomy is not necessary. There is some enthusiasm for even more conservative resection of lung cancers with curative intent. (See Wedge Resection of Lung Lesion, p. 179, and Thoracoscopy, p. 202)

The standard incision for lobectomy or pneumonectomy, or for any operation requiring safe access to the pulmonary hilar structures, is posterolateral with the patient in the lateral decubitus position. Latissimus dorsi and serratus anterior muscles are divided. A rib may or may not be resected. Exploration of the pleural cavity is carried out to determine resectability in the case of lung cancer and to further assess the pathologic process which is present. Safe dissection and division of appropriate hilar vessels and bronchi depend on the surgeon having a thorough knowledge of hilar anatomy, including its important variations (of which there are many). Complications are far better prevented than treated. Specific techniques for division of vessels and bronchi vary among surgeons. For the main PA and veins, staplers are used widely. Some thoracic surgeons still ligate vessels and staple bronchi. Fewer suture bronchi.

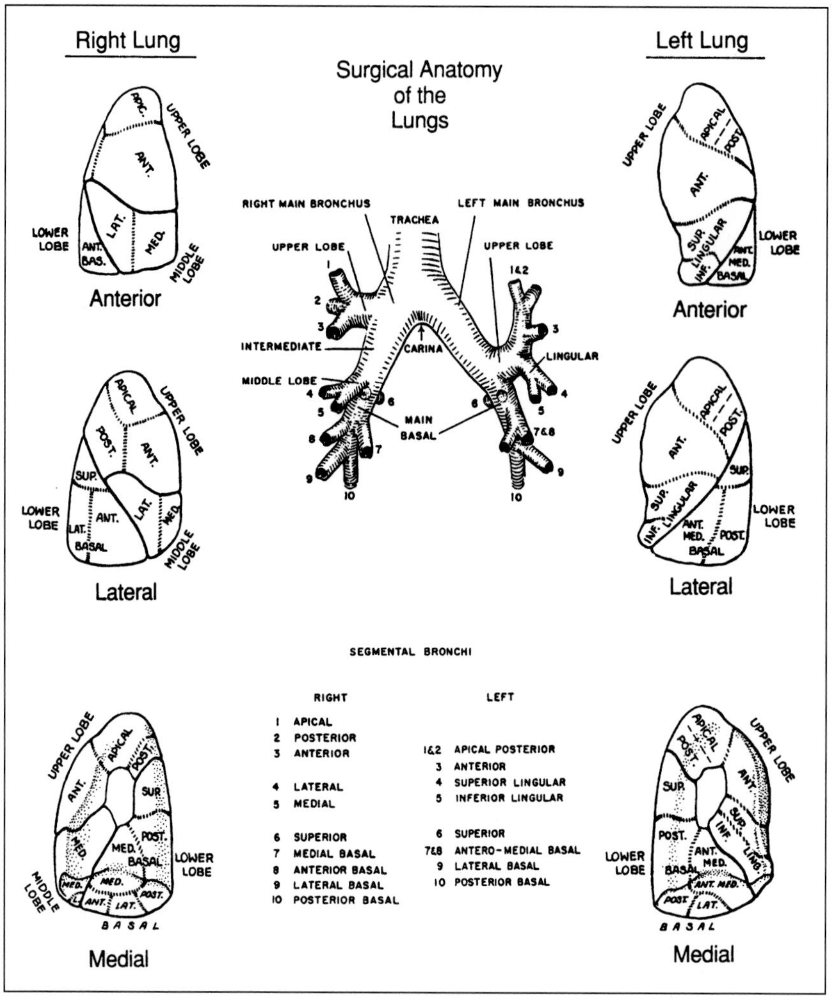

Figure 5-1. Segmental anatomy of the lungs. (Reproduced with permission from Waldhausen JA, Pierce WS: *Johnson's Surgery of the Chest.* Hill E, Beisel D, illustrators. Year Book Medical Pub: 1965.)

Standard chest drainage following lobectomy calls for the use of two tubes, usually 28-36 Fr, one positioned anteriorly and one posteriorly. The tubes are attached to an underwater seal apparatus. Suction is employed (usually at –20 cmH_2O) to encourage expansion of the remaining lobe or lobes, in addition to improving drainage of air and fluid. Pleural drainage following pneumonectomy is not practiced uniformly. A small (16 Fr) tube may be placed during closing in order to establish an intrapleural pressure of about –5 cmH_2O by removal of or instillation of air. At this point, the tube is removed. Our preference is to leave a 24-28 Fr tube in the empty pleural cavity for 18-24 hours with the tube attached to a special pneumonectomy Pleurevac, which balances the intrapleural pressures appropriately and does not allow suction. A more limited, muscle-sparing incision is sometimes used in an effort to cause less pain and, consequently, fewer postop pulmonary problems. Postop pain generally can be well controlled with epidural analgesia. The standard incision provides the safest access to structures deep in the chest. Median sternotomy can be used for pneumonectomy or lobectomy, although it has the disadvantage of providing less access to the posteriorly placed structures and particularly difficult access to the left inferior pulmonary vein.

Lobectomy and, less often, pneumonectomy are occasionally accompanied by bronchoplasty in order to preserve functioning pulmonary tissue while still completely removing the cancer. In special circumstances a median sternotomy approach is used for lobectomy or pneumonectomy.

Usual preop diagnosis: Carcinoma of the lung

SUMMARY OF PROCEDURE

	Lobectomy	Pneumonectomy
Position	Lateral/supine	⇐
Incision	Posterolateral/median sternotomy	⇐
Special instrumentation	DLT; SCD or TED hose	⇐
Antibiotics	Cefazolin 1 g	⇐

	Lobectomy	Pneumonectomy
Surgical time	2-3 h	⇐
EBL	< 500 ml (more in redo or inflammatory cases)	⇐
Postop care	ICU; careful attention to pulmonary toilet; chest tube output – tubes	Special balanced drainage – tube
Mortality	± 1%	± 5%
Morbidity	Dysrhythmias: 20-30%	⇐
	DVT: 5-20%	⇐
	PE	⇐
	MI	⇐
	Bronchopleural fistula	⇐
	Chylothorax	⇐
	Subcutaneous emphysema	⇐
	Phrenic nerve injury	⇐
	Recurrent laryngeal nerve injury	⇐
Pain score	7-8	7-8

PATIENT POPULATION CHARACTERISTICS

Age range	0-80 yr
Male:Female	15:1
Incidence	Common thoracic procedure; increasing in females.
Etiology	Smoking
Associated conditions	Cardiopulmonary disease; PVD

ANESTHETIC CONSIDERATIONS

PREOPERATIVE

Most patients presenting for these operations have either an infectious process or a lung neoplasm. They often have Hx of cigarette smoking with associated emphysema and/or chronic bronchitis. Selective lung isolation with or without OLV (with a DLT or a BB) is essential for this procedure.

Respiratory Question patient about dyspnea, productive cough and cigarette smoking. Examine patient for cyanosis, clubbing, RR and pattern. Listen to chest for wheezes, rhonchi, rales. Morbidity and mortality following thoracotomy increased with preexisting pulmonary, cardiovascular and neurologic disease.

Tests: PFT (see below and Table 5-1); CXR; if chest CT available, look for airway obstruction that could interfere with DLT placement; ABG.

Pulmonary function Establish a baseline and identify patients with advanced pulmonary disease who are unable to tolerate planned operation. Obtain whole-lung tests (ABG, spirometry), and single-lung tests (split-function lung tests = ventilation/perfusion studies) if pneumonectomy planned. A VC at least 3 × TV is necessary for effective cough postop. A VC < 50% predicted or < 1500 ml predicts increased risk for postop complications following pulmonary resection. Operative risk for pneumonectomy increases if patient is hypercapnic ($PaCO_2$ > 45 mmHg) on room air, FEV_1/FVC < 50% of predicted, FEV_1 < 2 L, if > 60-70% blood flow is to diseased lung, and if mean PA pressure increases > 30 mmHg with occlusion of PA. Mimic post pneumonectomy conditions by temporary unilateral occlusion of main PA. Patient may show improvement in PFTs following bronchodilator therapy.

Cardiovascular Prophylactic digitalization to reduce risk of postop heart failure is controversial and may be reserved for those at high risk of right heart failure. Consider subcutaneous heparin (5000 U) for DVT prophylaxis.

Tests: ECG—look for evidence of RV hypertrophy, conduction problems and prior ischemia; ECHO to evaluate RV function; others as indicated from H&P.

Neurological ✓ Hx of previous back surgery, peripheral neuropathy. Examine lumbar area for skin lesions, infection, deformities. Avoid placement of epidural catheter in patient with neurologic problems.

Table 5-1. Assessment of Risk of Postop Pulmonary Complications Following Thoracic and Abdominal Procedures

Category	Point
I. Expiratory Spirogram	
a. Normal (%FVC + %FEV_1/FVC >150)	0
b. %FVC + %FEV_1/FVC = 100-150	1
c. %FVC + %FEV_1/FVC < 100	2
d. Preop FVC < 20 ml/kg	3
e. Post-bronchodilator FEV_1/FVC < 50%	3
II. Cardiovascular System	
a. Normal	0
b. Controlled HTN, MI sequelae for more than 2 yr	0
c. Dyspnea on exertion, orthopnea, paroxysmal nocturnal dyspnea, dependent edema, CHF, angina	1
III. ABGs	
a. Acceptable	0
b. $PaCO_2$ >50 mm Hg or $PaCO_2$ < 60 mmHg on room air	1
c. Metabolic pH abnormality > 7.50 or < 7.30	1
IV. Nervous System	
a. Normal	0
b. Confusion, obtundation, agitation, spasticity, discoordination, bulbar malfunction	1
c. Significant muscular weakness	1
V. Postop Ambulation	
a. Expected ambulation (minimum, sitting at bedside) within 36 h	0
b. Expected complete bed confinement for at least 36 h	1

0 Points = Low Risk 1-2 Points = Moderate Risk 3 Points = High Risk

Shapira BA, Harrison RA, Kacmarek RM, Cane RD: *Clinical Application of Respiratory Care*, 3rd edition. Year Book Medical Publishers, Chicago: 1985. (With permission.)

Musculoskeletal Patients with lung cancer may have myasthenic (Eaton-Lambert) syndrome with increased sensitivity to nondepolarizing muscle relaxants. Monitor relaxation with peripheral nerve stimulator.

Hematologic Transfuse patient with preop Hct < 25%. Adequate O_2-carrying capacity essential. T&C 2-4 U of blood, or obtain 1-3 U of autologous blood during the month before surgery.
Tests: Hct; PT; PTT (if epidural anesthesia planned)

Laboratory Other tests as indicated from H&P.

Premedication Midazolam 1-2 mg iv if patient anxious. When epidural opioids are planned, avoid opioid or sedative premedication which can potentiate postop respiratory effects of spinal opioids.

INTRAOPERATIVE

Anesthetic technique: Combined epidural (lumbar or thoracic) and inhalational agent. Anesthesia for lobectomy/pneumonectomy relies upon OLV techniques to improve surgical exposure and minimize damage to the operative lung in the case of lobectomy or bilobectomy. The challenges to the anesthesiologist include maintaining oxygenation in patients with poor pulmonary reserve, and ensuring that the patient is comfortable, warm and awake at the end of surgery.

Preinduction A lumbar epidural catheter is placed and advanced 4-6 cm past needle in epidural space; secure with tape. Administer test dose: 3 ml lidocaine (1.5%) + 1:200,000 epinephrine. If no hypotension or tachycardia, administer 12-18 ml lidocaine (1.5-2.0%) and record evidence of anesthetic level. Confirm functioning epidural catheter preop to ensure predictable postop analgesia. Giving local anesthetics through the epidural catheter intraop reduces the amounts of general anesthetics and muscle relaxants required. Post thoracotomy analgesia is excellent with thoracic or lumbar epidural opioids. Placement of a lumbar catheter is safer than a thoracic catheter. Fentanyl (75-100 μg) or morphine (4 mg) are often used with local anesthetics (e.g., bupivacaine 0.125%, 4-6 ml).

Induction

Standard induction (p. B-2). Intubate with SLT (≥ 8 mm), which will be replaced with DLT after bronchoscopy (see below).

Maintenance

O_2 and isoflurane (1.0-1.5%); less anesthetic required when epidural local anesthetics used. Avoid N_2O, especially during OLV, since hypoxemia is unpredictable. Use FiO_2 = 1.0. Lidocaine (1.5% or 2.0%) 10-12 ml, administered via lumbar epidural every 45 min, or bupivacaine (0.5%) 10-12 ml every 1.5-2 h with hydromorphone (Dilaudid) (1.0-1.5 mg) or morphine (5.0-7.5 mg) in 10 ml NS through lumbar epidural during case. Epidural hydromorphone is preferred since, in equipotent doses, analgesia is equivalent to that with morphine, but with fewer side effects. Lung manipulation during surgery releases vasoactive substances that interfere with hypoxic pulmonary vasoconstrictive (HPV) reflex. Thus, clinically, the choice of anesthetic agent should not be influenced by experimental studies which indicated that the HPV reflex is maintained with iv agents, but may not be with inhalational agents. Inhalational anesthetics are potent bronchodilators and depress airway reflexes.

Emergence

Prior to closing of chest, lungs are inflated to 30 cmH_2O pressure to reinflate atelectatic areas and to check for significant air leaks. Surgeon inserts chest tubes to drain pleural cavity and aid lung reexpansion. Patient is extubated in OR. If postop ventilation is required (rare), DLT exchanged for ETT. Patient transferred in head-elevated position to PACU or ICU breathing mask O_2. If hemodynamically unstable, monitor ECG, pulse oximetry and arterial pressure during transfer.

Blood and fluid requirements

IV: 18 ga x 1 + 16 ga × 1
Restrict iv fluids; usually administer 1000-1500 ml NS/LR total.
Blood: ± 1 U autologous blood if available; use vasopressor (ephedrine 5-10 mg iv bolus or phenylephrine 50-100 μg iv bolus) if hypotensive.

Postop, PVR is increased proportionate to the amount of lung tissue removed. An overhydrated patient is at increased risk of right heart failure. Use of epidural local anesthetics can cause hypotension in a volume-restricted patient; vasopressor often needed.

Monitoring

Standard monitors (p. B-1)
Arterial line
Urinary catheter
± CVP line
± PA line

It is mandatory to follow oxygenation continuously during OLV. Typically this can be done with pulse oximetry, although continuous intraarterial PO_2 monitoring is now commercially available. CVP and/or PA line optional for pneumonectomy and for patients with coexisting cardiac disease. During open thoracotomy, CVP monitoring may be inaccurate. A PA line, placed immediately preop in the operated PA, may interfere with pneumonectomy. Central volume monitoring is useful for postop management.

Positioning

Axillary roll, "airplane" for upper arm; avoid hyperextending arms.
✓ and pad pressure points.
✓ eyes.

Fiber optic bronchoscopy

FOB performed immediately prior to thoracotomy to evaluate resectability of lesion. Patient intubated with large ETT (≥ 8 mm), replaced with DLT or BB following bronchoscopy (see Bronchoscopy, p. 196).

Use the largest plastic DLT that atraumatically passes through the glottis (typically, 41 Fr for men, 39 Fr for women).[2] DLT can be placed accurately by careful auscultation ± confirmation by FOB. If FOB is used, pass down tracheal lumen. Top of blue endobronchial cuff should be visible below carina in bronchus. For small children, the balloon of a Fogarty embolectomy catheter is used as a BB; for adults, use a Univent tube. FOB always needed to confirm BB placement. With BB, operated lung cannot safely be reinflated and collapsed periodically during surgery.

Lung isolation

Separate lungs to prevent contralateral contamination (infection, pus, blood, tumor), allow selective ventilation and facilitate operation.

One-lung ventilation (OLV)	Use large TV (10-12 ml/kg) during two-lung ventilation; do not change TV when OLV instituted.	Large TV during OLV prevents atelectasis of the dependent ("down," ventilated) lung. Ventilation rate adjusted to avoid hyperventilation. Compliance is reduced (same TV to one lung) and resistance is increased (1 lumen instead of 2); PIPs will be higher and some auto-PEEP may be generated, depending on size of DLT. Intraop hypoxemia during OLV is uncommon when FiO_2 = 1.0 and large TV used. If pulse oximetry < 94% or PO_2 < 100, recheck position of DLT or BB. The DLT endobronchial cuff can obstruct the upper lobe bronchus of the ventilated lung or the DLT or BB balloon can herniate into the carina, obstructing both lungs. PEEP to ventilated lung can be used, but with caution since overdistention of alveoli will increase shunt to the "up" lung, worsening hypoxemia. If hypoxemia persists, insufflate operated ("up," collapsed) lung with 100% O_2 and apply CPAP (5-10 cmH_2O) to the "up" lung to improve oxygenation without interfering with surgical field. The PA of the operated lung during pneumonectomy can be clamped completely, eliminating shunt.
Complications	Hypoxemia	✓ position of DLT and ensure adequate TV; correct ↓BP and dysrhythmias.
	Airway rupture	✓ integrity of intubated bronchus after reexpanding lung.
	Hypotension	✓ volume status, cardiac function. ✓ for mechanical compression of heart or vessels.

POSTOPERATIVE

Complications	Airway trauma from intubation, tracheobronchial rupture	Do not overdistend bronchial balloon or DLT cuffs. DLT bronchial cuff usually requires < 2 ml air for airtight seal if an appropriate (large) DLT is used.
	Injuries related to lateral positioning	Pressure damage to ear, eye, nose, deltoid muscle, iliac crest, brachial plexus, and radial, ulnar, common peroneal and sciatic nerves have all been reported.
	Structural injuries related to thoracotomy	Neurologic (phrenic and recurrent laryngeal nerves), thoracic duct, spinal cord; bronchopleural fistula, tracheobronchial disruption
	Surgical complications	Cardiac herniation, tension pneumothorax, bleeding, torsion of residual lobe, post pneumonectomy PE
	Cardiopulmonary complications	Supraventricular dysrhythmias, acute cor pulmonale, atelectasis, pneumonia, PE
Pain management	Neuraxial opioids – epidural or intrathecal Parenteral opioids (iv, im, continuous iv, PCA [p. C-3]). Intercostal blocks Interpleural analgesia Epidural local anesthetics Cryoanalgesia Transcutaneous nerve stimulation	Effective analgesia is essential for patient to cough, deep breathe and ambulate early. Thoracic epidural is often recommended, but lumbar route is as effective and safer. Intraop, administer a single bolus of hydromorphone (1.0-1.5 mg) in 10 ml NS through lumbar epidural catheter. In immediate postop period, 0.2-0.3 mg/h of hydromorphone infused through epidural. Fentanyl 50-100 μg bolus in 10 ml NS for breakthrough pain.
Tests	CXR, ABG and others as indicated.	

References

1. Baue AE, ed: *Glenn's Thoracic and Cardiovascular Surgery*, 6th edition, Volume II. Geha AS, Hammond GL, Laks H, Naunheim KS, assoc eds. Appleton & Lange, Norwalk, CT: 1996.
2. Brodsky JB, Macario A, Mark JBD: Tracheal diameter predicts double-lumen tube size: a method for selecting left double-lumen tubes. *Anesth Analg* 1996; 82: 861-64.

3. Cohen E, Eisenkraft JB, Thys DM, et al: Oxygenation and hemodynamic changes during one-lung ventilation: Effects of $CPAP_{10}$, $PEEP_{10}$, $CPAP_{10}/PEEP_{10}$. *J Cardiothorac Anesth* 1988; 2 (1): 34-40.
4. Kavanagh BP, Katz J, Sandler AN, et al: Pain control after thoracic surgery. A review of current techniques. *Anesthesiology* 1994; 81: 737-59.
5. Sabiston DC Jr, Spencer FC: *Surgery of the Chest*, 6th edition, Vol II. WB Saunders Co, Philadelphia: 1995.
6. Slinger P, Scott WAC: Arterial oxygenation during one-lung ventilation. A comparison of enflurane and isoflurane. *Anesthesiology* 1995; 82: 940-46.

WEDGE RESECTION OF LUNG LESION

SURGICAL CONSIDERATIONS

Description: Wedge resection (removal of a mass and 1 cm margins in a manner that does not remove an entire anatomical pulmonary segment) may be carried out for a number of reasons. A known or suspected cancer may be removed by this limited resection. There is general agreement that this is an appropriate operation for patients with limited pulmonary reserve who are unable to withstand lobectomy. Wedge resection is also used for resection of single- or multiple-metastatic lesions from various primary neoplasms. A single metastasis may be removed through a limited thoracotomy incision. At the other extreme, **sternotomy** may be carried out to remove bilateral lesions. Wedge resection is also indicated for diagnostic and therapeutic purposes in lesions which defy diagnosis by less invasive techniques. Incisions vary with location and number of lesions and technique employed. **Limited thoracotomy**, **standard thoracotomy** or **median sternotomy** may be used under different circumstances. **Stapling** (Fig 5-2), **clamp and suture** technique or **excision and suture** technique may be used for lesions in different locations. Chest tubes are used for postop drainage.

Variant approach: Video-assisted thoracoscopy (see p. 202).

Usual preop diagnosis: Metastatic tumor to the lungs; primary lung cancer (typically, lobectomy); unknown pulmonary lesion

SUMMARY OF PROCEDURE

Position	Lateral or supine
Incision	Limited and related to location of solitary lesion; sternotomy for bilateral lesions
Special instrumentation	DLT
Antibiotics	Cefazolin 1 g (or as indicated from culture and sensitivity)
Surgical time	< 1-3 h, depending on number of lesions
EBL	< 500 ml
Postop care	ICU; careful attention to pulmonary toilet, chest tube output
Mortality	Minimal
Morbidity	Air leaks
	Cardiac dysrhythmias
Pain score	2-6

PATIENT POPULATION CHARACTERISTICS

Age range	30-60 yr most common
Male:Female	1:1
Incidence	Common thoracic procedure
Etiology	Variable – neoplasm or inflammatory disease
Associated conditions	COPD; cardiovascular disease; malignancy; infection

ANESTHETIC CONSIDERATIONS

PREOPERATIVE

The anesthetic considerations for this procedure are very similar to those for lobectomy/pneumonectomy. Wedge resection of the lung is often reserved for patients with poor pulmonary reserve, e.g., an absolute FEV_1 < 1.2-1.4L or 40% predicted.

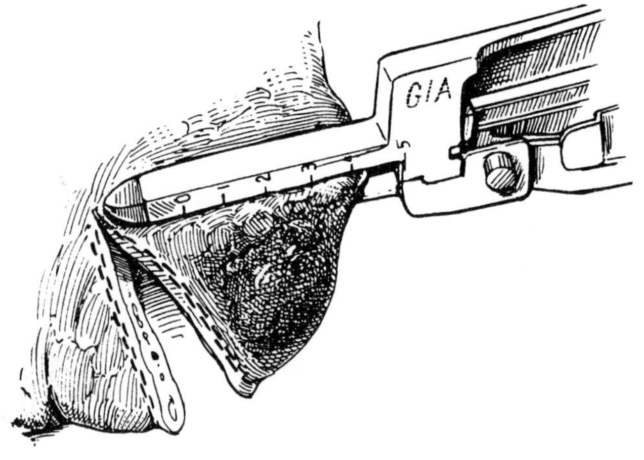

Figure 5-2. Stapler used to perform wedge incision. (Reproduced with permission from *Johnson's Surgery of the Chest*, 5th edition. Year Book Medical Pub: 1985.

Respiratory PFTs similar to major thoracotomy. Further evaluation directed toward an underlying disease (e.g., immunocompromised patient for open-lung biopsy, patient with metastatic lesions, etc.).
Tests: PFTs (see Pulmonary Resection, p. 173); CXR; if chest CT available, look for airway obstruction that could interfere with DLT placement; Hct; ABG.

Cardiovascular **Tests:** ECG—look for evidence of RV hypertrophy, conduction problems and prior ischemia.

Neurological Hx of previous back surgery, peripheral neuropathy. Examine lumbar area for skin lesions, infection, deformities. Avoid placement of epidural catheter in patient with neurologic problems.

Musculoskeletal Patients with lung cancer may have myasthenic (Eaton-Lambert) syndrome with increased sensitivity to nondepolarizing muscle relaxants. Monitor relaxation with peripheral nerve stimulator.

Hematologic Patients are often anemic from primary disease. Consider preop blood transfusion.
Tests: Hct

Laboratory Other tests as indicated from H&P.

Premedication Midazolam 1-2 mg iv if patient anxious. When epidural opioids are planned, avoid opioid or sedative premedication which can potentiate postop respiratory effects of spinal opioids.

INTRAOPERATIVE

Anesthetic technique: GETA, often combined with epidural for thoracotomy approach. Consider DLT if OLV needed.

Induction STP 3-5 mg/kg iv or propofol 1-2 mg/kg iv, succinylcholine 1 mg/kg or vecuronium 0.1 mg/kg for tracheal intubation.

Maintenance **Balanced technique:** O_2, isoflurane and iv opioids, usually fentanyl or remifentanil 0.05-2 μg/kg/min. N_2O used during two-lung ventilation but discontinued during OLV. Epidural catheter seldom used in thoracoscopic approach because pain from limited incision is easily treated by conventional analgesic therapy. If epidural used, follow same guidelines as for major thoracotomy (opioid dosage may be reduced). If an epidural is not utilized, a possible useful adjunct is local anesthetic infiltrated into the wound and also given through the chest tube once the lung is inflated. Bupivacaine 0.25% with epinephrine to a maximum of 0.5 ml/kg is appropriate.

Emergence Extubate in OR, transfer in head-up position to PACU or ICU breathing O_2 by mask.

Blood and fluid requirements IV: 18 ga × 1
NS/LR @ 2 ml/kg/h

Monitoring Standard monitors (p. B-1)
± Arterial line

Arterial line needed occasionally.

Positioning	Lateral decubitus or supine, with wedge under back on operated side. ✓ and pad pressure points. ✓ eyes.	
Ventilation	ETT; DLT or BB rarely needed; TV (12-15 ml/kg) during two-lung ventilation and OLV.	

POSTOPERATIVE

Complications	Atelectasis Pneumonia Fluid overload	
Pain management	Parenteral opioids (iv, im, continuous iv, PCA [p. C-3]). Intercostal blocks Interpleural analgesia	If lumbar epidural catheter available: bolus of bupivacaine 0.25% (0.5 ml/kg), followed by continuous infusion of 0.2 ml/kg/h).

References

1. Baue AE, ed: *Glenn's Thoracic and Cardiovascular Surgery*, 6th edition, Volume II. Geha AS, Hammond GL, Laks H, Naunheim KS, assoc eds. Appleton & Lange, Norwalk, CT: 1996.
2. Mitchell RL: The lateral limited thoracotomy incision: standard for pulmonary operations. *J Thorac Cardiovasc Surg* 1990; 99(4):590-5.
3. Sabiston DC Jr, Spencer FC: *Surgery of the Chest*, 6th edition, Vol II. WB Saunders Co, Philadelphia: 1995.

CHEST-WALL RESECTION

SURGICAL CONSIDERATIONS

Description: Removal of portions of the thoracic cage may be required under several circumstances. Perhaps the most common indication is lung cancer that has invaded the chest wall. Other indications include primary tumors of the chest wall and areas of radiation necrosis. If the tumor or other disease process involves the skin, an appropriate area of skin—sometimes as much as 4 or 5 cm around the tumor—must be resected along with the specimen. Underlying subcutaneous tissue and muscle should always be resected in continuity; however, the tumor itself must not be exposed. Wide skin flaps are frequently necessary as well. Resection of larger areas of the chest wall may require extensive reconstruction. Limited resection (1-5 cm segments of 1-3 ribs) generally requires limited chest-wall reconstruction (including the use of plastic mesh replacement with or without methylmethacrylate, rib grafts and muscle or myocutaneous flaps). Extensive reconstruction of the chest wall (procedures that are often complex and time-consuming) is usually carried out in conjunction with plastic surgeons. Removal of anterolateral or anterior portions of the chest wall, particularly resections that include the sternum, are associated with greater postop instability than are resections of posterior portions of the chest wall, which are protected by the back muscles and scapula. Thus, anterior resections may require more extensive reconstruction with wide preparation and draping.

Usual preop diagnosis: Lung cancer with chest-wall attachment; primary tumor of the chest wall (bone, cartilage or soft tissue); radiation necrosis

SUMMARY OF PROCEDURE

Position	Supine or lateral
Incision	Over mass to be resected
Special instrumentation	Bone instruments; Marlex (or other) mesh; methylmethacrylate
Antibiotics	Cefazolin 1 g (or as indicated by culture and sensitivity)
Surgical time	1-8 h
Closing considerations	May require help of plastic surgeon in extensive cases.
EBL	100-2000 ml
Postop care	PACU or ICU; some patients require temporary ventilatory support.
Mortality	< 5%
Morbidity	Paradoxical chest-wall motion (less in posterior resections) Pneumothorax Wound complications
Pain score	3-8

PATIENT POPULATION CHARACTERISTICS

Age range	Adults of all ages; children, rarely
Male:Female	1:1
Incidence	Relatively rare
Etiology	Unknown
Associated conditions	Lung cancer; metastatic disease; smoking-related diseases; cardiovascular disease

ANESTHETIC CONSIDERATIONS

See Anesthetic Considerations following Repair of Pectus Excavatum or Carinatum, p. 183.

References

1. Baue AE, ed: *Glenn's Thoracic and Cardiovascular Surgery*, 6th edition, Volume II. Geha AS, Hammond GL, Laks H, Naunheim KS, assoc eds. Appleton & Lange, Norwalk, CT: 1996.
2. Sabiston DC Jr, Spencer FC: *Surgery of the Chest*, 6th edition, Vol II. WB Saunders Co, Philadelphia: 1995.

REPAIR OF PECTUS EXCAVATUM OR CARINATUM

SURGICAL CONSIDERATIONS

Description: Standard bony and cartilaginous repair of a pectus excavatum (funnel chest) or carinatum (pigeon breast) is usually elective surgery to improve contour and body image. There is no documentation that these repairs have any positive effect on cardiopulmonary function, although some surgeons feel that it can be more than a cosmetic procedure. To repair pectus excavatum, enough pairs of costal cartilages—usually 4-6—must be removed to be able to mobilize and elevate the sternum. Depending on the severity of the defect and patient's age, fixation of the sternum in the corrected position may be necessary. Repair of pectus carinatum is somewhat more varied because the defects are more varied; however, removal of cartilages and correction of the position of the sternum are still the mainstays of treatment.

A midline incision provides the most satisfactory access to the cartilages and sternum. For cosmetic reasons, however, it may be important to use a curvilinear transverse incision, particularly in females. This incision requires extensive mobilization of subcutaneous and muscle flaps. The wound complication rate is somewhat greater after transverse incisions. The costal cartilages are moved by subperichondrial dissection. This may be tedious and time-consuming, especially since 4 or 5, or even more, pairs of cartilages need to be removed. The elevation of the sternum is usually fairly straightforward, and is usually accompanied by a transverse sternal osteotomy. Intercostal muscle bundles may be left attached to the sternum or may be detached and reattached for better positioning of the sternum. Sternal support normally is not used in infants, but may be used in older children. The most common method of support is the use of a transverse metal strut resting on the ribs, but beneath the sternum. This is removed at a later date. The final position of the sternum is easier to predict following repair of pectus carinatum than following repair of pectus excavatum. Because of the negative intrathoracic pressure it is easier to hold the sternum down than up. Ideally, patients for repair of pectus excavatum are just under school age. Satisfactory repair, however, may be carried out at almost any time during childhood. As full growth is attained, results tend to be less favorable. Pectus carinatum generally has its onset during adolescence, and it is well to let the patient complete his or her growth spurt prior to undertaking repair. In certain circumstances, particularly in teenage girls and patients who do not engage in strenuous sports, subcutaneous, custom-made implants may be placed to improve body contour without necessitating major bony and cartilaginous repairs. These are usually carried out by plastic surgeons.

Usual preop diagnosis: Pectus excavatum or carinatum

SUMMARY OF PROCEDURE

Position	Supine
Incision	Transverse or vertical
Special instrumentation	Bone instruments; sometimes metal struts or wires for reconstruction
Antibiotics	Cefazolin 1 g iv q 8 h × 36-48 h
Surgical time	2-3 h
Closing considerations	Pleural and wound drainage common
EBL	100-500 ml
Postop care	ICU
Mortality	Minimal
Morbidity	Pneumothorax: 5-10% Paradoxical chest-wall motion → hypoventilation/atelectasis
Pain score	4-5

PATIENT POPULATION CHARACTERISTICS

Age range	Usually children, 5-10 yr; teenagers, sometimes; adults, rarely
Male:Female	1:1
Incidence	Unusual
Etiology	Unknown
Associated conditions	Marfan syndrome; MVP

ANESTHETIC CONSIDERATIONS

(Procedures covered: chest-wall resection; repair of pectus excavatum/carinatum)

PREOPERATIVE

Patients for chest-wall resection often have extensive cancer and may be weak and debilitated. A very large resection may create a "flail chest" situation, compromising postop ventilation.

Respiratory Pectus seldom interferes with ventilation; no special studies indicated. Severe pectus deformity can be associated with restrictive pulmonary disease.
Tests: Consider CXR; PFT, if indicated from H&P.

Cardiovascular With severe pectus, the deformity results in right-ventricular-outflow-tract obstruction (RVOTO) with restriction of ventricular filling in the sitting position. Right-heart catheterization may demonstrate low cardiac index during upright exercise.
Tests: ECG; cardiac catheterization if indicated. Obtain ECHO if MVP suspected.

Hematologic **Tests:** Hct

Musculoskeletal Chest-wall resection performed for invasive or metastatic cancer; patient may be malnourished,

Musculoskeletal, cont.	anemic; pectus repair of chest-wall deformity for cosmetic, orthopedic or cardiopulmonary indications; pectus deformity usually asymptomatic.	
Laboratory	Other tests as indicated from H&P.	
Premedication	Midazolam 1-2 mg iv if patient anxious. When epidural opioids are planned, avoid opioid or sedative premedication which can potentiate postop respiratory effects of spinal opioids.	

INTRAOPERATIVE

Anesthetic technique: GETA, occasionally combined with epidural.

Induction	Standard induction (see p. B-2). If severe RVOTO, high-dose opioid/O_2 technique (e.g., fentanyl 25 μg/kg and midazolam 0.1-0.1 mg/kg). Avoid myocardial depressants; if RVOTO very severe, consider high-dose opioid anesthetic technique.	
Maintenance	Standard maintenance (see p. B-3) or high-dose opioid technique (fentanyl 50-100 μg/kg) for patient with severe RVOTO.	
Emergence	Extubate in OR; if high-dose opioid → ICU for later extubation.	
Blood and fluid requirements	IV: 18 ga × 1 NS/LR @ 1-2 ml/kg/h	Usually minimal blood loss. Fluid restriction unnecessary as this is extrapulmonary operation.
Monitoring	Standard monitors (p. B-1)	
Positioning	✓ and pad pressure points. ✓ eyes.	
Complications	Pneumothorax	Unintentional pleural tear can cause pneumothorax. Intraop deterioration with increased ventilatory pressure suggests pneumothorax. D/C N_2O. Insert chest tube immediately following operation.

POSTOPERATIVE

Complications	Hypoventilation Flail chest Atelectasis	Although most patients do not require postop ventilatory support, with extensive chest-wall resection patient may hypoventilate. Paradoxical chest-wall movement during spontaneous ventilation with flail chest; postop atelectasis from splinting.
Pain management	Depends on site and extent of chest wall resected. Parenteral or epidural opioids.	Epidural opioids particularly useful if flail chest present—reduces need for ventilatory support.

References

1. Baue AE, ed: *Glenn's Thoracic and Cardiovascular Surgery*, 6th edition, Volume II. Geha AS, Hammond GL, Laks H, Naunheim KS, assoc eds. Appleton & Lange, Norwalk, CT: 1996.
2. Garcia VF, Seyfer AE, Graeber GM: Reconstruction of congenital chest-wall deformities. *Surg Clin North Am* 1989; 69(5):1103-18.
3. Ghory MJ, James FW, Mays W: Cardiac performance in children with pectus excavatum. *J Pediatr Surg* 1989; 24(8):751-55.
4. McBride WJ, Dicker R, Abajian JC, et al: Continuous thoracic epidural infusions for postoperative analgesia after pectus deformity repair. *J Pediatr Surg* 1996; 31(1): 105-107.
5. Sabiston DC Jr, Spencer FC: *Surgery of the Chest*, 6th edition, Vol II. WB Saunders Co, Philadelphia: 1995.

THORACOPLASTY

SURGICAL CONSIDERATIONS

Description: The objective of a **thoracoplasty** (removal of several ribs) is to permanently obliterate an existing pleural space or to collapse a portion of the lung. Formerly, this operation was used in the treatment of tuberculosis (TB); however, because of better drug therapy, appropriate pulmonary resection and the decrease in incidence of TB, thoracoplasty is now rare. The procedure also was used for obliterating empyema spaces and helping to close bronchopleural fistulas (BPFs). The use of **pedicled muscle flaps** (serratus anterior, pectoralis major and latissimus dorsi are the most common) or an **omental transposition** have largely replaced thoracoplasty for filling empyema spaces and encouraging closing of BPFs. These operations are less deforming and better tolerated physiologically since they do not result in paradoxical motion of the chest wall.

Thoracoplasty is accomplished by removing several ribs in a subperiosteal fashion, allowing the underlying chest wall to collapse. This collapse is aided by the normally negative intrapleural pressure. Since the periosteum is left intact, the ribs will regenerate, resulting in a permanent, bony collapse of the chest wall. If the objective of the thoracoplasty is to obliterate a relatively small space (meaning that segments of only 2-3 ribs need be removed), the procedure may be done in a single stage, with little postop physiologic impairment of respiration. If extensive thoracoplasty is necessary, however, the procedure may be done in stages to minimize postop chest-wall instability and resultant respiratory problems.

Usual preop diagnosis: Pulmonary TB; BPF; empyema

SUMMARY OF PROCEDURE

Position	Usually lateral
Incision	Along rib line
Special instrumentation	Bone instruments
Unique considerations	TB or fungal infection may be present
Antibiotics	As indicated by culture and sensitivity
Surgical time	2-3 h
EBL	500 ml or more
Postop care	ICU
Mortality	Minimal
Morbidity	Paradoxical chest-wall motion → atelectasis → hypoxemia: 10% Pneumothorax: Rare
Pain score	7-8

PATIENT POPULATION CHARACTERISTICS

Age range	Middle-aged or older adults
Male:Female	1:1
Incidence	Rare
Etiology	TB; pneumococcal infection; neoplasm; complication of pneumonectomy
Associated conditions	Immunosuppression

ANESTHETIC CONSIDERATIONS

See Anesthetic Considerations following Drainage of Empyema, p. 186.

References

1. Baue AE, ed: *Glenn's Thoracic and Cardiovascular Surgery*, 6th edition, Volume II. Geha AS, Hammond GL, Laks H, Naunheim KS, assoc eds. Appleton & Lange, Norwalk, CT: 1996.
2. Sabiston DC Jr, Spencer FC: *Surgery of the Chest*, 6th edition, Vol II. WB Saunders Co, Philadelphia: 1995.

DRAINAGE OF EMPYEMA

SURGICAL CONSIDERATIONS

Description: Collections of pus in the pleural cavity require appropriate and adequate drainage. In the acute situation, and particularly if the fluid is thin, **tube thoracostomy** at the bedside may suffice. In other circumstances, more formal drainage in the OR environment may be required. In the acute situation, **thoracotomy** and **decortication of the pleura** may be indicated, accompanied by generous tube drainage. With chronic localized empyema, **resection of the rib**, **local debridement** and **tube drainage** may suffice. On rare occasions, construction of an **Eloesser flap** may be indicated. This is a permanent, skin-lined flap which creates an opening into a chronic empyema cavity. A tongue-shaped flap is based either superiorly or inferiorly over the rib immediately above or below (as the case may be) the intended area of localized rib resection. After elevation of the flap, resection of several-centimeter segments of 1 or 2 ribs is carried out and the chronic empyema space is entered. The flap is then sutured to the underlying parietal pleura or wall of the empyema cavity and the cavity is left open for permanent drainage. A variant of this procedure, called the **Clagett procedure,** is carried out for empyema (with or without bronchopleural fistula) following **pneumonectomy**, since closed drainage rarely suffices in such a situation. The principal is the same: that is, an epithelial-lined, permanent opening to achieve drainage of an empyema. In the Clagett procedure, the opening is generally made anterolaterally and dependently so that drainage is effective and the patient can handle dressing changes without assistance. Segments of 2 or 3 ribs are removed and the skin is sutured to the parietal pleura, leaving a permanent opening for drainage and irrigation. Without an underlying lung, and with a relatively fixed mediastinum, this procedure is well tolerated physiologically.

Usual preop diagnosis: Nontuberculosis empyema (typically pneumococcal)

SUMMARY OF PROCEDURE

	Eloesser or Clagett	Tube Thoracostomy
Position	Usually lateral	Lateral
Incision	Over empyema pocket for Eloesser; low anterolateral for Clagett	Lateral
Special instrumentation	None	Large tubes
Unique considerations	Patient may have BPF	Local or GA
Antibiotics	As indicated by culture and sensitivity	⇐
Surgical time	1 h; occasionally more	< 1 h
Closing considerations	Wound left open	None
EBL	100 ml	Minimal
Postop care	PACU → room	⇐
Mortality	Minimal	⇐
Morbidity	Fluid drainage Bleeding: Rare	Air leak
Pain score	3-4	2-3

PATIENT POPULATION CHARACTERISTICS

Age range	Usually adults
Male:Female	1:1
Incidence	Decreasing
Etiology	Pneumonia; esophageal or bronchial leak; lymphatic or hematogenous spread of infection; posttrauma or thoracic surgery
Associated conditions	Bronchopleural fistula (BPF); sepsis; malnutrition

ANESTHETIC CONSIDERATIONS

(Procedures covered: thoracoplasty; drainage of empyema)

PREOPERATIVE

The guiding principle in the anesthetic management of empyema is to protect the nonaffected lung from soiling by the affected side. These patients are often chronically ill with sepsis and cachexia; and there is usually an underlying BPF (which may require awake intubation).

Respiratory Patients usually have preexisting pulmonary disease. Procedure often is performed for empyema in the presence of BPF following lung resection (particularly pneumonectomy), penetrating injury to chest or rupture of a cyst or bulla. When possible, surgeon should drain empyema under local anesthesia before induction, with patient sitting upright. If empyema loculated, complete drainage may not be possible.

Tests: Consider PFTs; ABG; obtain CXR to determine efficacy of preop chest drainage; if chest CT available, look for airway obstruction that could interfere with DLT placement.

Cardiovascular There may be ECG changes because of mediastinal shift to the affected side.

Tests: As indicated from H&P.

Neurological ✓ Hx of back surgery, peripheral neuropathy. Examine lumbar area for skin lesions, infection, deformities. Avoid placement of epidural catheter in patient with neurologic problems or if obviously septic.

Musculoskeletal Patients with lung cancer may have myasthenic (Eaton-Lambert) syndrome with increased sensitivity to nondepolarizing muscle relaxants. Monitor relaxation with peripheral nerve stimulator.

Hematologic Transfuse patients with preop Hct < 25% (Hb level necessary to maintain adequate O_2 content). Obtain autologous blood during the month before surgery.

Laboratory Other tests as indicated from H&P.

Premedication Midazolam 1-2 mg iv if patient anxious. When epidural opioids are planned, avoid opioid or sedative premedication which can potentiate postop respiratory effects of spinal opioids.

INTRAOPERATIVE

Anesthetic technique: GETA; occasionally combined with epidural anesthesia/analgesia.

Induction Consider awake tracheal intubation with sedated, spontaneously breathing patient. Rapid-sequence induction with cricoid pressure is an alternative. Intubate with DLT; isolate lungs to protect from aspiration and tension pneumothorax. Use DLT with bronchial lumen to side opposite BPF. Contamination of the healthy lung from aspiration of pus is a major concern. Large DLT provides snug fit in bronchus and limits aspiration. Pus may appear in tracheal lumen (lumen to the diseased lung); suction frequently to avoid soiling good lung.

Maintenance O_2 and isoflurane (1.0-1.5%); less required if epidural local anesthetics used. Avoid N_2O, especially during OLV, since hypoxemia during OLV is unpredictable. Use FiO_2 = 1.0. Lidocaine (1.5% or 2%) 10-12 ml, administered via lumbar epidural every 45 min, or bupivacaine (0.5%) 10-12 ml every 1.5-2.0 h. Hydromorphone (1.0-1.5 mg) or morphine (5.0-7.5 mg) in 10 ml NS through epidural. Following intubation, isolate lung with DLT or BB. Chest tube is then removed while chest is prepped for operation. Ventilate only the healthy lung. Since BPF is an abnormal communication between bronchial tree and pleural cavity, if no chest tube present, conventional intubation with IPPV can produce tension pneumothorax. Keep unclamped and do not remove a functioning chest tube until lung is isolated and ventilation to diseased lung stopped. Once chest is opened, there is no chance of pneumothorax, but the large air leak through BPF may prevent satisfactory ventilation of that lung. High-frequency ventilation (HFV) is recommended by some, but studies show no benefit; in some patients the BPF is actually increased with HFV.

Emergence Prior to closing of the chest, lungs are inflated to 30 cmH_2O pressure to reinflate atelectatic areas and to check for significant air leaks. The surgeon will insert chest tubes to drain pleural cavity and aid lung reexpansion. Patient is extubated while still in OR. If postop ventilation is required (rare), the DLT is exchanged for an ETT. If BPF is still open, consider selective ventilation postop through DLT. Ventilate each lung separately; use smaller TVs to lung with BPF.

Blood and fluid requirements IV: 16-18 ga × 1

Restrict iv fluids; usually administer 1000-1500 ml NS/LR ± 1 U autologous blood if available; use vasopressor (ephedrine 5-10 mg iv bolus or phenylephrine 50-100 μg iv bolus) if hypotensive.

An overhydrated patient is at increased risk of right-heart failure. Use of epidural local anesthetics can cause hypotension in a volume-restricted patient; vasopressor often needed.

Monitoring	Standard monitors (p. B-1) ± CVP and/or PA line	It is mandatory to follow oxygenation continuously during OLV. Typically this is done with pulse oximetry, although continuous intraarterial PO_2 monitoring is now commercially available.
Positioning	Axillary roll, "airplane" for upper arm; avoid hyperextending arms. ✓ and pad pressure points. ✓ eyes.	

POSTOPERATIVE

Complications	Tension pneumothorax Aspiration pneumonia ("down" lung)	Functioning chest tube necessary to prevent tension pneumothorax.
Pain management	Analgesic requirements minimal	

References

1. Baue AE, ed: *Glenn's Thoracic and Cardiovascular Surgery*, 6th edition, Volume II. Geha AS, Hammond GL, Laks H, Naunheim KS, assoc eds. Appleton & Lange, Norwalk, CT: 1996.
2. Benjaminsson E, Klain M: Intraoperative dual-mode independent lung ventilation of a patient with bronchopleural fistula. *Anesth Analg* 1981; 60(2):118-19.
3. Bishop MJ, Benson MS, Sato P, Pierson DJ: Comparison of high-frequency jet ventilation with conventional mechanical ventilation for bronchopleural fistula. *Anesth Analg* 1987; 66(9):833-38.
4. Langston HT: Thoracoplasty: the how and the why. *Ann Thorac Surg* 1991; 52(6):1351-53.
5. Sabiston DC Jr, Spencer FC: *Surgery of the Chest*, 6th edition, Vol II. WB Saunders Co, Philadelphia: 1995.

RESECTION OF TRACHEA FOR STENOSIS OR TUMOR

SURGICAL CONSIDERATIONS

Description: Tracheal resection with **primary anastomosis** may be carried out for tracheal stenosis or for tumor. The approach to the trachea varies, depending on the nature of the lesion, its location and the extent of resection and reconstruction to be carried out. The simplest resection is of the **cervical** trachea for tracheal stenosis or localized tumor. This can be done through a cervical incision alone with primary tracheal anastomosis. Longer and/or more inferiorly located lesions may be approached through a cervical incision, combined with **sternotomy**.

When operating through a cervical incision, it is important that the dissection be carried out on the anterior and posterior surface of the trachea, leaving the vascular attachments laterally to assure good blood supply to the remaining trachea. This also minimizes the chance of injury to the recurrent laryngeal nerves. Generous amounts of trachea may be mobilized inferior to the incision by this method, so that the anastomosis may be carried out without tension. After the lesion is resected, the distal trachea is intubated across the operative field and maintained in this fashion, while the tracheal anastomosis is being done using interrupted sutures of absorbable material. The ETT, inserted from above, is left in the superior portion of the trachea. After the anastomosis is completed, the ETT is advanced into the distal trachea, while the tube which had crossed the field is removed (Fig 5-3). After the anastomosis is completed and the wound closed, it is important that tension be avoided on the suture line. Some surgeons prefer to put a suture from the skin of the chin to the anterior chest in order to hold the neck in flexion for a few days. Others use a plaster jacket for the same purpose.

For tumors of the mid-trachea, a **right thoracotomy** approach, either alone or combined with sternotomy, may be necessary. For particularly complex tracheal tumors requiring carinal resection and complex reconstruction, a transverse, or clam shell, incision may be necessary. All tracheal resections require excellent communication and cooperation between surgeon and anesthesiologist. Special anesthetic techniques, including intubation of the distal trachea across the surgical field and jet ventilation may be necessary. Rarely, CPB will be indicated for a complex tracheal resection and reconstruction.

Usual preop diagnosis: Tracheal stenosis or tumor (adenoid cystic carcinoma or squamous cell carcinoma most common)

SUMMARY OF PROCEDURE

	Cervical Approach	Sternotomy	Right Thoracotomy
Position	Supine	⇐	Left lateral decubitus
Incision	Transverse low cervical	Cervical plus sternotomy	Right thoracotomy
Antibiotics	Cefazolin 1 g	⇐	⇐
Surgical time	3 h	3-4 h	4 h
Closing considerations	Neck flexion (chin stitch)	⇐	⇐
EBL	200 ml	350 ml	350-500 ml
Postop care	ICU	⇐	⇐
Mortality	< 5%	5%	⇐
Morbidity	Retained secretions Dehiscence Recurrent stenosis Recurrent/superior laryngeal nerve injury Granuloma	⇐	⇐
Pain score	3-4	5-6	7-9

PATIENT POPULATION CHARACTERISTICS

Age range	Wide variation
Male:Female	1:1
Incidence	Rare
Etiology	Stenosis usually 2° to intubation or injury; tumor, either primary (e.g., smoking) or secondary (e.g., esophageal, lung, thyroid cancer)
Associated conditions	Carcinoid syndrome; cardiopulmonary disease; tracheoesophageal fistula (TEF)

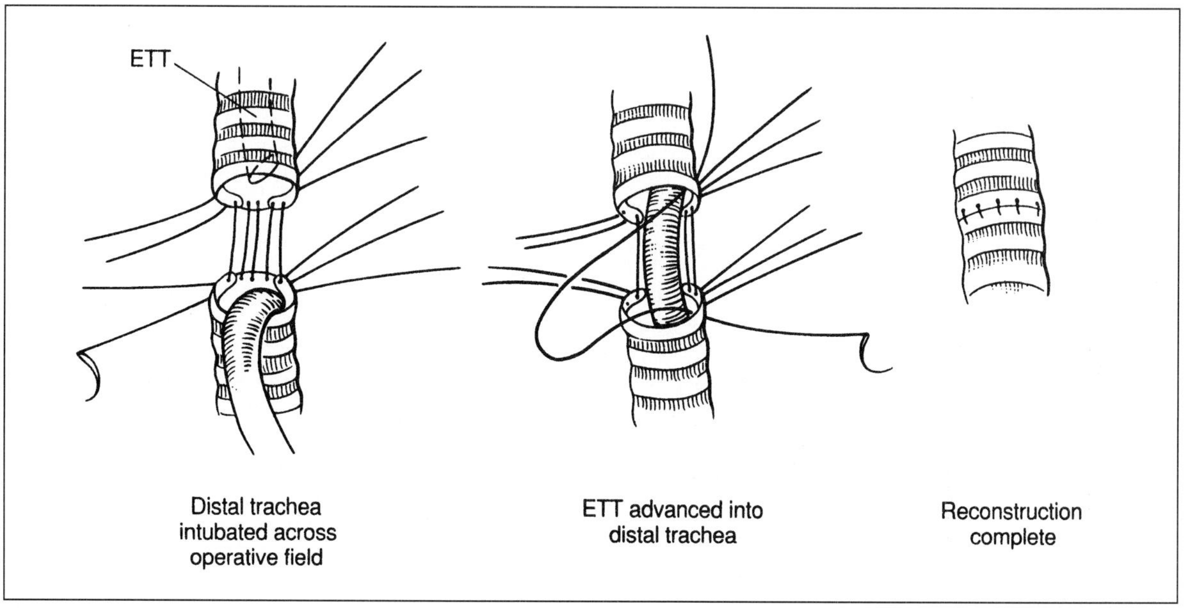

Figure 5-3. Stages of tracheal reconstruction. Note ETT in distal trachea. (Reproduced with permission from Grillo HC: *Current Problems in Surgery*. Year Book Medical Publishers: 1970.)

ANESTHETIC CONSIDERATIONS

PREOPERATIVE

Respiratory Initial presentation may involve Sx of airway obstruction (stridor, cough, dyspnea) which may be misdiagnosed as asthma or pneumonitis. A careful evaluation of the airway is usually followed by bronchoscopy. Lesion should be identified by site and size. Using this information, estimate what size ETT will easily pass lesion site.
Tests: PFTs; flow/volume loops; CT scan to determine extent of tracheal obstruction

Laboratory Other tests as indicated from H&P.

Premedication Patients with stridor or critical airway lesions should not receive preop sedation. It is probably best to avoid sedation in all patients.

INTRAOPERATIVE

Anesthetic technique: GETA

Induction Be prepared for airway emergency. Surgeon must be present and prepared for emergency rigid bronchoscopy and/or to perform tracheostomy below lesion. Mask inhalational induction or awake fiber optic intubation with spontaneous ventilation; avoid iv drugs that could depress ventilation. Avoid muscle relaxants; if necessary, consider small doses of succinylcholine. Sevoflurane/O_2 is preferred for smooth induction with depression of cough reflex; avoid N_2O. High concentrations of sevoflurane may be necessary. Helium has been recommended to decrease resistance to flow past the obstruction; however, helium is not usually available.

Have a variety of laryngeal blades and uncut ETTs of all sizes, including thin (5 mm) tubes. If ETT passes beyond lesion, can begin IPPV. If ETT cannot be passed, spontaneous ventilation with 100% O_2 and halothane or sevoflurane is required. For carinal resections, use armored ETTs, which can be placed by surgeon directly into each bronchus during resection. An armored tube is preferable because it is constantly being removed while the surgeon works; also, there is less kinking and less chance of obstructing.

Maintenance Standard maintenance (p. B-3). FiO_2 = 1.0 during apneic oxygenation; continuous monitoring with pulse oximetry mandatory. Consider HFV through a small-diameter catheter if ETT interferes with operation. HFV will require iv anesthesia since inhalational agents cannot be delivered predictably; CPB can be used (rare).

Emergence Early extubation; presence of ETT and IPPV can disrupt fresh suture line. Remove ETT as soon as patient is awake enough to protect airway, but before bucking and coughing occur.

Blood and fluid requirements IV: 18 ga × 1 (left arm)
NS/LR @ 3 ml/kg/h

Monitoring Standard monitors (p. B-1)
± Arterial line

Left radial artery cannulation permits uninterrupted monitoring of BP during periods of innominate artery compression. Placement of iv in left arm allows unimpeded infusion. Right-extremity pulse oximetry will help detect innominate artery occlusion (which otherwise could lead to stroke.)

Positioning ✓ and pad pressure points.
✓ eyes.

Airway management ETT replaced with sterile ETT and circuit intraop.

Once the trachea is divided, the surgeon places a sterile ETT in the distal trachea. The original ETT is withdrawn above the surgical site. The surgeon attaches a sterile anesthesia circuit to distal ETT for ventilation. Then, the surgeon places a suture through the distal tip of the original ETT. Prior to reanastomosis of trachea, the distal trachea is suctioned to remove accumulated blood and secretions. After a posterior suture line is completed, the original ETT is pulled through the trachea and the distal tube (which is below the resection) is removed. Reattach and ventilate patient through original ETT.

Complications	Tracheal edema	Corticosteroids (dexamethasone 6-8 mg iv) to reduce tracheal edema.
	Injury to neck	Any structure in the neck can be damaged, including superior and recurrent laryngeal nerves, trachea and thoracic duct.

POSTOPERATIVE

Complications	Tracheal disruption	Neck swelling, subcutaneous emphysema, and inability to ventilate, indicate loss of air-tight anastomosis. Immediate reexploration of neck is essential.
	Recurrent laryngeal nerve injury	Bilateral (occasionally unilateral) laryngeal nerve damage may result in airway obstruction, necessitating reintubation. Mask ventilation may be ineffective.
Position	Keep head flexed to reduce tension on tracheal suture line.	
Pain management	Parenteral opioids (p. C-1)	Once patient is fully awake.

References

1. Baue AE, ed: *Glenn's Thoracic and Cardiovascular Surgery*, 6th edition, Volume II. Geha AS, Hammond GL, Laks H, Naunheim KS, assoc eds. Appleton & Lange, Norwalk, CT: 1996.
2. Grillo HC, Mathisen DJ: Surgical management of tracheal strictures. *Surg Clin North Am* 1988; 68(3):511-24.
3. Perera ER, Vidic DM, Zivot J: Carinal resection with two high-frequency jet ventilation delivery systems. *Can J Anaesth* 1993; 40(1): 59-63.
4. Sabiston DC Jr, Spencer FC: *Surgery of the Chest*, 6th edition, Vol II. WB Saunders Co, Philadelphia: 1995.
5. Young-Beyer P, Wilson RS: Anesthetic management for tracheal resection and reconstruction. *J Cardiothoracic Anesth* 1988; 2(6):821-35.

EXCISION OF MEDIASTINAL TUMOR

SURGICAL CONSIDERATIONS

Description: Tumors in the anterior mediastinum are usually removed through a **median sternotomy**, while tumors in the middle and posterior mediastinum are usually removed through a **lateral thoracotomy**. Some cysts or small tumors may be excised using **video thoracoscopy** (see Video-Assisted Thoracoscopy, p. 202). Mediastinal tumors that are well encapsulated are generally removed in a straightforward fashion. If anterior mediastinal tumors are not well encapsulated and are attached to pericardium or lung on either side, appropriate portions of these attached structures may be removed in continuity with the tumor. If there is attachment to phrenic nerves on either side, one nerve may be sacrificed if necessary to remove the tumor completely. In patients with anterior mediastinal tumors, invasion of the major vascular structures, particularly the aorta and arch vessels, presents an even greater problem. Patients with large anterior mediastinal masses who have some evidence of intrathoracic obstruction (e.g., orthopnea, cough) may have airway obstruction at the time of induction. Although most mediastinal masses do not cause obstruction of the trachea or tracheobronchial tree, large mediastinal masses in the anterior mediastinum, in conjunction with muscle relaxation, can lead to complete obstruction of the airway with inability to ventilate the patient. Although rigid bronchoscopy may permit ventilation through the obstruction, it cannot be counted on to relieve the obstruction. Therefore, only short-acting or no muscle relaxants (spontaneous ventilation) should be used in these patients. In general, the surgical procedure is quite limited, involving a small anterior thoracotomy for a biopsy. Rarely is a large procedure undertaken for these masses as they are usually unresectable or are treated by other means. Posterior mediastinal tumors are usually benign. Even so, they may be densely adherent to the posterior chest-wall structures. On occasion, dissection can result in injury to an intercostal vessel. Mediastinal tumors sometimes cause tracheal compression and special anesthetic techniques may be necessary to safely secure the airway. Close communication between the surgeon and anesthesiologist is essential.

Usual preop diagnosis: Thymoma; teratodermoid; ganglioneuroma; lymphoma; schwannoma

SUMMARY OF PROCEDURE

Position	Supine or lateral
Incision	Median sternotomy or lateral thoracotomy
Special instrumentation	Sternal or rib retractors
Antibiotics	Cefazolin 1 g
Surgical time	≤ 2 h
EBL	< 500 ml
Postop care	Frequently ICU
Mortality	Minimal
Morbidity	Bleeding
Pain score	5-8

PATIENT POPULATION CHARACTERISTICS

Age range	All ages
Male:Female	1:1
Etiology	**Anterior mediastinum:** Thymoma; teratoma; pericardial cyst; lymphoma; parasternal (Morgagni) hernia; lipoma **Superior mediastinum:** Goiter; aneurysm; parathyroid tumor; esophageal tumor; angiomatous tumor **Middle mediastinum:** Lymphoma; lymph node inflammation; bronchogenic tumor; bronchogenic cyst **Posterior mediastinum:** Neurogenic tumor; aneurysm (enteric cyst); esophageal tumor; bronchogenic tumor
Associated conditions	SVC syndrome; myasthenia gravis; recurrent laryngeal nerve damage; airway obstruction; dyspnea; Horner's syndrome

ANESTHETIC CONSIDERATIONS

See Anesthetic Considerations following Mediastinoscopy, p. 194.

References

1. Baue AE, ed: *Glenn's Thoracic and Cardiovascular Surgery*, 6th edition, Volume II. Geha AS, Hammond GL, Laks H, Naunheim KS, assoc eds. Appleton & Lange, Norwalk, CT: 1996.
2. Lewer BM, Torrance JM: Anaesthesia for a patient with a mediastinal mass presenting with acute stridor. *Anaesth Intensive Care* 1996; 24(5): 605-8.
3. Sabiston DC Jr, Spencer FC: *Surgery of the Chest*, 6th edition, Vol II. WB Saunders Co, Philadelphia: 1995.
4. Viswabathans S, Campbell CE, Cork RC: Asymptomatic undetected mediastinal mass: A death during ambulatory anesthesia. *J Clin Anesth* 1995; 7(2): 151-55.

MEDIASTINOSCOPY

SURGICAL CONSIDERATIONS

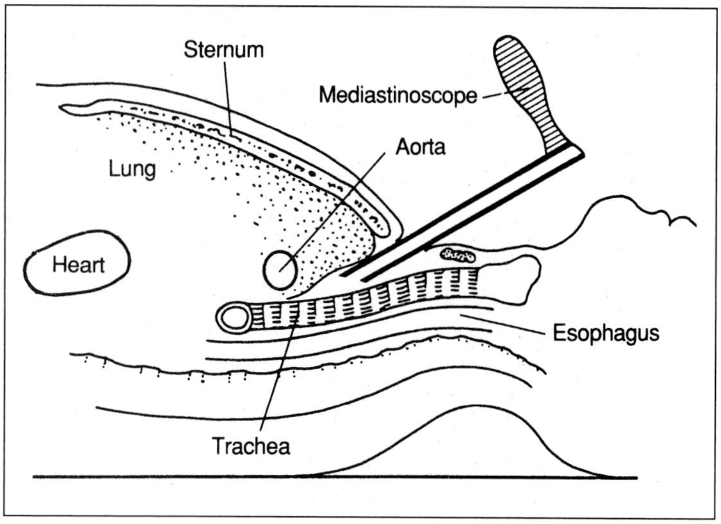

Figure 5-4. Insertion of mediastinoscope. (Reproduced with permission from Hurt R, Bates M: *Essentials of Thoracic Surgery*. Butterworths: 1986.)

Description: Mediastinoscopy is performed to ascertain extrapulmonary spread of pulmonary tumors, diagnose anterior mediastinal masses (neurogenic tumors, cysts, lymphomas, thymomas, parathyroid and substernal thyroid tissue). This technique also may be used for the placement of electrodes for atrial pacing of the heart. If a thoracic aneurysm is present or SVC is obstructed, mediastinoscopy is contraindicated as the anatomy is distorted and vessels can be punctured inadvertently by the mediastinoscope. Mediastinoscopy is performed by passing a short endoscope into the upper mediastinum through a small transverse incision just above the sternal notch (Fig 5-4). This procedure is used to biopsy mediastinal lymph nodes and masses as far down as the carina and upper mainstem bronchi. Blunt dissection is carried out in the pretracheal fascial plane. Nodes anterior to the trachea and in the right pretracheal region are readily accessible to biopsy by this technique (Fig 5-5); nodes on the left side are not so accessible. Occasionally, one can biopsy subcarinal nodes by this technique. The proximity of major vascular structures (Fig 5-6) leads to the potential for massive hemorrhage.

Variant procedure or approaches: For nodes on the left side of the mediastinum, an **anterior mediastinotomy (Chamberlain procedure**), usually in the second interspace, may be carried out instead of mediastinoscopy. Dissection may be transplural or retroplural, the objective being safe biopsy of the target node or mass. A tube is left during closure; it may be removed after closure of the chest or left overnight.

Usual preop diagnosis: Carcinoma of the lung with enlarged mediastinal nodes; mediastinal node enlargement 2° lymphoma, thymoma or other

SUMMARY OF PROCEDURE

Position	Supine
Incision	For mediastinoscopy, suprasternal; usually left 2nd interspace for anterior mediastinotomy.
Special instrumentation	Mediastinoscope for mediastinoscopy only; none for anterior mediastinotomy
Antibiotics	Cefazolin 1 g
Surgical time	≤ 1 h
EBL	Minimal (but risk of significant blood loss if major vascular injury occurs).
Postop care	PACU → room
Mortality	< 1%
Morbidity	Bleeding
	Pneumothorax: Rare
	Vocal cord paralysis: Rare
	Esophageal perforation: Rare
	Pleural tear: Rare
	Tracheal laceration: Rare
Pain score	2 (mediastinoscopy); 2-3 (anterior mediastinotomy)

PATIENT POPULATION CHARACTERISTICS

Age range	Adults, usually > 50 yr
Male:Female	Male > female
Incidence	Frequently part of evaluation for patients with lung cancer
Etiology	Lung cancer; lymphoma; thymoma; retrosternal goiter
Associated conditions	Airway obstruction

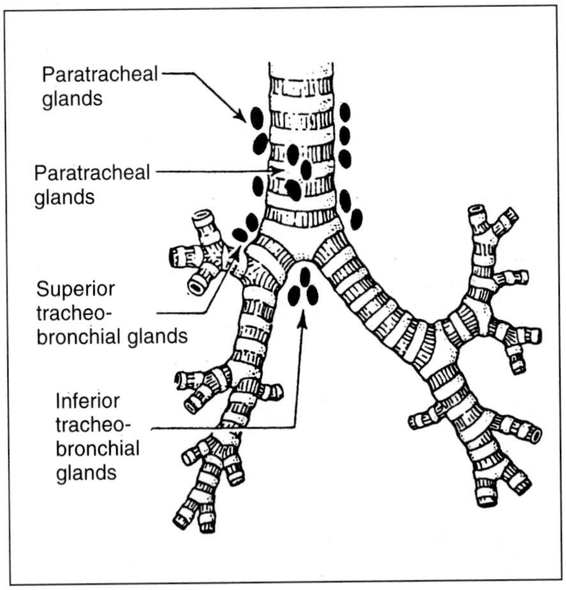

↑**Figure 5-5.** Common lymph node sites accessible to mediastinoscope biopsy. (Reproduced with permission from Hurt R, Bates M: *Essentials of Thoracic Surgery*. Butterworths: 1986.)

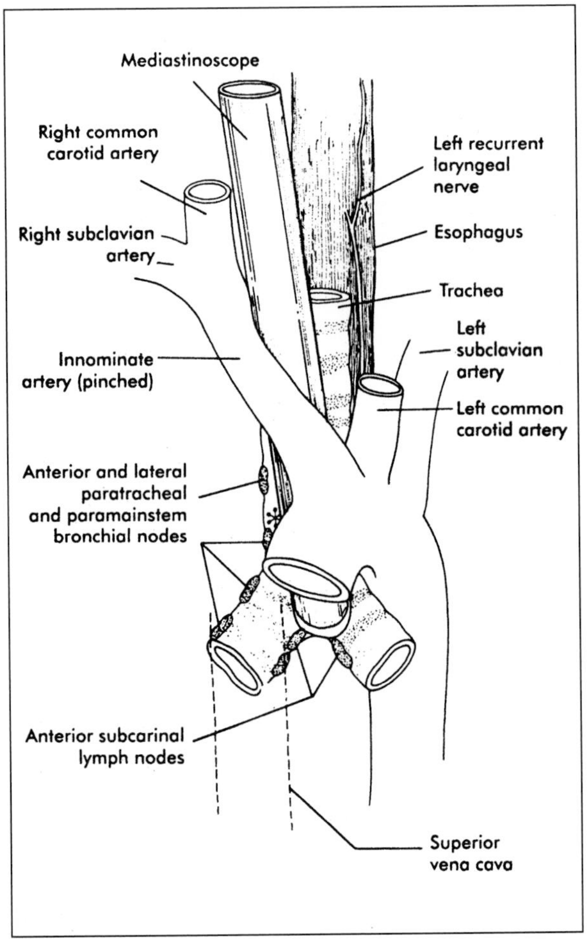

→**Figure 5-6.** Relationship of mediastinoscope to trachea and great vessels. (Reproduced with permission from Petty C: Right radial artery pressure during mediastinoscopy. *Anesth Analg* 1979; 58:428. Modified in Rogers MC: *Principles & Practices of Anesthesiology*. Mosby-Year Book, St Louis: 1993.)

ANESTHETIC CONSIDERATIONS

PREOPERATIVE

(Procedures covered: excision of mediastinal tumor; mediastinoscopy)

Typically, these patients can be divided into two populations, depending on the presence or absence of a significant mediastinal mass (with the potential for catastrophic airway obstruction or cardiovascular collapse on induction of anesthesia). The preop assessment must focus on the differentiation of these two populations. Close consultation with the surgeon is essential in formulating the anesthetic plan.

Respiratory Question patient with anterior mediastinal mass about ability to lie supine and the presence of cough or dyspnea; change in position may cause superior caval obstruction or cardiac and airway compression by mediastinal mass (may be apparent only following induction or on emergence from anesthesia). On PE, ✓ for presence of cyanosis, wheezing or stridor in the upright and supine positions. If significant airway compression or SVC obstruction is present, the surgeon may delay surgery for radiation or chemotherapy. Patients with SVC syndrome (edema, venous engorgement of head, neck and upper body, supine dyspnea, ± headache, mental status change) may have significant airway edema.

Tests: If airway compression is present, obtain PFTs with flow volume loops in upright and supine positions (Fig 5-7 shows flow volume loop). Order CT/MRI scan to determine airway distortion or compression and anatomic involvement with other intrathoracic structures.

Cardiovascular Intrathoracic vascular structures (e.g., heart, PA, SVC) may be compressed → ↓BP, hypoxia, SVC syndrome.

Tests: ECHO, CT/MR if indicated by H&P.

Musculoskeletal Patients with lung cancer may have myasthenic (Eaton-Lambert) syndrome with increased sensitivity to nondepolarizing muscle relaxants. Monitor relaxation with peripheral nerve stimulator.

Neurologic Patient may have ↑ICP if SVC is obstructed. Consider neurology consultation.

Laboratory Others tests as indicated from H&P.

Premedication Avoid sedation in patients with the potential for airway obstruction; otherwise, midazolam 1-2 mg iv may be appropriate.

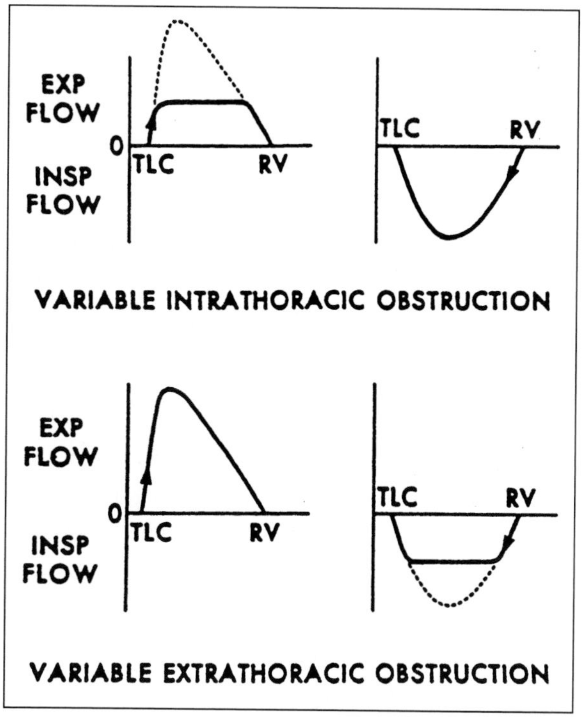

Figure 5-7. Flow loop volume: with variable extrathoracic lesion, the alteration in the flow volume loop is seen by flow limitation and a plateau on inspiration. The reverse occurs with variable intrathoracic lesions. (Reproduced with permission from Acres J, Kryger MH: Clinical significance of pulmonary function tests. *Chest.* 1981; 80:207-11.)

INTRAOPERATIVE

Anesthetic technique: GETA

Induction Consider awake FOB intubation (e.g., if symptomatic in supine position) or use short-acting muscle relaxant (e.g., succinylcholine). A mask induction with sevoflurane/O_2 in a spontaneously breathing patient may be a safe alternative. Complete or partial airway obstruction by anterior mediastinal mass can be due to changes in lung and chest-wall mechanics associated with changes in the patient's position (sitting to supine during procedure) or to muscle relaxation. A surgeon familiar with rigid bronchoscopy should be in the OR ready to bypass obstruction.

Maintenance O_2 (100%) and isoflurane (1-1.5%) or sevoflurane (1.5-2.5%). Avoid N_2O, especially during OLV. Short-acting muscle relaxant and opioid as required.

Emergence Extubation in OR

Blood and fluid requirements IV: 18 ga × 1
NS/LR @ 1-2 ml/kg/h
Blood in OR

Have blood for transfusion available in OR prior to surgery. With venous bleeding, fluids given through an iv in upper limb may enter mediastinum through a tear in the vein. A large-bore iv cannula should then be placed in lower limb for fluid and blood transfusions.

Monitoring Standard monitors (p. B-1)
± Arterial line
± CVP/PA

Invasive monitors are appropriate in patients with large mediastinal masses. In the presence of SVC syndrome, CVP/PA catheters should be placed, using the femoral vein. BP cuff on left arm; radial artery line (if used) and pulse oximeter on right. Mass or mediastinoscope can compress innominate artery, causing reduction in right-radial pulse and right-arm BP. If only right-arm BP is measured, patients may be treated inappropriately for "hypotension." Suspect great vessel compression if right-arm pressure is lower than left, or if right-arm BP disappears in the presence of a normal ECG. Arterial compression can compromise cerebrovascular perfusion → cerebral ischemia stroke.

Positioning Head-up position
✓ and pad pressure points.
✓ eyes.

In patients with an anterior mediastinal mass, the head-up position reduces mass compression effect on airway and vascular structures. Patients with SVC obstruction,

Positioning, cont.		if placed in head-down position with IPPV (further impedes venous return of thoracic cavity), are at ↑risk of airway edema and airway obstruction following extubation.
Complications	Bleeding	Surgical tamponade through mediastinoscope may be indicated. For major hemorrhage, emergency thoracotomy or median sternotomy may be required to stop bleeding. Can occur from laceration of mediastinal vein.
	Air embolism	Head elevation increases risk of embolism, particularly if patient breathes spontaneously. Monitor $ETCO_2$ and ETN_2.
	Airway rupture or obstruction	Requires immediate thoracotomy.
	Tracheal collapse	Acute obstruction may require rigid bronchoscope to reopen airway.

POSTOPERATIVE

Complications	Pneumothorax (see Postop Complications for Cervical Neurosurgical Procedures, p. 75). Phrenic/recurrent laryngeal nerve damage Bleeding	Bilateral laryngeal nerve damage may result in airway obstruction, necessitating reintubation. Mask ventilation may be ineffective.
Pain management	Parenteral opioids (p. C-1)	
Tests	CXR on all patients to r/o pneumothorax.	See Postop Complications for Thoracoscopy, p. 203.

References

1. Barash PG, Tsai B, Kitahata LM: Acute tracheal collapse following mediastinoscopy. *Anesthesiology* 1976; 44(1):67-8.
2. Baue AE, ed: *Glenn's Thoracic and Cardiovascular Surgery*, 6th edition, Volume II. Geha AS, Hammond GL, Laks H, Naunheim KS, assoc eds. Appleton & Lange, Norwalk, CT: 1996.
3. Neuman GG, Weingarten AE, Abramowitz RM, et al: The anesthetic management of the patient with an anterior mediastinal mass. *Anesthesiology* 1984; 60(2):144-47.
4. Petty C: Right radial artery pressure during mediastinoscopy. *Anesth Analg* 1979; 58(5):428-30.
5. Sabiston DC Jr, Spencer FC: *Surgery of the Chest*, 6th edition, Vol II. WB Saunders Co, Philadelphia: 1995.
6. Vaughan RS: Anesthesia for mediastinoscopy. *Anaesthesia* 1978; 33(2):195-98.
7. Vueghs PJ, Schurink GA, Vaes L, Langemeyer JS: Anesthesia in repeat mediastinoscopy: a retrospective study of 101 patients. *J Cardiothorac Vasc Anesth* 1992; 6(2):193-95.

BRONCHOSCOPY—FLEXIBLE AND RIGID

SURGICAL CONSIDERATIONS

Description: Most **flexible fiber optic bronchoscopy (FOB)** is done under topical anesthesia and does not require the services of an anesthesiologist. When flexible FOB precedes other surgery, it is usually carried out in an anesthetized patient through the ETT, using a special adaptor. **Rigid bronchoscopy**, alone or in combination with other procedures such as **mediastinoscopy** or **thoracotomy**, however, is usually done under GA. With the patient's eyes protected, and either a tooth guard or gauze pads protecting the upper lip, teeth and gums, the head and neck are extended. The bronchoscope is introduced through the right side of the mouth, following the contour of the tongue until the epiglottis is identified (Fig 5-8). As in laryngoscopy, the epiglottis is lifted to visualize the vocal cords and the bronchoscope is advanced into the upper airway; and the diagnostic or therapeutic procedure is carried out. Then the bronchoscope is carefully removed. Ventilation during rigid bronchoscopy under GA may be carried out using a special adaptor (Racine) or a Sander's attachment (see Anesthetic Considerations, below). **Laser bronchoscopy** can be carried out using flexible or rigid bronchoscopes. Carbon dioxide and neodymium:YAG lasers are commonly used in bronchoscopic procedures. The CO_2 laser is characterized by limited tissue penetration, which restricts its use to localized benign lesions of the upper airway. In contrast, the Nd:YAG laser, with its shorter wavelength, exhibits greatly enhanced depth penetration (several millimeters); therefore, it is much more effective than the CO_2 laser for the ablation of large masses. FiO_2 of 0.4 or less is necessary when laser is in use.

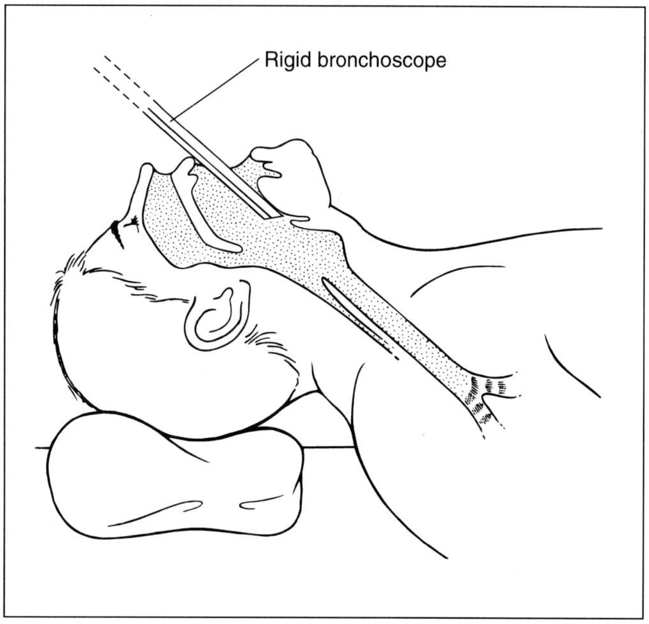

Figure 5-8. Patient positioning for rigid bronchoscopy.

Usual preop diagnosis: Carcinoma of the lung, primary or recurrent; hemoptysis; obstruction; foreign body; benign tumor

SUMMARY OF PROCEDURE

	Fiber Optic Bronchoscopy	Rigid Bronchoscopy	Laser Bronchoscopy
Position	Supine	⇐	⇐
Special instrumentation	FOB and instrument	Rigid bronchoscope and instruments	Nd:YAG laser and bronchoscope
Unique considerations	None	Shared airway	⇐ + Keep $FiO_2 \leq 0.4$ during use of laser.
Antibiotics	Usually none	± Cefazolin 1 g	⇐
Surgical time	< 30 min	⇐	1 h
EBL	Minimal	⇐	⇐
Postop care	PACU → room	⇐	⇐
Mortality	Minimal	⇐	5%
Morbidity	Barotrauma	⇐	⇐
	Airway obstruction	⇐	Airway fire
	Pneumothorax	⇐	Hemorrhage
		Tooth damage	Perforation
		Tracheal laceration	
		Pneumomediastinum	
		Esophageal perforation	
Pain score	1	1	1

PATIENT POPULATION CHARACTERISTICS

Age range	Usually adults > 50
Male:Female	1:1
Incidence	Common
Etiology	Smoking; hemoptysis; aspiration of foreign body
Associated conditions	Lung cancer or metastatic spread to tracheobronchial tree; airway obstruction 2° tumor or foreign body; lung infiltrates

ANESTHETIC CONSIDERATIONS

PREOPERATIVE

Patients presenting for bronchoscopy range from asymptomatic to those in severe respiratory distress. The fiber optic technique has virtually replaced rigid bronchoscopy for diagnostic procedures.

Respiratory H&P to focus on underlying condition. Evaluate for acute and chronic pulmonary problems by H&P and lab and radiologic studies.

Tests: Consider ABG (indicated if patient has Hx of heavy tobacco use, has SOB at rest or has poor exercise tolerance); PFT; CXR. Hypoxemia ($PaO_2 < 70$ mmHg) and/or hypercapnia ($PaCO_2 > 45$ mmHg) indicate significant respiratory impairment and predict increased risk.

Cardiovascular Many patients have Hx of cardiac disease. Cardiology consultation should be obtained for acute change in cardiac status or for patient with poorly controlled chronic disease.

Tests: Consider ECG; others as indicated from H&P.

Musculoskeletal Patients with lung cancer may have myasthenic (Eaton-Lambert) syndrome with increased sensitivity to nondepolarizing muscle relaxants. Monitor relaxation with peripheral nerve stimulator.

Hematologic Blood cross-match not necessary unless high risk of hemorrhage from biopsy. (Check with surgeon.) Adequate O_2-carrying capacity important.

Tests: Hb/Hct

Laboratory Other tests as indicated from H&P.

Premedication Antisialagogue (prefer glycopyrrolate 0.2 mg iv, no central anticholinergic effects); atropine or scopolamine also can be used. Light sedation with midazolam 1-2 mg iv and/or fentanyl, 50-100 μg iv. Avoid heavy sedation that might impair postop ventilation.

INTRAOPERATIVE

Flexible bronchoscopy: Anesthetic technique for flexible FOB requires sedation or GA. Anxious patients and those with respiratory compromise may not tolerate sedation for awake FOB; and patients with Hx of gastric reflux or aspiration are not candidates for awake FOB.

Sedation with topical anesthesia Sedate patient as necessary to ensure comfort and cooperation (midazolam 1-2 mg iv and/or fentanyl 50-100 μg iv. Spray palate, pharynx, larynx, vocal cords and trachea with lidocaine (4%), using nebulizer, or have patient gargle viscous lidocaine (4%).

Transtracheal local anesthesia: pass needle through cricothyroid membrane, aspirate air into syringe, and then inject lidocaine (2%), 2 ml. Remove needle quickly since injection causes cough (spreads the anesthetic). Perform superior laryngeal nerve blocks. Insert needle anterior to superior cornu of thyroid cartilage. After resistance is felt, aspirate gently, then inject lidocaine (2%) 2 ml; repeat on other side. Alternatively, hold base of tongue forward and, using Krause's forceps, place pledgets soaked in local anesthetic in each pyriform fossa to block the internal branch of superior laryngeal nerve. Patient can hold a suction catheter in the mouth to remove oral secretions and waste anesthetic gases. A special face mask (Patil-Syracuse) incorporates a diaphragm through which the FOB can pass while patient breathes $FiO_2 = 1$. Use a special oral airway (Ovassapian) to guide FOB over back of tongue into trachea to prevent damage to FOB by teeth. Limit amount of suctioning by surgeon since suctioning through FOB decreases FiO_2 and FRC, → ↓PaO_2.

General anesthesia: Almost any anesthetic technique is acceptable. A large ETT has less resistance to air flow; minimum size is 8 mm (I.D.) for adult FOB. If patient requires ETT < 8 mm, use a pediatric FOB. FOB through ETT causes PEEP effect, which can lead to hypotension in hypovolemic patient.

Rigid bronchoscopy: Anesthetic technique utilizing rigid bronchoscopy provides superior visualization and improved suctioning, and allows introduction of biopsy forceps. Requires GA.

Induction Preoxygenate to completely denitrogenate patient. Use only small amount of iv opioids since postop analgesic requirements are minimal; consider remifentanil (1μg/kg). Postop respiratory depression should be avoided. STP 3-5 mg/kg, succinylcholine 1 mg/kg or mivacurium 0.2 mg/kg.

Maintenance Isoflurane, sevoflurane or desflurane and 100% O_2; succinylcholine drip (1 g/250 ml NS, titrated to effect; be aware of onset of phase II block at doses > 5-6 mg/kg). A remifentanil infusion

(0.5-1 μg/kg/min) may be useful. Short-acting, nondepolarizing agents (atracurium, vecuronium or mivacurium) also can be used. Manual IPPV through side-arm of rigid bronchoscope. High flow (up to 20 L/min) to compensate for leak. Hyperventilate patient in preparation for periods of apnea. Ventilation must be interrupted whenever surgeon removes eyepiece to suction or biopsy. Manually ventilate to compensate for compliance changes that occur when bronchoscope is in trachea (ventilating both lungs) and when it is in bronchus (ventilating one lung). O_2 flush is used to compensate for leak; bypasses anesthetic vaporizer. Frequent flushing lowers anesthetic concentration. **Sanders Injection System**—jet ventilation using Venturi effect—is an alternative. Uninterrupted ventilation is possible since the presence of eyepiece is not necessary for ventilation. Fewer interruptions may shorten length of procedure. Requires iv anesthesia (e.g., propofol @ 100-200 μg/kg/min), remifentanil 0.5 μg/kg/min since high fresh-gas flow makes inhalational anesthetic concentrations unpredictable. Entrainment of air results in variable O_2 at distal tip. If total thoracic compliance is low, adequacy of ventilation is difficult to evaluate; patient easily hypoventilated. The greater need for muscle relaxation to move chest wall increases risk of residual weakness immediately postop.

Emergence

Reintubate with ETT after rigid bronchoscopy. Patient must be fully awake before extubation, with no residual neuromuscular blockade. Emergence can be "stormy." Patient may cough violently to clear secretions and blood. A smooth emergence may be facilitated by early suctioning of the airway, use of an antisialagogue and lidocaine (1 mg/kg iv) to decrease airway sensitivity. The sitting position improves breathing and clearance of secretions. Continue supplemental O_2.

Blood and fluid requirements	Blood usually not required. IV: 18 ga × 1 NS/LR @ 2 ml/kg/h	Transfusion unnecessary unless complicated by massive hemorrhage; be prepared for emergency thoracotomy. Usually restrict iv fluids to avoid fluid overload.
Monitoring	Standard monitors (p. B-1)	★ **NB:** $ETCO_2$ not accurate during rigid bronchoscopy because of dilution effect at sample port.
Positioning	✓ and pad pressure points. ✓ eyes. Shoulder roll for rigid bronchoscopy	
Complications	Hypoxemia	Monitor pulse oximetry continuously. If patient hypoxemic, surgeon must withdraw bronchoscope into trachea. If problem persists, remove bronchoscope and ventilate by mask or ETT.
	Hypercapnia	Common, due to hypoventilation. Ventricular dysrhythmias due to respiratory acidosis and "light" anesthesia. Treat by hyperventilation (increased rate) which lowers CO_2 and deepens inhalational anesthesia; iv lidocaine for dysrhythmias.
	Bleeding Tracheobronchial injury Aspiration of debris	Requires frequent suctioning. For major hemorrhage, place uncut ETT down healthy bronchus and ventilate good lung. May require thoracotomy using DLT or BB to isolate and/or tamponade bleeding site.

POSTOPERATIVE

Complications	Hypoxemia	Rx: Supplemental O_2
	Hypoventilation Dental damage Airway trauma Pneumothorax Hemorrhage	Incomplete reversal of muscle relaxants or opioid overdosage can cause hypoventilation. Obtain ABG if patient has difficulty breathing or is overly sedated. Be prepared to reintubate patient.
	Risk of aspiration Airway obstruction (bronchospasm, bleeding, dislodged tumor, foreign body)	If nerve blocks used to depress gag reflex, no eating or drinking for several h postbronchoscopy.
Pain management	Minimal pain; easily treated with iv opioids.	

Tests	CXR	Obtain CXR in recovery room to check for atelectasis, pneumothorax, mediastinal emphysema.

References

1. Baue AE, ed: *Glenn's Thoracic and Cardiovascular Surgery*, 6th edition, Volume II. Geha AS, Hammond GL, Laks H, Naunheim KS, assoc eds. Appleton & Lange, Norwalk, CT: 1996.
2. Brimacombe J, Tucker P, Simons S: The Laryngeal mask airway for awake diagnostic bronchoscopy. A retrospective study of 200 consecutive patients. *Eur J Anaesthesiol* 1995; 12(4):357-61.
3. Fraioli RL, Sheffer LA, Steffenson JL: Pulmonary and cardiovascular effects of apneic oxygenation in man. *Anesthesiology* 1973; 39(6):588-96.
4. Graham DR, Hay JG, Clague J, et al: Comparison of three different methods used to achieve local anesthesia for fiber optic bronchoscopy. *Chest* 1992; 102(3):704-7.
5. Sabiston DC Jr, Spencer FC: *Surgery of the Chest*, 6th edition, Vol II. WB Saunders Co, Philadelphia: 1995.

ANESTHETIC CONSIDERATIONS FOR LASER RESECTION

PREOPERATIVE

Typically, these patients present with a long Hx of smoking and consequent pulmonary dysfunction, complicated by an airway mass (endobronchial, carinal or tracheal) causing respiratory distress.

Respiratory It is important to define the exact location and magnitude of any tracheal mass, in order to estimate an appropriate size for the ETT and the likelihood of obstruction on induction. CXR and CT scan should be studied. PFTs and flow volume loops may help to characterize the lesion.
Tests: PFTs; ABGs; CXR; CT scan (to determine site of airway obstruction)

Musculoskeletal Although there may be no clinically detectable muscle weakness, some of these patients will have Eaton-Lambert syndrome → ↑sensitivity to muscle relaxants.

Hematologic Transfuse patients with preop Hct < 25% (or < 30% if CAD present).
Tests: Hct

Laboratory Other tests as indicated from H&P.

Premedication Minimal; avoid respiratory depressants.

INTRAOPERATIVE

Anesthetic technique: GETA or local anesthesia with heavy sedation. Unexpected patient movement may be disastrous. Nd:YAG laser can be transmitted through a flexible quartz monofilament passed through either a rigid bronchoscope or FOB. Rigid bronchoscope provides improved visibility and better debris retrieval. It also maintains the airway with less chance of fire since metal is nonignitable (it can reflect the laser beam, however, causing tissue damage), although manual ventilation through the side-arm may be more difficult. FOB is used with local anesthesia or through ETT under GA. Laser-safe ETTs (required for surgery in the proximal trachea) include regular ETTs wrapped in metallic tape or commercially available "laser" tubes (these are usually some combination of aluminum, stainless steel, Teflon and/or silicon. Fill cuff with saline (± methylene blue to facilitate leak detection). Steps must also be taken to protect the OR staff from laser injury.

Induction **Without airway obstruction:** Standard induction (see p. B-2).

With airway obstruction: Awake FOB may precede intubation in order to determine the feasibility of tracheal intubation. In patients with less severe obstruction, an inhalation induction with spontaneous ventilation may be appropriate. Avoid muscle relaxants until the airway has been secured. For FOB resections, a large, red rubber ETT is preferred as it is less flammable, and less combustible toxic products are released if ignited than if a plastic ETT is ignited. Special laser ETTs are not needed since Nd:YAG laser is fired distal to the tip of the ETT.

Maintenance Use isoflurane, air (N_2) and O_2 mixture. Keep $FiO_2 < 0.3$. Avoid N_2O, which supports combustion. Short-acting, nondepolarizing relaxant or succinylcholine infusion should be used since it is essential that the operating field be stationary to avoid damage to tissue from a misdirected laser beam. If the patient becomes hypoxemic, ventilate the lungs with higher FiO_2 and ask the surgeon to stop.

Emergence	Following rigid bronchoscopy, the patient usually is reintubated until awake and breathing well and protective airway reflexes have returned. Emergence can be "stormy," with bleeding and secretion clearance a problem. Patient should be recovered in the sitting position.	
Blood and fluid requirements	IV: 14-16 ga × 1-2 NS/LR @ 1-2 ml/kg/h	There is a potential for massive blood loss following inadvertent perforation of a major blood vessel.
Monitoring	Standard monitors (p. B-1)	Continuous pulse oximetry essential; monitor $ETCO_2$ to assess adequacy of ventilation. Keep alveolar $O_2 < 40\%$.
Positioning	✓ and pad pressure points. ✓ eyes.	
Complications	Airway obstruction	From tumor, blood, tissue debris, etc.
	Hypoxemia/hypercarbia	From inadequate ventilation.
	Bleeding	Can be massive from perforation of blood vessel by laser. Apply topical epinephrine following laser photocoagulation to control bleeding.
	Perforation of tracheobronchial tree	→ pneumothorax/mediastinum → cardiac arrest.
	Airway fire	Rx: stop ventilation, remove O_2 source, extubate trachea to decrease inhalation of toxic products. Suction all debris from airway. Ventilate patient by mask, then reintubate. Prior to extubation, perform bronchoscopy to reevaluate airway damage and suction debris.

POSTOPERATIVE

Complications	Airway edema	Only the surface of the affected tissue is visibly changed; there may be underlying edema formation. Patient may require emergency reintubation if airway obstruction due to edema occurs. Steroids usually given (dexamethasone 6-8 mg iv). Complications such as hemorrhage or obstruction can be delayed up to 48 h.
Pain management	Minimal pain; rarely requires analgesic.	
Tests	Continuous pulse oximetry monitoring. Frequent ABGs.	

References

1. Baue AE, ed: *Glenn's Thoracic and Cardiovascular Surgery*, 6th edition, Volume II. Geha AS, Hammond GL, Laks H, Naunheim KS, assoc eds. Appleton & Lange, Norwalk, CT: 1996.
2. Blomquist S, Algotsson L, Karlsson SE: Anaesthesia for resection of tumours in the trachea and central bronchi using the Nd:YAG-laser technique. *Acta Anaesthiol Scand* 1990; 34(6):506-10.
3. Chan AL, Tharratt RS, Siefkin AD, et al: Nd:YAG laser bronchoscopy. Rigid or fiber optic mode? *Chest* 1990; 98(2):271-75.
4. McCaughan JS Jr, Barabash RD, Penn GM, Glavan BJ: Nd:YAG laser and photodynamic therapy for esophageal and endobronchial tumors under general and local anesthesia. Effects on arterial blood gas levels. *Chest* 1990; 98(6):1374-78.
5. Sabiston DC Jr, Spencer FC: *Surgery of the Chest*, 6th edition, Vol II. WB Saunders Co, Philadelphia: 1995.
6. Vanderschueren RG, Westermann CJ: Complications of endobronchial neodymium:YAG (Nd:YAG) laser application. *Lung* 1990; 168 Suppl:1089-94.
7. Warner ME, Warner MA, Leonard PF: Anesthesia for Neodymium:YAG (Nd:YAG) laser resection of major airway obstructing tumors. *Anesthesiology* 1984; 60(3):230-32.

VIDEO-ASSISTED THORACOSCOPY (VAT)

SURGICAL CONSIDERATIONS

Description: While thoracoscopy itself is not new, **video-assisted thoracoscopy** (VAT) is a relatively new technique which is rapidly gaining popularity. Video thoracoscopy is most often used for assessment of pleural processes of unknown etiology, such as pleural effusion that has defied diagnosis. Its use is accepted for treatment of spontaneous pneumothorax due to apical blebs, for biopsy of peripheral infiltrates or nodules, and for drainage of pleural effusions and other fluid collections. Accessible, small lung cancers may be removed using the videoscope (wedge resections). VAT also has been used for lung-volume reduction surgery (see p. 210). **Heller myotomy** and **upper dorsal sympathectomy** can be done using video thoracoscopy. Less well accepted procedures using video capabilities include **lobectomy**, **pneumonectomy** and **esophagectomy**. Use of a DLT to provide collapse of the ipsilateral lung is mandatory, since satisfactory visualization of the pleural cavity is impossible without this collapse of the lung. The patient is usually in the lateral position. Several small incisions are used, usually 3; sometimes 4 or more. The video thoracoscope is placed through the first incision and the pleural cavity is inspected. Other small incisions are then made for insertion of instruments. The position of the video thoracoscope and instruments may be interchanged, depending on the location of the problem.

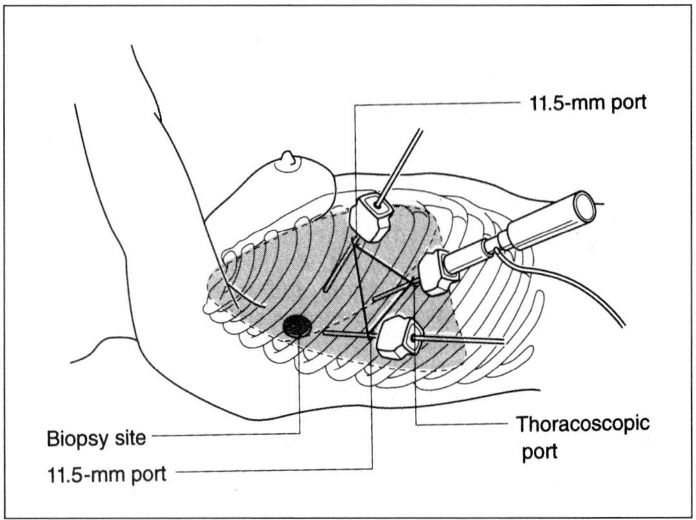

Figure 5-9. Example of thoracoscopic port placement. Positioning varies for individual need, but the principle of triangulation used for laparoscopic surgery is equally applicable in the thorax. (Reproduced with permission from Greenfield LJ, et al., eds: *Surgery Scientific Principles and Practice.* Philadelphia: Lippincott-Raven Publishers: 1997, 741.)

Usual preop diagnosis: Pleural disease (e.g., effusions); recurrent empyema; recurrent pneumothorax; localized lung masses; achalasia; pulmonary infiltrates; hyperhidrosis; reflex sympathetic dystrophy (RSD)

SUMMARY OF PROCEDURE

Position	Lateral
Incision	Usually 3 small incisions (portals) (Fig 5-9)
Special instrumentation	Video thoracoscope with thoracoscopy instruments; DLT required
Antibiotics	Cefazolin 1 g
Surgical time	1-3 h
Closing considerations	Chest tube placed
EBL	Minimal, although there is a risk for major bleeding.
Postop care	Chest tube
Mortality	Minimal
Morbidity	Major vascular injury: Rare Conversion to open thoracotomy: 4% Pneumothorax/persistent air leak
Pain score	2-3

PATIENT POPULATION CHARACTERISTICS

Age range	All age groups
Male:Female	1:1
Associated conditions	Pleural effusions; lung mass; pneumothorax

ANESTHETIC CONSIDERATIONS

PREOPERATIVE

As VAT is used for both diagnostic and therapeutic purposes, this patient population is quite diverse in symptomatology; however, it has in common some intrathoracic/respiratory disease process.

Respiratory	The preop evaluation should focus on the patient's ability to tolerate OLV as well as the postop effects of the planned surgery. PFTs and ABG are useful prognostic texts. Question patient about dyspnea, productive cough and cigarette smoking; examine for cyanosis, clubbing, RR and pattern. Listen to chest for wheezes, rhonchi and rales. Preop lung function may be improved by treating respiratory tract infections, stopping smoking, and treatment with bronchodilators and steroids as indicated. **Tests:** PFT; CXR; if chest CT available, look for airway obstruction that could interfere with DLT placement; ABG.
Cardiovascular	Directed at any underlying disease process.
Laboratory	As indicated from H&P.
Premedication	Standard premedication (see p. B-2). Avoid heavy sedation that might impair postop respiratory function.

INTRAOPERATIVE

Anesthetic technique: GETA, typically with OLV, using DLT or BB (see OLV, p. 176–178). Local or regional anesthetic technique ± sedation also may be used.

Regional anesthesia: The incision site is infiltrated with local anesthetics, and intercostal nerve blocks are performed at the level of incision and at several levels above and below incision. Alternatively, thoracic epidural anesthesia may be used. When the chest is opened, air enters pleural cavity, causing partial pneumothorax. Most patients usually tolerate this if warned in advance about the potential for dyspnea and visceral discomfort. Thoracoscope in chest-wall incision prevents complete lung collapse.

General anesthesia: The patient is intubated with DLT or BB to selectively collapse operated lung. Anesthetic choice optional, but FiO_2 = 1 during OLV. GA allows IPPV with complete reexpansion of lung without pain, if pleurodesis performed.

Induction	Standard induction (see p. B-2). (Placement of DLT is discussed on p. 178.)	
Maintenance	O_2 (100%) and isoflurane (1-1.5%). Avoid N_2O, especially during OLV. Short-acting muscle relaxant (e.g., mivacurium 0.01-0.1 mg/kg) and opioids as required. Consider remifentanil infusion (0.5 μg/kg/min).	
Emergence	Extubation in OR	
Blood and fluid requirements	IV: 18 ga × 1 NS/LR @ 2 ml/kg/h	
Monitoring	Standard monitors (p. B-1)	
Positioning	✓ and pad pressure points. ✓ eyes.	
Complications	Air leak from lung	Air leak obvious on reexpansion of lung.
	Hemorrhage	Excessive blood drainage via chest tube; falling Hct
	Injury to intrathoracic structures	Repair may require open thoracotomy.
	Air embolism	

POSTOPERATIVE

Complications	Tension pneumothorax	In the absence of chest tube, air leak can lead to pneumothorax (rare). This may manifest as wheezing, hyperresonance, decreased chest-wall movement, dyspnea, subcutaneous emphysema, tracheal shift, dysrhythmias, cardiovascular collapse, ↓PO_2 and ↓SaO_2.

Complications, cont.		CXR diagnostic. Requires immediate decompression of tension pneumothorax with large-bore iv cannula through chest wall, followed by chest tube and continuous suction.
Pain management	IV opioids, ketorolac (30 mg) Intrapleural anesthesia	Analgesic requirements less than for lateral thoracotomy. Intrapleural local anesthetics (0.25% bupivacaine + 1:200,000 epinephrine 0.5 ml/kg) via thoracostomy drainage tube after lung is reinflated but before chest tube suction applied.
Tests	CXR postop	

References

1. Baue AE, ed: *Glenn's Thoracic and Cardiovascular Surgery*, 6th edition, Volume II. Geha AS, Hammond GL, Laks H, Naunheim KS, assoc eds. Appleton & Lange, Norwalk, CT: 1996.
2. Kraenzler EJ, Hearn CJ: Anesthetic considerations for video-assisted thoracic surgery. *Semin Thorac Vasc Surg* 1993; 5(4):321-26.
3. Landreneau RJ, Hazelrigg SR, Ferson PF, et al: Thoracoscopic resection of 85 pulmonary lesions. *Ann Thorac Surg* 1992; 54(3):415-19.
4. Mault JR, Harpole DH, Douglas JM: Thoracoscopic pulmonary resection. In *Atlas of laparoscopic surgery.* Pappas TN, Schwartz LB, Eubanks S, eds. *Current Medicine*, 1996; 26:10.
5. Miller, DL, Allen MS, Trastek VF, et al: Videothoracoscopic wedge excision of the lung. *Ann Thorac Surg* 1992; 54(3): 410-14.
6. Rusch VW, Mountain C: Thoracoscopy under regional anesthesia for the diagnosis and management of pleural disease. *Am J Surg* 1987; 154(3):274-78.
7. Sabiston DC Jr, Spencer FC: *Surgery of the Chest*, 6th edition, Vol II. WB Saunders Co, Philadelphia: 1995.

THYMECTOMY

SURGICAL CONSIDERATIONS

Description: Thymectomy for myasthenia gravis is usually carried out through a median sternotomy incision. In these circumstances, the thymus may be grossly normal. The thymus is an H-shaped organ with long inferior tails heading toward the diaphragm and smaller superior ones extending up into the neck. The only major vascular structure usually encountered is the thymic vein, which enters the left brachiocephalic vein as it crosses anterior to the arterial structures in the anterior mediastinum. The thymus gland is anterior to all of this. Dissection is generally started inferiorly. It is important to remove the entire thymus gland, particularly in patients with myasthenia gravis. This may involve entry into one or both pleural cavities. The dissection is carried superiorly anterior to the left brachiocephalic vein and into the neck, removing the superior tails as well. Some surgeons prefer the **cervical approach** for thymectomy in myasthenia gravis. It is possible that part of the thymus gland might be left behind during the cervical approach. If there is any question about how much thymic tissue remains, a **sternotomy** is the procedure of choice. The cervical approach is not suitable if the patient has a thymoma (with or without myasthenia gravis).

Usual preop diagnosis: Myasthenia gravis; thymoma

SUMMARY OF PROCEDURE

	Sternotomy	Cervical Approach
Position	Supine	⇐
Incision	Median sternotomy	Suprasternal
Special instrumentation	None	Special sternal retractor
Antibiotics	Cefazolin 1 g	⇐
Surgical time	1-2 h	⇐

	Sternotomy	Cervical Approach
EBL	< 500 ml	⇐
Postop care	ICU – special attention to muscle strength related to respiratory function	⇐
Mortality	< 5%	⇐
Morbidity	Infection Pneumothorax Hemothorax	⇐
Pain score	5-7	2

PATIENT POPULATION CHARACTERISTICS

Age range	Usually young adults
Male:Female	Females > males
Incidence	Infrequent
Etiology	Unknown
Associated conditions	Myasthenia gravis; benign or malignant thymoma; other autoimmune diseases (e.g., rheumatoid arthritis)

ANESTHETIC CONSIDERATIONS

PREOPERATIVE

Typically, patients presenting for thymectomy may have myasthenia gravis. This is an autoimmune disease of the neuromuscular junction characterized by muscle weakness and easy fatiguability. Thymomas (benign or malignant) also may be associated with myasthenia gravis. The anesthesiologist needs to be aware of the possible compression effects of the tumor (see Excision of Mediastinal Tumor, p. 191), the potential for respiratory failure, as well as the interaction of various treatment modalities.

Respiratory Patient may have marked reduction in VC 2° muscle weakness; establish baseline spirometry values. Criteria necessary to predict need for postop ventilation include: duration of disease > 6 yr; chronic respiratory disease; pyridostigmine dose > 750 mg/d; VC < 2.9 L; preop use of steroids; and previous episode of respiratory failure.
Tests: PFTs, others as indicated from H&P.

Cardiovascular There is a rare association between myasthenia gravis and cardiomyopathy. Consider ECG and cardiac consult if indicated from H&P.

Neurological Review neurological assessment. Patients often exhibit diplopia, ptosis and easy fatiguability of muscles. Difficulties with swallowing and speaking are common. Review tests (EMGs, Tensilon) done by neurologist to evaluate the adequacy of drug therapy (steroids, anticholinesterases, azathioprine and cyclosporin A). Azathioprine (Imuran) may actually antagonize neuromuscular blockade by inhibiting phosphodiesterase. Cyclosporin A is reserved for severe disease because of the side effects of renal insufficiency and HTN. It may prolong neuromuscular blockade. 10-50% of the patients with thymomas will have myasthenia gravis and >85% of myasthenics will have thymus abnormalities.

Musculoskeletal Determine adequacy of anticholinesterase medication. Evaluate hand strength, inspiratory efforts and PFTs. Note that an excess of anticholinesterase agents can cause weakness and respiratory failure indistinguishable from myasthenia. A deleterious response to the Tensilon test (10 mg), as well as the presence of cholinergic side effects, distinguish cholinergic from myasthenic crises. Plasmapheresis may offer temporary (days to weeks) improvement in symptoms. Typically, patients with worsening symptoms receive 4-8 treatments prior to surgery. There should be a 24-h delay between the last plasmapheresis and surgery to restore clotting factors and immunoglobulins. Plasmapheresis also may transiently decrease plasma cholinesterase, which could prolong the effects of succinylcholine, mivacurium and ester-type local anesthetics.

Laboratory Other tests as indicated from H&P.

Premedication Avoid premedication; for the anxious patient, give a small dose of midazolam (1-2 mg); avoid opioids or any other sedatives that may depress ventilation. Current recommendations for

Premedication, cont. anticholinesterases suggest that, in mild disease without psychological dependence, the morning dose can be held or halved. Patients with severe disease or with marked anticholinesterase dependence should receive their regular morning dose. If patient is on steroids, give hydrocortisone (100 mg iv bolus) prior to induction, then 100 mg q 8 h × 24 h.

INTRAOPERATIVE

Anesthetic technique: GETA, combined with thoracic or lumbar epidural if transsternal thymectomy. DLT may be requested by surgeon.

Induction Mask inhalational induction with sevoflurane to avoid muscle relaxants entirely; or iv STP 2-4 mg/kg induction without muscle relaxants; succinylcholine may be used to facilitate intubation; however, the response to succinylcholine is unpredictable (myasthenia → ↓sensitivity; anticholinesterases → ↑sensitivity).

Maintenance Standard maintenance (see p. B-3). Patients with myasthenia gravis have increased sensitivity to nondepolarizing muscle relaxants, which usually are not required (especially during cervical thymectomy). If relaxants are needed, titrate small amounts of drug, using a peripheral nerve stimulator to maintain single twitch. Cisatracurium (20-30 μg/kg q 15-20 min or infusion 1-3 μg/kg/min) is useful since it is rapidly eliminated. Avoid drugs with neuromuscular blocking effects (e.g., antidysrhythmics, diuretics, aminoglycosides). If the patient has normal ventilatory function, then spontaneous ventilation during cervical thymectomy may be appropriate. Patients undergoing sternotomy, and any patient with decreased pulmonary reserve, require mechanical ventilation.

Emergence Criteria for extubation include: head lift (5 sec); MIF > –25 cmH_2O; TV > 5 ml/kg; and full reversal evidenced by twitch monitor. Extubate when fully awake; usually immediate postop ventilation is not necessary. Because of the variable response to muscle relaxation and delayed benefits of the surgery, some patients may require postop ventilation. Whether intubated or not, monitor patient for pulmonary function by measuring MIF and spirometry (TV). Avoid residual pharmacologic neuromuscular blockade, which will lead to hypoventilation and increase risk of gastric aspiration if protective airway reflexes are inadequate.

Blood and fluid requirements	IV: 18 ga × 1 NS/LR @ 1-2 ml/kg/h	
Monitoring	Standard monitors (p. B-1)	Avoid muscle relaxants if possible; if not, use neuromuscular twitch monitor.
Positioning	✓ and pad pressure points. ✓ eyes.	
Complications	Hemorrhage Dysrhythmia Compression of mediastinal structures Pneumothorax	

POSTOPERATIVE

Complications	Pneumothorax Respiratory failure Phrenic nerve damage Myasthenic or cholinergic crises	Pleura can be entered; if so, chest tube needed. (For Dx and Rx, see Thoracoscopy, pp. 203-204.)
Pain management	Parenteral opioids (p. C-1). Epidural opioids (p. C-1).	Avoid respiratory depression; parenteral opioids for cervical incision, epidural opioids for median sternotomy.
Drug management	Usually ↓anticholinesterase requirement in the immediate postop period.	Begin anticholinesterase drugs at half preop dose. Beware of "cholinergic" crisis. Sx include increased salivation, sweating, abdominal cramps, urinary frequency, fasciculations and weakness 2° anticholinesterase overdose. Rx: intubation and ventilation may be necessary.
Tests	Tensilon (edrophonium)	Neurologists can perform Tensilon test to differentiate between myasthenic and cholinergic crises.
	Muscle strength	Determine muscle strength postop (grip strength and sustained head lift).

References

1. Baraka A: Anaesthesia and myasthenia gravis. *Can J Anaesth* 1992; 39:476-86.
2. Baue AE, ed: *Glenn's Thoracic and Cardiovascular Surgery*, 6th edition, Volume II. Geha AS, Hammond GL, Laks H, Naunheim KS, assoc eds. Appleton & Lange, Norwalk, CT: 1996.
3. Burgess FW, Wilcosky B Jr: Thoracic epidural anesthesia for transsternal thymectomy in myasthenia gravis. *Anesth Analg* 1989; 69(4):529-31.
4. Naquib M, el Dawlatly AA, Ashour M, et al: Multivariate determinants of the need for postoperative ventilation in myasthenia gravis. *Can J Anaesth* 1996; 43(10):1006-13.
5. Sabiston DC Jr, Spencer FC: *Surgery of the Chest*, 6th edition, Vol II. WB Saunders Co, Philadelphia: 1995.
6. Smith CE, Donati F, Bevan DR: Cumulative dose-response curves for atracurium in patients with myasthenia gravis. *Can J Anaesth* 1989; 36(4):402-6.

EXCISION OF BLEBS OR BULLAE

SURGICAL CONSIDERATIONS

Description: Pulmonary blebs or bullae requiring surgical treatment may vary from small, apical blebs—most usually seen in young people with spontaneous pneumothorax—to expanding, giant bullae causing respiratory distress. The small blebs can be excised through **video thoracoscopy** (see p. 202), although some surgeons still prefer an open technique for this procedure. Giant bullae are generally removed by **open thoracotomy**, although these lesions also may be excised by video thoracoscopic techniques. Our preference is for **stapling** across the base and excising the lesion. **Clamp and suture** techniques may be used as well. It is important to ensure an airtight closure if possible. Particularly in patients with giant bullae and emphysema, prolonged air leaks may occur postop, and these can be very debilitating. Patients undergoing operation for giant bullae frequently have limited pulmonary reserve and present formidable operative risks. Since the operation is planned to improve their pulmonary function, however, these patients frequently do well following operation. Pleural abrasion or, rarely, **pleurectomy** may accompany the excision of blebs or bullae. The blebs in young patients with recurrent spontaneous pneumothorax are usually located at the apex of the upper lobe. Bullae in patients with emphysema are usually in the upper lobe but may be anywhere in the lung. Preop localization by CT scan is usually sufficient. If a thoracotomy is done, the approach is usually lateral.

Usual preop diagnosis: Spontaneous pneumothorax 2° ruptured blebs; giant bullae causing respiratory distress

SUMMARY OF PROCEDURE

Position	Usually lateral
Incision	Axillary
Special instrumentation	Staplers
Antibiotics	Cefazolin 1 g
Surgical time	1-3 h
EBL	< 500 ml
Postop care	PACU → room; ICU for giant bullae
Mortality	Minimal
Morbidity	Air leak: 20% or more in giant bullae
Pain score	5-7

PATIENT POPULATION CHARACTERISTICS

Age range	Young adults (blebs/small bullae); elderly (large bullae)
Male:Female	3:1
Incidence	Not uncommon
Etiology	Emphysema (usually 2° smoking); congenital; infection
Associated conditions	Spontaneous pneumothorax; emphysema; long smoking Hx; α-antitrypsin deficiency

ANESTHETIC CONSIDERATIONS

PREOPERATIVE

Older patients with this disease have significant COPD, often with pulmonary HTN and RV failure. Young patients are usually otherwise healthy. The risk of rupture of a bleb on the nonoperated side, with resultant tension pneumothorax, must be considered throughout the procedure.

Respiratory — Cysts may be bronchogenic, postinfective, infantile or emphysematous. Bullae usually result from destruction of alveolar tissue; they represent end-stage emphysematous disease associated with severe COPD. Patient may have incapacitating dyspnea. With blebs, elicit Hx of repeat pneumothoraces. Obtain PFTs and ABG for baseline. Patient may have little pulmonary reserve. CO_2 retention ± hypoxia may be present.
Tests: CXR; presence of pneumothorax; if chest CT available, look for airway obstruction that could interfere with DLT placement and also bilateral disease; Hct; ABG.

Cardiovascular — **Tests:** ECG

Neurological — ✓ Hx for previous back surgery, peripheral neuropathy. Examine lumbar area for skin lesions, infection, deformities. Avoid placement of epidural catheter in patient with neurologic problems.

Hematologic — Transfuse patient with preop Hct < 25%. T&C 2-4 U of blood or obtain 1-3 U of autologous blood during the month before surgery.
Tests: Hct

Laboratory — Other tests as indicated from H&P.

Premedication — Midazolam 1-2 mg iv if patient anxious. When epidural opioids are planned, avoid opioid or sedative premedication, which can potentiate postop respiratory effects of spinal opioids.

INTRAOPERATIVE

Anesthetic technique: GETA—may be combined with epidural.

Induction — Awake intubation or GA with patient breathing spontaneously. Awake intubation with a Univent or DLT is appropriate in cases with severe bilateral bullous disease with a past Hx of rupture. Ventilate those patients by hand with small TVs and a long expiratory time, minimizing peak pressures until the chest is open. Rapid placement of a chest tube is essential should a bulla rupture. If muscle relaxants are used to facilitate tracheal intubation, patient will need IPPV. If cyst or bleb ruptures, a tension pneumothorax can result on the operated side or on the opposite side if bilateral disease is present.

Maintenance — IPPV with small TVs until chest is opened. Inhalational anesthesia supplemented with epidural, local anesthetics or iv opioids. Avoid N_2O at all times since bullae may be filled with air.

Emergence — Reexpand lung under direct vision to check for major air leaks. Extubate patient early. Post-bullectomy, unlike other thoracotomy, patients have greater functional lung tissue than preop.

Blood and fluid requirements
IV: 16 ga × 1
NS/LR @ 1-2 ml/kg/h
Restrict iv fluids.
Use vasopressor (ephedrine 5-10 mg iv bolus or phenylephrine 50-100 μmg iv bolus) if hypotensive.

An overhydrated patient is at increased risk of right heart failure. Use of epidural local anesthetics can cause hypotension in a volume-restricted patient; vasopressor often needed.

Monitoring
Standard monitors (p. B-1)
Precordial stethoscope (nonoperated side)
Arterial line
± CVP and/or PA line

Optional CVP and/or PA line for patients with coexisting cardiac disease

Positioning
✓ and pad pressure points.
✓ eyes.
Axillary roll; "airplane" for upper arm

Ventilation	DLT or BB needed to separate the lungs.	Allows IPPV of the "good" lung. Use gentle IPPV with smaller, more frequent TVs than during routine thoracotomy. Inspiratory pressure should not exceed 10 cmH_2O to reduce likelihood of rupture of bullae in opposite lung. Treat intraop hypoxemia with CPAP to "up" lung. In extreme cases consider CPB (rare).
Complications	Tension pneumothorax	Can occur on either side during induction, only on non-operated side after chest is open and again on either side postop. Presents with increased ventilatory pressure, progressive tracheal deviation, wheezing, cardiovascular collapse. CXR to rule out tension pneumothorax. Rx: insertion of chest tube.
	Broncho-pleural-cutaneous fistula	Placement of a chest tube can create a broncho-pleural-cutaneous fistula. Rx: low TV; may require DLT.

POSTOPERATIVE

Complications	Hypoventilation Dental damage Airway trauma Pneumothorax Hemorrhage Risk of aspiration	Incomplete reversal of muscle relaxants or opioid overdosage can cause hypoventilation. Obtain ABG if patient has difficulty breathing or is overly sedated. Be prepared to reintubate patient.
	Airway obstruction (bronchospasm, bleeding, dislodged tumor, foreign body)	If nerve blocks used to depress gag reflex, no eating or drinking for several h postbronchoscopy.
Pain management	Epidural opioids (see p. C-1). Parenteral opioids	Parenteral opioids or intrapleural local anesthetics (0.5% bupivacaine + 1:200,000 epinephrine, 0.5 ml/kg) are adequate if procedure performed through a thoracoscope.
Tests	CXR	ABG if indicated.

References

1. Barker SJ, Clarke C, Trivedi N, et al: Anesthesia for thoracoscopic laser ablation of bullous emphysema. *Anesthesiology* 1993; 78(1): 44-50.
2. Baue AE, ed: *Glenn's Thoracic and Cardiovascular Surgery*, 6th edition, Volume II. Geha AS, Hammond GL, Laks H, Naunheim KS, assoc eds. Appleton & Lange, Norwalk, CT: 1996.
3. Benumof JL: Sequential one-lung ventilation for bilateral bullectomy. *Anesthesiology* 1987; 67(2):268-72.
4. Connolly JE, Wilson A: The current status of surgery for bullous emphysema. *J Thorac Cardiovasc Surg* 1989; 97(3):351-61.
5. Normandale JP, Feneck RO: Bullous cystic lung disease. Its anesthetic management using high frequency jet ventilation. *Anaesthesia* 1985; 40(12):1182-85.
6. Ohta M, Nakahara K, Yasumitsu T, et al: Prediction of postoperative performance status in patients with giant bulla. *Chest* 1992; 101(3): 668-73.
7. Sabiston DC Jr, Spencer FC: *Surgery of the Chest*, 6th edition, Vol II. WB Saunders Co, Philadelphia: 1995.

LUNG VOLUME REDUCTION SURGERY

SURGICAL CONSIDERATIONS

Description: Lung volume reduction surgery (LVRS) was reintroduced by Joel Cooper in 1995 for the treatment of severe emphysema. Typically, these patients are chronically ill, requiring steroids, bronchodilators and supplemental O_2. With appropriate perioperative care, these patients survive surgery and demonstrate improved pulmonary function. Physiologically, reducing the volume of the lung by resecting diseased tissue improves elastic recoil and decreases airway resistance. The chest cavity is also reduced in size, thereby improving chest-wall and diaphragmatic function.

The procedure can be carried out either through a median sternotomy or endoscopically via minithoracoscopies. The **open approach** begins with a median sternotomy. One-lung ventilation (OLV) is initiated following opening of the pleurae. Often the diseased portions of the lung remain inflated, while healthy areas develop absorption atelectasis. These diseased portions are resected with the aid of a linear stapler. The visceral pleura is very thin; the stapling is done with bovine pericardium to bolster the staple line; and high inspiratory pressures (> 20 cmH_2O) must be avoided. From 15% to 30% of the lung volume may be removed. Following careful examination for air leaks, the pleurae and chest wall are closed.

The **endoscopic approach** is carried out via minithoracotomies with instrumentation ports placed to facilitate manipulation of the lung. Diseased tissue will have been identified preop using V/Q and CT scans. Endoscopic forceps are used to guide this diseased tissue into the jaws of the stapler. Again, 15% to 30% of lung tissue may be removed by this means. At some centers the anesthesiologist may be asked to measure inspiratory and expiratory volumes. Any difference between these volumes may represent an air leak requiring further exploration. Following this, access ports and the thoracotomy are closed, and chest tubes are placed. The patient is turned over to the opposite side, reprepped and redraped, and the surgery is repeated. Patients should be extubated in the OR so that no unnecessary ventilatory pressures are put on the lungs. There is usually no suction on the chest tubes and, thus, a water seal is the primary method of controlling the pleural cavity pressures. A small pneumothorax (≤ 10%) is acceptable if the patient is not in respiratory distress. A functional epidural catheter, early extubation and the avoidance of chest tube suction are important to the success of this procedure, especially in the very ill patient. The short-term results have been encouraging. The long-term results are not yet known, but it is hoped that within the next few years more data will become available and we will have a better idea of the efficacy of this procedure.

Usual preop diagnosis: COPD (emphysema)

SUMMARY OF PROCEDURE

	Open LVRS	Endoscopic LVRS
Position	Supine	Lateral decubitus
Incision	Sternotomy	Minilateral thoracotomy
Special instrumentation	Stapling devices; DLT	⇐ + Endoscopic instrumentation
Unique considerations	Bovine pericardium to bolster staple line	⇐
Antibiotics	Cefazolin 1 g	⇐
Surgical time	2 h	45 min-1 h/side
Closing considerations	Avoid high PIPs (> 20 cmH_2O)	⇐
EBL	Minimal	⇐
Postop care	Extubated in OR; avoid chest tube suction	⇐
Mortality	≤ 5-10%	⇐
Morbidity	Pneumothorax	⇐
	Infection	⇐
	Tearing of suture line	⇐
	Wound healing problems	⇐
Pain score	6-8	4-6

PATIENT POPULATION CHARACTERISTICS

Age range	> 50 yr
Male:Female	Male > female
Incidence	Although the incidence of emphysema is high in the general population, only a fraction of these patients will be candidates for LVRS.
Etiology	Smoking; genetic factors
Associated conditions	CAD; pulmonary HTN; PVD; cerebrovascular disease

Table 5.2. Suggested Selection Criteria for LVRS

Medical history	Severe COPD (emphysema rather than chronic bronchitis) Age < 75 yr No cigarette smoking for 6 mo Lowest effective prednisone dose No previous chest surgery
Pulmonary function	FEV_1 > 30-35% of predicted $PaCO_2$ < 50 mmHg TLC > 120% of predicted
Cardiac function	Mean PAP < 35 mmHg (if pulmonary HTN is suspected). No evidence of LV dysfunction on dobutamine stress testing (if Hx of angina or CHF is present)
Radiographic	Hyperinflation, flattened diaphragm (CXR) Decreased upper lobe perfusion (Ventilation-Perfusion scan) Emphysema, with upper lobe predominance (CT scan)
Relative exclusion criteria	Continued smoking Illness other than emphysema that may cause severe dyspnea (e.g., CAD; CHF, cancer; interstitial lung disease; bronchiectasis) Severe malnutrition Obliteration of pleural space (e.g., pleurodesis or pleurectomy) Previous thoracic surgery Morbid obesity Severe pulmonary HTN (mean PAP > 35) Chest-wall deformity with restrictive lung disease (e.g., kyphoscoliosis; severe pectus deformity; $PaCO_2$ > 55 mmHg

ANESTHETIC CONSIDERATIONS

PREOPERATIVE

LVRS (also known as "**reduction pneumoplasty**") involves either laser thermal contraction or surgical resection of emphysematous lung tissue. Patients have advanced, severe COPD, often associated with other cardiorespiratory problems. These patients are a great challenge to the anesthesiologist since it may be difficult to maintain relatively normal physiologic parameters intraop, and to have a comfortable, spontaneously breathing patient at the completion of surgery.

Respiratory Patients for this procedure by definition have advanced pulmonary emphysema. Examine patient for cyanosis, clubbing, RR and pattern. Listen to chest—breath sounds are often very distant or absent. Hx should include use of O_2 supplementation, recent infection, prior surgery on the chest and other associated diseases such as CAD or CHF.

Tests: PFT (with and without bronchodilators). Hyperinflation is usually indicated by TLC and RV value > 120%; V/Q scan; CXR; chest CT scan; noninvasive exercise (6-min walk) test; preop ABG—check for hypoxemia, hypercarbia.

Cardiovascular These patients often have coexisting cardiac disease with pulmonary HTN.

Tests: Right heart function can be evaluated by dobutamine stress test or selective right heart catheterization and measurement of PA pressures.

Premedication Avoid premedication with sedative or opioids—cannot have respiratory depressants—patients have severe COPD, often CO_2 retainers.

INTRAOPERATIVE

Anesthetic technique: GETA (with DLT or BB) ± thoracic/lumbar epidural anesthesia. Place and test lumbar or thoracic epidural catheter before surgery.

Induction Standard induction (see p. B-2). DLT or BB absolutely necessary during surgery to selectively ventilate each lung (see Lobectomy, Pneumonectomy, p. 173).

Maintenance	Inhalational agent and/or propofol. IV opioids and sedative agents should not be used. Anesthesia may be supplemented by continuous or bolus administration of epidural anesthetics. Mechanical ventilation with O_2 and inhalation agent only. During 2-lung ventilation, VT = 8-12 ml/kg adjusted to limit PIP to < 25 cmH_2O. Respiratory rate and inspiratory flow should be adjusted to minimize air trapping. Beware of overinflation and "breath stacking," which can lead to pulmonary tamponade with severe hypotension and ↑airways resistance. Use ABG to maintain $PaCO_2$ at preop level. During OLV, VT is decreased by 25%; monitor PIP closely since ventilated lung has bullous disease also. Avoid overdistention with hyperinflation (→ pneumothorax) on ventilated, nonoperated lung. During OLV, moderate hypercapnia is tolerated, so long as there is no significant hemodynamic effect or hypoxemia. CPAP to nonventilated lung may be necessary to maintain oxygenation. Maintenance of hemodynamic stability may require pressor support (e.g., ephedrine, phenylephrine, dopamine). Lung hyperinflation during mechanical ventilation should be suspected if hypotension with ↑PIP occurs.	
Emergence	These patients should be extubated while deeply anesthetized to prevent coughing and straining which can exacerbate any air leak. These patients benefit from good analgesia, head elevation and suctioning to ↓mucous plugging (can be catastrophic). Immediate recovery from GA occurs in the OR and may take 1-2 h. Ventilatory assistance via face mask with supplemental O_2 is usually necessary. ABG and CXR may be necessary. When spontaneous ventilation and analgesia are satisfactory, the patient is transported to the ICU. If postop mechanical ventilation is required, consider using pressure support ventilation with low levels of CPAP. The CPAP may help minimize the inspiratory work of breathing caused by lung hyperinflation. The pressure support mode of ventilation will permit control of airway pressure while allowing patient control of $PaCO_2$.	
Blood and fluid requirements	IV 16 ga × 1 LR – 4 ml/kg/h Autologous PRBC	Fluid management to restore preop deficit and provide maintenance fluid. Replace blood loss with 3 ml of LR per ml blood. Transfuse autologous blood for Hct < 30.
Monitoring	Standard monitors (see p. B-1). Arterial line Urinary catheter	(See Lobectomy, p. 177). ✓ ABGs: baseline (preop) during sternotomy; 15 min after initiation of OLV; 15 min after initiation of OLV on the second lung; during closure of sternotomy; prior to extubation.
	CVP and/or PA line	Useful for postop fluid management.
Positioning	✓ and pad pressure points. ✓ eyes.	Axillary roll and support for upper airway is necessary for the lateral decubitus position.

POSTOPERATIVE

Complications	Hypercarbia Hypoxemia Air leak/pneumothorax Hemorrhage	
Pain management	Lumbar or thoracic epidural opioids with/without local anesthetics (see p. C-1).	Essential that patient be comfortable. Begin infusion of epidural opioids and local anesthetics (see Lobectomy, Pneumonectomy, p. 178). Breakthrough pain treatment options include iv morphine (1-2 mg) and/or ketorolac (30 mg).

General Thoracic/Anesthesia References

1. Brantigarn OC, Mueller E, Kress MB: A surgical approach to pulmonary emphysema. *Am Rev Respir Dis* 1959; 80:194-202.
2. Brodsky JB, ed: Thoracic anesthesia. In *Problems in Anesthesia*. JB Lippincott, Philadelphia: 1990.
3. Cohen E, ed: *The Practice of Thoracic Anesthesia*. JB Lippincott, Philadelphia, 1995.
4. Cooper JD, Trulock EP, Triantafillou AN, et al. Bilateral pneumonectomy (volume reduction). *J Thorac Cardiovasc Surg* 1995; 109:106-19.
5. Kaplan JA, ed: *Thoracic Anesthesia*. Churchill-Livingstone, New York: 1991.
6. Miller JI, Lee RB, Mansour KA: Lung volume reduction surgery: lessons learned. *Ann Thorac Surg* 1996; 61:1464-69.
7. Pearson FG, et al: *Thoracic Surgery*. Churchill Livingstone, New York, 1995.
8. Triantafillou AN: Anesthetic management for bilateral volume reduction surgery. *Sem Thorac Cardiovasc Surg* 1996; 8(1):94-8.
9. Wakabayashi A: Thoracoscopic laser pneumonectomy in the treatment of diffuse bullous emphysema. *Ann Thorac Surg* 1995; 60(4):936-42.

6.0 CARDIOVASCULAR SURGERY

Surgeons

R. Scott Mitchell, MD
Norman E. Shumway, MD, PhD

6.1 CARDIAC SURGERY

Anesthesiologists

Gordon R. Haddow, MB ChB, FFA(SA) (*Including port-access surgery*)
Lawrence C. Siegel, MD (*Port-access surgery*)

CARDIOPULMONARY BYPASS

SURGICAL CONSIDERATIONS

The development of cardiopulmonary bypass (CPB) technology has allowed the repair of many congenital and acquired lesions of the heart and great vessels. Designed to replace cardiac and pulmonary functions, full CPB requires a blood pump and oxygenator. The pump may be of the roller-head or centrifugal variety, with the latter producing less trauma to formed blood elements. The oxygenator may bubble gases (O_2 and CO_2) through a blood-filled reservoir (bubble oxygenator), or allow O_2 and CO_2 to diffuse through a thin membrane into the surrounding blood (membrane oxygenator). Utilization of any blood pump requires at least partial heparinization (ACT >180 sec), and introduction of an oxygenator mandates full heparinization (ACT > 400 sec).

Full CPB typically drains systemic venous return via the right atrium into a venous reservoir, from which the blood is pumped through an oxygenator and then returned to the aorta or femoral artery, completely bypassing the heart and lungs (Figs 6.1-1 and 6.1-2). **Partial CPB** usually supports only a portion of the body—typically the infradiaphragmatic portion—and may use the patient's lungs as an oxygenator (left atrium → femoral artery) or a mechanical oxygenator (femoral vein → femoral artery). Full CPB is utilized during a sternotomy for work on the heart, ascending aorta and transverse arch. Partial CPB, in which some systemic venous blood returns to the heart and is ejected into the aorta, is normally used for work on the descending or thoracoabdominal aorta. Heparin-coated components, which may partially or totally eliminate the necessity for any heparin, may soon become clinically available.

After exposure of the relevant organs (heart or descending thoracic aorta), and after heparinization, venous and arterial cannulae must be placed intraluminally. **Cannulation of the heart** usually involves venous drainage from the right atrium, with either two cannulae inserted through the atrium into the SVC and IVC (bicaval), or via a larger, dual-stage cannula draining the right atria and IVC. Bicaval cannulation reduces venous return (and rewarming) to the heart, and allows caval snares to be placed so that the right atrium can be opened without introducing air into the venous return. Occasionally, atrial manipulation for cannulation can depress CO, with resultant hypotension. This usually can be reversed with volume replacement. Aortic cannulation usually is not associated with any physiologic perturbation, although HTN must be avoided to minimize aortic complications. Once the cannulae are in place and connections are made to the bypass circuit, CPB may be instituted electively. Most cardiac operations are conducted under mild hypothermia (28°C),

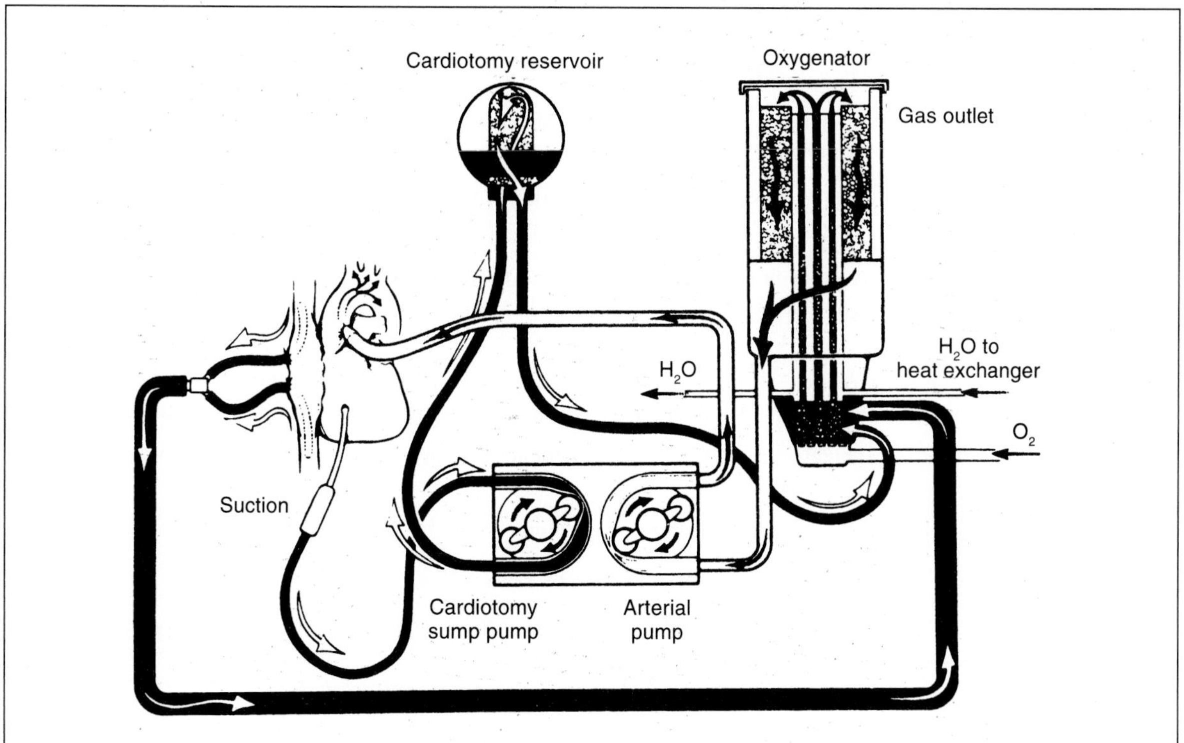

Figure 6.1-1. Schematic representation of the CPB circuit. (Reproduced with permission from Hardy JD: *Hardy's Textbook of Surgery*, 2nd edition. JB Lippincott: 1988.)

unless profound hypothermic circulatory arrest is to be utilized. In that case, a target temperature of 18°C is desirable. For operations on the descending thoracic aorta, normothermia is maintained.

Cessation of CPB is accomplished by gradually decreasing pump flows, allowing for right heart filling, and gradually replenishing the circulating blood volume. Pulmonary and coronary vasodilation are mandatory during this phase, as there appears to be heightened vasoreactivity after periods of ischemia and hypothermia. For periods of cardiac arrest, during which the heart is deprived of its arterial blood supply, the metabolic demands of the myocardium must be minimized. This usually is accomplished by achieving diastolic arrest with a hyperkalemic cardioplegic solution, and also by lowering myocardial temperature to < 15°C. Frequent reinfusions of cardioplegia maintain hypothermia, prevent lactic acid accumulation, and deliver some minimally available dissolved O_2.

The **physiologic response to CPB** is complex, and is associated with a massive catecholamine release which resolves after its cessation. Subsequent changes include abnormal bleeding tendencies, increased capillary permeability, leukocytosis, renal dysfunction and impairment of the immune response. Hemodilution, nonpulsatile flow, hypothermia, exposure of formed elements to nonendothelial surfaces, complement activation, protein denaturation, cascading effects within the coagulation and fibrinolytic system, and activation of the kallikrein-bradykinin cascade, all contribute to this unphysiologic state, and account for much of the morbidity and mortality after CPB.

Many physiologic variables are now controlled by the anesthesiologist, perfusionist and surgeon, including systemic flow and perfusion pressure, arterial O_2 and CO_2, temperature and Hct. Other physiologic parameters follow either directly or indirectly. Thus, physiologic monitoring for the anesthesiologist and perfusionist include, at a minimum, arterial pressure, CVP, ABG determination (preferably on-line during CPB), CO, UO and ECG. Constant communication among surgeons, perfusionist and anesthesiologist is mandatory for a smooth operation.

Secondary effects of CPB demand some special considerations during the final stages of the procedure and chest closure. Adverse effects on coagulation have already been mentioned, and vigorous attention to maintenance and replacement of coagulation factors is essential. The capillary leak phenomenon results in interstitial myocardial and pulmonary edema. Decreased myocardial performance and compliance mandate an increased preload, especially during the physical act of chest closure, where a transient rise in intramediastinal pressure may depress systemic venous return. Similarly, decreased pulmonary compliance and gas exchange mandate vigilance over inspiratory pressures and lung volumes during chest closure, as mediastinal volume is physically decreased.

ANESTHETIC CONSIDERATIONS FOR CARDIOPULMONARY BYPASS (CPB)

This segment is not meant to be a definitive text on CPB, but rather a guide to the anesthetic management of bypass. Communication among surgeons, anesthesiologists and pump technicians is of vital importance in carrying out this procedure.

PREPARATION FOR BYPASS

Prebypass/ anticoagulation — ✓ baseline ACT (normal = 90-130 sec). Heparin (3 mg[~300 U]/kg) is administered via a central vein (✓ back-bleeding to verify intravascular position) or by the surgeon directly into the atrium (preferred). ✓ ACT 3 min after heparin. It is essential to ensure adequate anticoagulation (ACT > 400 sec).

Aortic cannulation — Control MAP to ~70 mmHg for cannulation to ensure that the aortotomy does not extend. If needed, vasodilators may be used. The arterial line should be inspected for air bubbles.

Venous cannulation — Venous cannulation may be associated with atrial dysrhythmias. Blood loss can be excessive.

Pupils — Assess pupil symmetry for later comparison.

TRANSITION ONTO CPB

Stop ventilation — Commencing bypass is a dangerous period for the patient as a result of the many hemodynamic changes that occur. D/C ventilation once there is no pulmonary blood flow.

Withdraw PA catheter — Withdraw PA catheter 4-5 cm.

Stop infusions — Stop iv drugs and reduce iv fluid infusions to TKO.

Anticoagulation — ACT should be checked after 5 min on CPB to ensure anticoagulation (ACT > 400 sec).

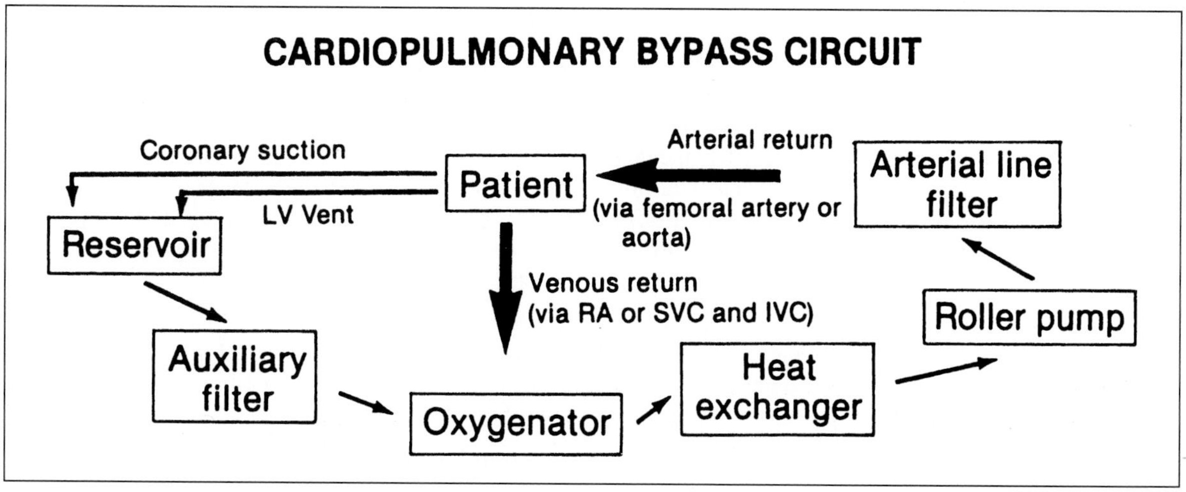

Figure 6.1-2. CPB circuit. (Reproduced with permission from Tinker JH: Technical aspects of cardiopulmonary bypass. In Thomas SJ, ed: *Manual of Cardiac Anesthesia*, 2nd edition. Churchill Livingstone: 1993.)

Oxygenation	Verify oxygenation by checking arterial inflow color, inline sensors and by ABG within 5 min of beginning CPB.
Flow	✓ for adequate venous drainage (CVP falls to a low level). Ensure adequate arterial inflow. Initial pressures may be very low, but will usually increase.
Anesthesia	Anesthetics (e.g., fentanyl and midazolam) may be needed. A repeat dose (e.g., 10 mg pancuronium) should be given to prevent movement or shivering (which increases O_2 requirements).
Pupils	Assess pupils. Unilateral dilation may indicate arterial inflow into the innominate artery (unilateral carotid perfusion).

BYPASS PERIOD

Anticoagulation	ACT levels should be checked regularly (q 20-30 min) and kept at > 400. Add heparin (5,000-10,000 U), if needed.
Pressure/flow	There is controversy about safe flows and pressures. Generally, flows of 1.2-3 L/m²/min are used, with pressures of 30-80 mmHg. A MAP of 50-60 mmHg is probably best for cerebral perfusion and does not result in excessive noncoronary blood flow.
Acid-base status	Alpha-stat (ABG measured and interpreted at 37° regardless of actual patient temperature) regulation of acid-base status is preferred because of maintenance of normal cerebral flow and autoregulation on CPB.
Hct/Electrolytes	Generally, Hct will fall to ~20, which is acceptable in most patients. Hypokalemia is common and should be corrected. A K^+ > 4.5 mEq/L is desirable.
UO	Keep UO >1 ml/kg/h. If needed, mannitol and/or furosemide should be given (assuming pump flow is adequate).
Temperature	During bypass the temperature is usually maintained at ~28°C.

TERMINATION OF BYPASS

Rewarming	Prior to discontinuing CPB, the patient should have a core temperature of at least 36.5°C.
Anesthesia/ relaxation	Patient awareness may be a problem during rewarming. Volatile agents ± benzodiazepine (e.g., diazepam 5-10 mg) ± a narcotic to prevent awareness. In addition, a muscle relaxant should also be given.
Acid-base/ electrolytes/Hct	✓ electrolytes, acid-base status and Hct. Correct acidosis. K^+ 4.5-5.5, normal ionized Ca^{++}, and Hct ≥ 20 should be assured.
Air maneuvers	Air maneuvers (to remove intracardiac and intraaortic air) are carried out when the heart is opened. Ventilation is commenced once there is pulmonary blood flow and will aid in the evacuation of air. Pleural fluid should be removed.

WEANING FROM BYPASS

Prior to weaning Prior to weaning from CPB, the aortic cross-clamp should have been off for 30 min to allow rewarming and reperfusion of the heart. Defibrillation is often needed and pacing may be required. NSR or A-V pacing is preferred. Vasoactive drugs should be available. Once normal temperature, ventilation, cardiac rhythm and reperfusion are established, bypass may be terminated. The heart is gradually volume-loaded (transfused from oxygenator) to adequate filling pressures and bypass flow slowly decreased over 15-45 sec until it is off. Return to bypass in the event of progressive cardiac distension or dysfunction. Assess CO and BP, and adjust vascular resistance as necessary. Inotropic agents are often required at this stage.

Reversal of anticoagulation Once patient is off CPB, anticoagulation must be reversed with protamine (1-1.3 mg/100 U heparin), administered slowly over 10-30 min, since rapid administration is associated with ↓BP. (Treat with α-agonists and volume.) Other reactions include pulmonary HTN and true allergic reactions. ✓ ACT to ensure that it has returned to control (90-130 sec).

BP management Vasoactive support is often needed in the postbypass period—the need varying with surgical procedure, disease process and underlying cardiac function. In general, SBP should be limited to 120 mmHg to avoid stress on the aortotomy site.

COAGULATION AND CPB

General Bleeding is common post CPB and may be considerable. Both preop and intraop factors contribute to this. A knowledge of these factors and the tests involved will aid with the management of these patients (Fig 6.1-3).

Preop factors Hx of previous bleeding during surgery is important. Many drugs may contribute to bleeding: ASA/NSAIDs (platelet dysfunction), anticoagulants (heparin, Coumadin) and fibrinolytic agents. These should be stopped preop, if possible, or their action reversed. Other pathological processes (e.g., liver failure/congestion, renal failure or hemophilia) also play a role. Preop testing is important and should include PT, PTT, Plt count and bleeding time, as a minimum.

Intraop factors CPB is associated with ↓platelet count and function. Circulating clotting factors are decreased and fibrinolysis occurs.

Post CPB bleeding The common causes of post CPB bleeding are: surgical causes, inadequate heparin reversal, ↓number of platelets and Plt dysfunction, ↓clotting factors, fibrinolysis, DIC, excessive BP. Surgical causes and inadequate heparin reversal (✓ ACT) should be ruled out. If no surgical cause is found and ACT is normal, platelets (10 U) should be infused. PT, PTT, Plt count, TT, reptilase time, fibrinogen and FSP should be checked. The TEG may prove very useful. (See Fig 7.12-8 and Table 7.12-3 in Liver/Kidney Transplantation, pp. 503, 504.)

References

1. Bowering J, Levy JH: The postcardiopulmonary period: a systems approach. In *A Practical Approach to Cardiac Anesthesia*, 2nd edition. Hensley FA, Martin DE, eds. Little, Brown, Boston: 1995, Ch 8, 231-45.
2. Campbell FW, Jobes DR, Ellison N: Coagulation management during and after cardiopulmonary bypass. In *A Practical Approach to Cardiac Anesthesia*, 2nd edition. Hensley FA, Martin DE, eds. Little, Brown, Boston: 1995, Ch 16, 434-63.
3. DiNardo JA: Management of cardiopulmonary bypass. In *Anesthesia for Cardiac Surgery*. DiNardo JA, Schwartz MJ, eds. Appleton & Lange, Norwalk CT: 1990, Ch 9, 217-52.
4. Hindman BJ, Lillehaug SI, Tinker JH: Cardiopulmonary bypass and the anesthesiologist. In *Cardiac Anesthesia*, 3rd edition. Kaplan J, ed. WB Saunders, Philadelphia: 1993, Ch 28, 191-50.
5. Horrow J: Management of coagulation and bleeding disorder. In *Cardiac Anesthesia*, 3rd edition. Kaplan J, ed. WB Saunders, Philadelphia: 1993, Ch 29, 951-94.
6. Larach DR: Anesthetic management during cardiopulmonary bypass. In *A Practical Approach to Cardiac Anesthesia*, 2nd edition. Hensley FA, Martin DE, eds. Little, Brown, Boston: 1995, Ch 6, 193-217.
7. Romanoff ME, Larach DR: Weaning from cardiopulmonary bypass. In *A Practical Approach to Cardiac Anesthesia*, 2nd edition. Hensley FA, Martin DE, eds. Little, Brown, Boston: 1995, Ch 7, 218-30.

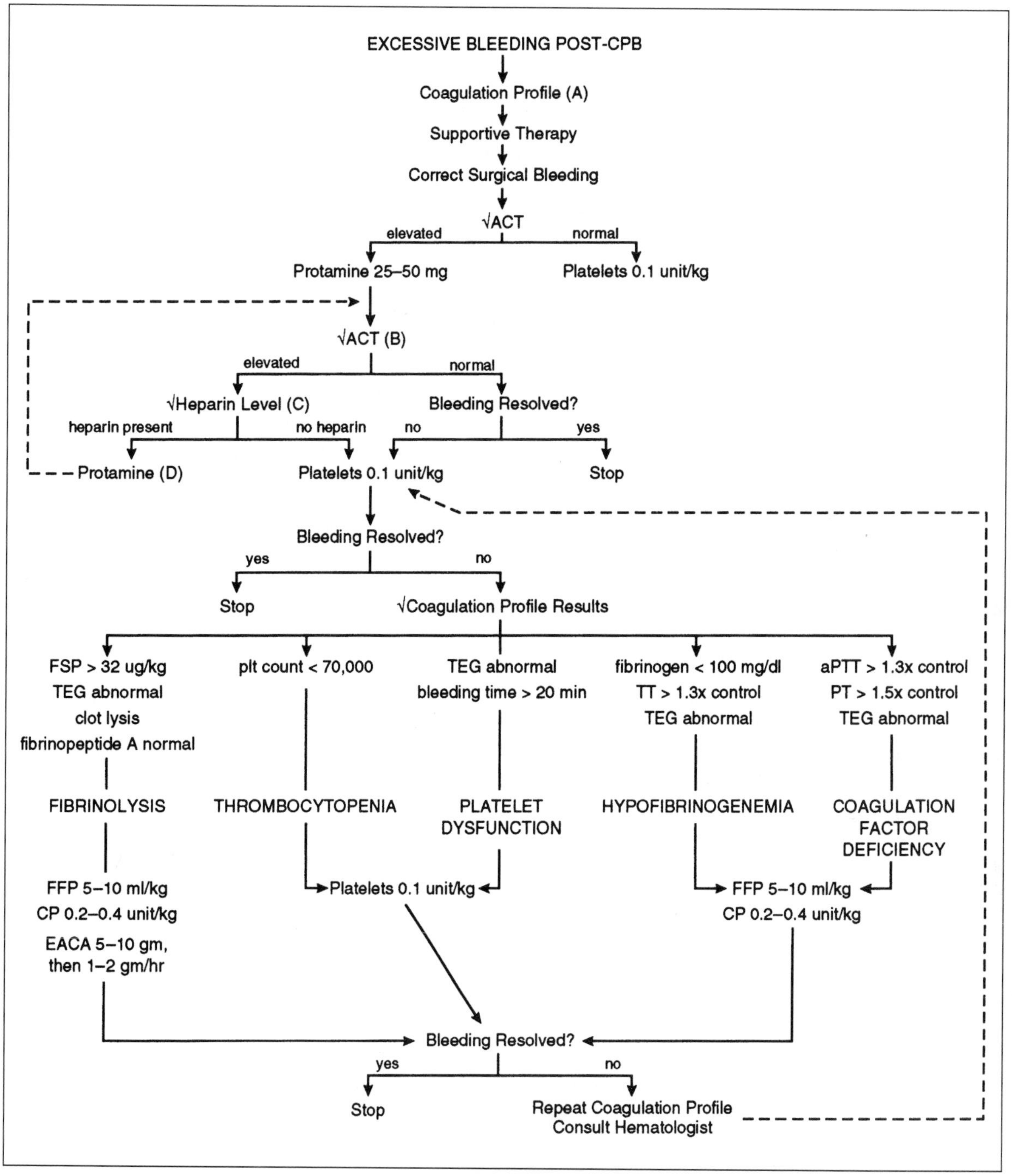

Figure 6.1-3. An algorithm for the treatment of patients bleeding excessively after CPB: (A) Commonly includes Plt count, PT, aPTT, TT, fibrinogen level, FSPs. Template bleeding time or TEG is desirable if available and feasible. (B) Heparin level may be checked at this step. (C) Most commonly by *in vitro* whole blood protamine titration (manual or automated); alternatively, by protamine-corrected TT. (D) Protamine dose determined by measured heparin level. Disseminated intravascular coagulation (DIC) is a rare cause of post CPB hemorrhage and, therefore, is not included in the outline of coagulation profile results and treatment of post CPB hemostatic abnormalities shown in the lower portion of the figure. It would be suspected on the occurrence of hypofibrinogenemia, thrombocytopenia, and elevated fibrinopeptides, in association with increased FSPs, clot lysis, or a TEG characteristic of fibrinolysis. The treatment of DIC includes identification and arrest of the inciting cause and coagulant replacement with FFP, CP, and platelets. EACA should not be administered to the patient with DIC and secondary fibrinolysis because of the risk of intravascular thrombosis.

ACT = activated coagulation time; aPTT = activated partial thromboplastin time; CP = cryoprecipitate; EACA = epsilon-aminocaproic acid; FFP = fresh frozen plasma; FSP = fibrin(ogen) split products; Plt count = platelet count, PT = prothrombin time; TEG = thromboelastogram; TT = thrombin time. (Reproduced with permission from Hensley FA Jr, Martin DE: *The Practice of Cardiac Anesthesia*. Little, Brown: 1990.)

CORONARY ARTERY BYPASS GRAFT SURGERY

SURGICAL CONSIDERATIONS

Description: **Coronary artery bypass grafting (CABG)** is the most frequently performed cardiac operation (Fig 6.1-4). Since the discovery that coronary thrombosis is the causative event for MI, many schemes have been devised to augment the restricted coronary blood flow, including collateral pericardial blood flow to epicardial arteries and implantation of the internal mammary artery with unligated side branches into the LV muscle. With the discovery by Favalaro that saphenous veins could be anastomosed to the epicardial coronary arteries, a new era of myocardial revascularization began. Basically, the technique involves bypass to a narrowed or occluded epicardial coronary greater than 1 mm in diameter with a small-diameter conduit (usually reversed saphenous vein or internal mammary artery) distal to the narrowed segment, with the proximal arterial inflow source being the ascending aorta. The mammary artery may be mobilized from the chest wall, leaving its proximal origin with the subclavian artery intact (pedicled graft), or the mammary may be transected and its proximal end anastomosed to the aorta or saphenous vein as a "free mammary graft."

The heart is approached through a median sternotomy, with the patient supported on full **CPB** (see separate section on CPB, p. 217). Although various operative strategies may be used, the most common regimen is for all distal (epicardial) anastomoses to be performed during a single period of aortic cross-clamping and cardiac arrest. During that period of induced asystole, myocardial protection is achieved by hypothermia and occasional reperfusion via antegrade or retrograde cardioplegia. Cardiac standstill and a bloodless field are mandatory to allow these very demanding small-diameter anastomoses to be constructed with no obstruction to flow in a minimal amount of time. The cross-clamp is then removed and the heart allowed to resume beating. A partially occluding aortic cross-clamp can then be applied to allow construction of the proximal aortic anastomoses. After a sufficient period of resuscitation, the patient is weaned from CPB, and decannulation, heparin reversal and chest closure are allowed to proceed as previously noted.

The choice of conduit depends on availability and durability. Historically, the saphenous vein was the first small vessel conduit with acceptable patencies, but with prolonged experience it appears that 50% of vein grafts will be significantly diseased or occluded at 10 yr. The internal mammary artery appears to have superior long-term performance, with approximately 90% 10-year patency rates. Other arterial conduits, such as the left gastroepiploic artery, superficial epigastric artery and the radial artery are being investigated as to their long- and short-term durability. Typical target

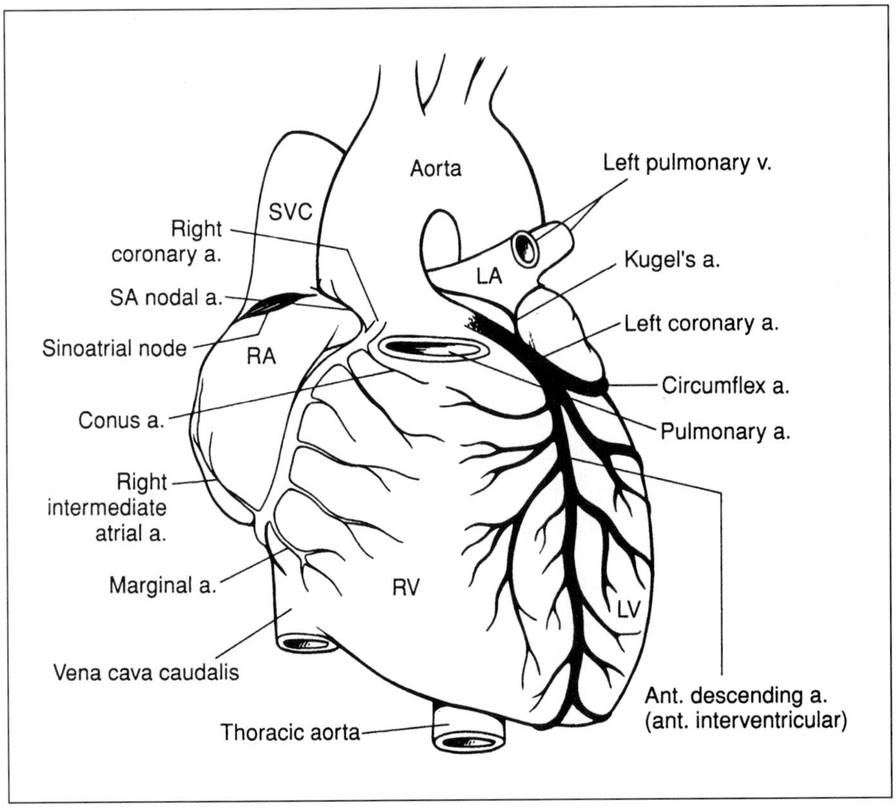

Figure 6.1-4. Coronary artery circulation—anterior view. (Reproduced with permission from Edwards EA, Malone PD, Collins JJ Jr: *Operative Anatomy of the Thorax*. Lea & Febiger, Philadelphia: 1972.)

arteries include the distal right coronary and its major terminal branch, the posterior descending artery. From the left circulation, the left anterior descending (LAD), with its diagonal and septal branches, is the most important, having been estimated to supply blood to 60% of the left ventricle.

The left circumflex coronary artery courses in the posterior atrioventricular groove, and is not easily accessible for bypass, which is usually performed to its obtuse marginal or posterolateral branches.

In a randomized study on coronary artery surgery (CASS)[3], coronary bypass was noted to be superior to medical management for relief of angina, and to prolong life in patients with left main CAD, and in patients with 3-vessel disease and impaired LV function. Other patients may receive bypass for intractable angina refractory to medical management.

Usual preop diagnosis: CAD with Class 3 or 4 angina (angina with minimal exertion or at rest)

SUMMARY OF PROCEDURE

Position	Supine
Incision	Median sternotomy with legs prepped for saphenous vein harvest
Special instrumentation	Complete hemodynamic monitoring
Unique considerations	Avoidance of cardiac ischemia
Antibiotics	Cefamandole 1 g iv at induction
Surgical time	3.5-4.5 h
Closing considerations	Prevention of coagulopathy; maintenance of preload
EBL	500-600 ml
Postop care	ICU: 1-3 d, intubated 6-24 h.
Mortality	2-4%
Morbidity	Overall: 3-6% MI: 3-6% Pneumonia: 5% CVA: 1-2%
Pain score	7-8

PATIENT POPULATION CHARACTERISTICS

Age range	60-80 yr (mean = 74 yr)
Male:Female	2:1
Incidence	Common
Etiology	Coronary atherosclerosis
Associated conditions	LV failure; pulmonary HTN; ischemic mitral regurgitation; diabetes mellitus; obstructive pulmonary disease

ANESTHETIC CONSIDERATIONS

(Procedures covered: coronary artery bypass graft surgery; left ventricular aneurysmectomy)

PREOPERATIVE

History, examination and tests will divide these patients broadly into two groups: (1) high-risk, characterized by poor LV function (cardiac failure; EF < 40%; LVEDP > 18 mmHg; CI < 2.0 L/min/m^2; ventricular dyskinesia; 3-vessel disease; occlusion of left main or left main equivalent; valvular disease; recent MI; ventricular aneurysm; VSD; MI in progress; and old age); and (2) low-risk, characterized by good LV function. The type of monitoring chosen will depend on which group the patient is in.

Respiratory Hx of smoking or COPD; patient should be encouraged to stop smoking at least 2 wk prior to surgery. Treat COPD and optimize therapy prior to surgery.
Tests: CXR; PFTs; as indicated by H&P.

Cardiovascular In the preop assessment, the following factors will affect patient management and surgical outcome:
- Hx of angina (stable, unstable at rest, and precipitating factors).
- The patient's exercise tolerance will provide a clue to LV functions and surgical outcome.
- The presence of CHF (Sx: SOB, PND, orthopnea, DOE, pulmonary edema, JVD, 3rd-heart sound).

Cardiovascular, cont.
- Recent (< 6 mo) MI, dysrhythmias, HTN, vascular disease (particularly carotid stenosis, aortic disease).
- Valvular disease (particularly MR or AS) or the presence of a VSD or LV aneurysm may portend increased risk of perioperative complications.

Tests: 12-lead ECG: ✓ ischemia (area involved), LVH, previous MI, dysrhythmias. Exercise stress testing: ✓ effort tolerance, area of ischemia, maximal HR and BP before ischemia occurs, dysrhythmias. Thallium scan: ✓ component of reversible ischemia. ECHO (may be combined with stress ECHO): ✓ LV function, wall motion abnormalities, valvular disease, VSD. Cardiac catheterization: ✓ extent and location of disease, LV function, valvular pathology, VSD, LVEDP, LV aneurysm.

Postinfarction VSD
The development of a postinfarction VSD is associated with high operative morbidity and mortality because of the difficulty in repairing the lesion due to friable tissue, difficulty in obtaining hemostasis, emergent nature of the condition and possible pulmonary edema. These patients effectively have poor LV function and should be considered as high risk. They often require support, including IABP, during induction, prebypass and postbypass.

LV aneurysm
LV aneurysm is usually a late complication of infarction; however, it can occur early, when it is usually associated with cardiac rupture (and high mortality). These patients usually have poor myocardial function and should be anesthetized with full monitoring, including PA catheterization. Postbypass, the LV cavity is reduced in size and compliance. To ensure an adequate CO, maintain adequate preload, a higher than normal HR (A-V pacing if needed) and sinus rhythm, and consider the use of inotropes. LV aneurysms are often associated with dysrhythmias and may require cardiac mapping (see Cardiac Mapping and Ablation Procedures, p. 240). Hemostasis is often difficult to obtain, and adequate iv access is a necessity. Treatment usually entails the use of blood and blood products.

Emergency revascularization
Emergency revascularization occurs in the setting of acute MI, often with acute LV failure or after failed PTCA, where the patient may be stable, suffering acute ischemia and hemodynamically unstable, or even in full cardiac arrest. Factors to consider in these cases are: full stomach (and the need for rapid-sequence induction in the face of ischemia); the prior use of fibrinolytic agents (with increased risk of hemorrhage); need for inotropes; antianginals; IABP; and dysrhythmias. These patients have a higher morbidity and mortality. In patients who have received fibrinolytic agents, consider the postbypass use of antifibrinolytic agents (e.g., aminocaproic acid).

Neurological
Previous stroke or carotid artery disease Hx/Sx should be documented and evaluated.

Endocrine
Diabetes is common and perioperative control of blood glucose is important.
Tests: Blood glucose

Renal
✓ baseline renal function, as CPB places these patients at risk for renal failure.
Tests: Creatinine; BUN; electrolytes (particularly K^+)

Hematologic
Patients are often on aspirin or other antiplatelet therapy, which may lead to increased intraop hemorrhage. These agents should be stopped 7-10 d before surgery, if possible. Some patients may be on anticoagulants (usually heparin in the immediate preop period). Heparin should be stopped 6-8 h preop; however, in some patients, heparin infusion is continued into the OR. Other patients may have received fibrinolytic agents which put them at increased risk for intraop hemorrhage.
Tests: Consider Plt count, PTT, if indicated

Laboratory
Hb/Hct; other tests as indicated from H&P. T&C 2-4 U PRBCs.

Premedication
Patients should be instructed to continue all medications (e.g., nitrates, β-blockers; Ca^{++} antagonists, antidysrhythmics and antihypertensives) prior to surgery, with the exception of diuretics on the day of surgery. Allaying anxiety may decrease the incidence of perioperative ischemia and help with the preinduction placement of lines. Typical preop sedation includes diazepam (10 mg po) or lorazepam (1-2 mg po) the night before and again 1-2 h before arrival in the OR, with the addition of morphine (0.1 mg/kg im) and scopolamine (0.3 mg im). Severely compromised patients will require less premedication.

INTRAOPERATIVE

Anesthetic technique: GETA

Induction
Generally, a moderate- to high-dose narcotic technique (e.g., fentanyl 10-100 μg/kg or sufentanil 2.5-20 μg/kg), supplemented by etomidate (0.1-0.3 mg/kg) or midazolam (50-350 μg/kg), is

Induction, cont.

appropriate. As with all cardiac cases, the speed of induction and total drug dose depends on the patient's cardiac function and pathology. Muscle relaxation may be obtained using pancuronium (0.1 mg/kg), given slowly to avoid tachycardia, or vecuronium (possibility of bradycardia, especially if the patient is β-blocked). It is important to avoid the sympathetic response to laryngoscopy. The use of high-dose narcotics (see above), esmolol (100-500 μg/kg over 1 min, followed by 40-100 μg/kg/min infusion), SNP (0.5-3 μg/kg/min), lidocaine (1-2 mg/kg) or a combination of these agents, may decrease or ablate this response. NTG (0.5-2 μg/kg/min) also may be used during induction if evidence of ischemia occurs.

Maintenance

Usually narcotic (total: fentanyl 10-100 μg/kg or sufentanil 5-20 μg/kg) with midazolam (50-350 μg/kg) for amnesia. Those patients with good LV function may benefit from the decreased myocardial O_2 demand associated with the use of volatile agents (2° ↓contractility). N_2O is generally avoided. Propofol infusion may be used while rewarming and postbypass.

Emergence

Transported to ICU, sedated, intubated and ventilated. Extubate when able—often < 6 h if lower-dose narcotic technique used (fast-track).

Blood and fluid requirements

IV: 14 ga × 1-2
NS/LR @ 6-8 ml/kg/h
UO 0.5-1 ml/kg/h
Warm all fluids.
Humidify gases.

Monitoring	Standard monitors (p. B-1)	Standard and invasive monitors placed prior to induction.
	Arterial line	✓ BP in both arms. Right radial preferred if left internal mammary artery (LIMA) graft, because retraction of the sternum may compress the left subclavian.
	CVP or PA catheter	In the low-risk/good LV function group, CVP is adequate; high-risk/poor LV function, a PA catheter is useful for hemodynamic monitoring, weaning from bypass and vasoactive therapy. Some groups use routine PA catheterization for all patients undergoing CABG surgery.
	ECG	5-lead monitoring II and V_5 (or area most at risk for ischemia).
	TEE	Will reflect regional wall motion abnormalities, papillary muscle dysfunction and MR.
Myocardial O_2 Balance	Supply – Coronary blood flow: Perfusion pressure (DP-LVEDP) Diastolic filling time (HR) Blood viscosity (optimal Hct = 30) Coronary vasoconstriction: Spasm $PaCO_2$ (hypocapnia → constriction) α-sympathetic activity Supply – O_2 delivery: O_2 sat Hct Oxyhemoglobin dissociation curve Demand – O_2 consumption: BP (afterload) Ventricular volume (preload) Wall thickness (↓subendocardial perfusion) HR Contractility	The balance of myocardial O_2 supply vs demand is important in the management of these patients. The goal of anesthesia is to ensure that this balance remains in equilibrium and that no ischemia occurs, or, if it does, that it is treated promptly. Those patients with poor LV function or complicated disease will benefit from maintenance of contractility (avoid volatile agents) and a high FiO_2, whereas those with good LV function may benefit from the mild cardiac depression (↓demand associated with the addition of low-dose volatile agents). Certain events are associated with increased risk of intraop ischemia: intubation, incision, sternotomy, cannulation, tachycardia, ↑BP or ↓BP, ventricular fibrillation or distension, inadequate cardioplegia, emboli, spasm or inadequate revascularization. Care should be taken to avoid these complications and to ablate responses to stimuli.
Detection of ischemia	ECG	ST segment depression or elevation or a new T-wave alteration may suggest ischemia. Monitoring 2 leads—one lateral (e.g., V_5) and one inferior (e.g., II)—give the best detection rate.
	PA catheter	Elevations of PCWP may be indicative of ischemia. A

Detection of ischemia, cont.	TEE	new V-wave on the PCWP trace is a better sign of possible ischemia (papillary muscle dysfunction). The appearance of a new regional wall motion abnormality is the most sensitive indicator of ischemia, but it requires constant monitoring.
Treatment of ischemia	Caused by tachycardia: Esmolol (100-500 μg/kg) ↑anesthesia Verapamil (2.5-10 mg iv) Caused by ↑BP: NTG (0.5-4 μg/kg/min) ↑anesthesia Caused by ↓BP: Phenylephrine (0.2-0.75 μg/kg/min) ↑preload Caused by ↓↓HR: A-V pacing	While avoidance of ischemia is the goal, when it does occur it should be treated aggressively. Treatment may include inotropic support (e.g., dopamine 1-5 μg/kg/min or dobutamine 0.5-30 μg/kg/min). If LV failure persists despite other therapy, an IABP may be inserted.
Positioning	✓ and pad pressure points. ✓ eyes.	

POSTOPERATIVE

Complications	Infarction Ischemia Tamponade Dysrhythmias Cardiac failure Coagulopathy Hemorrhage	Postop control of ischemia is important since hemodynamic instability may be associated with inadequate pain relief, awakening and ventilation.
Pain management	Parenteral opioids	Supplement with benzodiazepine for sedation.
Tests	ECG CPK CXR Electrolytes ABG Coagulation profiles	

References

1. Horrow JC, Hensley FA, Merin RG: Anesthetic management for myocardial revascularization. In *A Practical Approach to Cardiac Anesthesia*, 2nd edition. Hensley FA, Martin DE, eds. Little, Brown & Co, Boston: 1995, Ch 10, 275-95.
2. O'Connor JP, Ramsey JG, Wynands JE Kaplan JA: Anesthesia for myocardial revascularization. In *Cardiac Anesthesia*, 3rd edition. Kaplan JA, ed. WB Saunders, Philadelphia: 1993, Ch 19, 587-628.
3. Rogers WJ, Coggin CJ, Green B, et al: 10-year followup of quality of life in patients randomized to receive medical treatment or coronary artery bypass graft surgery. *Circulation* 1990; 82(5):1647-58.

LEFT VENTRICULAR ANEURYSMECTOMY

SURGICAL CONSIDERATIONS

Description: Extensive MI may result in large areas of myocardial necrosis, with subsequent aneurysm formation. LV failure may ensue as a result of continuous LV dilatation or mitral insufficiency 2° annular dilatation or involvement of papillary muscles. Indications for this surgery include worsening CHF and increased dysrhythmias. Typically, apical dilatation with maintenance of basilar myocardial contractility allows for aneurysm resection and preservation of both myocardial contractility and chamber size to produce an adequate CO. Operation is commenced in the usual manner, establishing CPB (see p. 217), cross-clamping the aorta, establishing myocardial protection, and then assessing the left ventricle. A thinned, dilated ventricular segment with full-thickness scar formation, can be resected and ventricular continuity restored with improvement of ventricular geometry and myocardial energy demands. Coronary bypass can be performed during this same period. Then air is removed from the left side of the heart, the cross-clamp is removed and coronary perfusion is reestablished. After a sufficient period of resuscitation and return of vigorous contractility, bypass is discontinued, not infrequently with the assistance of intraaortic balloon pump (IABP) to augment forward output. Decannulation, protamine administration and closure proceed as described in CPB, p. 217.

Usual preop diagnosis: LV aneurysm with CHF

SUMMARY OF PROCEDURE

Position	Supine
Incision	Median sternotomy, ± leg incision for saphenous vein harvest if coronary bypass is planned.
Unique considerations	Preparations (ECG leads) should be made for pre- or postop IABP or LV assist device (LVAD)
Antibiotics	Cefamandole 1 g iv at induction
Surgical time	Aortic cross-clamp: 40-100 min CPB: 70-130 min Total: 3-4 h
EBL	300-400 ml
Postop care	ICU × 1-3 d, intubated 6-24 h; usually requires inotropic support ± mechanical support (LVAD, IABP).
Mortality	5-7%
Morbidity	Overall: 8-10% Requirement for IABP: 10% Respiratory insufficiency: 5% CVA: 2-3%
Pain score	7-10

PATIENT POPULATION CHARACTERISTICS

Age range	50-70 yr
Male:Female	3:1
Incidence	Uncommon
Etiology	Usually the end result of MI 2° CAD
Associated conditions	Mitral insufficiency; pulmonary HTN; CAD

ANESTHETIC CONSIDERATIONS

See Anesthetic Considerations following Coronary Artery Bypass Graft Surgery, p. 223.

Reference

1. Mills NL, Everson CT, Hockmuth DR: Technical advances in the treatment of left ventricular aneurysm. *Ann Thorac Surg* 1993; 55:792-800.

AORTIC VALVE REPLACEMENT

SURGICAL CONSIDERATIONS

Description: Disease of the aortic valve may present as valvular stenosis, insufficiency, or a combination of the two. Valvular disease most commonly occurs as a result of rheumatic disease, but also may occur 2° calcific degeneration (aortic sclerosis) in the elderly. Congenitally bicuspid valves and endocarditis account for most of the remainder. Repair of the aortic valve is rarely possible, and most conditions require valve replacement. The three most commonly used **prostheses** are: porcine bioprostheses, especially in the older patient; mechanical prostheses, with the necessity for lifelong anticoagulation; and cryopreserved homografts, which unfortunately are expensive and in short supply. The operation, on full CPB, is usually performed through a median sternotomy. After routine bicaval and aortic cannulation, the patient is taken onto full CPB. Left heart drainage is accomplished through a pulmonary artery vent, and a left atrial vent usually is inserted through the right superior pulmonary vein, or via a LV vent inserted through the LV apex. Because of the LV hypertrophy, myocardial protection is of utmost importance. Stanford favors hyperkalemic, hypothermic cardioplegic arrest, augmented by topical cooling either with a continuous infusion of cold saline into the pericardial well or with a cooling jacket. Cardioplegic administration can be achieved either antegrade into the coronary ostia or retrograde via the coronary sinus. Myocardial temperature is monitored continuously.

After the heart is arrested, the aorta is opened to expose the aortic valve. The rheumatic, stenotic valve, including aortic annulus, is frequently heavily calcified, and all calcium must be debrided to allow the prosthetic valve to be securely seated. This is frequently a tedious and time-consuming procedure, but one which then allows the remainder of the procedure to proceed in a timely fashion. After excision of the valve leaflet and debridement of the annulus, assuring that no particulate debris embolizes into the ventricle or coronary arteries, the annulus is measured to assure a proper match between prosthetic valve and annulus and an appropriate valve prosthesis is selected. Interrupted sutures are then placed through the annulus for its entire circumference, then passed through the sewing ring of the prosthesis. The prosthesis is then lowered into the annulus and securely tied in place. Proper sizing and positioning are mandatory to prevent perivalve leaks or impingement on the coronary ostia. Systemic rewarming is initiated during the final stages of the valve implantation and the LV allowed to fill during aortic closure. With the patient in the head-down position, all remaining air is vented from the left heart and aorta, and the cross-clamp removed to allow myocardial perfusion. The heart is allowed to recover from this period of ischemia, and after sufficient resuscitation, with continuous venting of air from the aorta, the patient is weaned from CPB. Vasodilators are almost always utilized, as there appears to be excessive vasospasm present in both the coronary and pulmonary circulations after hypothermia. Decannulation and heparin reversal with protamine are then accomplished in the routine manner.

Usual preop diagnosis: Severe AS with syncope, chest pain or CHF; aortic insufficiency with CHF

SUMMARY OF PROCEDURE

	Valve Replacement with Prosthesis	Homograft Valve Replacement
Position	Supine	⇐
Incision	Median sternotomy	⇐
Special instrumentation	TEE; hemodynamic monitoring; CPB	TEE or surface ECHO
Unique considerations	ECHO assessment of valve function and regional wall motion intraop	ECHO assessment of annular size and intraop evaluation of valve function after implantation
Antibiotics	Cefamandole 1 g iv at incision	⇐
Surgical time	Aortic cross-clamp: 45 min	60 min
	CPB: 90 min	105 min
	Total: 3 h	⇐
EBL	300-400 ml	⇐
Postop care	ICU × 1-3 d, intubated 6-24 h; hypertrophied, noncompliant LV requiring high preload.	⇐
Mortality	5-8%	⇐
Morbidity	Pneumonia: 5-10%	⇐
	Neurological sequela: Transient: 3-7%; CVA: 1-2%; Permanent: 1-2%	⇐
	Infection: 1%	⇐
Pain score	7-10	7-10

PATIENT POPULATION CHARACTERISTICS

Age range	Bicuspid valves – 50-60 yr; rheumatic – 55-80 yr (mean = 58 ± 13 yr)
Male:Female	3:1
Incidence	70-100 cases/yr in tertiary care center
Etiology	Postrheumatic (majority of patients); aortic sclerosis; progressive stenosis of a bicuspid aortic valve; endocarditis
Associated conditions	Poststenotic dilatation of the ascending aorta (may require separate surgical attention); rheumatic mitral valvular involvement; CAD; CHF

ANESTHETIC CONSIDERATIONS

PREOPERATIVE

Respiratory

Respiratory compromise may occur 2° pulmonary congestion (LV failure) and pleural effusion. An effusion, if significant, should be drained prior to surgery as it may impair oxygenation and, with IPPV, may impair venous return → ↓CO + ↓myocardial perfusion.
Tests: CXR

Cardiovascular

Aortic stenosis (AS): Sx are those of angina pectoris (if at rest may indicate concurrent CAD), syncope and CHF (indicates severe disease with 2-yr life expectancy). The ejection murmur of AS is best heard at the 2nd right interspace. ECG shows LVH. Important points in the preop investigations include:

- Aortic orifice size: moderate AS = 0.7-0.9 cm^2; critical AS = < 0.5 cm^2 (normal = 2.6-3.5 cm^2)
- Aortic valvular gradient: severe = > 70 mmHg
- Ejection fraction (EF): ↓EF indicates evidence of LV failure (normal = > 0.6).
- Coronary angiography: associated CAD often demonstrated.
  AS → ↑LV work (↑pressure load) → LV concentric hypertrophy → ↓LV diastolic function + ↑risk for ischemia (MVO_2 + O_2 supply):
- Reliance on atrial "kick": important to maintain NSR.
- Sensitivity to changes in SVR: ↓SVR → ↓↓BP → ↓myocardial perfusion + ↓CO → ↓↓↓BP.
- Sensitivity to volume changes: hypovolemia → ↓preload → ↓↓CO.
- Sensitivity to rate changes: tachycardia → ↓ejection time → ↓myocardial perfusion.
- LV wall tension + ↑duration of systole → ↑MVO_2.
- ↑LVEDP + ↑wall thickness and tension + ↓diastolic aortic pressure → ↓O_2 supply.

Aortic regurgitation (AR): Sx include DOE, orthopnea, PND, palpitations and, less frequently, angina. Exercise tolerance may remain reasonably good, even with severe AR. Acute AR is very poorly tolerated. The pandiastolic murmur of AR is loudest over the sternum and left lower sternal border.

AR → chronic LV volume overload → LV eccentric hypertrophy → massive cardiomegaly → LV failure (CHF) → ↑LVEDP → ↑PA pressure and pulmonary congestion.

- Possibility of ischemia: ↑MVO_2 and ↓supply (↓diastolic pressure, ↑HR).
- Sensitivity to rate changes: ↓HR → ↑AR + ↓CO.
- Sensitivity to changes in SVR: ↑SVR → ↑regurgitation + ↓CO.

Tests: ECG: ✓ hypertrophy, LV strain, ischemia, rhythm. ECHO: ✓ LV function, valve area, regurgitant fraction. Angiography: ✓ LV function, right heart pressure, CAD, valve area, regurgitant fraction.

Hepatic

CHF may result in passive liver congestion with decrease in liver function and possible coagulopathy.
Tests: LFTs; PT; PTT

Neurological

Syncopal episodes may have resulted in neurologic deficits. These should be well documented.

Renal

Prerenal failure is often associated with AR 2° ↓CO.
Tests: BUN; creatinine, creatinine clearance, if indicated; electrolytes

Hematologic

Tests: Hb/Hct; clotting profile to investigate abnormalities. T&C for 8 U PRBCs.

Laboratory

✓ digitalis level and electrolytes; other tests as indicated from H&P.

Premedication

Beware of oversedation in patients with AS where ↓BP could be detrimental. Light premedication with an anxiolytic is usually sufficient. Digitalis and diuretics should be continued.

INTRAOPERATIVE

Anesthetic technique: GETA

Induction

AS: Typically, O_2 with moderate- to high-dose narcotic (e.g., fentanyl 10-100 μg/kg). Avoid sufentanil in AS because of ↓BP. Etomidate (0.1-0.3 mg/kg), midazolam (50-350 μg/kg) may be used to supplement the above. Paralysis with vecuronium or pancuronium (0.1 mg/kg, depending on desired HR). Induction is a critical period. CPB and surgeons should be available and ready to proceed. Danger is hypotension with a cycle of ischemia, further hypotension and more ischemia. Hypotension should be treated aggressively with fluid and α-adrenergic agonists (phenylephrine 50-100 μg iv bolus, infusion 0.1-0.75 μg/kg/min). Critical AS patients may benefit from the use of phenylephrine as an infusion during induction and prebypass. The avoidance of hypotension is even more critical in the presence of CAD. Drugs causing tachycardia should be avoided. Atrial fibrillation (AF) or SVT should be treated with cardioversion. β-blockers and other negative inotropes are generally contraindicated. Ventricular irritability should be treated early as ventricular fibrillation may be refractory to defibrillation. Beware of vasodilators, including NTG.

AR: Again, O_2 with moderate- to high-dose narcotic (e.g., fentanyl 10-100 μg/kg or sufentanil 2.5-10 μg/kg). Etomidate (0.1-0.3 mg/kg) or benzodiazepines (e.g., midazolam 50-350 μg/kg) may be used to supplement the opiates. Muscle relaxation with pancuronium (0.1 mg/kg). These patients benefit from fluid augmentation, high normal HR (90 bpm) with afterload reduction (e.g., SNP 0.25-2 μg/kg/min) to improve forward flow.

Maintenance

Narcotic (e.g., total fentanyl 10-100 μg/kg). Low-dose volatile agent/air/O_2. Relaxant. (See Anesthetic Considerations for Cardiopulmonary Bypass, p. 218.)

The following table summarizes the goals of intraop management:

Parameter	AS	AR
LV preload	↑	Normal to ↑
HR	Normal-to-slow ↓	Modest ↑
Rhythm	NSR	NSR
Contractility	Maintain	Maintain
SVR	Modest ↑	↓
PVR	Maintain	Maintain

Postbypass

AS: Postbypass, patients may be hyperdynamic and require vasodilators for HTN, although inotropes also may be needed. Because of the hypertrophied, noncompliant ventricle, filling pressure may be higher than normally required.

AR: In the immediate postbypass period, patients with AR may require inotropic support (e.g., dopamine 3-10 μg/kg/min, dobutamine 5-10 μg/kg/min; epinephrine 25-100 ng/kg/min) is often needed. Maintain LV filling. Other supportive measures (e.g., IABP) may be necessary.

Emergence

Transport to ICU sedated, intubated (6-24 h) and ventilated. Early extubation may be possible if a lower-dose narcotic technique is used (fast-track).

Blood and fluid requirements

IV: 14 ga × 1-2
NS/LR @ 6-8 ml/kg/h
UO 0.5-1 ml/kg/h
Warm all fluids.
Humidify gases.
2-4 U blood cross-match

Monitoring

Standard monitors (p. B-1).
Arterial line
CVP line
PA catheter
ECG
TEE
Urinary catheter

Standard and invasive monitors should be placed prior to induction.
CVP may underestimate left-side pressures. In acute AR, PCWP may underestimate true LVEDP.
V_5 lead should be monitored for ischemia.
TEE may be useful to estimate LV filling and regional wall motion abnormalities.

Positioning

✓ and pad pressure points.
✓ eyes.

Cardiovascular, cont.

symptomatology and valve area: mild = 1.5-2 cm^2; moderate = 1-1.5 cm^2; and severe = < 1.0 cm^2 (normal = 4-6 cm^2). AF is often the factor precipitating deterioration in these patients.

Because of the decreased LV filling, these patients are sensitive to:

- Loss of atrial "kick": maintain NSR.
- Volume changes: keep full.
- Rate changes: avoid ↑HR → ↓diastolic filling time → ↓CO.

Pathophysiology:

- MS → ↓LVH filling → ↓CO.
- MS → ↑LA pressure → pulmonary edema + ↑PA pressure → ↑PVR → RV failure + TR + left shift of iv septum → ↓CO → ↑LA pressure → ↑LA volume → AF and thrombi.

Mitral Regurgitation (MR): May be acute (MI/endocarditis) or chronic (often associated with MS). Chronic Sx include: palpitations, DOE, PND, fatigue and orthopnea. Acute MR may lead to sudden ↓↓CO and pulmonary edema. MR can be classified as mild (< 30% RF), moderate (30-60% RF); or severe (> 60% RF). The pansystolic murmur is loudest at the apex. The ECG may show LA and LV overload. MR patients are sensitive to:

- Changes in SVR: ↑SVR → ↑RF → ↓CO + ↓BP.
  ↓SVR → ↓RF → ↑CO + ↑BP.
- Change in HR: ↓HR → acute LA volume overload.
  Mild ↑HR → ↑CO.

Pathophysiology:

- Acute MR → ↑↑LA pressure → ↓CO + ↓BP → ↑HR → ↑contractility → ↑O_2 demand.
  → ↑LV diastolic volume → ↑LVEDP → ↑O_2 demand.
  → Pulmonary edema.
- Chronic MR → ↑LA volume + AF → pulmonary edema → RV failure.
  → LV volume overload → LVH → ↓CO + LV failure.

Tests: ECG: ✓ LVH, left and right atrial enlargement, rhythm. ECHO: ✓ RF, valve pressure gradients, LV function, valve pressure gradient and area.

Neurological

The large left atrium and AF may result in thrombus formation, with the possibility of embolism. Neurological deficits should be documented.

Gastrointestinal

Hepatic congestion may → decreased function, which may be reflected in coagulation problems.
Tests: Consider LFTs; PT; PTT

Renal

↓CO may lead to renal failure.
Tests: BUN; creatinine; electrolytes

Hematologic

Because of the potential for thromboembolism, these patients may be on anticoagulants, which may be given up to the day before surgery. In the case of Coumadin, anticoagulant effects can be reversed by the use of FFP and vitamin K.
Tests: Consider PT; PTT

Laboratory

T&C for 2-4 U PRBCs. Hb/Hct; coagulation profile; other tests as indicated from H&P.

Premedication

Premedication with an anxiolytic (e.g., lorazepam 1-2 mg po, midazolam 0.05-0.2 mg/kg im) or an analgesic (e.g., morphine 0.1-0.2 mg/kg), or a combination of these agents may be used, depending on patient status.

INTRAOPERATIVE

Anesthetic technique: GETA

Induction

Typically, moderate- to high-dose narcotic (fentanyl 10-100 μg/kg or sufentanil 2.5-20 μg/kg), supplemental midazolam (50-350 μg/kg) or etomidate (0.1-0.3 mg/kg). Use pancuronium (MR) or vecuronium (MS) (0.1 mg/kg), depending on the desired HR to facilitate intubation.

MS: Hypotension should be treated with fluid, but beware of precipitating pulmonary edema. Occasionally phenylephrine may be needed to maintain SVR. Tachycardia should be avoided; if it occurs it should be treated (↑ anesthesia, esmolol if ventricular function is preserved). Sinus rhythm should be maintained. New onset atrial flutter/AF should be treated with defibrillation. Avoid factors that may increase PVR (N_2O, acidosis, hypoxia, hypercarbia).

MR: Maintain or augment preload, depending on response to fluid load. Inotropic agents may be useful to maintain contractility. Afterload reduction will improve forward flow. Generally SNP

Induction, cont. (0.5-4 μg/kg/m) is used, but NTG (0.5-4 μg/kg/m) may be more appropriate in patients with ischemia-induced regurgitation. Avoid ↑PVR caused by N_2O, acidosis, hypoxia or hypercarbia. IABP may be useful perioperatively in those patients with acute MR due to MI (↓afterload, ↑coronary perfusion pressure).

Maintenance Narcotic (total: fentanyl 10-100 μg/kg, or sufentanil 5-20 μg/kg) with benzodiazepine (e.g., midazolam 50-350 μg/kg) for amnesia; low-dose isoflurane; O_2/air.
The following table summarizes the goals of intraop management:

Parameter	MS	MR
LV preload	Normal to ↑	Normal → ↑
HR	↓	↑
Rhythm	NSR	NSR
Contractility	Maintain	Maintain
SVR	Normal	↓
PVR	Avoid ↑	Avoid ↑

Postbypass Although patients with MS generally do well after valve replacement, inotropes (e.g., dopamine, dobutamine) occasionally are necessary. This is especially true late in the disease when cardiomyopathy may be present.

Emergence Transport to ICU, intubated and ventilated 6-24 h. Early extubation is possible if lower-dose narcotic technique is used (fast-track).

Blood and fluid requirements
IV: 14 ga × 1-2
NS/LR @ 6-8 ml/kg/h
Maintain UO 0.5-1 ml/kg/h.
Warm all fluids.
Humidify gases.

Monitoring
Standard monitors (p. B-1)
Arterial line
CVP line
PA catheter
Urinary catheter
TEE

Standard and invasive monitoring should be placed prior to induction. Care should be exercised with PA catheter insertion because the dilated PA may be susceptible to rupture with the catheter. In MS, PCWP may overestimate LV filling pressure because of stenosis.
TEE may help in volume management, regional wall motion abnormalities (postacute MI) and in assessing the success of mitral valve repair. Occasionally the use of a valve ring during repair may cause systolic anterior motion of the valve leaflet, with resultant regurgitation, which may be seen on ECHO.

Positioning
✓ and pad pressure points.
✓ eyes.

POSTOPERATIVE

Complications
Hemorrhage
Tamponade
Cardiac failure
Dysrhythmias
Conduction defects
Atrioventricular disruption

Inotropic support or vasodilator therapy may be needed. IABP for mitral incompetence, especially in the presence of acute MR as a result of infarction.

Pain management
Parenteral opioids for pain relief
Benzodiazepine for sedation

Tests
ECG
CXR
ABG
Coagulation profile
Electrolytes

References

1. Cobanoglu A, Grunkenmeier GL, Aru GM, McKinley CL, Starr A: Mitral replacement: clinical experience with a ball-valve prosthesis; twenty-five years later. *Ann Surg* 1985; 202(3):376-83.
2. Fann JI, Miller DC, Moore KA, Mitchell RS, Oyer PE, Stinson EB, Robbins RC, Reitz RA, Shumway NE: Twenty-year clinical experience with porcine bioprostheses. *Ann Thorac Surg* 1996; 62:1301-2.
3. Galloway AC, Colvin SB, Baumann FB, et al: A comparison of mitral valve reconstruction with mitral valve replacement: intermediate-term results. *Ann Thorac Surg* 1989; 47:655-62.
4. Jackson JM, Thomas SJ: Valvular Heart Disease. In *Cardiac Anesthesia*, 3rd edition. Kaplan JA, ed. WB Saunders, Philadelphia: 1993, Ch 20, 629-80.
5. Moore RA, Martin DE: Anesthetic management for the treatment of valvular heart disease. In *A Practical Approach to Cardiac Anesthesia*, 2nd edition. Hensley FA, Martin DE, eds. Little, Brown, Boston: 1995, Ch. 11, 295-325.
6. Scott WC, Miller DC, Haverich A, Mitchell RS, Oyer PE, Stinson EB, Jamieson SW, Baldwin JC, Shumway NE: Operative risk of mitral valve replacement: Discriminant analysis of 1329 procedures. *Circulation* 1985; 72(3P+2):II-108-19.

TRICUSPID VALVE REPAIR

SURGICAL CONSIDERATIONS

Description: Insufficiency of the tricuspid valve is almost always 2° left-sided valvular disease, with tricuspid annular dilatation and resultant valvular insufficiency usually 2° pulmonary HTN. Some congenital conditions (Ebstein's deformity) may persist into early adulthood, when replacement is usually necessary. Tricuspid repair is normally possible in the absence of primary involvement of tricuspid leaflets. The procedure is usually accomplished on CPB (see p. 217), either with the heart fibrillating or during a brief period of aortic cross-clamping and diastolic arrest. After instituting CPB and snaring the venous cannulae to prevent air entry into the pump circuit, the tricuspid valve is exposed through an incision in the right atrium. In the absence of leaflet involvement by the rheumatic process, repair usually can be accomplished by a simple **annuloplasty**. After atrial closure, evacuation of air and myocardial resuscitation, the patient is weaned from CPB with vasodilator agents. Temporary pacing wires are usually inserted and passed to the anesthesiologist in case inadvertent injury to the AV node or His bundle cause complete heart block.

Variant procedure or approaches: **Tricuspid valve replacement**

Usual preop diagnosis: Tricuspid regurgitation, 2° annular dilatation 2° pulmonary HTN and left-side failure

SUMMARY OF PROCEDURE

Position	Supine
Incision	Median sternotomy
Special instrumentation	Intraop ECHO; hemodynamic monitoring; CPB
Antibiotics	Cefamandole 1 g iv at induction
Surgical time	Aortic cross-clamp: 30-40 min CPB: 70-80 min Total: 3-4 h
EBL	400-800 ml (Long-standing tricuspid regurgitation may result in impaired hepatic production of coagulation factors.)
Postop care	ICU × 1-3 d, intubated 6-24 h; vasodilator therapy for pulmonary HTN
Mortality	2-3%
Morbidity	Third-degree heart block: 10% RV failure: 2-3%
Pain score	7-10

PATIENT POPULATION CHARACTERISTICS

Age range	50-75 yr
Male:Female	1:1
Incidence	Rare
Etiology	Rheumatic; congenital (Ebstein's anomaly)
Associated conditions	Rheumatic involvement of left-side valves with pulmonary HTN

ANESTHETIC CONSIDERATIONS

PREOPERATIVE

Cardiovascular Tricuspid regurgitation (TR) is usually well tolerated and Sx (↓CO) may go unnoticed, masked by Sx associated with left-side valvular disease and pulmonary HTN. Occasionally TR is 2° endocarditis and raises the suspicion of iv drug abuse. TR may be caused by pulmonary HTN → ↑RV afterload → RV dilation, ↑RV wall tension → dilation of tricuspid valve annulus and TR.

Pathophysiology:

- TR → ↓CO 2° ↑RV size → shift of the intraventricular septum to the left → ↓LV size, ↓LV compliance → LV underloading due to ↓LV size and ↓RV stroke volume.
- TR → atrial fibrillation (AF) 2° ↑right atrial size. In isolated insufficiency, the ↑ in right atrial pressure may result in shunting across a patent foramen ovale (PFO), leading to paradoxical embolization with potentially disastrous consequences.

Tests: ECG: ✓ AF. ECHO: ✓ relative chamber size, contractility, PFO, valve lesions. Cardiac catheterization: ✓ contractility, CO, pulmonary pressures and their response to vasodilators, other valvular pathology.

Respiratory Pulmonary HTN (> 25 mmHg mean pressure), pulmonary edema and effusions may be present.
Tests: CXR: ✓ pulmonary edema, pleural effusion.

Renal Chronic venous congestion may lead to prerenal failure.
Tests: BUN; creatinine; electrolytes

Hepatic Hepatic congestion may lead to impaired synthetic function, particularly coagulation factors.
Tests: Consider PT; PTT

Hematologic **Tests:** Hb/Hct; other tests as indicated from H&P and Sx. Consider viral testing (HIV, hepatitis in isolated tricuspid endocarditis or in iv drug abusers). T&C 2-4 U PRBCs.

Laboratory Other tests as indicated from H&P.

Premedication Standard premedication (p. B-2) is usually appropriate.

INTRAOPERATIVE

Anesthetic technique: GETA

Induction Typically, O_2 and moderate- to high-dose narcotic (fentanyl 10-100 μg/kg or sufentanil 2.5-20 μg/kg) with etomidate (0.1-0.3 mg/kg) or midazolam (50-150 μg/kg). Muscle relaxation is obtained with a nondepolarizing agent (e.g., pancuronium 0.1 mg/kg, vecuronium 0.1 mg/kg).

Maintenance The choice of narcotic/benzodiazepine/O_2 or volatile agent and O_2 will be determined by the underlying lesion and ventricular function. Avoid N_2O (pulmonary HTN). Low-dose isoflurane may be used. Benzodiazepines (e.g., midazolam 50-300 μg/kg, diazepam 0.3-0.5 mg/kg) may be used for amnesia. Exact choice of agents for maintenance depends on underlying lesion, ventricular function and coexisting disease. Management goals of TR are often those of coexisting valvular problems. The general principles, however, are: (1) Adequate preload (↓preload ↓RV stroke volume); (2) HR: normal-to-increased; (3) Contractility: normal. May require inotropic support for ↑PVR, anesthetic myocardial depression or IPPV. (4) PVR: normal or decreased (high PVR ↓RV stroke volume). (5) SVR: little effect unless it affects left-side pathology.

Emergence To ICU intubated and ventilated × 6-24 h. Early extubation may be possible if a lower-dose narcotic technique is used (fast-track).

Blood and fluid requirements IV: 14 ga × 1-2
NS/LR @ 6-8 ml/kg/h

Because of the possibility of PFO and R→L shunt, ensure that all venous lines are clear of air.

Blood and fluid requirements, cont.	UO 0.5-1 ml/kg/h Warm all fluids. Humidify gases. T&C 2-4 U PRBC.	
Monitoring	Standard monitors (p. B-1) Arterial line CVP or PA catheter Urinary catheter	Standard and invasive monitoring should be placed prior to induction. CVP may be a poor indicator of RV or LV filling. PA catheter may be helpful in the management of fluid balance, CO and management of pulmonary HTN, but may be difficult to place and will require removal while valve or annular ring is placed.
	TEE	Because RV distention may affect LV filling and stroke volume, TEE may be useful in judging filling and relative LV size.
Pulmonary HTN	↑PVR can result from: ↓PaO_2 ↑$PaCO_2$ ↓pH N_2O α-agonists Inadequate anesthesia	In TR, control of PVR is important because ↑PVR may result in ↓CO. Hypoxia, hypercarbia, acidosis, N_2O or α-agonists may increase PVR. PVR may be reduced with hypocarbia, inotropic support with dobutamine (5-10 μg/kg/min), isoproterenol (10-50 ng/kg/m) or amrinone (loading 0.75 mg/kg, infusion 2-20 μg/kg/min) and by using pulmonary vasodilators—NTG (1-4 μg/kg/min), SNP (0.5-4 μg/kg/min), prostaglandin E_1 (0.05-0.4 μg/kg/min), or NO (0.1-100 ppm inhaled).
Positioning	✓ and pad pressure points. ✓ eyes.	
Complications	Coagulopathy Hemorrhage RV failure	Coagulopathy 2° prolonged bypass time for multiple valve replacements. RV failure 2° ↑PVR (previously, RV decompressed by tricuspid incompetence). Rx includes inotropes dobutamine (5-10 μg/kg/min), isoproterenol (25-100 ng/kg/min), amrinone (loading 0.75 mg/kg, infusion 2-20 μg/kg/min), epinephrine (25-100 ng/kg/min), avoidance of factors causing ↑PVR, and the use of pulmonary vasodilators.

POSTOPERATIVE

Complications	Hemorrhage Coagulopathy Dysrhythmias RV failure Infection Renal impairment	Inotropic support and pulmonary vasodilators will need to be continued. Avoid those factors which ↑ PVR.
	Methemoglobinemia	Measure met-Hb levels during NO therapy.
Pain management	Parenteral opioids	Supplement with benzodiazepine for sedation.
Tests	ECG Coagulation profile Renal panel: BUN, creatinine ABG Electrolytes	

References

1. Jackson JM, Thomas SJ: Valvular heart disease. In *Cardiac Anesthesia*, 3rd edition. Kaplan JA, ed. WB Saunders, Philadelphia: 1993, Ch 20, 629-80.
2. Moore RA, Martin DE: Anesthetic management for the treatment of valvular heart disease. In *A Practical Approach to Cardiac Anesthesia*, 2nd edition. Hensley FA Jr, Martin DE, eds. Little, Brown, Boston: 1995, Ch 11, 295-325.

SEPTAL MYECTOMY/MYOTOMY

SURGICAL CONSIDERATIONS

Description: Patients with asymmetric septal hypertrophy usually present with symptoms 2° LV outflow tract obstruction (LVOTO), increased diastolic dysfunction and stiffness, or a combination of the two, manifested as syncope, CHF or severe chest pain. The systolic hemodynamic abnormality is caused by anterior leaflet of the mitral valve being drawn into the LV outflow tract (LVOT), and abutting the asymmetrically hypertrophied intraventricular septum, narrowing the LVOT, and producing a large intracavitary gradient. Additionally, severe mitral insufficiency may result. The most common surgical procedure for asymmetric septal hypertrophy is **septal myectomy/myotomy**. After institution of CPB, aortic cross-clamping and cardioplegic arrest, the aorta is opened, and visualization of the subvalvar ventricular septum attained. Bimanual palpation, as well as TEE visualization, can localize the asymmetric hypertrophy. Using the right coronary orifice as a landmark, the ventricular septum is longitudinally incised with two parallel incisions approximately 1 cm apart, with care being taken to avoid injury of the papillary muscle or mitral valve chordae. A trough of the hypertrophied septum is then excised, alleviating the LVOTO. Removal of a portion of the asymmetrically hypertrophied myopathic septum also usually reduces the systolic anterior motion (SAM) of the anterior mitral leaflet, reduces the intracavitary gradient and mitral regurgitation (MR). Infrequently, mitral valve replacement may be necessary for persistent MR.

Usual preop diagnosis: Asymmetric septal hypertrophy with CHF, chest pain, and/or syncope

SUMMARY OF PROCEDURE

Position	Supine
Incision	Median sternotomy
Special instrumentation	TEE; hemodynamic monitoring; CPB
Unique considerations	Because of LV hypertrophy, maintenance of adequate preload is essential. Afterload must also be maintained to prevent LVOTO.
Antibiotics	Cefamandole 1 g iv at induction
Surgical time	2.5 h
EBL	150 ml
Postop care	ICU, intubated on ventilator 6-24 h
Mortality	3-4%
Morbidity	Complete heart block: 5% Persistent MR: 5% New aortic insufficiency: 2-5% CVA: < 1% VSD: < 1%
Pain score	6-10

PATIENT POPULATION CHARACTERISTICS

Age range	20-80 yr (mean = 45 yr)
Male:Female	1:1
Incidence	10/yr at Stanford University Medical Center
Etiology	Asymmetric septal hypertrophy

ANESTHETIC CONSIDERATIONS

PREOPERATIVE

Respiratory Affected only 2° to cardiac failure.

Cardiovascular Patients with idiopathic hypertrophic subaortic stenosis (IHSS) often present with Sx of syncope, angina pectoris (CAD), CHF and palpitations. The main feature of IHSS is dynamic LVOTO 2° to septal hypertrophy and a possible venturi effect which draws the anterior mitral valve leaflet into the outflow tract. LVOTO → ↑LV hypertrophy → ↓compliance and ↓diastolic function → ↑LVEDP, making diastolic filling dependent on preload and atrial contraction. Obstruction is worsened by decreased preload or afterload, increased contractility or HR. IHSS also results in ↑MVO_2 and

Cardiovascular, cont.

↓coronary perfusion, especially to the septum and subendocardium, which increases the risk of ischemia. Hypertrophy occurs throughout the whole myocardium and may lead to further dysfunction. MR, caused by a venturi suction effect, is often present and is exacerbated by the same conditions that increase LVOTO. (Note that ↓afterload → ↑MR, unlike the usual [nonventuri-suction] form of MR.) Patients are often on β-blockers or Ca^{++} antagonists. These should be continued to day of surgery.

Tests: ECG: ✓ Q-waves (indicative of septal hypertrophy); short PR interval with slurred QRS complex; supraventricular tachycardia; LV hypertrophy.
ECHO: ✓ septal hypertrophy; MR; LV hypertrophy, myocardial dysfunction.
Cardiac catheterization: ✓ LVOT pressure gradient which may increase with provocation (e.g., Valsalva maneuver); obliteration of the LV cavity; MR; CAD.

Neurological

Document syncope and any neurological deficits.

Laboratory

Hb/Hct; electrolytes; other tests as indicated from H&P.

Premedication

Avoid activation of the sympathetic nervous system since this will cause ↑HR and ↓inotropy → ↓CO + ↓BP. Thus, adequate anxiolysis is essential and can be obtained by premedication with a benzodiazepine (e.g., midazolam 0.05-0.2 mg/kg im, lorazepam 1-2 mg po, or diazepam 5-10 mg po). Avoid ↓SVR, and maintain β-blockade and Ca^{++} channel blocker therapy.

INTRAOPERATIVE

Anesthetic technique: GETA

Induction

Typically, moderate- to high-dose narcotic (fentanyl 10-100 μg/kg; avoid sufentanil due to vasodilation). Supplement with etomidate (0.1-0.3 mg/kg), midazolam (50-350 μg/kg) or STP (2-4 mg/kg). Ketamine should be avoided due to the activation of the sympathetic nervous system. Introduction of a volatile agent prior to intubation may be helpful. Vecuronium (0.1 mg/kg) for muscle relaxation. Use pancuronium with caution (tachycardia) and avoid d-tubocurarine (hypotension).

Maintenance

O_2 and narcotic (total fentanyl 10-100 μg/kg) + volatile agent—most commonly, halothane because of decreased contractility and preservation of SVR. Halothane, however, may lead to loss of NSR. Isoflurane is relatively contraindicated (↓SVR). Midazolam (50-350 μg/kg) can be used for amnesia. The cornerstone of anesthesia for IHSS is to avoid factors which will increase LVOTO: (1) ↓preload; (2) ↓afterload; (3) ↑contractility; (4) loss of NSR; and (5) ↑HR.

Emergence

To ICU intubated and ventilated × 6-24 h. Early extubation is possible if a lower-dose narcotic technique is used (fast-track).

Blood and fluid requirements

IV: 14 ga × 1-2
NS/LR @ 6-8 ml/kg/h
Maintain UO 0.5-1 ml/h
Warm fluids.
Humidify gases.

Monitoring

Standard monitors (p. B-1) Arterial line PA catheter Urinary catheter	Standard and invasive monitors should be placed prior to induction. A PA catheter is useful for assessment of LV filling (keep high normal PCWP) and for monitoring SVR (normal-to-high). A pacing or pace port PA catheter may be useful for conduction problems occurring postop.
TEE	TEE is useful to judge LV filling, LV contractility, LVOTO, MR and VSD.

Intraoperative problems

↓Preload	Rx: volume, phenylephrine
↓Afterload	Rx: phenylephrine
↑Contractility	Rx: esmolol, halothane
↑HR	Rx: esmolol
Loss of NSR	Rx: cardioversion, verapamil
Complete heart block	Should have reliable means of pacing available, including temporary ventricular leads.
VSD	Septum may be damaged, resulting in VSD (diagnosed by TEE). If present, it should be repaired.

Position	✓ and pad pressure points. ✓ eyes.	

POSTOPERATIVE

Complications	Hemorrhage	Dx: from chest tube drainage. Rx with blood and factors as needed. ✓ coagulation status. May require reexploration.
	Complete heart block	Pacing should be available. Occasionally, inotropes of vasodilators required. β-blockers and Ca^{++} antagonists usually discontinued.
	Late VSD	Late VSD, indicated by development of a murmur, will require repair.
	Tamponade	Dx: by rising filling pressure, equalization of CVP and PADP, ↓CO, ↓UO and by ECHO. Rx: reexploration and drainage.
Pain management	Parenteral opioids	Supplement with benzodiazepine for sedation.
Tests	ECG: ✓ conduction problems ABG ECHO: ✓ LVOTO; VSD Coagulation profile Electrolytes	

References

1. Jackson JM, Thomas SJ: Valvular Heart Disease. In *Cardiac Anesthesia*, 3rd edition. Kaplan JA, ed. WB Saunders, Philadelphia: 1993, Ch 20, 629-80.
2. Maron BJ, Bonow RO, Cannon RO III, Leon MB, Epstein SE: Hypertrophic cardiomyopathy. Interrelations of clinical manifestations, pathophysiology, and therapy. *N Engl J Med* 1987; 316(13):780-89; 316(14):844-52.
3. Morrow AG, Reitz BA, Epstein SE, Henry WL, Conkle DM, Itscoitz SB, Redwood DR: Operative treatment in hypertrophic subaortic stenosis. Techniques, and the results of pre- and postoperative assessment in 83 patients. *Circulation* 1975; 52(1):88-102.
4. Oliver WC, DeCastro M, Strickland PA: Uncommon diseases and cardiac anesthesia. In *Cardiac Anesthesia*, 3rd edition. Kaplan J, ed. WB Saunders, Philadelphia: 1993, Ch 24, 819-64.

CARDIAC MAPPING, ABLATION AND AICD PROCEDURES

SURGICAL CONSIDERATIONS

Description: Cardiac dysrhythmias may occur 2° abnormal or accessory conduction pathways in the heart. Electrophysiologic testing can localize these abnormal pathways, evaluate their suppressibility by dysrhythmic medications, and even ablate, with radiofrequency, certain localized pathways. Surgical ablation is possible for those pathways not amenable to catheter-directed radiofrequency ablation. For polymorphic dysrhythmias not amenable to ablation or pharmacologic suppression, **automatic implantable cardiac defibrillators (AICD)** can be highly effective by delivering a depolarizing shock after detecting the dysrhythmia. The evaluation decision tree proceeds as follows: monomorphic ventricular tachycardia (VT) → pharmacologic suppression; if unsuccessful, mapping with catheter or surgical ablation. Polymorphic VT → pharmacologic suppression, if unsuccessful, mapping and catheter ablation, if still unsuccessful → AICD.

Surgical ablation is performed on CPB (see p. 217). After routine cannulation and implantation of electrophysiologic leads, an attempt is made to induce VT. If successful, and the patient remains stable, **electrophysiologic mapping** is performed. Avoidance of antidysrhythmics is important at this stage. If the patient is hemodynamically unstable, CPB is begun, and the mapping procedure completed. Once complete, the heart is arrested, and during hypothermic cardiac arrest, the dysrhythmogenic focus is excised or cryoblated. For polymorphic VT, an AICD is usually implanted. Initially, this was performed through a left anterior thoracotomy, but some lead systems have progressed so that only subcutaneous patches, a superior caval electrode, and RV pacing leads are necessary, as is an incision for the defibrillator. Defibrillator testing requires multiple episodes of VT or ventricular fibrillation (VF) with rescue "shocks," which may produce some cardiac instability. For polymorphic dysrhythmias not amenable to ablation or pharmacologic suppression, implantable automatic defibrillators can be highly effective in delivering a depolarizing shock after detecting the dysrhythmia.

Usual preop diagnosis: Supraventricular tachycardia (SVT); ventricular tachycardia or fibrillation; Wolff-Parkinson-White (WPW) syndrome; Lown-Ganong-Levine (LGL) syndrome

SUMMARY OF PROCEDURE

	Mapping and/or Ablation	AICD
Position	Supine	Supine, with slight elevation of left chest
Incision	Median sternotomy	Central venous access (left subclavian vein) with either pericardial defibrillator patches, placed through an anterior thoracotomy, or subcutaneous patches.
Special instrumentation	Electrophysiologic instrumentation; defibrillator patches on skin; CPB	External defibrillator; DLT to allow collapse of left lung; defibrillator patches/paddles on skin
Unique considerations	Avoid antidysrhythmic agents during induction, if possible.	None
Antibiotics	Cefamandole 1 g iv at induction	⇐
Surgical time	Aortic cross-clamp: 30-60 min CPB: 70-150 min Total: 3-4 h	Total: 2-3 h (no CPB)
EBL	300-400 ml	< 100 ml
Postop care	ICU × 2 d; ECG monitoring × 7 d	ICU × 1 d; ECG monitoring × 7 d
Mortality	5-15% (highly dependent on mechanism of dysrhythmia. If aberrant pathway (WPW), 1-2%; if 2° LV aneurysm with ischemic dysfunction, 5-15%)	1-2%
Morbidity	Overall: 10% Recurrent VT/VF: 20-30% MI: 2-5%	2% Respiratory complications: 2-5% CVA: 1%
Pain score	6-10	5-10

PATIENT POPULATION CHARACTERISTICS

Age range	30-70 yr in general WPW and other anatomical pathways: 2-50 yr Acquired dysrhythmias from ischemic damage: 50-75 yr
Male:Female	2:1
Incidence	Rare
Etiology	SVT, usually 2° congenital bypass tracts; VT and VF, usually 2° ischemia-induced changes such as LV aneurysm formation or an irritable peri-infarct zone

ANESTHETIC CONSIDERATIONS

PREOPERATIVE

Patients may be divided into two populations based on symptomatology, associated pathology and probable outcome: (1) **Supraventricular dysrhythmias**: e.g., WPW. These patients are usually young and otherwise healthy. May be associated with Ebstein's anomaly (tricuspid valve defect → RV failure), mitral valve disease or CAD. Low perioperative mortality (1%). (2) **Ventricular dysrhythmias**: usually older patients with significant ventricular dysfunction (EF = 10-35%) and other pathologies such as CAD or cardiac failure. Procedure is often accompanied by LV aneurysmectomy or myocardial revascularization (see Coronary Artery Bypass Graft Surgery, p. 222). Mortality is 15% for mapping/ablation, but much less for AICD implantation. Patients presenting for AICD implantation have either survived an episode of VT/VF or are otherwise at risk for sudden death.

Respiratory May have associated pulmonary disease 2° smoking.
Tests: CXR; consider PFT, as indicated from H&P.

Cardiovascular **Supraventricular dysrhythmias**: Occasionally associated disease as above. Look for precipitating factors in the dysrhythmia and any methods that have been used to terminate the dysrhythmia. Usually drug therapy is terminated prior to surgery to make the dysrhythmia inducible. Note type of drugs used, especially those used to terminate a dysrhythmia.
Ventricular dysrhythmias: Inquire about any methods that have been used to terminate the dysrhythmia. Look for associated conditions—CAD, CHF, cardiomyopathy, LV aneurysm, HTN, mitral insufficiency, diabetes. Generally these patients will have poor LV function with increased sensitivity to myocardial depressants. It is important to note that they may be on combinations of antidysrhythmics. Many of these drugs have significant negative inotropic effects. Of special note is amiodarone, which has been associated with intractable bradydysrhythmias, refractory vasodilation and difficulty in weaning from CPB.
AICD: AICD patients are left on full medication as it is usually impossible to wean them from antidysrhythmic medications before surgery. In most studies, patients have a mean LV ejection fraction of 35% and a New York Heart Association functional class II and III.
Tests: ECG: ✓ dysrhythmia, ischemia. Electrophysiologic report: ✓ type of dysrhythmia, means of termination—pharmacologic or electrical. ECHO: ✓ ventricular function, wall motion abnormalities, valvular problems. Cardiac angiography: ✓ventricular function, CAD, valvular disease, LV aneurysm.

Renal Patients with poor ventricular function may have associated renal compromise. Electrolyte abnormalities (K^+, Mg^{++}) may be associated with increased cardiac irritability and should be corrected preop.
Tests: BUN; creatinine; electrolytes

Hematologic Hb/Hct; T&C for 8 U (AICD patients are not T&C'd).

Laboratory Other tests as indicated from H&P.

Premedication Typically, a benzodiazepine (e.g., lorazepam 1-2 mg po, midazolam 0.05-0.2 mg/kg im), morphine (0.1-0.2 mg/kg), or a combination, depending on LV function.

INTRAOPERATIVE

Anesthetic technique: GETA

Induction **Supraventricular and ventricular dysrhythmias:** Exact type of induction depends on the planned surgery, need for CPB, ventricular function and whether prolonged (12+ h) postop ventilation will be necessary. For patients with supraventricular dysrhythmias and good LV function, early extubation in the ICU can be planned. For these patients, induction with STP (2-4 mg/kg) or etomidate (0.1-0.3 mg/kg), with low-to-moderate dose narcotic (e.g., fentanyl 5-20 μg/kg) and muscle relaxation with vecuronium (0.1 mg/kg) is often used. For patients with poor ventricular function, a high-dose narcotic (e.g., fentanyl 20-100 μg/kg), 100% O_2 and muscle relaxation with vecuronium (0.1 mg/kg) is appropriate.
AICD: Placement of most AICDs are done in the cardiac catheterization suite (see AICD, p. 1057). These devices are very small and are implanted in the same position as a pacemaker. Often, MAC with sedation (and short periods of GA during testing) is all that is required. Midazolam or a propofol infusion may be used. Alternatively, GETA or a LMA can be used. GA ± DLT required for thoracotomy, sternotomy and subcostal approaches.

Maintenance **Superventricular dysrhythmias:** Generally, mapping is done prior to bypass, but after cannulation. If the focus is left-side, cardioplegia is used after mapping; but right-side foci are usually done with normothermic bypass and a beating heart. This has relevance in the increased heparin requirements (↑metabolism), so that frequent ACTs should be performed. If rapid cardiac rates are induced, myocardial O_2 demand will be high. Ensure amnesia with a benzodiazepine (e.g., midazolam 50-350 μg/kg).

Maintenance, cont.	**Ventricular dysrhythmias:** These foci are usually left-side and 2° to CAD. Both epicardial and endocardial mapping often are needed and are carried out under normothermic bypass. The same consideration of increased heparin requirement and ↑MVO_2 during induced ventricular tachycardia apply. In addition, the ventricle may be open while the aorta is not cross-clamped. It is important that the aortic valve remain closed during this period to prevent air entering the aorta. Adequate aortic pressure is important and may be obtained with a phenylephrine infusion (0.15-0.75 μg/kg iv). During the procedure, ventricular tissue may be excised, and this, together with the already compromised ventricle, may result in difficulty in terminating CPB. Inotropes and IABP may be required. Coagulopathies, particularly 2° low platelets, may occur during prolonged normothermic bypass. Ensure amnesia with a benzodiazepine (e.g., midazolam 50-350 μg/kg). **AICD:** AICD devices have leads for sensing rate and for delivering a 10-30 J shock to prevent sustained ventricular fibrillation. These may be placed via a small anterior thoracotomy or (more frequently) via a transvenous route. Verification of placement involves the induction of ventricular fibrillation or tachycardia and the testing of the device's capability to restore NSR. External defibrillation should be available at all times, as should antidysrhythmics (e.g., bretylium). While the device is tested, the patient should be breathing 100% O_2. Multiple testing cycles can result in depressed LV function and inotropes may be needed.	
Emergence	**AICD:** These patients are extubated (if GETA or LMA is used). Recovery is in the PACU. If, however, multiple test shocks are needed or the heart displays evidence of injury (need for inotropes, ST segment abnormalities), then extubation may need to be deferred to ICU. Generally, with supraventricular and ventricular dysrhythmia patients (where sternotomy is performed), emergence is deferred to ICU. Electrophysiologic testing is usually repeated a few wk after surgery. AICD patients usually go to PACU; others to ICU and may be mechanically ventilated for 4-24 h.	
Blood and fluid requirements	IV: 14 ga × 1-2 NS/LR @ 6-8 ml/kg/min UO 0.5-1 ml/kg Warm all fluids. Humidify gases.	
Monitoring	Standard monitors (p. B-1) Arterial line CVP line PA catheter Urinary catheter	A CVP or PA catheter may be placed according to LV function. Generally, a PA sheath should be used. PA catheter should be advanced when the chest is open and access to the heart is available because of the potential for inducing dysrhythmias. AICD patients generally require only an arterial line.
	External defibrillation pads	Because antidysrhythmics may affect the mapping procedure, they should be avoided when possible. Defibrillation or cardioversion are treatments of choice.
	TEE	TEE is useful to assess LV function before and after mapping or ablation.
	Temperature	Normothermia should be maintained, since decreased temperature may affect conduction in aberrant pathways and, thus, the mapping procedure.
Positioning	Shoulder roll for median sternotomy; supine for AICD. ✓ and pad pressure points. ✓ eyes.	
Complications	Pneumo/hemothorax Pericardial effusion/tamponade ↓BP/CHF	

POSTOPERATIVE

Complications	Recurrent dysrhythmias Hemorrhage Coagulopathy Ischemia

Pain management	Parenteral opioids	Supplement with benzodiazepine for sedation.
Tests	CXR: ✓ line/lead placement, pneumothorax ECG: ✓ ischemia dysrhythmias Electrophysiologic testing Coagulation profile Electrolytes	

References

1. Cox JL: Anatomic-electrophysiologic basis for the surgical treatment of refractory ischemic ventricular tachycardia. *Ann Surg* 1983; 198(2):119-29.
2. Cox JL, Gallagher JJ, Cain ME: Experience with 118 consecutive patients undergoing surgery for the Wolff-Parkinson-White syndrome. *J Thorac Cardiovasc Surg* 1985; 90(4):490-501.
3. Lappis DG, Hogue CW, Cain ME, Cox JL: Anesthesia for electrophysiologic procedures. In *Cardiac Anesthesia*, 3rd edition. Kaplan JA, ed. WB Saunders, Philadelphia: 1993, Ch 23, 780-818.
4. Matthews EL, Atlee JL, Luck JC, Martin DE: Anesthesia for patients with electrophysiologic disorders. In *A Practical Approach to Cardiac Anesthesia*, 2nd edition. Hensley FA Jr, Martin DE, eds. Little, Brown, Boston: 1995, Ch 14, 392-415.

PACEMAKER INSERTION

SURGICAL CONSIDERATIONS

Description: **Pacemaker insertion** may be required for relief of abnormalities of the conduction system. A transvenous pacemaker lead may be placed via the subclavian vein, through the tricuspid valve into the right ventricle (single-chamber pacing); or two leads may be placed, one into the right atrium and the other into the right ventricle (dual-chamber pacing). Typically, 2nd- or 3rd-degree heart block is the diagnostic indication, although sick sinus syndrome (SSS) and other abnormalities also may be found. Access to the subclavian veins is usually attained percutaneously, although a cut-down may be used to expose the cephalic vein in the deltopectoral groove. Passage of a guide wire into the right ventricle may cause frequent premature ventricular beats which usually subside spontaneously with repositioning of the guide wire or lead. After ventricular and/or atrial lead placement, the pacing lead will have to be tested for sensing threshold, pacing threshold, depolarization amplitude and lead resistance. After satisfactory placement of the pacing leads, the actual pacemaker generator unit is connected and then placed in a subcutaneous pocket at the site of percutaneous lead placement.

Usual preop diagnosis: Abnormalities of S-A nodal function (SSS) or A-V nodal function (heart block)

SUMMARY OF PROCEDURE

Position	Supine
Incision	Left subclavicular; mostly percutaneous
Special instrumentation	Fluoroscopy with fluoro-table
Unique considerations	Patient usually awake with mild sedation
Antibiotics	Cefamandole 1 g iv at induction
Surgical time	1 h
EBL	Minimal
Postop care	PACU → CCU; ECG monitoring × 2-4 h; chest radiograph to document lead configuration.
Mortality	0-1%
Morbidity	Lead displacement: 1-2% Pneumothorax: 1-2%
Pain score	2

PATIENT POPULATION CHARACTERISTICS

Age range	50-80 yr
Male:Female	2:1
Incidence	Infrequent
Etiology	CAD; cardiac valve repair/replacement
Associated conditions	Complete heart block with syncope; SSS; paroxysmal tachycardia; SVT

ANESTHETIC CONSIDERATIONS

PREOPERATIVE

The indications for permanent pacemaker insertion are usually bradydysrhythmias (e.g., 3rd-degree heart block, sinus node dysfunction, etc.) or, less commonly, tachycardia (e.g., atrial flutter not responsive to medical therapy). There are many different types of pacemakers, which are classified according to the chamber paced, chamber sensed, response to sensing, programmability and antitachyrhythmia functions. The anesthesiologist should be aware of the type of pacemaker to be implanted and the means for external control.

Cardiovascular Evaluate patient for associated disease, including CAD (~50%), HTN (~20%), cardiomyopathy, CHF, valvular defect, and for any symptoms or recent changes related to the conduction problems (syncope, CHF). It is important to know the reason for pacemaker implantation and the patient's escape rhythm. These patients are often on antidysrythmics, diuretics, cardiac glycosides and a variety of other cardiovascular agents, which should be continued up to the day of surgery.
Tests: Exercise tolerance by Hx; ECG: ✓ rate, ischemic changes, rhythm. Other tests as indicated by H&P. ✓ serum digoxin and other antidysrhythmic levels.

Pacemaker If a permanent pacemaker is already in place, its type and present functional state should be assessed. (Sx of problems include chest pain, palpitations, syncope and weakness.) If no permanent pacemaker, a temporary transvenous pacemaker should be placed prior to surgery, except in unusual circumstances.
Tests: ECG: ✓ Valsalva maneuver or carotid sinus massage—may slow the heart sufficiently to allow the permanent pacemaker to fire and allow assessment of function. A rate lower than the set rate may indicate battery failure. CXR: ✓ lead continuity.

Hematologic Hct or Hb

Laboratory ✓ K^+ level, which can affect pacing threshold, lead to loss of pacemaker capture if low, or ventricular tachycardia, if high. Other tests as indicated from H&P.

Premedication Standard premedication (p. B-2).

INTRAOPERATIVE

Anesthetic technique: Permanent pacemakers are commonly placed via the transvenous route, requiring only local anesthesia and MAC with sedation. For epicardial pacemaker placement, GETA is required. These patients should be transported to OR monitored. Care is taken to avoid dislodging temporary pacing electrodes. The function of the temporary pacemaker should be checked prior to induction.

General anesthesia:

Induction Usually anesthesia can be induced with STP (3-5 mg/kg) or etomidate (0.2-0.3 mg/kg), in combination with an opiate (e.g., fentanyl 1-2 μg/kg) to attenuate the response to intubation. Vecuronium or pancuronium (0.1 mg/kg) will provide adequate muscle relaxation.

Maintenance Standard maintenance (p. B-3). Avoid excessive hyperventilation (→ ↓K^+) and use volatile agents with caution, as they may increase A-V conduction time.

Emergence Generally, patient is extubated at the end of the case.

Blood and Fluid requirements Minimal fluid requirements
IV: 16 ga × 1
NS/LR @ 4-6 ml/kg/h

Monitoring	Standard monitors (p. B-1). Urinary catheter	Rarely, arterial line if patient disease indicates.
Electrocautery interference	Minimize by: • Using bipolar cautery, if possible. • Grounding pad on leg. • Limiting cautery output. • Limiting cautery use.	The use of electrocautery may interfere with pacemaker function and result in dysrhythmias or failure of the pacemaker. Monitor ECG and pulse (since electrical activity does not mean CO) for interference. Have a magnet available to convert the pacemaker to asynchronous mode (check that this is possible and will not change the programming of the pacemaker).
Complications	Dysrhythmias Air embolism Cardiac tamponade Hemo/pneumothorax Hemorrhage	Availability of temporary pacing is important because complete heart block or dislodgement of leads may occur. In addition, pharmacologic agents (atropine, 0.5-2 mg; isoproterenol 10-100 ng/kg/min) to increase HR should be available.

POSTOPERATIVE

Complications	Dislodging of electrodes Dysrhythmias Pneumothorax Tamponade
Pain management	Parenteral opioids for pain relief Benzodiazepine for sedation
Tests	ECG CXR Electrolytes

References

1. Atlee J: Cardiac pacing and electroconversion. In *Cardiac Anesthesia*, 3rd edition. Kaplan J, ed. WB Saunders, Philadelphia: 1993, Ch 26, 877-904.
2. Matthews EL, Atlee JL, Luck JC, Martin DE: Anesthesia for patients with electrophysiologic disorders. In *A Practical Approach to Cardiac Anesthesia*, 2nd edition. Hensley FA, Martin DE, eds. Little, Brown, Boston: 1995, Ch 14, 392-415.

PERICARDIECTOMY

SURGICAL CONSIDERATIONS

Description: Constrictive pericarditis, either acute or chronic, interferes with ventricular filling, reducing stroke volume and depressing the cardiac index (CI). Although there are many possible etiologies (infectious, nephrogenic, postradiation), the cause remains unknown for a majority of patients. Typically, patients present with a progressive Hx of breathlessness, fatigability, or peripheral or abdominal swelling, often months to years after the inciting event. The diagnosis may be confirmed by cardiac catheterization, with equalization of end diastolic pressures, although volume loading may be necessary to demonstrate this in the patient under medical management. The differentiation between constrictive pericardial disease and restrictive myocardial disease may be difficult, if not impossible, and may coexist in a single patient. Once this diagnosis has been confirmed, surgical **pericardiectomy** should be undertaken, since the outlook without surgical relief is one of gradual, but persistent deterioration. Although surgical mortality remains in the 10-15% range, long-term relief for survivors is good. Since these patients are usually significantly hemodynamically compromised, intensive monitoring is indicated. Approach may be through a **median sternotomy** or left **anterolateral thoracotomy.** Removal of both visceral and parietal pericardium is essential for relief, but dense adhesions of these layers to underlying muscle may make this dissection very difficult, tedious and bloody, especially if the visceral pericardium and epicardium are involved in the constrictive process. CPB (see p. 217) may be utilized for hemodynamic instability, but it obviously increases bleeding complications. Complete excision from both ventricular surfaces is mandatory. Most perioperative difficulties evolve from cardiac failure.

Variant procedure or approaches: A limited **pericardial window**, draining fluid into the left hemithorax, may relieve tamponade, but will be of no benefit for a true constrictive process.

Usual preop diagnosis: Constrictive pericarditis

SUMMARY OF PROCEDURE

	Median Sternotomy	Anterolateral Thoracotomy
Position	Supine	Supine, with elevation of left hemithorax
Incision	Midline	Fifth interspace
Special instrumentation	TEE; full hemodynamic monitoring; CPB standby	⇐
Antibiotics	Cefamandole 1 g iv at induction	⇐
Surgical time	2-5 h, depending on tenacity of visceral peel	⇐
Closing considerations	Avoid volume overload and cardiac distention. Chronically depressed hearts may require inotropic or mechanical support (i.e., IABP) postop.	⇐
EBL	100-500 ml	⇐
Postop care	ICU; intubated × 4-6 h. Hemodynamic monitoring. Low CO state may persist postop.	⇐
Mortality	5-15%, predominantly from cardiac failure	⇐
Morbidity	Persistent CHF: 5% Transient phrenic nerve dysfunction: < 1%	⇐
Pain score	7-10	7-10

PATIENT POPULATION CHARACTERISTICS

Age range	10-80 yr (median = 45 yr)
Male:Female	2:1
Incidence	3-4 patients/yr at tertiary referral center
Etiology	Majority unknown. Infectious, radiation, prior cardiac operation, rheumatic pericarditis, amyloid deposition.
Associated conditions	Restrictive myocardial diseases

ANESTHETIC CONSIDERATIONS

PREOPERATIVE

Pericardiectomy is most commonly performed for patients with constrictive pericarditis, while pericardial window procedures are used for patients with cardiac tamponade.

Respiratory Restrictive disease may be present due to fibrosis (e.g., post TB) or pleural effusions. This may impair oxygenation and, if the effusions are significant, may ↓venous return on institution of IPPV, resulting in rapid decompensation (↓CO). Drain prior to surgery.

Tests: CXR: ✓ active disease, fibrosis, effusions, pericardial calcification. Consider ABG; PFT, as indicated by CXR and Sx, and if time permits.

Cardiovascular Of importance is the presence or absence of a pericardial effusion. A large effusion which develops slowly (chronic pericarditis) may cause little or no Sx. Conversely, a small and rapidly forming effusion may lead to cardiac tamponade. While the cardiovascular signs for both tamponade and constriction are similar (pulsus paradoxus, venous HTN, exaggerated venous pulsations, hypotension, tachycardia), it is important to differentiate between them as it may affect intraop

Cardiovascular, cont. management. Constrictive pericarditis can be differentiated from cardiac tamponade by ECHO, by pulsus paradoxus (frequent with tamponade; rare with constrictive pericarditis). Kussmaul's sign (distention of the jugular veins on inspiration) is rare with tamponade and common with constrictive pericarditis. Electrical alternans is present with tamponade and absent in constrictive pericarditis. Examination of the RV pressure wave form is unchanged in tamponade, but shows a dip and prominent Y descent in constrictive pericarditis.

Anesthetic management is influenced by the planned procedure, the underlying process (constriction or tamponade) and its severity. Clues to severity are the physical symptoms and the degree of tachycardia, hypotension and the filling pressure. (While it is not possible to give exact figures, a HR of >100 bpm, systolic BP < 100 mmHg and a filling pressure > 15 mmHg are probably significant.) In addition, it is important to assess concurrent cardiac problems: cardiomyopathy, CAD or valvular disease (especially in constrictive disease associated with TB, radiation therapy or in rheumatoid diseases such as lupus).

Tests: ECG: ✓ low-voltage complexes, electrical alternans. ECHO: ✓ pericardial effusion, calcification of pericardium, valvular lesions, myocardial function.

Gastrointestinal Chronic hepatic congestion may lead to decreased synthetic function (↓procoagulants). Development of ascites may result in ↑intraabdominal pressure. Because of this and the fact that these are sometimes emergency procedures, consider possible full stomach.

Tests: Consider LFTs; PT; PTT

Renal Renal failure may cause pericarditis and, conversely, pericarditis may cause renal failure (2° prerenal factors: ↑venous pressure, ↓perfusion pressure). This may affect the choice of drugs used for anesthesia that depend on renal clearance (particularly muscle relaxants).

Tests: BUN; creatinine, consider creatinine clearance; electrolytes

Hematologic Some renal or hepatic conditions may be associated with coagulation disorders. These include both procoagulant and Plt problems. If possible, any coagulopathy should be corrected prior to surgery with FFP, platelets or both. Consult with a hematologist if necessary.

Tests: Hb/Hct; PT; PTT; Plt count

Laboratory Other tests as indicated from H&P.

Premedication Little or no premedication may be indicated. Otherwise, a benzodiazepine may be used (e.g., midazolam 0.05-0.2 mg/kg im). Consider full-stomach precautions: H_2-antagonists (e.g., ranitidine 50 mg iv), metoclopramide (10 mg iv), antacids (e.g., Na citrate 0.3 M 30 ml po).

INTRAOPERATIVE

Anesthetic technique: GETA. Consider pericardiocentesis or pericardial window under local anesthesia prior to induction, as drainage of even a small amount of fluid may dramatically improve the patient's status. The considerable manipulation of the heart, extensive dissection, blood loss, dysrhythmias and unrelieved tamponade make pericardiectomy cases a challenge.

Induction Typically, ketamine 1-2 mg/kg or etomidate 0.2-0.3 mg/kg ± narcotic (fentanyl 2-30 μg/kg), depending on patient status. Consider maintaining spontaneous ventilation in tamponade patients until drained, as institution of IPPV may result in rapid decompensation and cardiac arrest due to ↓↓venous return. Otherwise, succinylcholine (1 mg/kg) with cricoid pressure (full stomach) or pancuronium (0.1 mg/kg) for muscle relaxation.

Maintenance Narcotic (total fentanyl 5-50 μg/kg), low-dose volatile agent, midazolam (50-350 μg/kg), or a combination of these agents in 100% O_2. CO is dependent on maintaining a high preload to ensure adequate cardiac filling, avoiding and treating bradycardia and preserving myocardial contractility. The use of inotropes (dobutamine, isoproterenol or epinephrine) may be necessary. α-agonists should be avoided but, on occasion, may be needed to increase coronary perfusion. These anesthetic considerations apply to both tamponade and constrictive disease.

Emergence In general, plan for extubation in the OR in the case of pericardial window and transport to ICU for postop ventilation 4-24 h following pericardiectomy.

Blood and fluid requirements

IV: 14 ga (or 7 Fr) × 1-2
UO: 0.5-1 ml/kg/h
Warm fluids and humidify gases.
T&C 2-4 U for pericardiectomy.

During pericardiectomy, anticipate rapid blood loss (a major cause of mortality). For this reason, CPB should be available on standby for all pericardiectomy procedures.

Monitoring	Standard monitors (p. B-1) Arterial line CVP line PA catheter TEE Urinary catheter	All monitors should be placed prior to induction. PA catheters aid the management of filling pressures, CO and afterload. TEE may be useful to gauge filling volume and degree of relief of pericardial constriction.
Complications	Cardiac tamponade Dysrhythmias	Intrathoracic pressure associated with IPPV may produce a ↓↓CO in these patients (because of ↓venous return). Spontaneous ventilation, therefore, is preferred until the tamponade is drained.
	Hemorrhage Coagulopathy	Hemorrhage is not usually a problem unless penetrating trauma is the cause of the tamponade.
	Heart failure	Once constriction is relieved, myocardial function does not return to normal quickly. Inotropes are often needed. Due to extensive dissection and hemorrhage, coagulopathies may develop and should be treated aggressively.
Positioning	✓ and pad pressure points. ✓ eyes.	

POSTOPERATIVE

Complications	Hemorrhage Coagulopathy Ventricular hypofunction Dysrhythmias Ischemia	Following pericardial window surgery, patients improve with the relief of the tamponade. Postpericardiectomy patients, however, may have a continuation of intraop dysrhythmias and myocardial depression. Inotropes (e.g., dopamine 5-10 μg/kg/min) may be needed for 24-48 h. Normal cardiac function can take 4-6 wk to return.
Pain management	Parenteral opioids	Supplement with benzodiazepine for sedation.
Tests	ECG CXR ABG Coagulation profile Electrolytes	

References

1. Lake CL: Anesthesia and pericardial disease. *Anesth Analg* 1983; 62(4):431-43.
2. McCaughan BC, Schaff HV, Piehler JM, Danielson GK, Orszulak TA, Puga JR, Connolly DC, McGoon DC: Early and late results of pericardiectomy for constrictive pericarditis. *J Thorac Cardiovasc Surg* 1985; 89:340.
3. Oliver WC, DeCastro M, Strickland PA: Uncommon diseases and cardiac anesthesia. In *Cardiac Anesthesia*, 3rd edition. Kaplan JA, ed. WB Saunders, Philadelphia: 1993, Ch 24, 819-64.
4. Reich DL, Brooks JL, Kaplan JA: Uncommon cardiac disease. In *Anesthesia and Uncommon Diseases*, 3rd edition. Katz J, Benumof JL, Kadis LB, eds. WB Saunders Co, Philadelphia: 1990, Ch 8, 356-61.

MINIMALLY INVASIVE AND PORT-ACCESS CORONARY REVASCULARIZATION

SURGICAL CONSIDERATIONS

Description: Along with advances in videoscopic technology, a less invasive approach has become the treatment of choice for many general and thoracic surgical diseases. Progress in less invasive surgery has led to the development of alternative methods of cardiac surgery.[2,6,8,9,13,14,16,17] One technique—**minimally invasive coronary artery bypass grafting (MICABG)**—involves the use of a small, anterior mediastinotomy or a limited left thoracotomy to access the target coronary artery with the anastomosis performed on a beating heart. In this manner, cardiopulmonary bypass (CPB) and cardioplegic arrest are unnecessary,[2,6,12,15] and the complications associated with those procedures are avoided. Another method employs an **endovascular or port-access system** (Heartport, Inc., Redwood City, CA) that uses CPB (femoral artery-to-femoral vein, Fig 6.1-5) and cardioplegic arrest, allowing the surgeon to perform various cardiac procedures in a still and bloodless field through similarly small mediastinotomy or thoracotomy incisions.[8,9,16,17] The safety and efficacy (in terms of graft patency and survival data) of these less invasive approaches to coronary artery bypass grafting (CABG) await long-term follow-up evaluations.

CABG without CPB: Since the early 1960s, coronary artery grafting has been performed via a median sternotomy incision on a beating heart without CPB.[7,11,18] Although this technique was employed for first-time and reoperative coronary revascularization, it was later abandoned by most surgeons as cardiac procedures became more complex and the technique of CPB with cardioplegic arrest became safer to use.[1,10] Because of concern for the ill effects of CPB, and with the availability of newer drugs to decrease the heart rate, CABG on a beating heart has been reexamined as an alternative to the conventional approach.[3-5] In the last 15 to 20 years, more than 2,000 cases of coronary revascularization without CPB via a median sternotomy have been performed.[3,4]

In order to decrease the invasiveness of a median sternotomy, many surgeons have employed a **limited thoracotomy exposure** (or MICABG).[2,6,12,15] Through this incision, the internal mammary artery is mobilized under direct vision or, occasionally, with thoracoscopic assistance, and the internal mammary artery-to-coronary anastomosis performed (Figs 6.1-6, 6.1-7). Currently, single-vessel coronary artery disease (CAD), involving the left anterior descending artery, appears to be the primary indication for MICABG.[5] Reported advantages of coronary revascularization without CPB in-

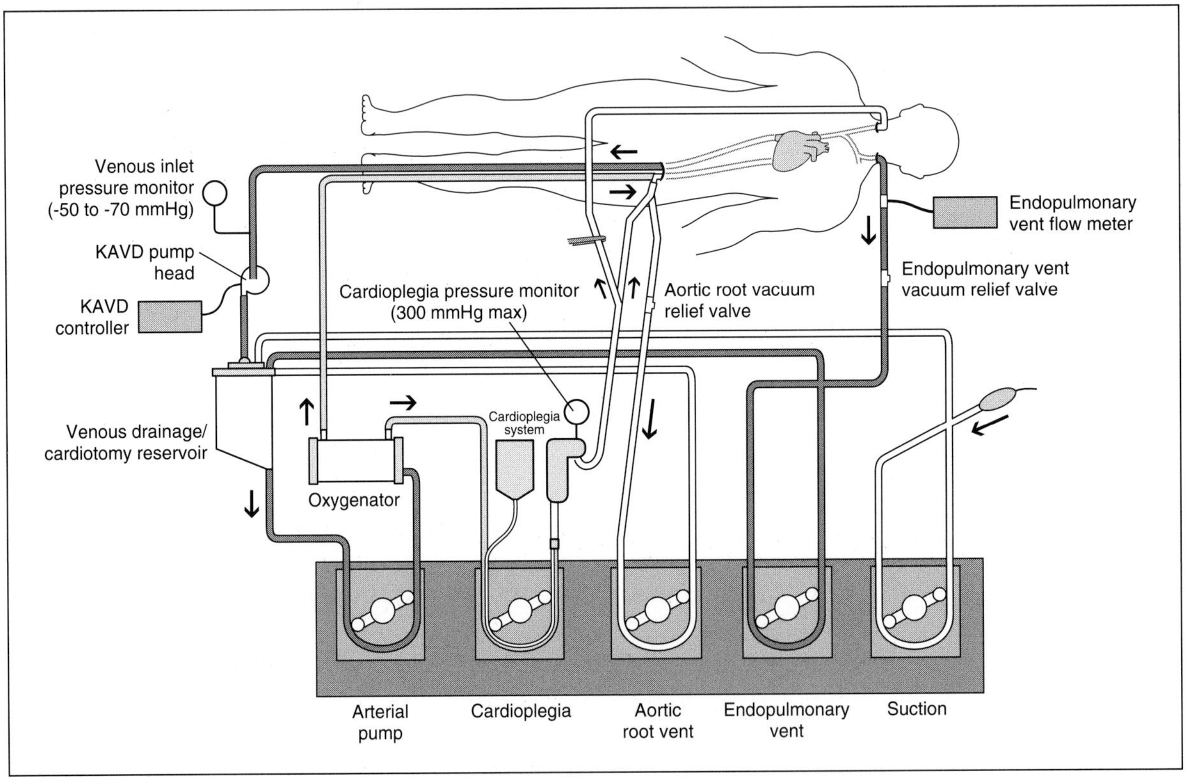

Figure 6.1-5. Schematic diagram of femoral vein-to-femoral artery (fem-fem) bypass.

clude decreased transfusion requirements, shorter hospitalization, and decreased cost.[3,5,6] Additionally, patients with compromised left ventricular function, the elderly and those requiring a reoperation may benefit from this technique. Coronary revascularization without CPB, however, may be technically more demanding than conventional methods; also, it may not be possible in some patients, and may be associated with variable results[4-6] A small left anterior descending artery and a small left internal mammary artery contribute to the technical difficulty of this approach. Although temporary occlusion of left anterior descending artery during the anastomosis is usually not problematic,[6] hemodynamic instability or arrhythmias can develop. A technically satisfactory result is critically dependent on the size of the coronary artery and satisfactory hemodynamics during cardiac retraction for exposure.[4] Hemodynamic instability from cardiac manipulation to expose the posterior descending artery and the obtuse marginal artery likely requires the use of CPB.

Port-access CABG: Peters devised a method of minimally invasive cardiac surgery using an aortic balloon catheter that provides aortic occlusion, cardioplegia delivery and aortic root venting.[13] Modifications of this design provide the basis for the present endovascular system for CPB and cardioplegic arrest (Fig. 6.1-8). Utilizing the port-access system, the surgeon can perform various cardiac operations, including coronary revascularization and intracardiac procedures (e.g., valve surgery), through smaller chest incisions, avoiding a median sternotomy.

The endoaortic clamp is a peripherally inserted, triple-lumen catheter with an inflatable balloon at its distal end (Heartport,

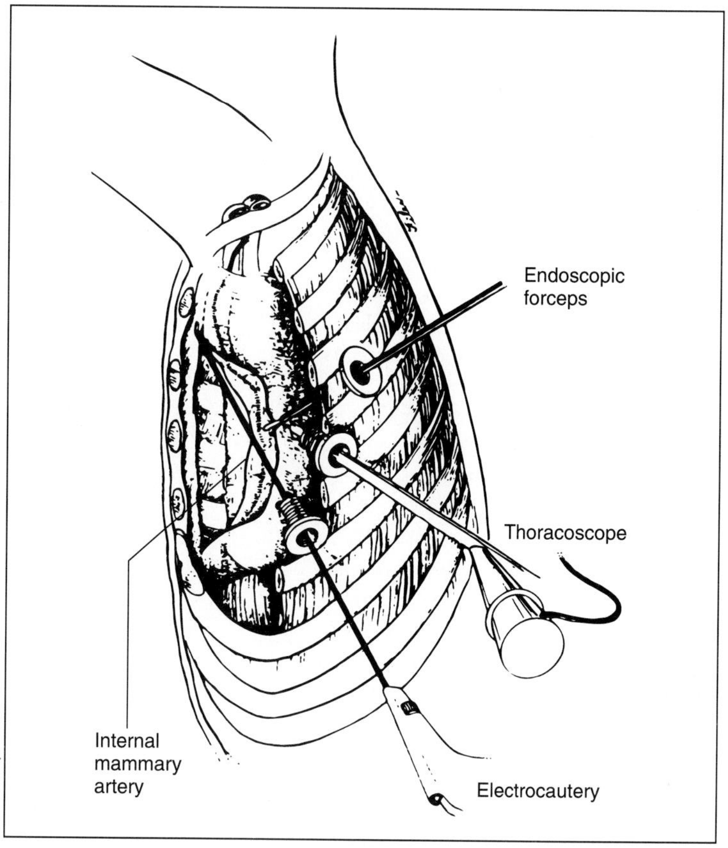

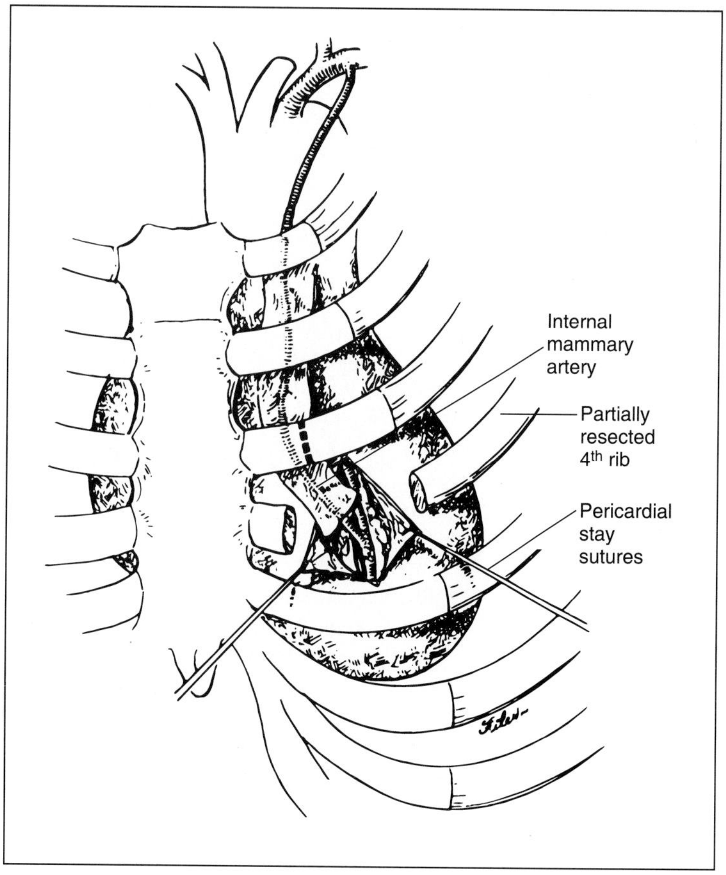

Figure 6.1-6. (Top) Dissection and harvesting of the left internal mammary artery using a thoracoscopic approach. (Redrawn with permission from Acuff TE, et al: Minimally invasive coronary artery bypass grafting. *Ann Thorac Surg* 1996; 61:135-7.)

Figure 6.1-7. (Right) The left internal mammary artery-to-left anterior descending artery anastomosis is performed under direct vision. Stay sutures suspend the pericardium and bring the heart into view. (Redrawn with permission from Acuff TE, et al: Minimally invasive coronary artery bypass grafting. *Ann Thorac Surg* 1996; 61:135-7.)

Inc.)[9,16,17] The endoaortic balloon "clamp" is positioned in the ascending aorta using fluoroscopy and transesophageal echocardiography guidance. The lumen used for balloon inflation is connected to a manometer to monitor balloon pressure. Cardioplegic solution is delivered through a central lumen, which also acts as an aortic root vent after cardioplegia delivery. A third lumen serves as an aortic root pressure monitor. Percutaneously placed through the jugular vein, the pulmonary artery venting catheter assists in ventricular decompression. The left internal mammary artery is grafted to the left anterior descending artery, and is harvested under direct vision and with video-assisted thoracoscopy. After peripheral CPB is achieved, the endoaortic clamp provides aortic occlusion and cardioplegic arrest. Recent experience with port-access coronary revascularization has been extended experimentally and clinically into multivessel CABG.[8,9] With cardioplegic arrest, better exposure of the lateral and posterior aspects of the heart is achieved, thereby permitting two- and three-vessel port-access coronary revascularization.

Usual preop diagnosis: CAD

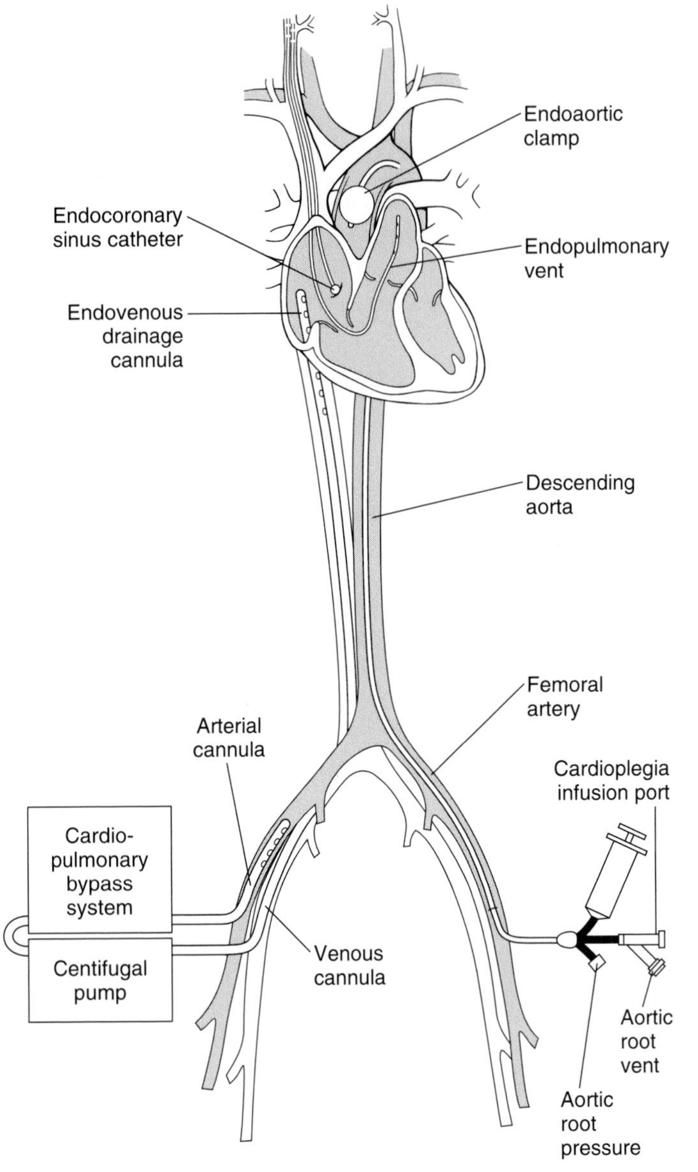

Figure 6.1-8. The port-access cardiopulmonary bypass (CPB) system. Femoro-femoral (fem-fem)CPB is utilized, and a centrifugal pump augments venous drainage. The endoaortic balloon occlusion catheter is inflated in the ascending aorta, and antegrade cardioplegia is delivered through the central lumen. The endopulmonary vent assists in ventricular decompression. (Redrawn with permission from Fann JI, et al: Port-access cardiac operations with cardioplegic arrest. *Ann Thorac Surg* 1997; 63:S35-9.)

SUMMARY OF PROCEDURE

	MICABG	Port-access CABG
Position	Supine	⇐
Incision	4th interspace, left anterior mediastinotomy for left coronary bypass; right-sided approach for right coronary artery bypass. May resect 4th rib; ports for possible thoracoscopy; internal mammary artery harvested.	4th interspace, left anterior mediastinotomy for left coronary bypass; right-sided approach for right coronary artery bypass. May resect 4th rib; ports for possible thoracoscopy; internal mammary artery harvested.
Special instrumentation	Specially designed retractors and cardiac stabilizing instruments.	⇐ TEE and fluoroscopy are necessary to guide endoaortic clamp.
Unique considerations	CPB unnecessary; coronary anastomosis is performed with beating heart. Hemodynamic instability may occur during cardiac retrac-	CPB used with peripheral femoral cannulation; coronary anastomosis performed on still, nonbeating heart. Monitor for effects of

	MICABG	Port-access CABG
Unique considerations, cont.	tion. May require conversion to open procedure with sternotomy. Pharmacologic intervention (β-blockers, adenosine, etc.) may be needed to assist in cardiac stabilization.	CPB. May require conversion to open procedure with sternotomy.
	OLV may be required during internal mammary takedown (IMA).	⇐
Antibiotics	Cefazolin 1-2 g iv at induction	⇐
Surgical time	2-3 h	3-6 h
Closing considerations	Assess chest wall for hemorrhage; chest tube inserted.	⇐
EBL	50-250 ml	250-500 ml
Postop care	ICU monitoring; early extubation; may require inotropic support.	⇐
Mortality	1-2%, depending on comorbidities.	⇐
Morbidity	2-5% (overall)	⇐
	Myocardial infarction (MI)	⇐
	Kinking or thrombosis of graft (graft failure)	⇐
	Chest-wall hemorrhage	⇐
	Arrhythmias	Problems associated with femoral artery/vein cannulation (e.g., arterial dissection) and CPB.
Pain score	1-4	1-4

PATIENT POPULATION CHARACTERISTICS

Age range	40-80 yr (mean age, mid 60s)
Male:Female	3-4:1
Incidence	Common
Etiology	Atherosclerosis
Associated conditions	LV dysfunction; chronic obstructive pulmonary disease; PVD; ischemic mitral regurgitation; diabetes mellitus

---

ANESTHETIC CONSIDERATIONS FOR MICABG

PREOPERATIVE

Preop assessment is similar to that used for standard CABG patients (see p. 223). Relative contraindications for MICABG include: low EF, morbid obesity, previous cardiac surgery and COPD. Atrial fibrillation makes MICABG very difficult and is a strong relative contraindication.

Premedication Adequate control of preop anxiety using midazolam (titrated to effect) may reduce the dose of β-blocker required intraop for rate control.

INTRAOPERATIVE

Anesthetic technique: GETA. Double-lumen ETT or Univent ETT.

Induction As for CABG surgery (p. 224). These patients will undergo a small anterior thoracotomy, and the aim is to extubate them at the end of the procedure or shortly thereafter. Thus, the dose of narcotic should be reduced (e.g., fentanyl 5-15 μg/kg). Long-acting muscle relaxants should be avoided for the same reason. Consider spinal narcotics (e.g., morphine 0.3-0.5 mg).

Maintenance Since early extubation is planned, volatile agents or propofol should be used, and the overall dose of narcotic reduced.

Emergence If the patient is not suitable for extubation in the OR, the double-lumen ETT may be exchanged for a conventional ETT (over a tube changer) prior to transport to ICU.

Blood and fluid requirements	See CABG surgery (p. 225).	
Monitoring	See CABG surgery (p. 225).	PA catheters are useful in patients with poor LV function to detect ischemia.
	TEE	Useful to detect ischemia and LV dysfunction.
Special considerations	Temporary occlusion → ischemia Vessel immobilization → ↓CO Need for ↓HR	During grafting, the vessel is temporarily occluded by surgeon to avoid blood flooding the field. The myocardium distal to this may become ischemic. ✓ ECG, TEE. In addition, the surgeon will place instruments to immobilize the vessel being grafted. Pressure from these instruments may impair cardiac function. It may be necessary to ↓ HR to facilitate the anastomosis. This is done with esmolol (titrated to effect), diltiazem (5-25 mg over 10 min), adenosine (6-45 mg) or a combination of these drugs.
Positioning	✓ and pad pressure points. ✓ eyes.	

POSTOPERATIVE

Complications	See CABG surgery (p. 226). Premature extubation	
Pain management	Same as CABG surgery (p. 226).	Intrathecal narcotics or intercostal blocks placed at the end of surgery may aid in early extubation.
Tests	See CABG surgery (p. 226).	

References–Surgeon's

1. Ankeney LJ: To use or not to use the pump oxygenator in coronary bypass operations. *Ann Thorac Surg* 1975; 19:108-9.
2. Benetti FJ, Ballester C, Sani G, Doonstra P, Grandjean J: Video assisted coronary bypass surgery. *J Card Surg* 1995; 10:620-25.
3. Benetti FJ, Naselli G, Wood M, Geffner L: Direct myocardial revascularization without extracorporeal circulation. Experience in 700 patients. *Chest* 1991; 100:312-16.
4. Buffolo E, deAndrade JCS, Branco JNR, Teles CA, Aguiar LF, Gomes WJ: Coronary artery bypass grafting without cardiopulmonary bypass. *Ann Thorac Surg* 1996; 61:63-6.
5. Calafiore AM, Angelini GD, Bergsland J, Salerno TA: Minimally invasive coronary artery bypass grafting. *Ann Thorac Surg* 1996; 62:1545-48.
6. Calafiore AM, DiGiammarco G, Teodori G, Bosco G, D'Annunzio E, Barsotti A, Maddestra N, Paloscia L, Vitolla G, Sciarra A, Fino C, Contini M: Left anterior descending coronary artery grafting via left anterior small thoracotomy without cardiopulmonary bypass. *Ann Thorac Surg* 1996; 61:1658-65.
7. Demikhov VP: *Experimental transplantation of vital organs* (authorized translation from Russian). New York: Consultant Bureau Enterprises, 1962; 220-27.
8. Fann JI, Peters WS, Burdon TA, Stevens JH, Pompili MF, Rosenfeldt FI, Reitz BA: Port-access two-vessel coronary revascularization in the dog (abst). *J Am Coll Cardiol* 1997; 29(A):466A.
9. Fann JI, Pompili MF, Stevens H, Siegel LC, StGoar FG, Burdon TA, Reitz BA: Port-access cardiac surgery with cardioplegic arrest. *Ann Thorac Surg* 1997; 63:S-35-9.
10. Favaloro RG, Effler DB, Groves LK, Sheldon WC, Sones FM: Direct myocardial revascularization by saphenous vein graft. Present operative technique and indication. *Ann Thorac Surg* 1970; 10:97-111.
11. Kolesov VI: Mammary artery-coronary artery anastomosis as method of treatment of angina pectoris. *J Thorac Cardiovasc Surg* 1967; 54:535-44.
12. Nataf P, Lima L, Regan M, Benarim S, Pavie A, Cabrol C, Gandjbakch I: Minimally invasive coronary surgery with thoracoscopic internal mammary artery dissection: Surgical technique. *J Card Surg* 1996; 11:288-92.
13. Peters WS: Minimally invasive cardiac surgery by cardioscopy. *Australas J Cardiac Thorac Surg* 1993; 2(3):152-54.
14. Robinson MC, Gross DR, Zeman W, Stedje-Larson E: Minimally invasive coronary artery bypass grafting: A new method using an anterior mediastinotomy. *J Card Surg* 1995; 10:529-36.
15. Shennib H, Lee AGL, Akin J: Safe and effective method of stabilization for coronary artery bypass grafting on the beating heart. *Ann Thorac Surg* 1997; 63:988-92.
16. Stevens JH, Burdon TA, Peters WS, Siegel LC, Pompili MF, Vierra MA, StGoar FG, Ribakove GH, Mitchell RS, Reitz BA: Port-access coronary artery bypass grafting: A proposed surgical method. *J Thorac Cardiovasc Surg* 1996; 111:567-73.
17. Stevens JH, Burdon TA, Siegel LC, Petes WS, Pompili MF, StGoar FG, Berry GJ, Ribakove GH, Vierra MA, Mitchell RS, Toomasian JM, Reitz BA: Port-access coronary artery bypass with cardioplegic arrest: Acute and chronic canine studies. *Ann Thorac Surg* 1996; 62:435-41.
18. Trapp WG, Bisary R: Placement of coronary artery bypass graft without pump oxygenator. *Ann Thorac Surg* 1975; 19:1-9.

References–Anesthesiologist's

1. Gayes JM, Emery RW: The MIDCAB experience: A current look at evolving surgical and anesthetic approaches. *J Cardiothorac Vasc Anesth* 1997; 11:625-28.
2. Gayes JM, Emery RW, Nissen M: Anesthetic considerations for patients undergoing minimally invasive coronary bypass surgery: ministernotomy and minithoracotomy approaches. *J Cardiothorac Vasc Anesth* 1996; 10:531-35.
3. Greenspun HG, Adourian UA, Fonger JD, Fann JS: Minimally invasive direct coronary artery bypass (MIDCAB): surgical techniques and anesthetic considerations. *J Cardiothorac Vasc Anesth* 1996; 10(4):507-9.

LIMITED THORACOTOMY AND PORT-ACCESS APPROACH TO MITRAL VALVE SURGERY

SURGICAL CONSIDERATIONS

Description: Although the field of mitral valve surgery has seen marked advances in biomaterials and innovative repair techniques since the early 1960s,[2,4,6,8] the conventional median sternotomy approach to access and expose the mitral valve has not changed substantially. Because of the progress in video-assisted surgery, a less invasive approach to cardiac surgery has been proposed, and various techniques of mitral valve surgery through limited thoracotomy or upper sternotomy incisions and a port-access technique (Heartport, Redwood City, CA) to achieve cardioplegic arrest are currently being evaluated in the clinical setting.[1,3,5,7,10-17]

Limited thoracotomy: The right thoracotomy incision is a less invasive approach (compared to median sternotomy) for mitral valve procedures (Fig 6.1-9).[3,9,10,12,18] Utilizing hypothermic fibrillatory or cardioplegic arrest, the mitral valve, annulus and subvalvular apparatus can be visualized directly and the valve procedure carried out. The recent addition of video-assisted thoracoscopy to mitral valve surgery has resulted in even smaller thoracotomy incisions for mitral valve procedures.[3,10]

Chitwood, et al, reported a **"micro-mitral" approach** to mitral valve replacement, using video-assisted thoracosopy through a 5-cm thoracotomy.[3] Peripheral cardiopulmonary bypass (fem-fem) is used and a catheter placed in the coronary sinus for retrograde cardioplegia delivery. An external aortic cross-clamp is introduced through a separate incision. After achieving cardioplegic arrest, the mitral valve is replaced with thoracoscopic assistance. Proposed advantages of the micro-mitral approach include the avoidance of a sternotomy with decreased chest-wall trauma and patient discomfort.[3]

Navia and Cosgrove described a **right parasternal approach** for mitral valve surgery,[12] using a 10-cm parasternal incision and right internal mammary artery ligation to enhance exposure. Cardiopulmonary bypass (CPB) is established with femoral artery and femoral vein cannulations, along with direct cannulation of the SVC. The aorta is cross-clamped externally and antegrade cardioplegia administered; supplemental retrograde cardioplegia is given through a catheter placed in the coronary sinus.

Arom and Emery presented an alternative **partial sternotomy approach** to mitral and aortic valve surgery.[1] The 7-cm partial sternotomy permits aortic and right atrial cannulation for CPB; the external aortic cross-clamp is positioned and a left ventricular vent is placed through the right superior pulmonary vein. Mitral valve exposure is achieved through the dome of the left atrium.

Port-access mitral valve surgery: The port-access system has been used successfully in mitral valve surgery.[5,7,11,13-15] To facilitate dissection and to provide adequate exposure of the left atrium, double-lumen endobronchial intubation for single-lung ventilation is used. Under fluoroscopic and TEE guidance, a retrograde cardioplegia catheter is directed into the coronary sinus via an introducer placed in the jugular vein; a pulmonary artery-venting catheter is inserted through another jugular vein introducer. A limited right thoracotomy is made with or without resection of a short segment of the fourth rib, followed by the placement of a soft-tissue retractor. A separate port is placed in the 6th interspace for introduction of a thoracoscope, if necessary. The pericardium is opened anterior to the phrenic nerve. After systemic heparinization, the femoral artery and vein are cannulated. The endoaortic clamp is introduced through the side limb of the femoral arterial cannula and its tip positioned in the ascending aorta. CPB is initiated and systemic hypothermia achieved. The balloon of the endoaortic clamp is inflated, achieving effective aortic occlusion. Cold blood cardioplegia is delivered using the distal port of the endoaortic clamp; retrograde cardioplegia is administered via the coronary sinus catheter. A left atriotomy is made, and an atrial retractor is placed through a separate port. Valve repair or replacement is carried out using specially designed instruments. Prior to completion of atriotomy closure, deairing maneuvers are accomplished. These include temporarily discontinuing pulmonary and aortic root venting, inflating the lungs to displace residual air and increasing the patient's blood volume from the venous reservoir. Also, the patient is placed in a Trendelenburg and left lateral decubitus position for further deairing. The balloon of the endoaortic catheter is deflated, and the catheter is left in place for further deairing through the aortic vent lumen. Temporary ventricular pacing wires are placed. After being weaned from CPB, the patient is decannulated and the anticoagulation reversed.

The overall safety and efficacy of less invasive mitral valve surgery await long-term evaluations and followup.

Usual preop diagnosis: Mitral valve disease

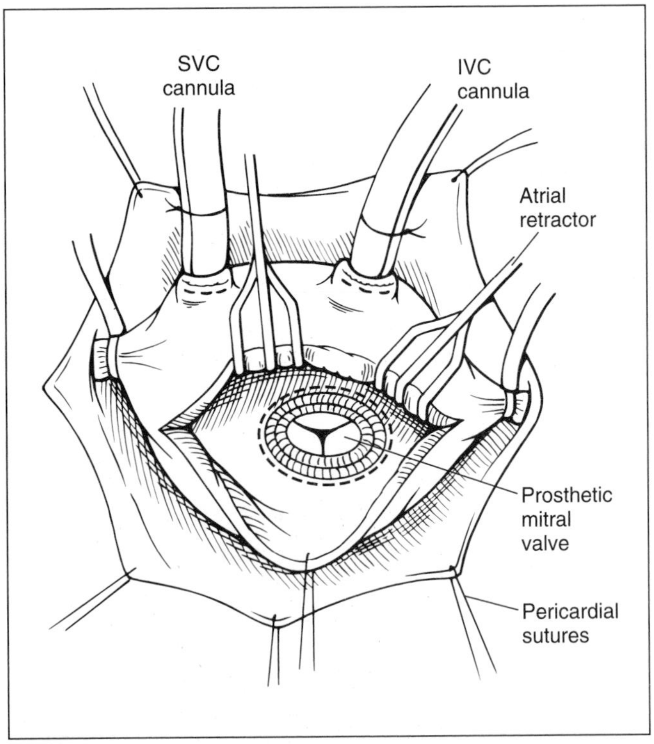

Figure 6.1-9. The right thoracotomy approach with left atriotomy and exposure of the mitral valve area with prosthetic valve in place. (Reproduced with permission from Tribble, et al: Anterolateral thoracotomy as an alternative to repeat median sternotomy for replacement of the mitral valve. *Ann Thorac Surg* 1987; 43:380-82.)

SUMMARY OF PROCEDURE

	Port-Access	Limited Thoracotomy
Position	Supine, with right side slightly elevated	⇐
Incision	4th interspace right thoracotomy; 4th rib may be resected; ports for possible thoracoscopy; port for atrial retractor.	⇐ ± Port for aortic cross-clamp
Special instrumentation	Specially designed retractors; TEE and fluoroscopy for guiding placement of endopulmonary vent, retrograde cardioplegia catheter and endoaortic clamp.	Specially designed instruments ± thorascopic instruments
Unique considerations	CPB is achieved with peripheral femoral cannulation; placement of endopulmonary vent; placement of retrograde cardioplegia catheter; may require conversion to open procedure.	CPB via femoral artery and vein
Antibiotics	Cefazolin 1-2 g iv at induction	⇐
Surgical time	3-5 h	⇐
Closing considerations	Assess chest wall for hemorrhage.	⇐
EBL	250-500 ml	⇐
Postop care	ICU monitoring; early extubation; may require inotropic support.	⇐
Mortality	5%, depending on comorbidities.	⇐
Morbidity	2-5% (overall)	⇐
	Chest-wall hemorrhage	–
	Vascular injury	–
	Pneumonia	⇐
	Atrial fibrillation	⇐

	Port-Access	Limited Thoracotomy
Morbidity, cont.	Stroke	–
	Renal failure	–
Pain score	1-4	4-7

PATIENT POPULATION CHARACTERISTICS

Age range	40-70 yr
Male:Female	1:1
Incidence	Unknown (new procedures)
Etiology	Myxomatous mitral valve; rheumatic valve disease; endocarditis; ischemic (papillary muscle dysfunction); mitral annular calcification
Associated conditions	Pulmonary HTN; atrial arrhythmias; CAD; aortic valve disease; tricuspid regurgitation

ANESTHETIC CONSIDERATIONS FOR PORT-ACCESS CARDIAC SURGERY (VALVULAR AND CABG PROCEDURES)

PREOPERATIVE

As with all anesthetic procedures, the use of the port-access system should not be attempted without appropriate training. Catheter placement and monitoring relies heavily on TEE. The evaluation of the patient for port-access cardiac surgery should parallel that of patients having conventional cardiac surgery. (For mitral valve surgery, see p. 232; for CABG surgery, see p. 223.) There are, however, a number of specific conditions which preclude the use of the port-access system:

1. Aortic regurgitation (AR): While mild-to-moderate AR is not a contraindication, it may make the delivery of anterograde cardioplegia via the endoaortic clamp catheter (EAC) problematic; therefore, insertion of the endocoronary sinus catheter (ESC) is very important. Severe AR is a contraindication.
2. Atheromatous disease of the aorta: The retrograde perfusion system may be associated with embolization of atheromatous plaques (particularly pedunculated lesions).
3. Peripheral vascular disease (PVD): Femoral bypass may be associated with retrograde arterial dissection. PVD and tortuous femoral and iliac vessels are contraindications.
4. Thoracic aortic aneurysm/Marfan syndrome: Port-access procedures require passage of the EAC into the thoracic aorta and inflation of the EAC balloon; therefore, aneurysms or a weakened aortic wall are contraindications.
5. Scarring of the pleural cavity (e.g., chest trauma, previous thoracotomy) may make surgical access difficult.
6. Inability to obtain TEE imaging, since monitoring and placement of catheters relies on TEE.

Preop evaluation should focus on the underlying pathophysiology (valvular disease vs CAD). In addition, the following aspects should be considered:

Respiratory	Single-lung ventilation is used to facilitate surgical exposure; thus, evaluation of patients with severe lung disease may include CXR, ABG, PFTs (see Thoracic Surgery, p. 178).
Cardiovascular	The vascular system should be evaluated with respect to insertion of the catheters and cannulae for endovascular CPB. Severity of arterial occlusive or atherosclerotic disease should be evaluated (embolization/dissection risk). The possible presence of a persistent left SVC should be considered. **Tests:** CXR; aortography; iliofemoral arteriography; vascular MRI/MRA; vascular ultrasound; TEE
Premedication	As for the underlying condition. Usually, a mild anxiolytic (e.g., midazolam 1-3 mg iv) is sufficient.

INTRAOPERATIVE

Anesthetic technique: GETA (DLT or BB). Anesthetic technique depends on the underlying pathophysiology (e.g., valvular disease vs CAD). Early extubation and postop pain relief can be facilitated by using intrathecal narcotics (e.g., Duramorph 10 μg/kg intrathecal) injected prior to induction.

Induction Typically, induction can be accomplished with etomidate (0.1-0.3 mg/kg), propofol (0.5-2 mg/kg) or STP (2-4 mg/kg), fentanyl (5-20 μg/kg) and pancuronium or vecuronium (0.1 mg/kg). The overall length of port-access procedures is similar to or slightly longer than conventional approaches so that a long-acting muscle relaxant can be used. Intubation is accomplished with a double-lumen tube, and its placement is checked by auscultation or bronchoscopy.

Maintenance With the goal of early extubation, it is important to avoid oversedation. The use of volatile agents or a propofol infusion (25-100 μg/kg/min) before, during and after CPB will facilitate early extubation. During dissection of the IMA or exposure of the left atrium, one-lung anesthesia is needed.

Emergence At the end of the procedure, intercostal blocks with ropivacaine or bupivacaine may be placed, and infiltration of the skin incision also may be helpful. Extubation in the OR may be appropriate for stable patients. Alternatively, the patient may be transported to the ICU and ventilated. The DLT may be exchanged for a single-lumen tube when postop mechanical ventilation is required.

Special considerations: Placement/ monitoring of endocardio-pulmonary system The port-access system consists of fem-fem bypass via an endovenous drain (EVD) and an endoaortic return cannula (EARC) which is Y-ed to accept the EAC. These are placed by the surgeon with the aid of fluoroscopy and TEE. Additional drainage of the right side of the heart is accomplished via an endopulmonary vent (EPV) placed by the anesthesiologist. Immediately after intubation and before CVP insertion, a TEE exam should be performed to exclude any contraindication to endoCPB (e.g., severe AR, aortic atheromatous disease, aortic aneurysm); the size of the ascending aorta should be measured (aids the surgeon in inflation of the aortic balloon); and the coronary sinus should be identified to aid placement of the ESC (coronary sinus catheter). The right IJ vein is then cannulated with 2 sheaths (9 Fr for EPV and 11 Fr for the ESC). Cardioplegia is delivered in an anterograde fashion via the EAC or retrograde via an ESC also placed by the anesthesiologist (Fig. 6.1-8).

Placement of ESC The ESC can be placed with fluoroscopy and/or TEE. The coronary sinus is identified on TEE (transverse view of the right atrium or longitudinal bicaval view). Prior to placement, the patient should be partially anticoagulated with 70 U/kg of heparin. The ESC is placed through the 11 Fr sheath. Once the tip of the catheter engages the coronary sinus, the catheter is advanced either directly or over a guiding wire until the occlusion balloon is 2-4 cm inside the sinus. Position is confirmed by inflating the balloon and obtaining ventricularization of the pressure tracing. Careful note should be taken of the volume of fluid required to occlude the coronary sinus (1-2 ml) so that overinflation and possible coronary sinus trauma does not occur. Contrast injection will define the correct positioning of the ESC in the coronary sinus. Care should be taken to avoid injecting contrast too quickly, thus pushing the ESC out of the coronary sinus. A time limit should be set to pass this catheter (20-30 min) as repeated attempts increase the risk of cardiac injury (e.g., right ventricular perforation).

Placement of EPV The EPV (pulmonary vent) is positioned by passing the catheter over a guiding 5 Fr balloon flotation catheter using pressure monitoring (as with a Swan-Ganz catheter, fluoroscopy and/or TEE.

Placement of EVD The EVD (venous drain) cannula is placed via the femoral vein into the right atrium over a guide wire. Fluoroscopy or TEE is used to ensure that the wire enters the SVC prior to advancing the EVD into position. The tip of the EVD should be at the SVC/RA junction or just inside the SVC.

Placement of EARC A guide wire is advanced under fluoroscopy and no resistance to its passage should be felt. The guide wire is advanced into the descending aorta and its intraluminal position confirmed on TEE prior to advancing the EARC (aortic return cannulation) into its final position. The perfusionist should confirm normal line pressures with a test bolus of fluid and ✓ that normal arterial pulsation is present. These precautions will decrease the likelihood of arterial dissection.

Placement of EAC Under fluoroscopy, the EAC (endoaortic clamp) is advanced over a guide wire into the ascending aorta so that the tip of the catheter is just proximal to the sinotubular ridge (2-3 cm above the aortic valve). Position is confirmed by contrast injection and/or TEE. It is also useful to identify the takeoff of the innominate artery in relation to the balloon. Migration of the balloon proximally or distally can occur and, thus, its position needs to be monitored. Monitoring of the pressure in the aortic root via this catheter should show that the mean aortic root pressure is the same as mean radial artery pressure prior to the initiation of bypass.

Sequence of events during endoCPB

After initiation of bypass, the anesthesiologist should observe the descending aorta to exclude retrograde aortic dissection and open the EPV to allow the perfusionist to drain the heart. EPV pressures during bypass should be negative (positive pressures may indicate inadequate decompression of the heart or kinking of the EPV). Once adequate CPB is established and the heart drained, the EAC balloon can be inflated (balloon pressure = 250-350 mmHg). CPB is restarted and occlusion of the aorta confirmed by a differential between the radial and aortic root pressures and by an aortic root contrast injection. Anterograde cardioplegia is delivered via the EAC with careful monitoring to ensure that the balloon is not displaced distally, thus occluding the innominate artery (see Monitoring of endoCPB: regional perfusion, below)

After cardioplegic arrest, retrograde cardioplegia may be delivered via the ESC and the left side of the heart may be vented via the EAC. Avoid overventing, high systemic pressures or high CPB flow, which could displace the EAC toward the aortic valve. Initiation of retrograde cardioplegia should begin using a low flow to avoid displacing the ESC, followed by inflation of the ESC balloon until the pressure in the coronary sinus just starts to rise, indicating coronary sinus occlusion. No further inflation of the balloon should take place. Normal coronary sinus perfusion pressure is < 40 mmHg. After retrograde cardioplegia is delivered, the ESC balloon is deflated. Once the surgery is completed, the EAC balloon is deflated (after deairing procedures as needed), the heart is reperfused and the EAC is removed. Prior to weaning from CPB, mobility of the ESC and EPV should be assessed in mitral procedures to ensure that they have not been incorporated in the atrial suture line. Weaning from bypass is routine. The ESC should be removed prior to heparin reversal and the EPV can be replaced with a pulmonary artery catheter if needed.

Blood and fluid requirements

As for underlying condition:
For mitral valve surgery, see p. 234.
For CABG, see p. 225.

Monitoring

As for underlying condition:
For mitral valve surgery, see p. 234.
For CABG, see p. 225.

Special monitoring considerations for port-access are discussed below.

Positioning

Supine
Roll under left chest for CABG and under right chest for mitral valve.

External defibrillator pads should be placed on all patients.

Monitoring of endoCPB

Regional perfusion

Distal migration of the EAC (innominate artery occlusion $\rightarrow \downarrow$cerebral blood flow) is possible, especially while cardioplegia is being delivered when pressure in the aortic root exceeds that in the systemic arterial system. Monitoring for regional perfusion includes:
(1) Right-sided arterial pressure—radial, brachial or axillary. The pump-induced artifact may be of use if roller heads are being used.
(2) Bilateral arterial lines—right-sided, plus a second line in the left radial or in the femoral vessels to allow comparison.
(3) TEE—EAC visible in the ascending aorta proximal to the innominate artery.
(4) Transcranial or carotid artery Doppler.

Proximal EAC balloon migration

Most likely to occur during aortic root venting when the systemic pressure exceeds aortic root pressure. Monitored by TEE.

Cardiac decompression

TEE can be useful in monitoring for adequate decompression of the heart.

EAC balloon pressure

This is usually monitored by the perfusionist and ranges from 250-550 mmHg. Decreases in pressure may be 2° proximal migration of the balloon into a wider area of the ascending aorta, rupture of the balloon or prolapse into the left ventricle. Loss of balloon occlusion is indicated

Monitoring of endoCPB, cont.		by blood in the surgical field, return of cardiac activity, cardiac distension, increased root venting and TEE evidence.
	Aortic root pressure	Less than 80 mmHg while giving cardioplegia; 0-10 mmHg, during venting. Overventing should be avoided, as should venting when the left side of the heart is open, to avoid drawing air into the aortic root.
	Intracardiac air	TEE is very useful for determining that adequate deairing of the heart has occurred.
Complications of endoCPB	Retrograde aortic dissection	
	Coronary sinus damage	
	Right ventricular perforation	During ESC or EPV placement
	EAC balloon migration	
	EAC balloon rupture	Especially 2° sutures placed in the mitral valve annulus.
	Retained EPV in atrial suture line	
	Chest-wall hemorrhage	It is important that the surgeon check the chest wall prior to closure.
	Limb ischemia	May follow femoral cannulation.

POSTOPERATIVE

Complications	As for the primary procedure Low CO Chest-wall hemorrhage Problems associated with peripheral cannulation (e.g., dissection, embolization) Perivalvular leak Heart block	See mitral valve surgery (p. 234) or CABG (p. 226).
Pain management	Parenteral narcotics NSAIDs	Pain control is important to facilitate early extubation. Intrathecal narcotics and/or intercostal blocks with wound infiltration may be useful.
Tests	ECG; electrolytes; ABG	

References–Surgeon's

1. Arom KV, Emery RW: Minimally invasive mitral operations (let). *Ann Thorac Surg* 1997; 63:1219-20.
2. Baudet EM, Puel V, McBride JT, Grimaud JP, Roques F, Clerc F, Roques X, Laborde N: Long-term results of valve replacement with St. Jude Medical prosthesis. *J Thorac Cardiovasc Surg* 1995; 109:858-70.
3. Chitwood WR, Elbeery JR, Chapman WHH, Moran JM, Lust RL, Wooden WA, Deaton DH: Video-assisted minimally invasive mitral valve surgery: The "micro-mitral" operation. *J Thorac Cardiovasc Surg* 1997; 113:413-14.
4. Deloche A, Jebara VA, Relland JY, Chauvaud S, Fabiani JN, Perier P, Dreyfus G, Mihaileanu S, Carpentier A: Valve repair with Carpentier techniques. The second decade. *J Thorac Cardiovasc Surg* 1990; 99:990-1002.
5. Fann JI, Pompili MF, Burdon TA, Stevens JH, StGoar FG, Reitz BA: Minimally invasive mitral valve surgery. *Semin Thorac Cardiovasc Surg* 1997; 9(4):320-30.
6. Galloway AC, Colvin SB, Baumann FG, Exposito R, Vohra R, Harty S, Freedberg R, Kronzon I, Spencer FC: Current concepts in mitral valve reconstruction for mitral insufficiency. *Circulation* 1988; 78(I):97-105.
7. Glower DD, Landolfo K, Clements F, Debruijn NP, Stafford-Smith M, Smith PK, Duhaylongsod F: Mitral valve operation via port-access versus median sternotomy. Abstract presented at the World Congress on Minimally Invasive Cardiac Surgery, Paris, May 1997.
8. Khan S, Chaux A, Matloff J, Blanche C, DeRobertis M, Kass R, Tsai TP, Trento A, Nessim S, Gray R, Czer L: The St. Jude Medical Valve: experience with 1000 cases. *J Thorac Cardiovasc Surg* 1994; 108:1010-20.
9. Kumar AS, Prasad S, Rai S, Saxena DK: Right thoracotomy revisited. *Texas Heart J* 1993; 20:40-1.
10. Lin PJ, Chang CH, Chu JJ, et al: Video-assisted mitral valve operations. *Ann Thorac Surg* 1996; 61:1781-87.
11. Mohr FW, Falk V, Diegeler A, Walther T, vanSon JAM, Autschbach R: First results with video-assisted minimally invasive mitral valve repair using the port-access system. Abstract presented at the American Association for Thoracic Surgery, Washington DC, April 1997.
12. Navia JL, Cosgrove DM: Minimally invasive mitral valve operations *Ann Thorac Surg* 1996; 62:1542-44.
13. Peters WS: Minimally invasive cardiac surgery by cardioscopy. *Australas J Cardiac Thorac Surg* 1993; 2(3):152-54.

14. Pompili MF, Stevens JH, Burdon TA, Siegel LC, Peters WS, Ribakove GH, Reitz BA: Port-access mitral valve replacement in dogs. *J Thorac Cardiovasc Surg* 1996; 112:1268-74.
15. Pompili MF, Yakub A, Siegel LC, Stevens JH, Awang Y, Burdon TA: Port-access mitral valve replacement: Initial clinical experience. *Circulation* 1996; 94(I):I-533.
16. Reitz BA, Stevens JH, Burdon TA, StGoar FG, Siegel LC, Pompili MF: Port-access coronary artery bypass grafting: Lessons learned in a Phase I clinical trial (abst). *Circulation* 1996; 94:1294.
17. Stevens JH, Burdon TA, Peters WS, Siegel LC , Pompili MF, Vierra MA, StGoar FG, Ribakove GH, Mitchell RS, Reitz BA: Port-access coronary artery bypass grafting: A proposed surgical method. *J Thorac Cardiovasc Surg* 1996; 111:567-73.
18. Tribble CG, Killinger WA, Harman PK, et al: Anterolateral thoracotomy as an alternative to repeat median sternotomy for replacement of the mitral valve. *Ann Thorac Surg* 1987; 43:380-82.

References–Anesthesiologist's

1. Fann JI, Pompili MF, Burdon TA, Stevens JH, StGoar FG, Reitz BA: Minimally invasive mitral valve surgery. *Semin Thorac Cardiovasc Surg* 1997; 9(4):320-30.
2. Peters WS, Siegel LC, Stevens JH, StGoar FG, Pompili MF, Burdon TA: Closed-chest cardiopulmonary bypass and cardioplegia for less invasive cardia surgery. *Ann Thorac Surg* 1997; 63:1748-54.
3. Schwartz DS, Ribakove GH, Grossi EA, Buttenheim PA, Schwartz JD, Applebaum RM, Kronzon IK, Baumann FG, Colvin SB, Galloway AC: Minimally invasive mitral valve replacement: port-access techniques, feasibility, and myocardial functional preservation. *J Thorac Cardiovasc Surg* 1997; 113:1022-31.
4. Schwartz DS, Ribakove GH, Grossi EA, Stevens JH, Siegel LC, StGoar FG, Peters WS, McLaughlin P, Baumann FG, Colvin SB, Galloway AC: Minimally invasive cardiopulmonary bypass and cardioplegic arrest: a closed chest technique with equivalent myocardial protection. *J Thorac Cardiovasc Surg* 1996; 111:556-66.
5. Siegel LC, StGoar FG, Stevens JH, Pompili MF, Burdon TA, Reitz BA, Peters WS: Monitoring considerations for port-access cardiac surgery. *Circulation* 1997; 96:562-68.
6. Stevens JH, Burdon TA, Peters WS, Siegel LC, Pompili MF, Vierra MA, StGoar FG, Ribakove GH, Mitchell RS, Reitz BA: Port-access coronary artery bypass grafting: a proposed surgical method. *J Thorac Cardiovasc Surg* 1996; 111:567-73.
7. Toomasian JM, Peters WS, Siegel LC, Stevens JH: Extracorporeal circulation for port-access cardiac surgery. *Perfusion* 1997;12:83-91.

Surgeons

James I. Fann, MD
R. Scott Mitchell, MD
Stephen T. Kee, MD (*Endovascular stent-grafting*)
Michael D. Dake, MD (*Endovascular stent-grafting*)

6.2 VASCULAR SURGERY

Anesthesiologists

Kristi L. Peterson, MD (*General vascular surgery*)
Gordon R. Haddow, MB, ChB, FFA(SA)
(*Repair of thoracic aortic aneurysms, aortic dissections*)

CAROTID ENDARTERECTOMY (VASCULAR)

SURGICAL CONSIDERATIONS

Description: Carotid endarterectomy (CEA) is one of the most commonly performed vascular surgery procedures in the U.S. Because of presumed microemboli from stenotic/ulcerated plaques at the carotid bifurcation, CEA has been championed as an effective procedure to reduce the risk of subsequent stroke. Recently, the NASCET trial has determined, in a prospective, randomized, blinded trial, that CEA is more effective than medical therapy for symptomatic patients with internal carotid artery narrowing between 60-90%.[1] Symptoms are usually hemispheric (contralateral, upper or lower extremity paresis or numbness) or retinal (unilateral monocular blindness). Symptoms may be transient (TIA or reversible ischemic neurological deficit [RIND]) or permanent (CVA). The Asymptomatic Carotid Atherosclerosis Study (ACAS) has shown benefit from prophylactic CEA in asymptomatic patients with > 60% stenosis of the internal carotid artery. Although some surgeons routinely prefer local anesthesia, most prefer GA with careful hemodynamic monitoring because of the frequent concomitant CAD.

The carotid artery is approached through an oblique neck incision along the anterior border of the sternocleidomastoid muscle. After division of the common facial vein, the carotid sheath is opened and the carotid artery is exposed, avoiding injury to the phrenic, vagus, ansa hypoglossi and hypoglossal nerves. After controlling the internal, external and common carotid arteries, heparin is administered, and the internal, external and common carotid arteries are clamped sequentially. An indwelling shunt may be utilized, at the discretion of the surgeon. An endarterectomy plane is established proximally, and developed distally into both the external and internal branches, with establishment of a fine tapered end point. After removal of all thrombus, loose smooth muscle fibers, and endothelium, the arteriotomy is closed, with or without a patch, the artery flushed and flow restored. The incision is then closed, after meticulous hemostasis has been assured.

Usual preop diagnosis: Carotid artery disease

SUMMARY OF PROCEDURE

Position	Supine, with neck extended and turned away from the side of the lesion.
Incision	Anterior to sternocleidomastoid from earlobe to base of neck, or curvilinear in a skin crease over the carotid bifurcation.
Special instrumentation	Complete hemodynamic monitors; EEG monitors; ± shunt
Unique considerations	Capability to measure stump pressure may be needed. This can be accomplished by a high-pressure arterial line being passed off the field to a pressure transducer. During carotid cross-clamping, it is imperative that there be no intraop hypotension. An indwelling shunt may be utilized to restore carotid perfusion during CEA. Heparin 5,000-10,000 U 5 min prior to cross-clamping, and protamine may be given after restoration of flow.
Antibiotics	Cefazolin 1 g iv at induction of anesthesia
Surgical time	Carotid cross-clamp: 30 min
	Total operating time: 90 min
Closing considerations	In order to assess the patient's neurologic status, it is best to be able to awaken and extubate the patient at the conclusion of the procedure. Avoidance of HTN is also critical during this period, since the endarterectomy tissues are thin and friable.
EBL	100-200 ml
Postop care	ICU × 12-24 h; BP control; cardiac monitoring
Mortality	1%
Morbidity	MI: Major cause of postop mortality
	Cranial nerve injury (recurrent and superior laryngeal nerves): 39%
	Restenosis
	Asymptomatic: 9-12%
	Symptomatic: < 3%
	Neurologic complications: < 2%
	Hemorrhage: 1%
	False aneurysm: < 0.5%
Pain score	3-5

PATIENT POPULATION CHARACTERISTICS

Age range	55-80 yr
Male:Female	3:1
Incidence	Second most common vascular surgical procedure (after AAA repair)
Etiology	Arteriosclerosis; fibromuscular dysplasia
Associated conditions	Significant CAD coexists with carotid artery disease in at least 30% of patients, necessitating careful cardiac and hemodynamic monitoring.

ANESTHETIC CONSIDERATIONS

See Anesthetic Considerations for Carotid Endarterectomy (Neurosurgical) in Other Neurosurgery, p. 82.

References

1. NASCET Collaborators: *N Engl J Med* 1991; 325:445-53.
2. Moore WS, Barnett HS, Beebe HG, et al: Guidelines for carotid endarterectomy. A multidisciplinary consensus statement from the Ad Hoc Committee, American Heart Association. *Circulation* 1995; 91:566-79.
3. Young B, Moore WS, Robertson JT, et al: An analysis of perioperative surgical mortality and morbidity in the Asymptomatic Carotid Atherosclerosis Study. ACAS Investigators. *Stroke* 1996; 27:2216-24.

REPAIR OF THORACIC AORTIC ANEURYSMS

SURGICAL CONSIDERATIONS

Description: Repairs of aneurysms of the ascending, transverse arch and descending thoracic aorta are performed to repair expanding or leaking aneurysms or prophylactically to prevent rupture. Patients with Sx of rapid expansion or aneurysm leaking[7] may require urgent repair. Each surgical type—ascending, arch and descending—is considered separately, as follows. Aneurysms of the **ascending aorta** may arise 2° the degenerative changes of atherosclerosis (exacerbated by old age, HTN, tobacco use), from inborn errors of metabolism (Marfan syndrome), or from poststenotic dilatation and continued expansion of a chronic dissection. Diseases of the entire aorta, including the sinuses of Valsalva, as in Marfan syndrome and annuloaortic ectasia, require replacement of the entire aorta with a composite, valved conduit, while acquired diseases usually allow replacement of the aorta distal to the sinotubular ridge. Repair of the ascending aorta is usually accomplished on full CPB with an aortic cross-clamp placed just proximal to the innominate artery, and arterial inflow through the femoral artery. The aneurysmal ascending aorta is replaced with a Dacron tube graft from the sinotubular ridge to the innominate artery. Dilatation of the sinuses of Valsalva mandates replacement with a valved conduit sewn proximally to the aortic annulus and distally to the aorta at the innominate, with coronary ostia reimplanted in the side of the tube graft.

Aneurysms of the **aortic arch** are the least common of the thoracic aorta. Because of the need for concomitant replacement of the arch vessels, however, they are the most complex to repair. Total CPB is utilized, and cerebral protection is accomplished either by CPB perfusion of one or all cerebral vessels, or by profound hypothermic circulatory arrest at 15-18°C. Repair can originate from the aortic annulus and extend distally to the mid descending thoracic aorta at the level of the carina. Routine caval cannulation is accomplished via a median sternotomy, and arterial access is gained via the femoral artery. If circulatory arrest is to be used, the patient is cooled to 15-18°C, the heart is arrested and, with no distal cross-clamp, distal anastomosis is accomplished, followed by implantation of the head vessels attached to an island of aorta. Perfusion is then reinstituted, the graft clamped proximal to the innominate artery and the proximal anastomosis performed, while the patient is being rewarmed. Alternatively, if one elects to perfuse the cerebral vessels, the innominate and left carotid arteries can be individually cannulated and perfused via a "Y" connection from the femoral arterial perfusion line. The necessity for profound hypothermic circulatory arrest is thus avoided. After completion of the distal aortic, arch vessel island, and proximal aortic anastomoses, weaning from CPB and subsequent steps proceed in a routine fashion.

Repair of aneurysms of the **descending thoracic aorta** is usually performed for symptomatic and leaking aneurysms, enlarging aneurysms and aneurysms of sufficient size to warrant prophylactic repair. **Aneurysmorrhaphy** is accomplished through a left posterolateral thoracotomy on partial CPB. After entry into the left thorax, venous drainage for CPB may be obtained from the PA or the femoral vein; and arterial return is via the femoral artery. If partial bypass without an oxygenator is elected, thus minimizing the amount of heparin necessary, venous access can be gained via the pulmonary veins or left atrium, and arterial return via the femoral artery or distal thoracic aorta. After institution of bypass, the aorta is cross-clamped above and below the aneurysm, the aorta divided, a tube graft interposed and clamps removed. The patient is weaned from bypass, and the operation is terminated in the routine fashion.

Usual preop diagnosis: Enlarging or symptomatic aortic aneurysm

SUMMARY OF PROCEDURE

	Ascending Aorta	Transverse Arch	Descending Aorta
Position	Supine	⇐	Lateral decubitus with left side up
Incision	Median sternotomy	⇐	Left posterolateral thoracotomy with access to femoral artery and vein
Special instrumentation	CPB, if used.	Complete hemodynamic monitors; CPB	⇐ + DLT; lower extremity BP monitor
Unique considerations	Routine CPB hemodynamic monitoring	If profound hypothermic arrest is utilized, neuroprotective adjuncts, including local hypothermia, barbiturates and steroids, should be used.	One-lung ventilation (OLV); partial CPB
Antibiotics	Cefazolin 1 g iv	⇐	⇐
Surgical time	Aortic cross-clamp: 40-120 min CPB: 70-150 min Total: 2.5-5 h	Aortic cross-clamp: 75-120 min Circulatory arrest: 30-45 min CPB: 3-4.5 h Total: 4-6 h	Aortic cross-clamp: 25-45 min CPB: 30-60 min Total: 2.5-4.5 h
Closing considerations	Aggressive management of coagulopathy, if a long pump run is necessary.	Aggressive management of coagulopathy	Replacement of DLT with single-lumen tube
EBL	300-400 ml	400-700 ml	200-300 ml
Postop care	ICU, intubated 5-20 h, depending on preop condition	ICU, intubated 6-24 h	ICU, intubated 5-25 h
Mortality	5-10%	10-15%[4]	⇐
Morbidity	Renal failure: 5-10%[5]	–	10-15%
	CVA: 4-6%	2-5%	2-4%
	Respiratory insufficiency: 3-5%	10%	10-15%
	MI: 2-5%	⇐	2-4%
Pain score	7-10	7-10	9-10

PATIENT POPULATION CHARACTERISTICS

Age range	23-80 yr (mean = 55 yr)	50-75 yr	34-79 yr (mean = 65 yr)
Male:Female	3:1	2:1	2.5:1
Incidence	15-20/yr at tertiary center	10-15/yr at tertiary center	10-20/yr at tertiary center
Etiology	Degenerative disease	⇐	⇐
	Atherosclerotic disease	⇐	⇐
		Chronic dissections	⇐
Associated conditions	CHF (50%); angina (30%); HTN (30%); COPD (15%)	Aortic valve disease (30%); COPD (20%); CAD (15%)	HTN (65%); CAD (50%); COPD (30%); CHF (10%)

ANESTHETIC CONSIDERATIONS

PREOPERATIVE

In contrast with thoracic aortic dissections, Sx of thoracic aortic aneurysms may be of a more chronic nature. A ruptured or leaking aneurysm, however, may have a more precipitous presentation. Patients may be asymptomatic; however, most will have coexisting CAD, PVD, and/or cardiovascular disease.

Cardiovascular — **Arch and ascending aneurysms** (60-70% of aneurysms): commonly associated with HTN, syphilis, cystic medial necrosis or connective tissue disorder (e.g., Marfan syndrome, atherosclerosis). CHF may occur 2° to dilation of the aortic annulus and aortic incompetence. Aneurysmal compression or intrinsic disease of the coronary arteries may result in myocardial ischemia.
Descending (30%): usually associated with HTN, cystic medial necrosis, Marfan syndrome, atherosclerosis.
Tests: ECG: ✓ for LVH, ischemia. ECHO: ✓ for valvular disease, size and extent of aneurysm, LV function. Angiography: ✓ exact extent of aneurysm (allows planning of procedure and sites for arterial monitoring), coronary artery anatomy and degree of occlusion.

Respiratory — Recurrent laryngeal nerve palsy may lead to hoarseness (ascending/arch aneurysms). Stridor or dyspnea may be present 2° tracheal or bronchial compression. Hemoptysis or a hemorrhagic pleural effusion suggest aneurysmal leakage or rupture. The implications include the possibility of compromised oxygenation, risk of massive hemorrhage on thoracotomy, increased intrathoracic pressure and consequent decreased venous return (especially when IPPV is instituted).
Tests: CXR: ✓ for widened mediastinum, distortion of trachea and left main bronchus (because it may affect the placement of DLT); others as indicated from H&P.

Neurologic — Any deficit should be well documented as neurologic sequelae frequently occur after surgery.

Renal — Renal problems may occur 2° to AR and heart failure, HTN, or involvement of renal arteries in the aneurysm.
Tests: BUN; creatinine; consider creatinine clearance; electrolytes

Gastrointestinal — Descending aneurysms that involve the coeliac or superior mesenteric arteries may result in bowel ischemia.
Tests: Consider ABG: ✓ persistent metabolic acidosis. If indicated by H&P, consider abdominal x-ray: ✓ ileus.

Hematological — If time permits, consider autologous blood donation; preexisting coagulopathy increases risk of the procedure.
Tests: PT; PTT; Hct/Hb

Laboratory — Consider syphilis serology; others as indicated from H&P.

Premedication — Pain and anxiety may significantly contribute to HTN and should be treated (e.g., morphine 0.1 mg/kg im ± midazolam 0.025-0.1 mg/kg iv or 0.05-0.2 mg/kg im); but avoid obtundation. Since many of these patients present emergently, consider full-stomach precautions—H_2 antagonists (e.g., ranitidine 50 mg iv), metoclopramide (10 mg iv), antacids (e.g., Na citrate 0.3 M 30 ml po).

INTRAOPERATIVE

Anesthetic technique: The anesthetic management of patients with aortic dissections and aortic aneurysms are similar in many respects. For intraop and postop management of these conditions, see Anesthetic Considerations for Repair of Acute Aortic Dissections and Dissecting Aneurysms, p. 274.

References

1. Cammarata BJ: Anesthesia for surgery of the thoracic aorta. In *Anesthesia for Cardiac Surgery,* 2nd edition. DiNardo JA, ed. Appleton & Lange, Stamford: 1998, 259-76.
2. Crawford ES, Snyder DM: Treatment of aneurysms of the aortic arch. *J Thorac Cardiovasc Surg* 1983; 85:237-46.
3. Fann JI, Miller DC: Descending thoracic aortic aneurysms. In *Glenn's Thoracic and Cardiovascular Surgery*, 6th edition. Baue AE, Geha AS, Hammond GL, Laks H, Naunheim KS, eds. Appleton & Lange, Stamford: 1996, 2255-72.
4. Galloway AC, Colvin SB, Mendola CL, Hurwitz JB, Baumann FG, Harris LJ, Culliford AT, Grossi EA, Spencer FC: Ten-year operative experience with 165 aneurysms of the ascending aorta and aortic arch. *Circulation* 1989; 80(Suppl 1): I-249-56.

5. Moreno-Cabral CE, Miller DC, Mitchell RS, Stinson EB, Oyer PE, Jamieson SW, Shumway NE: Degenerative and atherosclerotic aneurysms of the thoracic aorta. *J Thorac Cardiovasc Surg* 1984; 88:1020-32.
6. Pressler BA, McNamara JJ: Thoracic aortic aneurysm. Natural history and treatment. *J Thorac Cardiovasc Surg* 1980; 79:489-98.
7. Skeehan TM; Cooper JR Jr: Anesthetic management for thoracic aneurysms and dissections. In *The Practice of Cardiac Anesthesia.* Hensley FA Jr, Martin DE, eds. Little, Brown and Co, Boston: 1990, Ch 15, 461-92.

ENDOVASCULAR STENT-GRAFTING OF AORTIC ANEURYSMS

SURGICAL CONSIDERATIONS

Description: The standard treatment for descending **thoracic aortic aneurysm** is surgical resection of the aneurysm and replacement with a segment of prosthetic graft material. While resection of aneurysms often can be performed without the need for extracorporeal circulation, the procedure has a reported mortality rate of up to 50% in emergency cases and 12-15% in elective cases. Transluminal endovascular stent-grafting offers an alternative treatment that is less invasive, less hazardous and potentially less expensive than standard operative repair.

In the initial workup, all patients have contrast-enhanced spiral CT scans of the thorax and thoracic aortography to assess the dimensions of the aneurysms. The most important features to consider in evaluating an aortic aneurysm for endovascular stent-graft treatment is the presence of an adequate proximal and distal neck. A minimum neck length of at least 1.5 cm is required to allow secure anchoring of most stent-grafts. The distance from the origins of the left subclavian artery and celiac axis to the aneurysm should be at least 1.5-3 cm to ensure that the stent-graft does not inadvertently block these arteries. In an effort to reduce the incidence of paraplegia, and to limit exclusion of intracostal arteries, the overall length of the stent-graft is kept to a minimum.

Another important anatomic consideration is the size of the proposed conduit vessels (e.g., iliac) for introduction of the stent-graft to ensure that they are adequate for accommodation of the device-introducer system, which usually requires at least an 8-mm-diameter vessel. Where the pelvic vessels are less than 8 mm, either a retroperitoneal iliac or retroperitoneal aortic approach is utilized. The stent is the metallic framework to which the graft material is applied. Various balloon-expandable or self-expanding stents are available. For application in the thoracic aorta, stents of 30-40 mm in diameter (mean 35 mm) are required.

Presently, all thoracic aortic aneurysm stent-graft procedures are performed in the OR, with the patient intubated and under general anesthesia. The OR is prepared as for aortic surgery, with the patient placed on the table in a shallow right decubitus position. The patient's thorax is prepped and draped as for a left thoracotomy. For an approach via the common femoral artery, the groin area is prepped for a femoral artery cut-down. When the iliac arteries are of insufficient size, the left lower abdomen is prepped for a retroperitoneal approach to either the aorta or the common iliac artery. High-quality fluoroscopic equipment is essential to assure accurate placement of the device, and a portable C-arm with digital subtraction capability is moved into position and centered over the thorax. When the iliac vessels are of sufficient size, a cut-down is performed on a femoral artery, the artery is punctured, and a guide wire is advanced into the thoracic aorta. A pigtail catheter is placed, and aortogram performed. The patient is then fully anticoagulated with iv heparin (300 IU/kg). A long, stiff guide wire is placed, and the 24 Fr sheath and dilator assembly is advanced over the wire until the sheath tip is proximal to the proximal aneurysm neck. The dilator and guide wire are withdrawn, and the stent-graft is introduced into the sheath from its loading cartridge using the Teflon pusher. The device is pushed through the sheath until the stent-graft approaches the tip of the sheath.

In order to reduce the likelihood of inadvertent downstream deployment of the stent-graft caused by the force of blood flow during initial delivery, the arterial BP may be lowered to a mean of 50-60 mmHg using SNP. Holding the pusher firmly in position, the sheath is rapidly withdrawn, and the stent-graft expands into position. Rapid deployment helps to minimize distal migration of the stent-graft. Immediately following deployment, the SNP is discontinued, allowing the BP to normalize. Repeat aortogram is performed, and any early leakage of contrast into the aneurysm is treated either with balloon angioplasty of the stent-graft or further stent-graft placement. Occasionally a faint, persistent leak of contrast is caused by leakage through the graft material. This typically ceases when the patient's coagulation status returns to normal. Following removal of the delivery sheath, heparin is reversed with protamine sulfate and the arteriotomy is repaired surgically. For stent placement through the retroperitoneal aorta, the procedure has a more extensive surgical component; however, the technique is similar.

The basic concept of **abdominal aortic aneurysm (AAA)** repair via an endovascular route is similar to the preceding section on thoracic aneurysm repair, with some notable exceptions. AAAs commonly arise inferior to the renal arteries, and 80-90% of cases involve either one or both iliac arteries. For this reason, stent-grafts that can accommodate this more complicated anatomy are required. The superior aneurysm neck needs to be of sufficient length (1.5-2 cm) inferior to the most inferior renal artery to provide for stable anchoring. Inferiorly the stent-graft must accommodate either or both iliac arteries. The procedure is performed in a two-stage fashion. Initially an aorta-to-single-iliac-artery device is placed from the infrarenal aortic neck into one of the iliac vessels. A contralateral femoral artery puncture is then performed and a catheter and guide wire are used to access an open stump of the stent-graft from the contralateral limb. At this stage, a modular section of stent-graft is placed from the aortic component into the contralateral limb; in this way, an aorta-to-bi-iliac graft is placed.

Usual preop diagnosis: Aortic aneurysm

SUMMARY OF PROCEDURE

	Thoracic Aortic Aneurysms	Abdominal Aortic Aneurysms
Position	Left decubitus	Supine
Incision	Femoral artery cut-down	Bilateral femoral artery cut-downs
Special instrumentation	Catheters, guide wires, sheaths, dilators and stent-grafts	⇐
Unique considerations	May require adjunctive procedure (e.g., brachial artery catheterization, balloon angioplasty, possible left subclavian-to-common-carotid-artery bypass procedure); iv heparin 300 IU/kg	⇐
Antibiotics	Cefazolin 1 g iv	⇐
Surgical time	1-3 h	⇐
Closing considerations	None	⇐
EBL	Usually minimal; however, can be up to 2-3 U	⇐
Postop care	ICU × 1 d	⇐
Mortality	3-5%	2-3%
Morbidity	Paraplegia: 2-3%	Acute rupture: < 1%
	Infection: 1%	⇐
	Surgical conversion: < 1%	⇐
Pain score	3-4	3-4

PATIENT POPULATION CHARACTERISTICS

Age range	30-90 yr	40-90 yr
Incidence	1/10,000 of the population in U.S.	1/1000 of the population in U.S.
Etiology	Atherosclerosis; HTN; trauma; aortic dissection; infection	Atherosclerosis; infection
Associated conditions	CAD; aneurysmal disease elsewhere	⇐

ANESTHETIC CONSIDERATIONS

The anesthetic considerations for thoracic and abdominal stent-grafting are similar since the surgical techniques, complications, patient concurrent disease and stent-graft deployment techniques are similar. Patients may be asymptomatic; most will have coexisting CAD, PVD and/or cardiovascular disease.

PREOPERATIVE

Preop considerations for these patients are the same as for any patient undergoing repair of a descending thoracic aneurysm, abdominal aortic aneurysm or aortobifemoral aneurysm. Many of these patients, however, are not suitable for conventional repair via a thoracotomy because of respiratory disease (e.g., FEV_1 < 1L, severe COPD, $PaCO_2$ > 60 mmHg), CAD, renal failure, CHF or a combination of these factors. As such, they generally are at very high risk of perioperative morbidity and mortality. Prior to surgery the anesthesiologist should consult with the surgical and radiological team to decide what will be done should a complication such as penetration or rupture of the aneurysm occur during surgery; i.e., will a thoracotomy or laparotomy be performed?

INTRAOPERATIVE

Anesthetic technique: Usually GETA with or without DLT. It also may be possible to perform this procedure under epidural anesthesia and, on occasion, it may be carried out in the interventional radiology suite with local anesthesia or MAC. In that case, the patient will come to the OR for removal of the introducer system and repair of the femoral artery.

Induction Since these patients are typically extubated in the OR, the dose of fentanyl (5-10 μg/kg) is limited to that which will suppress the hypertensive response to laryngoscopy, while still allowing for early extubation. The same considerations apply to the use of muscle relaxants (e.g., vecuronium [0.1 mg/kg]). A DLT or a Univent ETT should be used unless the team decides that a thoracotomy will not be performed under any circumstance.

Maintenance Usually a balanced anesthetic technique of O_2/N_2O/isoflurane, supplemented with fentanyl (or remifentanil infusion) as needed. Hemodynamic control of the BP (esmolol, SNP, NTG) to avoid HTN and myocardial ischemia is important.

Anesthetic management during stent-graft deployment: During stent-graft deployment the aorta is momentarily occluded. This may result in a rapid ↑BP. The full force of CO will act against the deploying stent-graft with the potential for its being moved from its intended position. To avoid this, BP is lowered to 50-65 mmHg (SNP) just prior to deployment. In addition, the CO and force of contractility may be decreased with the use of a short-acting β-blocker (esmolol), or adenosine (12-48 mg iv bolus) may be used to induce asystole or very low HR during deployment. Alternatively, a Valsalva maneuver or temporary occlusion of the IVC will ↓ CO during deployment. Immediately after deployment, BP needs to be increased to preop baseline levels to aid with graft expansion. Phenylephrine or ephedrine are normally used for this purpose. Aortobifemoral stent-grafting involves the placement of 3 components (1 aortic and 2 iliac stent-grafts). Hence, BP may need to be lowered on 3 occasions.

Emergence Extubation in the OR is desirable, although hypothermia (< 34° C) often prevents this. Otherwise, aim for early extubation in the ICU. DLT may be replaced with a standard ETT at end of procedure if the patient is not extubated in the OR. Recovery is usually in the ICU.

Blood and fluid requirements	IV: 14-16 ga × 1 NS/LR @ 4-8 ml/kg/h PRBC available	Although usually minimal, blood loss can be considerable.
Monitoring	Standard monitors (p. B-1). Arterial line CVP catheter Urinary catheter	Arterial line placement should be on the right as the radiologists may require access to the left brachial artery. CVP monitoring is usually sufficient. Central access for vasoactive drugs is needed.
	TEE	TEE is used to aid in the identification of the thoracic aneurysm necks, to monitor deployment of the stent-graft and to identify any continued flow of blood into the aneurysmal sac after deployment.
Positioning	✓ and pad pressure points. ✓ eyes.	Supine with roll under left chest
Complications	Hemorrhage	Hemorrhage at the groin site can be considerable and may be concealed. A Cell Saver should be used.
	Vessel damage	Damage to the vessels (femoral, iliac or abdominal aorta) during passage of the insertion system can occur with attendant massive hemorrhage.
	Rupture of aorta	Rupture or penetration of the thoracic aneurysm also can occur, necessitating rapid conversion to open thoracotomy.
	Deployment failure/incorrect position	The stent-graft may deploy in an incorrect position or fail to fully deploy. This may need either positioning of further stent-grafts, balloon expansion of the stent-graft or conversion to thoracotomy.
	Hypothermia	Hypothermia can be a problem as a warming blanket cannot be used on the operating table (use of fluoroscopy).

Complications, cont.		Much of the patient is exposed (leaving little room for a Bair Hugger) and a lower-body warming blanket cannot be used as the lower limbs may be ischemic during insertion of the stent-graft. Other complications as with any descending thoracic or abdominal aortic aneurysm.

POSTOPERATIVE

Complications	Aortic perforation/rupture	
	Migration of grafts	→ Loss of distal pulses, mesenteric ischemia, acute renal insufficiency.
	Femoral artery dehiscence Distal embolization Paraplegia	
Pain management	Minimal analgesic requirements	If groin incision, local anesthetic infiltration may be used.
Tests	As indicated by patient condition.	CT scan, angiogram prior to discharge and at regular intervals following discharge.

References

1. Blum U, Voshage G, Lammer J, Beyersdorf F, Tollner D, Kretschmer G, Spillner G, Polterauer P, Nagel G, Holzenbein T: Endoluminal stent-grafts for infrarenal abdominal aortic aneurysms [see comments]. *N Engl J Med* 1997; 336(1):13-20.
2. Chuter TA, Malina M, Brunkwall J, Lindh M, Ivancev K, Lindblad B, Risberg B: A telescopic stent-graft for aortoiliac implantation. *Eur J Vasc Endovasc Surg* 1997; 13(1):79-84.
3. Dake MD, Miller DC, Semba CP, Mitchell RS, Walker PJ, Liddell RP: Transluminal placement of endovascular stent-grafts for the treatment of descending thoracic aortic aneurysms. *N Engl J Med* 1994: 331(26):1729-34.
4. Dorros G, Cohn JM. Adenosine-induced transient cardiac asystole enhances precise deployment of stent-grafts in the thoracic or abdominal aorta [see comments]. *J Endovasc Surg* 1996; 3(3):270-2.
5. Fann JI, Dake MD, Semba CP, Liddell RP, Pfeffer TA, Miller DC: Endovascular stent-grafting after arch aneurysm repair using the "elephant trunk." *Ann Thorac Surg* 1995; 60:1102-05.
6. Fann JI, Miller DC: Descending thoracic aortic aneurysms. In: *Glenn's Thoracic and Cardiovascular Surgery,* 6th edition. Baue AE, Geha AS, Hammond GL, Laks H, Naunheim KS, eds. Appleton and Lange, Stamford: 1995, 2255-72.
7. Fann JI, Miller DC: Results of endovascular stent-grafting in patients with descending thoracic aortic aneurysm. In: *Progress in Vascular Surgery.* Yao JST, Pearce WH, eds. Appleton and Lange, Stamford: 1997, 241-54.
8. Kato N, Semba CP, Dake MD: Embolization of perigraft leaks after endovascular stent-graft treatment of aortic aneurysms. *J Vasc Interv Radiol* 1996; 7(6):805-11.
9. Liston SM: Stent-graft placement procedures for descending thoracic aortic aneurysms. *AORN J* 1997; 66(3):433-38, 400, 442.
10. Mitchell RS: Endovascular stent-graft repair of thoracic aortic aneurysms. *Semin Thorac Cardiovasc Surg* 1997; 9(3):257-68.
11. Mitchell RS, Dake MD, Semba CP, Fogarty TJ, Zarins CK, Liddel RP, Miller DC: Endovascular stent-graft repair of thoracic aortic aneurysms. *J Thorac Cardiovasc Surg* 1996; 111(5):1054-62.
12. Moon MR, Mitchell RS, Dake MD, Zarins CK, Fann JI, Miller DC: Simultaneous abdominal aortic replacement and thoracic aortic stent-graft placement for multilevel aortic disease. *J Vasc Surg* 1997; 25:332-40.
13. Semba CP, Kato N, Kee ST, Lee GK, Mitchell RS, Miller DC, Dake MD: Acute rupture of the descending thoracic aorta: repair with use of endovascular stent-grafts. *J Vasc Interv Radiol* 1997; 8(3):337-42.
14. Taylor PR: Vascular stents and stent-grafts: a vascular surgeon's view. *Cardiovasc Intervent Radiol* 1997; 20(1):1-4.

REPAIR OF ACUTE AORTIC DISSECTIONS AND DISSECTING ANEURYSMS

SURGICAL CONSIDERATIONS

Description: Repair of acute aortic dissection is performed to prevent life-threatening complications such as hemorrhage, tamponade and heart failure secondary to acute aortic valvular insufficiency, and to redirect flow into the true lumen. Emergent repair of acute ascending dissections is generally accepted therapy to prevent rupture of the aortic root with exsanguination or pericardial tamponade. Mortality for acute ascending dissection is estimated at 1% per hour, for the first 48 hours. The management of descending thoracic aortic dissections remains controversial, but surgical intervention probably should be recommended only for younger patients, patients with uncontrolled pain or evidence for continued expansion or extravasation, and those with branch-vessel compromise.

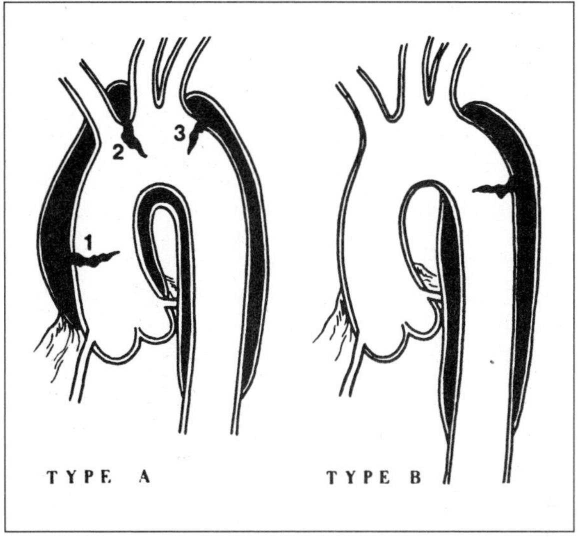

Figure 6.2-1. Types of dissections: Type A = ascending aortic dissection; Type B = descending aortic aneurysm. (Reproduced with permission from Miller DC, Stinson EB, et al: Aortic dissections. *J Thorac Cardiovasc Surg* 1979; 78:367.)

Ascending dissections typically produce sharp, tearing retrosternal pain that penetrates straight through to the subscapular area. The presentation, however, is so frequently variable that for any patient in extremis, especially with migratory pain or vacillating findings, and even asymptomatic patients with valvular aortic regurgitation (AR), should be considered for the diagnosis. With a suggestive history, a new murmur or a pulse deficit, an enlarged mediastinal shadow on chest radiography should prompt further diagnostic efforts. CT scanning, MRI and aortography may all be diagnostic, but no diagnostic modality has 100% sensitivity. Recently, TEE has enjoyed popularity for it appears highly sensitive in detecting a mobile intimal flap in the ascending or descending aorta. In addition, TEE can provide useful information regarding AR, periaortic hematoma and flow within a false channel. It is usually available at the bedside, or in the emergency ward, and does not subject the patient to a contrast load.

Once diagnosed, these patients are transported immediately to the OR. Through a median sternotomy, venous access is gained via the right atrium, and arterial inflow is supplied through a femoral artery. CPB is established, the patient cooled to 18°C, and circulatory support discontinued. During a period of profound circulatory arrest, the ascending aorta is opened, and the tear localized. The repair is carried distally into the arch, if the entire dissection can be resected, and the distal aortic layers are reapproximated with a Teflon felt strip supporting the medial and adventitial layers. The distal graft anastomosis is then completed, the graft clamped, the bypass pump restarted and systemic warming commenced. Proximally, the aortic root is reconstructed, again using Teflon felt to support the medial and adventitial layers and to resuspend the aortic valve, which can be salvaged in approximately 85% of cases. The heart is then cleared of air, and the cross-clamp removed to allow reperfusion of the coronary circulation. After a sufficient period of resuscitation, the patient is weaned from CPB. Aggressive management of an acquired coagulopathy is not unusual prior to chest closure.

Repair of dissections involving the descending thoracic aorta is accomplished through a left thoracotomy utilizing partial CPB. Venous drainage is usually via the femoral vein, although the PA or pulmonary vein may be used. Arterial access is via the femoral artery. After institution of CPB, the dissected aorta above and below the most damaged area is cross-clamped and the aorta transected. After oversewing patent intercostal arteries, the medial and adventitial layers are buttressed with Teflon felt, and an interposition Dacron graft is sewn into place. After evacuation of air, clamps are removed, and the patient weaned from CPB. Heparin reversal, decannulation and closure are accomplished in the usual manner.

Usual preop diagnosis: Acute dissection of the aorta (see Fig 6.2-1 for types of dissection).

SUMMARY OF PROCEDURE

	Ascending Aorta	Descending Aorta
Position	Supine	Lateral decubitus, left side up
Incision	Median sternotomy	Left lateral thoracotomy
Unique considerations	Full hemodynamic monitoring, with provisions for circulatory arrest, topical hypothermia, barbiturates and steroids; TEE	DLT; CPB; TEE
Antibiotics	Cefazolin 1 g iv	⇐
Surgical time	Cross-clamp: 30-50 min Circulatory arrest: 20-30 min CPB: 60-100 min Total: 3-5 h	30-60 min – 35-60 min ⇐
Closing considerations	Aggressively treat coagulopathy (frequently 2° ↓Plt).	Replace DLT with single-lumen ETT.
EBL	400-800 ml	600-800 ml
Postop care	ICU: 1-2 d, intubated	⇐
Mortality	10-25%	⇐
Morbidity	Bleeding: 3-8% Respiratory insufficiency: 2-5% CVA: 2-4%	Paraplegia: 5% CVA: 1-2% MI: 1-2%
Pain score	7-10	9-10

PATIENT POPULATION CHARACTERISTICS

Age range	40-70 yr
Male:Female	3:2
Incidence	10/100,000
Etiology	Degenerative aortic disease
Associated conditions	HTN; secondary aortic regurgitation; bicuspid aortic valve; Marfan syndrome

ANESTHETIC CONSIDERATIONS

PREOPERATIVE

Sx are usually of sudden onset and depend on the site of dissection and specific organ involvement. Aortic dissections are divided into 2 types, depending on the site of initial dissection: **Type A**—ascending and arch aorta, and **Type B**—descending aorta. Initial treatment involves the use of antihypertensive medications (e.g., SNP) to control BP and β-blockers (e.g., esmolol) to ↓ contractility. Type A dissections usually require urgent surgery.

Respiratory ✓ for recurrent laryngeal nerve palsy with chronic aneurysmal dilation. Tracheal and left main bronchus compression → difficult intubation, atelectasis; hemoptysis 2° rupture into lung; hemothorax → compromised oxygenation, ↑intrathoracic pressure → ↓ venous return, especially with IPPV.

Tests: CXR: ✓ for widened mediastinum, tracheal or left main bronchus compression and distortion (affects DLT placement), atelectasis, pleural effusion (or hemothorax 2° rupture).

Cardiovascular Aortic dissections may be associated with chronic HTN, cystic medial necrosis or other connective tissue disorder (e.g., Marfan syndrome) and trauma. Dissection may result in cardiac tamponade, acute aortic valve incompetence, acute cardiac failure, angina, MI or rupture of the aorta. Dissection of major arteries may result in ↓ or absent peripheral pulses which may affect the placement sites for intraarterial monitoring and central venous access. Pain and anxiety may result in HTN, while rupture or leakage may result in hypotension and shock.

Tests: ECG: ✓ for Sx of LVH, ischemia or infarction, low voltage (tamponade). ECHO: ✓ for site of dissection, valvular competence, LV function, pericardial effusion or tamponade. Angiography: ✓ for site of dissection (Type A or B), valvular function, involvement of coronary and other major arteries, sites of rupture, LV function. CT scan: ✓ site and extent of dissection.

Neurological Deficits are not uncommon, especially with Type B dissections where the blood supply to the spinal cord may be jeopardized. Document carefully.

Renal Renal failure 2° renal artery involvement in dissection, shock or cardiac failure. UO should be closely monitored during initial medical therapy.
Tests: UO; BUN; creatinine; electrolytes

Gastrointestinal Compromised blood supply to the bowel or liver may result in ischemia → metabolic acidosis and ↓liver function.
Tests: Consider ABG: ✓ persistent metabolic acidosis; LFTs, if indicated by H&P.

Hematologic Coagulopathy may be present 2° massive hemorrhage or liver involvement, and can increase risk of the surgery.
Tests: PT; PTT; Hct/Hb

Laboratory Other tests as indicated from H&P.

Premedication Since many of these patients present emergently, consider full-stomach precautions: H_2-antagonists (ranitidine 50 mg iv), metoclopramide (10 mg iv), antacids (Na citrate 0.3 M 30 ml po). Alleviate anxiety and pain, which may worsen HTN, but avoid obtundation (e.g., morphine 0.1 mg/kg im, ± midazolam 0.025-0.1 mg/kg iv or 0.05-0.2 mg/kg im).

INTRAOPERATIVE

Anesthetic technique: GETA. Preinduction control of BP and contractility (NTG or SNP to SBP = 105-115 and esmolol to HR = 60-80) is important in preventing extension of the dissection or rupture of the aneurysm. Fluid resuscitation may be necessary prior to induction. If present, cardiac tamponade should be relieved by pericardiocentesis.

Induction Control of hypertensive response to laryngoscopy is important and may be accomplished with moderate- to high-dose narcotic (fentanyl 10-100 μg/kg or sufentanil 0.5-20 μg/kg) with etomidate (0.1-0.3 mg/kg) or midazolam (50-350 μg/kg) and esmolol (100-500 μg/kg over 1 min, followed by 50-100 μg/kg/min infusion). SNP (0.5-3 μg/kg/min) and/or pretreatment with lidocaine (1.5 mg/kg) also may be required to further control the hypertensive response to laryngoscopy. Avoid ketamine because of its hypertensive effect. Muscle relaxation may be obtained using vecuronium or pancuronium (0.1 mg/kg). Remember the possibility of a full stomach in this patient population. Hence a modified rapid-sequence induction (cricoid pressure with manual ventilation and nondepolarizing muscle relaxant) may achieve the two goals of relatively rapid induction and intubation and tight control of BP. Usually a left DLT is used in patients with descending lesions to improve surgical access; however, it may be difficult to place due to aneurysmal compression of the trachea and left mainstem bronchus, and it is associated with a small risk of aneurysmal rupture. For these reasons, a right DLT may be preferred. FOB is useful to verify ET placement.

Maintenance O_2/narcotic/benzodiazepine: low-dose volatile agent may be used to control BP (MAP = 60-80), although infusion of vasopressors, vasodilators or inotropes may be necessary. Control HR (< 80; anesthesia, esmolol), and contractility (β-blockade or inotropes, depending on circumstances). Benzodiazepines may be used for amnesia (midazolam 50-350 μg/kg; diazepam 0.3-0.5 mg/kg). Most type A aneurysms and ascending/arch aneurysms require hypothermic CPB (see Anesthetic Considerations for Cardiopulmonary Bypass, p. 218). Intraop anesthetic considerations are governed primarily by the site of the aortic pathology. These considerations are discussed below.

Emergence Transported to ICU, sedated, intubated and ventilated × 24-48 h. Following repairs of the descending aorta (thoracotomy incision), weaning from ventilator may be aided by epidural narcotics after documentation of normal spinal cord function and coagulation.

Blood and fluid requirements
Anticipate large blood loss.
IV: 14 ga - 7 Fr × 2
NS/LR @ 6-8 ml/kg/h
Warm all fluids.
Humidify gases.
Cross-match 2-4 U of blood.
UO 0.5-1 ml/kg/h

In Type A dissections and arch aneurysms, if possible, avoid iv placement in the left arm or left IJ/subclavian veins because of the possibility of innominate vein ligation. Mannitol (0.5-1 g/kg iv) should be given if renal perfusion is compromised by dissection or before cross-clamping. Consider normovolemic hemodilution if the patient is stable and the Hct > 35.

Monitoring
Standard monitors (p. B-1).
Arterial line

Arterial line site is dependent on type of surgery and location of the lesion. Because the right subclavian artery

Monitoring, cont.	PA catheter Urinary catheter	may be compromised in patients with ascending lesions, the left radial or femoral arteries may need to be used. Aortic arch lesions may involve the vascular supply to both upper extremities; hence, femoral artery catheterization may be necessary. In ascending lesions, two artery lines may be required—right radial (above clamp pressure) and left femoral (below clamp pressure). Consult with surgeon as to best site.
	TEE	TEE is useful to assess cardiac function, regional wall motion abnormalities, valvular pathology, aortic valvular repair (if required as part of a Type A repair). Probe passage may increase compression of the trachea, impeding ventilation. Caution should be used in the presence of aneurysmal compression of the esophagus.
	Temperature	Monitor both core (rectal/bladder) and nasopharyngeal/tympanic membrane temperature (as indicative of brain temperature)—important in deep hypothermic arrest.
	EEG (arch/ascending lesions)	EEG may help in assessing effectiveness of cerebral protection (silent EEG) or adequacy of cerebral perfusion.
	SSEPs (descending lesions)	SSEPs may detect posterior spinal perfusion problems, but cannot detect anterior cord dysfunction or predict postop paraplegia. Both EEG and SSEP may require expert help to set up, monitor and interpret.
Complications	Hemorrhage Coagulopathy	Both are common. Hemorrhage should be treated with crystalloid, colloid or blood, as indicated.
Ascending lesions	CPB AR Coronary arteries	Usual site of cannulation for CPB is the femoral artery. Aortic valve replacement may be necessary. Patients may have myocardial ischemia 2° coronary artery occlusion; may require CABG or reimplantation of vessels.
	Deep hypothermic arrest	Cerebral protective measures and selective perfusion of cerebral vessels may be required. (See below.)
Arch lesions	CPB Deep hypothermic arrest	Usual site of cannulation for CPB is femoral artery. Cerebral protection relies on hypothermia (15-18°C) and drugs (methylprednisolone [Solu-Medrol] 1 g, mannitol 0.5-1 g/kg, STP 15-30 mg/kg) to reduce $CMRO_2$ and neuronal injury. The head is surface cooled (protect eyes and ears from cold injury). Monitor EEG to ensure absence of brain electrical activity. Monitor tympanic membrane or nasopharyngeal temperatures as an indication of brain temperature. Avoid hyperglycemia and maintain normal pH and $PaCO_2$ when measured at 37°C (alpha stat). Maintain muscle relaxation.
Descending lesions	Pre cross-clamping	Mannitol (0.5-1 g/kg) should be given prior to clamp application to provide renal protection, even if a shunt is placed. Hypothermia (32-34°C) may protect spinal cord.
	Shunt	A heparin-bonded shunt may be used from the aortic arch to the femoral artery to provide distal perfusion.
	Partial bypass	Partial CPB may be used to provide distal perfusion. In this arrangement, the heart perfuses the head and upper extremities, while CPB is used to perfuse and oxygenate the lower body. Venous drainage is from the femoral vein, PA or left atrium and returned via the femoral artery. Distal and proximal pressures are altered by controlling cardiac filling, pump flow and vasodilators.
	Cross-clamping	Application of clamp may → acute HTN with ischemia and LV failure. This may be controlled by partial bypass,

Descending lesions, cont.		shunting or use of vasodilators (SNP 0.5-4 μg/kg/min, NTG 0.5-4 μg/kg/min). During cross-clamping, monitor UO and ✓ metabolic acidosis (renal or bowel ischemia) with serial ABGs. Cross-clamp time should be < 30 min to reduce incidence of paraplegia. Occasionally, the surgeons may request that a lumbar CSF drain be inserted to ↓ CSF pressure in the spine and thus improve spinal cord blood flow.
	Unclamping	Unclamping may result in severe hypotension and myocardial depression. Hypovolemia, acidosis, vasodilator factors and reactive hyperemia have been implicated as the cause. Prior to unclamping, ensure adequate volume status (PCWP 2-5 mmHg above patient's normal); treat acidosis; have vasopressors available, and the clamp should be released slowly over 1-2 min. Use of partial bypass or a shunt to ensure distal perfusion will mitigate unclamping shock.
Positioning	✓ eyes. ✓ and pad pressure points. Arch and ascending: supine, shoulder roll Descending: lateral decubitus, axillary roll, pillow between knees	

POSTOPERATIVE

Complications	Myocardial ischemia, CHF Dysrhythmias Hemorrhage Coagulopathy Renal failure Bowel ischemia Respiratory failure	A DLT may be required in lesions of the descending aorta, if hemorrhage continues from left lung; otherwise, the tube may be replaced at the end of procedure by a single-lumen ETT. BP should be controlled to MAP 60-80 and HR < 100 to decrease the likelihood of repeat dissection or graft dehiscence.
	Paraplegia	Anterior spinal artery syndrome
Pain management	Parenteral opioids for pain relief Benzodiazepines for sedation	
Tests	ECG: ischemia, infarction, dysrhythmias CXR: line and ETT placement, pulmonary contusion Coagulation profile Renal: BUN, creatinine ABG: Respiratory, gut ischemia CT scan: CNS or spinal neurologic deficits Electrolytes	

References

1. Brodkin IA, Murkin, JM: Protection of the brain during cardiac surgery. In *The Practice of Cardiac Anesthesia*, 2nd edition. Hensley FA Jr, Martin DE, eds. Little, Brown: 1995, 581-602.
2. Cammarata BJ: Anesthesia for surgery of the thoracic aorta. In *Anesthesia for Cardiac Surgery,* 2nd edition. DiNardo JA, ed. Appleton & Lange, Stamford: 1998, 259-76.
3. Fann JI, Smith JA, Miller DC, et al: Surgical management of aortic dissection over a 30-year period. *Circulation* 1995; 92(II):113-21.
4. Hickey PR; Anderson NP: Deep hypothermic circulatory arrest: a review of pathophysiology and clinical experience as a basis for anesthetic management. *J Cardiothorac Anesth* 1987; 1(2):137-55.
5. Kwitka G, Kidney SA, Nugent M: Thoracic and abdominal aortic aneurysm resections. In *Vascular Anesthesia.* Churchill-Livingstone, New York: 1991, 363-94.
6. Miller DC, Mitchell RS, Oyer PE, et al: Independent determinants of operative mortality for patients with aortic dissections. *Circulation* 1984; 70(Suppl I):I-153-64.

REPAIR OF ANEURYSMS OF THE THORACOABDOMINAL AORTA

SURGICAL CONSIDERATIONS

Description: Aneurysms of the thoracoabdominal aorta (TAAA) may occur because of degenerative aortic disease (atherosclerosis), as a consequence of hereditary disorders of metabolism (Marfan syndrome), or as a sequela of chronic aortic dissections. These aneurysms are classified into four types that occur with equal frequency: Type I consists of aneurysms that involve most of the descending thoracic and upper abdominal aorta. Type II involves most of the descending thoracic aorta and most or all of the abdominal aorta. Type III involves the distal thoracic and varying segments of the abdominal aorta. Type IV involves most or all of the abdominal aorta, including the origins of the visceral vessels.

Repair of these aneurysms is an extensive, difficult and demanding procedure, as blood flow to the entire body below the neck is interrupted, with resultant renal and visceral ischemia. Additionally, the blood supply to the spinal cord may arise from lumbar and/or intercostal vessels in the affected aortic segment, producing critical cord ischemia during cross-clamping and postop paraplegia.

Almost all thoracoabdominal aneurysm repairs are performed through a thoracoabdominal incision using the **inclusion technique** as advocated by **Crawford**, et al.[3] After opening the chest, the incision is extended across the costal cartilage onto the abdomen. The diaphragm is radially incised to the aortic hiatus, and the retroperitoneal dissection plane established anterior to the psoas musculature. All intraabdominal contents, as well as the left kidney, are reflected anteriorly. Only proximal aortic control is established. After minimal heparinization, single-lung anesthesia is established to allow collapse of the left lung, the proximal aorta at the aneurysm neck is cross-clamped, and the aneurysm incised. Back-bleeding from patent intercostal, mesenteric and renal vessels can be controlled by balloon catheters; and aggressive blood salvage with autotransfusion devices is mandatory. The repair entails suturing a tube graft proximally to the divided aorta, and then sewing islands of aortic tissue containing intercostal visceral vessels onto appropriate sized holes in the side of the tube graft to allow reperfusion of important intercostal, celiac axis, superior mesenteric, renal arteries and, finally, the distal aorta or iliac arteries. Since there is obligate visceral ischemia during the period of cross-clamping (which must be limited to less than 60-75 minutes), the operation must proceed expeditiously.

Alternatively, in an effort to afford both spinal cord and visceral protection through hypothermia, the operation may be performed on CPB during a period of profound hypothermic circulatory arrest, but with marked exacerbation of hemorrhagic complications.

After aortic cross-clamping, the aneurysm is opened and the repair performed from within the aneurysm, sewing on-lay patches of the intercostal, mesenteric and renal vessels to openings created in the tube graft. This no-clamp technique allows reasonable management of these very extensive aneurysms, but results in an obligatory and ongoing blood loss through back-bleeding of visceral vessels until the anastomoses are complete.

Usual preop diagnosis: Expanding, painful or large thoracoabdominal aneurysm

SUMMARY OF PROCEDURE

Position	Right lateral decubitus; hips rotated posteriorly to 45° and left arm draped forward over an airplane sling. Axillary roll placed.
Incision	Posterolateral thoracotomy incision, in appropriate interspace, extended across the costal margin to midline, then extended inferiorly as a midline abdominal incision. The incision is one of the largest incisions in surgery, necessitated by the absolute need for exposure in this difficult area, and is, unfortunately, associated with a lot of postop pain.
Special instrumentation	DLT; CPB; NG tube
Unique considerations	OLV with collapse of left lung necessary for most cases. Cold LR may be injected into renal or visceral arteries for organ preservation. Alternatively, operation can be performed under profound hypothermic circulatory arrest for spinal cord protection in patients with chronic dissections. Cell Savers and rapid-infusion devices used to augment red-cell salvage and rapid-transfusion requirements. Frequently, operation is performed with only proximal cross-clamping; so there may be an obligate ongoing blood loss from visceral arterial orifices, as well as from distal aorta and iliac arteries.
Antibiotics	Cefazolin 1 g iv
Surgical time	6 h. Proximal aortic cross-clamping until completion of visceral revascularization may extend to 60 min. Longer cross-clamp times may be anticipated in patients with chronic aortic dissections for which profound hypothermic circulatory arrest is frequently utilized.
Closing considerations	OR → ICU, intubated × 24-48 h.

EBL Ongoing back-bleeding from visceral and iliac vessels results in substantial volume loss during cross-clamping, approaching 5-7 L. Most red-cell volume may be salvaged and returned through a RBC salvage system.

Postop care ICU, intubated and ventilated × 24-72 h. Rewarming, hemodynamic monitoring and volume resuscitation are often required in ICU.

	Aneurysm Group:	Type I	Type II	Type III	Type IV
Mortality	Overall: 9%	–	10-25%	–	5%
Morbidity	Paraplegia/spinal cord ischemia	6%	15%	3%	2%
	Other neurological complications	6%	12%	2%	1%
	Renal insufficiency	–	2-5%	–	–
	Respiratory failure	–	10%	–	–
	Graft infection	–	1-6%	–	–
	MI	–	–	–	–
	Graft failure	–	Rare	–	–
	Graft thrombosis	–	–	–	–
	False aneurysm	–	–	–	–
	Embolization	–	–	–	–
	Bowel ischemia	–	2-10%	–	–
	Impotence	Rare	⇐	⇐	⇐
	Ureteral injury	Rare	⇐	⇐	⇐
	Hemorrhage	Common	⇐	⇐	⇐
Pain score	6-10				

PATIENT POPULATION CHARACTERISTICS

Age range Non-Marfan: 55-75 yr; Marfan: 35-55 yr

Male:Female 3:1

Incidence < 5 cases/yr in most hospitals, except major referral centers

Etiology Predominantly atherosclerotic. Patients with Marfan syndrome may present with a progressive dilatation of a chronic dissection.

Associated conditions HTN (75%); CAD (30%); COPD (30%); renal insufficiency (15%)

ANESTHETIC CONSIDERATIONS

PREOPERATIVE

Respiratory Chronic pulmonary disease is associated with postop morbidity. Preop preparation with bronchodilators, cessation of smoking, incentive spirometry and chest physiotherapy may decrease the risk of postop problems.
Tests: CXR: ✓ for distortion of the left mainstem bronchus which may affect placement of the DLT. May need PFTs, ABG to determine severity of pulmonary disease.

Cardiovascular CAD is the most frequent cause of perioperative and late death in elective thoracoabdominal aortic aneurysm repair. It is commonly associated with HTN.
Tests: ECG: ✓ for LVH and ischemia.

Neurological Increased risk of spinal cord ischemia with cross-clamping of the aorta; therefore, any preop neurologic deficits should be well documented. The use of deep hypothermic circulatory arrest may be used in patients with chronic aortic dissections.

Renal Preop renal dysfunction increases the potential for postop renal problems. Aneurysmal involvement of the renal arteries also may occur.
Tests: BUN; creatinine; consider creatinine clearance

Gastrointestinal Aneurysmal involvement of the inferior mesenteric and superior mesenteric arteries may cause visceral ischemia.
Tests: Consider abdominal x-ray (ileus) and ABG (metabolic acidosis)

Hematologic Preexisting coagulopathy increases risk. Many patients have been on aspirin preop. Excessive alcohol use is associated with anemia, thrombocytopenia and low production of vitamin K-dependent factors. Rarely, a DIC process may occur within the lumen of the aneurysm.
Tests: PT; PTT; Plt count; Hct

Laboratory Electrolytes; radiologic assessment of aneurysm (ultrasonography, CT and arteriography)

Premedication Anxiety and pain may contribute to HTN and risk of aneurysmal rupture. Morphine 0.1 mg/kg im and midazolam 0.07 mg/kg im. Full-stomach precautions for emergent procedures (e.g., metoclopramide 10 mg iv, ranitidine 50 mg iv, Na citrate 30 ml po).

INTRAOPERATIVE

Anesthetic technique: GETA. The goals of anesthesia for this procedure are to: (1) preserve myocardial, renal, pulmonary, CNS and visceral organ function; (2) maintain adequate intravascular volume so that CO is not impaired; (3) control BP so that the transmural pressure across the aneurysm does not increase, thereby increasing the risk of rupture; and (4) provide good perfusion of other organs. CPB is used to accomplish deep hypothermic circulatory arrest. The rationale for this use is controversial. Deep hypothermic cardiac arrest (DHCA) may confer spinal cord protection and is usually reserved for patients with chronic dissections. In addition, removal of CSF has been proposed as a means of protecting the spinal cord against ischemic injury. CPB also may be used for distal perfusion of organs and afterload protection of the left ventricle. Partial CPB is usually reserved for suprarenal or supraceliac aneurysms in order to perfuse bowel and kidneys. (See Anesthetic Considerations for Cardiopulmonary Bypass, p. 218, and Repair of Acute Aortic Dissections, p. 274, for more discussion on CPB and DHCA.)

Induction Prevent hypertensive response to laryngoscopy with high-dose narcotic technique (fentanyl 10-50 μg/kg or sufentanil 5-15 μg/kg) and the use of benzodiazepine (midazolam 50-300 μg/kg) or etomidate (0.1-0.3 mg/kg). Esmolol 100-500 μg/kg over 1 min, NTP 0.5-3 μg/kg, or lidocaine administered either by topical spray or an iv dose of 1.5 mg/kg will also decrease the cardiovascular response to intubation. Muscle relaxation for intubation may be achieved with vecuronium (beware of ↓HR) or pancuronium (0.1 mg/kg). Etomidate is useful in unstable patients for emergent repair following rupture or ongoing dissection. A modified rapid-sequence induction may be necessary in emergent cases. A DLT is mandatory for this procedure; however, it may be difficult to position due to distorted anatomy. FOB may be helpful to position DLT.

Maintenance O_2/air/narcotic, ± low-dose volatile agent. Benzodiazepines may be used for amnesia (e.g., midazolam 50-300 μg/kg, diazepam 0.3-0.5 mg/kg). In hemodynamically unstable patients, scopolamine (400 μg) provides amnesia. Maintain CO and control of BP at preop levels. These patients may have increased hemodynamic variability on cross-clamping aorta, 2° bleeding and coexisting disease. Keeping the patient warm may be difficult due to large incision and visceral exposure.

Emergence Deferred to ICU. Postop ventilation 24-72 h. DLT may need to be maintained postop 2° to facial, oral and airway edema.

Blood and fluid requirements

Anticipate large blood loss.
IV: 14 ga or 7 Fr × 2
Rapid infuser
Cell Saver
PRBCs cross-match 8-10 U.
Warm fluids and humidify gases.
Maintain UO 0.5-1 ml/kg/h.

Large incision and visceral exposure requires administration of large volumes of fluid. Consider use of mannitol, furosemide, ACE inhibitors or low-dose dopamine 1-3 μg/kg/min if concerned about renal function and UO.

Monitoring

Standard monitors (p. B-1)
PA catheter
ST segment analysis
Arterial line
UO

✓ for ↑ PA pressures and PCWP, ↓ in CO, TEE wall motion abnormalities and changes in EF. Consult with surgeon regarding placement of cross-clamp so arterial line will not be affected.

TEE

TEE is a good monitor for ventricular filling and myocardial ischemia.

Core temperature

Monitor core temperature (rectal, bladder). Nasopharyngeal or tympanic membrane temperature (indicative of brain temperature) is monitored for circulatory arrest cases.

Monitoring, cont.	± EEG, SSEP	EEG, SSEPs may be useful in assessment of cerebral protection and spinal cord perfusion problems.
Cross-clamping	Clamping	Application of cross-clamp at supraceliac level probably produces the greatest hemodynamic stress experienced by surgical patients. Application of the clamp may result in HTN and ischemia. Preload, afterload and HR can be controlled with SNP (0.25-5 μg/kg/min) and esmolol (100-500 μg/kg/min) infusions.
	Unclamping	Ensure adequate volume; replace blood loss. Just before removal of the cross-clamp, filling volumes are allowed to rise gradually, avoiding the occurrence of myocardial ischemia. Dilators are D/C. Hypotension may occur with removal of cross-clamp 2° hypovolemia, reactive hyperemia, acidosis or myocardial dysfunction. If necessary, surgeon can reclamp or occlude the aorta.
Positioning	Right axillary roll ✓ and pad pressure points. ✓ eyes.	Right lateral decubitus with hips rotated posteriorly. Left arm placed in airplane sling or supported by pillows.
Complications	Myocardial ischemia HTN Coagulopathy Hemorrhage Hemostasis Hypothermia Other organ ischemia	Coagulopathy due to dilutional and consumptive processes. Hypothermia may exacerbate coagulopathy, cause dysrhythmias and depress cardiac contractility.

POSTOPERATIVE

Complications	Myocardial ischemia Neurologic deficits 2° cerebral or spinal cord ischemia Renal failure Respiratory failure	BP should be closely controlled postop to decrease bleeding from graft site and raw surfaces.
Pain management	Epidural narcotics (p. C-1).	Epidural is placed only after normal neurologic and coagulation status is determined.
Tests	CXR line and ETT placement Coagulation profile ABG analysis	

References

1. Bailin MT, Davison KJ: Amnesia for abdominal aortic reconstruction: One approach at Massachusetts General Hospital. In *Anesthesia for Vascular Surgery*. Churchill Livingstone, New York: 1990, Ch 12.
2. Coselli JS: Thoracoabdominal aortic aneurysms: experience with 372 patients. *J Card Surg* 1994; 9(6):638-4.
3. Crawford ES, Crawford JL, Safi HJ, Coselli JS, Hess KR, Brooks B, Norton HJ, Glaeser DH: Thoracoabdominal aortic aneurysms: Preoperative and intraoperative factors determining immediate and long-term results of operations in 605 patients. *J Vasc Surg* 1986; 3(3):389-404.
4. Crawford ES, Walker HSJ III, Solen SA, Normann NA: Graft replacement of aneurysm in descending thoracic aorta: results without bypass or shunting. *Surgery* 1981; 89: 73-85.
5. Kazama S, Masaki Y, Maruyma S, Ishihara A: Effect of altering cerebrospinal fluid pressure on spinal cord blood flow. *Ann Thorac Surg* 1994; 58(1):112-5.
6. Moore W: *Vascular Surgery*, 5th edition. WB Saunders Co, Philadelphia: 1998.
7. Roizen MF, Beaupre PN, Alpert RA, et al: Monitoring with two-dimensional transesophageal echocardiography. Comparison of myocardial function in patients undergoing supracelias, suprarenal-infraceliac, or infrarenal aortic occlusion. *J Vasc Surg* 1984; 1:300-5.

SURGERY OF THE ABDOMINAL AORTA

SURGICAL CONSIDERATIONS

Description: Operations on the abdominal aorta are generally performed for aneurysmal or occlusive diseases. Although aortic aneurysms may involve the suprarenal aorta, the majority are infrarenal in origin, and may extend into the iliac arteries (Fig 6.2-2). Most (> 95%) are asymptomatic, and are discovered incidentally during investigation of another medical problem. Because of the associated increased risk for rupture as the aneurysm increases in size, most vascular surgeons recommend prophylactic repair for aneurysms > 5 cm in cross-section dimension. Repair also is indicated for painful aneurysms, those that have been associated with atheroembolism, and when there is documented recent increase in size, or evidence of leak or rupture. CAD coexists in 30-40% of these patients, and should be assessed preop.

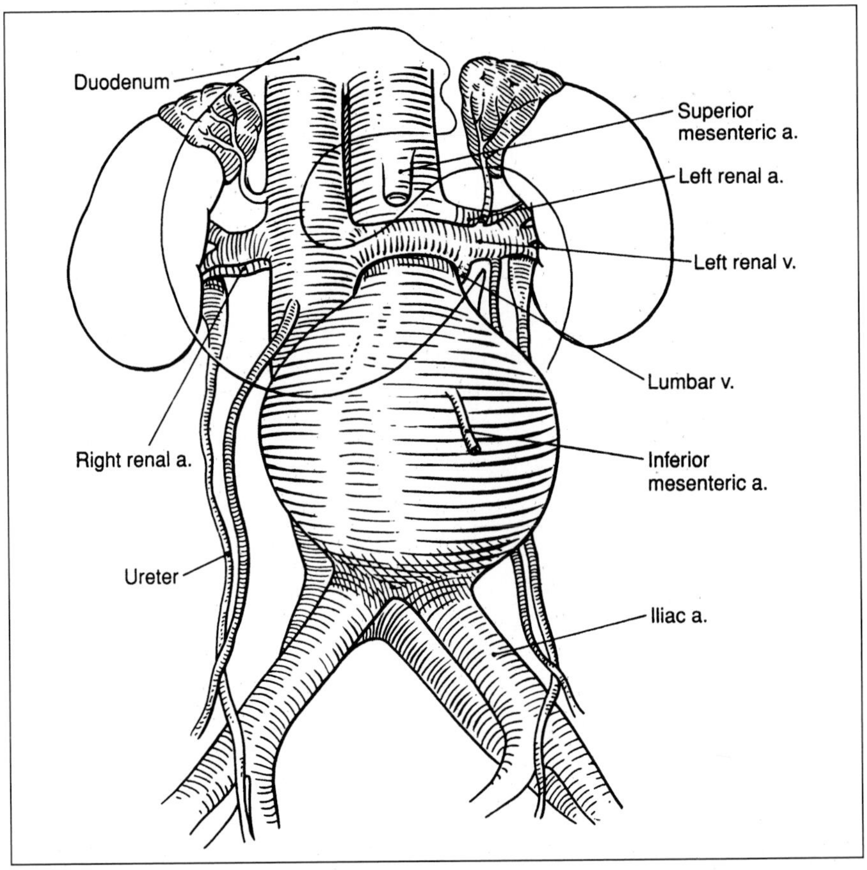

Figure 6.2-2. Aneurysm of the abdominal aorta. (Reproduced with permission from Calne R, Pollard SG: *Operative Surgery*. Gower Medical Pub: 1992.)

The operative repair may be either transperitoneal or retroperitoneal. After exposure of the abdominal aorta from the level of the renal vein distally to the iliac arteries, the aorta is cross-clamped, distally at first to prevent atheroembolism, and then proximally. Graft origin is usually from the infrarenal aorta, but may arise from the inframesenteric aorta or even the supraceliac aorta. Graft termination may be to the distal aorta above the bifurcation (tube graft), to the common or external iliac arteries (Y graft), or the femoral arteries. Immediately prior to cross-clamping, vasodilators are increased to reduce afterload, which is significantly increased with application of the aortic cross-clamp. The aorta is then incised, lumbar vessels oversewn, and the aorta transected to allow an interposition graft to be sewn into place. The retroperitoneal approach has many advocates, as it may require less volume intraop, may be associated with less temperature loss, and may result in a shorter period of postop adynamic ileus. In a randomized, prospective study, however, no significant difference could be detected between these two approaches as regards blood loss or postop recovery time.

Aortoiliac occlusive disease can be a significant cause of lower extremity arterial insufficiency. Although the operative approach may be similar to that for aneurysmal disease, there exists a significant difference intraop in that there are not such profound changes associated with aortic clamping, since there is already some element of increased afterload 2° the occlusive disease. Nevertheless, hemodynamic monitoring is mandatory to allow for rapid volume shifts, and to assure adequate preload and sufficient afterload reduction, especially during the period of aortic cross-clamping.

Variant procedure or approaches: In the rare patient with COPD severe enough to preclude weaning from the ventilator postop, extraanatomic grafts (e.g., axillofemoral, iliofemoral and fem-fem bypass) can be constructed under local anesthesia.

Usual preop diagnosis: Abdominal aortic aneurysm (AAA); severe aortoiliac stenosis sufficient to cause debilitating buttock, thigh or calf claudication; isolated-inflow (aortoiliac) disease (rarely the sole cause for ischemic symptoms at rest or for tissue loss, except as a result of embolic complications)

SUMMARY OF PROCEDURE

	Transperitoneal Approach	Retroperitoneal Approach
Position	Supine	Supine with mild elevation of left flank
Incision	Midline abdominal	Left subcostal, left oblique, along 10th rib toward umbilicus
Special instrumentation	Self-retaining retractor; TEE	⇐
Unique considerations	Will need pharmacologic manipulation to ↓ afterload or ↑ preload coincident with clamping or unclamping of aorta.	⇐ (The retroperitoneal approach is not used for emergency cases.)
Antibiotics	Cefazolin 1 g iv	⇐
Surgical time	3-5 h	⇐
EBL	500 ml	⇐
Postop care	ICU 8-16 h, intubated. Requires aggressive volume administration to allow for 3rd-space loss in 1st 12 h postop. Patient comfort and respiratory management markedly improved by epidural catheter for postop analgesia. Careful cardiac monitoring.	⇐
Mortality	2-5% elective; 50% emergent	⇐
Morbidity	MI: 10-15% (3% fatal) Respiratory insufficiency/pneumonia: 5-10% Lower extremity ischemia: 2-5% Renal insufficiency: 2-5% Bowel complications: 3-4% Hemorrhage: 2-4% CVA: < 1% Infection: < 1% Paraplegia: < 0.4%	⇐
Pain score	8-10	7-10

PATIENT POPULATION CHARACTERISTICS

Age range	55 yr +
Male:Female	4:1
Incidence	3% of males > 55 yr; > 5% of patients > 50 yr in a general cardiology clinic[2,9]; 30-66/1000
Etiology	Atherosclerosis; Marfan syndrome; Ehlers-Danlos syndrome; dissection; infection, including syphilis
Associated conditions	HTN; CAD; COPD; cerebrovascular disease; renal insufficiency

ANESTHETIC CONSIDERATIONS

PREOPERATIVE

Respiratory Many patients have COPD and a long Hx of smoking. Preop preparation including bronchodilators, cessation of smoking, incentive spirometry and chest physiotherapy will decrease the risk of postop complications.

Tests: CXR. May need PFTs and ABG to determine severity of pulmonary disease.

Cardiovascular CAD is the most common cause of morbidity and mortality in this patient population. HTN increases risk of aneurysmal rupture; hence, preop control of BP is essential. ✓ BP in both arms to determine placement of arterial line intraop (arterial line should be placed in arm with higher BP).

Tests: Radiologic assessment of aneurysm using ultrasonography, CT, arteriography and MRI. ECG: ✓ for evidence of ischemia, infarction and LVH.

Renal Chronic renal insufficiency occurs frequently in this patient population 2° HTN, diabetes mellitus (DM) and atherosclerotic renovascular disease. Hypovolemia 2° radiographic dye studies and bowel prep → renal failure.

Renal, cont.	**Tests:** BUN, creatinine; consider creatinine clearance; electrolytes
Hematologic	Preop coagulation disorders should be corrected. Many patients are on aspirin, which should be D/C 7 d preop. Alcohol abuse can be associated with anemia, thrombocytopenia and ↓ vitamin K-dependent factors. Preop autologous blood donation ↓ transfusion risks. **Tests:** PT; PTT; Hct; Plt
Laboratory	Other tests as indicated from H&P.
Premedication	Anxiety and pain may cause HTN and ↑ risk of aneurysmal rupture. Sedatives and analgesics should be used as indicated (p. B-2). Full-stomach precautions for emergent procedures (p. B-5).

INTRAOPERATIVE

Anesthetic technique: GETA, combination of epidural and GA. The goals of anesthesia are to: (1) preserve myocardial, renal, pulmonary and CNS perfusion; (2) maintain adequate intravascular volume and CO; (3) anticipate the surgical maneuvers that will affect BP and blood volume; and (4) control BP to minimize risk of rupture while ensuring perfusion of other organs.

Induction	Undesirable cardiovascular responses may be minimized by using a high-dose narcotic technique (e.g., fentanyl 10-50 μg/kg or sufentanil 5-15 μg/kg) if the patient is to remain intubated postop. This can be used in conjunction with a benzodiazepine (midazolam 50-300 μg/kg). If it is planned to extubate the patient postop, anesthesia should be induced using less narcotic (e.g., fentanyl 5 μg/kg) in conjunction with STP (2-4 mg/kg) or etomidate (0.2-0.4 mg/kg). If an epidural will be used for postop pain relief, no further iv doses of narcotic should be given intraop. Patients with an epidural typically receive 10 ml of 2% lidocaine or 10 ml of 0.5% bupivacaine intraop. A sensory block is obtained and induction is begun. Muscle relaxants are chosen to minimize tachycardia or hypotension (e.g., vecuronium 0.1 mg/kg). If there is a hemodynamic response to oral airway insertion, tracheal lidocaine or further anesthetic is given before gentle laryngoscopy and intubation. Etomidate is useful for induction in hemodynamically unstable patients. Full-stomach precautions may be necessary.
Maintenance	O_2/air/narcotic and volatile agent. N_2O can be used, but it may cause bowel distention. Combining epidural and GA offers good abdominal relaxation. Patients receiving epidural local anesthesia may require phenylephrine to treat ↓BP 2° sympathetic blockade. Epidural catheter placement before systemic anticoagulation is a safe technique. Narcotic epidural analgesia should be given within 1 h of skin incision if morphine 3-8 mg is used. If hydromorphone (0.5-0.8 mg) is given epidurally, it is given within 1 h of abdominal closure. Patient may become hypothermic 2° large incision with visceral exposure and prolonged operation.
Emergence	Patients who have had uneventful surgery, especially utilizing a retroperitoneal approach, are frequently extubated in the OR, or shortly after arrival in the ICU. Patients with severe cardiac or pulmonary disease generally are mechanically ventilated for 24-48 h. Prevention of HTN and tachycardia during emergence may require titration of ß-adrenergic-blocking drugs (e.g., esmolol 50-300 μg/kg/min) and/or vasodilators (e.g., SNP 0.25-5.0 μg/kg/min) or NTG (0.25-5.0 μg/kg/min). It is important to assure full reversal from neuromuscular blockade.

Blood and fluid requirements	Major blood loss IV: 14 ga (or 7 Fr) × 2 4 U PRBC UO 0.5-1 ml/kg/h Warm all fluids. Humidify all gases.	Use of rapid infusion and blood-salvaging devices helpful. Consider acute normovolemic hemodilution. Hemorrhage should be treated with crystalloid, colloid or blood as appropriate.
Monitoring	Standard monitors (p. B-1)	Monitor for cardiac ischemia. Automated ST segment analysis is useful.
	CVP line	The measurement of CVP may be sufficient in patients with good ventricular function and exercise tolerance.
	PA catheter	In patients with recent MI, Hx of CHF, Hx of unstable angina, multisystem disease or in those presenting emergently (without the benefit of a complete workup), however, a PA catheter is appropriate.

Monitoring, cont.	TEE	TEE is invaluable for assessing cardiac changes 2° cross-clamping and unclamping the aorta.
	Arterial line Urinary catheter	The arterial line is generally placed in the radial artery of the arm having the higher BP (if difference exists).
Cross-clamping	↑↑ Afterload—HTN ↓ Preload ↑ Filling pressures ± ↓ Spinal cord perfusion ± ↓ Renal perfusion ↓ Perfusion to viscera below the clamp	Application of aortic cross-clamp causes HTN proximal to the clamp. In a healthy heart, this is well tolerated with minimal increase in filling pressure. In hearts with poor ventricular function, filling pressures generally rise. Control of preload, afterload and HR can be accomplished with vasodilators and β-blockers. Negative inotropic agents, like β-blockers and inhalational anesthetics, are used cautiously. Occlusion of infrarenal aorta decreases renal blood flow. Ensure adequate intravascular volume and CO. Consider use of mannitol, furosemide or low dose of dopamine 1-3 mg/kg/min to maintain UO.
Aortic unclamping	↓↓ Afterload Volume loading Lactate washout ± Phenylephrine	Immediately before unclamping, D/C dilators and negative inotropic agents. Gradually increase filling pressures (volume loading) to avoid myocardial ischemia. ↓↓BP may occur with removal of cross-clamp 2° to hypovolemia, reactive hyperemia or myocardial dysfunction. Reperfusion of lower limbs and washout of lactate does not usually require use of HCO_3. Patients with an epidural sympathetic block often require phenylephrine support during unclamping. The surgeon can reclamp or occlude the aorta, if ↓↓BP persists.
Positioning	✓ and pad pressure points. ✓ eyes.	
Complications	Myocardial ischemia HTN Hemorrhage Coagulopathy Hypothermia Organ ischemia	Hypothermia may cause dysrhythmias, depress contractility and exacerbate coagulopathy.

POSTOPERATIVE

Complications	Myocardial ischemia Renal failure Respiratory failure	
Pain management	Epidural narcotics (p. C-1)	
Tests	CXR to ✓ line and ETT placement ABG Coagulation profile BUN; creatinine	BP should be closely controlled postop to decrease bleeding from graft site and raw surfaces.

References

1. Brimacombe J, Berry A: A review of anaesthesia for ruptured abdominal aortic aneurysm with special emphasis on preclamping fluid resuscitation. *Anaesthes Intensive Care* 1993; 21(3):311-23.
2. Darling RC, Messina CR, Brewster DC, Ottinger LW: Autopsy study of unoperated abdominal aortic aneurysms. The case for early resection. *Circulation* 1977; 56(3 Suppl):II-161-64.
3. Dunn E, Prager RL, Fry W, Kirsh MM: The effect of abdominal aortic cross-clamping on myocardial function. *J Surg Res* 1977; 22:463-68.
4. Falk JL, Rackow EC, Blumenberg R, et al: Hemodynamic and metabolic effects of abdominal aortic cross-clamping. *Am J Surg* 1981; 142:174-77.
5. Foster JH, Bolasny BL, Gobbel WG Jr, Scott HW Jr: Comparative study of elective resection and expectant treatment of abdominal aortic aneurysm. *Surg Gynecol Obstet* 1969; 129:1-9.

6. Gold MS, DeCrosta D, Rizzuto C, Ben-Itarari RR, Ramanathan S: The effect of lumbar epidural and general anesthesia on plasma catecholamines and hemodynamics during abdominal aortic aneurysm repair. *Anesth Analg* 1994; 78(2):225-30.
7. Gooding JM, Archie JP Jr, McDowell H: Hemodynamic response to infrarenal aortic cross-clamping in patients with and without coronary artery disease. *Crit Care Med* 1980; 8:382-85.
8. Story RJ, Wylie EJ: Surgical management of arterial lesions of the thoracoabdominal aorta. *Am J Surg* 1972; 126:157-64.
9. Taylor LM Jr, Porter JM: Basic data related to clinical decision-making in abdominal aortic aneurysms. *Ann Vasc Surg* 1987; 1(4):502-4.

INFRAINGUINAL ARTERIAL BYPASS

SURGICAL CONSIDERATIONS

Description: Due to the limited durability of distal bypass procedures, bypass to the infrainguinal arteries is indicated only for salvage of the severely ischemic lower extremity, as manifest by gangrene, ischemic ulceration or ischemic rest pain. Less frequently, it is used to alleviate functional ischemia of claudication, or leg discomfort with exercise. Its use is predicated on the preexistence of adequate inflow to the level of the groin or femoral artery. Other necessary components include an adequate target vessel, preferably in continuity with runoff into the plantar arch of the foot, and an adequate conduit, preferably autologous saphenous vein. Long-term patency rates of nonautologous conduits to the below-knee arteries is distinctly inferior to that of saphenous vein, and should be avoided whenever possible. This population, almost by definition, includes patients with diabetes mellitus (DM), CAD and cerebrovascular disease, all of which must be assessed preop.

The operative repair usually involves incisions at the groin distal bypass sites to expose the donor and recipient arteries, and to harvest leg or arm venous conduit. The operative approaches are rather similar. An unobstructed inflow source—usually the common femoral, superficial femoral or deep femoral artery—is exposed in the groin. The target distal artery, usually at the level of the knee or below, can be approached through a medial incision. More distally, the peroneal and anterior tibial arteries can be approached laterally at the midtibial level. At the level of the malleolus, both the dorsalis pedis and posterior tibial arteries can be revascularized. After control of donor and recipient vessels, an anatomic tunnel is created, and the bypass conduit (saphenous vein, prosthetic graft) passed through its length. After administration of 10,000 U of heparin, the distal anastomosis is constructed first, followed by the proximal anastomosis. A completion arteriogram confirms unobstructed flow. Heparin is then partially reversed and meticulous hemostasis obtained, and the wounds are closed.

Although conventional wisdom has held that the anesthetic and operative risks for these patients undergoing distal reconstructions are low, recent data have shown little difference in postop morbidity and mortality when compared with patients undergoing a major inflow procedure within the abdomen.[11]

Usual preop diagnosis: Severe peripheral vascular disease; CAD; DM; HTN; obstructive PA disease. (These are almost ubiquitous comorbidities.)

SUMMARY OF PROCEDURE

Position	Supine
Incision	Groin, medial knee, ± distal leg incisions; + incision to harvest venous conduit
Antibiotics	Cefazolin 1 g iv at induction of anesthesia
Surgical time	2-5 h
Closing considerations	Optimization of coagulation status
EBL	200-300 ml
Postop care	Possible ICU × 24 h; careful monitoring is mandatory as patients are at risk for myocardial ischemia.
Mortality	2-4%[20]
Morbidity	MI: 5-12% Respiratory insufficiency: 5% Infection: 2-5% Amputation: 2-4% CVA: < 1%
Pain score	4-6

PATIENT POPULATION CHARACTERISTICS

Age range	> 55 yr (mean age = > 70 yr)
Male:Female	4:1
Incidence	Claudication fairly common in elderly; however, 75% will remain untreated, but stable, over 2-5 yr, with < 5% requiring amputation.
Etiology	Arteriosclerosis (primarily); chronic embolic disease (rare); vasculitis; popliteal artery entrapment; cystic adventitial disease of popliteal artery
Associated conditions	CAD; cerebrovascular disease; DM; HTN; COPD

ANESTHETIC CONSIDERATIONS

(Procedures covered: infrainguinal arterial bypass; lumbar sympathectomy; venous thrombectomy or vein excision)

PREOPERATIVE

Patients presenting for peripheral vascular surgery may suffer from major systemic diseases, including CAD, HTN and DM. Three types of occlusive vascular disease have been described: Type 1—isolated to the aortic and iliac bifurcations; is not associated with CAD. Type 2—diffuse pattern involving coronary and cerebral circulations, associated with a higher incidence of diabetes and HTN. Type 3—involves small vessels, especially of the lower limbs, and is associated with higher postop morbidity and mortality.

Respiratory Vascular patients frequently have Hx of smoking and COPD. Preop evaluation of pulmonary function helps to determine whether regional vs GA is appropriate, while providing baseline values for postop comparison.
Tests: CXR; consider PFTs; ABG

Cardiovascular Vascular surgery of the lower extremities is often associated with ↑morbidity and mortality 2° ↑incidence of CAD and HTN in this patient population.
Tests: ECG: ✓ for LVH and ischemia; other tests as indicated from H&P.

Neurological Increased incidence of cerebrovascular disease. Careful neurological assessment is necessary to document existing deficits.

Endocrine Increased incidence of DM, which may be associated with peripheral and autonomic neuropathies (silent MI, labile BP) and delayed gastric emptying. Insulin requirements for most diabetic patients can be managed by administering one-half the usual a.m. dose of insulin once a dextrose-containing iv (e.g., D5LR) has been established. Frequent blood glucose measurements should be made perioperatively.

Renal There is a higher incidence of renal artery disease and renal insufficiency in this patient population.
Tests: BUN; creatinine; consider creatinine clearance; electrolytes; UA

Hematologic Many patients presenting for this surgery are taking anticoagulant/anti Plt medications. Inquire as to bleeding or bruising tendency.
Tests: Hct; Plt; consider PT, PTT

Laboratory As indicated from H&P.

Premedication Continue usual medications up to time of surgery. Anxiety can contribute to HTN and tachycardia. Premedicate conservatively (midazolam 5 mg im) for elderly patients. If ischemic pain is present, a narcotic such as morphine (3-7 mg im) can be given. Avoid im administration in patients on anticoagulant therapy.

INTRAOPERATIVE

Anesthetic technique: Either regional anesthesia or GETA may be used. For infrainguinal arterial bypass, there is evidence that regional anesthesia is superior for promoting graft survival. To date, no study has shown a difference in patient mortality between these anesthetic techniques. **Lumbar sympathectomy** may be accomplished with regional or GA. For **thrombectomy**, GETA with IPPV may reduce the risk of pulmonary emboli.

General anesthesia:

Induction Hemodynamic stability is important; therefore, a slow, gradual induction is carried out.

Induction, cont.	Preoxygenation is followed by smooth iv induction using small, incremental doses of fentanyl (1-2 μg/kg), then STP is given in divided doses (50-75 mg at a time) until the patient is asleep. A full dose of muscle relaxant is given and ventilation is controlled. Muscle relaxation is not necessary during the procedure, but muscle relaxant is given to facilitate intubation. The muscle relaxant is chosen to avoid undesirable effects on HR. Alternatively, if the LV function is poor, and the depressant effects of STP cannot be tolerated, a high-dose narcotic technique (e.g., fentanyl 10-50 μg/kg) is appropriate.
Maintenance	Standard maintenance (p. B-3). If high-dose narcotic technique is used, benzodiazepines are given for amnesia. Continued muscle relaxation is unnecessary. These surgical procedures are associated with minimal hemodynamic instability.
Emergence	Tracheal extubation should be based on standard criteria, such as adequacy of ventilation, return of airway reflexes and reversal of muscle relaxation. Control of BP is accomplished with vasodilators (e.g., NTG 0.1-4.0 μg/kg/min or SNP 0.25-5.0 μg/kg/min). Esmolol can be given in incremental doses of 10 mg or by infusion (50-200 μg/kg/min).

Regional anesthesia: Patients presenting for regional anesthesia must have a normal coagulation profile; also, they cannot be on heparin (including low molecular weight), urokinase or streptokinase. The important goals in regional anesthesia are to achieve hemodynamic stability while establishing an adequate block. An epidural or spinal catheter (multiorifice) is frequently used to infuse local anesthetic for a gradual onset and to prevent an excessively high block. Hemodynamic stability can be improved by infusing 500-1000 ml of crystalloid before performing the block. The patient may be placed in the lateral decubitus position (with operative side down), which may provide a denser and more prolonged block on that side. Achieving a T8-T10 level is optimal. Overzealous hydration may → CHF in this patient population, when the vasodilation 2° regional sympathectomy dissipates. The use of regional anesthesia in patients receiving intraop anticoagulation is controversial. We feel it is a relatively safe procedure and have not had a complication with this technique. If blood is aspirated after placement of an epidural, we remove the catheter and then replace it at a different interspace. Patients on minidose heparin should have a normal PTT before use of regional anesthesia.

Spinal	**One-shot spinal:** 1% hyperbaric tetracaine (6-10 mg) or 0.75% bupivacaine (10-15 mg). Add epinephrine 0.2 mg (generally increases duration of block about 50%) or phenylephrine 5 mg (generally increases duration of block about 100%). Do not add vasoconstrictor if patient is diabetic. Large doses of hyperbaric local anesthetic should be avoided as they may cause postop cauda equina syndrome. **Continuous spinal:** A 20-ga catheter is placed via an 18-ga Tuohy needle. 0.5% hyperbaric tetracaine or 0.75% bupivacaine is titrated to desired anesthetic level (T8-T10). Catheters should be redosed every 60-80 min or as soon as BP trends upward. The risk of spinal headache is very low with continuous spinals.
Epidural	Lidocaine 2% with 1:200,000 epinephrine or 0.5% bupivacaine is used. Titrate to desired anesthetic level (T8-T10).

Blood and fluid requirements	IV: 14 or 16 ga × 1 NS/LR @ 3-5 ml/kg/h Warm fluids. Humidify gases. Maintain UO 0.5-1 ml/kg/h	Minimal-to-moderate blood loss
Monitoring	Standard monitors (see p. B-1). ST-segment analysis Arterial line	An arterial line is most often used in patients with severe cardiopulmonary disease or brittle diabetics. Blood sampling for ABGs, electrolytes, glucose and Hct is facilitated by the use of an arterial line.
	± CVP/PA catheters	CVP and PA catheters are not used routinely because large changes in intravascular volumes are uncommon. Patients with poor LV function, recent MI or severe valvular disease may need PA monitoring.
Positioning	✓ and pad pressure points. ✓ eyes.	Diabetic patients may be at risk of skin ischemia due to poor positioning or inadequate padding of limbs, etc.
Complications	HTN Ischemia	

Complications, cont.	Hypothermia Hemorrhage	

POSTOPERATIVE

Complications	CHF Hypothermia Graft occlusion	Infrainguinal bypass: Avoid overhydration; when epidural sympathectomy fades, these patients are at increased risk for CHF. Maintain normovolemia so that peripheral vasoconstriction (which may limit outflow to the graft) does not occur. Hypothermia causes vasoconstriction and also may limit outflow to the graft.
Pain management	Epidural/spinal opiates (p. C-1) PCA	Epidural (or spinal) catheter may be used for postop analgesia (p. C-1).
Tests	CXR if central line placed Hct	

References

1. Bernards CM: Epidural and spinal anesthesia. In *Clinical Anesthesia,* 3rd edition. Barash PG, Cullen BF, Stoelting RK, eds. Lippincott-Raven, Philadelphia: 1997, 645-68.
2. Carli F, Gabrielczyk M, Clark MM, Aber VR: An investigation of factors affecting postoperative rewarming of adult patients. *Anaesthesia* 1986; 41(4):363-69.
3. Christopherson R, Beattie C, Meinert CL, Gottlieb SO, Frank SM, Norris EJ, Yates H, Rock P, Parker SD, Perler BA, Williams GM: Perioperative Ischemia Randomized Anesthesia Trial Study Group: Perioperative morbidity in patients randomized to epidural or general anesthesia for lower extremity vascular surgery. *Anesthesiology* 1993; 79:422-34.
4. Collin GJ, Rich HM, Clagett GP: Clinical results of lumbar sympathectomy. *Am Surg* 1981; 47:31-35.
5. Concepciono M, Maddi R, Francis D, Rocco AG, Murray E, Covino BG: Vasoconstrictors in spinal anesthesia with tetracaine—a comparison of epinephrine and phenylephrine. *Anesth Analg* 1984; 63(2):134-38.
6. Cousins MJ, Wright CJ: Graft; muscle, skin blood flow after epidural block in vascular surgical procedures. *Surg Gynecol Obstet* 1971; 133(1):59-64.
7. Covino BG: *Reasons to preferentially select regional anesthesia.* IARS Review Course Lectures, 60th Congress. International Anesthesia Research Society, Cleveland: 1986, 61-5.
8. Dalessandri KM, Carson SN, Tillman P, et al: Effect of lumbar sympathectomy in distal arterial obstruction. *Arch Surgery* 1983; 118:1157-60.
9. Damask MC, Weissman C, Barth A, et al: General vs epidural—which is the better anesthetic technique for femoral-popliteal bypass surgery? *Anesth Analg* 1986; 65:539.
10. Denny N, Masters R, Pearson D, Rend J, Sihota M, Selander D: Postdural puncture headache after continuous spinal anesthesia. *Anesth Analg* 1987; 66(8):791-94.
11. Krupski WC, Layug EL, Reilly LM, Rapp JH, Mangano DT: Comparison of cardiac morbidity between aortic and infrainguinal operations. Study of Perioperative Ischemia (SPI) Research Group. *J Vasc Surg* 1992; 15(2):354-65.
12. McKenzie PJ, Wishart HY, Dewar KM, Gray I, Smith G: Comparison of the effects of spinal anaesthesia and general anaesthesia on postoperative oxygenation and perioperative mortality. *Br J Anaesth* 1980; 52(1):49-54.
13. Park WY, Balingit BE, MacNamara TE: Effects of patient age, pH of cerebrospinal fluid, and vasopressors on onset and duration of spinal anesthesia. *Anesth Analg* 1975; 54(4):455-58.
14. Rao TL, El-Etr AA: Anticoagulation following placement of epidural and subarachnoid catheters: an evaluation of neurologic sequelae. *Anesthesiology* 1981; 55(6):618-20.
15. Rosenfeld BA, Beattie C, Christopherson R, Norris EJ, Frank SM, Breslow MJ, Rock P, Parker SD, Gottlieb SO, Perler BA, Williams GM, Seidler A, Bell W: Perioperative Ischemia Randomized Anesthesia Trial Study Group: The effects of different anesthetic regimens on fibrinolysis and the development of postoperative arterial thrombosis. *Anesthesiology* 1993; 79:435-43.
16. Rutherford RB: Role of sympathectomy in the management of vascular disease. In *Vascular Surgery*, 5th edition. Moore WS, ed. WB Saunders, Philadelphia: 1998, 349-60.
17. Terry HJ, Allan JS, Taylor GW: The effect of adding lumbar sympathectomy to reconstructive arterial surgery in the lower limb. *Br J Surg* 1970; 57(1):51-5.
18. Varkey GP, Brindle GF: Peridural anaesthesia and anti-coagulant therapy. *Can Anaesth Soc J* 1974; 21(1):106-9.
19. Vaughan MS, Vaughan RW, Cork RC: Postoperative hypothermia in adults: relationship of age, anesthesia, and shivering to rewarming. *Anesth Analg* 1981; 60(10):746-51.
20. Veith FJ, Gupta SK, Samson RH, et al: Progress in limb salvage by reconstructive arterial surgery combined with new or improved adjunctive procedures. *Ann Surg* 1981; 194:386-401.

LUMBAR SYMPATHECTOMY

SURGICAL CONSIDERATIONS

Description: The role of **lumbar sympathectomy** is not well defined.[2,5] The procedure is used selectively in patients with causalgia, inoperable lower limb ischemia with rest pain or toe gangrene, symptomatic vasospastic disorders (e.g., Raynaud's phenomenon, frostbite), and sometimes as an adjunct to distal revascularization procedures.[1,2,5] Causalgia responds well to lumbar sympathectomy, especially if performed early in the clinical course. There may be some benefit of the procedure in 50-60% of patients with rest pain or ischemic ulceration.[4] Sympathectomy may increase collateral blood flow and local skin blood flow.[3] Scleroderma with impending "minor" amputation may benefit from sympathectomy with improved wound healing.[2] Sympathetic denervation involves the division of preganglionic fibers along their segmental origins and resection of corresponding relay ganglia.[5] For most clinical indications, L2 and L3 **ganglionectomy** sufficiently sympathectomizes the lower extremity.

The **anterolateral retroperitoneal approach** (**Flowthow**) is most commonly performed because of the adequate exposure and a relatively well tolerated incision.[5] For this approach, an oblique incision is made through the abdominal musculature, extending from the lateral border of the rectus abdominus to the anterior axillary line. Cephalad and caudad blunt dissection is performed between the transversalis fascia and peritoneum. The dissection is continued in a retroperitoneal fashion. The psoas muscle is identified, with care being taken to leave the ureter and gonadal vessels attached to overlying peritoneum. The sympathetic chain is identified between the psoas muscle and the vertebra (medial to psoas and overlying the transverse process of lumbar vertebra). The sympathetic chain is dissected free from surrounding tissue, clipped proximally and distally and resected. On the left side, the sympathetic chain is lateral to the abdominal aorta; on the right, the sympathetic chain is beneath the IVC. Hemostasis is achieved and the abdominal wall is closed in layers.

A **posterior approach** (**Royle**) is used less often because of significant postop paraspinous muscle spasms. In this approach, a transverse lumbar incision is made, and the paraspinous muscles are partially divided and retracted to expose the vertebra. The sympathetic chain is identified and resected as described. The anterior/transperitoneal approach is performed in conjunction with an abdominal aortic or intraperitoneal procedure. Dissection is carried to the psoas muscle; the retroperitoneum is entered and the sympathetic chain is isolated in the groove between the psoas and the vertebra. The sympathetic chain is clipped proximally and distally and resected. **Adson's anterior transperitoneal approach** is used when combined with an abdominal aortic or other intraperitoneal procedure.

Usual preop diagnosis: Causalgia; inoperable arterial occlusive disease with limb-threatening ischemia causing rest pain, ulceration or superficial digital gangrene; symptomatic vasospastic disorders (e.g., Raynaud's phenomenon or frostbite)

SUMMARY OF PROCEDURE

	Anterolateral Retroperitoneal (Flowthow)	Posterior (Royle)	Anterior Transperitoneal (Adson)
Position	Supine (flank slightly raised); widen distance between costal margin and iliac crest.	Prone	Supine
Incision	Oblique (lateral edge of rectus to ribs at anterior axillary line)	Posterior transverse over midlumbar region	Transverse or midline abdominal
Special instrumentation	Self-retaining retractor	⇐	⇐
Unique considerations	May use frozen section to confirm specimen.	⇐	
Antibiotics	Cefazolin 1g iv	⇐	⇐
Surgical time	2-3 h	3 h	4 h
Closing considerations	Flex table to facilitate abdominal wall closure; occasionally drain is placed.	⇐	⇐
EBL	50-100 ml (unless complicated)	50-100 ml	⇐
Postop care	PACU → ward. (May require cardiac and hemodynamic monitoring in high-risk patients, or if combined with distal revascularization.	⇐	⇐

	Anterolateral Retroperitoneal (Flowthow)	Posterior (Royle)	Anterior Transperitoneal (Adson)
Mortality[1,3,4]	Minimal	⇐	⇐
Morbidity	Postsympathectomy neuralgia: 50%	~50%	⇐
	Sexual derangement—retrograde ejaculation (usually bilateral L1 sympathectomy): 25-50%	~25-50%	⇐
	Wound hematoma: 10%	~10%	⇐
	Wound infection: 1-3%	~1-3%	⇐
		Paraspinous muscle spasms	
Pain score	5	5	5 (related to primary procedure)

PATIENT POPULATION CHARACTERISTICS

Age range	38-91 yr; younger patients with vasospastic disease; older patients with PVD
Male:Female	2:1
Incidence	Unknown. Approximately 30 cases/yr at SUMC, mainly for inoperable lower extremity ischemia or as an adjunct to revascularization procedures.
Etiology	PVD (rest pain and tissue loss); vasospastic disorders; causalgia
Associated conditions	PVD (rare); vasospastic disorders (rare)

ANESTHETIC CONSIDERATIONS

See Anesthetic Considerations following Infrainguinal Arterial Bypass, p. 287.

References

1. Abu Rahma AF, Robinson PA: Clinical parameters for predicting response to lumbar sympathectomy in patients with severe lower limb ischemia. *J Cardiovasc Surg* 1990; 31(1):101-6.
2. Boltax RS: Lumbar sympathectomy: a place in clinical medicine. *Conn Med* 1989; 53(12):716-17.
3. Norman PE, House AK: The early use of operative lumbar sympathectomy in peripheral vascular disease. *J Cardiovasc Surg* 1988; 29(6):717-22.
4. Repelaer van Driel OJ, van Bockel JH, van Schilfgaarde R: Lumbar sympathectomy for severe lower limb ischaemia: results and analysis of factors influencing the outcome. *J Cardiovasc Surg* 1988, 29(3):310-14.
5. Rutherford RB: Role of sympathectomy in the management of vascular disease. In *Vascular Surgery*, 5th edition. Moore WS, ed. WB Saunders Co, Philadelphia: 1998, 349-60.

UPPER EXTREMITY SYMPATHECTOMY

SURGICAL CONSIDERATIONS

Description: **Upper extremity sympathectomy** is the surgical treatment for hyperhidrosis, reflex sympathetic dystrophy (RSD), posttraumatic pain syndromes and certain vasospastic disorders affecting the hands and digits.[2,3,5] Palmar hyperhidrosis is especially responsive to surgical sympathectomy.[3] The results achieved with sympathectomy for upper extremity ischemic and posttraumatic pain syndromes are less favorable. It is recommended that T2 and T3 ganglia be excised and the stellate ganglion spared. Manipulation of the stellate ganglion is associated with increased incidence of Horner's syndrome.[3] The **supraclavicular approach** was introduced in 1935[5] and is still used commonly. The **axillary, extrapleural approach** of **Atkins** was designed to provide an anatomic approach to the sympathetic chain. **Roos'**

modification of the Atkins technique includes an extrapleural approach to the sympathetic chain after resection of the first rib. This is very useful for identifying the exact level of the sympathetic chain, and is associated with less postop pain because rib retraction is unnecessary. The **anterior thoracic approach** involves a limited thoracotomy through the third interspace, which provides excellent exposure. It is, however, associated with the morbidity and mortality of a thoracotomy. Part of the sympathetic chain below the stellate ganglion may be excised more readily via this approach. All of these methods have intrinsic advantages and disadvantages, but only the supraclavicular and axillary methods are used widely. Newer techniques, such as **CT-guided phenol sympathetic block** and **transthorascopic sympathectomy**, have been developed and may yield comparable short- and long-term results.[3,6]

Usual preop diagnosis: Hyperhidrosis; RSD; ischemia; posttraumatic pain syndromes; vasospastic disorders; various forms of arteritis

SUMMARY OF PROCEDURE

	Supraclavicular	Axillary Transthoracic Or Extrapleural	Anterior Transthoracic
Position	Supine	Lateral decubitus (arm supported to avoid brachial plexus traction)	Supine (slight lateral decubitus)
Incision	Above medial 1/3 of clavicle	For **transthoracic:** transverse lower axilla (enter thorax at 2nd or 3rd interspace); for **extrapleural:** transverse axillary (resect 1st rib)	Anterior thoracotomy (enter thorax at 3rd interspace and divide 3rd-costal cartilage)
Special instrumentation	DLT	⇐	⇐
Antibiotics	Cefazolin 1 g iv	⇐	⇐
Surgical time	3-4 h	⇐	⇐
Closing considerations	May need drain.	Chest tube placed and connected to water seal for transthoracic approach.	Chest tube placed and connected to water seal.
EBL	100-200 ml	⇐	⇐
Postop care	PACU → ward	⇐	⇐
Mortality	Minimal	⇐	⇐
Morbidity	Postsympathectomy neuralgia: Common	⇐	⇐
	Pleurotomy: 10%	–	–
	Pleural effusion: 7%	~7%	⇐
	Gustatory sweating: 6%	~6%	⇐
	Horner's syndrome: 4%	~4%	⇐
	Pneumonia: 3%	~3%	⇐
	Atelectasis: 2%	~2%	⇐
	Phrenic nerve injury: 2%	–	–
	Pneumomediastinum: 2%	–	–
	Subclavian artery injury: 2%	–	–
	Lymphocele: 1%	–	–
	Wound hematoma: 1%	–	–
	Chylous fistula: Rare	⇐	–
	Winged scapula: Rare	⇐	–
Pain score	4	5	5

PATIENT POPULATION CHARACTERISTICS

Age range	11-45 yr
Male:Female	1:1
Incidence	Hyperhidrosis ≤ 1% of the population (palmar hyperhidrosis in 0.15-0.25%)
Etiology	Hyperhidrosis (strong family Hx); vasospasm and arteritides (idiopathic); ischemia—PVD, trauma, autoimmune disease
Associated conditions	PVD; trauma; autoimmune disease

ANESTHETIC CONSIDERATIONS

PREOPERATIVE

Patients are often young and generally healthy, although they may have associated autoimmune diseases and PVD.

Respiratory	Patients may require single-lung ventilation during surgery. ✓ for Hx of asthma, pneumonia, respiratory disease and recent Sx of dyspnea or productive cough. **Tests:** PFT and CXR, if indicated from H&P.	
Musculoskeletal	Avoid BP cuff and iv placement in affected limb.	
Laboratory	Other tests as indicated by H&P.	
Premedication	Midazolam 1-2 mg iv	

INTRAOPERATIVE

Anesthetic technique: GETA ± epidural. A thoracic epidural is beneficial for postop pain management.

Induction	Standard induction (p. B-2). DLT placement may be requested (see discussion of one-lung ventilation, p. 178).	
Maintenance	Standard maintenance (p. B-3)	
Emergence	No special considerations	
Blood and fluid requirements	Minimal blood loss IV: 18 ga × 1	
Monitoring	Standard monitors (p. B-1)	Arterial line needed occasionally.
Positioning	✓ and pad pressure points. ✓ eyes.	Avoid brachial plexus traction.
Complications	Pneumothorax Subclavian artery injury	

POSTOPERATIVE

Complications	Atelectasis Pneumothorax Pneumomediastinum Pleural effusion Chylous effusion Phrenic nerve injury Horner's syndrome	
Pain management	Epidural PCA (p. C-3)	Local anesthetic opioid (p. C-1)
Tests	CXR; Hct	As indicated

References

1. D'Haese J, Camu F, Noppen M, Herregodts P, Claeys MA: Total intravenous anesthesia and high-frequency jet ventilation during transthoracic endoscopic sympathectomy for treatment of essential hyperhidrosis palmaris: a new approach. *J Cardiothorac Vasc Anesth* 1996; 10(6):767-71.
2. Hartrey R, Poskitt KR, Heather BP, Durkin MA: Anaesthetic implications for transthoracic endoscopic sympathectomy. *Eur J Surg* (Suppl) 1994; (572):33-6.
3. Hashmonai M, Kopelman D, Kein O, Schein M: Upper thoracic sympathectomy for primary palmar hyperhidrosis: long-term follow-up. *Br J Surg* 1992; 79(3):268-71.
4. Moore WS: *Vascular Surgery,* 5th edition. WB Saunders, Philadelphia: 1998.
5. Moran KT, Brady MP: Surgical management of primary hyperhidrosis. *Br J Surg* 1991; 78(3):279-83.
6. Pace RF, Brown PM, Gutelius JR: Thoracoscopic transthoracic dorsal sympathectomy. *Can J Surg* 1992; 35(5):509-11.
7. Rutherford RB. Role of sympathectomy in the management of vascular disease. In *Vascular Surgery*, 5th edition. Moore WS, ed. WB Saunders, Philadelphia: 1998, 349-60.

VENOUS SURGERY—THROMBECTOMY OR VEIN EXCISION

SURGICAL CONSIDERATIONS

Description: Standard therapy for acute DVT consists of anticoagulation, bed rest and elevation of the extremity.[4,8] Surgical thrombectomy for acute iliofemoral DVT remains controversial. **Venous thrombectomy** is recommended for patients with threatened limb loss or venous gangrene caused by massive DVT associated with high compartment pressures and arterial insufficiency (phlegmasia cerulea dolens).[4,8] Venous thrombectomy requires exposure of the femoral vein via a groin cut-down. The common femoral vein is isolated (located medial or posteromedial to the femoral artery) and controlled proximally and distally. The patient is given iv heparin at this stage, if not already heparinized. A transverse venotomy is followed by extraction of the thrombus, using forceps and Fogarty embolectomy catheters. Distal thrombi are expressed through the same incision with the aid of an Esmarch bandage placed on the extremity.[4] After complete removal of the thrombus, the venotomy is closed with nonabsorbable sutures and flow through the femoral vein is reestablished. The femoral incision is closed in layers. A plastic/Silastic drain may or may not be used. The best results of thrombectomy are obtained in young patients with the first episode of proximal (iliofemoral) thrombosis.

Nonsuppurative thrombophlebitis of the superficial veins may develop due to local trauma, prolonged inactivity, fungal infection or the use of oral contraceptives.[4] Suppurative thrombophlebitis may occur as a complication of iv line placement or iv drug abuse. Underlying varicose veins may predispose to thrombophlebitis. Migratory superficial thrombophlebitis may be associated with chronic ischemia of the extremities in Buerger's disease, or it may develop in patients with a malignancy.[4] Conservative management with hot compresses, nonsteroidal anti-inflammatory medications, and elevation of the extremity is effective in most cases. Rarely, **excision** of the acutely thrombosed greater saphenous vein is indicated to prevent progression of thrombosis to the saphenofemoral junction and into the deep venous system.[4] Vein excision is simply approached by a longitudinal incision directly over the affected vein. The phlebitic vein is dissected from the surrounding tissue, ligated proximally and distally, and removed. The surrounding fibrotic tissue is debrided gently. The wound is irrigated and packed open with moist gauze. Suppurative phlebitis is treated with iv antibiotics and complete excision of the involved vein segment through multiple small incisions.

Usual preop diagnosis: Lower-limb venous thrombosis threatening viability; femoral thrombosis < 10 d; iliac thrombosis < 3 wk; floating thrombi at hip level; acute deep or superficial venous thrombosis; suppurative thrombophlebitis

SUMMARY OF PROCEDURE

	Thrombectomy	Vein Excision
Position	Supine	⇐
Incision	Ipsilateral longitudinal or oblique groin incision	Multiple small incisions along the course of vein to be excised
Special instrumentation	Fogarty embolectomy catheters; RBC salvage system	None
Unique considerations	IPPV during thrombectomy may decrease chance of PE 2° ↓venous return → more complete extraction of the thrombus.	None
Antibiotics	Cefazolin 1 g iv. If the patient has a septic thrombus, antibiotic is dependent on blood culture.	Dependent on culture of aspirate. Usually a septic patient is on broad-spectrum antibiotics (guided by culture).
Surgical time	2-3 h	1-3 h
Closing considerations	None	Wound packed open for drainage
EBL	50-250 ml	⇐
Postop care	PACU → ward; ICU in high-risk patients; heparin administered before and after procedure, followed by Coumadin for 1-6 mo.[8]	PACU → ward; support stockings
Mortality	Minimal (depending on underlying illness)	Minimal
Morbidity	Postthrombotic syndrome: < 10-44%[8] Venous stasis Nonpitting edema Brawny induration Aching pain	Minimal
Pain score	3	2

PATIENT POPULATION CHARACTERISTICS

Age range	Young adult–elderly
Male:Female	1:2
Incidence	6-7 million in U.S. have adverse effects from chronic venous stasis[7]; 500,000 have complications of leg ulceration.
Etiology	Chronic primary varicose veins; defective venous valves; impaired pumping action of muscles in leg; previous iliofemoral thrombophlebitis; obstruction of venous return
Associated conditions	Multifactorial: varicose veins; underlying malignancy; altered coagulation status (hypercoagulability, acquired or congenital); Hx of DVT/thrombophlebitis

ANESTHETIC CONSIDERATIONS

See Anesthetic Considerations following Infrainguinal Arterial Bypass, p. 287.

References

1. Angle N, Bergan JJ: Varicose veins: Chronic venous insufficiency. In *Vascular Surgery*, 5th edition. Moore WS, ed. WB Saunders, Philadelphia: 1998, 800-7.
2. Bergan JJ, Yao JS, et al. Surgical treatment of venous obstruction and insufficiency. *J Vasc Surg* 1986; 3(1):174-81.
3. Friedell ML, Samson RH, Cohen MJ, Simmons GT, Rollins DL, Mawyer L, Semrow CM: High ligation of the greater saphenous vein for treatment of lower extremity varicosities: the fate of the vein and therapeutic results. *Ann Vasc Surg* 1992; 6(1):5-8.
4. Gloviczki P, Merrell SW: Surgical treatment of venous disease. *Cardiovasc Clin* 1992; 22(3):81-100.
5. Greenfield LJ: Venous thromboembolic disease. In *Vascular Surgery,* 5th edition. Moore WS, ed. WB Saunders, Philadelphia: 1998, 787-99.
6. Large J: Surgical treatment of saphenous varices, with preservation of the main great saphenous trunk. *J Vasc Surg* 1985; 2(6):886-91.
7. Lofgren KA: Surgical management of chronic venous insufficiency. *Acta Chir Scand Suppl* 1988; 544:62-8.
8. Lord RS, Chen FC, et al: Surgical treatment of acute deep venous thrombosis. *World J Surg* 1990; 14(5):694-702.
9. Sottiurai VS: Surgical correction of recurrent venous ulcer. *J Cardiovasc Surg* 1991; 32(1):104-9.

SURGERY FOR PORTAL HYPERTENSION

SURGICAL CONSIDERATIONS

Description: Alcoholic liver disease is the major cause of portal HTN. End-stage liver disease with cirrhosis is the 10th leading cause of death in the U.S. (exceeding 23,000/year). 15-20% of patients with portal HTN have variceal hemorrhage during the first year of diagnosis (additional 5-10 % incidence of bleeding per year), and the initial episode of variceal hemorrhage is associated with 50% mortality. Portal HTN (>15 mmHg) develops when splanchnic venous flow to the right heart becomes impeded.[1,2,11,16] Medical and surgical therapeutic interventions are directed not at portal HTN per se, but at its complications, notably bleeding esophageal varices. Intractable ascites and hypersplenism are less common indications for operative therapy. Presinusoidal portal HTN, unlike sinusoidal or postsinusoidal obstruction, is not associated with severe hepatocellular disease; thus, the prognosis for patients with presinusoidal block is better than those with sinusoidal or postsinusoidal disease. Shunt procedures can be classified as **total shunts** (decompression of the portal venous system) or **selective shunts** (decompression of only the varix-bearing area).[12]

There are two general types of total shunt **(portosystemic shunt)** procedures.[13] The **end-to-side portacaval shunt** (Fig 6.2-3A) is technically simpler and may be more appropriate in emergency situations. It is associated with immediate control of hemorrhage in the majority of cases. The portacaval shunt, however, does eliminate portal perfusion of the liver and does not decompress the hepatic sinusoids. Alternatively, the **functional side-to-side shunt** (Fig 6.2-3B) allows decompression of hepatic sinusoids and may preserve some degree of portal perfusion of the liver. Also, it is more effective in controlling ascites. Variations of the side-to-side shunt include: **portacaval**, **splenorenal**, **mesocaval** (**Clatworthy**), and **portarenal** (rarely used).

For the **end-to-side** and **side-to-side portacaval shunts**, the approach is via an extended right subcostal incision. **Cholecystectomy** usually is not performed because of the likelihood of profuse bleeding from the liver bed. The hepatoduodenal ligament is identified, and the portal vein is exposed from the hilum of the liver to the pancreas. The gastroduodenal and right gastric branches may be divided to provide additional exposure of the portal vein. The IVC is exposed by incising the peritoneum just beneath the hepatic triad. Proximal and distal control of the portal vein is achieved; a side-biting clamp is placed on the IVC. In order to perform an end-to-side portacaval shunt, the portal vein is divided and oversewn proximally; the end-to-side anastomosis is performed from the portal vein to the IVC. The alternative is to perform a side-to-side anastomosis of the portal vein to the IVC without division of the portal vein.

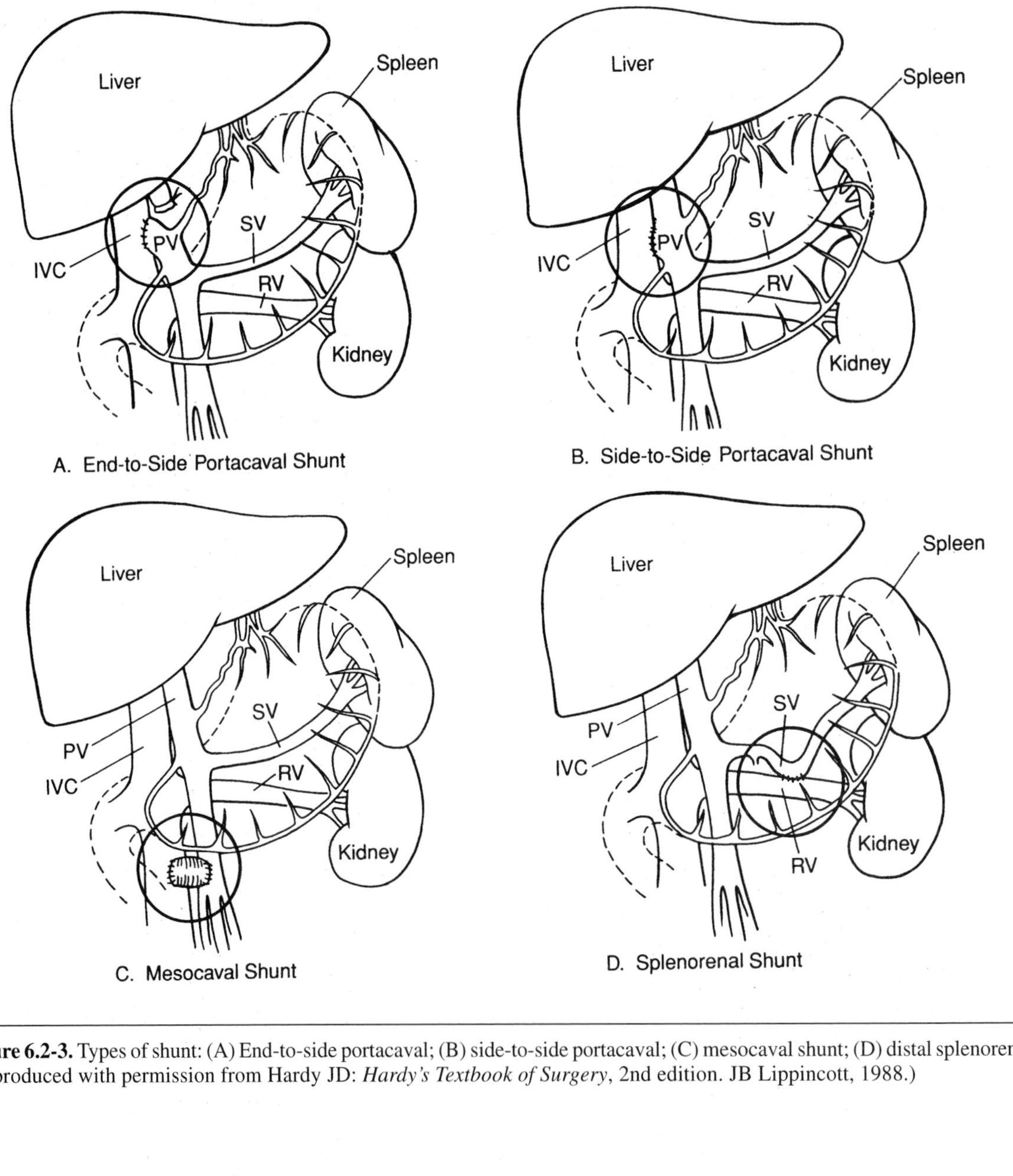

Figure 6.2-3. Types of shunt: (A) End-to-side portacaval; (B) side-to-side portacaval; (C) mesocaval shunt; (D) distal splenorenal. (Reproduced with permission from Hardy JD: *Hardy's Textbook of Surgery*, 2nd edition. JB Lippincott, 1988.)

The **proximal splenorenal shunt** is approached through a left thoracoabdominal or transabdominal incision. The spleen is isolated and removed, and the distal splenic vein is mobilized from the distal pancreatic bed. The left renal vein is exposed and controlled. The distal splenic vein is then anastomosed in an end-to-side fashion to the mid renal vein. The **mesocaval shunt** (Fig 6.2-3C) is indicated in cases of ascites, periportal fibrosis, portal vein thrombosis and Budd-Chiari syndrome.[1] The mesocaval shunt is approached through a vertical midline incision. The colon is retracted cephalad and the superior mesenteric vein (SMV) is identified at the root of the mesentery. A length of the SMV is isolated and encircled. A **Kocher maneuver** (mobilization of the duodenum) is performed and the IVC is exposed anteriorly and laterally. A side-biting clamp partially occludes the IVC and a 14-20 mm Dacron graft is anastomosed in an end-to-side fashion to the IVC. The graft is clamped and the side-biting clamp removed from the IVC, thereby restoring flow via the IVC. The SMV is clamped and an end-to-side anastomosis created from the graft to the SMV. Flow is thus reestablished from the SMV through the graft to the IVC.

Selective shunts are designed to decompress esophageal varices, while some portal perfusion of the liver is maintained.[7,8] The hallmark example of this approach is the **distal splenorenal shunt** (**Warren**) (Fig 6.2-3D), which is seldom used in emergency situations. The principal feature of this shunt is disconnection of the splenic and superior mesenteric venous drainage systems. The distal splenorenal shunt is approached through a left chevron or extended left subcostal incision. The lesser sac is entered after division of the gastroepiploic vessels and mobilization of the splenic flexure of the colon. The stomach is retracted cephalad and the peritoneum overlying the inferior aspect of the pancreas incised. The splenic vein is identified and controlled proximally and distally. The inferior mesenteric vein is divided. The splenic vein is divided proximally and the proximal stump oversewn. Then the splenic vein is mobilized from the pancreatic bed. The left renal vein is identified and 5-7 cm of the vein is isolated. The splenic vein is anastomosed in an end-to-side fashion to the renal vein. The coronary vein is ligated close to its origin. The distal splenorenal shunt decompresses the stomach, distal esophagus and spleen and controls variceal hemorrhage in 85% of patients.[7]

Variant procedure or approaches: **Total shunt** (e.g., portacaval, proximal splenorenal, mesocaval); **selective shunt** (e.g., Warren); **non-shunt procedures** (e.g., **Sugiura**, **Hassab** and **esophageal transection with stapling**)

Usual preop diagnosis: Bleeding esophageal varices (as a result of portal HTN); ascites; hypersplenism

SUMMARY OF PROCEDURES (TOTAL AND SELECTIVE SHUNTS)

	Portacaval	Proximal Splenorenal	Mesocaval (Clatworthy)	Distal Splenorenal (Warren)
Position	Supine	Supine ± left flank elevated	Supine	Supine, left side elevated slightly
Incision	Extended right subcostal–may be lengthened or converted to left thoracoabdominal.	Left thoracoabdominal or left subcostal, or vertical midline	Vertical midline abdominal	Left chevron or left subcostal with midline extension
Special instrumentation	Self-retaining retractor	⇐	⇐	⇐
Unique considerations	May need FFP; consider Cell Saver.	⇐	⇐	⇐
Antibiotics	Cefazolin 1 g iv	⇐	⇐	⇐
Surgical time	4-6 h	⇐	⇐	⇐
Closing considerations	None	⇐	⇐	⇐
EBL	1000-2000 ml	⇐	⇐	⇐
Postop care	Patient → ICU; careful fluid management; consider Na restriction; may require PA catheter.	⇐	⇐	⇐
Mortality[1,2,7,11-13,17,20]	Emergency: 38% 5-10% Elective: 3% Child's A: 0-15% Child's B: 1-43% Child's C: 6-58%	5-10%	⇐	1-16%

	Portacaval	Proximal Splenorenal	Mesocaval (Clatworthy)	Distal Splenorenal (Warren)
Morbidity[1,9,11,12,13]	Late liver failure: 50%	~50%	⇐	–
	Encephalopathy: 32%	~32%	⇐	5-47% (overall)
	Child's A: 8%			5% at 2 yr
	Child's B: 20%			12% at 3-6 yr
	Child's C: 30%			27% at 10 yr
	Early rebleeding: 0-19%	~0-19%	⇐	–
	Shunt thrombosis: 1-10%	20%	9-30%	–
			Duodenal obstruction	Loss of selectivity: 60% (@ 2 yr)
			Erosion through bowel wall	Recurrent variceal hemorrhage (shunt occlusion): 3-19%
				Portal vein thrombosis: 4-10%
Pain score	6	6	6	6

Note: In addition to the shunt procedure itself, other factors that determine postop morbidity and mortality include: severity of hepatocellular disease, degree of hepatic reserve, and urgency of the procedure. Although the specific numbers may vary, several comparative series have shown no difference in operative mortality rate or long-term survival rate among the various shunt procedures.[12]

NONSHUNT PROCEDURES

Nonshunt procedures are designed to devascularize the esophagogastric region, thus eliminating acute variceal hemorrhage. Procedures of this type include: **portazygous disconnection**; **splenectomy**; **coronary vein ligation**; and **transesophageal** or **transgastric varix ligation**.

The **Sugiura** operation, approached via abdominal and thoracic incisions, includes esophageal transection and devascularization, splenectomy and pyloromyotomy. This procedure is usually performed in two operative stages, with the second stage sometimes delayed. The **Hassab** procedure involves devascularization of the upper half of the stomach and splenectomy, thus effectively disconnecting the esophageal varices.[6] This operation has been reserved in some centers for the failures of sclerotherapy. Finally, **esophageal transection**, using a stapling device, disconnects the varices in the lower esophagus. This is accomplished by placing a row of staples at the esophagus just above the esophagogastric junction.[2,9,10,18] Because portal perfusion of the liver is maintained after the nonshunt procedures, hepatic function is preserved.[2]

SUMMARY OF NONSHUNT PROCEDURES

	Sugiura (2 Stages)	Hassab	Esophageal Transection
Position	Supine, left side elevated	Supine	⇐
Incision	Abdominal stage: midline; thoracic stage: left thoracotomy	Vertical midline	⇐
Special instrumentation	Self-retaining retractor	⇐	⇐
Antibiotics	Cefazolin 1 g iv	⇐	⇐
Surgical time	4-6 h for both stages	4 h	⇐
EBL	1000-2000 ml	⇐	⇐
Postop care	ICU; careful hemodynamic monitoring; PA catheterization	⇐	⇐
Mortality[1,5,12,18]	Overall: 5-14%	12-38%	10-83%
	Emergent: 14% (≤ 60%)	10%	
	Elective: 3%		
Morbidity[5,18]	Recurrent hemorrhage: 2-50%	7%	0-50%
	Esophagopleural leak: 6%	–	3%
	Encephalopathy: 3%	1-25%	33%
	Ascites: 2%	4%	11%
	Wound infection: 2%	–	11%
Pain score	6	5	5

PATIENT POPULATION CHARACTERISTICS

Age range	11-72 yr (mean age = 48 yr); depending on etiology: pediatric (e.g., congenital hepatic fibrosis) to adult (e.g., alcoholic liver disease)
Male:Female	2-8:1
Incidence	Rare
Etiology	Alcoholic liver disease (alcoholic hepatitis, chronic alcoholism, cirrhosis); postnecrotic cirrhosis; portal vein thrombosis; splenic vein occlusion; hematologic diseases; hepatic vein occlusion; schistosomiasis; congenital hepatic fibrosis; sarcoidosis; sinusoidal occlusion (vitamin A toxicity, Gaucher's disease); venoocclusive disease
Associated conditions	Alcohol dependency; cirrhosis/liver failure; poor nutritional status; coagulopathy; encephalopathy

ANESTHETIC CONSIDERATIONS

(Procedures covered: shunt and nonshunt procedures for portal HTN surgery)

PREOPERATIVE

Respiratory Hypoxemia may be present 2° ascites, V/Q mismatch, ↑R→L pulmonary shunting, atelectasis, pulmonary infections and ↓pulmonary diffusing capacity.
Tests: Consider ABG; PFTs, as indicated; CXR

Cardiovascular Patients presenting with portal HTN often have a hyperdynamic circulatory state with ↑plasma volume, ↑CO and ↓SVR with a decreased ability to ↑ SVR or ↑ HR in response to stimuli. Ventricular performance may be abnormal (CHF) especially in patients with alcoholic liver disease. Ascites → ↑intrathoracic pressure, ↓FRC, ↓venous return and ↓CO. Older patients in this population usually have CAD.
Tests: ECG. If LV function in question, ECHO or angiography.

Hepatic The physical manifestations of hepatic disease include palmar erythema, caput medusae, spider angiomas and gynecomastia. Albumin and other products of liver synthesis (e.g., coagulation factors) may be decreased. Encephalopathy may be present as a result of impaired ammonia metabolism.
Tests: Bilirubin; albumin; PT; SGOT; SGPT; ammonia; alkaline phosphatase

Gastrointestinal Portal HTN eventually results in esophageal and gastric varices. Patients may present emergently with profuse GI bleeding. Ascites occurs in approximately 80% of patients with portal HTN and splenomegaly is invariably present. As a result of elevated intraabdominal pressure from ascites, and slow gastric emptying, a rapid-sequence induction with full-stomach precautions will be necessary (see p. B-5).

Renal Portal HTN → ↓GFR and ↓renal blood flow → renal failure.
Tests: Consider UA; creatinine clearance as indicated from H&P

Hematologic These patients are often anemic as a result of poor nutrition, malabsorption, and intestinal tract blood loss. Hypersplenism may be present (Plt count < 50,000 and WBC < 2,000). Synthesis of all coagulation factors is decreased except factor VIII and fibrinogen. A low-grade DIC may be present. Cross-match for 8-10 U PRBC.
Tests: CBC; Plt count; PT; PTT; consider DIC screen.

Pharmacologic The liver is the major site of drug biotransformation; however, the effects of hepatic dysfunction on drug elimination and disposition are inconsistent.

Laboratory These patients may have significant electrolyte disturbances (e.g., ↓↓Na^+, ↓K^+).
Tests: Electrolytes and others as indicated from H&P.

Premedication If premedication is appropriate, small doses of anxiolytic such as midazolam (0.5-1 mg iv) are preferable. Avoid im medications in patients with possible coagulopathy. Full-stomach precautions are necessary. Metoclopramide (10 mg iv) and ranitidine (50 mg iv) may be given 60 min before surgery.

INTRAOPERATIVE

Anesthetic technique: GETA. Preservation of intravascular volume and myocardial stability can be a challenge in these patients.

Induction Rapid-sequence induction with STP (3-5 mg/kg) and succinylcholine (1-2 mg/kg) should be used. Replace blood loss and ensure normovolemia before induction (if possible). Etomidate (0.2 mg/kg) or ketamine (1 mg/kg) may be preferable for induction in hemodynamically unstable patients.

Maintenance High-dose narcotic technique with fentanyl (50-100 μg/kg) or sufentanil (10-15 μg/kg) and low-dose isoflurane. Midazolam (0.1-0.2 mg/kg) is often given in conjunction with the narcotic to ensure amnesia during times of hemodynamic instability when isoflurane cannot be tolerated. N_2O is avoided to prevent bowel distention. Muscle relaxation is needed (e.g., vecuronium 0.1 mg/kg or less, titrated using a nerve stimulator).

★ **NB:** After drainage of ascitic fluid, there may be a precipitous drop in BP requiring rapid volume replacement ± vasopressor.

Emergence Generally deferred to ICU due to large fluid shifts and transfusion requirements. Patients who have undergone uneventful and nonemergent surgery may be candidates for extubation.

Blood and fluid requirements

IV: 14 ga × 2 or 7 Fr × 2
Anticipate large blood loss.
Rapid infuser
RBC salvage device
8-10 U PRBC
Warm all fluids.
Humidify all gases.
Warming blanket
Bair-Hugger warmer

FFP, Plt and cryoprecipitate should be available to treat coagulopathy.

Monitoring

Standard monitors (p. B-1) — Arterial and central pressure monitoring are essential.
Arterial line
CVP or PA catheter — A PA catheter is useful in this setting because most patients are cirrhotic and may have excessive blood loss and large fluid shifts.
UO — In these procedures, prevention of hypothermia is important. UO is measured and is helpful as a monitor of renal perfusion. Mannitol (0.25-1 g/kg iv) may be needed to maintain UO.
In patients with large varices, avoid esophageal placement of temperature probes or stethoscopes.
ABGs — Serial ABGs to determine adequacy of ventilation and normal acid base status should be done.
Hct, coags, Ca^{++} — Hct, coagulation, and Ca^{++} should be measured following replacement of large blood volumes.
Electrolytes — Electrolytes and glucose also should be monitored.
Blood glucose — Glucose metabolism in liver disease may be impaired → ↓glucose.

Positioning

✓ and pad pressure points.
✓ eyes.

Complications

Coagulopathy
Hemorrhage
Hypothermia

POSTOPERATIVE

Complications

Coagulopathy
Hypothermia
Encephalopathy
Renal failure

Pain management

PCA (p. C-3)
Parenteral opiates

Tests

CXR: line placement — DIC screen, if continued bleeding.
Hct
Electrolytes
Glucose

References

1. Collini FJ, Brener B: Portal hypertension. *Surg Gynecol Obstet* 1990; 170(2):177-92.
2. Gelabert HA: Portal hypertension. In *Vascular Surgery*, 5th edition. Moore WS, ed. WB Saunders, Philadelphia: 1998, 754-86.
3. Gelman S, Fowler KC, Smith: Liver circulation and function during isoflurane and halothane anesthesia. *Anesthesiology* 1984; 6:726.
4. Gusberg RJ: Selective shunts in selected older cirrhotic patients with variceal hemorrhage. *Am J Surg* 1993; 166(3): 274-78.
5. Haberer JP, Schoeffler P, Couderc E, Duraldestin P: Fentanyl pharmacokinetics in anesthetized patients with cirrhosis. *Br J Anaesth* 1982; 54:1267.
6. Hassab MA: Nonshunt operations in portal hypertension without cirrhosis. *Surg Gynecol Obstet* 1970; 131(4):648-54.
7. Henderson JM: The distal splenoral shunt. *Surg Clin North Am* 1990; 70(2):405-23.
8. Henderson JM, Millikan WJ Jr, Galloway JR: The Emory perspective of the distal splenorenal shunt in 1990. *Am J Surg* 1990; 160(1):54-9.
9. Hoffmann J: Stapler transection of the oesophagus for bleeding oesophageal varices. *Scand J Gastroenterol* 1983; 18(6):707-11.
10. Huizinga WK, Angorn IB, Baker LW: Esophageal transection versus injection sclerotherapy in the management of bleeding esophageal varices in patients at high risk. *Surg Gynecol Obstet* 1985; 160(6):539-46.
11. Johansen K, Helton WS: Portal hypertension and bleeding esophageal varices. *Ann Vasc Surg* 1992; 6(6):553-61.
12. Langer B, Taylor BR, Greig PD: Selective or total shunts for variceal bleeding. *Am J Surg* 1990; 160(1):75-9.
13. Levine BA, Sirinek KR: The portacaval shunt. Is it still indicated? *Surg Clin North Am* 1990; 70(2):361-78.
14. Martella AT, Levine BA: Portal hypertension: Nonshunting procedures. In *Current Surgical Therapy*, 5th edition. Cameron JL, ed. Mosby Year Book, St Louis: 1995, 305-8.
15. Orozco H, Mercado MA, Takahashi T, Hernandez-Ortiz J, Capellan JF, Garcia-Tsao G: Elective treatment of bleeding varices with the Sugiura operation over 10 years. *Am J Surg* 1992; 163(6):585-89.
16. Rikkers LF: New concepts of pathophysiology and treatment of portal hypertension. *Surgery* 1990; 107(5):481-88.
17. Smith GW: Use of hemodynamic selection criteria in the management of cirrhotic patients with portal hypertension. *Ann Surg* 1974; 179(5):782-90.
18. Takasaki T, Kobayashi S, Muto H, Suzuki S, Harada M, Nakayama K: Transabdominal esophageal transection by using a suture device in cases of esophageal varices. *Int Surg* 1977; 62(8):426-28.
19. Turcotte JG: Variceal hemorrhage, hepatic cirrhosis and portocaval shunts. *Surgery* 1973; 73:810-17.
20. Turcotte JG, Lambert MJ III: Variceal hemorrhage, hepatic cirrhosis, and portacaval shunts. *Surgery* 1973; 73(6):810-17.

ARTERIOVENOUS ACCESS FOR HEMODIALYSIS

SURGICAL CONSIDERATIONS

Description: **Peripheral subcutaneous arteriovenous (AV) fistula**, or **prosthetic graft**, is the current procedure of choice for patients requiring permanent hemodialysis access.[1-3] The blood flow in the autogenous AV fistula increases with time, and the resulting vein wall thickening prevents venous tears and infiltration during dialysis.

The standard AV fistula is usually constructed by anastomosing the cephalic vein to the radial artery at the wrist level (**Brescia-Cimino** fistula). Other locations include the "snuff box," or antebrachium. Vascular access using vascular substitutes or prosthetic grafts is performed when there is a lack of suitable veins in patients who have had failed access procedures, peripheral vein sclerosis, or severe arterial disease involving the upper extremity. Forearm grafts are constructed as a direct communication between the radial or ulnar artery and the antecubital or brachial vein, or as a "loop" between the brachial artery and these veins. Similarly, an access can be constructed in the upper arm as a communication between the brachial artery above the elbow and the basilic or axillary vein in a straight fashion.[1] The polytetrafluoroethylene (Teflon) graft has become the mainstay for hemodialysis access in patients who are not candidates for Brescia-Cimino fistula placement. These grafts are associated with a primary patency rate of 50-60% at 2-3 years.[2,3]

Variant procedure or approaches: **Forearm AV fistula** (Brescia-Cimino fistula), **loop or straight graft** using vascular substitute in forearm, and **upper arm straight graft**

Usual preop diagnosis: End-stage renal failure requiring graft hemodialysis

SUMMARY OF PROCEDURE

	Forearm AV Fistula	Forearm Loop or Straight Graft	Upper Arm Straight Graft
Position	Supine, arm abducted	⇐	⇐
Incision	Longitudinal or transverse at wrist or "snuff box"	Transverse at antecubital fossa and/or at wrist; counterincision in forearm	Transverse or longitudinal in upper arm
Special instrumentation	Arm/hand table (for arm abduction); Doppler flow probe may be used.	⇐	⇐
Unique considerations	Local anesthesia; consider brachial plexus block (increased incidence of hematoma); heparinization	⇐	⇐
Antibiotics	None	Vancomycin 1 g iv	⇐
Surgical time	1-2 h	⇐	⇐
Closing considerations	Use of Doppler to ✓ shunt patency	⇐	⇐
EBL	25-50 ml	25-100 ml	⇐
Postop care	Hemodynamic monitoring for poor-risk patients; can be done as outpatient.	⇐	⇐
Mortality	Minimal, depending on associated risk factors	⇐	⇐
Morbidity	Thrombosis: 20%	8-32%	~8-32%
	Technical failure: 10-15%	⇐	⇐
	Arterial steal: Rare	Similar	⇐
	Cardiac failure: Rare	Similar	⇐
	Infection: Rare	10%	⇐
	No-venous-outflow: Rare	6%	~6%
	Seroma: Rare	⇐	⇐
	Venous aneurysm: Rare	⇐	⇐
	Venous HTN: Rare	Similar	⇐
Pain score	1	2	2

PATIENT POPULATION CHARACTERISTICS

Age range	Pediatric and adult population (mean age = 56 yr in one series)
Male:Female	1:1
Incidence	Hemodialysis access is one of the most commonly performed procedures by vascular surgeons.
Etiology	Glomerulonephritis; diabetes; HTN; pyelonephritis
Associated conditions	Diabetes mellitus; PVD/CAD

ANESTHETIC CONSIDERATIONS

See Anesthetic Considerations following Permanent Vascular Access, p. 304.

References

1. Bennion RS, Wilson SE: Hemodialysis and vascular access. In *Vascular Surgery*, 5th edition. Moore WS, ed. WB Saunders, Philadelphia: 1998, 626-47.
2. Hill SL, Donato AT: Complications of dialysis access: a six-year study. *Am J Surg* 1991; 162(3):265-67.
3. Schuman ES, Gross GF, Hayes JF, Standage BA: Long-term patency of polytetrafluoroethylene graft fistulas. *Am J Surg* 1988; 155(5):644-46.

PERMANENT VASCULAR ACCESS

SURGICAL CONSIDERATIONS

Description: Silastic or plastic catheters are placed in patients who require venous access for chronic antibiotic therapy, TPN, chemotherapy or hemodialysis.[1,4,5,7,11,13] **Hickman**, **Broviac** and **Groshong catheters** are made of silicone rubber or plastic with a cuff near the skin exit site, which, in theory, serves as a barrier to infection. Access is generally achieved via subclavian, IJ or femoral vein puncture. These catheters are available in various sizes and in single- or double-lumen configurations. Larger diameter (13 Fr) Hickman or Permacath DL catheters have been introduced for hemodialysis.[4,7,13] **Mediport** and **Portacath devices** have a metallic or plastic reservoir connected to the catheters and are intended for complete subcutaneous implantation. These catheters are used in chronically ill patients, particularly those requiring chemotherapy. The implantable access ports have been associated with improved patient comfort and reduced infection rates.[5] Long-term catheter survival is limited by infection. Removal and replacement of the catheter is the only way to eradicate the infection.

Variant procedure or approaches: Two major distinctions: Hickman/Broviac catheters (no reservoir) vs Mediport/Portacath catheters (subcutaneous with reservoir). Subclavian, IJ or femoral vein puncture, depending on vein status, previous operations and patient comfort.

Usual preop diagnosis: Chronic antibiotic therapy; TPN; chemotherapy; end-stage renal failure

SUMMARY OF PROCEDURE

	Hickman/Broviac/Groshong	Mediport/Portacath
Position	Supine, slight Trendelenburg	⇐
Incision	Puncture site (subclavian, IJ or femoral vein); subcutaneous tunnel for passage of catheter. Alternative: cephalic or IJ vein cut-down to achieve access.[2]	Puncture site (subclavian, IJ or femoral vein); subcutaneous pocket for port. Alternative: cephalic or IJ vein cut-down to achieve access.[2]
Special instrumentation	Image intensifier or fluoroscope	⇐
Unique considerations	Local anesthesia; may need iv sedation; monitor for ectopy during placement.	⇐
Antibiotics	Cefazolin 1 g iv	⇐
Surgical time	30-90 min	45-90 min
EBL	10-25 ml	25-50 ml
Postop care	CXR in recovery room; may be outpatient.	⇐
Mortality[7,13]	Minimal	⇐
Morbidity[1,4,5,7,13]	Catheter thrombosis: 25%	4%
	Skin exit site infection: 13%	–
	Poor flow: 10-13%	~10-13%
	Catheter sepsis: 5-8%	2%
	Arterial puncture: 6%	~6%
	Local bleeding: 5%	–
	SVC thrombosis: 5%	~5%
	Catheter displacement: 3%	~3%
	Subclavian thrombosis: 2%	~2%
	Pneumothorax 1-2%	~1-2%
	Failed attempt: 1%	~1%
	Infection: 3-5/1000 cath days	–
		Pocket hematoma: 2%
		Pocket infection: 3%
		Catheter leakage: 1%
Pain score	1	2

PATIENT POPULATION CHARACTERISTICS

Age range	Pediatrics and adults, 8-80 yr
Male:Female	1:1
Incidence	Depending on underlying disease
Etiology	Access for chemotherapy; infections; hemodialysis; chronic TPN
Associated conditions	Malignancy; chronic illness/infection; renal failure

ANESTHETIC CONSIDERATIONS FOR VASCULAR ACCESS

(Procedures covered: arteriovenous access for hemodialysis; permanent vascular access)

PREOPERATIVE

The patient populations presenting for vascular access surgery are extremely diverse. Patients requiring vascular access for chemotherapy, TPN and chronic antibiotic therapy frequently can be done with MAC (p. B-4). Also presenting for these procedures are end-stage renal failure patients who need arteriovenous access for hemodialysis (generally involving the upper extremity). These patients return to the OR frequently for revising or replacing of fistulas. They are often ASA III & IV patients who may require GA or an upper extremity block. Anesthetic considerations for the chronic renal patient are discussed below.

Respiratory Pulmonary edema may be present from fluid overload. CHF and uremic pleuritis can occur. Pneumonia occurs more frequently in these patients due to depressed immune systems. Hemodialysis contributes to hypoxemia due to V/Q mismatch and hypoventilation.
Tests: CXR; consider ABG.

Cardiovascular Often have HTN related to hypervolemia and a disorder of the renin-antiogensin system. May have LVH 2° to HTN. Cardiomyopathy, pericarditis and pericardial effusion occur with uremia. Hypervolemia and hypoalbuminemia can contribute to CHF. Uremic patients often have defective aortic and carotid body reflex arcs. Ejection murmurs are common.
Tests: ECG; others as indicated from H&P.

Renal A comprehensive preop evaluation should include an assessment of renal function and adequacy of recent dialysis therapy. Ascertaining the patient's usual and recent weights is useful. Dialysis is usually advisable shortly before anesthesia and surgery. The symptoms of uremia (Plt dysfunction, electrolyte/fluid abnormalities, CNS and GI disturbances) improve with dialysis. If a transfusion is needed, it is best done during dialysis so intravascular volume can be controlled.
Tests: Serum BUN; creatinine. If patient produces urine, consider creatinine clearance, UA.

Hematologic Chronic anemia with Hct ranging from 15-21 g/dL. Normochromic, normocytic anemia present due to bone marrow depression, lack of erythropoietin, nutritional deficiency and diminished red-cell survival time. Patients adjust to chronic anemia through ↑CO and ↑2,3-DPG levels. Accumulation of waste products inhibit Plt function. Defects do occur in the coagulation cascade, but PT and PTT are usually normal.
Tests: CBC; Plt; PT; PTT

Gastrointestinal Uremic patients commonly have hiccups, anorexia, N/V and diarrhea. They are very prone to developing GI bleeds. Renal failure causes ↓gastric emptying. Premedication with metoclopramide (10 mg po) and ranitidine (150 mg po) will ↓ gastric volume and pH.

Nervous system CNS Sx of uremia range from malaise to seizures to coma. Fatigue and intellectual impairment commonly occur. Peripheral and autonomic neuropathies exist. Peripheral neuropathy presents as itching and paresthesia of the lower extremities. Autonomic dysfunction can cause postural hypotension. Document deficits carefully.

Endocrine Diabetes frequently may be the cause of renal failure, with its attendant problems.
Tests: Glucose

Immune system Often depressed. Patients prone to sepsis. Hepatitis and HIV infections from blood products may exist.

Metabolic and biochemical Accumulation of K^+ urea, parathyroid hormone (hypercalcemia), Mg, aluminum (neurotoxicity), acid metabolites and phosphate occurs. Knowing hyperkalemia exists is of importance because of the potential for fatal cardiac dysrhythmias. Shift of the oxyhemoglobin curve to the right occurs due to the metabolic acidosis and increased 2,3-DPG (improves tissue oxygenation). Hyponatremia is a common electrolyte disturbance in chronic renal failure.

Premedication If warranted, it is best to use light premedication with sedatives or opioids due to the possibility of exaggerated effects (p. B-2).

INTRAOPERATIVE

Anesthetic technique: GA, upper extremity block or MAC.

Regional anesthesia: May be advantageous due to decreased number of drug effects. See section on upper extremity blocks (Anesthetic Considerations for Wrist Procedures, p. 683). If the patient was very recently dialyzed, there may be a residual heparin effect. Regional anesthesia is contraindicated if coagulopathy is present.

General anesthesia: The duration of action and elimination of many anesthetic drugs is altered in the patient with renal failure.

Induction Renal failure reduces protein binding; therefore, highly protein-bound drugs may produce prolonged and exaggerated effects. Acidemia increases the proportion of agent existing in the nonionized, unbound state, which increases its availability to effector sites (e.g., brain). In addition, renal failure patients require a lower dose of STP for induction due to the increased permeability of the blood-brain barrier 2° uremia. Because ketamine and benzodiazepines are less heavily protein-bound than barbiturates, the induction dose does not need to be decreased as much. Ketamine may exaggerate preexisting HTN. Succinylcholine is not associated with greater than normal increases in K^+ in renal-failure patients. It should be avoided, however, if the $K^+ > 5.5$ mEq/L. Repeated doses of succinylcholine do not prolong muscle relaxation, since serum cholinesterase levels are normal in renal failure. Nondepolarizing muscle relaxants, such as pancuronium and d-tubocurarine, have delayed excretion and increased duration of action. Atracurium elimination is not significantly affected in renal failure. Similarly, vecuronium does not have a significantly increased duration of action.

Maintenance Inhalation anesthesia offers the advantage of not being renally eliminated. Biotransformation may produce some inorganic fluoride (nephrotoxin); however, this is not an issue in dialysis patients. There is less fluoride released with halothane than isoflurane, but because of myocardial depression with halothane, isoflurane may be a better choice of inhalation anesthesia. Opioids can produce an increased magnitude and duration of effect. Increased accumulation of morphine glucuronides → prolonged respiratory depression. An accumulated metabolite of meperidine (normeperidine) can cause seizures. Fentanyl and remifentanil are good choices, 2° rapid tissue redistribution (fentanyl) or rapid metabolism (remifentanil).

Emergence Prolonged effect of anticholinesterases (e.g., neostigmine and edrophonium) effectively offsets prolongation of blockade. Other factors affecting reversal of nondepolarizers should be taken into account. These include acid-base status, depth of blockade, temperature and use of drugs such as diuretics or antibiotics, which can potentiate blockade.

Blood and fluid requirements	IV: 18-20 ga × 1 NS @ 1-2 ml/kg/h	IV access may be difficult; avoid iv placement in operated arm. Minimize fluids in renal-failure patients.
Monitoring	Standard monitors (p. B-1)	Avoid BP cuff placement on operated arm.
Positioning	✓ and pad pressure points. ✓ eyes.	
Complications	Local anesthetic toxicity	

POSTOPERATIVE

Complications	Nerve damage Hematoma	These are rare complications of brachial plexus blocks.
Pain management	PO analgesics	

References

1. Bour ES, Weaver AS, Yang HC, Gifford RR: Experience with the double lumen Silastic catheter for hemoaccess. *Surg Gynecol Obstet* 1990; 171(1): 33-9.
2. Chuter T, Starker PM: Placement of Hickman-Broviac catheters in the cephalic vein. *Surg Gynecol Obstet* 1988; 166(2): 163-64.
3. Don HF, Dieppa RA, Taylor P: Narcotic analgesics in anuric patients. *Anesthesiology* 1975; 42:745.
4. Donnelly PK, Hoenich NA, Lennard TW, Proud G, Taylor RM: Surgical management of long-term central venous access in uraemic patients. *Nephrol Dial Transplant* 1988; 3(1):57-65.
5. Franceschi D, Specht MA, Farrell C: Implantable venous access device. *J Cardiovasc Surg* 1989; 30(1):124-29.
6. Ghoneim MM, Pandya H: Plasma protein binding of thiopental in patients with impaired renal or hepatic function. *Anesthesiology* 1975; 42:545.
7. Gibson SP, Mosquera D: Five years' experience with the Quinton Permacath for vascular access. *Nephrol Dial Transplant* 1991; 6(4):269-74.

8. Kaufman BS, Contreras J: Preanesthetic assessment of the patient with renal disease. *Anesth Clin North Am* 1990; 8:677.
9. Mazze RI, Calverley RK, Smith NT: Inorganic fluoride nephrotoxicity: prolonged enflurane and halothane anesthesia in volunteers. *Anesthesiology* 1977; 46:1265.
10. Monk TG, Weldon BC: The renal system and anesthesia for urologic surgery. In *Clinical Anesthesia,* 3rd edition. Barash PG, Cullen BF, Stoelting RK, eds. Lippincott-Raven Publishers, Philadelphia: 1997, 941-74.
11. Silberman H, Berne TV, Escandon R: Prospective evaluation of a double-lumen subclavian dialysis catheter for acute vascular access. *Am Surg* 1992; 58:443-45.
12. Wilson SE, Connall TP, White R, Connolly JE: Vascular access surgery as an outpatient procedure. *Ann Vasc Surg* 1993; 7(4)325-29.
13. Wisborg T, Flaatten H, Koller ME: Percutaneous placement of permanent central venous catheters: experience with 200 catheters. *Acta Anaesthesiol Scand* 1991; 35(1):49-51.

VENOUS SURGERY—VEIN STRIPPING AND PERFORATOR LIGATION

SURGICAL CONSIDERATIONS

Description: Chronic venous insufficiency results from static blood flow in the deep, superficial and perforating veins of the lower extremity.[7] Clinical manifestations include pathologic changes in the skin and subcutaneous tissues, such as pigmentation, dermatitis, induration and ulceration around the lower portion of the leg.[3,4] The condition is most commonly caused by defective venous valves, and less often by obstruction to the venous return or impaired pumping action of the muscles in the leg.[7] The disorder is sometimes the residual of previous iliofemoral thrombophlebitis. Varicose veins of the primary type, particularly those of long duration, are a common cause of chronic venous insufficiency of milder degrees.[7] Most symptoms respond well to conservative management, which includes compression stockings, elevation of the extremity and topical treatment of ulcerations. Failure of medical management is an indication for surgical intervention. Split-thickness skin grafting is indicated for large ulcers to accelerate healing and shorten hospitalization time.[4,7] **Ligation of perforators** is best performed when the ulcer has completely healed. The classic approach of **Linton** is rarely used today. If the quality of the skin overlying the perforators prevents a direct approach, **subfascial ligation** of the perforators may be performed through a short, posterior midline incision.[9] The incompetent greater or lesser saphenous veins are resected only if patency of the deep system is confirmed. Venous ulcers recur in 30% of patients after surgical therapy, and ulcerations persist for prolonged period in 15% of patients.[4] Adjunctive procedures include: **valvuloplasty**, **vein transposition** and **venous valve transplant**.[2,9]

Usual preop diagnosis: Chronic deep venous insufficiency

SUMMARY OF PROCEDURE

Position	Supine
Incision	**Vein stripping:** longitudinal or oblique groin incision and transverse incision at medial malleolus; transverse incision over posterior lower leg for lesser saphenous vein stripping. **Perforator ligation:** longitudinal incision along medial aspect of tibia to posterior medial malleolus.
Special instrumentation	Vein stripper
Antibiotics	If patient has an associated venous ulcer, preop antibiotics should be based on culture results; generally, cefazolin 1 g iv, if culture results are not available.
Surgical time	3 h
EBL	50-250 ml
Postop care	PACU → ward; antiembolism stockings and SCDs
Mortality	Minimal
Morbidity[7,10]	Persistence of nonhealing ulcer: 20-53%
Pain score	3

PATIENT POPULATION CHARACTERISTICS

Age range	Young adult–elderly (generally older adults, although present in younger patients as well).
Male:Female	1:2
Incidence	6-7 million people in U.S. have adverse effects from chronic venous stasis;[7] 500,000 have complications of leg ulceration.
Etiology	Chronic primary varicose veins; defective venous valves; impaired pumping action of muscles in leg; previous iliofemoral thrombophlebitis; obstruction of venous return
Associated conditions	Varicose veins; Hx of DVT/thrombophlebitis

ANESTHETIC CONSIDERATIONS

See Anesthetic Considerations following Varicose Vein Stripping, p. 308.

References

See references for Venous Surgery—Thrombectomy or Vein Excision, p. 295.

VARICOSE VEIN STRIPPING

SURGICAL CONSIDERATIONS

Description: In patients with primary varicose veins, no definite cause has been identified, although age, female sex, pregnancy, obesity and positive family history are predisposing factors.[4,5] The causes of secondary varicosity include incompetence or obstruction of the deep veins as a result of previous DVT, tumor, trauma or congenital or acquired arteriovenous fistulas.[2] Usual indications for operative therapy include aching, swelling, heaviness, cramps, itching, cosmesis, stasis dermatitis, pigmentation, burning and ulcers.[1,4,5,7,9] Surgical treatment is contraindicated in: pregnant patients; elderly patients who are considered high risk; and patients with arterial insufficiency of the lower extremities, lymphedema, skin infection or coagulopathy.[4,7]

There are two principal approaches: the **stab avulsion technique** and **high ligation and stripping.**[1,6] With **stab avulsion,** the varicosities are marked preop. Small transverse or longitudinal incisions are made directly over these varicosities, which are dissected from the surrounding subcutaneous tissue (with undermining of the skin) and bluntly removed or avulsed. Firm pressure over the region being operated on will achieve hemostasis. After removal of all marked varicosities, sterile dressings are placed and a compression bandage wrapped around the affected leg. The patient is instructed to keep the leg elevated as much as possible while convalescing at home. The chief advantage of the stab avulsion technique is preservation of the saphenous vein when it is not directly involved with varicosities.

If there is valvular incompetence of the saphenous vein, the treatment of choice is **stripping (avulsion)** of the incompetent portion of the greater and lesser saphenous veins, together with avulsion of the superficial varicose veins of the thigh and calf.[4] **High ligation and stripping** refers to the removal of the greater saphenous vein from the level of medial malleolus to the saphenofemoral junction. A small transverse incision is made at the level of the ankle and the saphenous vein is dissected free. A longitudinal or oblique incision at the groin permits isolation of the saphenous vein at the saphenofemoral junction. The greater saphenous vein is ligated proximally and distally. After a **venotomy,** a plastic or metallic vein stripper is passed and the vein is removed or stripped in a distal-to-proximal fashion. Sterile dressings are applied, followed by a compressive dressing.

If all varicose veins are removed and the incompetent segment of the saphenous vein is stripped, 85% of the patients will have good-to-excellent results at late follow-up.[4] These procedures can be performed with regional or GA.

Usual preop diagnosis: Varicose veins; symptoms of venous insufficiency; cosmetic considerations

SUMMARY OF PROCEDURE

	Stab Avulsion Technique	High Ligation and Stripping
Position	Supine	⇐
Incision	Varicosities marked preop; short stab incisions made and veins avulsed with small forceps.	Varicosities marked preop; small transverse incision over saphenous vein proximal to medial malleolus; proximal saphenous vein exposed via groin incisions and stripper passed.
Special instrumentation	None	Vein stripper
Unique considerations	May be facilitated by tourniquet.	⇐
Antibiotics	None	⇐
Surgical time	2-3 h	⇐
Closing considerations	Leg compressed with elastic wrap	⇐
EBL	50-250 ml	50-150 ml
Postop care	PACU → ward; support stockings	⇐ + Elevate foot of bed 10°; short periods of ambulation.
Mortality	Minimal	⇐
Morbidity[3,6]	Recurrence: < 10%	⇐
	Hematoma: Rare	⇐
	Infection: Rare	⇐
	Postop DVT: Rare	5%
	Nerve injury: Rare	⇐
	Lymph fistula: Rare	⇐
	Femoral artery injury: Nil	Very rare
Pain score	2	2

PATIENT POPULATION CHARACTERISTICS

Age range	Wide range, young adult–elderly (average = 48 yr)
Male:Female	1:3
Incidence	24,000,000 in U.S.
Etiology	Primary varicose veins: no definite cause (predisposing factors include age, female sex, pregnancy, obesity and positive family Hx) Secondary varicose veins: incompetence or obstruction of the deep veins from DVT, tumor, trauma or high venous pressures due to congenital or acquired arteriovenous fistulas
Associated conditions	Older age; pregnancy; obesity; DVT; tumor; trauma

ANESTHETIC CONSIDERATIONS

(Procedures covered: vein stripping and perforator ligation; varicose vein stripping)

PREOPERATIVE

Patients presenting for varicose vein surgery are a generally healthy patient population (ASA I & II). Preop considerations and tests, therefore, should be guided by the H&P.

Hematologic If regional anesthesia planned, check patient's coagulation status.
Tests: Plt count; Hct

Laboratory Tests as indicated from H&P.

Premedication If necessary, standard premedication (p. B-2).

INTRAOPERATIVE

Anesthetic technique: General, regional or local anesthesia ± sedation are all appropriate anesthetic techniques. Choice depends on factors such as extent of surgery, patient physical status and patient and surgeon preference.

Regional anesthesia:

Spinal Single-shot vs. continuous: Patient in sitting or lateral decubitus position (operative site down) for placement of hyperbaric subarachnoid block. Doses of local anesthetics are as follows for T10-

Spinal, cont.	T12 level: 0.75% bupivacaine in 8% dextrose 7-10 mg; 0.5% tetracaine in 5% dextrose 10-12 mg. For continuous spinal (multiorifice catheter), titrate local anesthetic to desired surgical level (T12). Large doses of hyperbaric local anesthetic should be avoided as they may cause postop cauda equina syndrome.	
Epidural	Patient in sitting or lateral decubitus position for placement of epidural catheter. After locating the epidural space, administer a test dose (e.g., 3 ml of 1.5% lidocaine with 1:200,000 epinephrine) to elucidate whether the catheter is subarachnoid or intravascular. Titrate local anesthetic until desired surgical level is obtained (3-5 ml at a time) usually < 15 ml.	
Local	Requires gentle surgical technique. Surgical field block, plus ilioinguinal and iliohypogastric nerve blocks using 0.5% bupivacaine with 1:200,000 epinephrine. Usually done by surgeon.	
General anesthesia:		
Induction	LMA/mask vs ETT: Standard induction (p. B-2). LMA or mask GA may be suitable for many patients.	
Maintenance	Standard maintenance (p. B-3)	
Emergence	No special considerations	
Blood and fluid requirements	Minimal blood loss IV: 18 ga × 1 NS/LR @ 5-8 ml/kg/h	
Monitoring	Standard monitors (see p. B-1).	
Positioning	✓ and pad pressure points. ✓ eyes.	

POSTOPERATIVE

Complications	Cauda equina syndrome	The diagnosis of cauda equina syndrome (urinary and fecal incontinence, paresis of lower extremities, perineal hyperesthesias) should be sought in the postop period in patients who have received large doses of intrathecal local anesthetic during continuous spinal techniques. ✓ patients for bowel or bladder dysfunction and perineal sensory deficits. If present, consider a neurology consultation and continue followup of the patient's neurologic dysfunction.
	Urinary retention common with regional anesthesia	Patients with urinary retention may require intermittent catheterization until urinary function resumes.
Pain management	PO analgesics: Acetaminophen and codeine (Tylenol #3 1-2 tab q 4-6 h) Oxycodone and acetaminophen (Percocet 1 tab q 6 h)	Regional anesthesia should provide sufficient analgesia postop.

Reference

1. Vloka JD, Hadzic A, Mulcare R, Lesser JB, Kitain E, Thys DM: Femoral and genitofemoral nerve blocks versus spinal anesthesia for outpatients undergoing long saphenous vein stripping surgery. *Anesth Analg* 1997; 84(4):749-52.

Surgeons

Bruce A. Reitz, MD
James I. Fann, MD

6.3 HEART/LUNG TRANSPLANTATION

Anesthesiologist

Lawrence C. Siegel, MD

SURGERY FOR HEART TRANSPLANTATION

SURGICAL CONSIDERATIONS

Description: Although heart transplantation has been practiced since 1967, it has had its greatest expansion since the early 1980s with the introduction of cyclosporine immunosuppression. Currently, there are approximately 150 transplant centers and 2,200 heart transplant procedures performed yearly in the U.S. Indications for heart transplantation range from hypoplastic left heart syndrome in the neonate to cardiomyopathy and ischemic heart disease in the adult. Recipients usually have end-stage heart disease manifested by CHF and a prognosis of less than 1-year survival. Many patients are on inotropic drugs or on some type of additional mechanical assist, such as the use of an intraaortic balloon pump (IABP) or an implanted LV assist device. Current immunosuppressive protocols consist of a combination of cyclosporine with prednisone and azathioprine. Immunosuppression begins either immediately preop or perioperatively and will continue throughout the life of the patient. Current 1-year survival averages 85% in most centers, with 5-year survival of > 60%.

In **adult heart transplantation**, following median sternotomy, the pericardium is opened, with care being taken to preserve the phrenic nerve. The aorta and vena cava are cannulated, the aorta is cross-clamped and caval tapes (tourniquets to prevent VAE) are applied. The aorta and PA are then transected. This is followed by an incision through the atria, and the recipient heart is removed. The donor heart is prepared by opening the left atrium through the pulmonary veins, separating the aorta and PA. The donor heart is attached by a long, continuous suture line around the left atrium, followed by a similar suture line around the right atrium. Next, the PA and aorta are anastomosed to their respective recipient vessels. Multiple deairing maneuvers are followed by aortic unclamping and rewarming and resuscitation of the heart. Normal sinus rhythm (NSR) is established and CPB discontinued. Heparin is reversed, hemostasis is secured, and the chest is closed in a routine manner.

Neonatal heart transplantation differs in that the PA is cannulated if the ductus arteriosus is patent. Reconstruction of the aortic arch in the patient with **hypoplastic left heart syndrome** requires CPB with deep hypothermia (< 18°C) and circulatory arrest. The heart is then excised and the transverse aortic arch is opened beyond the ductus arteriosus to minimize risk of late coarctation. The donor heart is prepared, with special attention given to trimming the transverse aortic tissue for subsequent reconstruction. The left and right atrium, PA and aorta are sutured in place. The new ascending aorta and right atrium are cannulated and CPB with rewarming is reinstituted. Chest closure is routine.

Usual preop diagnosis: Cardiomyopathy; CAD with ischemic cardiomyopathy; CHD (e.g., hypoplastic left heart syndrome or anomalous left coronary artery); end-stage valvular heart disease

SUMMARY OF PROCEDURE

	Adult Heart Transplantation	Neonatal Heart Transplantation
Position	Supine	⇐
Incision	Median sternotomy	⇐
Special instrumentation	Ascending aortic, SVC and IVC cannulae	Ascending aortic and right atrial cannulae
Unique considerations	Due to complete excision of the heart, use of a PA catheter is usually not feasible.	Deep hypothermia with circulatory arrest
Antibiotics	Erythromycin 500 mg + cefamandole 1 g iv	Erythromycin 5-10 mg/kg + cefamandole 10-30 mg/kg iv
Surgical time	Cross-clamp: 45-60 min Surgery: 3-4 h	Circulatory arrest: 45-60 min Surgery: 3-4 h
Closing considerations	Temporary AV pacing wires are usually placed. A PA catheter may be advanced, especially if there are concerns about residual pulmonary HTN and donor right heart function. An isoproterenol infusion is started intraop to keep HR = 100-110, and to help improve right heart function and ↓ PVR.	Temporary ventricular pacing wire is usually placed. Temporary transthoracic left atrial line may be placed. Extensive aortic suture line requires avoidance of postop hypertensive episodes.
EBL	500-1500 ml	50-100 ml
Postop care	Cardiac ICU: 1-2 d of assisted ventilation; 2-3 d stay.	Pediatric ICU × 1-2 d of assisted ventilation; 4-5 d stay, with attention to pulmonary care.
Mortality	< 5%	⇐

	Adult Heart Transplantation	Neonatal Heart Transplantation
Morbidity	Early acute rejection episodes from 10-21 d: 50%	⇐
	Infection, particularly pulmonary: 10%	Respiratory problems: 20%
	Pulmonary HTN with right heart dysfunction: < 10%	Infection: 10%
	Dysrhythmias with nodal rhythms: 5%	Pulmonary vasospasm with right heart dysfunction: < 10%
	Bleeding: 2-4%	Bleeding: 2-4%
	Hyperacute rejection: Rare (< 1%)	
	Intracoronary air emboli	
Pain score	8-10	8-10

PATIENT POPULATION CHARACTERISTICS

Age range	18-65 yr (average 45-50 yr)	1 d-2 mo
Male:Female	7:3	1:1
Incidence	2200/yr (U.S.)	Rare
Etiology	Cardiomyopathy: 50% CAD with multiple previous infarcts: 48% Others: 2%	No apparent correlation with any specific genetic disorder. Cardiomyopathy: 49% CHD: 42% Other: 7%
Associated conditions	CHF	Other congenital anomalies

ANESTHETIC CONSIDERATIONS

PREOPERATIVE

Patients scheduled for heart transplantation are terminally ill, typically with CHF, which has a mortality of > 50% in 2 yr. (Studies have shown that patients with severe CHF have a mortality of 50% in 6 mo.) The progression of cardiovascular disease is usually well documented in these patients. A history of recent exacerbation of cardiac dysfunction should be sought and all data should be interpreted in light of interval changes.

Respiratory The presence of pulmonary HTN and elevated PVR may be disclosed by catheterization. The severity of the abnormality and the responsiveness to specific vasodilators must be determined.

Tests: Right heart catheterization

Cardiovascular Indicators to consider include: hemodynamic status; LV EF (mortality is rapid in patients with EF < 10% and is worse for patients with EF of 10-20%, as compared with those with EF > 20%); myocardial structure and morphology, symptoms and functional capacity; neuroendocrine status; serum sodium; and dysrhythmia. Unfortunately, while these measures show trends with mortality, they are not individually strong enough to predict a particular patient's course. Low maximum O_2 consumption (< 10 ml/kg/min) is associated with poor survival. Normal O_2 consumption is 40 ml/kg/min. In practice, however, this measure is too severe, as many patients awaiting heart transplantation have maximum O_2 consumption of 20 ml/kg/min. Dysrhythmia is a major cause of death, and electrophysiology studies of these patients may not be helpful because dysrhythmia tends to be noninducible in them. This phenomenon frustrates efforts to select and test antidysrhythmic drug therapy. The effectiveness of past antidysrhythmic therapy should be reviewed.

Tests: ECG; cardiac catheterization; ECHO

Hematologic Patients with dilated cardiomyopathy or previous cardiac surgery are frequently treated with anticoagulants to reduce the risk of thrombus formation, although the efficacy of this therapy has not been studied. Hepatic dysfunction may result from RV failure and may reduce synthetic function. Mild hepatic dysfunction and chronic anticoagulation may contribute to postop bleeding. The anticoagulant effect of warfarin should be reversed with FFP.

Tests: Hct; PT; PTT; fibrinogen; Plts

Endocrine

Neuroendocrine abnormalities are often present in severe CHF cases. The cardiomyopathy produces low CO → compensatory sympathetic activation and renin-angiotensin activity. The result is excessive vasoconstriction with salt and H_2O retention, which further impair myocardial performance. Markedly worse survival is seen in CHF patients with serum sodium < 130. This may indicate the importance of neuroendocrine pathophysiology, or may simply be evidence of the severity of the CHF. It may also simply indicate that patients with more severe CHF are treated with more diuretics. When patients are treated with an angiotensin-converting enzyme inhibitor such as enalapril, the serum sodium is normalized and survival chances are improved because of the slowing of the progression of CHF, not from alteration in the incidence of sudden death.
Tests: Electrolytes; creatinine

Laboratory

Evidence of renal and hepatic dysfunction should be sought by H&P and lab studies. Hypokalemia is generally not treated in view of the potassium in the graft.

Premedication

Although anxious, these patients are usually well informed and psychologically prepared to undergo heart transplantation. They respond well to the reassurance of the preop visit, and pharmacologic premedication usually is not necessary. O_2 therapy should commence prior to transport of the patient to the OR. Reassuring the family of a patient who suffers from rapidly progressive cardiac dysfunction also is valuable. The patient may be at increased risk for pulmonary aspiration of gastric contents because of the unscheduled nature of the surgery, and use of oral cyclosporine immediately preop may be appropriate. Ranitidine (50 mg) and metoclopramide (10 mg) may be administered iv, most efficiently accomplished in the OR.

INTRAOPERATIVE

Anesthetic technique: GETA. After the patient is placed on operating table, O_2 and noninvasive monitors are applied. Dyspnea (a complication of the supine position) can be treated by raising the back of the table. As infection is a much-feared complication in the immunosupressed transplant patient, aseptic technique is extremely important. Airway equipment is presterilized, and a disposable circle system and bacterial filters are used. Aseptic technique is used in inserting and securing all vascular catheters. The anesthesia machine should be equipped with a supply of air to control the FiO_2.

Induction

A CVP catheter is usually inserted prior to induction of anesthesia. Anesthesia is not induced until the team harvesting the graft reports that the donor heart appears to be normal. The patient is denitrogenated ($FiO_2 = 1.0$), and cricoid pressure is applied just before induction. Induction agents include fentanyl (5-20 μg/kg) or sufentanil (1-4 μg/kg). Etomidate (0.1-0.2 mg/kg) is useful in permitting rapid control of the airway and for assuring lack of patient awareness. Midazolam also may be used. Vecuronium (0.15 mg/kg), pancuronium (0.1 mg/kg), or a combination of these two agents should be administered immediately to permit airway control.
Care must be taken to avoid bradycardia, which often results in low CO in these patients. Immediate control of the airway is crucial, as hypercarbia and hypoxia must be avoided. The patient can be expected to have a low CO, resulting in a delayed induction of anesthesia, which must be anticipated to avoid anesthetic overdosage. Low CO and a volume-contracted condition make the patient initially very sensitive to anesthetics. High preload is often necessary, and iv fluid is often administered to compensate for the vasodilating effect of anesthetic-mediated sympatholysis. Inotropic support may be necessary when induction is poorly tolerated.
Patient should be ventilated by mask, and cricoid pressure released only after the airway has been secured with a cuffed ETT. The usual aids for managing the unexpectedly difficult airways should be readily available. Antibiotics are administered, and additional monitors (urinary catheter with thermistor, nasopharyngeal temperature probe, TEE or esophageal stethoscope) are set up. If there is a delay in the anticipated arrival of the graft, the donor should be covered and kept warm and skin prep should be delayed. Additional narcotics should be administered only in immediate anticipation of the commencement of surgery.

Maintenance

Typical cumulative anesthetic doses for the entire intraop course are: fentanyl 50 μg/kg or sufentanil 10-15 μg/kg; midazolam 0.2 mg/kg; vecuronium 0.3 mg/kg or pancuronium 0.2 mg/kg; scopolamine 0.07 mg/kg.

Termination of CPB

Junctional rhythm is common in the denervated transplanted heart. Isoproterenol 10-75 ng/kg/min is used to achieve a HR of 100-120 bpm. Isoproterenol is also useful in providing inotropic support

Termination of CPB, cont. and pulmonary vasodilation (see below). When sinus rhythm is achieved, it is common to observe 2 P-waves. The original atrial tissue produces nonconducting P-waves. Responses mediated by vagal tone will be observed in the rate of the original atrial tissue and have no clinical importance beyond the ease with which the ECG is interpreted. Atropine and neostigmine do not affect HR. HTN does not produce reflex bradycardia. The graft atrium produces normally conducted P-waves. The graft-conductive tissue contains adrenergic receptors and responds normally to norepinephrine, epinephrine and isoproterenol.

Inotropic support with dopamine (2-10 μg/kg/min), isoproterenol (10-150 ng/kg/min) and epinephrine (20-100 ng/kg/min) may be necessary, especially if pulmonary HTN promotes RV failure. A PA catheter may be helpful in guiding the use of inotropes and vasodilators.

After termination of CPB, TEE may be of particular value in assessing RV dysfunction and guiding appropriate fluid therapy, pharmacologic support and mechanical support as necessary. RV failure may be produced by the presence of air in the RCA. Visual inspection may demonstrate this problem, and one should wait for the passage of the air and the resolution of ischemia before terminating CPB. SNP (0.2-2.0 μg/kg/min) is used for afterload reduction. NO, prostaglandin E_1 (PGE_1) (20-100 ng/kg/min) and NTG (0.2-2.0 μg/kg/min) may be used for pulmonary vasodilation, especially if a preop catheterization study demonstrates responsiveness of the pulmonary circulation. Isoproterenol infusion (10-100 ng/kg/min) may provide appropriate pulmonary vasodilation, chronotropy and inotropy. IV fluid and vasodilators must be given with particular care, as the flow produced by the denervated heart is quite sensitive to preload.

Postbypass hemorrhage Postbypass bleeding is a common problem brought on by the preop use of anticoagulants, the depressed synthetic function of the liver in chronic heart failure, and the trauma of CPB. Following administration of protamine, infusion of Plts, FFP and RBCs may be necessary. Cryoprecipitate is occasionally needed, especially for patients with previous chest surgery. The use of aprotinin, epsilon amino caproic acid (EACA) or tranexamic acid may be appropriate in some cases.

Immunosuppression Methylprednisolone 500 mg is given after bypass is terminated.

Diuresis There may be little urine production, especially if patient received high-dose diuretics preop. Cyclosporine may exacerbate renal dysfunction. Mannitol and furosemide may be needed to induce diuresis.

Transport A Jackson-Rees system is used in transporting the patient to the ICU.

Blood and fluid requirements

Possible severe bleeding
IV: 14-16 ga × 1-2
NS/LR @ 4-6 ml/kg/h

Bleeding is often a major problem after termination of CPB. A second iv catheter is inserted in patients with previous chest surgery.

Monitoring

Standard monitors (see p. B-1).
Arterial line
CVP/PA catheter
UO

Typically, invasive monitors are placed prior to induction; however, if the patient is very dyspneic in the supine position, it may be advantageous to insert the CVP catheter immediately following induction. A triple-lumen CVP catheter is used for those patients who do not have significant pulmonary HTN. An 8.5 Fr introducer is used for patients with ↑PVR in anticipation that a PA catheter may be necessary to manage right heart failure following the transplantation. The left IJ vein is the preferred site of cannulation, which leaves the right IJ unscarred for repeated endomyocardial biopsy of the transplanted heart.

± TEE

TEE is used to optimize fluid therapy, inotropic agents, vasodilators and chronotropic agents.

Positioning

✓ and pad pressure points.
✓ eyes.
Arms padded at sides
Chest roll

POSTOPERATIVE

Complications

RV dysfunction

RV failure may occur in patients with pulmonary HTN and high RV afterload (see pulmonary HTN, below).

Complications, cont.	Pulmonary HTN	Maneuvers which exacerbate pulmonary HTN should be avoided. These include hypoxia, hypercarbia, acidosis and extremes of lung volume. NO can be used to treat pulmonary HTN (0.1-100 ppm inspired concentration); however, it must be used with caution in patients with severe heart failure. Efforts to treat pulmonary HTN with vasodilator therapy may be complicated by impaired V/Q matching with hypoxemia and by systemic hypotension producing poor coronary perfusion and RV ischemia. Inotropic support of the RV may be necessary. Isoproterenol infusion (10-150 ng/kg/min) is attractive because it combines inotropy, pulmonary vasodilation and chronotropy.
	Oliguria Drug side effects: • Cyclosporine: HTN, nephrotoxicity, hepatotoxicity • Corticosteroids: glucose intolerance, HTN, obesity, hyperlipidemia, aseptic necrosis of hip, bowel perforation, infection • Azathioprine: anemia, thrombocytopenia, leukopenia, hepatotoxicity	Preexisting impairment may → chronic ↓UO state. Other renal problems may be related to cyclosporine toxicity, diuretic toxicity or CPB. Rx by optimizing hemodynamics. Consider reduction or elimination of nephrotoxins and continuing use of diuretics. Cyclosporine nephrotoxicity occurs in most patients. A functional toxicity with ↓GFR occurs at low dose and is reversible. Tubular toxicity with morphologic changes occurs at high doses and is generally clinically unimportant and reversible. The most serious damage is vascular interstitial toxicity, which occurs over months at high doses and is not reversible.
Pain management	PCA (see p. C-3) after weaning from mechanical ventilation.	
Tests	Creatinine, Hct	

References

1. Babir M, Lazem F, Banner N, Mitchell A, Yacoub M: The prognostic significance of noninvasive cardiac tests in heart transplant recipients. *Eur Heart J* 1997; 18:692-96.
2. Baumgartner WA, Reitz BA, Achuff SA, eds: *Heart and Heart-Lung Transplantation.* WB Saunders Co, Philadelphia: 1990.
3. Cannon DS, Rider AK, Stinson EB, Harrison DC: Electrophysiologic studies in the denervated transplanted human heart. II. Response to norepinephrine, isoproterenol and propranolol. *Am J Cardiol* 1975; 36(7):859-66.
4. Cirella VN, Pantuck CB, Lee YJ, Pantuck EJ: Effects of cyclosporine on anesthetic action. *Anesth Analg* 1987; 66(8):703-6.
5. CONSENSUS Trial Study Group: Effects of Enalapril on mortality in severe congestive heart failure. Results of the Cooperative North Scandinavian Enalapril Survival Study. *N Engl J Med* 1987; 316(23):1429-35.
6. Costard A, Hill I, Schroeder J, Fowler M: Response to nitroprusside-Predictor of early post transplant mortality. *J Am Coll Cardiol* 1989; 14:62A.
7. Demas K, Wyner J, Mihm FG, Samuels S: Anesthesia for heart transplantation. A retrospective study and review. *Br J Anaesth* 1986; 58(12):1357-64.
8. Govier AV: Anesthesia and cardiac transplantation. In *Anesthesia and the Heart Patient.* Estafanous FG, ed. Butterworths, Boston: 1989, 99-107.
9. Grebenik CR, Robinson PN: Cardiac transplantation at Harefield. A review from the anaesthetist's standpoint. *Anaesthesia* 1985; 40(2):131-40.
10. Keogh AM, Freund J, Baron DW, Hickie JB: Timing of cardiac transplantation in idiopathic dilated cardiomyopathy. *Am J Cardiol* 1988; 61(6):418-22.
11. Kieler-Jensen N, Ricksten SE, Stenqvist O, Bergh CH, Lindelov B, Wennmalm A, Waagstein F, Lundin S: Inhaled nitric oxide in the elevated pulmonary vascular resistance. *J Heart Lung Transplant* 1994; 13:366-75.
12. Kormos RL, Thompson M, Hardesty RL, et al: Utility of preoperative right heart catheterization data as a predictor of survival after heart transplantation. *J Heart Transplant* 1986; 5:391.
13. Kriett JM, Kaye MP: The Registry of the International Society for Heart and Lung Transplantation: eighth official report – 1991. *J Heart Lung Transplant* 1991; 10(4):491-98.
14. Lee WH, Packer M: Prognostic importance of serum sodium concentration and its modification by converting-enzyme inhibition in patients with severe chronic heart failure. *Circulation* 1986; 73(2):257-67.
15. Loh E, Stamler JS, Hare JM, Loscalzo J, Colucci WS: Cardiovascular effects of inhaled nitric oxide in patients with left ventricular dysfunction. *Circulation* 1994; 90:2780-85.
16. Massie BM, Conway M: Survival of patients with congestive heart failure: past, present, and future prospects. *Circulation* 1987; 75(5 P+2):IV11-9.

17. Ouseph R, Stoddard MF, Lederer ED: Patent foramen ovale presenting as refractory hypoxemia after heart transplantation. *J Am Soc Echocardiogr* 1997; 10:973-76.
18. Propst J, Siegel L, Feeley T: Aprotinin reduces transfusions during repeat sternotomy for heart transplantation. *Anesthesia Analgesia* 1993; 76(25):5337.
19. Ream AK, Fowles RE, Jamieson S: Cardiac transplantation. In *Cardiac Anesthesia*, 2nd edition. Kaplan JA, ed. WB Saunders Co, Philadelphia: 1987, 881-91.
20. Ryffel B, Foxwell BM, Gee A, Greiner B, Woerly G, Mihatsch MJ: Cyclosporine – relationship of side effects to mode of action. *Transplantation* 1988; 46(2 Suppl):90S-96S.
21. Schulte-Sasse Y, Hess W, Tarnow J: Pulmonary vascular response to nitrous oxide in patients with normal and high pulmonary vascular resistance. *Anesthesiology* 1982; 57(1):9-13.
22. Starling RC, Cody RJ: Cardiac transplant hypertension. *Am J Cardiol* 1990; 65(1):106-11.
23. Waterman PM, Bjerke R: Rapid-sequence induction technique in patients with severe ventricular dysfunction. *J Cardiothorac Anesth* 1988; 2:602-6.

SURGERY FOR LUNG AND HEART/LUNG TRANSPLANTATION

SURGICAL CONSIDERATIONS

Description: With the availability of cyclosporine, the ability to successfully transplant the heart and both lungs was proven in monkeys and then successfully applied in a patient in March, 1981. Subsequently, single-lung transplantation was successfully performed in 1984 and an *en bloc*, double-lung transplant in 1986. Clinical lung transplantation of these various types has increased markedly in the last few years, and, currently, approximately 700 single-lung transplants, 200 bilateral lung transplants, and 60 heart/lung transplants are performed in the U.S. each year.

Current indications for heart/lung transplantation are primarily those of combined heart and lung disease, including Eisenmenger's syndrome due to a congenital heart defect with irreversible pulmonary HTN. Certain types of diffuse lung disease, such as cystic fibrosis and primary pulmonary HTN without significant heart failure, also are treated in some centers by heart/lung transplantation. Recipients for single-lung transplant usually have end-stage pulmonary disease without significant sepsis. This includes patients with interstitial fibrosis, emphysema, and lymphangioleiomyomatosis. Some patients with pulmonary vascular disease, such as primary pulmonary HTN or pulmonary HTN associated with an ASD, have undergone single-lung transplantation with or without cardiac repair. Bilateral lung transplantation is now performed usually as a sequential single-lung transplant, with the major indications being septic lung disease, such as cystic fibrosis, chronic bronchiectasis, severe bullous emphysema, or pulmonary vascular disease with or without cardiac repair. Current immunosuppressive protocols consist of a combination of cyclosporine with prednisone and azathioprine, with or without early induction therapy, using a cytolytic agent such as antithymocyte globulin. Immunosuppression may begin preop and continue throughout the life of the patient. Current 1-year survival averages between 60% and 70% for the various types of lung transplants.

Heart/lung transplants are usually performed through a median sternotomy, although occasionally bilateral, transsternal thoracotomy has been employed. **Single-lung transplants** (usually left side) and **bilateral sequential lung transplants** use a lateral thoracotomy or transsternal bilateral thoracotomy. Single- and double-lung transplants are greatly facilitated with single-lung (one-lung) ventilation (OLV), which is essential for the procedures. If this type of ventilation is not feasible, a bronchial-blocker must be inserted through the operative field during pneumonectomy and reimplantation. CPB is routinely used for heart/lung transplantation, and is used for either single- or bilateral-lung transplantation, depending on the stability of the patient during OLV and/or clamping of the PA. Patients with severe pulmonary HTN undergoing single- or double-lung transplantation will almost always require CPB to reduce PA pressure during clamping. For combined transplants, the recipient heart is removed as for standard heart transplantation (see Surgery for Heart Transplantation, p. 313). A portion of the PA near the ligamentum arteriosum, however, is left intact in order to preserve the recurrent laryngeal nerve. Next, each recipient lung is excised and the trachea is transected above the carina. For single-lung transplant, usually the left recipient lung is excised, leaving a bronchial stump and vascular pedicles for the PA and veins (left atrium). For bilateral lung transplants, both recipient lungs are removed, the trachea transected just above the carina, and the main PA and left atrium prepared for subsequent anastomosis.

Implantation of the grafts involves a tracheal anastomosis, aortic and right atrial anastomosis for heart/lung transplants, and a bronchial anastomosis with PA and pulmonary venous anastomosis for single-lung transplantation. **Bilateral sequential lung transplants** are performed as if they were single-lung transplants. CPB requires heparinization and protamine reversal. Prior to closure, extensive exploration for potential bleeding sites within the posterior mediastinum is carried out with placement of right and left pleural and mediastinal drainage. Thoracotomies are closed in standard fashion with routine chest tube drainage.

Usual preop diagnosis: End-stage heart and lung disease, such as Eisenmenger's syndrome; cystic fibrosis; primary pulmonary HTN; emphysema; bronchiectasis; lymphangioleiomyomatosis; interstitial pulmonary fibrosis; sarcoidosis; and other unusual forms of lung disease

SUMMARY OF PROCEDURE

	Heart/lung Transplantation	Single-Lung Transplantation	Bilateral Lung Transplantation
Position	Supine	Lateral thoracotomy	Supine (arm above head)
Incision	Median sternotomy, usual; bilateral anterior thoracotomy, occasionally	Posterolateral thoracotomy	Transsternal bilateral thoracotomy
Special instrumentation	Ascending aortic, SVC and IVC cannulae	Occasional need for BB to be inserted through the operative field.	± Aortic, SVC and IVC cannulation; occasional need for BB.
Unique considerations	CPB. If recipient has had previous thoracotomies, mediastinal collaterals may cause troublesome bleeding. Some patients with cystic fibrosis have severe bilateral scarring, requiring extensive dissection in order to remove the recipient lung.	± CPB. Patient may become severely hypoxic or hypercarbic during OLV, requiring need for CPB. During right thoracotomy, cannulation can be performed through the thorax, but left thoracotomy may require femoral artery and vein cannulation.	CPB. Thoracotomy is usually performed on left side first, with implantation of lung on this side, followed by completion of right-side thoracotomy and right-lung transplantation. If patient becomes unstable, cannulation in the thorax is usually possible to facilitate transplantation.
Antibiotics	Continue specific antibiotic regime. Coverage for pseudomonas is suggested in patients with cystic fibrosis.	Cefazolin 1 g iv	⇐ With appropriate coverage for pseudomonas in patients with cystic fibrosis.
Surgical time	4-5 h	2-3 h	5-6 h
Closing considerations	Temporary pacing wire applied and isoproterenol infusion is usually started intraop to keep HR between 100-110, as with a cardiac transplant.	Ventilation with as low an FiO_2 as possible to maintain a PO_2 > 90. Minimize iv fluids.	⇐
EBL	500-2000 ml	< 500 ml (more if CPB is used)	500-2000 ml
Postop care	Cardiac ICU: 3-7 d; 1-2 d assisted ventilation	⇐	⇐
Mortality	10-15%	10%	10-15%
Morbidity	Early acute rejection episodes from 10-21 d: 75%	–	–
	Infection, particularly pulmonary: 30-40%	⇐	⇐
	Pulmonary interstitial edema: 20%	Bleeding: 2-4%	⇐
		Bronchial leak or stenosis: 2-4%	⇐
	Return for bleeding: 4-6%		
	Hyperacute rejection: Rare		
Pain score	8-10	8-10	8-10

PATIENT POPULATION CHARACTERISTICS

	Heart/lung Transplantation	Single-Lung Transplantation	Bilateral Lung Transplantation
Age range	3 mo-55 yr (average 30-40 yr)	1-65 yr	⇐
Male:Female	1:1	⇐	⇐
Incidence	60/yr (U.S.) 200/yr (worldwide)	600/yr (U.S.) 1000/yr (worldwide)	200/yr (U.S.) 400/yr (worldwide)
Etiology	Eisenmenger's syndrome; CHD; cystic fibrosis; PVD; other lung diseases	Acquired chronic lung disease; PVD	Cystic fibrosis; interstitial fibrosis; emphysema
Associated conditions	Severe cyanosis and polycythemia; diabetes in patients with cystic fibrosis; sinus infections in patients with cystic fibrosis	Right heart dysfunction; pulmonary valve insufficiency and tricuspid valve insufficiency	Diabetes mellitus; sinus infections in patients with cystic fibrosis

ANESTHETIC CONSIDERATIONS FOR HEART/LUNG TRANSPLANTATION

PREOPERATIVE

Patients scheduled for heart/lung transplantation are terminally ill, although they may still be able to maintain limited activity. Indications include primary pulmonary HTN, Eisenmenger's syndrome, cystic fibrosis and combined cardiac and pulmonary disease. The standard preanesthetic evaluation is supplemented with considerations particular to these patients. The progression of disease is usually well documented.

Respiratory Patients with severe pulmonary HTN (80/50 mmHg) have enlarged PAs. Vocal cord dysfunction (Sx: hoarseness, inability to phonate "e") may occur when the left recurrent laryngeal nerve is stretched by an enlarged PA, making these patients at increased risk for pulmonary aspiration. Appropriate precautions to avoid aspiration should be taken (see Induction, below).
Tests: ABG; cardiac catheterization

Cardiovascular Hx of recent exacerbation of symptoms should be sought and cardiac catheterization data interpreted in light of interval changes. The severity of pulmonary HTN and the responsiveness to specific vasodilators during catheterization should be reviewed.
Tests: ECG; cardiac catheterization; ECHO

Neurological R → L intracardiac shunting may be present in patients with pulmonary HTN, and Hx of embolic episodes should be sought. Extra care should be used to avoid injection of even small quantities of intravenous air.

Hematologic The medication schedule should be verified with particular attention to the recent use of anticoagulants.
Tests: Hct; PTT; PT (special tubes required if severe polycythemia present 2° ↓plasma volume); Plt count; fibrinogen

Laboratory Evidence of renal and hepatic dysfunction should be sought by H&P and lab studies. Hypokalemia is generally not treated because the heart/lung graft is preserved with K^+ and implantation will reverse hypokalemia.

Premedication Although anxious, these patients are usually well informed and psychologically prepared. They respond well to the reassurance of the preop visit and pharmacologic premedication usually is not necessary. O_2 therapy should commence prior to transport of patient to the OR. Patient may be at increased risk for pulmonary aspiration of gastric contents because of the unscheduled nature of the surgery, the use of oral cyclosporine immediately preop and the presence of recurrent laryngeal nerve damage. Ranitidine (50 mg) and metoclopramide (10 mg) may be administered iv preop.

INTRAOPERATIVE

Anesthetic technique: GETA. Infection is a much feared complication in the immunosupressed transplant patient; thus, aseptic technique is important. Airway equipment is presterilized. A disposable circle system and bacterial filters are used. Aseptic technique is used in inserting and securing all vascular catheters. The anesthesia machine should be equipped with a supply of air to permit control of the FiO_2. Anesthesia is not induced until the team harvesting the graft reports that it appears to be normal to direct inspection.

Induction	Once in OR, the patient should be placed on the operating table and O_2 and noninvasive monitors applied. A patient who is dyspneic in the supine position may be treated by raising the back of the table. Cricoid pressure must be used when the patient is at risk for aspiration of gastric contents. A major goal of anesthetic induction is the avoidance of further increases in PVR by guarding against respiratory acidosis, hypoxia, N_2O, light anesthesia and extremes of lung volume. When hemodynamically tolerated, fentanyl (30 μg/kg) is useful in blunting the pulmonary vascular response to intubation. Etomidate (0.1-0.2 mg/kg) may be used when hypotension limits administration of narcotics. Vecuronium (0.15 mg/kg), pancuronium (0.1 mg/kg), or a combination of the 2, should be administered early to permit rapid airway control. Midazolam and scopolamine produce amnesia. N_2O is not used because it exacerbates pulmonary HTN, reduces FiO_2 and expands intravascular air bubbles. Patient should be ventilated by mask, and cricoid pressure released only after the airway has been secured with a cuffed ETT. Excessive pressure of the cuff on the trachea should be avoided. An ETT of internal diameter of 8.0 mm will facilitate FOB postop.
Maintenance	Typical total anesthetic doses for the entire intraop course are: fentanyl 50 μg/kg or sufentanil 10-15 μg/kg; midazolam 0.2 mg/kg; vecuronium 0.3 mg/kg or pancuronium 0.2 mg/kg; scopolamine 0.07 mg/kg.
Termination of CPB	After tracheal anastomosis is completed, lungs are ventilated with $FiO_2 = 0.21$ at 5 breaths/min and a TV of 6 ml/kg. When bladder temperature reaches 36°C, ventilation is increased to 10 breaths/min and TV of 12 ml/kg. TV should be adjusted to eliminate atelectasis and to achieve a peak inflation pressure of 25-30 cmH_2O with the chest open. The FiO_2 is increased to 0.4 and may be altered in response to pulse oximetry and blood gas data. FiO_2 is limited in the hope of curtailing free radical injury. PEEP may be used to enhance oxygenation and is adjusted with an appreciation of the effect of lung volume on PVR. Hypoxemia must be avoided. Hyperkalemia may be treated with Ca^{++} (e.g., 3-5 ml 10% CaCl q 30 min), glucose (50 g), insulin (10 U) and diuresis. Junctional rhythm is common in the denervated transplanted heart. Isoproterenol (10-75 ng/kg/min) is used to achieve a HR of 100-120. When sinus rhythm is achieved, it is common to see 2 P-waves. The residual atrial tissue produces nonconducting P-waves. Responses mediated by vagal tone will be seen in the rate of the original atrial tissue and have no clinical importance beyond the ease with which the ECG is interpreted. In the denervated heart, atropine and neostigmine will not affect HR, and HTN will not produce reflex bradycardia. The graft atrium produces normally conducted P-waves. The transplanted heart contains adrenergic receptors and responds normally to norepinephrine, epinephrine and isoproterenol. The CO of the denervated heart is quite sensitive to preload; thus, iv fluid and vasodilators must be given with particular care. SNP is used for afterload reduction. TEE may be of particular value in assessing RV dysfunction and guiding appropriate fluid therapy, pharmacologic support and mechanical support as necessary. NO, PGE_1 (20-100 ng/kg/min), isoproterenol and NTG (0.2-2.0 μg/kg/min) also may be used for pulmonary vasodilation. Inotropic support with dopamine (2-10 μg/kg/min), isoproterenol and epinephrine (20-100 ng/kg/min) may be necessary, especially if pulmonary HTN and RV failure occur.
Immuno-suppression	Methylprednisolone 500 mg iv is given after bypass is terminated.
Diuresis	There may be little urine production, especially if patient received high-dose diuretics preop. Cyclosporine may exacerbate renal dysfunction. Mannitol and furosemide may be needed to induce diuresis.
Transport	A sterile, disposable Jackson-Rees system is used in transporting the patient to the ICU.

Blood and fluid requirements	Anticipate large blood loss. IV: 14-16 ga × 2	Bleeding is often a major problem after termination of CPB. Patients with intracardiac defects are at increased risk for cerebral embolic events. Care must be taken to remove all air bubbles from intravascular lines.
Control of blood loss	Postbypass bleeding is a common problem.	Postbypass bleeding is exacerbated by preop use of anti-coagulants, depressed synthetic liver function, trauma of CPB; and/or previous chest therapy.

Control of blood loss, cont.	Coagulation therapy necessary.	Coagulation therapy may include: protamine (30 mg/kg); Plts; FFP; RBCs; EACA (300 mg/kg); DDAVP; aprotinin (500,000 U/h after loading dose).
	Possible severe bleeding	Severe bleeding prompts further therapy: cryoprecipitate, factor IX concentrate.
Monitoring	Standard monitors (see p. B-1). Arterial line CVP/PA catheter UO	Typically, invasive monitors are placed prior to induction; however, if patient is very dyspneic in the supine position, it may be advantageous to insert the CVP catheter following anesthetic induction. An introducer permits the rapid insertion of a PA catheter when necessary. The left IJ vein is the preferred site of cannulation, leaving the right IJ unscarred for repeated endomyocardial biopsies of the transplanted heart.
	± TEE	TEE is used to optimize the selection of fluid therapy, inotropic agents, vasodilators and chronotropic agents.

POSTOPERATIVE

Complications	Oliguria Pulmonary edema	Diuresis may be induced with mannitol and furosemide. Given the lack of lymphatic drainage in the transplanted lung, pulmonary edema may occur. Diuresis and restriction of iv fluid may be required.
	RV dysfunction	RV failure may occur in patients with pulmonary HTN and high RV afterload (see pulmonary HTN Rx, below).
	Pulmonary HTN	Maneuvers which exacerbate pulmonary HTN should be avoided. These include hypoxia, hypercarbia, acidosis and extremes of lung volume. NO can be used to treat pulmonary HTN (0.1-100 parts per million inspired concentration); however, it must be used with caution in patients with severe heart failure. Efforts to treat pulmonary HTN with vasodilator therapy may be complicated by impaired V/Q matching with hypoxemia and by systemic hypotension producing poor right coronary perfusion and RV ischemia. Inotropic support of the RV may be necessary. Isoproterenol is attractive because it combines inotropy, pulmonary vasodilation and chronotropy.
	Rejection Infection	Monitor rejection Sx with transvenous endomyocardial biopsy and transbronchial biopsy.
	Drug side effects: • Cyclosporine: HTN, nephrotoxicity, hepatotoxicity • Corticosteroids: glucose intolerance, HTN, obesity, hyperlipidemia, aseptic necrosis of hip, bowel perforation, infection • Azathioprine: anemia, thrombocytopenia, leukopenia, hepatotoxicity	Cyclosporine nephrotoxicity occurs in most patients. A functional toxicity with reduced GFR occurs at low dose and is reversible. Tubular toxicity with morphologic changes occurs at high doses and generally is clinically unimportant and reversible. The most serious damage is vascular interstitial toxicity, which occurs over months at high doses and is not reversible.
Pain management	PCA (see p. C-3).	

References

1. Baumgartner WA, Reitz BA, Achuff SA, eds: *Heart and Heart-Lung Transplantation*. WB Saunders Co, Philadelphia: 1990.
2. Boscoe M: Anesthesia for patients with transplanted lungs and heart and lungs. *Int Anesthesiol Clin* 1995; 33:21-44.
3. Cirella VN, Pantuck CB, Lee YJ, Pantuck EJ: Effects of cyclosporine on anesthetic action. *Anesth Analg* 1987; 66(8):703-6.
4. Peterson KL, DeCampli WM, Feeley TW, Starnes VA: Blood loss and transfusion requirements in cystic fibrosis patients undergoing heart-lung or lung transplantation. *J Cardiothorac Vasc Anesth* 1995; 9:59-62.
5. Propst JW, Siegel LC, Feeley TW: Effect of aprotinin on transfusion requirements during repeat sternotomy for cardiac transplantation surgery. *Transplant Proc* 1994; 26:3719-21.

6. Pucci A, Forbes RD, Berry GJ, Rowan RA, Billingham ME: Accelerated post-transplant coronary arteriosclerosis in combined heart-lung transplantation. *Transplant Proc* 1991; 23(1P+2):1228-29.
7. Reitz BA, Wallwork JL, Hunt SA, Pennock JL, Billingham ME, Oyer PE, Stinson EB, Shumway NE: Heart-lung transplantation: successful therapy for patients with pulmonary vascular disease. *N Engl J Med* 1982; 306(10):557-64.
8. Royston D: Aprotinin therapy in heart and heart-lung transplantation. *J Heart Lung Transplant* 1993; 12:S19-S25.
9. Scott JP, Sharples L, Mullins P, Aravot DJ, Stewart S, Otulana BA, Higenbottom TW, Wallwork J: Further studies on the natural history of obliterative bronchiolitis following heart-lung transplantation. *Transplant Proc* 1991; 23(1P+2):1201-2.
10. Shaw JH, Kirk AJ, Conacher ID: Anesthesia for patients with transplanted hearts and lungs undergoing non-cardiac surgery. *Br J Anesth* 1991; 67:772-78.

ANESTHETIC CONSIDERATIONS FOR LUNG TRANSPLANTATION

PREOPERATIVE

The patient presenting for lung transplantation typically has end-stage pulmonary fibrosis or emphysema, although other diseases such as pulmonary HTN also may be treated by single-lung transplantation. Double-lung transplantation can be used to treat cystic fibrosis and bronchiectasis. The progression of the disease is usually well documented; however, Hx of recent exacerbation of symptoms should be sought.

Respiratory Assess the patient's ability to undergo OLV by review of the ventilation-perfusion scan. If little perfusion of the nonoperative lung is present, anticipate the need for CPB.[10] The extent of the restrictive lung disease and diffusion abnormality must be assessed preop. For example, room-air PaO_2 < 45 mmHg predicts the need for CPB.
Tests: PFT; V/Q scan; ABG

Airway Patients with severe pulmonary HTN (80/50 mmHg) have enlarged pulmonary arteries. Vocal cord dysfunction (Sx: hoarseness, inability to phonate "e") may occur when the left recurrent laryngeal nerve is stretched by an enlarged PA, making these patients at increased risk for pulmonary aspiration; therefore, appropriate precautions to avoid aspiration should be taken (see Induction, below).

Cardiovascular Evidence of RV dysfunction with tricuspid regurgitation should be sought by physical exam, ECHO and cardiac catheterization. RV ejection fraction (EF) may be estimated with radionuclide ventriculography (normal EF = > 50%). Pulmonary HTN is considered to be severe and may produce RV failure when pressure is > 2/3rds of systemic arterial pressure. Note response to specific vasodilators recorded during catheterization.
Tests: Preview cardiac catheterization data; ECG; mean PAP > 40 mmHg and PVR > 5 mmHg/min/L may predict the need for partial CPB.

Neurological R→L intracardiac shunting may be present in patients with pulmonary HTN, and Hx of embolic episodes should be sought. Extra care should be used to avoid injection of even small quantities of intravenous air.

Musculoskeletal Chronic cachexia precludes the procedure.

Hematologic Polycythemia 2° chronic hypoxemia is common. Autologous blood is collected as CPB is initiated.
Tests: Hct; coagulation studies require special blood tubes to correct for low plasma volume in patients with severe polycythemia.

Laboratory Other tests as indicated from H&P.

Premedication Patients awaiting lung transplantation are generally well informed about the planned perioperative course. These patients respond well to the reassurance of the preop visit, and pharmacologic premedication is usually not necessary. O_2 therapy, with the usual home O_2 regimen, should commence prior to transport to the OR. Patient may be at ↑risk for pulmonary aspiration of gastric contents because of the unscheduled nature of the surgery, the use of oral cyclosporin immediately prior to surgery and the presence of recurrent laryngeal nerve damage. Ranitidine (50 mg) and metoclopramide (10 mg) may be administered iv prior to surgery.

INTRAOPERATIVE

Anesthetic technique: GETA. Typically, OLV through a DLT is required for single-lung transplants. Consider ETT/BB in cystic fibrosis patients with tenacious sputum. Infection is a much feared complication in the immunosuppressed transplant patient; thus, aseptic technique is important. Airway equipment is presterilized. A disposable circle system and bacterial filters are used. Aseptic technique is used in inserting and securing all vascular catheters.

Induction Typically, fentanyl 30 mg/kg (incremental doses) after invasive monitors placed, ± etomidate 0.1-0.2 mg/kg when rapid control of the airway is desirable; vecuronium 0.15 mg/kg or pancuronium 0.1 mg/kg (avoid succinylcholine 2° ↓HR); midazolam 0.1 mg/kg or scopolamine 0.005 mg/kg for amnesia. Cricoid pressure must be used when the patient is at risk for aspiration because of the unscheduled nature of the surgery, use of preop oral cyclosporin and possible vocal cord dysfunction associated with stretch injury of the recurrent laryngeal nerve. Avoid further increases in PVR by guarding against hypoxemia, acidosis, hypercarbia, light anesthesia and extremes of lung volume.

Maintenance Typically, narcotic/O_2/air/± isoflurane (in absence of hypoxemia and right heart failure). Typical total anesthetic doses for the entire intraop course: fentanyl 50-75 μg/kg or sufentanil 10-15 μg/kg, midazolam 0.2 mg/kg, vecuronium 0.3 mg/kg, or pancuronium 0.2 mg/kg or pipecuronium 0.2 mg/kg, scopolamine 0.07 mg/kg.

Emergence Prior to closure of the chest, lungs are inflated to 35 cmH_2O, in order to reinflate atelectatic areas and check adequacy of bronchial closure. At the conclusion of surgery, both lumens of the DLT should be aspirated and the tube replaced with a single-lumen 8.0 mm ETT. The patient is transported to the ICU intubated and ventilated.

Blood and fluid requirements

IV: 14 or 16 ga × 1-2
NS/LR @ 4 ml/kg/h

Patients with intracardiac defects are at increased risk for cerebral embolic events; take care to remove all air bubbles from intravascular lines.

Monitoring

Standard monitors (see p. B-1).
Arterial line
PA catheter
Urinary catheter with thermistor

ECG leads should be covered with tape to insure that electrical contact is not degraded by prep solution or blood. An 8.5 Fr introducer and a thermodilution PA catheter are inserted prior to induction of anesthesia. Mixed venous oximetry may be desirable during OLV, and with partial CPB. Be careful of air embolization during catheter insertion. Patients who are profoundly dyspneic (→ high negative intrathoracic pressure) are at high risk for VAE; consider inserting the catheter after GA and IPPV have been instituted. Oxygenation must be watched closely. Blood gases are sampled at 10-min intervals.

TEE

RV EF measurement may be useful for evaluating RV function (normal LEF = 0.5-0.7).

OLV

DLT: 41 Fr (men); 39 Fr (women)
Use large TV (12-15 ml/kg) during regular and OLV.

A DLT is inserted in the left mainstem bronchus to permit surgical access. Verification of tube position by auscultation may be difficult due to the severity of the lung disease. FOB is used to verify proper tube placement. Positioning of the bronchial cuff in the proximal left mainstem bronchus does not interfere with surgical access to the bronchus. The position of the DLT should be verified after the patient is moved to the lateral position. Finally, verify ventilation and proper functioning of the tube, then eliminate volatile anesthetic or vasodilators which may blunt hypoxic pulmonary vasoconstriction. Apply O_2 with CPAP at 5 cmH_2O to the nondependent lung. Further adjustment of CPAP may enhance oxygenation. The nondependent lung may be reinflated with O_2 if necessary to achieve adequate oxygenation. If adequate oxygenation cannot be achieved, CPB should be initiated.

Frequent suctioning

Frequent suctioning is necessary in patients with tenacious secretions.

PA clamping

Improve V/Q mismatch.
Improve oxygenation.
PAP ↑↑ → RV failure

Clamping of the PA will improve V/Q mismatch and oxygenation; however, severe pulmonary HTN and RV failure may develop. Vasodilators, such as NTG (0.2-2

PA clamping, cont.		μg/kg/min), SNP (0.2-10 μg/kg/min) or PGE_1 (20-100 ng/kg/min), should be used to treat pulmonary HTN and reduce RV afterload; however, care must be taken to avoid systemic hypotension. Inotropic support for the RV may be necessary (dopamine [2-10 μg/kg/min] or epinephrine [20-100 ng/kg/min]). The right atrial pressure should be monitored for evidence of tricuspid regurgitation associated with RV dilation.
PA unclamping	PIP: 20-25 cmH_2O O_2 sat: 95-100% PEEP: 5-10 mmHg	Temporary unclamping of the PA may be necessary to allow further pharmacologic therapy. If RV failure cannot be controlled pharmacologically, CPB should be initiated. The PA should not be unclamped until ventilation is possible to the transplanted lung. Perfusion without oxygenation of the transplanted lung would produce profound shunt and hypoxemia. TV should be adjusted to eliminate atelectasis and to achieve a PIP of 20-25 cmH_2O with the chest open. The FiO_2 (0.35) is limited in the hope of curtailing free radical injury. PEEP may be used to enhance oxygenation.
Positioning	For single-lung (OLV): • Supine to lateral decubitus • Axillary roll • Airplane splint • Avoid hyperextension (> 90°).	Verify correct position of DLT or BB after moving patient to the lateral position.
	For double-lung: • Supine with arms above head for bilateral subcostal incision. ✓ and pad pressure points. ✓ eyes.	Difficult access to airway after patient positioned. ★ **NB:** potential for kinking of iv and arterial lines

POSTOPERATIVE

Complications	Pulmonary edema Infection: bacterial, viral, fungal or protozoan	Given the lack of lymphatic drainage in the transplanted lung, pulmonary edema may occur. Diuresis and restriction of iv fluid may be required. Mannitol and furosemide can be used to induce diuresis.
	Side effects of immunosuppressive agents: • Cyclosporine: hepatotoxicity, HTN nephrotoxicity, seizures • Corticosteroids: HTN, osteoporosis, glucose intolerance, hyperlipidemia • Azathioprine: anemia, thrombocytopenia, leukopenia	Immunosuppression drugs typically include: cyclosporin, azathioprine and corticosteroids. Polyclonal antilymphocyte globulin or monoclonal antilymphocyte antibodies also may be used.
Pain management	Epidural narcotics (see p. C-1). Parenteral narcotics (see p. C-1).	Postop analgesia may be provided by infusion of narcotics through an epidural catheter. If CPB is used, the insertion of the epidural catheter should be delayed until normal coagulation function is documented in the ICU.

References

1. Adatia I, Lillehei C, Arnold JH, Thompson JE, Palazzo R, Fackler JC, Wessel DL: Inhaled nitric oxide in the treatment of postoperative graft dysfunction after lung transplantation. *Ann Thorac Surg* 1994; 57:1311-18.
2. Benumof JL, Partridge BL, Salvatierra C, Keating J: Margin of safety in positioning modern double-lumen endotracheal tubes. *Anesthesiology* 1987; 67(5):729-38.
3. Capan LM, Turndorf H, Chandrankant P, et al: Optimization of arterial oxygenation during one-lung anesthesia. *Anesth Analg* 1980; 59(1):847-51.

4. Carere R, Patterson GA, Liu P, Williams T, Maurer J, Grossman R: Right and left ventricular performance after single and double lung transplantation. The Toronto Lung Transplant Group. *J Thorac Cardiovasc Surg* 1991; 102(1):115-23.
5. Colley PS, Cheney FW: Sodium nitroprusside increases Qs/Qt in dogs with regional atelectasis. *Anesthesiology* 1977; 47(4):388.
6. Della Rocca G, Pugliese F, Antonini M, Coccia C, Pompei L, Vizza CD, Rendina EA, Ricci C, Cortesini R: Hemodynamics during inhaled nitric oxide in lung transplant candidates. *Transplant Proc* 1997; 29:3367-70.
7. DeMajo WAP: Anesthetic technique for single lung transplantation. In *The transplantation and replacement of thoracic organs*. Cooper DKC, Novitsky D, eds. Kluwer Academic Publishers, Boston: 1990.
8. DeMajo WAP: Pulmonary transplantation. In *Thoracic Anesthesia*, 2nd edition. Kaplan J, ed. Churchill Livingstone, New York: 1991, 555-62.
9. Eishi K, Takazawa A, Nagatsu M, Hirata K, et al: Pulmonary flow-resistance relationships in allografts after single lung transplantation in dogs. *J Thorac Cardiovasc Surg* 1989; 97(1):24-9.
10. Hurford WE, Kolker AC, Strauss W: The use of ventilation/perfusion lung scans to predict oxygenation during one-lung anesthesia. *Anesthesiology* 1987; 67(5):841-44.
11. Kramer MR, Marshall SE, McDougall IR, Kloneck A, Starnes VA, Lewiston NJ, Theodore J: The distribution of ventilation and perfusion after single-lung transplantation in patients with pulmonary fibrosis and pulmonary hypertension. *Transplant Proc* 1991; 23(1 P+2):1215-16.
12. Limbos MM, Chan CK, Kesten S: Quality of life in female lung transplant candidates and recipients. *Chest* 1997; 112:1165-74.
13. Macdonald P, Mundy J, Rogers P, Harrison G, Branch J, Glanville A, Keogh A, Spratt P: Successful treatment of life-threatening acute reperfusion injury after lung transplantation with inhaled nitric oxide. *J Thorac Cardiovasc Surg* 1995; 110:861-63.
14. Mair P, Balogh D: Anaesthetic and intensive care considerations for patients undergoing heart or lung transplantation. *Acta Anaesthesiol Scand* Suppl 1997; 111:78-9.
15. Marshall SE, Lewiston NJ, Kramer MR, Sibley RK, Berry G, Rich JB, Theodore J, Starnes VA: Prospective analysis of serial pulmonary function studies and transbronchial biopsies in single-lung transplant recipients. *Transplant Proc* 1991; 23(1 P+2):1217-19.
16. Maurer JR, Winton TL, Patterson GA, Williams TR: Single-lung transplantation for pulmonary vascular disease. *Transplant Proc* 1991; 23(1 P+2):1211-12.
17. Patterson GA: Indications. Unilateral, bilateral, heart-lung, and lobar transplant procedures. *Clin Chest Med* 1997; 18:225-30.
18. Gasparetto A: Intraoperative inhaled nitric oxide during anesthesia for lung transplant. *Transpl Int* 1997; 10:439-45.
19. Sekela ME, Noon GP, Holland VA, Lawrence EC: Differential perfusion: potential complication of femoral-femoral bypass during single lung transplantation. *J Heart Lung Transplant* 1991; 10(2):322-24.
20. Siegel LC: Selection of anesthetic agent for thoracic surgery. In *Problems in Anesthesia*, Vol 4. Brodsky JB, ed. JB Lippincott, Philadelphia: 1990, 249-63.
21. Siegel LC, Brodsky JB: Choice of anesthetic agents for intrathoracic surgery. In *Thoracic Anesthesia*, 2nd edition. Kaplan JA, ed. Churchill Livingstone, New York: 1991.
22. Smith CM: Patient selection, evaluation, and preoperative management for lung transplant candidates. *Clin Chest Med* 1997; 18:183-97.
23. Thomas BJ, Siegel LC: Anesthetic and postoperative management of single-lung transplantation. *J Cardiothoracic Vasc Anesth* 1991; 5(3):266-67.
24. Toronto Lung Transplant Group: Experience with single-lung transplantation for pulmonary fibrosis. *JAMA* 1988; 259(15):2258-62.
25. Williams EL, Jellish WS, Modica PA, Eng CC, Tempelhoff R: Capnography in a patient after single lung transplantation. *Anesthesiology* 1991; 74(3):621-22.

7.0 GENERAL SURGERY

Surgeon

Harry A. Oberhelman, MD, FACS

7.1 ESOPHAGEAL SURGERY

Anesthesiologist

Steven K. Howard, MD

ESOPHAGOSTOMY

SURGICAL CONSIDERATIONS

Description: Esophagostomy is performed to divert oral secretions away from the esophagus to a stoma pouch in certain types of esophageal perforation. In addition, it may be utilized for feeding purposes when the patient cannot swallow due to obstructive lesions of the pharynx. Through a left cervical incision, the sternocleidomastoid muscle and carotid sheath are retracted laterally and the thyroid medially, exposing the cervical esophagus (Fig 7.1-1). The esophagus is mobilized, with care being taken not to injure the recurrent laryngeal nerve. The esophagus is brought to the skin surface as a loop or end stoma and sutured to the skin with absorbable sutures.

Variant procedure or approaches: The procedure is usually performed via a left cervical approach; the right side is an alternative.

Usual preop diagnosis: Esophageal perforation; nasopharyngeal cancer; esophageal atresia

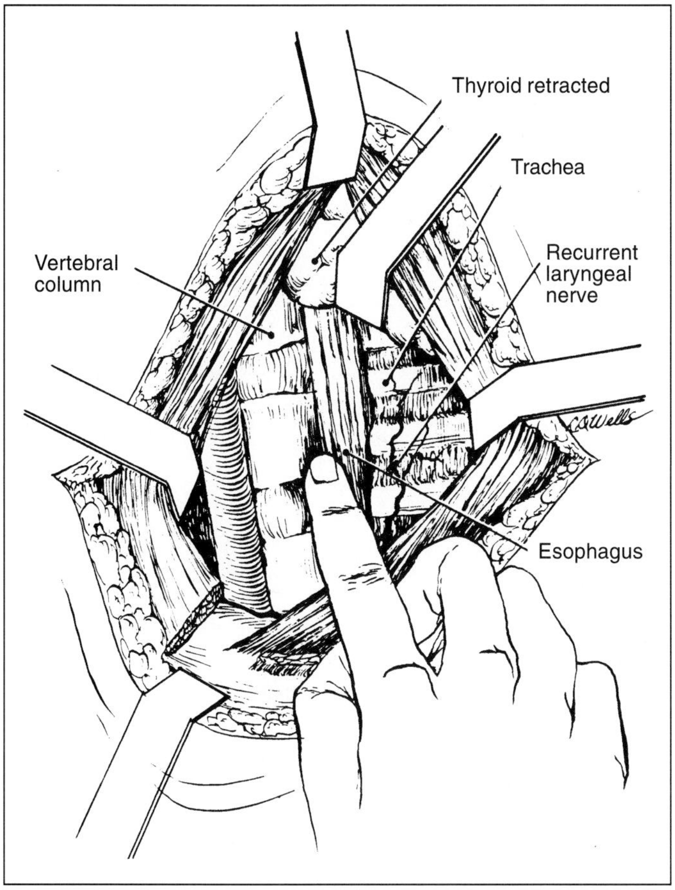

Figure 7.1-1. Surgical anatomy for cervical esophagostomy. (Reproduced with permission from Nora PF, ed: *Operative Surgery Principles and Techniques*. WB Saunders Co: 1990.)

SUMMARY OF PROCEDURE

Position	Supine, with head rotated to right
Incision	Cervical
Antibiotics	Cefazolin 1 g iv 30 min preop
Surgical time	45 min
EBL	25-50 ml
Postop care	Stoma pouch to collect saliva; PACU → room
Mortality	< 0.1%
Morbidity	Skin irritation: 15-20% Saliva leakage: 5-10% Wound infection: < 5%
Pain score	5-7

PATIENT POPULATION CHARACTERISTICS

Age range	Variable: 20-60 yr
Male:Female	1:1
Incidence	Not uncommon
Etiology	Surgically created
Associated conditions	Esophageal perforation or atresia (50%); pharyngeal cancer (50%)

ANESTHETIC CONSIDERATIONS

See Anesthetic Considerations for Esophageal Surgery following Esophagectomy, p. 339.

Reference

1. Jones WG, Ginsberg RJ: Esophageal perforations: a continuing challenge. *Ann Thorac Surg* 1992; 53:534.

ESOPHAGEAL DIVERTICULECTOMY

SURGICAL CONSIDERATIONS

Description: Diverticula of the esophagus may be of congenital or acquired origin. The most common sites are **hypopharyngeal** (**Zenker's**), just above the cricopharyngeal sphincter, and in the **epiphrenic** area just above the distal high-pressure zone. The usual treatment consists of excision of the diverticulum, combined with a cricopharyngeal myotomy or a lower esophagomyotomy (Fig 7.1-2). Care must be taken not to enter the esophageal lumen. If this occurs, the mucosal tear is approximated with fine Maxon or Dexo sutures. The **hypopharyngeal diverticulum** is approached through either side of the neck. The upper esophagus is exposed by retracting the sternocleidomastoid muscle and carotid sheath laterally and the thyroid gland medially. The diverticulum is located in the prevertebral space. Care is taken not to injure the recurrent laryngeal nerve. Following excision of the diverticulum, a **myotomy** is performed, starting on the upper esophagus and curving across the cricopharyngeal muscle near the neck of the diverticulum. The epiphrenic diverticulum is approached through the left chest and the dissection started at the pulmonary hilum. Care is taken not to injure the vagus nerves as the esophagus is mobilized downward. The diverticulum is freed from the right pleura and posterior mediastinum. Once the diverticulum has been freed, an **esophagomyotomy** is performed on the side opposite the diverticulum. The diverticulum is then excised, leaving a cuff of tissue to suture the mucosa. The muscle layer is then approximated over this mucosal closure.

Variant procedure or approaches: The hypopharyngeal diverticulum is approached through either side of the neck, while the epiphrenic diverticulum is approached via a left thoracotomy.

Usual preop diagnosis: Esophageal diverticulum

SUMMARY OF PROCEDURE

	Hypopharyngeal	Epiphrenic
Position	Supine	Right lateral decubitus
Incision	Left or right cervical	Left thoracotomy
Special instrumentation	None	Chest retractor
Unique considerations	Care not to injure recurrent laryngeal nerve	10 cm myotomy
Antibiotics	Cefazolin 1 g iv preop	⇐
Surgical time	1-2 h	⇐
Closing considerations	Inspect for perforation	⇐
EBL	50-100 ml	100-200 ml
Postop care	PACU	ICU × 1-2 d
Mortality	< 1%	⇐
Morbidity	Recurrent nerve paralysis: < 5% Temporary phonetic problems: < 5% Esophageal stricture: < 3% Esophageal fistula: < 2%	Atelectasis: 5-10% Esophageal stricture: < 5% Esophageal perforation: < 2%
Pain score	6-7	7-9

PATIENT POPULATION CHARACTERISTICS

Age range	38-92 yr (50% of patients > 70 yr)
Male:Female	2:1
Incidence	Uncommon
Etiology	Uncoordinated cricoesophageal muscle and lower esophageal sphincter (100%); weakness of esophageal wall (100%)
Associated conditions	Cachexia (25-30%); hiatus hernia with or without reflux (25%); chronic pulmonary infection (15-20%); aspiration (30-40%)

ANESTHETIC CONSIDERATIONS

See Anesthetic Considerations for Esophageal Surgery following Esophagectomy, p. 339.

Reference

1. Little AG, Ferguson MK, Skinner DB: *Diseases of the Esophagus*, Vol. II, Benign Diseases. Futura Publishing, New York: 1990.

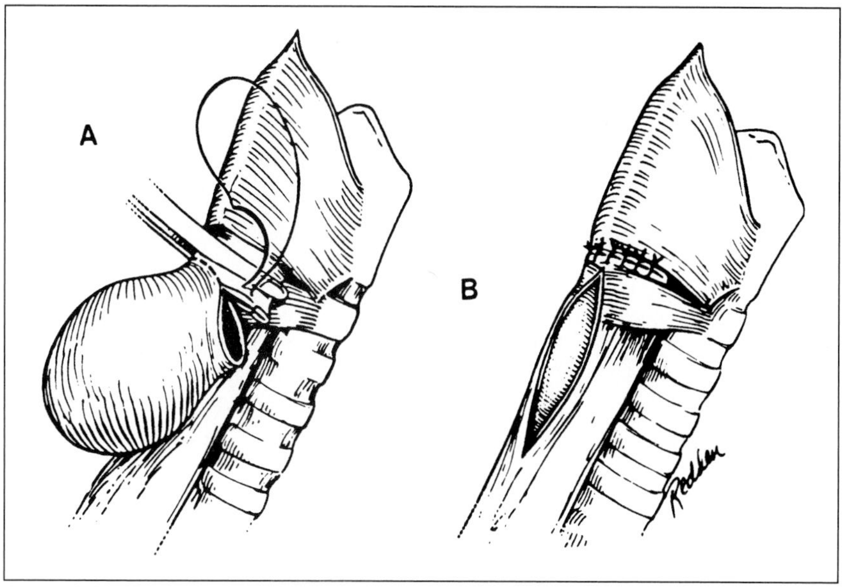

Figure 7.1-2. Esophageal diverticulectomy: (A) Excision of Zenker's diverticulum; (B) Division of the cricopharyngeus (myotomy) reduces the chance of recurrence or postop dysphagia. (Reproduced with permission from Hardy JD: *Hardy's Textbook of Surgery*, 2nd edition. JB Lippincott: 1988.)

CLOSURE OF ESOPHAGEAL PERFORATION

SURGICAL CONSIDERATIONS

Description: Esophageal perforation may be spontaneous, instrumental, traumatic or 2° intrinsic esophageal disease. Spontaneous perforations commonly occur in the lower third of the esophagus. Instrumental perforations may occur at any level, but are most common just above the cardia and in the cervical esophagus. The level of traumatic perforation depends on the location of the penetrating wound. Symptoms of esophageal perforation at the cricopharyngeal sphincter include neck pain, fever and crepitations in the substernal and neck areas. Perforation in the mediastinum may result in hydropneumothorax, mediastinitis, fever and substernal pain. Cervical perforations are managed with antibiotics and drainage in the cervical area. Therapy for thoracic esophageal perforation generally requires drainage of the pleural cavity and antibiotics. Open thoracotomy with closure of the perforation and an onlay patch of pleura may be indicated, depending on the size of the perforation and the patient's condition.

Variant procedure or approaches: Cervical or right thoracic drainage are indicated when the perforation occurs in the neck or high in the mediastinum.

Usual preop diagnosis: Esophageal perforation

SUMMARY OF PROCEDURE

	Left Thoracotomy	Cervical or Thoracic Drainage
Position	Left lateral decubitus	Supine or right lateral decubitus
Incision	Left thoracotomy	Cervical or right chest
Antibiotics	Cefazolin 1 g iv	⇐
	Fluconazole 200 mg/d	⇐
Surgical time	2 h	1 h
Closing considerations	Chest drain	Cervical or thoracic drain
EBL	100-200 ml	50-100 ml
Postop care	Chest tube to suction; PACU → room	⇐
Mortality	5-10%	2-5%

	Left Thoracotomy	Cervical or Thoracic Drainage
Morbidity	Pneumonia: 5-10%	–
	Esophageal leak: 2-5%	10%
	Pericarditis: 1-3%	–
Pain score	8-10	8-10

PATIENT POPULATION CHARACTERISTICS

Age range	Variable: 20-80 yr
Male:Female	1:1
Incidence	1 in 8,000 admissions
Etiology	Instrumental (endoscopy, dilatation, intubation); traumatic (penetrating, foreign body, caustic agents); intrinsic disease (carcinoma, peptic ulceration); spontaneous
Associated conditions	Esophageal stricture (75%); cancer (25%)

ANESTHETIC CONSIDERATIONS

See Anesthetic Considerations for Esophageal Surgery following Esophagectomy, p. 339.

Reference

1. Orringer MB: The Mediastinum. In *Operative Surgery*, 3rd edition. Nora PF, ed. WB Saunders Co, Philadelphia: 1990, 370-73.

ESOPHAGOMYOTOMY

SURGICAL CONSIDERATIONS

Description: Esophagomyotomy is performed for achalasia and other motility disorders to facilitate esophageal emptying into the stomach. It consists of incising the muscular layer of the distal esophagus and continuing down across the gastroesophageal junction for at least 1 cm (Heller).[2] The muscle is dissected back from the mucosa so that roughly 180° is exposed (Fig 7.1-3). The distal esophagus is mobilized either from below the diaphragm or via a left thoracic approach. Care is taken not to injure the vagus nerve.

When approached from the abdomen, the esophagus is exposed by incising the gastroesophageal ligament. The distal esophagus is mobilized and pulled downward to perform the myotomy.

Variant procedure or approaches: The procedure is usually performed through a left thoracotomy, but some surgeons prefer a **transabdominal approach**. More recently, laparoscopic or thoracoscopic approaches are being employed to perform esophagomyotomy (see p. 417).

Usual preop diagnosis: Achalasia; diffuse esophageal spasm; nutcracker esophagus

SUMMARY OF PROCEDURE

	Thoracic Approach	Abdominal Approach
Position	Right lateral decubitus	Supine
Incision	Left thoracotomy in 6th interspace	Midline upper abdomen
Special instrumentation	Chest retractor	Denier retractor

Figure 7.1-3. Surgical anatomy for esophagomyotomy. (Reproduced with permission from Hardy JD: *Hardy's Textbook of Surgery*, 2nd edition. JB Lippincott: 1988.)

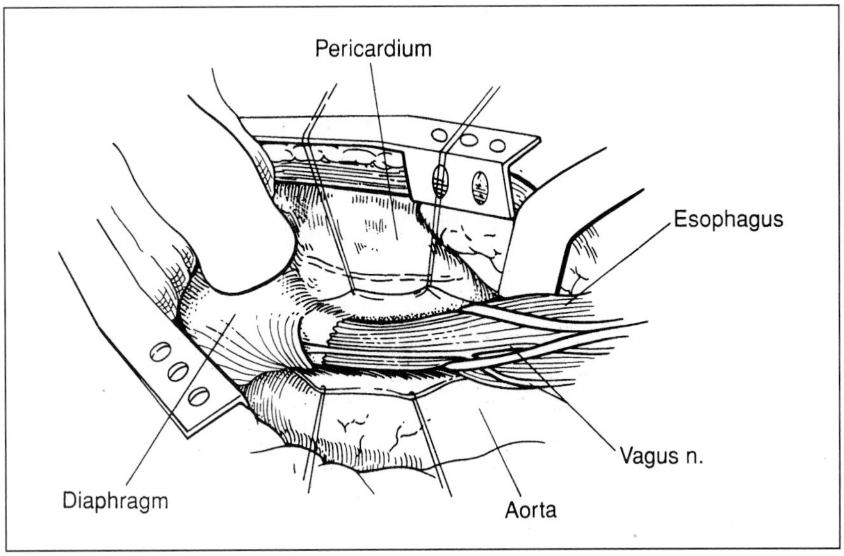

	Thoracic Approach	Abdominal Approach
Unique considerations	Care should be taken to avoid extending gastric myotomy too far to prevent esophageal reflux.	⇐
Antibiotics	Cefazolin 1-2 g iv 30 min preop	⇐
Surgical time	1-2 h	⇐
Closing considerations	✓ for perforation. Consider fundoplication to prevent esophageal reflux.[2]	⇐
EBL	150-200 ml	100-150 ml
Postop care	ICU × 1-2 d	PACU → room
Mortality	< 0.5%	⇐
Morbidity	Esophagitis: ≤ 20%	⇐
	Transient dysphagia/reflux: 5%	⇐
	Esophageal leak: 1-2%	⇐
Pain score	7-9	6-8

PATIENT POPULATION CHARACTERISTICS

Age range	30-50 yr
Male:Female	1:1
Incidence	0.6/100,000
Etiology	Neuromuscular disorder of unknown etiology often characterized by absence of ganglion cells of Auerbach's plexus (100%)
Associated conditions	Predisposition to development of carcinoma (1-20%); pulmonary complications 2° aspiration (5-10%)

ANESTHETIC CONSIDERATIONS

See Anesthetic Considerations for Esophageal Surgery following Esophagectomy, p. 339.

References

1. Ellis FH Jr, Crozier RE, Watkins E Jr: Operation for esophageal achalasia. Results of esophagomyotomy without an antireflex. *J Thorac Cardiovasc Surg* 1984; 88(3):344-51.
2. Pellegrini C, Wetters LA, Palti M, et al: Thorascopic esophagomyotomy. *Ann Surg* 1992; 216:29.
3. Stuart RC, Hennessy TP: Primary motility disorders of the esophagus. *Br J Surg* 1989; 76:111.

ESOPHAGOGASTRIC FUNDOPLASTY

SURGICAL CONSIDERATIONS

Description: Esophagogastric fundoplasty represents a variety of operations designed to prevent esophageal reflux by wrapping the fundus of the stomach around a 3-4 cm segment of the lower esophagus. This fundal wrapping acts to reinforce the lower esophageal sphincter. Surgery may be performed transabdominally, transthoracically or laparoscopically, depending on surgeon's preference. The most commonly employed is the open or laparoscopic **Nissen fundoplication**, utilizing both the anterior and posterior walls of the stomach. They are sutured together around the lower esophagus with nonabsorbable sutures (Fig 7.1-4A). This is accomplished by incising the gastrosplenic ligament and ligating 3 or 4 short gastric vessels. Care must be taken not to injure the spleen or vagus nerves during the repair.

Variant procedure or approaches: Modifications of the Nissen fundoplication include the **Toupet procedure**, a posterior partial fundoplication, and the **Hill procedure**, in which the gastroesophageal junction is sutured to the median arcuate ligament of the diaphragm or to the preaortic fascia (Fig 7.1-4B). Another modification is the **Belsey Mark IV** repair, in which there is a 240° semifundoplication between the stomach and esophagus, making it easier for the patient to overcome the resistance of the wrap. There are proponents of each repair, although the Nissen fundoplication remains the procedure most widely used. The laparoscopic approach is being used with increasing frequency (see p. 415).

Usual preop diagnosis: Sliding hiatus (hiatal) hernia or free reflux

SUMMARY OF PROCEDURE

	Nissen (Toupet) Fundoplication	Hill Procedure[3]	Belsey Mark IV[1]
Position	Supine	⇐	Right lateral decubitus
Incision	Midline abdominal or laparoscopic ports	⇐	Left posterolateral thoracotomy
Special instrumentation	#40-50 Hurst dilators; NG tube	NG tube	Chest retractor; NG tube
Unique considerations	Fundoplication should be loose; parietal cell vagotomy performed if peptic ulcer disease present. Fundoplication may be limited to 180-280° posterior wrap (Toupet)	⇐	⇐
Antibiotics	Cefazolin 1-2 g iv 30 min preop	⇐	⇐
Surgical time	1-2 h	⇐	⇐
Closing considerations	Inspect spleen for bleeding	⇐	⇐
EBL	100-150 ml	⇐	100-200 ml
Postop care	PACU → room	⇐	ICU × 1-2 d
Mortality	< 0.5%	⇐	⇐
Morbidity	Recurrent hernia: 20%	⇐	⇐
	Gas-bloat syndrome: 10-20%	< 5%	⇐
	Temporary dysphagia: 5-10%	5%	2%
	Gastric fistula: < 2%	⇐	⇐
Pain score	6-8	7-8	7-9

PATIENT POPULATION CHARACTERISTICS

Age range	46-60 yr
Male:Female	1:2
Incidence	Not uncommon
Etiology	Esophagogastric reflux (100%); esophageal hiatus hernia (80-90%)
Associated conditions	Diverticulosis of colon (30-35%); cholelithiasis (25-30%)

ANESTHETIC CONSIDERATIONS

See Anesthetic Considerations for Esophageal Surgery following Esophagectomy, p. 339.

References

1. Belsey R: Mark IV repair of hiatal hernia by the transthoracic approach. *World J Surg* 1977; 1(4):475-81.
2. Cuschieri, A: Laparoscopic antireflux surgery and repair of hiatal hernia. *World J Surg* 1993; 17(1): 40-45.
3. Hill LD: Progress in the surgical management of hiatal hernia. *World J Surg* 1977; 1(4):425-36

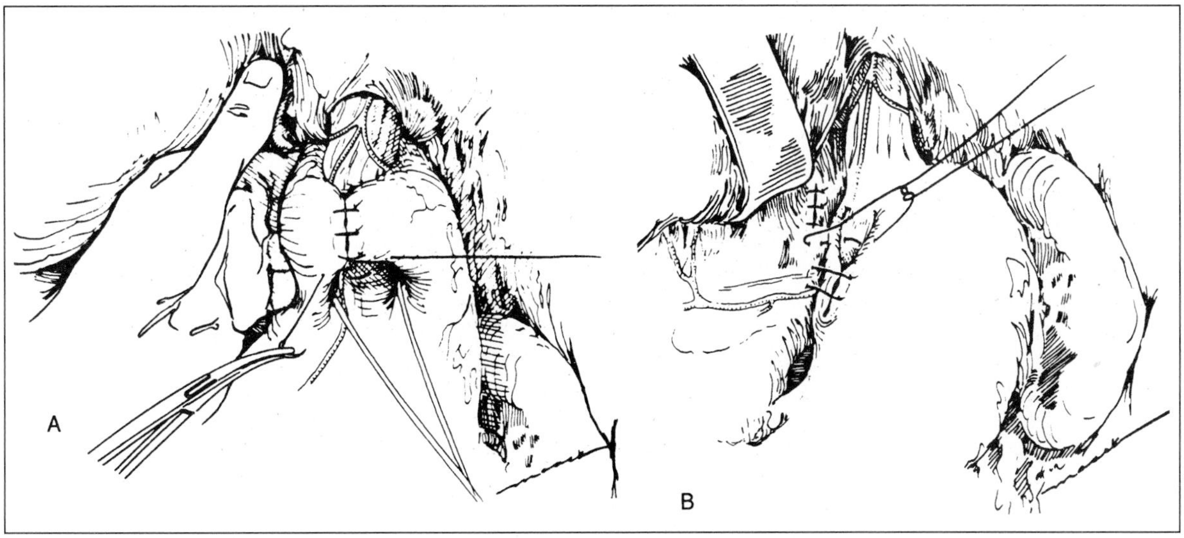

Figure 7.1-4. (A) Nissen fundoplication may be performed via either the transabdominal or transthoracic approach; (B) Hill repair is performed through the abdomen. (Reproduced with permission from Hardy JD: *Hardy's Textbook of Surgery*, 2nd edition. JB Lippincott: 1988.)

ESOPHAGECTOMY

SURGICAL CONSIDERATIONS

Description: Esophagectomy is commonly performed for malignant disease of the middle and lower thirds of the esophagus. It may also be indicated for Barrett's esophagus (peptic ulcer of lower esophagus ± stricture) and for peptic strictures that fail dilatation. Lesions in the lower third are usually approached via a left thoracoabdominal incision, while middle-third lesions are best approached via the abdomen and right chest (**Ivor Lewis**). Resections of the esophagogastric junction for malignant disease are best performed through a left thoracoabdominal approach, in which a portion of the proximal stomach is removed, along with a celiac node dissection.

The esophagus is removed *en bloc*, along with its pleural coverings, adjacent lymph nodes, subcarinal lymph nodes and thoracic duct. The azygos vein is divided and a segment removed where it courses close to the wall of the esophagus. Mobilization of the stomach is achieved by dividing the short gastric vessels to the spleen and the left gastric artery. The celiac axis is cleaned free of all lymph nodes and the gastric-colic ligament incised. Following the **Kocher maneuver** (reflecting duodenum) and a **Ramstedt-Fredet** or **Heineke-Mikulicz pyloroplasty**, the stomach is pulled into the chest and anastomosed to the proximal cut end of the esophagus. This is usually done with an EEA stapling instrument.

Variant procedure or approaches: Orringer introduced the so-called "**blind esophagectomy**" approached via the abdomen and neck by blunt dissection. This is useful primarily for benign esophageal lesions or malignant lesions of the pharynx and larynx where the pharynx and/or upper esophagus require resection. In addition, malignant lesions of the mid or distal esophagus are treated in this fashion following chemoradiation neoadjunctive Rx in increasing numbers.

Total esophagectomy may be done via an abdominal and right thoracotomy approach with colonic interposition and anastomosis in the neck (Fig 7.1-5). Either the right or left side of the colon can be mobilized for interposition. Both depend on the middle colic artery and the marginal artery of the colon for their vascular supply. When the proximal portion of the right colon is utilized, the interposed segment of bowel is isoperistaltic, but when the left colon is brought up, the segment is antiperistaltic. Although the colonic interposition is said to function primarily as a conduit for food, it is found that the isoperistaltic colonic segment functions better. In either case, the colonic segment is connected to the body of the stomach after suturing the esophageal-colonic anastomosis.

Usual preop diagnosis: Carcinoma of esophagus or gastroesophageal junction; Barrett's esophagus; benign strictures

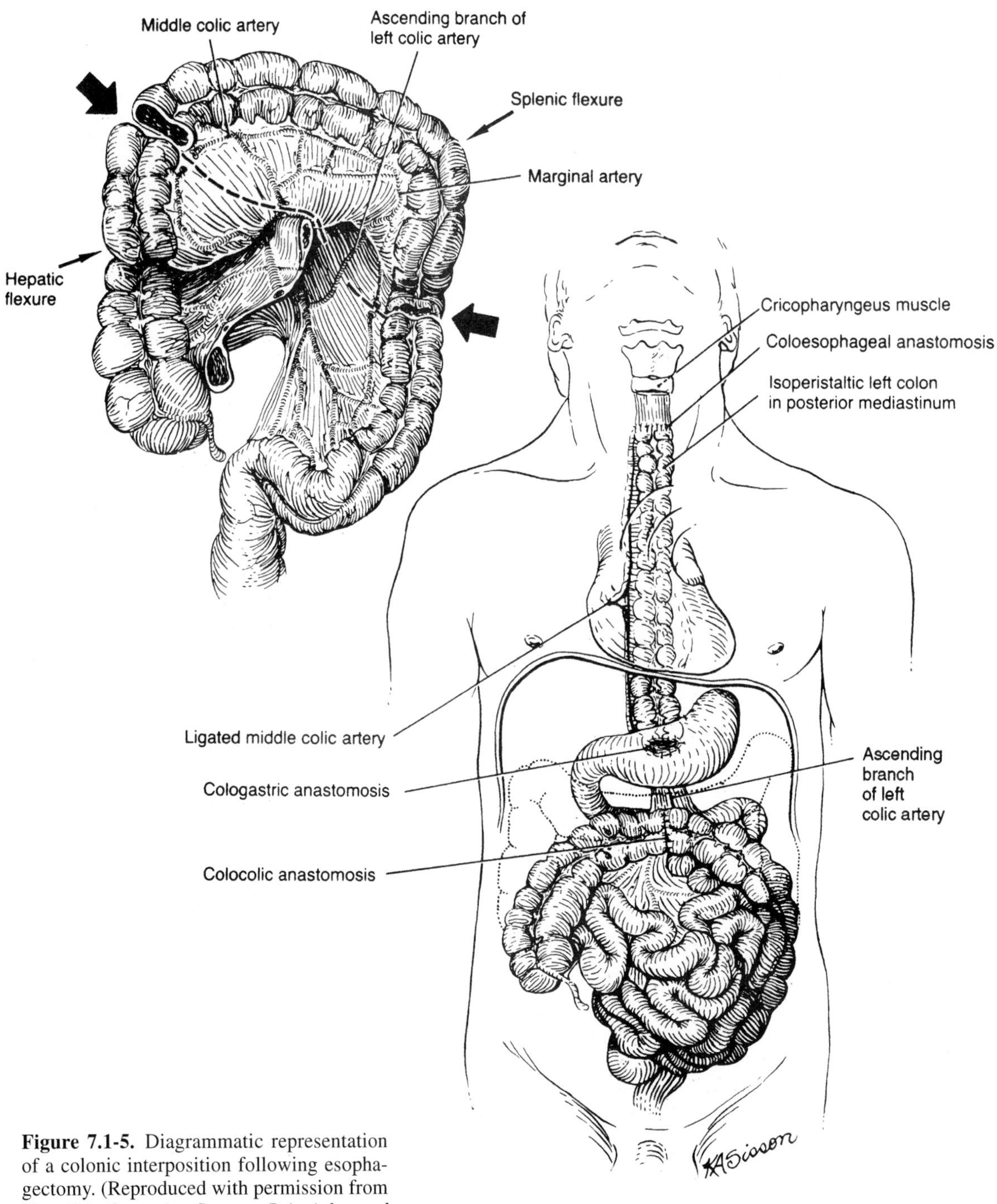

Figure 7.1-5. Diagrammatic representation of a colonic interposition following esophagectomy. (Reproduced with permission from Nora PF: *Operative Surgery Principles and Techniques*. WB Saunders: 1990.)

SUMMARY OF PROCEDURE

	Esophagectomy	Blind Esophagectomy	Esophago-gastrectomy	Total Esophagectomy + Colonic Interposition
Position	Supine and left lateral decubitus	Supine	Left lateral decubitus	Supine and right lateral decubitus
Incision	Midline abdominal + right or left chest and/or cervical incisions	Cervical and midline abdominal	Thoracoabdominal across costal margin	Midline + right thoracic and cervical
Special instrumentation	Chest retractor ± EEA stapler	Denier retractor	Chest retractor ± EEA stapler	Chest retractor
Unique considerations	DLT	None	DLT	⇐
Antibiotics	Cefazolin 2 g iv preop	⇐	⇐	⇐
Surgical time	3-4 h	4-5 h	3-4 h	5-6 h
Closing considerations	Lung reexpansion	Pneumothorax	Lung reexpansion	Vascular integrity of colonic interposition
EBL	200-300 ml	500-600 ml	200-300 ml	500-600 ml
Postop care	ICU × 1-2 d	⇐	⇐	ICU × 2-3 d
Mortality	5-10%	⇐	⇐	10%
Morbidity	Respiratory complications: 15-20%	⇐	⇐	⇐
	Anastomotic leakage: < 5%	5-10%	< 5%	10%
	Anastomotic stricture: < 5%	⇐	⇐	10%
	Wound infection: < 5%	⇐	⇐	⇐
Pain score	7-9	6-8	7-9	7-9

PATIENT POPULATION CHARACTERISTICS

Age range	4-80 yr
Male:Female	2:1 for carcinoma
Incidence	1-2% of malignant disease
Etiology	Alcohol and tobacco; dietary factors – hot spicy foods; lye burns
Associated conditions	Barrett's esophagus; hiatus hernia; reflux esophagitis; radiation esophagitis; caustic burns

ANESTHETIC CONSIDERATIONS FOR ESOPHAGEAL SURGERY

(Procedures covered: esophagostomy; esophageal diverticulectomy; closure of esophageal perforation; esophagomyotomy; esophagogastric fundoplasty; esophagectomy)

Patients presenting for esophageal surgery typically are those with carcinoma, motility disorders, strictures, hiatal hernia, reflux esophagitis, diverticula and/or perforation. Some forms of esophageal disorders will predispose the patient to aspiration pneumonitis.

PREOPERATIVE

Respiratory Hx of gastric reflux suggests the possibility of recurrent aspiration pneumonia: ↓pulmonary reserve and ↑risk of regurgitation/aspiration during anesthetic induction. (See Premedication, below.) If thoracic approach is planned, patient should be evaluated to insure that OLV can be tolerated (see below). Determine if patient has been exposed to bleomycin, which may cause pulmonary toxicity (above a total dose of 300 U/m^2); toxicity may be made worse by high concentrations of O_2. Many patients with esophageal cancer have a long history of smoking, with consequent respiratory impairment. Mediastinal lymphadenotomy → tracheal compression.

Tests: Consider PFTs (FEV_1, FVC), ABG, if indicated by H&P. They can be helpful in predicting likelihood of perioperative pulmonary complications and probability that patient may require postop mechanical ventilation. Patients with baseline hypoxemia/hypercarbia on room air will have a higher likelihood of postop complications and need for postop ventilatory support. Severe restrictive or obstructive lung disease also will increase the chance of pulmonary morbidity in the perioperative period, A-P, lateral CXR (if suggestive of tracheal compression → MRI/CT).

Cardiovascular Patient may be hypovolemic and malnourished from dysphagia or anorexia. Chemotherapeutic drugs (daunorubicin, Adriamycin) may cause cardiomyopathies. Often seen if total dose is >550 mg/m². Chronic alcohol abuse also may produce a toxic cardiomyopathy. CHF, if present, may be refractory to treatment; however, preop optimization of cardiac status is essential. (Consider cardiac consultation.)
Tests: If cardiomyopathy suspected, ECHO or MUGA scan will provide data on ejection fraction. ECG, to rule out myocardial ischemia as cause of pain/heartburn.

Hematologic Encourage preop autologous blood donation.
Tests: CBC with differential

Laboratory Tests as indicated from H&P.

Premedication Midazolam titrated to effect. Consider H_2-antagonists (e.g., ranitidine 50 mg iv), metoclopramide (10 mg iv 1 h preop), and Na citrate (30 ml po 10 min preop).

INTRAOPERATIVE

Anesthetic technique: GETA (with or without epidural for postop analgesia). If postop epidural analgesia is planned, placement and testing of the catheter prior to anesthetic induction is helpful. (This is accomplished by injecting 5-7 ml of 1% lidocaine via the epidural catheter and eliciting a segmental block.) If a thoracic or abdominothoracic approach is performed, placement of a DLT is indicated, as one-lung anesthesia provides excellent surgical exposure. (For additional discussion, see Anesthetic Considerations in Lobectomy and Pneumonectomy in Thoracic Surgery, p. 175.)

Induction Patients with esophageal disease are often at risk for pulmonary aspiration; therefore, the trachea should be intubated with the patient awake or after rapid-sequence induction with cricoid pressure. Awake intubation: (1) **Blind nasal:** topical vasoconstrictor to nose (1% phenylephrine or 4% cocaine on cotton-tipped applicators). Advance ETT until at laryngeal inlet; when patient inspires, advance ETT into trachea. Manipulation of ETT or head may be necessary for successful placement. (2) **Fiber optic intubation** (see p. B-6). If patient is clinically hypovolemic, restore intravascular volume prior to induction and titrate induction dose of sedative/hypnotic agents.

Maintenance Standard maintenance (p. B-3), without N_2O. Alternatively, a combined technique may be used. A local anesthetic (2% lidocaine with 1:200,000 epinephrine) can be injected into a thoracic (3-5 ml) or lumbar (5-10 ml q 60 min) epidural catheter to provide both anesthesia and optimal surgical exposure (contracted bowel and profound muscle relaxation). A continuous infusion of local anesthetic (e.g., 2% lidocaine or 0.25% bupivacaine @ 5-10 ml/h [lumbar]; 5 ml/h [thoracic]) may enhance hemodynamic stability. Be prepared to treat hypotension with fluid and vasopressors. GA is administered to supplement regional anesthesia and for amnesia. Systemic sedatives (droperidol, opiates, benzodiazepines, etc.) should be minimized during epidural opiate administration as they increase the likelihood of postop respiratory depression. If epidural opiates are used for postop analgesia, a loading dose (e.g., hydromorphone 1.0-1.5 mg [lumbar]; 0.5-1 mg [thoracic]) should be administered at least 1 h before conclusion of surgery.

Emergence The decision to extubate at the end of surgery depends on patient's underlying cardiopulmonary status and the extent of the surgical procedure. Patient should be hemodynamically stable, warm, alert, cooperative and fully reversed from any muscle relaxants prior to extubation. Patients who may require prolonged postop ventilation should have the DLT changed to a single-lumen ETT (use airway exchange catheter) prior to transport to ICU. Weaning from mechanical ventilation should begin when patient is awake and cooperative, able to protect the airway, and have adequate return of pulmonary function (as measured by VC of ≥ 15 ml/kg, MIF of -25 cmH_2O, respiratory rate < 25 and ABG that approaches preop baseline).

Blood and fluid requirements
IV: 14-16 ga × 1
NS/LR @ 8-12 ml/kg/h
Fluid warmer
T&C for 4 U PRBC.

Plt, FFP and cryoprecipitate (if required) should be administered according to lab tests (Plt count, PT, PTT, DIC screen, thromboelastography [TEG]).

Monitoring Standard monitors (p. B-1)

CVP cannulation site determined by surgical approach.

Monitoring, cont.	Urinary catheter Arterial line ± CVP	Attempt to prevent hypothermia during long operations. Consider forced air warmer, heated humidifier, warming blanket, warming room temperature, keeping patient covered until ready for prep, etc.
Positioning	If lateral decubitus position, use axillary roll, airplane arm holder. ✓ pressure points, including ears, eyes and genitals. ✓ radial pulses to ensure correct placement of axillary roll (if misplaced, will compromise distal pulses).	Problems that can arise include brachial plexus injuries, damage to soft tissues, ears, eyes, genitals from malpositioning. Check "down" eye at frequent intervals. Placing the oximeter probe on the down arm may assist in monitoring adequacy of perfusion.
Complications	Hypoxemia DVT	Hypoxemia during OLV may result from malposition of DLT → ↓vent. Rx: ✓position and adjust. 100% FiO_2, PEEP to ventilated lung, CPAP to nonventilated lung, return to double-lung ventilation. Temporary clamping of the PA may be necessary to ↑ O_2 saturation.

POSTOPERATIVE

Complications	Aspiration Atelectasis Hemorrhage Pneumothorax Hemothorax	For patients at risk for atelectasis or aspiration, recover in the Fowler position (lateral). For hemorrhage, ✓ coags; replace factors as necessary. Dx for pneumothorax and hemothorax: wheezing, coughing, ↓PO_2, ↑PCO_2. Confirm by CXR. Rx: chest tube drainage as necessary. In emergency (e.g., tension pneumothorax) use needle aspiration. Supportive Rx: O_2, vasopressors, volume, ± ETT and IPPV.
	Hypoxemia Hypoventilation	For hypoxemia and hypoventilation, adequate analgesia, supplemental O_2.
	Recurrent laryngeal nerve injury	For laryngeal nerve injury, indirect visualization of vocal cords; patient usually will be hoarse.
	Esophageal anastomotic leak DVT	Surgical repair for esophageal anastomotic leak
Pain management	Lumbar-thoracic epidural analgesia: hydromorphone (0.5-1.5 mg load; 0.1-0.3 mg/h infusion) PCA (p. C-3)	Patient should recover in ICU or hospital ward that is accustomed to treating side effects of epidural opiates (e.g., respiratory depression, breakthrough pain, nausea, pruritus).
Tests	CBC; ABG; CXR (rule out pneumothorax, atelectasis).	

References

1. Belsey R: Reconstruction of the esophagus with left colon. *J Thorac Cardiovasc Surg* 1965; 49:33-55.
2. Eisenkraft JB, Cohen E, Neustein SM: Anesthesia for thoracic surgery. In *Clinical Anesthesia*, 3rd edition. Barash, PG, Cullen BF, Stoelting RK eds. JB Lippincott Co, Philadelphia: 1997, 769-804.
3. Orringer MB: Tumors, injuries, and miscellaneous conditions of the esophagus. In *Surgery: Scientific Principles and Practice*, 2nd edition. Greenfield LJ, Mulholland M, Oldham KT, Zelenock GB, Lillemoe KD, eds. Lippincott-Raven Publishers, Philadelphia: 1997, 694-734.
4. Orringer MB, Orringer JS: Esophagectomy without thoracotomy: a dangerous operation? *J Thorac Cardiovasc Surg* 1983; 85(1):72-80.
5. Patterson GA, Cooper JD: Complications of thoracotomy. In *Anesthesia for Thoracic Procedures*. Marshall BE, Longnecker DE, Fairley HB, eds. Blackwell Scientific Publications, Boston: 1988, 559-79.

Surgeon

Mark A. Vierra, MD

7.2 STOMACH SURGERY

Anesthesiologist

Steven K. Howard, MD

GASTRIC RESECTIONS

SURGICAL CONSIDERATIONS

Description: Total gastrectomy is performed most commonly for gastric cancer, and may include **omentectomy**, **lymph node dissection** and/or **splenectomy**, depending on the extent of the tumor, condition of the patient and surgeon's preference. Occasionally it is performed for uncontrollable symptoms due to Zollinger-Ellison syndrome. Rarely, this procedure may be used for control of hemorrhage from diffuse gastritis. Even more rarely, patients with intractable post gastrectomy symptoms may eventually require total gastrectomy.

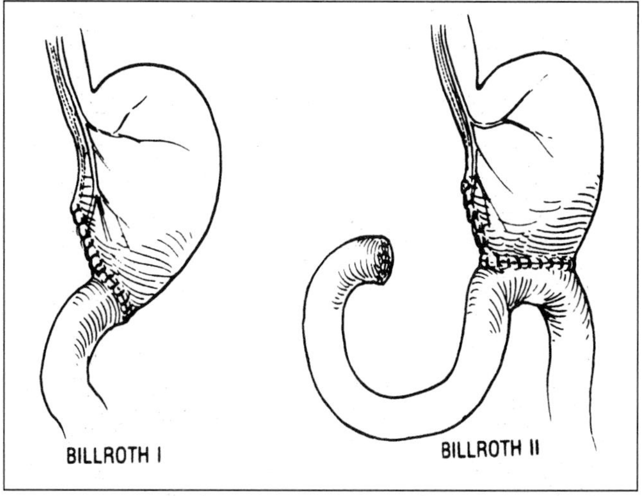

Figure 7.2-1. Anatomy of duodenostomy (Billroth I) and gastrojejunostomy (Billroth II). (Reproduced with permission from Hardy JD: *Hardy's Textbook of Surgery*, 2nd edition. JB Lippincott: 1988.)

In a gastric resection, the abdomen is entered through an upper midline incision and the lateral segment of the left lobe of the liver is retracted to the patient's right, exposing the esophagogastric junction. The omentum is taken off of the colon and the spleen is delivered; then the splenic vessels are divided, leaving the spleen attached to the stomach by the short gastric vessels. The vessels to the stomach are individually ligated and divided; then the duodenum is divided just distal to the pylorus. The stomach is divided at or near the esophagogastric junction. The jejunum is divided just beyond the Ligament of Treitz, and the distal end is brought up through a hole in the mesentery of the colon and anastomosed to the esophagus. The duodenum is closed with either sutures or staples. Intestinal continuity is established by anastomosing the end of the proximal limb of the jejunum to a Roux limb of jejunum, approximately 60 cm distal to the anastomosis with the esophagus. A drain is then placed. Occasionally, following total gastrectomy, the surgeon may choose to create a jejunal reservoir to simulate a stomach. This does not add appreciably to the duration, difficulty or morbidity of the operation, but its efficacy is not widely accepted. A nasogastric tube is advanced across the esophagojejunal anastomosis, and the abdomen is closed. Total gastrectomy has traditionally been associated with a morbidity and mortality out of proportion to the operation's apparent magnitude. This is most likely a consequence of the patient's underlying condition, which often includes advanced malignancy and, almost invariably, some degree of malnutrition.

Variant procedure or approaches: Exposure for a **hemigastrectomy** is similar to, but less extensive than that required for a total gastrectomy. The abdomen is entered through an upper midline or right subcostal incision, but the lateral segment of the left lobe of the liver is simply retracted superiorly. If the resection is performed for cancer, an **omentectomy** may still be performed; however, it would be unusual to intentionally perform a **splenectomy**. The blood supply to the distal stomach is divided, and the duodenum is divided just beyond the pylorus. The body of the stomach is divided, using either clamps and sutures or staples, at a level appropriate for the pathology. If the resection is for cancer, an adequate proximal margin will dictate the proximal line of resection; if for a benign gastric ulcer, approximately half of the distal stomach is resected (preferably excising the ulcer itself). Reconstruction may be either to the duodenum (**Billroth I**), loop of jejunum (**Billroth II**) (Fig 7.2-1), or to a **Roux-en-Y loop of jejunum**. The anastomoses may be stapled or sewn; then the abdomen is closed.

Usual preop diagnosis: Total gastrectomy: gastric malignancy; Zollinger-Ellison syndrome; hemorrhage 2° diffuse gastritis. Hemigastrectomy: gastric cancer; gastric ulcers

SUMMARY OF PROCEDURE

	Total Gastrectomy	Hemigastrectomy
Position	Supine	⇐
Incision	Upper midline or bilateral subcostal	Upper midline or right subcostal
Special instrumentation	Upper hand or other self-retaining costal retractor	Upper hand or other costal retractor
Antibiotics	Cefotetan 1 g iv	⇐

	Total Gastrectomy	Hemigastrectomy
Surgical time	2-4 h	1.5-2 h
Closing considerations	Muscle relaxation required; NG suction	⇐
EBL	500+ ml, with potential for significantly more	100-500 ml
Postop care	PACU	⇐
Mortality	0-22%	0-1.8% (may be >10% if emergency)
Morbidity	Pulmonary complications: 15% Reoperation: 0-5% Esophagojejunal leak Sepsis Late anastomotic stricture Cardiac complications	Anastomotic leak Wound infection Cardiopulmonary complications
Pain score	7-8	7-8

PATIENT POPULATION CHARACTERISTICS

Age range	Mostly elderly
Male:Female	Male predominance
Incidence	Declining, due to declining incidence of gastric cancer and gastric ulcer and medical treatment for Zollinger-Ellison syndrome
Etiology	Gastric cancer and ulcer associated with: advanced age, alcohol and tobacco use, geographic location
Associated conditions	Weight loss (common); anemia (common); malnutrition (common); Zollinger-Ellison syndrome (rare)—avoid H_2-antagonists preop, if intraop gastric pH monitoring is planned by surgeon.

ANESTHETIC CONSIDERATIONS

See Anesthetic Considerations following Operations for Peptic Ulcer Disease, p. 350.

References

1. Dent DM, Madden MB, Price SK: Randomized comparison of R1 and R2 gastrectomy for gastric carcinoma. *Br J Surg* 1988; 75(2):110-12.
2. Heberer G, Teichmann RK, Kramlin HJ, Gunther B: Results of gastric resection for carcinoma of the stomach: the European experience. *World J Surg* 1988; 12(3):374-81.
3. Herrington LL Jr: Vagotomy and antrectomy. In *Surgery of the Stomach, Duodenum and Small Intestine*, 2nd edition. Scott HW Jr, Sawyers JL, eds. Blackwell Scientific Publications, Boston: 1992, 524-39.
4. Kauffman GL Jr, Conter RL: Stress ulcer and gastric ulcer. In *Surgery: Scientific Principles and Practice*, 2nd edition. Greenfield LJ, et al, eds. Lippincott-Raven Publishers, Philadelphia: 1997, 773-87.
5. Longmire WP Jr: Gastric carcinoma: is radical gastrectomy worthwhile? *Ann R Coll Surg Engl* 1980; 62(1):25-30.
6. Mulholland MW: Gastric neoplasms. In *Surgery: Scientific Principles and Practice*, 2nd edition. Greenfield LJ, et al, eds. Lippincott-Raven Publishers, Philadelphia: 1997, 795-804.

OVERSEW GASTRIC OR DUODENAL PERFORATION

SURGICAL CONSIDERATIONS

Description: Oversew operations are usually emergencies, and patients usually have peritonitis at presentation. Closure of the perforation alone, as opposed to performance of a definitive ulcer operation, is performed based on the surgeon's assessment of the patient's ability to tolerate a more extensive operation and the risk of recurrent ulceration.

In the younger patient with duodenal perforation (and where there is no delay in the diagnosis), a **highly selective vagotomy** may be added to closure of the perforation. Stomach or duodenum perforation is almost always a consequence of peptic ulcer disease, although on rare occasion, it may be caused by penetrating trauma. While perforation of the duodenum is almost never a consequence of malignant ulceration, perforation of the stomach due to malignant ulceration must always be considered. For this reason, the preferred treatment of a perforated gastric ulcer includes **resection**. If the general condition of the patient is poor or local inflammation is present, a biopsy of the ulcer, followed by closure, may be prudent. Biopsy of a perforated duodenal ulcer, on the other hand, is seldom necessary. In patients who are not systemically ill at the time of operation and who do not have severe peritonitis, some surgeons prefer to do a definitive ulcer operation such as a **vagotomy and pyloroplasty** or **highly selective vagotomy** at the time of closure of the perforation. Under other circumstances, closure of the perforation alone may be appropriate.

For closure of perforations, an upper midline incision commonly is used, although a right subcostal incision may be appropriate. The liver is retracted superiorly and the area of perforation identified. A nasogastric tube will have been placed preop and should remain on suction throughout the case to minimize ongoing leakage from the perforation. Perforation of the stomach may be handled either by resection (see Gastric Resections, p. 345), or by biopsy and simple suture closure. Perforation of the duodenum is usually repaired by simple suture of the site. Omentum is often used to buttress the area of closure of the stomach or duodenum. Closed suction drains are placed near the area of perforation and the abdomen is irrigated. Abdominal closure is routine, and the skin may be closed either primarily or packed open, depending on surgeon's preference.

Variant procedure or approaches: In certain patients, **nonoperative management** of perforated ulcer may be appropriate. In general, this has a relatively high likelihood of success in otherwise healthy patients with sealed duodenal perforation, but is much less reliable in frailer patients. While this may be a reasonable approach in some patients, there is no data to suggest that it is safer than traditional operative treatment.

Usual preop diagnosis: Perforated peptic ulcer

SUMMARY OF PROCEDURE

Position	Supine
Incision	Midline
Special instrumentation	Costal retractor
Unique considerations	Patients usually have peritonitis.
Antibiotics	Cefazolin or cefotetan 1 g iv
Surgical time	1 h
Closing considerations	Muscle relaxation required for closure; NG suction
EBL	Minimal
Postop care	PACU
Mortality	5-15%, largely dependent on patient population
Morbidity	Pneumonia Intraabdominal abscess Sepsis Wound infection Reperforation
Pain score	7

PATIENT POPULATION CHARACTERISTICS

Age range	Adult, increasingly elderly, especially women
Male:Female	Previous heavy male predominance still exists for duodenal ulcer, but large increase in incidence in gastric perforation in women > 65.
Incidence	Fairly common. Stable incidence, but with change in distribution, especially more elderly women.
Etiology	Peptic ulcer disease (PUD); nonsteroidal medications; malignancy (if gastric)
Associated conditions	Malignancy (if perforation is gastric); nonsteroidal medications; steroid use, especially during pulse therapy; other risk factors for PUD (e.g., alcoholism, smoking, etc.)

ANESTHETIC CONSIDERATIONS

See Anesthetic Considerations following Operations for Peptic Ulcer Disease, p. 350.

References

1. Debas HT, Mulvihill SJ: Complications of peptic ulcer: In *Maingot's Abdominal Operations*, 10th edition, Vol. I. Zinner MJ, Schwartz SI, Ellis H, eds. Appleton & Lange, Stamford, CT: 1997, 981-998.
2. Jick SS, Perera DR, Walker AM, Jick H: Non-steroidal anti-inflammatory drugs and hospital admission for perforated peptic ulcer. *Lancet* 1987; 2(8555):380-82.
3. Johnston D, Martin I: Duodenal ulcer and peptic ulceration. In *Maingot's Abdominal Operations*, 10th edition, Vol. I. Zinner MJ, Schwartz SI, Ellis H, eds. Appleton & Lange, Stamford, CT: 1997, 941-970.
4. Kauffman GL Jr, Conter RL: Stress ulcer and gastric ulcer. In *Surgery: Scientific Principles and Practice*, 2nd edition. Greenfield LJ, et al, eds. Lippincott-Raven Publishers, Philadelphia: 1997, 773-787.
5. Mulholland MW: Duodenal ulcer. In *Surgery: Scientific Principles and Practice*, 2nd edition. Greenfield LJ, et al, eds. Lippincott-Raven Publishers, Philadelphia: 1997, 759-72.
6. Sawyers JL: Acute perforation of peptic ulcer. In *Surgery of the Stomach, Duodenum and Small Intestine*. Scott HW Jr, Sawyers JL, eds. Blackwell Scientific Publications, Boston: 1992, 566-72.

OPERATIONS FOR PEPTIC ULCER DISEASE

SURGICAL CONSIDERATIONS

Description: Gastric ulcers are commonly associated with advanced age, and patients often have other medical problems, particularly cardiovascular and pulmonary. Currently there is a trend toward more emergency operations for bleeding gastric ulcers, particularly in elderly women and perhaps related to increasing use of nonsteroidal medications. All operations for peptic ulcer disease (PUD) require exposure of the upper abdomen and may be performed using either an upper midline or a long, right subcostal incision. The choice of surgical procedure depends on a number of considerations, including whether it is performed as an emergency or electively; the reason for performing the procedure (common factors include bleeding, perforation, intractability or gastric outlet obstruction); duration of symptoms; condition of the patient; and experience of the surgeon.

Vagotomy and antrectomy (V&A): This is the most extensive of the operations performed for peptic ulcer disease, and is generally reserved for healthy patients with significant intractable symptoms. The esophageal hiatus is exposed either by taking down the lateral segment of the left lobe of the liver and reflecting it to the patient's right, or by retracting this segment of the liver superiorly to gain exposure. The phrenoesophageal ligament is divided and the anterior and posterior vagus nerves (there may be more than one of each) are identified by feel. Division of all vagal trunks at the esophageal hiatus is performed, and specimens of the nerves are sent for pathology. The blood supply to the antrum is then divided, usually by dividing the right gastric and gastroepiploic vessels first. The gastrohepatic ligament is divided and the stomach elevated off of its attachments to the transverse colon. The gastric antrum is resected, leaving the duodenum just beyond the pylorus and dividing the stomach just above the junction of the body with the antrum. Reconstruction may be as a **Billroth I** (stomach-to-duodenum) or **Billroth II** (stomach-to-jejunal loop) (Fig 7.2-1). The anastomosis may be stapled or hand-sewn. Drains are not commonly used if a Billroth I is performed, but may be used in Billroth II because of the concern for a leak from the duodenal stump.

Vagotomy and pyloroplasty (V&P): This is the most commonly performed operation for PUD in the U.S. and is especially common for emergency operations. It is generally accepted to be simpler and safer to perform than V&A, but not as effective at preventing recurrence of ulcer disease. The abdominal incision and exposure of the hiatus to perform a vagotomy is the same as for V&P. After division of both vagal trunks (Fig 7.2-2), a longitudinal incision is made through the pylorus. The incision is then sutured together transversely, completing the pyloroplasty.

Parietal cell vagotomy (PCV): This operation requires even more meticulous exposure of the esophageal hiatus than that needed for a truncal vagotomy. The hiatus is exposed as above, and the main vagal trunks supplying the stomach are identified, but not divided. The stomach is retracted downward, and it is often helpful to divide a portion of the gastrocolic omentum to facilitate grasping the stomach. Branches supplying the body of the stomach (Fig 7.2-2), are individually divided and ligated with fine ligatures. Because the nerve fibers run with the blood vessels to the stomach, this necessarily involves division of the blood supply to the proximal lesser curvature of the stomach. This dissection is carried to the region of the "crow's foot" of the stomach, which is preserved. By denervating only the acid-producing portion of the stomach, while preserving innervation to the antrum, gastric acidity is diminished without significantly impairing gastric motility or emptying. A pyloroplasty is, therefore, not necessary. The operation is relatively tedious compared to the other procedures, and is usually performed electively or, rarely, urgently if there is a recent perforation and minimal soilage. It can be recommended only for duodenal ulcer disease, not gastric ulcer. Side-effects of this operation are generally less than with other ulcer operations.

Variant procedure or approaches: At the time of this writing, there have been several attempts to perform vagotomy, particularly PCV and V&P, **laparoscopically**. There is not enough experience to date, however, to describe its usefulness.

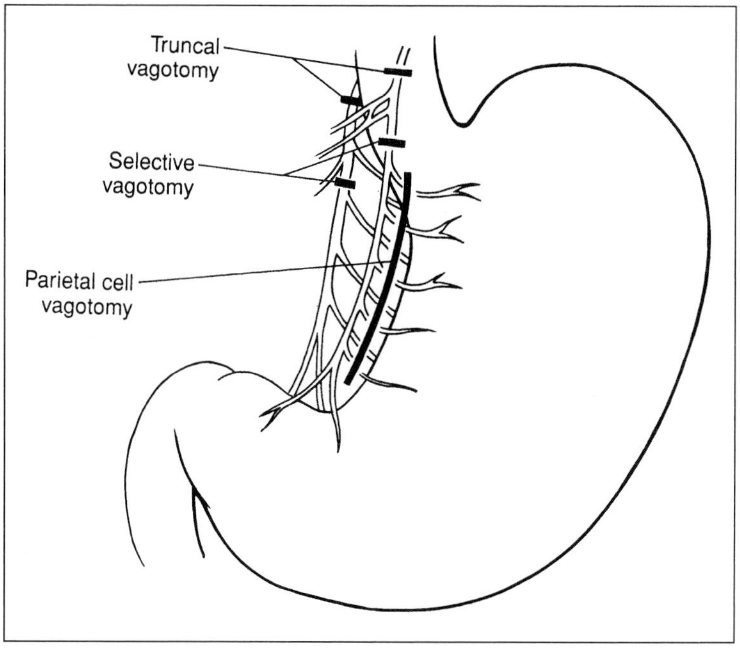

Figure 7.2-2. Types of vagotomy. Heavy lines indicate where vagal trunks are cut.

Usual preop diagnosis: V&P: complications of duodenal ulcer disease (bleeding, perforation and gastric outlet obstruction). V&A: duodenal and prepyloric ulcer disease. PCV: isolated duodenal ulcer disease; recent perforation and minimal peritoneal soilage

SUMMARY OF PROCEDURE

	V&P	V&A	PCV
Position	Supine	⇐	⇐
Incision	Midline or long subcostal	⇐	Midline
Special instrumentation	Costal margin retractor	⇐	⇐
Antibiotics	Cefotetan 1 g iv	⇐	Cefazolin 1 g iv
Surgical time	1-2 h	1.5-3 h	1.5-2.5 h
Closing considerations	Muscle relaxation required for closure; NG suction	⇐	⇐
EBL	< 250 ml; greater for emergency surgeries	250-500 ml	< 250 ml
Postop care	PACU	⇐	⇐
Mortality	0-2% (most series include emergencies)	0-1.6% (most series do not include emergencies)	0-0.4%
Morbidity	Dumping and diarrhea: 6-20% Recurrence: 4.9-12.3%	17-27% 0-2%	– 5-15% Impaired gastric emptying: 0.3% Necrosis, lesser curve: < 0.3% PE: rare
Pain score	6	6	6

PATIENT POPULATION CHARACTERISTICS

Age range	Adults
Male:Female	Male > female
Incidence	Declining
Etiology	Acid hypersecretion; abnormal mucosal permeability and repair mechanisms; Helicobacter pylori
Associated conditions	Gastrinoma (rare); hyperparathyroidism (rare)

ANESTHETIC CONSIDERATIONS

(Procedures covered: gastric resections; oversew gastric/duodenal perforation operations for peptic ulcer disease; duodenotomy)

PREOPERATIVE

Patients presenting for gastric surgery generally comprise 2 groups: (1) those presenting for emergency surgery following GI bleeding or perforation, and (2) those presenting with gastric carcinoma or elective treatment of PUD. Patients in the first group are often hemodynamically unstable and require rapid preop assessment and appropriate fluid therapy. It is prudent to consider full-stomach precautions in both patient groups (see p. B-5).

Respiratory — Patients with GI bleeding are prone to aspiration of blood and gastric contents. If this has occurred, patient may have significant respiratory insufficiency (in urgent need of tracheal intubation for "protection" of airway).
Tests: CXR; consider ABG.

Cardiovascular — Hypovolemia may be severe due to N/V, diarrhea, poor po intake or GI blood loss. Sx include ↓skin turgor, ↑HR, ↓BP, ↓UO. Correct hypovolemia prior to inducing anesthesia.
Tests: Orthostatic vital signs; ECG, if indicated from H&P.

Renal — GI fluid loss can lead to renal and electrolyte abnormalities.
Tests: Consider electrolytes; BUN; creatinine.

Hematologic — Polycythemia 2° GI fluid loss may be present; patients with GI bleeding will likely be anemic and may have a coagulopathy.
Tests: CBC with Plts

Laboratory — Other tests as indicated from H&P.

Premedication — Standard premedication (p. B-2) for elective procedures. Consider H_2-antagonist (ranitidine 10 mg iv), metoclopramide (10 mg iv 1 h preop), and Na citrate (30 ml po 10 min preop).

INTRAOPERATIVE

Anesthetic technique: GETA ± epidural for postop analgesia. If postop epidural analgesia is planned, placement of catheter prior to anesthetic induction is helpful to establish correct placement in the epidural space (accomplished by injecting 5-7 ml of 1% lidocaine via the epidural catheter, eliciting a segmental block).

Induction — The patient with gastric disease or upper GI bleeding is often at risk for pulmonary aspiration, and the trachea should be intubated with the patient awake or after rapid-sequence induction with cricoid pressure. (See Rapid-Sequence Induction, p. B-5.) If patient is clinically hypovolemic, restore intravascular volume (colloid, crystalloid or blood) prior to induction, and titrate induction dose of sedative/hypnotic agents.

Maintenance — Standard maintenance (p. B-3) without N_2O. **Combined epidural/GA**: A local anesthetic (2% lidocaine with 1:200,000 epinephrine) can be injected into a thoracic (3-5 ml) or lumbar (5-10 ml q 60 min) epidural catheter to provide both anesthesia and optimal surgical exposure (contracted bowel and profound muscle relaxation). A continuous infusion of local anesthetic (e.g., 2% lidocaine or 0.25% bupivacaine at 5-10 ml/h [lumbar]; 5 ml/h [thoracic]), may enhance hemodynamic stability. Be prepared to treat hypotension with fluid and vasopressors. GA is administered to supplement regional anesthesia and for amnesia. Systemic sedatives (droperidol, opiates, benzodiazepines, etc.) should be minimized during epidural opiate administration as they increase the likelihood of postop respiratory depression. Treat hypotension with fluid and vasopressors. If epidural opiates are used for postop analgesia, a loading dose (e.g., hydromorphone 1.0 mg [lumbar]; 0.5 mg [thoracic]) should be administered at least 1 h before conclusion of surgery.

Emergence — The decision to extubate at the end of surgery depends on the patient's underlying cardiopulmonary status and extent of the surgical procedure. Patient should be hemodynamically stable, warm, alert, cooperative and fully reversed from any muscle relaxants prior to extubation.

Blood and fluid requirements — Anticipate large third-space losses.
IV: 14-16 ga × 1
NS/LR @ 8-12 ml/kg/h
Fluid warmer

T&C for 4 U PRBC. Plts, FFP and cryoprecipitate should be administered according to lab tests (Plt count, PT, PTT, DIC screen, thromboelastography).

Monitoring	Standard monitors (p. B-1) UO ± Arterial line ± CVP catheter	+ Others as indicated by patient's status. Prevent hypothermia: Consider heated humidifier, forced air warmer, warming blanket, warming room temperature, keeping patient covered until ready for prep, etc.
Positioning	✓ and pad pressure points. ✓ eyes.	
Complications	Acute hemorrhage Hypoxemia	 2° abdominal packs → ↓FRC.

POSTOPERATIVE

Complications	Atelectasis Hemorrhage Ileus Hypothermia
Pain management	Epidural analgesics (p. C-1) PCA (p. C-3)
Tests	CXR if CVP placed perioperatively.

References

1. Clark CG, Fresini H, Aranjo JG, Boulos PB: Proximal gastric vagotomy or truncal vagotomy and drainage for chronic duodenal ulcer? *Br J Surg* 1986; 73(4):298-300.
2. Goligher JC, Pulvertaft CN: Comparison of different operations. In *After Vagotomy*. Williams JA, Cox AG, eds. Butterworths, London: 1969, 83-118.
3. Goligher JC, Pulvertaft CN, De Dombal FT, Congers JH, Duthie HL, Fether DB, Latchmore AJ, Shoesmith JH, Smiddy FG, Willson-Pepper J: Five-to-eight-year results of Leeds-York controlled trial of elective surgery for duodenal ulcer. *Br Med J* 1968; 2(608):781-87.
4. Gorey TF, Lennon F, Heffernan SJ: Highly selective vagotomy in duodenal ulceration and its complications. A 12-year review. *Ann Surg* 1984; 200(2):181-84.
5. Hoffmann J, Jensen HE, Christiansen J, Olesen A, Loud FB, Hauch O: Prospective controlled vagotomy trial for duodenal ulcer. Results after 11-15 years. *Ann Surg* 1989; 209(1):40-5.
6. Johnston D, Martin I: Duodenal ulcer and peptic ulceration: In *Maingot's Abdominal Operations*, 10th edition, Vol. I. Zinner MJ, Schwartz SI, Ellis H, eds. Appleton & Lange, Stamford, CT: 1997, 941-70.
7. Jordan PH Jr, Condon RE: A prospective evaluation of vagotomy-pyloroplasty and vagotomy-antrectomy for treatment of duodenal ulcer. *Ann Surg* 1970; 72(4):547-63.
8. Jordan PH Jr, Thornby J: Twenty years after parietal cell vagotomy or selective vagotomy antrectomy for treatment of duodenal ulcer: final report. *Ann Surg* 1994; 220(3): 283-93.
9. Moreno GE, Narbona AB, Charo DT, Figueroa AJ: Proximal gastric vagotomy. A prospective study of 829 patients with four-year follow-up. *Acta Chir Scand* 1983; 149(1):69-76.
10. Passaro EP Jr, Stabile BE: Gastric ulcers: In *Maingot's Abdominal Operations*, 10th edition, Vol. I. Zinner MJ Schwartz SI, Ellis H, eds. Appleton & Lange, Stamford, CT: 1997, 971-980.
11. Soybel DI, Zinner MJ: Complications following gastric operations: In *Maingot's Abdominal Operations*, 10th edition, Vol. I. Zinner MJ, Schwartz SI, Ellis H, eds. Appleton & Lange, Stamford, CT: 1997, 1029-1056.
12. Thompson JC, Wiener I: Evaluation of surgical treatment for duodenal ulcer: short- and long-term effects. *Clin Gastroenterol* 1984; 13(2):569-600.

OPERATIONS FOR MORBID OBESITY

SURGICAL CONSIDERATIONS

Description: Procedures devised to promote weight loss are of two fundamental types: (1) **gastric partitioning procedures**, which work by decreasing the size of the gastric pouch, thereby limiting the amount of food that can be consumed at one time; and (2) **malabsorptive procedures**, which work by bypassing most of the small bowel and creating a state of chronic malabsorption. Of these two general types of procedures, the partitioning procedures are generally less effective at promoting weight loss than are the malabsorptive procedures, but are much more popular because they are associated with far fewer serious side-effects.

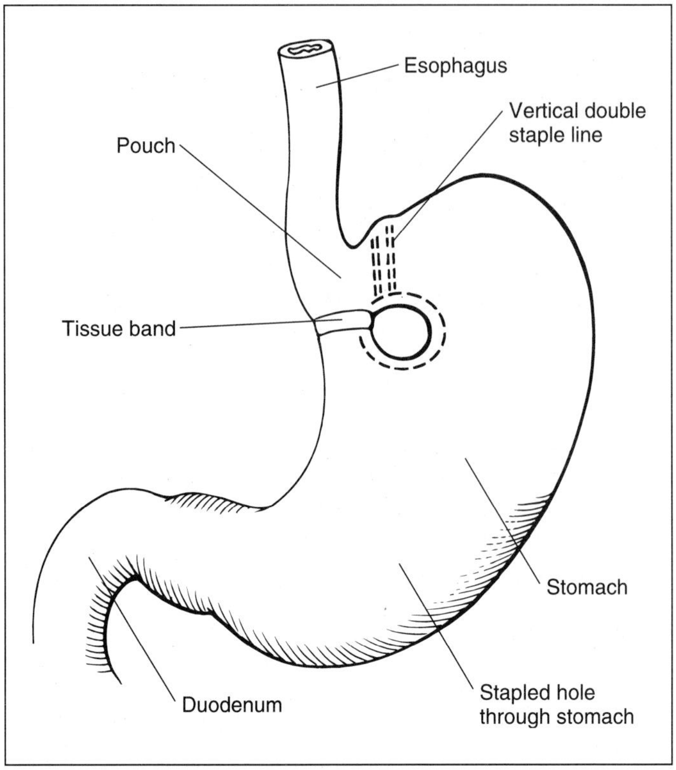

Figure 7.2-3. Vertical banded gastroplasty.

The partitioning procedure most commonly used today is the **vertical banded gastroplasty (VBG)**. The abdomen is entered through an upper midline incision, and the esophagogastric junction is exposed either by retracting the liver superiorly or by taking down the ligamentous attachments of the lateral segment of the left lobe of the liver and retracting this down and to the patient's right. The vessels to the lesser curvature are taken down for a short distance near the esophagogastric junction, and the posterior attachments of the stomach are taken down. A large bougie is passed by the anesthesiologist into the stomach and an EEA circular stapler is used to create a hole in the stomach adjacent to the bougie near the esophagogastric junction. Through this, a special stapler with thick, strong staples is passed and is fired up along the esophagus, creating a pouch of approximately 30 ml in volume (Fig 7.2-3). This leaves an outlet to the remainder of the stomach of only 1-2 cm, which is reinforced with a band of mesh. A nasogastric tube is placed through the gastroplasty into the distal stomach and the abdomen is closed without drains.

Perhaps more commonly performed today than the gastroplasty is the **Roux-en-Y gastric bypass** (Fig 7.2-4). Exposure is similar to that for a VBG. The upper stomach is mobilized and two rows of staples are used to partition the stomach into a small proximal and large distal pouch. A Roux segment of jejunum is then anastomosed to the small proximal pouch to provide drainage of it. A nasogastric tube is placed and the abdomen is closed without drains.

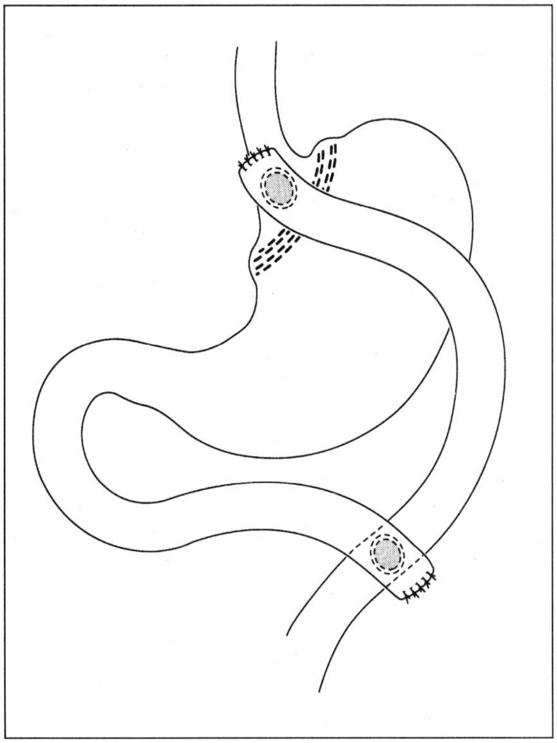

Figure 7.2-4. Proximal Roux-en-Y gastric bypass. (Reproduced with permission from Greenfield LJ, et al, eds: *Surgery: Scientific Principles and Practice*, 2nd edition. Lippincott-Raven Publishers, Philadelphia: 1997, 792.)

Variant procedure or approaches: An alternative to these procedures is the **jejunoileal (JI) bypass** (Fig. 7.2-5), in which the proximal jejunum is anastomosed to the terminal ileum. Exposure may be through a short, midabdominal or right, transverse incision and is generally less than is needed for a gastroplasty. The proximal jejunum is anastomosed to the terminal ileum, creating a chronic state of malabsorption. A nasogastric tube is placed and the abdomen is closed without drains.

Usual preop diagnosis: Morbid obesity (100 lbs above ideal body weight or 100% over ideal body weight), generally in combination with some medical condition felt to be worsened by the obesity (e.g., osteoarthritis, diabetes, respiratory insufficiency, CHF)

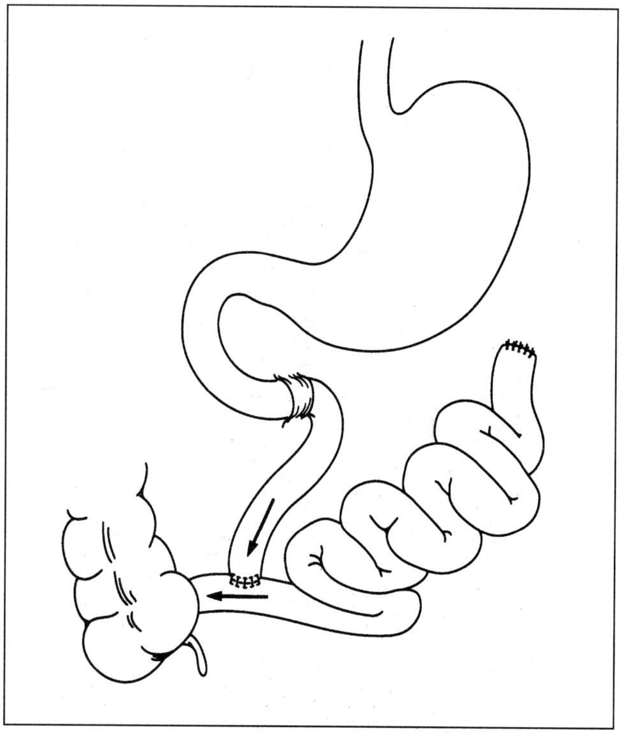

Figure 7.2-5. Schematic representation of jejunoileal bypass. (Reproduced with permission from Greenfield LJ, et al, eds: *Surgery: Scientific Principles and Practice*, 2nd edition. Lippincott-Raven Publishers, Philadelphia: 1997, 791.)

SUMMARY OF PROCEDURE

	Gastroplasty	JI Bypass
Position	Supine (Fig 7.2-6)	⇐
Incision	Midline	⇐
Special instrumentation	Large OR tables; heavy-duty retractors; special stapling devices	Large OR tables, heavy-duty retractors
Unique considerations	Prophylactic cholecystectomy often advocated. Pneumatic compression boots may not be large enough; heparin (5,000 U sc 2 h before surgery then q 12 h) used commonly.	⇐
Antibiotics	± Cefazolin 1 g iv	⇐
Surgical time	2-3 h	~1.5-3 h
Closing considerations	Anticipate 1+ h closure time; NG suction	⇐
EBL	< 500 ml	⇐
Postop care	Postop ventilation may be necessary; DVT precautions.	⇐
Mortality	0.5-1.6%	⇐
Morbidity	PE: 1-1.6%	⇐
	Wound infection: 4-8%	⇐
	Anastomotic leak: 3%	⇐
	Dehiscence: 1.6%	⇐
Pain score	7	5-6

PATIENT POPULATION CHARACTERISTICS

Age range	Adult
Male:Female	< 1:1
Incidence	4.9% of males and 7.2% of females in U.S. population considered morbidly obese
Etiology	Multifactorial
Associated conditions	Respiratory insufficiency ± CO_2 retention; CHF/cardiomyopathy; pulmonary HTN/systemic HTN; diabetes; unusually high risk of DVT and PE

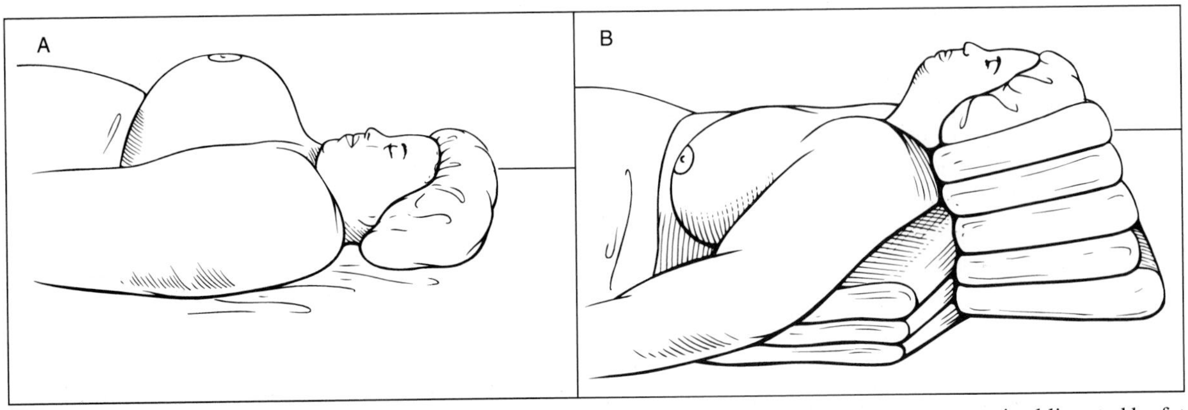

Figure 7.2-6. (A) In standard supine position, the atlantooccipital gap of morbidly obese pregnant woman is obliterated by fat and access for laryngoscope is hindered by large breasts. (B) By elevating the shoulders and occiput so that head is in the "sniffing" position, airway access is greatly facilitated.

ANESTHETIC CONSIDERATIONS

PREOPERATIVE

Morbid obesity is variably defined (>100 pounds over ideal body weight or 2 times ideal body weight), and may be associated with increased perioperative mortality and morbidity. Obstructive sleep apnea (OSA) is common in the morbidly obese patient.

Respiratory Increased O_2 consumption and CO_2 production (e.g., increased basal metabolic rate). Decreased chest wall compliance (↓20-60%) with normal lung compliance. Reduced ERV and FRC, so that tidal breathing may fall within the range of closing capacity → V/Q abnormalities. Supine position decreases FRC further → worsening hypoxemia. Increased minute ventilation is required to remain normocarbic. There is a normal response to CO_2 unless patient develops the obesity hypoventilation ("Pickwickian") syndrome (↑$PaCO_2$, ↓PaO_2, loss of hypercarbic drive, sleep apnea, hypersomnolence, polycythemia, pulmonary HTN, CHF). Tracheal intubation often is difficult in this patient population.
Tests: CXR; PFTs (FVC, FEV_1, $MMEF_{25\text{-}75}$ ± bronchodilators; room-air ABG)

Cardiovascular Blood volume and CO increase with rising weight. HTN is very common (use correct size BP cuff). LV dysfunction may be present; patient unable to increase CO or tolerate ↑blood volume. Pulmonary HTN may be present in OSA. Obesity is a risk factor for CAD and sudden death. Anticipate problems with vascular access. Patients with a Hx of phentermine/fenfluramine treatment should be evaluated for the presence of valvular disease. Consider cardiology consult.
Tests: ECG; others as indicated from H&P. (Patient with SOB may require MUGA scan and ECHO for LV function, as SOB can have a cardiac or pulmonary etiology.)

Endocrine Glucose intolerance and diabetes mellitus (DM) common.
Tests: Fasting glucose

Hepatic Liver function is often abnormal and drug metabolism may be significantly affected. Combined with altered pharmacokinetics, many drugs (e.g., midazolam and vecuronium) may have unpredictably prolonged action.

Gastrointestinal Increased intraabdominal pressure, gastric volume and acidity, with an increased incidence of hiatal hernia, make this patient population at risk for pulmonary aspiration of gastric contents.

Musculoskeletal Higher incidence of airway problems in obese patients. Careful airway examination is paramount. These patients are excellent candidates for fiber optic intubation. Establish availability of OR table large enough to accommodate morbidly obese patient.

Hematologic Polycythemia may occur 2° chronic hypoxemia
Tests: CBC

Laboratory Other tests as indicated from H&P.

Premedication Sedatives are best given either orally or iv in monitored environment. The sleep apneic patient may be especially sensitive to sedatives and narcotic drugs. Intramuscular medications can be erroneously injected into adipose tissues. Consider anticholinergics if performing awake fiber optic intubation (glycopyrrolate 0.2 mg iv 30 min preop). Take full-stomach precautions: metoclopramide (10 mg iv 60 min preop); H_2-antagonist (ranitidine 50 mg iv); nonparticulate antacid (3 M Na citrate) 30 ml, 10 min prior to induction.

INTRAOPERATIVE

Anesthetic technique: GETA ± epidural for postop analgesia.

Induction Patient at risk for aspiration of gastric contents and should be intubated either awake (p. B-6) or after rapid-sequence induction with cricoid pressure. Err on the side of caution (awake intubation) as the incidence of difficult mask ventilation and intubation is high in obese patients. Following successful intubation and induction of anesthesia, a NG tube should be placed and the stomach contents suctioned. Lipophilic drugs (e.g., STP) will have a greater volume of distribution, necessitating increased dosage. If using combined anesthetic approach, placement of an epidural catheter should be accomplished with the patient in the sitting position. A bilateral sensory block (using 5-7 ml 2% lidocaine) prior to induction will help confirm correct placement of the catheter within the epidural space. Verification of placement is particularly important in this population since regional anesthesia in the obese patient is technically more difficult.

Maintenance Standard maintenance (p. B-3). N_2O is best avoided to minimize bowel distention. Obese patients metabolize volatile anesthetics to a greater extent than their nonobese counterparts. Thus, isoflurane, desflurane or sevoflurane may be the volatile anesthetic of choice.

Combined epidural/GA: A local anesthetic (2% lidocaine with 1:200,000 epinephrine) can be injected into a thoracic (3-5 ml) or lumbar (5-10 ml q 60 min) epidural catheter to provide both anesthesia and optimal surgical exposure (contracted bowel and profound muscle relaxation). A continuous infusion of local anesthetic (e.g., 2% lidocaine or 0.25% bupivacaine at 5-10 ml/h [lumbar]; 5 ml/h [thoracic]) may enhance hemodynamic stability. The dose of local anesthetic administered via the epidural catheter should be decreased to 75% of normal dose. Be prepared to treat hypotension with fluid and vasopressors (ephedrine 5-10 mg iv, phenylephrine 50-100 μg iv). GA is administered to supplement regional anesthesia and for amnesia. Sedative drugs (droperidol, opiates, benzodiazepines, etc.) should be minimized in the presence of epidural opiates, as they increase the likelihood of postop respiratory depression. If epidural opiates are used for postop analgesia, a loading dose (e.g., hydromorphone 0.5-1.0 mg) should be administered 1-2 h before conclusion of surgery.

Emergence Elective ICU admission for postop care is common. The decision to extubate at the end of surgery depends on patient's underlying cardiopulmonary status and the extent of the surgical procedure. Patients should be hemodynamically stable, warm, alert, cooperative and fully reversed from any muscle relaxants prior to extubation.

Blood and fluid requirements	Anticipate large fluid loss. IV: 14-16 ga × 1-2 NS/LR @ 10-15 ml/kg/h Warm all fluids. Humidify gases.	Third-space losses greatly exceed blood loss. Guide fluid management by UO, filling pressure. T&S for 2 U PRBCs.
Monitoring	Standard monitors (p. B-1) UO ± Arterial line	Invasive monitoring as clinically indicated. Arterial line if noninvasive BP unreliable 2° extremity size.
Positioning	✓ and pad pressure points. ✓ eyes. Supine position = ↓FRC Avoid Trendelenburg.	Supine positioning → ↓lung volumes, which may ↑ V/Q, resulting in hypoxemia. This is exacerbated by use of the Trendelenburg position, which usually is not well tolerated by morbidly obese patients.
Complications	Hypoxemia 2° ↓FRC	100% O_2 → absorption atelectasis

POSTOPERATIVE

Complications	Hypoxemia Hypercarbia	Recover patient in sitting position to improve ventilatory mechanics. Give supplemental O_2.

Complications, cont.	DVT PE Atelectasis	Verify DVT prophylaxis preop.
Pain management	Epidural analgesia: hydromorphone (0.8-1.5 mg load, 0.2-0.3 mg/h infusion) PCA (p. C-3)	Patient should be recovered in ICU or hospital ward accustomed to treating side effects of epidural opiates (e.g., respiratory depression, breakthrough pain, nausea, pruritus).
Tests	ABG CXR	Others as clinically indicated. CXR for line placement

References

1. Buckley FP: Anesthesia and obesity and gastrointestinal disorders. In *Clinical Anesthesia.* Barash PG, Cullen BF, Stoelting RK, eds. Lippincott-Raven Publishers, Philadelphia: 1997, 975-90.
2. Buckley FP: Anesthetizing the morbidly obese patient. *ASA Annual Refresher Course Lectures* 1992; 163:1-6.
3. Buckley FP, Robinson NB, Simonowitz DA, Dellinger EP: Anaesthesia in the morbidly obese. A comparison of anaesthetic and analgesic regimens for upper abdominal surgery. *Anaesthesia* 1983; 38(9):840-51.
4. Flickinger DG, Pories WJ: Gastric bypass and other gastric restrictive procedures for morbid obesity. In *Surgery of the Stomach, Duodenum, and Small Intestine*, 2nd edition. Scott HW, Sawyers JL, eds. Blackwell Scientific Publications, Boston: 1992, 638-52.
5. Fox GS, Whalley DG, Bevan DR: Anaesthesia for the morbidly obese. Experience with 110 patients. *Br J Anaesth* 1981; 53(8):811-16.
6. Gastrointestinal surgery for severe obesity: Proceedings of a National Institutes of Health Consensus Development Conference. March 25-27, 1991, Bethesda, MD. *Am J Clin Nut* Feb 1992; 55(2 Suppl):487S-619S.
7. Griffen WO Jr: Gastric bypass. In *Surgical Management of Morbid Obesity.* Griffen WO Jr, Printen KJ, eds. Marcel Dekker, New York: 1987, 27-45.
8. Lechner GW, Callender AK: Subtotal gastric exclusion and gastric partitioning: a randomized prospective comparison of one hundred patients. *Surgery* 1981; 90(4):637-44.
9. Linner JH: Comparative effectiveness of gastric bypass and gastroplasty: a clinical study. *Arch Surg* 1982; 117(5):695-700.
10. Rawal N, Sjostrand V, Christofferson E, et al: Comparison of intramuscular and epidural morphine for postoperative analgesia in the grossly obese. Influence on postoperative ambulation and pulmonary function. *Anesth Analg* 1986; 63:583.

GASTROSTOMY PLACEMENT

SURGICAL CONSIDERATIONS

Description: A **gastrostomy** is a tube placed through the abdominal wall directly into the stomach. Such tubes can be used for gastric decompression or for feeding, and they may be permanent or temporary. Patients undergoing gastrostomy placement often have neurologic impairment which compromises their ability to handle oral secretions and increases their risk of aspiration. **Percutaneous gastrostomy**, in contrast to the other techniques, is most commonly performed using intravenous sedation and local anesthesia.

Variant procedure or approaches: The traditional **Stamm gastrostomy** is most commonly placed at the time of a laparotomy performed for another purpose, or may be performed through a separate, small laparotomy incision in patients in whom endoscopic placement is not possible for technical reasons. The incision may be upper midline or transverse directly over the stomach. The anterior wall of the stomach is identified and two pursestring sutures are placed in the stomach around the site at which the tube will enter. The gastrostomy tube is introduced through the abdominal wall directly over the intended site of entry into the stomach. A small hole is made in the stomach in the center of the pursestring sutures, the tube is introduced into the stomach, and the pursestrings are tied securely around the tube. The wound is then closed. General anesthesia is usually preferred, but the operation may be performed under local anesthesia in thin patients.

The **Janeway gastrostomy** is a technical modification, also requiring performance of a laparotomy. The greater curvature of the stomach is identified and a stapler placed across a portion of this, creating a tube that arises from the main body of the stomach. The staple line may be oversewn and then the end of the tube is brought through the abdominal wall and matured to the skin as a small stoma. This allows for permanent access to the stomach with removal of the tube between feedings, and is useful in patients with long-term dependence on gastrostomy access. The Janeway gastrostomy is rarely used, though young patients with neurologic impairment who are expected to need lifetime gastrostomy feeding are good candidates.

In **percutaneous (endoscopic) gastrostomy**, the stomach is intubated endoscopically and the gastric and abdominal walls punctured under endoscopic guidance. The gastrostomy tube is introduced through the mouth and passed through the stomach and abdominal wall from inside out. In most centers this has become the most common technique of gastrostomy placement due to its simplicity and because, in most patients, it can be performed under local anesthesia with MAC. Previous gastric operations may make endoscopic placement difficult or dangerous, as may some obstructing lesions of the esophagus or pharynx.

Usual preop diagnosis: Temporary gastrostomies are often used after major abdominal surgery as an alternative to NG suction. Percutaneous gastrostomies are often placed in patients with advanced malignancy and intestinal obstruction or inadequate oral intake, and in patients with neurologic impairment and difficulty in eating.

SUMMARY OF PROCEDURE

	Stamm	Janeway	Percutaneous
Position	Supine	⇐	⇐
Incision	Midline or transverse	⇐	Puncture
Special instrumentation	None	⇐	Endoscope, percutaneous gastrostomy kit
Antibiotics	± Cefazolin 1 g iv	⇐	⇐
Surgical time	45 min	1 h	0.5-1 h
Closing considerations	Muscle relaxation for closure	⇐	None
EBL	Minimal	⇐	⇐
Mortality	Minimal	⇐	⇐
Morbidity	Wound infection: 2.1-9%	⇐	–
	Hemorrhage: 0.9-1.1%	⇐	⇐
	Aspiration pneumonia: 2.2%	⇐	1.6%
	Failure to function: 2.2%	⇐	–
Pain score	4-5	5	1-2

PATIENT POPULATION CHARACTERISTICS

Age range	All ages, though with peaks in infancy and the elderly
Male:Female	~1:1
Incidence	Common
Etiology	See Preop Diagnosis, above.
Associated conditions	Gastrostomy placed at time of laparotomy, when NG drainage is anticipated for prolonged period. For feeding in the neurologically impaired or in those with complex upper digestive difficulties. Advanced malignancy (for either feeding or palliative decompression).

ANESTHETIC CONSIDERATIONS

See Anesthetic Considerations for Ostomy Procedures in Intestinal Surgery, p. 366.

References

1. Gauderer MW, Stellato TA: Gastrostomies: evolution, techniques, indications and complications. *Curr Probl Surg* 1986; 23(9):657-719.
2. Grant JP: Comparison of percutaneous endoscopic gastrostomy with Stamm gastrostomy. *Ann Surg* 1988; 207(5):598-603.
3. Shellito PC, Malt RA: Tube gastrostomy. *Ann Surg* 1985; 201(2):180-85.
4. Webster MW Jr, Carey LC, Ravitch MM: The permanent gastrostomy: use of the gastrointestinal anastomotic stapler. *Arch Surg* 1975; 110(5):658-60.

Surgeon

Harry A. Oberhelman, MD, FACS

7.3 INTESTINAL SURGERY

Anesthesiologist

Steven K. Howard, MD

DUODENOTOMY

SURGICAL CONSIDERATIONS

Description: A duodenotomy is performed to ligate a bleeding vessel at the base of a duodenal ulcer or to perform some procedure on the ampulla of Vater. It is important to be familiar with the anatomy of the proximal duodenum in relation to the major and minor pancreatic duct orifices. The duodenotomy may be made longitudinally or transversely, depending on the surgeon's preference. A transverse opening allows one to close the duodenotomy without tension; however, it must be placed very accurately for the purpose of exposure. Bleeding vessels at the base of an ulcer must be secured with suture ligatures. Care must be taken to avoid perforating the duodenum when performing a sphincterotomy.

Usual preop diagnosis: Duodenal ulcer; impacted common duct stone

SUMMARY OF PROCEDURE

Position	Supine
Incision	Midline abdominal or subcostal
Unique considerations	Magnifying glasses if operation involves lesser pancreatic sphincter
Antibiotics	Cefazolin 1 g iv preop
Surgical time	1-2 h
Closing considerations	Secure closure of duodenum
EBL	Minimal
Postop care	NG decompression
Mortality	< 0.5%
Morbidity	Duodenal leak: < 5% Postop pancreatitis: < 3%
Pain score	6-8

PATIENT POPULATION CHARACTERISTICS

Age range	Any age
Male:Female	1:1
Incidence	Not uncommon
Etiology	Duodenal ulcer; impacted common duct stone; villous tumors of ampulla
Associated conditions	Bleeding duodenal ulcer (50-60%); chronic pancreatitis (20-25%); impacted common duct stones (10-15%)

ANESTHETIC CONSIDERATIONS

See Anesthetic Considerations following Operations for Peptic Ulcer Disease, Stomach Surgery, p. 350.

Reference

1. Nora PF: *Operative Surgery: Principles and Techniques*, 3rd edition. WB Saunders Co, Philadelphia: 1990.

APPENDECTOMY

SURGICAL CONSIDERATIONS

Description: Appendectomy is performed for appendicitis or suspected appendicitis. The negative laparotomy rate has been reduced by the judicious use of ultrasonography, laparoscopy, barium enema and CT examination. Through a RLQ (**McBurney**) or right paramedian incision, the cecum is exposed and pulled into the wound (Fig 7.3-1). The appendix is then delivered through the wound, and the mesoappendix is clamped, cut and ligated. The appendix is removed by crushing and ligating, and then transecting the base. The appendiceal stump may be invaginated into the wall of the cecum or left alone. In some instances it may be easier to divide the base of the appendix before delivering the appendix into the wound. The wound should be left open and soft drains used in cases of perforated appendix. In children, the appendix may be inverted and allowed to slough off internally. Open appendectomy has been largely replaced by a laparoscopic approach (see p. 429).

Variant procedure or approach: Laparoscopic appendectomy (see p. 429).

Usual preop diagnosis: Appendicitis

SUMMARY OF PROCEDURE

Position	Supine
Incision	RLQ (McBurney's[2]) or right paramedian
Unique considerations	Variation in stump closure; NG tube if prolonged ileus expected.
Antibiotics	Cefazolin 1 g preop
Surgical time	1 h
Closing considerations	Skin wound should not be closed when appendix is perforated. Drain in presence of well defined abscess cavity.
EBL	< 75 ml
Postop care	Wound care when left open
Mortality	Perforated: 2% Nonperforated: < 0.1%
Morbidity	Pelvic, subphrenic or intraabdominal abscess (perforation): 20% Wound abscess: < 5% Fecal fistula: < 1% Wound hematoma: < 0.5% Ileus: Variable
Pain score	5-7

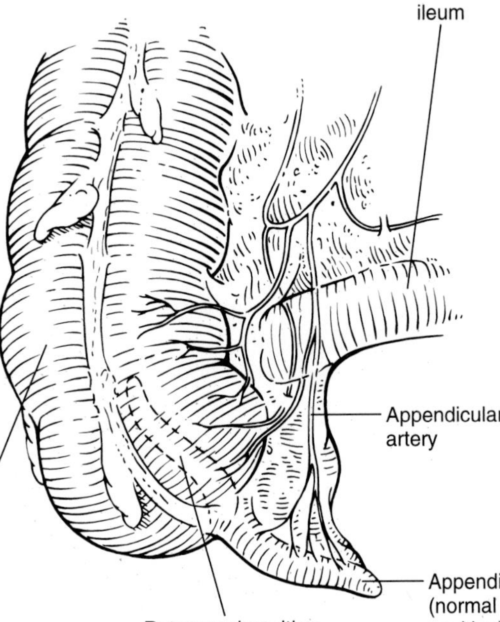

Figure 7.3-1. Relevant anatomy for appendectomy. (Reproduced with permission from Calne R, Pollard SG: *Operative Surgery*. Gower Medical Pub: 1992.)

PATIENT POPULATION CHARACTERISTICS

Age range	Any age
Male:Female	1:1
Incidence	1/15 persons
Etiology	Obstruction[5] (80-90%); fecaliths (75%); carcinoid tumors (< 5%)
Associated conditions	None

ANESTHETIC CONSIDERATIONS

See Anesthetic Consideration following Excision of Meckel's diverticulum, p. 363.

EXCISION OF MECKEL'S DIVERTICULUM

SURGICAL CONSIDERATIONS

Description: Meckel's diverticulum is a true congenital diverticulum, usually arising within two feet of the ileocecal valve. It was first described by Meckel[3] in 1809. Excision of a Meckel's diverticulum is indicated for bleeding, obstruction, perforation, inflammation, intussusception, and when there is a palpable mass near the base of the diverticulum. Ectopic mucosa is present in roughly 50% of symptomatic patients, with gastric mucosa the most frequent.[4] After entering the peritoneal cavity, the distal ileum, along with the diverticulum, is delivered into the wound. The diverticulum is excised and the wound closed in two layers. Following excision of the diverticulum, care must be taken not to narrow the bowel lumen during closure. If a diagnosis can be made preop, a laparoscopic approach may be used (see Laparoscopic Bowel Resection p. 426).

Usual preop diagnosis: Meckel's diverticulum

SUMMARY OF PROCEDURE

Position	Supine
Incision	Midline abdominal or RLQ (McBurney's)
Antibiotics	Cefazolin 1-2 g iv preop
Surgical time	1 h
EBL	< 100 ml
Mortality	< 0.5%
Morbidity	Wound infection: 5% Pulmonary complication: < 5% Anastomotic leak: < 1%
Pain score	6-8

PATIENT POPULATION CHARACTERISTICS

Age range	< 40 yr
Male:Female	3:1
Incidence	0.3%-2.5%
Etiology	Congenital
Associated conditions	Exomphalos; esophageal atresia; anorectal atresia; gross malformations of CNS or CV system

ANESTHETIC CONSIDERATIONS

(Procedures covered: appendectomy; excision of Meckel's diverticulum)

PREOPERATIVE

This patient population is generally fit and healthy apart from their acutely presenting illness. Full-stomach precautions are appropriate in these patients.

Respiratory — Respiratory impairment can occur 2° acute abdominal pain and splinting. Tachypnea and hyperpnea can be heralding Sx of appendiceal perforation and sepsis. Patients with acute abdomen should be treated as if they have full stomachs. Consider administration of metoclopramide (10 mg iv) and H_2 blocker (ranitidine 50 mg iv), and Na citrate 0.3 M 30 ml po.
Tests: As indicated from H&P.

Cardiovascular — May be dehydrated from fever, emesis and decreased oral intake. Assess volume status with vital signs in the supine and standing positions (if possible) and hydrate adequately prior to proceeding with anesthetic induction.
Tests: ECG, if indicated from H&P.

Gastrointestinal — Patient typically has abdominal pain with N/V. Muscular resistance to palpation of abdominal wall frequently parallels the severity of the inflammatory process. With spreading peritoneal irritation (as with perforation), patient will develop abdominal distension and paralytic ileus.
Tests: Electrolytes

Hematologic	Moderate leukocytosis (10,000-18,000) with moderate left shift. Hemoconcentration is probable, if patient is dehydrated. **Tests:** CBC
Laboratory	Other tests as indicated from H&P.
Premedication	Full-stomach precautions (see p. B-5). Opiate premedication (morphine 0.03-0.15 mg/kg iv) is indicated after patient is scheduled for surgery. If surgical intervention is still in question, administration of opiates may mask Sx of appendicitis.

INTRAOPERATIVE

Anesthetic technique: GETA, with rapid-sequence iv induction, followed by ET intubation (see full-stomach precautions, p. B-5). If systemic sepsis absent, hydration adequate, patient cooperative, and high abdominal exploration unlikely, then regional anesthetic can be considered.

Induction	Rapid-sequence induction of anesthesia (see p. B-5). Restore intravascular volume prior to anesthetic induction if patient is clinically hypovolemic.	
Maintenance	Standard maintenance (see p. B-3), without N_2O.	
Emergence	Patient should be extubated awake after return of airway reflexes.	
Blood and fluid requirements	IV: 16-18 ga × 1 NS/LR @ 5-8 ml/kg/h	
Monitoring	Standard monitors (see p. B-1).	Others, as indicated by patient's status.
Positioning	✓ and pad pressure points. ✓ eyes.	
Complications	Sepsis	

POSTOPERATIVE

Complications	Sepsis (possible with appendiceal rupture)	Adequate antibiotic coverage
	Paralytic ileus Atelectasis	Adequate pain control, incentive spirometry, early ambulation
Pain management	PCA (see p. C-3).	
Tests	As indicated clinically.	

References

1. McBurney C: Experience with early operative interference in cases of disease of the vermiform appendix. *NY Med J* 1889; 50:676-84.
2. Meckel JF: Ulcer die divertikel an darmkanal. *Arch Physiol* 1809; 9:421-53.
3. Merritt WT: Anesthesia for gastrointestinal surgery. In *Principles and Practice of Anesthesiology,* 2nd edition. Longnecker DE, et al, eds. Mosby-Year Book, Inc. St. Louis: 1998, 1881-1903.
4. Söderlund S. Meckel's diverticulum. A clinical and histologic study. *Acta Chir Scand* 1959 (Suppl 248); 13-233.
5. Van Zwalenburg C: The relation of mechanical distention to the etiology of appendicitis. *Ann Surg* 1905; 41:437-50.

ENTEROSTOMY

SURGICAL CONSIDERATIONS

Description: Enterostomy is performed for stenting the small intestine with a long tube, for feeding purposes, for bypassing small or large bowel obstructions, and following total proctocolectomy. An intestinal tube is either purse-stringed into the small bowel and brought through the abdominal wall, or the intestine itself is brought to the exterior and fashioned into a stoma. Different tubes are used for feeding, according to surgeon's preference. After purse-stringing the tube in the bowel, the seromuscular layer of the jejunum is sutured over the tube for a distance of 3-4 cm before exiting through the abdominal wall. The **Brooke ileostomy** is created by bringing a 2" segment of ileum through an abdominal wall stab wound. The ileum is folded back on itself and sutured to the skin edge or dermis (Fig 7.3-2). Some surgeons secure the ileum to the underlying peritoneum, but this is not necessary.

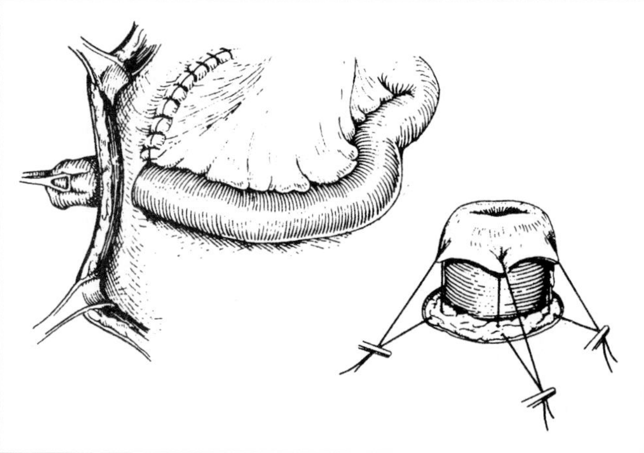

Figure 7.3-2. Brooke ileostomy. (Reproduced with permission from Hardy JD: *Rhoad's Textbook of Surgery*, 5th edition. JB Lippincott: 1977.)

Variant procedure or approaches: There are various intestinal or drainage tubes that may be inserted into the bowel, depending on the function required. For example, certain tubes are used for feeding, while others may be used for drainage or decompression.

Usual preop diagnosis: Intestinal obstruction due to extensive adhesions; following removal of the large intestine (including the rectum); for enteral feedings

SUMMARY OF PROCEDURE

	Enterostomy	Ileostomy
Position	Supine	⇐
Incision	Midline abdominal	⇐
Antibiotics	Cefazolin 1-2 g iv preop	⇐
Surgical time	1-1.5 h	⇐
Closing considerations	Securing tube to abdominal wall	Viable stoma
EBL	< 100 ml	⇐
Postop care	Tube irrigation	Stoma care
Mortality	< 0.5%	⇐
Morbidity	Ileus: 60-70%	⇐
	Wound infection: < 5%	⇐
		Stoma necrosis: < 2%
Pain score	5-6	5-6

PATIENT POPULATION CHARACTERISTICS

Age range	20-65 yr
Male:Female	1:1
Incidence	Common
Etiology	Intestinal obstruction (60-70%); diseases resulting in total proctocolectomy (10-15%); inability to eat (5-10%)
Associated conditions	Inflammatory bowel disease; intestinal adhesions; inability to eat orally

ANESTHETIC CONSIDERATIONS FOR OSTOMY PROCEDURES

(Procedures covered: enterostomy; continent ileostomy; gastrostomy; gastrojejunostomy)

PREOPERATIVE

This patient population is very diverse and includes those with inflammatory bowel disease, cancer or post CVA, and those presenting following trauma. Thus, the patient population ranges from the otherwise healthy to the critically ill. Many of these patients will have abnormal protective airway reflexes and are at risk of aspiration of gastric contents.

Respiratory — Patients post CVA or head trauma may have abnormal laryngeal reflexes and difficulty swallowing, making them prone to aspiration of gastric contents and associated pneumonitis; decreased pulmonary reserve and hypoxemia can be seen in patients with pulmonary infections.
Tests: Consider CXR to rule out pneumonia. Consider ABG.

Cardiovascular — Patients are likely to be hypovolemic 2° chronically poor po intake and malnutrition.
Tests: ECG; orthostatic vital signs

Musculoskeletal — Patients often sick and debilitated (e.g., post CVA).

Laboratory — CBC with differential; others as indicated from H&P.

Premedication — Depends on patient status. Titrate small doses of benzodiazepines (midazolam 0.25-0.5 mg iv) or opiate (fentanyl 25-50 μg iv). Consider H_2-antagonists (e.g., ranitidine 50 mg iv) and metoclopramide (10 mg iv 60 min preop).

INTRAOPERATIVE

Anesthetic technique: MAC with local anesthesia to area of incision typical for gastrostomy; otherwise, GA is appropriate for ostomy procedures.

Induction — Patient may be at risk for pulmonary aspiration. If GA is planned, the trachea should be intubated while patient is awake or after rapid-sequence induction with cricoid pressure. If patient is hypovolemic, volume status should be restored before induction, and doses of sedative/hypnotic should be titrated to effect.

Maintenance — **MAC:** Titration of sedatives (e.g., propofol 50-100 μg/kg/min) and analgesics (fentanyl 25-50 μg iv). **GA:** Standard maintenance (see p. B-3).

Emergence — Trachea should be extubated after return of protective laryngeal reflexes, if patient at risk for aspiration of gastric contents.

Blood and fluid requirements — Minimal blood loss
IV: 16-18 ga × 1
NS/LR @ 5-8 ml/kg/h

Monitoring — Standard monitors (see p. B-1). Others as clinically indicated.

Positioning — ✓ and pad pressure points.
✓ eyes.

POSTOPERATIVE

Complications — Atelectasis
Aspiration
Hypoxemia
Hypercarbia

Pain management — PCA (see p. C-3).

CONTINENT ILEOSTOMY POUCH (KOCK)

SURGICAL CONSIDERATIONS

Description: A **Kock pouch**[2] consists of an internal reservoir fashioned from the distal ileum and an intussuscepted nipple valve used to provide continence. Approximately 45 cm of small bowel are required for construction of the pouch and valve. After suturing two limbs of the ileum together over a distance of 15 cm, the distal segment is intussuscepted over itself to form the nipple valve. The pouch is then sutured closed and mounted beneath the abdominal wall stoma site (Fig 7.3-3). The stoma is made flush with the skin for cosmetic reasons and left intubated for 1 month with a special plastic catheter. The pouch requires catheterization for evacuation of its contents 3-4 times a day. The continent ileostomy reservoir has been modified by **Barnett**[1] to include the construction of an isoperistaltic valve with an intestinal collar around its base to prevent deintussusception and valve prolapse. These procedures are typically performed following total proctocolectomy or to replace conventional ileostomies.

Usual preop diagnosis: Inflammatory bowel disease; familial polyposis or malfunctioning ileostomies

SUMMARY OF PROCEDURE (KOCK OR BARNETT POUCH)

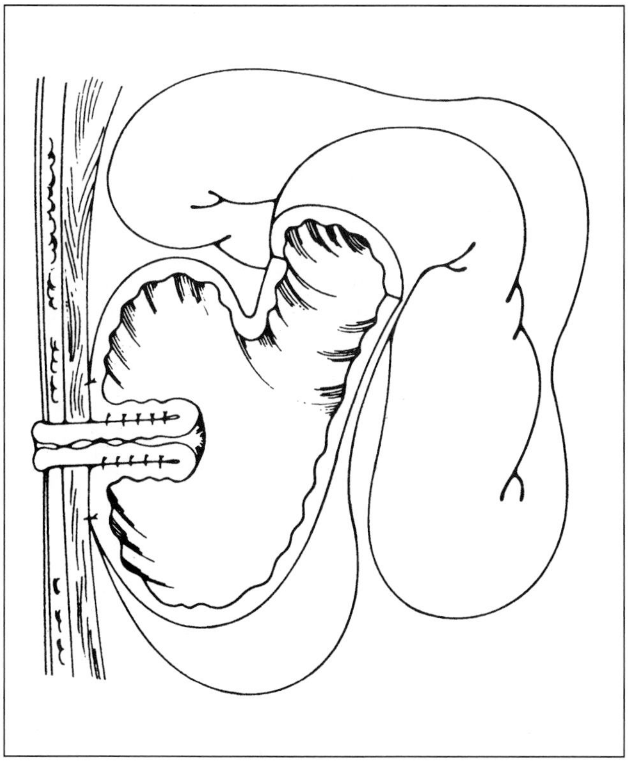

Figure 7.3-3. Continent ileostomy or Kock pouch. (Reproduced with permission from Hardy JD: *Hardy's Textbook of Surgery*, 2nd edition. JB Lippincott: 1988.)

Position	Supine
Incision	Midline abdominal
Special instrumentation	GIA or TA staplers
Antibiotics	Usual bowel prep with antibiotics; cefazolin 2 g iv preop
Surgical time	2-3 h
Closing considerations	Valve vascularity
EBL	200-300 ml
Postop care	Maintain pouch decompression
Mortality	< 1%
Morbidity	Intestinal ileus: 5% Wound infection: < 5% Intestinal obstruction: 2-3% Pouch fistula: 1-3% Valve necrosis: < 0.5%
Pain score	6-8

PATIENT POPULATION CHARACTERISTICS

Age range	18-80 yr
Male:Female	1:1
Incidence	Common
Etiology	Ileostomy (50%); proctocolectomy (5%)
Associated conditions	Extracolonic inflammatory bowel manifestations (10%)

ANESTHETIC CONSIDERATIONS

See Anesthetic Considerations for Ostomy Procedures, p. 366.

References

1. Barnett WO: Modified techniques for improving the continent ileostomy. *Am Surg* 1984; 50(2):66-9.
2. Becker JM: Ulcerative colitis. In *Surgery: Scientific Principles and Practice,* 2nd edition. Greenfield LJ, et al, eds. Lippincott-Raven Publishers, Philadelphia: 1997, 1093-1108.

SMALL-BOWEL RESECTION WITH ANASTOMOSIS

SURGICAL CONSIDERATIONS

Description: Resection of the small bowel is performed for a number of diseases (listed below). After entering the peritoneal cavity, the involved small bowel is delivered into the wound and the lesion resected between bowel clamps (Fig 7.3-4). Varying amounts of mesentery are included, depending on the diagnosis. More extensive resections indicated for malignant disease include regional lymph nodes. Reanastomosis may be accomplished by various suturing techniques or stapling. The peritoneal cavity may be accessed through vertical or transverse incisions. Operative techniques include **open end-to-end**, **closed end-to-end**, **side-to-side**, or **stapled, functional end-to-end anastomoses**.

Usual preop diagnosis: Intestinal obstruction, complicated by intestinal gangrene due to adhesions, internal hernia, volvulus, intussusception, mesenteric vascular occlusion, Crohn's disease, radiation enteritis, intestinal fistulae, small bowel tumors, and trauma[1]

SUMMARY OF PROCEDURE

Position	Supine
Incision	Vertical or transverse
Unique considerations	Adequate fluid resuscitation; NG tube
Antibiotics	Cefazolin 1-2 g iv preop
Surgical time	1-3 h
EBL	50-100 ml
Postop care	NG or long intestinal tube decompression
Mortality	Varies according to etiology: 1-5%
Morbidity	Atelectasis: < 10% Intestinal ileus: < 10% Wound infection: < 5% Intestinal leak, fistula: < 3%
Pain score	7-9

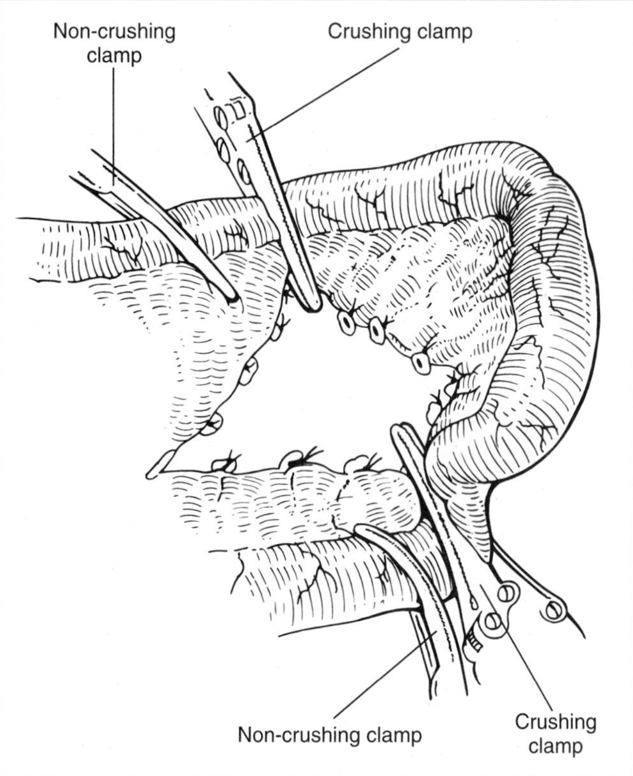

Figure 7.3-4. Application of bowel clamps. (Reproduced with permission from Calne R, Pollard SG. *Operative Surgery*. Gower Medical Pub: 1992.)

PATIENT POPULATION CHARACTERISTICS

Age range	20-70 yr
Male:Female	1:1
Incidence	Common
Etiology	Interference with blood supply (obstruction, strangulated hernia, volvulus, mesenteric thrombosis); trauma; tumors; Crohn's disease
Associated conditions	Multiple, depending on etiology (see Preop Diagnosis).

ANESTHETIC CONSIDERATIONS

See Anesthetic Considerations for Intestinal and Peritoneal Procedures, p. 370.

Reference

1. Zollinger RM Jr, Zollinger RM: *Atlas of Surgical Operations*, 7th edition. MacMillan, New York: 1993.

ENTEROLYSIS

SURGICAL CONSIDERATIONS

Description: Enterolysis consists of separating loops of bowel adhesed to other loops or the abdominal wall by sharp dissection, and excising adhesive bands. Care must be taken to avoid producing enterotomies. In recurrent cases of intestinal obstruction, small bowel plication or intraluminal tube stenting may be utilized. Plication is achieved by suturing the bowel or its mesentery so that the small bowel is aligned in an orderly manner without kinks. This also can be accomplished by threading a long, intraabdominal tube orally down through the small intestine.[1] This has the effect of holding the bowel in a nonobstructed position while new adhesions form.

Usual preop diagnosis: Intraabdominal adhesions

SUMMARY OF PROCEDURE

Position	Supine
Incision	Midline abdominal
Special instrumentation	A long intestinal tube may be necessary for decompression and fixation of bowel loop.
Unique considerations	Bowel decompression
Antibiotics	Cefazolin 1 g iv preop
Surgical time	1-4 h
Closing considerations	Adequate decompression to permit wound closure
EBL	150-500 ml
Postop care	PACU; continued intestinal decompression 2-5 d
Mortality	1-3%
Morbidity	Wound abscess: 15-20% Prolonged ileus: 10-20% Fistula formation: < 10% Pulmonary complications: 5-10% Recurrent intestinal obstruction: 5-8%
Pain score	5-7

PATIENT POPULATION CHARACTERISTICS

Age range	Any age
Male:Female	1:1
Incidence	Common
Etiology	Previous intraabdominal operative procedure (> 90%); malignant tumors (15-20%); hernias (10-15%); volvulus (5-10%); inflammatory bowel disease (5%); gallstone ileus (< 5%); intussusception (< 5%)

ANESTHETIC CONSIDERATIONS

See Anesthetic Considerations for Intestinal and Peritoneal Procedures, p. 370.

References

1. Brolin RE, Krasna MJ, Mast BA: Use of tubes and radiographs in the management of small bowel obstruction. *Ann Surg* 1987; 206:126.
2. Close MB, Christensen NM: Transmesenteric small bowel plication or intraluminal tube stenting. Indications and contraindications. *Am J Surg* 1979; 138(1):89-96.

CLOSURE OF ENTERIC FISTULAE

SURGICAL CONSIDERATIONS

Description: Enteric fistulae may occur between the bowel and abdominal wall (enterocutaneous), between loops of the intestine (enteroenteric or enterocoelic), or between the bowel and bladder or vagina (enterovesical or enterovaginal). Surgical repair is usually reserved for fistulae to the abdominal wall, bladder and vagina, and consists of excising the fistula and repairing the bowel and the other organ separately. Most fistulae are characterized by the adherence of the two visceral organs with a communication between their lumens.

The organs involved are separated by blunt-sharp dissection and repaired locally after excision of the indurated margins of the defect. In the case of both the small and large intestines, it may be necessary to resect a segment of bowel with the defect and to perform an end-to-end anastomosis. If the repair sites involved lie close together, it is important to interpose tissue, such as the omentum, between the viscera to minimize chance of recurrence. Occasionally a fistula may be bypassed rather than surgically resected.

Usual preop diagnosis: Enteric fistula

SUMMARY OF PROCEDURE

Position	Supine
Incision	Midline abdominal
Unique considerations	Preop nutritional support and fistula wound care
Antibiotics	Cefazolin 2 g iv preop
Surgical time	2-4 h
Closing considerations	Separation of repairs by interposition of omentum and other tissue
EBL	50-300 ml
Postop care	NG decompression until bowel function returns; TPN support
Mortality	0-5%
Morbidity	Ileus: 60-70% Pulmonary complications: 10% Recurrent fistula: 5-10% Wound infection: 5-10%
Pain score	6-8

PATIENT POPULATION CHARACTERISTICS

Age range	Any age
Male:Female	1:1
Incidence	Common
Etiology	Anastomotic leaks (60-70%); carcinoma (10-15%); Crohn's disease (5-10%); iatrogenic bowel injury (5-10%); perforative diverticulitis (5-10%); radiation enteritis (5%); foreign body perforation (< 5%)
Associated conditions	Malnutrition (30%); inflammatory bowel disease (25%); cancer (15%)

ANESTHETIC CONSIDERATIONS FOR INTESTINAL AND PERITONEAL PROCEDURES

(Procedures covered: small bowel resection; enterolysis; closure of enteric fistulae; excision of intraabdominal and retroperitoneal tumor; drainage of subphrenic abscess)

PREOPERATIVE

Patients requiring exploratory laparotomy are often at risk for aspiration of gastric contents. Precautions to prevent this are necessary to help assure safe patient outcome (see p. B-5).

Respiratory Respiratory insufficiency can be present due to intraabdominal pathology; ↓FRC → ↑A-a gradient and arterial hypoxemia; diaphragmatic impairment and splinting → ↑respiratory insufficiency.
Tests: Consider CXR; consider ABG.

Cardiovascular	Patient is likely to be critically ill and should be evaluated for presence of hypovolemia (hypotension, tachycardia) and should receive adequate volume replacement before anesthetic induction. **Tests:** ECG; orthostatic vital signs	
Musculoskeletal	Abdominal rigidity may be present; abdominal pain is common.	
Gastrointestinal	Diarrhea, vomiting and prolonged npo status can lead to electrolyte abnormalities. **Tests:** Electrolytes	
Renal	Renal insufficiency/failure may be present, especially in elderly and/or chronically ill patients, and in those who are hypovolemic. **Tests:** Consider BUN; creatinine; electrolytes.	
Laboratory	CBC with differential; Plt count	
Premedication	Standard premedication (see p. B-2). Consider H_2-antagonists (e.g., ranitidine 50 mg iv 1 hr preop), metoclopramide (10 mg iv 1 h preop, although contraindicated in bowel obstruction/perforation) and Na citrate (30 ml po 10 min preop).	

INTRAOPERATIVE

Anesthetic technique: GETA ± epidural for postop analgesia. If postop epidural analgesia is planned, placement of catheter prior to anesthetic induction is helpful to establish correct placement in the epidural space (accomplished by injecting 5-7 ml of 2% lidocaine via the epidural catheter, eliciting a segmental block).

Induction	The patient with abdominal pathology is often at risk for pulmonary aspiration and the trachea should be intubated with patient awake or after rapid-sequence iv induction with cricoid pressure. (See Rapid-Sequence Induction, p. B-5.) If patient is clinically hypovolemic, restore intravascular volume (colloid, crystalloid or blood) prior to induction and titrate induction dose of sedative/hypnotic agents.	
Maintenance	**Balanced anesthesia** without N_2O. (See Standard Maintenance Techniques, p. B-3) Complete muscle relaxation should be assured. **Combined epidural and GA:** Local anesthetic (2% lidocaine with 1:200,000 epinephrine 5-10 ml q 60 min) can be injected into the epidural catheter to provide both anesthesia and optimal surgical exposure (contracted bowel and profound muscle relaxation). A continuous infusion of local anesthetic (e.g., 2% lidocaine or 0.25% bupivacaine) at 5-10 ml/h. Be prepared to treat hypotension with fluid and vasopressors. GA is administered to supplement regional anesthesia and for amnesia. If epidural opiates are used for postop analgesia, a loading dose (e.g., hydromorphone 1.0 mg) should be administered at least 1 h before the conclusion of surgery. Systemic sedatives (droperidol, opiates, benzodiazepines, etc.) should be minimized during this type of anesthetic as they increase the likelihood of postop respiratory depression. An NG tube should be placed and kept on intermittent suction.	
Emergence	The decision to extubate at the end of surgery depends on the patient's underlying cardiopulmonary status and the extent of the surgical procedure. Patients should be hemodynamically stable, warm, alert, cooperative, and fully reversed from any muscle relaxants prior to extubation. If the above criteria are not met, patient should remain intubated and transported to ICU for further care.	
Blood and fluid requirements	Anticipate large fluid shift. IV: 14-16 ga × 1-2 T&C for 4 U RBCs. NS/LR @ 10-15 ml/kg/h Fluid warmer	Plts, FFP and cryoprecipitate should be administered according to lab tests (Plt count, PT, PTT, DIC screen, thromboelastography).
Monitoring	Standard monitors (see p. B-1). UO ± Arterial line ± CVP/PA catheter	Invasive monitors, as indicated by patient's status. Prevent hypothermia: consider heated humidifier, forced-air warmer, warming blanket, warm room temperature, keeping patient covered until ready for prep, etc.
Positioning	✓ and pad pressure points. ✓ eyes.	
Complications	Hemorrhage Sepsis	Acute septic shock may require PA catheter and aggressive hemodynamic support.

POSTOPERATIVE

Complications	Sepsis Hemodynamic instability Atelectasis Hypoxemia Hemorrhage Ileus	Pulmonary function abnormalities may persist for 1 wk postop (↓vital capacity and ↓FRC).
Pain management	Epidural analgesia (see p. C-1). PCA (see p. C-3).	Patient should be recovered in ICU or ward accustomed to treating the side-effects of epidural opiates (e.g., respiratory depression, breakthrough pain, nausea, pruritus).
Tests	CBC; CXR (if central line placed); electrolytes; glucose	Others as directed by intraop course.

References

1. Aguirre A, Fischer JE, Welch CE: The role of surgery and hyperalimentation in the therapy of gastrointestinal-cutaneous fistulae. *Ann Surg* 1974; 180(4):393-401.
2. Merritt WT: Anesthesia for gastrointestinal surgery. In *Principles and Practice of Anesthesiology*, 2nd edition. Longnecker DE, et al, eds. Mosby-Year Book, Inc. St. Louis: 1998, 1881-1903.

Surgeon

James M. Stone, MD

7.4 COLORECTAL SURGERY

Anesthesiologist

Steven K. Howard, MD

TOTAL PROCTOCOLECTOMY

SURGICAL CONSIDERATIONS

Description: Total proctocolectomy involves excision of the entire colon, rectum and anus (Fig 7.4-1). The end of the ileum may be fashioned into an **end ileostomy** (**Brooke ileostomy**), **continent ileostomy** (**Kock pouch**) or an **ileoanal pouch**. Most patients request the ileoanal pouch procedure to avoid the need for a stoma. The bacterial load of the colon is greatly diminished by mechanical cleaning, which may be accomplished by cathartics or nonabsorbed, lavage solutions. As a result of this bowel prep, patients are frequently hypokalemic and hypovolemic. Oral antibiotics are also given the night before surgery to further diminish the bacterial load. Neomycin 1 g and erythromycin base 1 g taken at 1 pm, 2 pm and 11 pm on the day before surgery are commonly used. Many other regimens of absorbed and/or nonabsorbed antibiotics, however, are equally effective. The efficacy of parenteral broad spectrum antibiotics, given at the time of induction, has not been established, although it is widely practiced.

Total proctocolectomy is performed through a midline incision. In the setting of ulcerative colitis, the small bowel is inspected for Crohn's disease or evidence of an unexpected colon cancer. In the setting of familial adenomatous polyposis (FAP), a search is made for unexpected intestinal cancers, metastases or desmoid tumors. The right colon is mobilized first and then the small bowel mesentery is mobilized to allow for creation of an ileostomy. The transverse colon may be mobilized by separating it from the greater omentum, or the greater omentum may be resected along with the specimen. The descending colon is mobilized, and the splenic flexure is taken down from both the transverse and descending colon sides. The sigmoid colon is then mobilized to the level of the sacral promontory. At this time, the ileum is transected at the ileocecal valve and the vascular supply to the colon is divided between clamps. Unless a malignancy is present, the mesentery may be taken at a convenient level near the bowel wall. At the level of the sacral promontory, the superior rectal artery and vein are divided between clamps. The dissection continues close to the rectal wall to avoid injury to the presacral sympathetic and the pelvic parasympathetic nerves. This diminishes the chances of postop impotence or retrograde ejaculation.

When the dissection reaches the pelvic floor, the perineal phase of the operation begins. A circumferential incision is made at the anal verge, and the intersphincteric space is identified. The dissection proceeds cephalad in the intersphincteric plane until the abdominal dissection is encountered and the specimen is removed. The abdomen and perineum are irrigated and a presacral drain is brought out of a stab wound adjacent to the perineal incision. The levator, external sphincter muscles, and skin are closed in layers. (If a second operating team is available, time may be saved by performing

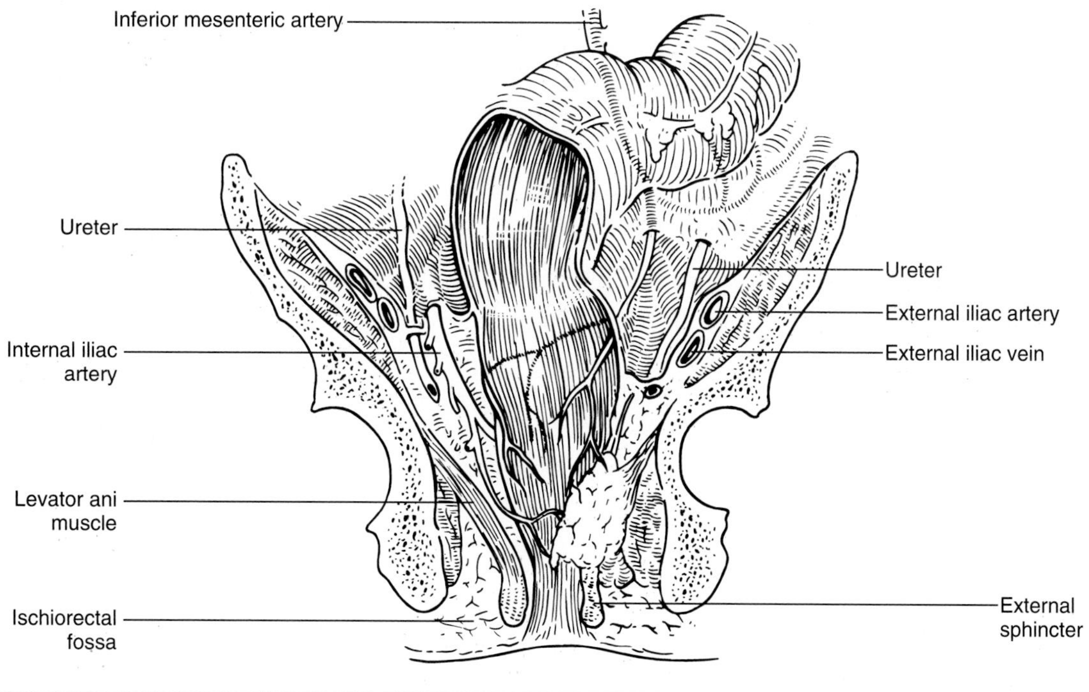

Figure 7.4-1. Relevant anatomy for proctocolectomy, colectomy. (Reproduced with permission from Calne R, Pollard SG: *Operative Surgery*. Gower Medical Pub: 1992.)

the perineal dissection while the abdominal colon is being mobilized.) A circular incision is made over an ileostomy site (which was marked preop) and a muscle-splitting incision is carried through the rectus fascia and muscle. The terminal ileum is mobilized and cleaned of its mesentery sufficiently to allow 5 cm to project above the skin when it is led through the stoma site. With the stoma projecting through the abdominal wall, the midline fascia and skin are closed. Retention sutures may be used in malnourished patients, as well as those taking chronic, high-dose corticosteroids. After the skin is closed, an everting, **Brooke ileostomy** is performed.

Variant procedure or approaches: With the **continent ileostomy procedure**, removal of the colon, rectum and anus is unchanged from above. The terminal ileum is used to create an intraabdominal reservoir as well as a sphincter mechanism (nipple valve). This is accomplished by sewing two loops of ileum together to form a pouch. A nipple valve is formed by intussuscepting ileum into itself and the pouch. The walls of the adjacent intussuscepted ileum are fixed together with several rows of staples. The patient does not wear an ileostomy appliance because stool collects in the ileal reservoir. The reservoir is emptied 3 to 4 times/day by passing a catheter through the nipple valve.

With the **ileoanal pouch procedure**, the anus and sphincter mechanism are preserved. A short segment of the distal rectal muscle tube is also preserved after the mucosa has been surgically removed. A reservoir (pouch), made from the terminal ileum, is anastomosed to the top of the anus. A temporary ileostomy is commonly performed at the same time. After the ileoanal pouch procedure, patients have 5-7 bowel movements in a 24-hour period. The ileoanal pouch procedure is contraindicated in patients with Crohn's disease or anal incontinence. Obesity, advanced age and severe underlying medical problems are relative contraindications. These operations may be performed more rapidly by two teams working simultaneously in the abdomen and perineum.

Usual preop diagnosis: Ulcerative colitis; familial adenomatous polyposis; Crohn's colitis

SUMMARY OF PROCEDURE

	Total Proctocolectomy With End Ileostomy	Total Proctocolectomy With Continent Ileostomy	Total Colectomy, Mucosal Proctectomy, Ileoanal Pouch
Position	Modified lithotomy	⇐	⇐
Incision	Long midline	⇐	⇐
Special instrumentation	2-table setup (separate abdominal and perineal instruments); deep pelvic instruments	2-table setup; long, noncutting linear staplers; Kock catheters; deep pelvic instruments	2-table setup; anal retractors; spinal needle; 1:2000,000 epinephrine; deep pelvic instruments
Unique considerations	Patients frequently on chronic high-dose corticosteroids	⇐	⇐+ Epinephrine solutions injected under the rectal mucosa to facilitate dissection and reduce bleeding.
Antibiotics	Cefotetan 1 g iv	⇐	⇐
Surgical time	3-4 h	3-7 h	⇐
Closing considerations	Ileostomy completed after skin closed (15-30 min).	None	Temporary ileostomy commonly used, completed after skin closure.
EBL	300-1000 ml (most blood loss during pelvic and perineal dissections)	⇐	⇐
Postop care	Transient inability to void common.	Maintain patency of catheter draining pouch; transient inability to void common.	Small bowel mesentery lengthened by dissection around duodenum. This frequently necessitates use of postop NG tube. Transient inability to void common.
Mortality	2-5% (older patients and those with underlying medical problems)	0-2%	⇐
Morbidity	Dyspareunia: 30%	⇐	5-10%
	Stoma complications: 20%	–	–
	SBO: 10-15%	⇐	⇐
	Impotence: 2-4%	⇐	⇐

	Total Proctocolectomy With End Ileostomy	Total Proctocolectomy With Continent Ileostomy	Total Colectomy, Mucosal Proctectomy, Ileoanal Pouch
Morbidity, cont.		Nipple valve failure: 20-50%	–
		Persistent perineal wound: 30%	–
		Pouchitis: 20-30%	⇐
		Intraabdominal sepsis: 5%	–
		Pouch incontinence 5%	–
			Nocturnal incontinence: 20%
			Poor function: 5%
			Pelvic sepsis: 0-4%
Pain score	8	8	8

PATIENT POPULATION CHARACTERISTICS

	Ulcerative colitis	Familial adenomatous polyposis
Age range	3rd-5th decade	2nd-4th decade
Male:Female	1:1	⇐
Incidence	6-10/100,000	100-150 cases/yr
Etiology	Unknown	Genetic
Associated conditions	Cushing's syndrome; anemia; malnutrition; colorectal cancer; sclerosing cholangitis	Colorectal cancer; desmoid tumors; adenomas or cancers of the duodenum and small intestine; brain tumors (Turcot's syndrome); adrenal adenomas; osteomas

ANESTHETIC CONSIDERATIONS

See Anesthetic Considerations for Large Bowel Surgery, p. 383.

References

1. Condon RE, Wittmann DH: The use of antibiotics in general surgery. *Curr Probl Surg* 1991; 28(2):801-949.
2. Francois Y, Dozois RR, Kelly KA, Beart RW Jr, Wolff BG, Pemberton JH, Ilstrup DM: Small intestinal obstruction complicating ileal pouch-anal anastomosis. *Ann Surg* 1989; 209(1):46-50.
3. Jarvinen HJ, Makitie A, Sivula A: Long-term results of continent ileostomy. *Int J Colorectal Dis* 1986; 1(1):40-3.
4. Kelly KA, Pemberton JH, Wolff BG, Dozois RR: Ileal pouch-anal anastomosis. *Curr Probl Surg* 1992; 29(2):57-131.
5. Metcalf AM, Dozois RR, Kelly KA: Sexual function in women after proctocolectomy. *Ann Surg* 1986; 204(6):624-7.
6. Wexner SD, Wong WD, Rothenberger DA, Goldberg SM: The ileoanal reservoir. *Am J Surg* 1990; 159(1):178-85.

PARTIAL COLECTOMY WITH ANASTOMOSIS

SURGICAL CONSIDERATIONS

Description: This procedure is used for resection of any portion of the abdominal colon with primary anastomosis (Fig 7.4-2). The most common types of partial colectomy are: **total abdominal colectomy**, **right hemicolectomy**, **sigmoid colectomy** and **left hemicolectomy**. Occasionally, **cecectomy** or **short segmental resections** are performed. Most patients presenting for elective colectomy undergo preop bowel preparation that consists of mechanical cleaning of the colon, and administration of preop oral antibiotics. As a result of the bowel prep, patients are frequently hypovolemic and hypokalemic when they come to the OR.

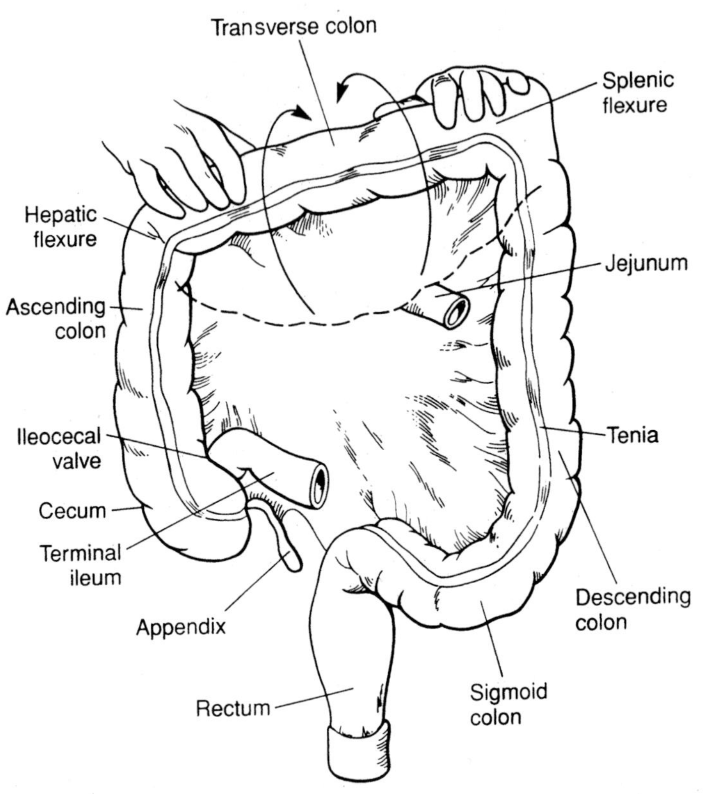

Figure 7.4-2. Anatomy of the colon. (Reproduced with permission from Hardy JD: *Hardy's Textbook of Surgery*, 2nd edition. JB Lippincott: 1988.)

Partial colectomy may be performed via midline or transverse abdominal incisions, depending on the underlying disease, portion of colon to be resected and surgeon's preference. In general, midline incisions are preferred when: a high-lying splenic flexure must be mobilized; inflammatory bowel disease is present; the extent of colon resection is not known preop; and/or combined hepatic resection is anticipated. Transverse incisions are commonly used for right hemicolectomy or sigmoid colectomy. The anastomosis may be handsewn or stapled; in the abdominal colon, there is no clear advantage to either anastomotic technique. The modified lithotomy position—thighs abducted and extended, knees flexed and legs supported by stirrups (Allen universal, Lloyd-Davies)—is useful when intraop lower endoscopy is planned, and when an anastomosis to the distal sigmoid or rectum is anticipated (e.g., sigmoid resection for diverticular disease). In this position, a stapling device may be passed through the anus to perform the anastomosis. Ureteral stents may be placed prior to laparotomy when an inflammatory mass is present in the pelvis (sigmoid diverticulitis, ileocolic or sigmoid Crohn's disease), when there has been prior irradiation of the operative field and when a bulky or recurrent pelvic cancer is resected.

The sequence of steps in partial colectomy is the same for all parts of the colon. The first step is mobilization, performed along the line of Toldt (separating the retroperitoneum from the peritoneum) for the right, left and sigmoid colon, and among the greater omentum for the transverse colon. Proximal and distal sites for resection are selected and the intervening mesentery is taken between clamps. Finally, the bowel is transsected and an anastomosis is effected. During mobilization of the pelvic colon, care must be exercised to identify and preserve the ureter. During mobilization of the hepatic flexure, care is taken not to injure the duodenum.

Creation of a **colostomy** may be desirable in patients who are hemodynamically unstable, or when local conditions such as inflammation, carcinomatosis, ischemia or unprepped bowel are present. The distal end of the resected colon may be brought through the skin as a mucous fistula, or it may be oversewn and placed within the peritoneal cavity.

Usual preop diagnosis: Colon cancer; diverticular disease; Crohn's disease; ulcerative colitis; trauma; ischemic colitis; lower GI hemorrhage; intractable constipation; colon volvulus

SUMMARY OF PROCEDURE

Position	Supine or modified lithotomy
Incision	Transverse or vertical midline
Unique considerations	Bowel prep, or underlying disease may result in dehydration, electrolyte abnormalities or anemia.
Antibiotics	Cefotetan 1 g iv
Surgical time	1-3 h
Closing considerations	Colostomy or ileostomy matured after wound is closed (requires 10-20 min).
EBL	100-300 ml (500-2000 ml if splenic injury, loss of major vascular pedicle or repeat operation for cancer, Crohn's disease)
Postop care	ICU for underlying disease; NG tube for distention or vomiting. Avoid use of long-lasting anticholinergics (e.g., Phenergan).
Mortality	0.5-2% (mostly related to underlying disease)
Morbidity	SBO: 5-10% Wound infection: 4-10% For anastomosis-anastomotic leak: 2-4% Wound dehiscence: 1-2% Bleeding: 1% Splenic injury: 1%
Pain score	8

PATIENT POPULATION CHARACTERISTICS

	Crohn's Disease	Colon cancer	Trauma	Diverticula
Age range	2nd-4th decade	5th-7th decade	2nd-4th decades	> 40 yr
Male:Female	1:1	1.3:1	3:1	1:1
Incidence	1-6/100,000	30/100,000	1-2/100,000	10/100,000
Etiology	Unknown	Genetic: 5%	Trauma	Western: low-fiber diet
Associated conditions	Malnutrition; anemia; intraabdominal sepsis; intestinal fistulae; perianal disease; nephrolithiasis; sclerosing and ankylosing spondylitis	Iron deficiency; colonic obstruction; colonic perforation	Liver fracture; spleen fracture; rib fracture; closed-head injury; penetration of viscera adjacent to colon injury	Hemorrhoids; chronic constipation

ANESTHETIC CONSIDERATIONS

See Anesthetic Considerations for Large Bowel Surgery, p. 383.

References

1. Benn PL, Wolff BG, Ilstrup DM: Level of anastomosis and recurrent colonic diverticulitis. *Am J Surg* 1986; 151(1):269-71.
2. Corman ML, Veidenheimer MC, Coller JA: Colorectal carcinoma: a decade of experience at the Lahey Clinic. *Dis Colon Rectum* 1979; 22(7):477-79.
3. Flint LM, Vitale GC, Richardson JD, Polk HC Jr: The injured colon: relationships of management to complications. *Ann Surg* 1981; 193(5):619-23.
4. Lock MR, Fazio VW, Farmer RG, Jagelman DG, Lavery IC, Weakly FL: Proximal recurrence and the fate of the rectum following incisional surgery for Crohn's disease of the large bowel. *Ann Surg* 1981; 194(6):754-60.

REPAIR OF CECAL OR SIGMOID VOLVULUS

SURGICAL CONSIDERATIONS

Description: Cecal volvulus occurs only in people with an abnormally mobile right colon. It accounts for 30-40% of colon volvulus in the U.S. Patients characteristically present with symptoms of intestinal obstruction, dehydration and a "coffee-bean" deformity arising from the RLQ seen on a plain abdominal radiograph. If there is clinical evidence of bowel necrosis, the patient must be taken directly to the OR for resection of nonviable bowel. In the case of cecal volvulus, a primary anastomosis usually can be performed but, with sigmoid volvulus, a colostomy normally is created. On occasion, a contrast enema is required to confirm the diagnosis. The treatment consists of correction of fluid and electrolyte disturbances, NG tube decompression, as well as detorsion and fixation of the colon. A related condition known as cecal bascule is said to exist when a mobile cecum folds in an anterior direction on top of a fixed ascending colon. The treatment for cecal bascule is identical to that of cecal volvulus.

Cecal volvulus may be treated by **resection** of the right colon, **detorsion and cecopexy**, or **detorsion and tube cecostomy**. **Right hemicolectomy** for cecal volvulus is performed in a similar manner to the way it is performed for any other condition. In cecal (or sigmoid) volvulus with ischemia, an attempt should be made to ligate the vascular supply to the colon prior to detorsion. This is done to avoid a sudden washout of the toxic byproducts of ischemia and bacterial overgrowth into the circulation. The intent of **cecopexy** is to recreate the normal situation of short, nonmobile peritoneal attachments to the right colon. Cecopexy is performed by suturing the colon to the parietal peritoneum in the right gutter. Some authors have advocated creating a flap of parietal peritoneum from the hepatic flexure to the cecum along the right gutter. The flap is lifted and the right colon is placed under the flap and against the denuded area of retroperitoneum. The flap is sutured to the anterior wall of the right colon with serosal sutures. Presumably, dense adhesions from the deperitonealized gutter will further fix the colon in place. The advantage of cecopexy is that there is no need to open the colon; the disadvantages are that the greatly distended cecum is not decompressed and that the fixation often fails and recurrent volvulus ensues. **Tube cecostomy**, on the other hand, allows decompression of the cecum and provides a more secure point of fixation. Tube cecostomy is performed by placing a pursestring suture in the anterior wall of the cecum, opening the cecum through the center of the pursestring and placing a large (> 32 Fr) mushroom catheter in the cecum. The tube exits the abdominal wall through a stab wound separate from the incision. The disadvantages are that leakage and irritation around the tube invariably occur and that the colon must be opened.

Sigmoid volvulus occurs in people with abnormally elongated sigmoid colons, along with narrowly based mesenteric attachments. It accounts for 60-70% of colon volvulus in the U.S. The majority of patients will come from chronic nursing facilities and are usually elderly or on chronic neuropsychiatric medications. Most cases of sigmoid volvulus can be reduced with a rigid proctoscope or a flexible sigmoidoscope. After detorsion (reduction), a bowel prep can be performed, followed by definitive surgery.

If a bowel prep can be performed, sigmoid volvulus is treated by **resection** of the redundant sigmoid with a **colorectal anastomosis**. This resection is performed in the typical fashion, with attention given to early ligation of the vascular supply. If a bowel prep cannot be performed, or if the patient is already completely dependent on nursing care for bowel function or is so frail that an absolutely minimal operation must be done, a sigmoid colostomy can be very simply created at the most redundant part of the sigmoid colon. If there is a question about the viability of the colon, the nonviable colon is resected, the distal sigmoid colon is oversewn and dropped into the pelvis (**Hartmann's procedure**) and the proximal end of the sigmoid is exteriorized as an end colostomy. Operative detorsion alone should not be performed because the recurrence rate is prohibitively high.

Usual preop diagnosis: Cecal volvulus; sigmoid volvulus

SUMMARY OF PROCEDURE

	Cecopexy	Tube Cecostomy	Sigmoid Resection, Anastomosis
Position	Supine	⇐	Supine or modified lithotomy
Incision	Transverse RLQ or lower midline	⇐	Transverse LLQ or lower midline
Special instrumentation	None	Large (> 32 Fr) drainage tubes; mushroom; Depezzar or Foley catheters	Surgical staplers

	Cecopexy	Tube Cecostomy	Sigmoid Resection, Anastomosis
Unique considerations	Detorsion may result in hypotension, wheezing or other manifestations of the sudden influx of the by-products of ischemia and bacterial overgrowth into the circulation.	⇐	⇐
Antibiotics	Cefotetan 1 g iv	⇐	⇐
Surgical time	60 min	⇐	60-90 min
Closing considerations	Abdomen will be distended; vital capacity may be limited by closure.	None	⇐
EBL	< 200 ml	⇐	200-400 ml
Postop care	Watch for respiratory compromise from distension.	Irrigate with cecostomy tube with 30 ml saline TID.	None
Mortality	30% (gangrenous cecum); 5-10% (viable cecum)	⇐	60-80% (gangrenous sigmoid); 5-15% (viable sigmoid)
Morbidity	Recurrent volvulus: 20%	5% Tube irritation and fecal soilage: 80-100%	Anastomotic leaks: 5-10% PE: 2-5% MI: 2-4%
Pain score	8	8	8

PATIENT POPULATION CHARACTERISTICS

	Cecal Volvulus	Sigmoid Volvulus
Age range	Peak in 7th-8th decade	⇐
Male:Female	1:2	1:1
Incidence	≤ 60 yr old: 0.45/100,000 > 60 yr old: 5.6/100,000	⇐ > 60 yr old: 8.8/100,000
Etiology	Lack of fixation of the right colon	Elongated sigmoid colon with short mesenteric attachment
Associated conditions	Dehydration	Chronic constipation; mental retardation; neuropsychiatric conditions

ANESTHETIC CONSIDERATIONS

See Anesthetic Considerations for Large Bowel Surgery, p. 383.

STOMA CLOSURE AND REPAIR SURGERIES

SURGICAL CONSIDERATIONS

Description: The intestine may be exteriorized as a loop, divided loop or end stoma. With an end stoma, the defunctionalized bowel distal to the stoma also may be exteriorized as a mucous fistula, dropped back into the abdomen as a **Hartmann's procedure** or totally resected as in a **proctectomy**. With loop stomas, both the afferent and efferent ends of bowel exit the abdominal wall through the same opening; therefore, these stomas may be closed (anastomosed) with a circumstomal incision. The closure of an end stoma with mucous fistula or Hartmann's procedure requires a formal **laparotomy**.

The most frequent indications for stomal revision are stomal stenosis, stomal retraction, parastomal hernia, parastomal fistula and poorly sited stomas. Many cases of stomal stenosis and retraction may be corrected with local operations through circumstomal incisions. A formal abdominal incision is generally required for the correction of parastomal hernia, which frequently requires resiting the stoma. The repair of peristomal fistula, which generally requires resection of the involved bowel, also requires a formal laparotomy. On occasion, a stoma may be resited or diseased bowel may be resected through a parastomal incision. These patients frequently receive a bowel prep and, as a result, are frequently hypovolemic and hypokalemic when they come to the OR.

Closure of a loop stoma is performed through a circular incision, placed just outside the mucocutaneous junction of the stoma and the skin. The proximal and distal ends of the bowel are separated from the subcutaneous tissue, the anterior fascia and then the posterior fascia. The bowel is cleaned of adherent skin and the previously opened antimesenteric border of the bowel is simply closed with sutures. Alternatively, the previously exteriorized portion of bowel is resected and the two ends are anastomosed with either sutures or staples. On rare occasion, it is necessary to extend the incision transversely through the abdominal wall to safely effect an anastomosis. The fascia is closed in the standard fashion. The time-honored practice of leaving the skin and subcutaneous tissues open has been challenged by many surgeons.

Closure of an end stoma with a mucous fistula generally requires a midline abdominal incision. After entering the peritoneal cavity, the functioning stoma and mucous fistula are identified and then freed from their attachment to the abdominal wall via circumstomal incisions. Intervening structures are moved out of the way and an anastomosis is created via sutured or stapled technique. The procedure is nearly identical for closure of a stoma with a long, defunctionalized, intraperitoneal Hartmann's procedure (resection of a diseased portion of colon with proximal colostomy and distal stump closure). On occasion, retrograde passage of a flexible endoscope via the rectum helps to identify the Hartmann's limb (distal stump). When the defunctionalized limb consists of only the pelvic rectum, it is frequently helpful to pass a rigid proctoscope into the rectum to help identify the distal end. It is only necessary to clean enough of the rectal wall to accommodate the head of an EEA stapler. The stapler is passed per rectum with the sharp trocar retracted inside the stapler. When the abdominal surgeon confirms proper placement of the stapler by feeling the outline of the staple-containing ring throughout the rectal wall, the perineal operator advances the trocar through the rectal wall. The abdominal operator then removes the trocar and locks the anvil (pursestringed within the proximal bowel) to the stapler shaft. The perineal operator closes and fires the stapler, while the abdominal operator holds the adjacent viscera out of the way. The anastomosis is tested by infusing air into the rectum after filling the pelvis with NS.

In **paracolostomy hernia repair,** the abdomen may be entered via a midline or a transverse parastomal incision. The stoma is freed from the abdominal wall and the hernia is repaired via direct suture approximation of the fascial edges or placement of a prosthetic mesh. Although most surgeons prefer to move the stoma to a fresh location, some have advocated simply closing the fascia around the stoma or placing the stoma via a hole cut through a piece of prosthetic mesh used to bridge the hernia gap. Since colostomy closure is at best a clean-contaminated case, the risk of periprosthetic infection is very real.

Simple closure of the internal opening of a parastomal fistula is rarely successful; in nearly all situations, resection of the diseased bowel will be done and either an anastomosis will be performed or the resected end will be used to form a new stoma. The external fistula track(s) will be unroofed or excised. This creates an open wound adjacent to the stoma and may impair bag fit to the point that resiting the stoma is necessary.

Usual preop diagnosis: Stomal stenosis; retraction; parastomal hernia; fistula

SUMMARY OF PROCEDURE

	Closure of Loop Stoma	Closure of End Stoma	Repair of Parastomal Hernia
Position	Supine	Supine or modified lithotomy*	Supine
Incision	Circumstomal	Midline or transverse abdominal	Midline or circumstomal
Special instrumentation	Anastomotic staplers	Endoscope for closure of Hartmann's procedure	Prosthetic mesh
Antibiotics	**Cefotetan 1 g iv	⇐	⇐
Surgical time	60-90 min	1-3 h	⇐
Closing considerations	Requires only a few fascial staples; skin may be left open.	None	Stoma matured after abdomen closed.
EBL	< 100 ml	100-500 ml	< 100 ml
Mortality	1%	2-4%	1%
Morbidity	Anastomotic leak	⇐	Recurrent hernia
	SBO	⇐	Peristomal infection
	Wound infection	⇐	Stomal ischemia

	Closure of Loop Stoma	Closure of End Stoma	Repair of Parastomal Hernia
Pain score	5	8	6

* The modified lithotomy position is used for closure of a Hartmann's procedure when an endoscope or stapling device may need to be passed through the anus.

** Bowel prep consists of mechanical cleaning of the colon, accomplished with cathartics or lavage solutions, as well as oral antibiotics. A commonly used regimen is: neomycin 1 g po and erythromycin base 1 g po, given at 1 pm, 2 pm and 10 pm on the night before surgery.

PATIENT POPULATION CHARACTERISTICS

Age range Variable

Male:Female 1:1

Incidence Not uncommon

Etiology Protection or avoiding an insecure anastomosis; traumatic injuries to the colon; complete colonic obstruction; colonic infections such as diverticulitis; inflammatory processes such as Crohn's disease or ulcerative colitis; after-emergency resection for ischemic colitis

Associated conditions Multiple trauma; inflammatory bowel disease; colon cancer; gut ischemia

---

ANESTHETIC CONSIDERATIONS FOR LARGE BOWEL SURGERY

(Procedures covered: total proctocolectomy; partial colectomy with anastomosis; colostomy; repair of cecal or sigmoid volvulus; stoma closure and repair surgeries)

PREOPERATIVE

Patients presenting for this group of surgical procedures have in common an increased risk for pulmonary aspiration. In addition, patients with bowel obstruction must be treated urgently as the obstruction may rapidly progress to bowel necrosis, perforation and septic shock. Patients with inflammatory bowel disease (IBD) (e.g., ulcerative colitis, Crohn's disease) may be on chronic steroid therapy and require perioperative steroid supplementation. These patients may have extracolonic manifestations of the disease (e.g., ankylosing spondylitis, liver disease, anemia), requiring modification of their anesthetic plan.

Respiratory Respiratory insufficiency 2° pulmonary metastases (colon cancer) or acute abdominal process (e.g., pain, splinting, sepsis, metabolic acidosis) and bowel distention limiting diaphragmatic excursion (↓TV, ↓FRC). IBD (arthritis) → ↓neck ROM → difficult intubation.
Tests: Consider CXR, ABG.

Cardiovascular Hemodynamic instability 2° sepsis or pain (↑HR, labile BP). Hypovolemia 2° fever, poor po intake, vomiting, diarrhea and bowel prep. Restoring intravascular volume and hemodynamic stability are goals prior to induction of anesthesia.
Tests: Orthostatic vital signs; ECG

Renal Electrolyte abnormalities common and may be worsened by bowel prep.
Tests: Electrolytes

Gastrointestinal A NG tube is usually in place and the stomach should be emptied before induction of anesthesia. IBD may be associated with impaired liver function → altered drug metabolism.

Musculoskeletal Abdominal musculature may be rigid due to acute abdominal process.

Hematologic Hemoconcentration due to GI fluid loss; anemia due to acute/chronic GI bleeding
Tests: CBC with Plt

Laboratory Other tests as indicated from H&P.

Premedication Light standard premedication (p. B-2) is usually appropriate. For aspiration prophylaxis, ranitidine 50 mg iv 1 h before induction, followed by Na citrate (30 ml, 0.3 M po) 10 min before induction, will significantly decrease the acidity of gastric contents. Metoclopramide is contraindicated in patients with bowel obstruction or perforation.

INTRAOPERATIVE

Anesthetic technique: GETA ± epidural for postop analgesia. If postop epidural analgesia is planned, placement of catheter prior to anesthetic induction is helpful to establish correct placement in the epidural space (accomplished by injecting 5-7 ml of 1% lidocaine via the epidural catheter, eliciting a segmental block).

Induction The patient with an acute abdominal process is at risk for pulmonary aspiration; trachea should be intubated with patient awake or after rapid-sequence induction with cricoid pressure (p. B-5). A NG tube may be left in place (does not interfere with cricoid pressure). If patient is clinically hypovolemic, restore intravascular volume (colloid, crystalloid or blood), prior to induction and titrate induction dose of sedative/hypnotic agents.

Maintenance Standard maintenance (p. B-3) without N_2O. **Combined epidural/GA:** local anesthetic (1.5-2% lidocaine with 1:200,000 epinephrine (5-10 ml q 60 min) can be injected into the epidural catheter to provide both anesthesia and optimal surgical exposure (contracted bowel and profound muscle relaxation). A continuous infusion of local anesthetic (e.g., 2% lidocaine or 0.25% bupivacaine at 5-10 ml/h may enhance hemodynamic stability. Be prepared to treat hypotension with fluid and vasopressors. If epidural opiates are used for postop analgesia, a loading dose (e.g., hydromorphone 1.0 mg) should be administered at least 1 h before conclusion of surgery. Systemic sedatives (droperidol, opiates, benzodiazepines, etc.) should be minimized during epidural opiate administration as they increase the likelihood of postop respiratory depression.

Emergence The decision to extubate at the end of surgery depends on the patient's underlying cardiopulmonary status and extent of surgical procedure. Patient should be hemodynamically stable, warm, alert, cooperative, fully reversed from any muscle relaxants prior to extubation, and have adequate return of pulmonary function (as measured by VC of 15 ml/kg, MIF of -25 cmH_2O, RR < 25 and ABG that approaches patient's baseline).

Blood and fluid requirements	Anticipate large 3rd-space losses. IV: 14-16 ga × 1 NS/LR @ 10-15 ml/kg/h Fluid warmer T&C for 4 U PRBCs.	Plt, FFP and cryoprecipitate should be administered according to lab tests (Plt count, PT, PTT, DIC screen, thromboelastography).
Monitoring	Standard monitors (p. B-1) UO	
	± Arterial line ± CVP	Arterial line and CVP, as indicated by patient's status.
	Hypothermia	Prevent hypothermia during long operations. Consider heated humidifier, warming blanket, warming room temperature, keeping patient covered until ready for preop, etc. Forced air warmer.
Positioning	✓ and pad pressure points. ✓ eyes.	
Complications	Septic shock	Hemodynamic instability 2° hemorrhage, sepsis

POSTOPERATIVE

Complications	Hypoxemia Hemodynamic instability Sepsis	Hypoxemia may be 2° atelectasis.
Pain management	Epidural analgesia (p. C-1) PCA (p. C-3)	
Tests	CBC; CXR (if central line placed); electrolytes; glucose	

Reference

1. Condon RE, Wittmann DH: The use of antibiotics in general surgery. *Curr Probl Surg* 1991; 28(12):801-949.

OPERATIONS FOR RECTAL PROLAPSE

SURGICAL CONSIDERATIONS

Description: Rectal prolapse (procidentia) is intussusception of the full thickness of the rectal wall beyond the anal canal. It must be distinguished from rectal mucosal prolapse, caused by elongation of the mucosal attachments to the underlying sphincter muscle, and internal intussusception, where the upper rectum folds into the lower rectum, but does not descend into the sphincter mechanism. Rectal mucosal prolapse is treated as part of the spectrum of hemorrhoidal disease, and internal intussusception rarely benefits from surgery. Procidentia is frequently associated with anal incontinence. The surgical approaches to procidentia are determined by patient age, concurrent medical disease, sphincter function and the amount of prolapsed tissue.

Surgical treatment of procidentia may be undertaken through an abdominal or a perineal approach. The **abdominal approaches** have a lower recurrence rate and, because they do not diminish the capacity of the rectal reservoir, are generally preferable for maintaining fecal continence. The primary abdominal approach is **rectopexy**, in which the rectum is mobilized in the posterior plane from the sacral promontory to the levator muscles. The rectum is then pulled cephalad and sutured to the presacral fascia with multiple nonabsorbable sutures. Many surgeons routinely perform **sigmoid resection** along with rectopexy. They contend that removal of the redundant sigmoid further diminishes the chance of late recurrence and may improve constipation; and that it avoids the possibility of sigmoid volvulus. (Pulling the rectum up creates a long sigmoid colon on a short mesenteric base, the anatomic condition necessary for volvulus.) The rectum may also be suspended by use of a sling attached to the rectum and secured to the presacral fascia. A number of approaches have been described, the most popular being the **Ripstein procedure**. **Sling procedures** have equivalent recurrence rates but higher complication rates. They also require that mobilization of the rectum along the presacral plane is carried to the level of the levators. A band of Marlex mesh is sewn to the presacral fascia below the level of the sacral promontory, upward traction is placed on the rectum, and several interrupted sutures are placed from the rectum to the mesh.

When patients are deemed too feeble to undergo laparotomy, prolapse may be repaired via a **perineal approach**. The most common of these is **perineal rectosigmoidectomy** (or **Altmeir procedure**). The prolapsed rectum is withdrawn through the anal canal to its full extent, and a circumcision is made in the outer tube of the prolapsed bowel just distal to the dentate line. This exposes the inner tube of prolapsed bowel, along with its mesentery, which is transected at the level of the anal verge. A primary anastomosis is made between the cut ends of the inner and outer bowel. Prior to anastomosis, the levator muscles are often approximated in the midline in an effort to aid continence. When the volume of prolapsed tissue is small, the **Delorme procedure** is often performed. During this procedure, the mucosa is stripped off the prolapsed rectum, and the prolapsed rectal muscle is foreshortened by plication until it resides above the sphincters.

Usual preop diagnosis: Full-thickness rectal prolapse (procidentia)

SUMMARY OF PROCEDURE

	Rectopexy	Rectopexy with Sigmoid Resection	Perineal Recto-sigmoidectomy	Delorme Procedure
Position	Supine, modified lithotomy; deep Trendelenburg	⇐	Prone jackknife; lithotomy	⇐
Incision	Low transverse; low midline	⇐	No external incision	⇐
Special instrumentation	Deep pelvic instruments; Teflon mesh if sling planned; sterile titanium thumbtacks (for bleeding from presacral venous plexus)	Deep pelvic instruments; sterile titanium thumbtacks (useful for bleeding from presacral venous plexus)	Hip-roll for jackknife position; anastomosis may be created with EEA stapler.	Hip-roll for jackknife position
Unique considerations	Presacral venous plexus bleeding may occur in procedures for recurrence; bowel prep may cause dehydration or hypokalemia.	⇐	Epinephrine solutions may be used to diminish bleeding; bowel prep may cause dehydration or hypokalemia.	⇐
Antibiotics	Cefotetan 1 g iv	⇐	⇐	⇐

	Rectopexy	Rectopexy with Sigmoid Resection	Perineal Recto-sigmoidectomy	Delorme Procedure
Surgical time	1-2 h	1-3 h	⇐	⇐
EBL	< 100 ml; more if re-operation	100-300 ml; more if reoperation	100-200 ml	100 ml
Postop care	No rectal probes or medications	⇐	⇐	⇐
Mortality	0-2%	0-4%	1-4%	0-1%
Morbidity	Rectal stricture (with sling): 5-10%	–	–	–
	Recurrent prolapse: 2-8%	2-5%	20-40%%	5-10%
	Pelvic infection: 5%	–	–	–
		Anastomotic leak: 2-4%	–	–
Pain score	7	7	2	2

PATIENT POPULATION CHARACTERISTICS

Age range	Women: peak incidence in 6th-7th decade; men: evenly distributed through age range
Male:Female	1:4
Incidence	Unknown
Etiology	Decreased pelvic muscular support; congenital deficiency of rectal support; pudendal neuropathy; chronic constipation and straining; multiparity; myelomeningocele; spina bifida; cystic fibrosis (children); acute parasitic diarrheal illness (children)
Associated conditions	Fecal incontinence; urinary stress incontinence; rectocele; cystocele

ANESTHETIC CONSIDERATIONS

See Anesthetic Considerations following Operations for Rectal Incontinence, p. 393.

References

1. Freidman R, Muggia-Sulam M, Freund HR: Experience with the one-stage perineal repair of rectal prolapse. *Dis Colon Rectum* 1983; 26(2):789-91.
2. Gordon PH, Hoexter B: Complications of the Ripstein procedure. *Dis Colon Rectum* 1978; 21(4):277-80.
3. Wassef R, Rothenberger DA, Goldberg SM: Rectal prolapse. *Curr Probl Surg* 1986; 23(6):397-451.
4. Watts JD, Rothenberger DA, Buls JG, Goldberg SM, Nivajvongs S: The management of procidentia. 30 years' experience. *Dis Colon Rectum* 1985; 28:(2)96-102.

RECTAL SURGERY

SURGICAL CONSIDERATIONS

Description: Many lesions within the distal two-thirds of the rectum can be excised through a **transanal approach**. Most benign lesions are amenable to a local transanal approach, and the application of local excision is increasing in the treatment of favorable, early-stage adenocarcinomas of the rectum. The most common benign tumors treated by local excision are adenomas. Lesions such as carcinoid tumor, endometrioma and solitary rectal ulcer also may be locally excised. **Transanal excision** of benign lesions may be performed in the submucosal plane, while suspected malignancies are excised by removing the entire thickness of the rectal wall. A full antibiotic and mechanical bowel prep is given preop. Transanal excision is usually performed in the prone jackknife position, although the lithotomy position may be used when the lesion is located on the posterior rectal wall. A local anal block, usually 0.25% marcaine, with 1:200,000 epinephrine, is performed to relax the sphincter mechanism and minimize sphincter injury, aid in hemostasis and diminish postop pain. A short bivalve anoscope is inserted into the anal canal. Stay sutures are placed adjacent to the area of resection, and the lesion is pulled into the operative field. On occasion, lesions may be prolapsed all the way through the anus and excised outside of the body. If prolapse is not possible, the dissection starts at the distal end of the lesion and proceeds proximally. The proctotomy incision is enlarged on each side of the lesion in 1-2 cm increments; after each increment, the previous incision is closed with full-thickness, absorbable sutures. These sutures are then grasped and used for further traction. When the specimen is removed, a few final sutures are needed to close the proximal-most incision. When large tumors are resected, **rigid proctoscopy** is performed to confirm preservation of an adequate lumen.

Variant procedure or approaches: The **transsacral (Kraske)**[1] **approach** to rectal tumors offers wider exposure than the transanal approach, but is more painful and has a substantially greater likelihood of complications (wound infection, fecal fistula, incontinence). A transsacral approach is advantageous when the lesion is located behind the rectum (retrorectal tumors) and when resection of the lower sacrum or coccyx is anticipated. Transsacral resection is generally performed in the prone jackknife position. An incision is made from the posterior commissure of the anus to the base of the sacrum. The sphincter muscles are spared, but the levator muscles are divided to expose the posterior wall of the rectum. The coccyx may be disarticulated and removed at this point to improve exposure without adding to operative morbidity. It is also possible to remove the lower sacral segments through this approach, but increasing morbidity accrues as the sacral nerve roots are sacrificed. The posterior wall of the rectum is opened and the lesion, along with a full-thickness disc of rectal wall, is excised. If the lesion is on the anterior wall, two proctotomy incisions are necessary. The proctotomy incisions are closed in one or two layers with standard anastomotic techniques. The levator muscles are reapproximated and the skin is closed. Some surgeons place a drain within the retrorectal space prior to closing. The transsacral approach may be combined with an abdominal approach (abdominal-transsacral resection) in some cases of low rectal cancer.

The **transsphincteric (Mason)**[7] **approach** to rectal lesions also gives wider exposure than does the transanal approach, but at the expense of a substantially greater risk of fecal incontinence. Transsphincteric excision is performed with the patient in the prone jackknife position. An incision is made at the posterior commissure of the anus and is extended along the lateral border of the coccyx and sacrum. The external sphincter, internal sphincter and levator ani muscles are sequentially transsected in the posterior midline. As each muscle is cut, the cut edges are tagged with sutures to facilitate accurate reapproximation. The rectal wall is incised and the lesion is excised. The proctotomy incision is closed via standard anastomotic suturing techniques, and the individual components of the sphincter muscle are reapproximated with interrupted sutures. The overlying skin is closed in a standard fashion.

Usual preop diagnosis: Villous adenoma; tubular adenoma; adenocarcinoma; carcinoid tumor; endometrioma; solitary rectal ulcer; retrorectal tumors (in decreasing frequency)

SUMMARY OF PROCEDURE

	Transanal Excision	Transsacral Excision	Transsphincteric Excision
Position	Prone jackknife or lithotomy	Prone jackknife	⇐
Incision	Intrarectal	Anus-to-lateral sacral wall	⇐
Special instrumentation	Rigid proctoscope; headlight and/or fiber optic retractors; Foley catheter	Gigli or power saw if sacral resection contemplated; headlight and/or fiber optic retractors; Foley catheter	Headlight and/or fiber optic retractors; Foley catheter
Unique considerations	Bowel prep may result in dehydration and hypokalemia.	⇐	⇐
Antibiotics	Cefotetan 1 g iv	⇐	⇐
Surgical time	15-120 min	1-2 h	⇐
EBL	< 100 ml	< 100 ml (500 ml if sacral resection)	⇐
Postop care	No rectal temperatures, suppositories or enemas	⇐	⇐
Mortality[1,2,5,6]	0-2%	⇐	⇐
Morbidity[1,2,5,6]	Tumor recurrence: 5-50%	50%	5-50%
	Urinary retention: 10-20%	⇐	⇐
	Bleeding: 2-5%	⇐	⇐
	Pelvic sepsis: 0-4%	⇐	⇐

	Transanal Excision	Transsacral Excision	Transsphincteric Excision
Morbidity cont.	Ureteral injury: < 1% (minimized by use of Foley)	⇐	⇐
		Fecal fistula: 10-30%	–
		Fecal incontinence: 5-10%	10-40%
Pain score	3	7	7

PATIENT POPULATION CHARACTERISTICS

Age range	Rectal adenomas – 5th-7th decades; rectal adenocarcinoma – 6th-9th decades; endometrioma – 2nd-4th decades; solitary rectal ulcer syndrome – 4th-8th decades; carcinoid tumors – 5th-8th decades
Male:Female	1:1
Incidence	Varies with disease; not uncommon
Etiology	Varies with disease
Associated conditions	Preexisting anorectal pathology, such as fecal incontinence, may require concurrent treatment

ANESTHETIC CONSIDERATIONS

See Anesthetic Considerations following Operations for Rectal Incontinence, p. 393.

References

1. Allgöwer M, Dürig M, Hochstetter A, Huber A: The parasacral sphincter-splitting approach to the rectum. *World J Surg* 1982; 6(5):539-48.
2. Biggers OR, Beart RW Jr, Ilstrup DM: Local excision of rectal cancer. *Dis Colon Rectum* 1986; 29(6):374-77.
3. Condon RE, Wittmann DH: The use of antibiotics in general surgery. *Curr Probl Surg* 1991; 28(12):801-949.
4. Corman ML: *Colon and Rectal Surgery*, 3rd edition. JB Lippincott Co, Philadelphia: 1993.
5. Hager TH, Gall FP, Hermanek P: Local excision of cancer of the rectum. *Dis Colon Rectum* 1983; 26(3)149-51.
6. Localio SA, Eng K, Gouge TH, Ranson JH: Abdominosacral resection for carcinoma of the midrectum: ten years' experience. *Ann Surg* 1978; 188(4):475-80.
7. Mason AY: Surgical access to the rectum—a transsphincteric exposure. *Proc R Soc Med* 1970; 63(Suppl)91-4.

ANAL FISTULOTOMY/FISTULECTOMY

SURGICAL CONSIDERATIONS

Description: The great majority of perianal fistulae arise as a result of infection within the anal glands located at the dentate line (cryptoglandular fistula). Fistulae may also arise as the result of trauma, Crohn's disease, inflammatory processes within the peritoneal cavity, neoplasms or as a consequence of radiation therapy. The ultimate treatment of fistula-in-ano is determined by the etiology and the anatomic course of the fistula. The principle behind treatment of cryptoglandular fistulae is to excise the offending gland and lay open or excise all infected tissue. Fistulae that track above the majority of the sphincter mechanism must be treated by procedures that either do not cut the overlying sphincter, cut the sphincter and repair it, or cut the sphincter very gradually (**seton**, see below). A fistula may be treated at the time of drainage of a perianal abscess or as a separate, elective operation. The route of a fistula tract is best determined by exploration at the time of operation. While local anesthesia is acceptable for simple fistulas with known routes, many fistula operations require regional or general anesthesia because the ultimate route and depth of the fistula will not be known. Special consideration is given to fistulae that arise in the setting of Crohn's disease. Poor wound healing, the likelihood of recurrent or multiple fistulae and the premium on sphincter function in patients with chronic diarrhea dictate that only the most superficial fistulae can be laid open. The primary goal is palliation; specifically, to drain abscesses and prevent their recurrence. This is often accomplished by placing a Silastic seton (a ligature placed around the sphincter muscles) around the fistula tract and leaving it in place indefinitely. In the absence of active Crohn's disease in the rectum, attempts at fistula cure may be undertaken.

Variant procedure or approaches: Fistulotomy involves cutting all tissues superficial to a fistula so that the fistula tract is brought to the skin level. The opened, fibrotic fistula wall is often sewn to the skin edge (marsupialized). **Fistulectomy** involves excision of the entire fistula tract. When conventional fistulotomy would cause incontinence, a **seton** may be used. The seton may be gradually tightened to transect the sphincter over a matter of weeks. Setons also may be placed loosely and left in place for several weeks with the intention of creating enough local fibrosis that the sphincter will not separate when it is cut at a second operation. Other approaches that may be used to avoid fecal incontinence are **complete fistulotomy with immediate reconstruction** of the sphincter and fistulectomy with closure of the internal opening by an **endorectal advancement flap** technique.

Usual preop diagnosis: Fistula-in-ano

SUMMARY OF PROCEDURE

	Fistulotomy or Fistulectomy	Fistulotomy with Seton	Endorectal Advancement Flap
Position	Prone jackknife; occasionally lithotomy	⇐	Prone jackknife
Incision	Perianal	⇐	⇐
Antibiotics	Cefotetan 1 g iv	⇐	⇐
Surgical time	15-60 min	⇐	60-90 min
EBL	< 50 ml	⇐	⇐
Mortality	Minimal	⇐	⇐
Morbidity	Fecal incontinence: 0-30%	10-30%	0-10%
	Nonhealing, or recurrent fistula: 5%	10-20%. (This procedure used only in complex fistulae, so complication rate appears higher.)	10-40%. (This procedure used only in complex fistulae, so complication rate appears higher.)
Pain score	6	6	6

PATIENT POPULATION CHARACTERISTICS

Age range	2nd-7th decades
Male:Female	2:1
Incidence	Common
Etiology	Infection within anal glands located at dentate line (cryptoglandular fistula); trauma; Crohn's disease; inflammatory processes within the peritoneal cavity; neoplasms; consequence of radiation therapy
Associated conditions	See above.

ANESTHETIC CONSIDERATIONS

See Anesthetic Considerations following Operations for Rectal Incontinence, p. 393.

References

1. Fazio VW: Complex anal fistulae. *Gastroenterol Clin North Am* 1987; 16(1):93-114.
2. Parks AG, Gordon PH, Hardcastle JD: A classification of fistula-in-ano. *Br J Surg* 1976; 63(1):1-12.
3. Stone JM, Goldberg SM: The endorectal advancement flap procedure. *Int J Colorectal Dis* 1990; 5(4)232-35.

HEMORRHOIDECTOMY

SURGICAL CONSIDERATIONS

Description: Hemorrhoids are normally occurring vascular tissues, located in discrete aggregations known as hemorrhoidal cushions within the distal rectum and anus. They are thought to play a role in the fine control of enteric continence, and are only treated if they cause a symptom that persists after conservative therapy. Hemorrhoids may cause bleeding, prolapse, mucous drainage, itching or pain (when thrombosed). The primary pathophysiologic event in the development of symptomatic hemorrhoids is thought to be mucosal prolapse caused by degeneration of the fibroelastic tissue that tethers the vascular cushions and overlying mucosa to the submucosa. All modern treatments for hemorrhoidal disease diminish prolapse by fixing the mucosa to the submucosa with scar tissue. Hemorrhoids are classified as internal, when they arise above the dentate line, or external, when they arise from below. Internal hemorrhoids are further classified by the degree of prolapse: I–protrude into lumen; II–prolapse and spontaneously reduce; III–prolapse and require manual reduction; IV–prolapsed and incarcerated. The most common symptom from external hemorrhoids is pain caused by acute thrombosis. The surgical treatment involves excision of the thrombosed hemorrhoid, usually under local anesthetic, in the office. Internal hemorrhoids may be treated by nonexcisional or excisional techniques. Nonexcisional techniques are generally used in the office or outpatient clinic. They do not require an anesthetic because their use is limited to the insensate tissues above the dentate line. Examples of nonexcisional treatments are **rubber-band ligation**, **infrared coagulation**, **sclerotherapy** and **cryotherapy**.

Surgical hemorrhoidectomy may be performed in the lithotomy or prone jackknife position. An operating anoscope is placed in the anal canal and a hemorrhoid column is grasped and tented up into the lumen. An incision is started at the anal verge and a plane is developed deep to the hemorrhoidal tissue and superficial to the sphincter muscles. When the internal sphincter is identified, the dissection proceeds in the avascular space along its luminal surface. The dissection is continued up into the rectum to include all redundant tissue. Lateral incisions along the redundant tissue are completed to excise the hemorrhoid. Care is taken to leave healthy bridges of mucosa between adjacent hemorrhoidal columns. Hemostasis is obtained with cautery and the mucosal defect may be closed with a running, absorbable suture. It is also acceptable to leave the mucosal wound open. The procedure is repeated over the other enlarged hemorrhoid columns, removing redundant tissue and leaving long, vertical scars to prevent further mucosal prolapse.

Variant procedure or approaches: The **Whitehead hemorrhoidectomy** is similar, except that instead of discrete vertical incisions, the hemorrhoidal tissue is dissected off of the sphincter circumferentially, redundant tissue is excised, and the rectal mucosa is brought down to the dentate line and sewn in place. Lasers have not been shown to improve results in the treatment of hemorrhoids, and they typically increase cost. Sphincter stretch for symptomatic hemorrhoids (**Lord procedure**) should be abandoned, because of the high incidence of incontinence associated with it.

Rubber-band ligation requires no anesthesia because the band is placed on the insensate, distal rectal mucosa. A slotted anoscope is inserted into the anal canal and a hemorrhoid column is visualized. The most proximal area of redundant mucosa is grasped with a clamp and pulled into the barrel of the ligation gun. The trigger is pulled, forcing the rubber band onto the base of the tented-up hemorrhoid tissue. The encompassed tissue sloughs over a 4- to 7-day period, and a scar is formed between the mucosa and the underlying muscle.

Usual preop diagnosis: Symptomatic hemorrhoids; bleeding, prolapse or pain

SUMMARY OF PROCEDURE

	Hemorrhoidectomy	Whitehead Hemorrhoidectomy
Position	Prone jackknife, lithotomy or left lateral decubitus	⇐
Incision	Series of vertical incisions from anal verge to top of hemorrhoid columns at the dentate	Circumferential intraanal incision line
Special instrumentation	Headlight or lighted anoscope; operating anoscope	⇐
Antibiotics	None	⇐
Surgical time	45-90 min	⇐
EBL	< 100 ml	⇐
Postop care	Sitz baths, oral fluids, fiber supplements	⇐
Mortality	Rare	⇐
Morbidity	Urinary retention: 15-30%	⇐
	Incontinence: 1-6%	⇐
	Bleeding: 2-5%	⇐

	Hemorrhoidectomy	Whitehead Hemorrhoidectomy
Morbidity, cont.	Stricture: 2-5% Infection: 1-2%	⇐ ⇐ Mucosal ectropion: 2-20%
Pain score	9	9

PATIENT POPULATION CHARACTERISTICS

Age range	Peak prevalence 45-65 yr
Male:Female	1:1
Incidence	Prevalence 75/1,000
Etiology	Low-fiber diet; genetic; pregnancy
Associated conditions	Constipation

ANESTHETIC CONSIDERATIONS

See Anesthetic Considerations following Operations for Rectal Incontinence (p. 393).

References

1. Barron J: Office ligation of internal hemorrhoids. *Am J Surg* 1963; 105(4):563-70.
2. Buls JG, Goldberg SM: Modern management of hemorrhoids. *Surg Clin North Am* 1978; 58(3):469-78.
3. Burchell MC, Thow GB, Mannson RR: A "modified Whitehead" hemorrhoidectomy. *Dis Colon Rectum* 1976; 19(3):225-32.
4. Johanson JF, Sonnenberg A: The prevalence of hemorrhoids and chronic constipation. An epidemiologic study. *Gastroenterology* 1990: 98(2)380-86.
5. Smith LE: Hemorrhoids. A review of current techniques and management. *Gastroenterol Clin North Am* 1987; 16(1)79-91.

OPERATIONS FOR RECTAL INCONTINENCE

SURGICAL CONSIDERATIONS

Description: The majority of patients with rectal (enteric) incontinence will not be helped by surgery. In these patients, incontinence is caused by a combination of pudendal neuropathy and atrophy of the muscles of the pelvic floor. When an anatomic defect in the sphincter mechanism can be identified, surgery is likely to be beneficial.

Sphincteroplasty is performed in the prone jackknife position after a full mechanical and antibiotic bowel prep, which may leave patient hypovolemic and hypokalemic. An incision is placed at the anal verge, centered over the area of injured sphincter, and extended sufficiently around the anus to reach the retracted, cut edges of the sphincter. The anoderm and rectal mucosa are dissected off of the internal surface of the sphincter. The external surface of the sphincter mechanism is then dissected free to the level of the pelvic diaphragm. Care must be taken not to injure the inferior hemorrhoidal nerves during dissection around the posterior-lateral sphincter. The fibrotic portion linking the two ends of sphincter is cut, and the ends are overlapped and secured in place with two layers of interrupted horizontal mattress sutures. In women with obstetric injuries, the transverse perineal muscles are reapproximated. The anoderm is pulled down and resecured to the skin at the anal verge. The remainder of the skin is closed as completely as possible.

Variant procedure or approaches: The surgical options for patients without anatomic defects in their sphincters are generally unsuccessful. The **posterior anoplasty of Parks** was designed to passively enhance continence by increasing the normally occurring angle between the rectum and the anal canal, and to increase the mechanical efficiency of weak sphincter muscle by shortening the fiber length. Lack of efficacy has limited its use, although some surgeons still perform the Parks procedure in the setting of continued incontinence after abdominal repair of rectal prolapse. The operation is performed in the prone jackknife position after a standard bowel prep. A hemispherical incision is placed at the level of the intersphincteric groove over the posterior half of the anus. The plane between the internal and external anal sphincters is identified and developed proximally to above the puborectalis musculus. The puborectalis fibers are "reefed," or pulled together, as far as possible with nonabsorbable suture. The external sphincter is plicated together in the midline with a series of nonabsorbable sutures that start at the deep external sphincter and progress to the subcutaneous sphincter. Skin is closed with absorbable sutures.

The **Thiersch operation (pinch graft)** has poor efficacy and a high complication rate and should be considered only as a procedure of last resort in patients with symptomatic rectal prolapse or fecal incontinence. As originally described, the anal canal was encircled with a silver wire which served as a passive obstacle to prolapse or defecation. In more recent years, an elastic sheet of Dacron-impregnated Silastic mesh has been used. Two small incisions are made on opposite sides of the anal verge. A pathway around the anal canal is created by blunt dissection and a 1.5 cm-wide piece of mesh is led around the anal canal. The ends of the mesh are overlapped in one of the incisions and either sutured or stapled together at an appropriate level of tension. The wounds are irrigated with antibiotic solution and the incisions are closed.

Usual preop diagnosis: Rectal (enteric) incontinence

SUMMARY OF PROCEDURE

	Overlapping Sphincteroplasty	Parks Repair	Modified Thiersch Procedure
Position	Prone jackknife	⇐	Prone jackknife or lithotomy
Incision	Circumanal	⇐	2 small incisions lateral to the anus
Special instrumentation	Headlight	⇐	Headlight; Silastic mesh
Unique considerations	Urinary catheter preop	⇐	None
Antibiotics	Standard bowel prep	⇐	⇐+ Cefotetan 1 g iv; antibiotic in irrigation fluid
Surgical time	1-2 h	1 h	30-45 min
EBL	< 100 ml	⇐	⇐
Postop care	Early: Sitz baths, "medical colostomy"*	⇐	⇐
	Late: fiber supplement, stool softener	⇐	⇐
Mortality	Rare	⇐	⇐
Morbidity	Unimproved incontinence: 20%	60-80%	20%
	Improved, but minor incontinence: 30%	–	Erosion of prosthesis: 30-60%
	Prolonged wound healing: 20%	–	Obstructed defecation: 20-40%
	Infection: 1-2%	–	
Pain score	8	7	6

* "Medical colostomy" is performed to prevent patients from having bowel movements for several days after the procedure. It involves a clear liquid diet and around-the-clock codeine pills for their constipating effect. This regimen is maintained for 3-4 d. After this period, the goal is to avoid constipation, so stool softeners and a fiber supplement are administered. Patients are instructed to take a laxative if they go more than 24 h without a bowel movement.

PATIENT POPULATION CHARACTERISTICS

Age range	Bimodal: 3rd-5th decades for obstetric injury, fistulotomy and perineal trauma; 6th-8th decades for pudendal neuropathy/pelvic floor atrophy
Male:Female	1:4
Incidence	Not uncommon
Etiology	Pudendal neuropathy; pelvic floor atrophy; obstetric injury; injury during anal surgery (fistulotomy, sphincterotomy, hemorrhoidectomy); perineal trauma; neurologic disease; congenital anomalies
Associated conditions	Urinary incontinence; chronic constipation; multiparity

ANESTHETIC CONSIDERATIONS

(Procedures covered: excision or repair of rectal prolapse; rectal surgery; anal fistulotomy/fistulectomy; anal sphincterotomy/sphincteroplasty; hemorrhoidectomy; operations for rectal incontinence)

PREOPERATIVE

Respiratory A careful evaluation of respiratory status is important. If patient has ↓respiratory reserve, the lithotomy position may be better tolerated than the prone or jackknife positions.
Tests: As indicated from H&P.

Musculoskeletal Pain is likely to be present at the surgical site and should be considered when positioning patient for anesthetic induction (e.g., if patient has pain while sitting, perform regional anesthesia in the lateral decubitus position). Evaluate bony landmarks if regional anesthetic is planned.

Hematologic If regional anesthesia is planned and patient is taking aspirin, NSAIDs, D/C these drugs at least 1 wk before surgery, if appropriate.
Tests: CBC with differential; Plt, as indicated from H&P.

Laboratory Other tests as indicated from H&P.

Premedication Standard premedication (p. B-2)

INTRAOPERATIVE

Anesthetic technique: GA, spinal or epidural techniques may be used.

General anesthesia:

Induction **General (LMA vs ETT):** Standard induction (p. B-2). Procedures done in the jackknife position may require ET intubation for airway control if a regional technique is not performed.

Maintenance Standard maintenance (p. B-3)

Emergence No special considerations

Regional anesthesia:

Spinal **Single-shot vs continuous:** Patient in either sitting, lateral decubitus, prone or jackknife position for placement of a subarachnoid block. Doses of local anesthetics should be adequate to provide high lumbar level of sensory anesthesia (e.g., lidocaine 5%, 50-75 mg; tetracaine 10-14 mg; bupivacaine 8-12 mg). For continuous spinal anesthesia, use a multiorifice catheter as single-orifice microcatheters have been associated with cauda equina syndrome. Large doses of local anesthetic (especially hyperbaric lidocaine) should be avoided as they also are associated with an increased incidence of cauda equina syndrome.

Epidural Patient in sitting or lateral decubitus position for placement of epidural catheter. A test dose (e.g., 3 ml of 1.5% lidocaine with 1:200,000 epinephrine) is administered and patient is observed for development of a subarachnoid block or symptoms of an intravascular injection. Then titrate 2% lidocaine with epinephrine (3-5 ml at a time) until desired T10 level is obtained.

Caudal Patient in prone, jackknife or lateral position for placement of caudal block. After needle has been positioned properly in the caudal canal, a 3 ml test dose of 1.5% lidocaine with 1:200,000 epinephrine is injected (as above). To obtain sacral levels of anesthesia, a volume of 10 ml should be sufficient (0.25% bupivacaine or 2% lidocaine with 1:200,000 epinephrine).

Blood and fluid requirements	IV: 16-18 ga × 1 NS/LR @ 5-8 ml/kg/h	Blood not likely to be required.
Monitoring	Standard monitors (p. B-1)	Others as clinically indicated.
Positioning	✓ and pad pressure points. ✓ eyes.	Chest support or bolsters to optimize ventilation in the jackknife position; care in positioning the patient's extremities and genitals after turning into jackknife position. Avoid pressure on eyes and ears after turning patient.
Complications	Foot drop Reflex laryngeal spasm	Lithotomy position can lead to damage to peroneal nerve. Laryngospasm will occur if inadequate depth of anesthesia during anal dilation.

POSTOPERATIVE

Complications	Urinary retention Cauda equina syndrome Poor wound healing Atelectasis	Catheterize until return of urinary function. Cauda equina syndrome is characterized by varying degrees of urinary/fecal incontinence, sensory loss in the perineal area and lower extremity motor weakness.
Pain management	PCA (p. C-3) Epidural analgesia (p. C-1)	PO analgesics may be suitable: acetaminophen and codeine (Tylenol #3 1-2 tab q 4-6 h) or oxycodone and acetaminophen (Percocet 1 tab q 6 h).
Tests	As indicated by patient status.	

References

1. Dershwitz, M: Local Anesthetics. in *Clinical Anesthesia Procedures of the Massachusetts General Hospital*, 3rd edition. Firestone LL, Lebowitz PW, Cook CE eds; Little, Brown and Co, Boston: 1988, 185-98.
2. Horn HR, Schoetz DJ Jr, Coller JA, Veidenheimer MC: Sphincter repair with a Silastic sling for anal incontinence and rectal procidentia. *Dis Colon Rectum* 1985; 28(11):868-72.
3. Parks AG: Anorectal incontinence. President's Address. *Proc R Soc Med* Meeting 27. 1975; 68(11):681-90.
4. Rigler ML, Drasner K, Krejcie TC, Yelich SJ, Scholnick FT, DeFontes J, Bohner D: Cauda equina syndrome after continuous spinal anesthesia. *Anesth Analg* 1991; 72(3):275-81.
5. Slade MS, Goldberg SM, Schottler JL: Sphincteroplasty for acquired anal incontinence. *Dis Colon Rectum* 1977: 20(1):33-5.
6. Snooks SJ, Swash M, Henry MM, Setchell M: Risk factors in childbirth causing damage to the pelvic floor innervation. *Int J Colorectal Dis* 1986; 1(1):20-4.

Surgeon

Harry A. Oberhelman, MD, FACS

7.5 HEPATIC SURGERY

Anesthesiologist

Steven K. Howard, MD

HEPATIC RESECTION

SURGICAL CONSIDERATIONS

Description: For major lobar resections (Fig 7.5-1) the corresponding hepatic artery, portal vein and bile duct are isolated and ligated in the porta hepatis. If possible, the major hepatic vein of the involved lobe is ligated at its entry into the vena cavae.

Transection of the liver is done by blunt dissection utilizing the Cavitron ultrasonic suction aspirator (CUSA), the harmonic scalpel, or by finger fracture. During dissection through the liver substance, the visible vessels and bile ducts should be clipped or ligated. During the transection, minor-to-moderate bleeding may occur, particularly if larger veins are torn, and these must be controlled with suture ligatures. Smaller vessels are controlled by the argon beam laser coagulator and/or by electrocautery. Total vascular isolation may be used to control bleeding, if necessary. This involves clamping the vena cava above and below the liver, as well as cross-clamping the porta hepatis. Following resection, suction drains are placed and the omentum is tacked to the cut surface of the liver for hemostasis.

As the principles and techniques of hepatic surgery have evolved, the overall mortality and morbidity have improved considerably. Since the normal liver is capable of regeneration, it is possible to resect the right or left lobe, along with a major segment of the contralateral lobe. This procedure is known as a **trisegmentectomy**. In patients afflicted with cirrhosis, the regeneration process is limited; thus, uninvolved liver should be preserved.

Partial resection of the liver for metastatic disease may be performed at the same time as surgical resection for the primary lesion. Although most major resections can be performed by a transabdominal approach, some surgeons prefer a thoracoabdominal approach.

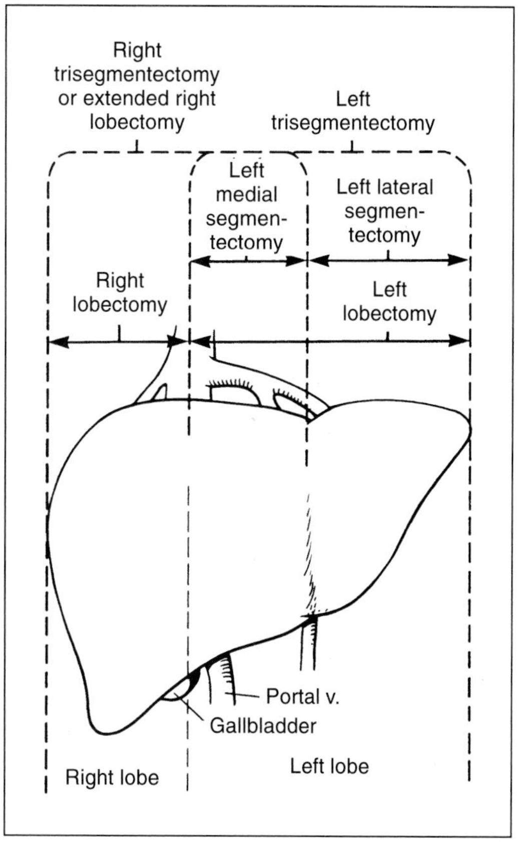

Figure 7.5-1. Types of liver resection. (Reproduced with permission from Hardy JD: *Hardy's Textbook of Surgery*, 2nd edition. JB Lippincott: 1988.)

Usual preop diagnosis: Benign and malignant primary or metastatic tumors of the liver

SUMMARY OF PROCEDURE

	Right/Left Lobectomy	Trisegmentectomy	Partial Resection
Position	Supine	⇐	⇐
Incision	Midline abdominal	⇐	⇐
Special instrumentation	Denier retractor (lifts anterior chest wall); CUSA; harmonic scalpel; argon beam laser; ± Cell Saver	⇐	⇐
Unique considerations	Correct abnormal PT; intraop ultrasound	⇐	⇐
Antibiotics	Cefazolin 1- 2 g preop	⇐	⇐
Surgical time	3-4 h	4-5 h	1-2 h
Closing considerations	Secure adequate hemostasis	⇐	⇐
EBL	500-1000 ml	⇐	300-500 ml
Postop care	ICU × 1-3 d	⇐	PACU → room
Mortality	3-10%	⇐	< 3%
Morbidity	Bile leak: 10-30%	⇐	⇐
	Intraabdominal infection: 10-15%	⇐	5-10%
	Pleural effusion: 10%	⇐	5%
	Wound infection: 5-10%	⇐	2-5%

	Right/Left Lobectomy	Trisegmentectomy	Partial Resection
Morbidity, cont.	Hepatic failure: 5%	⇐	< 1 %
	Postop hemorrhage: 2-3%	⇐	⇐
Pain score	7-9	7-9	7-9

PATIENT POPULATION CHARACTERISTICS

Age range	14-80 yr[3]
Male:Female	2:1
Incidence	Primary liver cancer 4/100,000
Etiology	Metastatic to liver from primary cancer; environmental and chemical carcinogens; chronic hepatitis and/or cirrhosis[2]; parasitic infection (Clonorchis sinensis)
Associated conditions	Chronic hepatitis; cirrhosis

ANESTHETIC CONSIDERATIONS

See Anesthetic Considerations following Hepatorrhaphy, p. 399.

References

1. Oberfield RA, Steele G Jr, Gollan JL, Sherman D: Liver cancer. *CA Cancer J Clin* 1989; July-August. 39(4):206-18.
2. Parker GA et al: Intraoperative ultrasound of the liver affects operative decision making. *Ann Surg* 1989; 209(5):569-77.
3. Sitzman RJV et al: Preoperative assessment of malignant hepatic tumors. *Am J Surg* 1990; 159(1):137-42.

HEPATORRHAPHY

SURGICAL CONSIDERATIONS

Description: Although most liver lacerations have stopped bleeding by the time a surgeon sees them, others require suturing or partial liver resection to control bleeding. Various techniques are available to control hemorrhage, including packing, suturing, inflow occlusion and resection. Small lacerations that have stopped bleeding require no specific therapy other than possible drainage. Lacerations that continue to bleed usually can be sutured and drained. Extensive tears of the liver that are actively bleeding may require temporary occlusion of the porta hepatis, containing the hepatic artery, portal vein and bile duct (**Pringle maneuver**) in order to excise deviated parenchyma and control bleeding with sutures, clips, coagulators, etc. Occasionally, the hepatic vein draining the involved lobe will require clamping to control back-bleeding. When the bleeding cannot be controlled, it is expedient to pack the wound, drain the abdomen and close. The pack can be removed without much risk of rebleeding within 48-72 hours.

Usual preop diagnosis: Trauma with CT evidence of hepatic laceration

SUMMARY OF PROCEDURE

Position	Supine
Incision	Midline abdominal
Special instrumentation	Denier retractor
Antibiotics	Cefazolin 1 g iv
Surgical time	1-2 h
EBL	~300-2000 ml
Mortality	1-2%

Morbidity	Continued bleeding: 2-3% Biliary fistula Perihepatic abscess Intrahepatic hematoma Arteroportal fistula Hepatic and renal failure
Pain score	7-9

PATIENT POPULATION CHARACTERISTICS

Age range	Variable
Male:Female	1:1
Incidence	Rare
Etiology	Trauma (blunt vs penetrating); surgical; hepatic adenomas; needle biopsies of liver
Associated conditions	See Etiology, above.

ANESTHETIC CONSIDERATIONS FOR HEPATIC PROCEDURES

(Procedures covered: hepatic resection; hepatorrhaphy; other hepatic surgery)

PREOPERATIVE

Patients presenting for hepatic surgery may have primary or metastatic tumors from GI and other sources. Liver function may be entirely normal in these patients. Hepatocellular carcinoma is seen commonly in males > 50 yr, and is associated with chronic active hepatitis B and cirrhosis. The preop considerations listed below describe patients without cirrhosis. (See Preoperative Considerations for Surgery for Portal Hypertension, p. 299) for evaluation of patients with cirrhosis).

Respiratory Respiratory function is typically normal; however, patients with ascites may have respiratory compromise.
Tests: CXR; others as clinically indicated.

Cardiovascular Patients may be hypovolemic, and volume status should be carefully assessed before induction of anesthesia (skin turgor, UO, orthostatic BP, HR, etc). Tumors may surround major vascular structures and impede venous return. Consider evaluation with CT/MRI scan.

Hepatic Liver resection can be indicated for hemangiomas, hydatid cysts and tumors. It is important to determine the size of the tumor and involvement of vascular structures preop so as to be adequately prepared for major intraop blood and fluid losses.
Tests: LFTs; albumin; ultrasound/CT/MRI

Hematologic The liver produces all clotting factors except VIII and the degree of hepatic insufficiency determines the extent of any coagulopathy. T&C 4 U PRBCs.
Tests: CBC; PT; PTT; Plt count; others as indicated from H&P.

Laboratory Tests as indicated from H&P. **NB:** For elective cases, if abnormal LFTs are present on preop labs, it is important to perform a complete medical workup. This can include reviewing old lab data, hepatitis serology and an abdominal ultrasound to rule out cholestatic causes of liver dysfunction. Surgery and anesthesia in the presence of acute hepatitis is associated with a high mortality.

Premedication Standard premedication (p. B-2). Consider administering vitamin K (e.g., 10 mg iv/sc) if PT is prolonged. (Beneficial results from vitamin K usually occur within 24 h. Consider FFP for rapid correction of PT.)

INTRAOPERATIVE

Anesthetic technique: GETA ± epidural for postop analgesia. If postop epidural analgesia is planned, establish correct placement of the catheter in the epidural space by injecting 5-7 ml of 1% lidocaine, eliciting a segmental block. The initial incision is usually right subcostal, but it may have to be extended into the right chest if surgical resection necessitates. If known beforehand, placement of a left DLT may improve surgical exposure.

Induction Standard induction (p. B-2). Restore intravascular volume prior to anesthetic induction. Trauma patients require awake intubation or rapid-sequence induction (p. B-5) with cricoid pressure

Induction, cont.	until intubation has been confirmed. If patient is hemodynamically unstable, consider etomidate (0.2-0.4 mg/kg) or ketamine (1-3 mg/kg) in place of STP.	
Maintenance	Standard maintenance (p. B-3); N_2O can be used if bowel distention will not impede surgical exposure/closure. **Combined epidural/GA:** Local anesthetic (2% lidocaine with 1:200,000 epinephrine (5-10 ml q 60 min) can be injected into the lumbar epidural catheter to provide both anesthesia and optimal surgical exposure (contracted bowel and profound muscle relaxation). Be prepared for possible cross-clamping of vena cava, and treat hypotension with fluid and vasopressors. If epidural opiates are used for postop analgesia, a loading dose (e.g., hydromorphone 1.0 mg) should be administered at least 1 h before the conclusion of surgery. Systemic sedatives (droperidol, opiates, benzodiazepines, etc.) should be minimized during this type of anesthetic as they increase the likelihood of postop respiratory depression.	
Emergence	For major hepatic resections, the patient will be best cared for in an ICU. Consider keeping the patient mechanically ventilated until hemodynamically stable and ventilatory status is optimized. If surgical resection was minimal, the patient can be extubated awake after return of airway reflexes.	
Blood and fluid requirements	Anticipate large blood loss. IV: 14-16 ga × 2 NS/LR @ 10-20 ml/kg/h Fluid warmer Humidify gases. Consider utilizing rapid-transfusion device.	Blood loss can be significant; keep at least 2 U PRBC ahead. Lobectomies are often associated with more blood loss than wedge resections. Massive transfusions may be required and appropriate blood products should be available (e.g., 2 FFPs + 6 PLT per 10 U PRBC). If procedure does not involve cancer, blood salvage devices can be utilized.
Control of blood loss	Surgical control Pringle maneuver Grafts Sealants	Surgical control of the main blood vessels entering the hilar area (Pringle maneuver). Grafts (omental or peritoneal) or rapidly polymerizing adhesives can be applied to the raw surface of the resected segment to provide a means of hemostasis.
Monitoring	Standard monitors (p. B-1) UO CVP Arterial line	Others as clinically indicated. If the extent of the resection is not known at the beginning of surgery, appropriate monitoring (CVP, arterial line, additional iv's) should be established prior to beginning resection. Forced air warmer.
Positioning	✓ and pad pressure points. ✓ eyes.	
Complications	Massive hemorrhage	Ensure adequate vascular access. Consider rapid-transfusion device.

POSTOPERATIVE

Complications	↓liver function Hemorrhage Electrolyte imbalance Hypoglycemia Hypothermia, shivering DIC	Patients with normal liver function preop may have significant postop impairment of liver function 2° loss of liver mass or surgical trauma.
	Pulmonary insufficiency	> 90% of patients will develop some form of respiratory complication (atelectasis, effusion, pneumonia).
Pain management	Epidural analgesia: (p. C-1) PCA (p. C-3)	Patient should be recovered in ICU or hospital ward that is accustomed to treating the side effects of epidural opiates (e.g., respiratory depression, breakthrough pain, nausea, pruritus).
Tests	ABG; CXR; others as clinically indicated.	

References

1. Feliciano DV, Jordan GL Jr, Bitondo CG, Mattox KL, Burch JM, Cruse PA: Management of 1000 consecutive cases of hepatic trauma. *Ann Surg* 1986; 204:438-45.
2. Merritt WT, Gelman S: Anesthesia for liver surgery. In *Principles and Practice of Anesthesiology*. Longnecker DE, Tinker JH, Morgan GE, eds. Mosby Year Book, St Louis: 1998, 1904-47.

Surgeon

Mark A. Vierra, MD

7.6 BILIARY TRACT SURGERY

Anesthesiologist

Steven K. Howard, MD

OPEN CHOLECYSTECTOMY

SURGICAL CONSIDERATIONS

Description: With the advent of laparoscopic cholecystectomy, the traditional **open cholecystectomy** has become a rarity, generally reserved for gallbladders that are expected to be difficult to remove due to inflammation, previous operations and adhesions, or because of other medical problems, such as coagulopathy or cirrhosis. In most institutions, fewer than 10% of cholecystectomies will be begun as open procedures, and perhaps 5% of laparoscopic cholecystectomies will be converted to open cholecystectomies during the course of the operation due to technical difficulties, complications or unexpected findings. The open cholecystectomy of the 90s is, in general, a substantially more challenging operation, for both surgeon and anesthesiologist, than it was in previous decades.

The **open cholecystectomy** is usually performed through a right subcostal or midline incision. Upward traction is applied to the liver or gallbladder, while downward traction on the duodenum exposes the region of the cystic duct and artery and common duct. Depending on local conditions and the surgeon's preference, the gallbladder may be removed from the top down, excising the gallbladder from the liver bed and isolating the cystic duct and artery as the final stage of the operation, or the cystic duct and artery may be isolated and divided first, and the gallbladder removed retrograde from the gallbladder bed as the final step of the procedure. The anatomy of the biliary tree is quite variable, and few surgeons always remove the gallbladder in exactly the same way every time. (Fig 7.6-1 shows biliary tree anatomy.)

Cholangiography may be performed in either laparoscopic or open cholecystectomy and is performed at the discretion of the surgeon—some surgeons perform it in all patients and others perform it only in patients in whom there is some clinical evidence of choledocholithiasis. The cystic duct is opened and a catheter placed into the duct and secured with a ligature, tie or special cholangiogram clamp. Dye is injected into the biliary tree via the catheter, and x-rays are taken. If stones are found, a common duct exploration may be performed. Alternatively, an endoscopic retrograde cholangiogram (ERCP) with stone extraction may be carried out postop. Cholangiography usually adds about 10-15 minutes to the procedure.

Choledochotomy, or **"common duct exploration,"** is the opening and exploration of the common duct for the purpose of extracting stones. The need for this may be anticipated preop or performed based on findings at operation, particularly

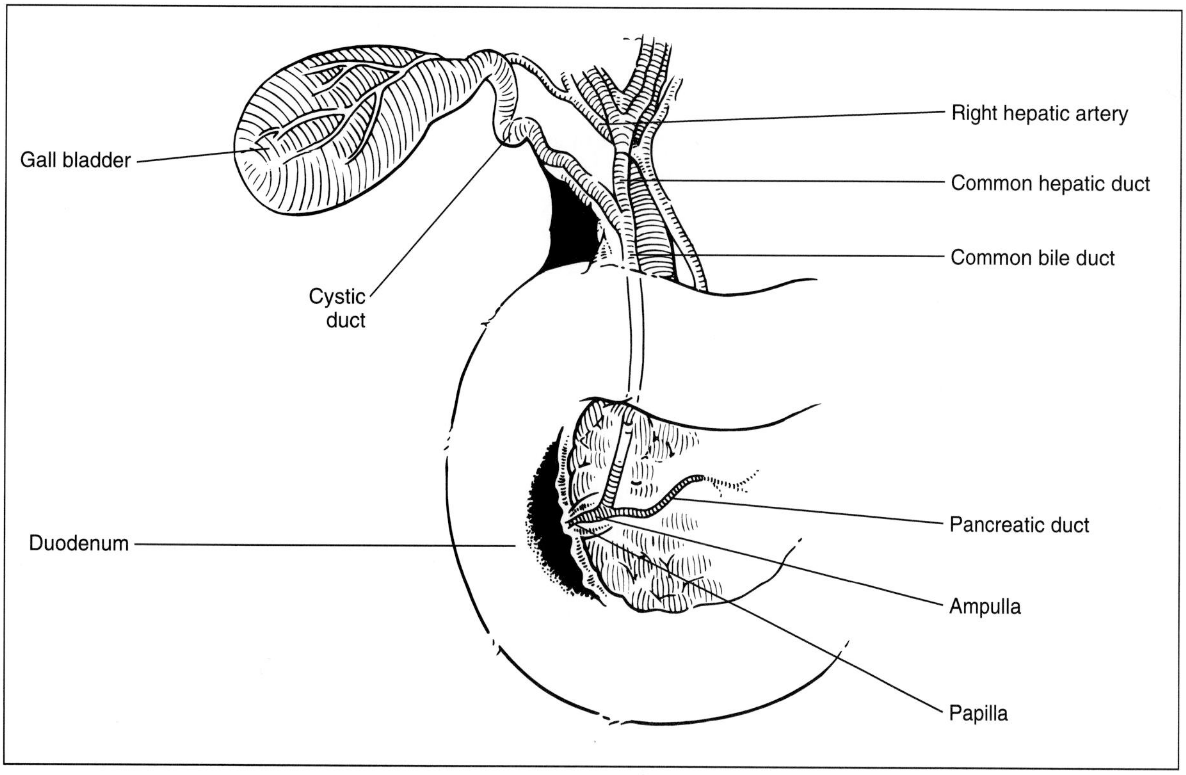

Figure 7.6-1. Anatomy of the biliary tree. (Reproduced with permission from Calne R, Pollard SG: *Operative Surgery*. Gower Medical Pub: 1992.)

the finding of common duct stones by cholangiography. A longitudinal incision approximately 1 cm long is made in the duct and exploration is carried out through this incision. The duct may be irrigated with NS, balloon catheters may be passed and various instruments introduced to grasp, remove or crush retained stones. The duct may be biopsied by this approach, and **choledochoscopy**—the direct visualization of the duct's interior using a small flexible scope—can be performed. Depending on the complexity of the findings, a common duct exploration can be expected to add from 30 minutes to more than an hour to the cholecystectomy. In general, the mortality of patients undergoing common duct exploration is approximately 2-5 times that of a simple cholecystectomy. This difference can be explained by the fact that patients undergoing common duct exploration tend to be older and sicker—the opening of the duct itself is not necessarily a significant physiologic insult.

Variant procedure or approaches: Cholecystectomy remains the mainstay of treatment for symptomatic biliary stone disease. **Nonsurgical treatment** of cholelithiasis, particularly by **oral dissolution** and/or **lithotripsy**, have very limited usefulness and are rarely used in clinical practice. **Laparoscopic cholecystectomy** (see p. 418) has largely replaced the open approach.

Usual preop diagnosis: Symptomatic cholelithiasis; acute cholecystitis; choledocholithiasis

SUMMARY OF PROCEDURE

	Cholecystectomy	Cholecystectomy/ Common Duct Exploration
Position	Supine	⇐
Incision	Right subcostal or midline	Midline
Special instrumentation	Costal margin retractor ± cholangiogram catheter	Choledochotomy instruments
Unique considerations	Requires intraop x-ray for cholangiogram.	May include choledochoscopy.
Antibiotics	Ampicillin, piperacillin or mezlocillin, 1-3 g iv ± gentamicin; or cefotetan 1-2 g iv	⇐
Surgical time	45-90 min	1-2.5 h
Closing considerations	Muscle relaxation	⇐
EBL	< 250 ml	⇐
Postop care	PACU	⇐
Mortality	0.7%	0-1.5% < 60 yr; ≤ 5% in advanced age
Morbidity	Postop bile leak: 0-9%	⇐
	Pancreatitis: 0-4.6%	2-5%
	Bile duct injury: 0-0.25%	
	Cardiac and respiratory complications: Rare, but leading cause of death	
	Hemorrhage: Rare	
Pain score	6	6-7

PATIENT POPULATION CHARACTERISTICS

Age range	Mostly adult; increases with age
Male:Female	1:2-3
Incidence	600,000/yr in U.S.; 90+% performed laparoscopically.
Etiology	See Associated Conditions, below.
Associated conditions	Ileal disease; cirrhosis; hemolytic disorders; choledocholithiasis; cholangitis or active pancreatitis

ANESTHETIC CONSIDERATIONS

See Anesthetic Considerations for Biliary Tract Surgery, p. 410.

References

1. Brooks JR: Acute and chronic cholecystitis. In *Current Surgical Therapy*. Cameron J, ed. BC Decker, Philadelphia: 1989, Vol III, 257-62.

2. Cuschieri A, Dubois F, Mouiel J, Mouret P, Becker H, Buess G, Trede M, Troidl H: The European experience with laparoscopic cholecystectomy. *Am J Surg* 1991; 161(3):385-87.
3. McSherry CK, Glenn F: The incidence and causes of death following surgery for nonmalignant biliary tract disease. *Ann Surg* 1980; 191(3):271-75.
4. Peters JH, Ellison EC, Innes JT, Liss JL, Nichols KE, Lomano JM, Roby SR, Front ME, Carey LC: Safety and efficacy of laparoscopic cholecystectomy. A prospective analysis of 100 initial patients. *Ann Surg* 1991; 213(1):3-12.
5. Voyles CR, Petro AB, Meena AL, Haick AJ, Koury AM: A practical approach to laparoscopic cholecystectomy. *Am J Surg* 1991; 161(3):365-70.

BILIARY DRAINAGE PROCEDURES

SURGICAL CONSIDERATIONS

Description: Biliary drainage procedures may be performed for malignant and nonmalignant indications, and the type of drainage procedure performed depends on factors such as the nature of the biliary obstruction, the patient's overall condition and prognosis, the need for other surgical procedures and institutional expertise. **Endoscopic** and **transhepatic techniques** are increasing in use and, today, most drainage procedures of the biliary tree are performed with these techniques. There remain a significant number of patients, however, for whom a traditional surgical procedure is the most appropriate. In general, the complexity of the different operations that may be performed and the morbidity attendant to these has more to do with the indications for operation than with which procedure is performed.

All of these operations are performed under GA through an upper midline or right subcostal incision. Self-retaining retractors are used to retract the liver superiorly to expose the region of the porta hepatis. If the gallbladder will not be used for the bypass procedure (**cholecystojejunostomy**), then it is usually removed as the first step in the procedure (see Open Cholecystectomy, p. 403). If the patient has had previous upper right quadrant surgery, the complexity and duration of the procedure and blood loss may increase significantly. Any associated hepatic cirrhosis may make the procedure particularly demanding.

Transduodenal sphincteroplasty is usually performed for benign obstruction of the ampulla of Vater or for extensive choledocholithiasis. **Endoscopic sphincterotomy** is the most commonly performed technique for opening the ampulla, and is most commonly performed by gastroenterologists outside of the OR with iv sedation. **Open sphincteroplasty** is usually reserved for patients in whom endoscopic retrograde cholangio-pancreatogram (ERCP) has been unsuccessful or in whom a laparotomy is required for other reasons. For these open procedures, the second portion of duodenum is incised over the region of the ampulla, and the ampulla is cannulated. A longitudinal incision is made over the course of the ampulla and the mucosa of the ampulla is sutured to the mucosa of the duodenum with fine interrupted sutures, with care being taken not to compromise the pancreatic duct. The duodenum is closed with suture, a small closed suction drain is placed, and the wound is closed. A postop stay of 5-7 days can be expected.

Cholecystojejunostomy is usually performed as palliation for malignant obstruction of the distal bile duct. Its advantage is that it does not require dissection of the portal triad, but the long-term results are less reliable than with the other two drainage procedures. This is partly because the gallbladder may not drain as well as the common duct, and partly because the tumor may grow to occlude the junction of the common and cystic ducts. The abdomen is opened as described above, and the region of the porta hepatis examined to assure that the cystic duct is not imminently compromised by tumor. The jejunum is then brought up to the gallbladder, usually by passing the jejunum through the transverse mesocolon. The anastomosis may be performed either to an intact loop of jejunum (**loop cholecystojejunostomy**) or to a Roux-en-Y loop of jejunum (**Roux-en-Y cholecystojejunostomy**), and is carried out with one or two layers of sutures, depending on surgeon's preference. If a Roux-en-Y is created, a second jejunojejunal anastomosis must be performed.

In **choledochoduodenostomy** or **choledochojejunostomy**, an anastomosis is fashioned between the common duct and the duodenum or the common duct and Roux loop of jejunum. This is often a relatively more demanding operation than cholecystojejunostomy because it requires dissection deep in the porta hepatis to gain access to the common duct. Long-term results are more reliable, however, and these are preferred for benign disease. Exposure of the biliary tree is the same as for the above procedures. The gallbladder is always removed (if it is still present). The common duct is dissected free from the surrounding structures in the porta hepatis and an anastomosis is constructed between the common duct and the duodenum or jejunum. If the jejunum is used, it is almost always brought up as a Roux-en-Y, requiring a second jejunojejunal anastomosis.

Variant procedure or approaches: Endoscopic or transhepatic placement of temporary or permanent **biliary stents** is an increasingly common alternative to surgical drainage in patients with incurable pancreatic or biliary tract disease.

Usual preop diagnosis: Transduodenal sphincteroplasty: extensive choledocholithiasis, often after failed attempt at ERCP; rarely, malignant disease. Cholecystojejunostomy: malignant obstruction of distal common bile duct, usually due to pancreatic cancer. Choledochojejunostomy or choledochoduodenostomy: benign strictures of the distal bile duct; longstanding stone disease; pancreatitis; iatrogenic injury; Oriental cholangiohepatitis; after resection of some tumors of the pancreas or distal bile duct.

SUMMARY OF PROCEDURE

	Cholecysto-jejunostomy	Choledocho-jejunostomy	Choledocho-duodenostomy	Transduodenal sphincteroplasty
Position	Supine	⇐	⇐	⇐
Incision	Midline or right subcostal	⇐	⇐	⇐
Special instrumentation	Costal retractor	⇐	⇐	⇐
Unique considerations	Consider usual prep for patients with obstructive jaundice.	⇐	⇐	⇐
Antibiotics	Ampicillin, piperacillin or mezlocillin, 1-3 g iv ± gentamicin; or cefotetan 1-2 g iv	⇐	⇐	⇐
Surgical time	1 h; may be significantly greater if resection of tumor is considered.	1.5-3 h	⇐	⇐
Closing considerations	Muscle relaxation; NG suction	⇐	⇐	⇐
EBL	< 250 ml (greater if tumor resection performed, or in presence of portal HTN).	250-500 ml (greater if tumor resection performed, or in presence of portal HTN).	⇐	< 250 ml (transfusion rarely needed).
Postop care	PACU	⇐	⇐	⇐
Mortality[1,3,6]	≤ 35% in advanced pancreatic cancer; otherwise, < 10%	≤ 29%, with pancreatic cancer; 0.5% for benign disease	0-5.4%[1,2,6] (usually for benign disease)	0-7%
Morbidity[3,6]	Sepsis	⇐	⇐	Pancreatitis: Rare
	Respiratory complications	⇐	⇐	Recurrent cholangitis: Rare
	Renal failure	⇐	⇐	
	Hemorrhage	⇐	⇐	
	Wound infection	⇐	⇐	
	Breakdown of biliary anastomosis	⇐	⇐	
	Thrombotic complications	⇐	⇐	
Pain score	7	7	7	6

PATIENT POPULATION CHARACTERISTICS

Age range	5th-7th decade; may be younger for sphincterotomy
Male:Female	1.1:2.1
Incidence	Procedure-related incidence not available, but clearly declining in favor of techniques by interventional gastroenterology and radiology.
Etiology	See Usual Preop Diagnosis, above.
Associated conditions	Jaundiced (very common); fat-soluble vitamin deficiencies; malignancy, especially pancreatic (common); malnutrition (common)

ANESTHETIC CONSIDERATIONS

See Anesthetic Considerations for Biliary Tract Surgery, p. 410.

References

1. Baker AR, Neoptolemos JP, Carr-Locke DL, Fossard DP: Sump syndrome following choledochoduodenostomy and its endoscopic treatment. *Br J Surg* 1985; 72(6):433.
2. Birkenfeld S, Serour F, Levi S, Abulafia A, Balassiano M, Krispin M: Choledochoduodenostomy for benign and malignant biliary tract diseases. *Surgery* 1988; 103(4):408-10.
3. Hines LH, Burns RP: 10 years' experience treating pancreatic and periampullary cancer. *Am Surg* 1976; 42(6):441-47.
4. Karan JA, Roslyn JJ: Cholelithiasis and cholecystectomy. In *Maingot's Abdominal Operations*, 10th edition. Zinner MJ, Schwartz SI, Ellis H, eds. Appleton & Lange, Stanford CT: 1997, 1717-38.
5. Nahrwold DL, Dawes LG: Biliary Neoplasms. In *Surgery: Scientific Principles and Practice*, 2nd edition. Greenfield LJ, et al, eds. Lippincott-Raven Publishers, Philadelphia: 1997, 1056-66.
6. Sarr MG, Cameron JL: Surgical palliation of unresectable carcinoma of the pancreas. *World J Surg* 1984; 8(6):906-18.
7. Thompkins RK: Choledocholithiasis and cholangitis. In *Maingot's Abdominal Operations*, 10th edition. Zinner MJ, Schwartz SI, Ellis H, eds. Appleton & Lange, Stanford, CT: 1997, 1739-54.

EXCISION OF BILE DUCT TUMOR

SURGICAL CONSIDERATIONS

Description: Primary tumors of the extrahepatic bile ducts, including the hepatic bifurcation (Klatskin tumors) are uncommon malignancies, with the only curative treatment for them being surgical excision. Such tumors are usually classified as being proximal bile duct tumors, involving the hepatic bifurcation and above; middle bile duct tumors, involving the midportion of the common hepatic and common bile duct; and distal bile duct tumors which involve the distal bile duct, including the intrapancreatic or intraduodenal portion of the bile duct (Fig 7.6-1). The gallbladder will usually be removed in any such operation.

Distal bile duct tumors, which carry a significantly higher cure rate than either proximal bile duct or pancreatic tumors, may be treated by **pancreaticoduodenectomy**. (See p. 442 for discussion of this operation.)

Mid bile duct tumors are usually excised by removing a generous portion of the mid bile duct, resecting the ducts up to the hepatic bifurcation and sometimes performing a pancreaticoduodenectomy. Biliary drainage is usually established by anastomosing the proximal bile duct to a Roux loop of jejunum. For proximal bile duct tumors, most of the extrahepatic bile ducts are excised and biliary drainage is established by anastomosis of the right and left hepatic ducts to a Roux loop of jejunum. These are often technically demanding operations with the potential for major blood loss. It may be necessary to perform a major hepatic resection at the same time, and the possibility of this should always be assumed when an operation of this sort is carried out.

Surgical exposure for any of these operations is usually achieved through a long midline or transverse subcostal incision and the use of self-retaining retractors. Often, a transhepatic catheter will have been placed radiographically preop to provide relief of jaundice and to facilitate identification of the bile ducts. The liver and gallbladder are retracted superiorly while downward traction is placed on the duodenum. If the gallbladder is still in place, a cholecystectomy is performed (see p. 403). For proximal bile duct tumors and mid bile duct tumors not requiring pancreaticoduodenectomy, the bile duct is divided distally, just above the duodenum, and the pancreatic portion of the bile duct is oversewn. The bile duct is then resected proximally to the level of the bifurcation of the hepatic ducts. A Roux-en-Y loop of jejunum is anastomosed to the hepatic ducts to establish biliary drainage. Drains are placed and most surgeons place a NG tube for such cases.

Variant procedure or approaches: Endoscopic or transhepatic stenting of areas of stricture is often used as a palliative alternative to surgical excision. These are usually performed radiographically and do not require GA. They may be used as an alternative to resection or in preparation for surgery.

Usual preop diagnosis: Cholangiocarcinoma (common); benign strictures of the bile ducts (infrequent); sclerosing cholangitis (rare)

SUMMARY OF PROCEDURE

Position	Supine
Incision	Midline or subcostal
Special instrumentation	Costal retractor
Unique considerations	Many cases prove unresectable at operation. Intraop radiation therapy may be used.
Antibiotics	Ampicillin, piperacillin or mezlocillin, 1-3 g iv, ± gentamicin; or cefotetan 1-2 g iv
Surgical time	3-8 h
Closing considerations	Muscle relaxation required for closure; NG suction
EBL	500-5000 ml, depending on need for liver resection and presence of portal HTN.
Postop care	ICU postop
Mortality	5-10%
Morbidity	Sepsis; hemorrhage; anastomotic leakage; wound infection; liver failure; PE
Pain score	7-8

PATIENT POPULATION CHARACTERISTICS

Age range	50s-70s
Male:Female	Male > female
Incidence	4500 cases of bile duct cancer/yr in U.S.
Etiology	Multifactorial
Associated conditions	Ulcerative colitis; sclerosing cholangitis; typhoid carrier state; clonorchis sinensis; choledochal cyst; Caroli's disease; gallstones

ANESTHETIC CONSIDERATIONS

See Anesthetic Considerations for Biliary Tract Surgery, p. 410.

References

1. Yeo CJ, Cameron JL: Tumours of the gallbladder and bile ducts. In *Maingot's Abdominal Operations*, 10th edition. Zinner MJ, Schwartz SI, Ellis H, eds. Appleton & Lange, Stanford, CT: 1997, 1835-54.
2. Zinner MJ: Bile duct tumors. In *Current Surgical Therapy*, Vol III. Cameron JL, ed. BC Decker, Philadelphia: 1989, 289-91.

CHOLEDOCHAL CYST EXCISION OR ANASTOMOSIS

SURGICAL CONSIDERATIONS

Description: This rare congenital anomaly includes various types of dilatation of the biliary tree, and patients may present with cholangitis, pancreatitis or, rarely, malignancy. Although four types of cyst are commonly recognized, the vast majority consist of fusiform dilatation of much or most of the extrahepatic biliary tree. While the traditional description of choledochal cyst is that of an infant with a palpable abdominal mass and jaundice or cholangitis, this is a relatively rare presentation today. Today, many cysts are found in adults undergoing evaluation for symptoms thought to be due to gallbladder disease. These patients may present with biliary colic, pancreatitis or cholangitis. Recommended treatment consists of **excision of the cyst**, when technically safe. **Cyst-enteric bypass**, usually to a Roux loop of jejunum, is almost never performed today because of the small, but real risk of developing malignancy in these cysts. Only in an elderly patient under unusual technical circumstances would this be appropriate.

The operation is performed through a midline or right subcostal incision. The liver is retracted superiorly and the duodenum inferiorly, exposing the biliary tree. The gallbladder is excised, along with as much of the cyst as possible. The duct is divided as distally as possible, just above the duodenum, and the cyst reflected superiorly. It is usually excised to the hepatic bifurcation, and an anastomosis is performed at this level, often between the common orifice of the right and left hepatic ducts and a Roux loop of jejunum.

Reoperative cases are not uncommon; most follow a cyst-enteric bypass. These cases may be significantly more difficult than first-time operations.

Variant procedure or approaches: There is an increasing tendency among gastroenterologists to perform **endoscopic sphincterotomy** in these patients, rather than to refer them for surgical resection, particularly in older patients. It remains to be seen if these patients will develop cancer in the retained cysts.

Usual preop diagnosis: Choledochal cyst, the most common type involving fusiform enlargement of the entire extrahepatic biliary tree

SUMMARY OF PROCEDURE

Position	Supine
Incision	Midline or right subcostal
Special instrumentation	Costal retractor
Antibiotics	Ampicillin, piperacillin or mezlocillin, 1-3 g iv ± gentamicin; or cefotetan 1-2 g iv
Surgical time	2-4 h
Closing considerations	NG suction
EBL	250 ml, with potentially greater blood loss in reoperations
Postop care	PACU
Mortality	Very rare
Morbidity	Anastomotic leak Wound infection Pulmonary complications Pancreatitis
Pain score	5-7

PATIENT POPULATION CHARACTERISTICS

Age range	Classically, 60% < 10 yr of age, although this may be changing; also adults of all ages
Male:Female	1:3
Incidence	Rare in U.S.; more common in Japan
Etiology	Unclear
Associated conditions	Jaundice; pancreatitis; malignancy within the cyst

ANESTHETIC CONSIDERATIONS FOR BILIARY TRACT SURGERY

(Procedures covered: open cholecystectomy; cholangiography; choledochotomy; biliary drainage procedures; transduodenal sphincterotomy or sphincteroplasty; cholecystojejunostomy; excision of bile duct tumor; choledochal cyst excision/anastomosis)

PREOPERATIVE

Patients presenting for biliary tract surgery are an extremely diverse group, ranging from the otherwise healthy to the extremely ill. With the increasing popularity of laparoscopic surgery, most open cholecystectomies will be performed only on the sickest patients or when it is not possible to complete the laparoscopic procedure. These patients, therefore, may be sicker than those undergoing open cholecystectomy in the mid 1980s. Cirrhosis, even of a mild degree, substantially increases the risk of cholecystectomy, with hemorrhage being the greatest danger. Patients with bile duct tumors are usually jaundiced at presentation and have undergone transhepatic and/or endoscopic studies for diagnostic purposes. Often an external transhepatic biliary drain may be present and jaundice may have been relieved in this way. Rarely, a hepatic resection may be performed as part of the procedure. Prior operation or the presence of portal HTN will substantially increase the duration, complexity and blood loss of the procedure.

Respiratory Pain 2° an acute abdominal process may cause splinting which, in turn, may impair respiratory function (↓FRC, hypoventilation, atelectasis). For patients undergoing laparoscopic cholecystectomy, intraabdominal CO_2 insufflation may → atelectasis, ↓FRC, ↑PIP, and ↑$PaCO_2$. Studies comparing patients undergoing open vs laparoscopic cholecystectomy reveal that respiratory function is less impaired and function is recovered more quickly in patients undergoing laparoscopic cholecystectomy. Tachypnea, hyperpnea and acute respiratory alkalosis can be signs of sepsis, or due solely to pain associated with inflammation of the gall bladder.
Tests: Consider CXR and others as indicated from H&P.

Cardiovascular Patients may be dehydrated from fever, vomiting and decreased oral intake; assess hemodynamic status by evaluating BP and HR in the supine and standing positions. Fluid resuscitate if patient shows Sx of orthostatic hypotension until hemodynamic status improves. Patients undergoing laparoscopic cholecystectomy may experience hemodynamic compromise 2° positioning (reverse Trendelenburg), excessive intraabdominal pressure with subsequent impairment of venous return. Epigastric discomfort is common with biliary tract disease and can mimic symptoms of myocardial ischemia.
Tests: ECG; others as indicated from H&P.

Renal In patients with obstructive jaundice, preop administration of bile salts po may prevent renal insufficiency following surgery.[1]
Tests: UA and others as indicated from H&P.

Gastrointestinal Patients with peritonitis will exhibit guarding and may develop abdominal distention and paralytic ileus. Therefore, full-stomach precautions are warranted. Laparoscopic approach is contraindicated in these patients.
Tests: Bilirubin; AST (SGOT); ALT (SGPT); alkaline phosphatase; albumin

Hematologic Leukocytosis is often present with a moderate left shift. ✓ coags. Administer vitamin K as needed (10 mg iv/sc).
Tests: CBC, with differential and Plt

Laboratory Other tests as indicated from H&P.

Premedication Meperidine (0.5-0.6 mg/kg iv) is thought to cause less sphincter of Oddi spasm than other opiates. Sphincter spasm can interfere with intraop cholangiograms and cause pain; reverse opiate-induced spasm with naloxone in 40 μg increments. Atropine (0.4-0.6 mg im or iv) or glycopyrrolate (0.2-0.3 mg im or iv) may help decrease spasm of the sphincter, and can be given in combination with the opiate. Parenteral vitamin K is indicated if PT is prolonged (10 mg/d im for 3 d). Administer H_2 antagonists (ranitidine 50 mg iv); metoclopramide (10 mg iv) may be given if patient is at risk for gastric aspiration.

INTRAOPERATIVE

Anesthetic technique: GETA. In patients at risk for aspiration of gastric contents, ET intubation should be accomplished either awake or following a rapid-sequence iv induction (see p. B-5).

Induction	Standard induction (see p. B-2) if no aspiration risk. In patients at risk of aspiration, a rapid-sequence induction should be performed (see p. B-5).	
Maintenance	Standard maintenance (see p. B-3). Muscle relaxants facilitate surgery and are indicated.	
Emergence	If there is a risk for aspiration of gastric contents, patient should be extubated awake after return of protective airway reflexes; otherwise, no special considerations.	
Blood and fluid requirements	Minimal blood loss Possible 3rd-space loss IV: 16-18 ga × 1 NS/LR @ 5-8 ml/kg/h	Blood products usually not required. Anticipate that patient may be dehydrated and require generous iv hydration prior to anesthetic induction (e.g., 10-15 ml/kg).
Monitoring	Standard monitors (see p. B-1).	Others as clinically indicated.
Positioning	✓ and pad pressure points. ✓ eyes.	A steep, reverse Trendelenburg position may be required, causing cardiorespiratory impairment: ↓venous return → ↓CO.
Complications	Atelectasis 2° surgical retraction Hypotension	These complications are unique to laparoscopic procedures.

POSTOPERATIVE

Complications	Ventilatory impairment Pneumothorax Atelectasis 2° splinting N&V	Monitor patients for hypoxemia in the postop period. Administer supplemental O_2 and consider a portable CXR to aid in the diagnosis.
Pain management	PCA: meperidine; loading dose, 20-100 mg; incremental dose, 10 mg; lockout, 10 min.	Intercostal nerve blocks, intrapleural analgesia, or epidural analgesia are also useful techniques. Prolonged PCA meperidine is associated with ↑normeperidine → CNS disorder.
	Shoulder pain	2° subdiaphragmatic gas trapping

References

1. Cahill CJ: Prevention of postoperative renal failure in patients with obstructive jaundice–the role of bile salts. *Br J Surg* 1983; 70(10):590.
2. Crittenden SL, McKinley MJ: Choledochal cyst–clinical features and classification. *Am J Gastroenterol* 1985; 80(8):643-47.
3. Giurgiu DIN, Roslyn JJ: Calculous biliary disease. In *Surgery: Scientific Principles and Practice*, 2nd ediition.Greenfield LJ, et al, eds. Lippincott-Raven Publishers, Philadelphia: 1997,1033-55.
4. Lippsett PA, Yeo CJ: Choledochal cysts. In *Maingot's Abdominal Operations*, 10th edition. Zinner MJ, Schwartz SI, Ellis H, eds. Appleton & Lange, Stanford, CT: 1997,1701-16.
5. Marco AP, Yeo CJ, Rock P: Anesthesia for a patient undergoing laparoscopic cholecystectomy. *Anesthesiology* 1990; 73:1268-70.
6. Nagorney DM, McIlrath DC, Adson MA: Choledochal cysts in adults: clinical management. *Surgery* 1984; 96(4):656-63.
7. Taylor E, Feinstein R, White PF, Soper N: Anesthesia for laparoscopic cholecystectomy. Is nitrous oxide indicated? *Anesthesiology* 1992; 76:541-43.
8. Venu RP, Geenen JE, Hogan WJ, Dodds WJ, Wilson SW, Stewart ET, Soergel KH: Role of endoscopic retrograde cholangiopancreatography in the diagnosis and treatment of choledochocele. *Gastroenterology* 1984; 87(5):1144-49.
9. Wesley JR, Oldham KT, Coran AG: Pediatric Abdomen. In *Surgery: Scientific Principles and Practice*, 2nd edition.Greenfield LJ, et al, eds. Lippincott-Raven Publishers, Philadelphia: 1997, 2082-2100.

Surgeon

Mark A. Vierra, MD

7.7 LAPAROSCOPIC GENERAL SURGERY

Anesthesiologist

Steven K. Howard, MD

LAPAROSCOPIC ESOPHAGEAL FUNDOPLICATION

SURGICAL CONSIDERATIONS

Description: Surgical procedures to treat gastroesophageal reflux disease (GERD) have become much more common in the past 5 years because of the introduction of laparoscopic techniques. Symptoms of esophageal reflux are among the most common complaints heard by gastroenterologists. A small minority of these patients may be best managed with a surgical antireflux procedure; the vast majority may be performed laparoscopically. Indications for these procedures are not well defined. Most patients can be effectively managed with medication and lifestyle changes alone, although this may require the lifelong use of proton pump inhibitors (e.g., Prilosec) prokinetic agents (e.g., Reglan) and dietary restrictions. The unwillingness to submit to a lifetime of medication, therefore, constitutes the most common indication to proceed with surgery. Less commonly, medication intolerance or inadequate control of symptoms with medication alone may constitute an indication for surgery.

The patient is placed in the supine lithotomy position and the surgeon stands between the patient's legs. One assistant, or a mechanical liver retractor, is at the patient's right and another assistant stands at the patient's left. The abdomen is usually entered with a Veress needle at the umbilicus and 5 laparoscopic ports are placed across the upper abdomen—2 beneath the left costal margin, 2 beneath the right costal margin, and one in the midline either at the umbilicus or midway between the umbilicus and the xiphoid. The liver is elevated using a laparoscopic retractor, and the ligamentous attachments of the esophagus are divided. The esophagus is encircled, with care being taken to avoid injury to the vagus nerves. If there is a hiatal hernia, it is reduced into the abdomen and the crura are approximated with sutures. The short gastric vessels to the fundus of the stomach are then divided. The fundus is brought around behind the esophagus to create a fundoplication. The most common is a Nissen fundoplication, in which the anterior and posterior walls of the fundus are approximated for a distance of about 2 cm using sutures between the stomach and stomach, and between stomach and esophagus (Fig. 7.7-1A). During this portion of the procedure, a large esophageal dilator (bougie), typically 54-60Fr, is passed by the anesthesiologist to prevent the fundoplication from being made too tight. Passage of the dilator is possibly the most hazardous part of the procedure, as it may cause perforation of the esophagus at the gastroesophageal junction. As the dilator approaches the stomach, it is important to watch the junction on the video monitors to ensure that it is not being held at an angle that will risk perforation. The dilator is then withdrawn. An NG tube may be placed at this time. The ports are withdrawn and the procedure is terminated.

Variant procedure or approaches: In some instances, a partial fundoplication may be performed. Terminology is evolving, but these are sometimes referred to as **Toupet procedures**. We prefer the term **"posterior hemifundoplication**." These are most commonly performed in patients with impaired esophageal peristalsis with the risk of postop dysphagia. All parts of the procedure are identical to those of a Nissen, but the two walls of the fundus do not actually meet one another. Instead, the stomach is sewn to the walls of the esophagus and anchored to the right and left crura (Fig 7.7-1B). This requires more suturing than the Nissen fundoplication, and adds about 20-30 min to the procedure, but does not otherwise alter the procedure significantly. Some surgeons may not require passage of a dilator during a partial fundoplication.

Usual preop diagnosis: GERD, with or without esophagitis, esophageal stricture or Barrett's esophagus

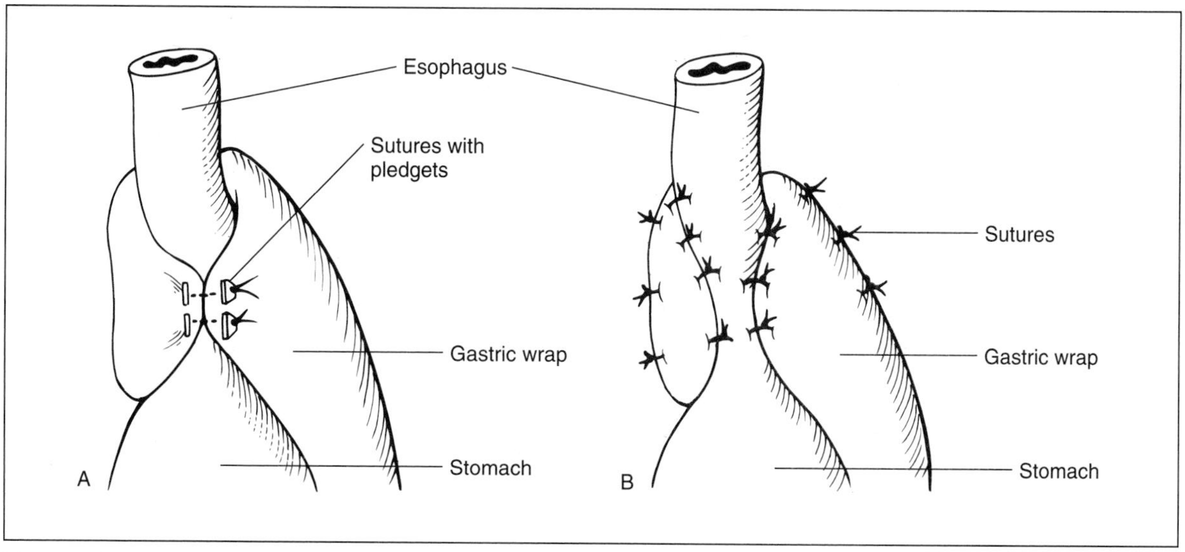

Figure 7.7-1. (A) Nissen fundoplication. (B) Partial fundoplication (Toupet procedure).

SUMMARY OF PROCEDURE

Position	Supine lithotomy
Incision	5 ports, upper abdomen
Special instrumentation	Harmonic Scalpel; bipolar cautery or endoscope. Esophageal dilators should be available.
Antibiotics	At surgeon's discretion
Surgical time	1.5-4 h
Closing considerations	Port closures only
EBL	Minimal
Postop care	2-d hospital stay; liquids on POD 1
Mortality	Rare
Morbidity	Atelectasis: Common Esophageal or gastric perforation: Rare (most commonly associated with passage of NG tube or esophageal dilator) Pneumothorax (does not usually require treatment) Transfusion: Very rare
Pain score	4

PATIENT POPULATION CHARACTERISTICS

Age range	May be performed in infants; next peak occurs in adulthood; rare in children and adolescents
Male:Female	1:1
Incidence	Increasing significantly over past 5 yr
Etiology	Unknown
Associated conditions	Aspiration risk; reactive airway disease

ANESTHETIC CONSIDERATIONS

See Anesthetic Considerations following Laparoscopic Cholecystectomy, p. 419.

References

1. Coster DD: Laparoscopic partial fundoplication vs laparoscopic Nissen-Rosetti fundoplication. Short-term results of 231 cases. *Surg Endosc* 1997; 11(6):625-31.
2. DeMeester TR, Peters JH, eds: *Minimally Invasive Surgery of the Foregut*. Quality Medical Publishing; St Louis: 1995.
3. Humphrey GM: Laparoscopic Nissen fundoplication in disabled infants and children. *J Pediatr Surg* 1996; 31(4):596-99.
4. Laine S: Laparoscopic vs conventional Nissen fundoplication. A prospective randomized study. *Surg Endosc* 1997; 11(5): 441-4.
5. Rosati R: Laparoscopic treatment of paraesophageal and large mixed hiatal hernias. *Surg Endosc* 1996; 10(4):429-431.
6. Swanstrom LL. Laparoscopic Collis gastroplasty is the treatment of choice for the shortened esophagus. *Am J Surg* 1996; 171(5):477-81.
7. Trus TL. Intermediate follow-up of laparoscopic antireflux surgery. *Am J Surg* 1996; 171(10): 32-5.
8. Trus TL. Minimally invasive surgery of the esophagus and stomach. *Am J Surg* 1997; 173(3):242-55.
9. Zucker KA, ed: *Surgical Laparoscopy Update*. Quality Medical Publishing, Inc; St. Louis: 1993.

LAPAROSCOPIC HELLER'S MYOTOMY AND ANTIREFLUX PROCEDURE

SURGICAL CONSIDERATIONS

Description: Laparoscopic and thoracoscopic esophageal myotomies have become much more common over the last 5 years as confidence in laparoscopic esophageal surgery—particularly antireflux surgery—has increased. These procedures are performed for achalasia, an uncommon condition in which the lower esophageal sphincter fails to relax with swallowing, and in which the body of the esophagus simultaneously loses its peristalsis. The patient complains of dysphagia and the esophagus dilates. The etiology of this condition remains unknown.

Treatment options consist of pneumatic dilatation, botulinum toxin injection of the lower esophageal sphincter or surgical myotomy. **Pneumatic dilation** remains the most common procedure performed for achalasia, and is effective as a single procedure in about 60% of patients. Many gastroenterologists are reluctant to perform these procedures, however, because of the risk of esophageal perforation, which is generally considered to be about 3-5%, but may be as high as 10%. **Botulinum toxin injection** is a newer technique that is effective to some degree in most patients, but the duration of its effectiveness is short. Most patients require retreatment within 1 1/2 years and the efficacy of retreatment may diminish over time. In many centers, **surgical myotomy** (**Heller's operation**) has become the procedure of choice for the treatment of achalasia.

The patient is positioned as for a laparoscopic antireflux procedure—supine in the lithotomy position with reverse Trendelenburg. The abdomen is usually entered with a Veress needle at the umbilicus and 5 laparoscopic ports are placed across the upper abdomen—2 beneath the left costal margin, 2 beneath the right costal margin, and one in the midline either at the umbilicus or midway between the umbilicus and the xiphoid. The liver is elevated, and the ligamentous attachments anterior to the esophagus are divided. The esophagus is not usually encircled; and, as hiatal hernias are uncommon with achalasia, crural repair is seldom necessary.

The myotomy is begun at the gastroesophageal junction using monopolar cautery, bipolar scissors or a Harmonic Scalpel. It is carried proximally until normal musculature is encountered. Some surgeons perform intraop esophagoscopy to ensure that the myotomy has been carried proximally enough and that there has not been a mucosal perforation. Generally, a myotomy of 5-8 cm is adequate, although sometimes a longer myotomy may be necessary. Some surgeons then perform a very loose, partial fundoplication to prevent reflux. This can be performed as an anterior or posterior fundoplication, bringing the fundus either anterior (our preference) or posterior to the esophagus. The stomach is secured to the esophageal wall and crural with sutures, and an NG tube may be passed. The ports are removed and port closure carried out.

Variant procedure or approaches: While most of these procedures are being performed laparoscopically, they also can be performed thoracoscopically or by thoracoscopy or thoracotomy. If a laparotomy or thoracotomy is performed, a DLT is required to allow collapse of the left lung.

Usual preop diagnosis: Achalasia

SUMMARY OF PROCEDURE

Position	Supine lithotomy, reverse Trendelenburg
Incision	5 ports, upper abdomen
Special instrumentation	Laparoscopic instrumentation ± gastroscope
Antibiotics	At surgeon's discretion
Surgical time	1.5-2 h
Closing considerations	None
EBL	Minimal
Postop care	2-d hospital stay; liquids on POD 1
Mortality	Rare
Morbidity	Insignificant atelectasis: Common Esophageal or gastric perforation: Rare Pneumothorax (does not usually require treatment) Transfusion required: Very rare Gastroesophageal reflux: > 15%
Pain score	4

PATIENT POPULATION CHARACTERISTICS

Age range	Adult
Male:Female	1:1
Incidence	Uncommon but not rare
Etiology	Unknown
Associated conditions	None. Chagas' disease may produce identical esophageal findings.

ANESTHETIC CONSIDERATIONS

See Anesthetic Considerations following Laparoscopic Cholecystectomy, p. 419.

References

1. Anselmino M: One-year follow-up after laparoscopic Heller-Dor operation for esophageal achalasia. *Surg Endosc* 1997; 11(1):3-7.
2. Esposito PS: Laparoscopic management of achalasia. *Am Surg* 1997; 63(3):221-23.
3. Holzman MD: Laparoscopic surgical treatment of achalasia. *Am J Surg* 1997; 173(4):308-11.
4 Pellegrini CA: Thoracoscopic esophageal myotomy in the treatment of achalasia. *Ann Thorac Surg* 1993; 56(3):680-82.
5. Slim K: Laparoscopic myotomy for primary esophageal achalasia: prospective evaluation. *Hepatogastroenterology* 1997; 44(13):11-15.
6. Swanstrom LL: Laparoscopic esophagomyotomy for achalasia. *Surg Endosc* 1995; 9(3):286-90.
7. DeMeester TR and Peters JH, eds: *Minimally Invasive Surgery of the Foregut.* Quality Medical Publishing, St Louis: 1995.

LAPAROSCOPIC CHOLECYSTECTOMY, WITH OR WITHOUT COMMON DUCT EXPLORATION

SURGICAL CONSIDERATIONS

Description: More than 90% of cholecystectomies are performed laparoscopically today. In laparoscopic cholecystectomy, 4 abdominal punctures are used to complete the procedure—one in the umbilicus, one in the upper midline and two beneath the right costal margin. Insufflation to a pressure of approximately 15 mmHg is routine. The liver is grasped and elevated, and the cystic duct and artery clipped and divided. Monopolar cautery is most commonly used to remove the gallbladder from the gallbladder fossa. The gallbladder is then usually removed through the umbilical port site, which may require slight enlargement of this site. The port is usually closed with fascial and skin sutures. Muscular relaxation is helpful during this portion of the procedure, even though it typically requires only 1 or 2 fascial sutures.

Cholangiography can be added easily to the laparoscopic cholecystectomy. A clip is placed high on the cystic duct; then a small incision is made in the duct just beneath the clip. A cholangiocatheter may be introduced and dye injected into the biliary tree. X-rays—either fluoroscopy or, more commonly, hard copy—are used to assess the biliary anatomy and to look for stones within the ductal system. Cholangiography carries few risks, generally adds about 10-15 min to the procedure and can be used to successfully identify the important anatomy ~85% of the time. Some surgeons perform it routinely during all cholecystectomies; others perform it selectively and only if there is evidence that the patient has had common duct stones or if the anatomy is in question.

In rare circumstances, **laparoscopic common duct exploration** may be carried out to treat common duct stones. A number of techniques have been used, most employing a thin fiber optic choledochoscope passed through the cystic duct into the common duct. This remains an uncommon procedure, performed in only a relatively few centers. More commonly, **endoscopic retrograde cholangiopancreaticotography (ERCP)** will be used, either preop or postop to demonstrate the presence or absence of stones and to remove any stones that might be found.

Variant procedure or approaches: Open cholecystectomy remains the major alternative to laparoscopic cholecystectomy, either because the cholecystectomy is predicted to be technically difficult or because of the illness of the patient. About 5% or less of laparoscopic cholecystectomies are converted to open cholecystectomy intraop because of difficulties with the procedure. ERCP remains the most common means of treating choledocholithiasis in the industrialized world, with laparoscopic techniques used in a relatively small number of centers and by a small number of surgeons. **Open common duct exploration** is occasionally necessary for stones not retrievable by ERCP (generally < 5%).

Usual preop diagnosis: Acute or chronic cholecystitis, usually with cholelithiasis, with or without choledocholithiasis

SUMMARY OF PROCEDURE

Position	Supine
Incision	4 upper abdominal ports
Special instrumentation	Routine laparoscopic instruments. May require fluoroscopy and choledochoscopes for cholangiography, common duct exploration
Antibiotics	Cefazolin 1 g
Surgical time	0.5-2 h; may be longer for common duct exploration.
Closing considerations	Muscular relaxation helpful for closure of umbilical port site
EBL	Minimal
Postop care	Usual discharge within 24 h
Mortality	< 1/1000
Morbidity	Common duct injury: 1/350 cases Hemorrhage (requiring transfusion) Infection Bile leak Injury to bowel Major vascular injury: Uncommon
Pain score	3

PATIENT POPULATION CHARACTERISTICS

Age range	Adult, increasing with age
Male:Female	Female > Male
Incidence	Common
Etiology	Stone disease
Associated conditions	Female gender; age; parity; obesity

ANESTHETIC CONSIDERATIONS

(Procedures covered: laparoscopic esophageal fundoplication; laparoscopic Heller's myotomy and antireflux surgery; laparoscopic cholecystectomy)

PREOPERATIVE: LAPAROSCOPIC CHOLECYSTECTOMY

The preop evaluation of patients undergoing laparoscopic removal of the gallbladder is discussed under Anesthetic Considerations for Biliary Tract Surgery, p. 410. Laparoscopic cholecystectomy is being performed much more commonly than the open procedure and can be accomplished quickly and safely even in very sick patients.

Respiratory Intraabdominal CO_2 insufflation → atelectasis, ↓FRC, ↑PIP, ↑$PaCO_2$ and ↓PaO_2; therefore, laparoscopic procedures may be contraindicated in patients with severe respiratory or cardiovascular disease. Postop respiratory function, however, is less impaired and is recovered more quickly in patients undergoing laparoscopic cholecystectomy then in the open procedure.

Laboratory CBC; others as indicated from H&P.

Premedication See Anesthetic Considerations for Biliary Tract Surgery, p. 410.

PREOPERATIVE: LAPAROSCOPIC FUNDOPLICATION/HELLER'S MYOTOMY

In general, this patient population is healthy, with the exception of those with gastroesophageal reflux disease (GERD). Patients often present with intractable heartburn, which is the reason for undergoing these surgical procedures.

Respiratory Patients may have Hx of recurrent aspiration with subsequently impaired pulmonary function or chronic pneumonitis. Intraabdominal CO_2 insufflation → atelectasis, ↓FRC, ↑PIP, ↑$PaCO_2$ and ↓PaO_2; therefore, laparoscopic procedures may be contraindicated in patients with severe respiratory impairment. These patients are at risk for aspiration of gastric contents during anesthetic induction and emergence.
Tests: Consider PA & lateral CXR; consider PFTs if Sx of impaired pulmonary function.

Cardiovascular Heartburn may mimic angina, and a cardiac origin for the pain should have been excluded prior to scheduling surgery.
Tests: ECG (r/o MI as cause of pain); others as indicated from H&P.

Laboratory As indicated from H&P.

Premedication These patients are at risk for aspiration and should be treated with full-stomach precautions. H_2 antagonists (e.g., ranitidine 50 mg iv, metoclopramide 10 mg iv, both 30 min before induction of anesthesia). Na citrate 30 ml po immediately before induction.

INTRAOPERATIVE

Anesthetic technique: GETA

Induction **Laparoscopic cholecystectomy**: Standard induction (see p. B-2). **Laparoscopic fundoplication** and **Heller's myotomy**: Given the patient's risk for aspiration, the trachea should be intubated after rapid-sequence induction with cricoid pressure (see p. B-5).

Maintenance Standard maintenance (see p. B-3) without N_2O, to prevent distension of the bowel. Continue muscle relaxation. Intraabdominal CO_2 insufflation will → ↑intraabdominal pressure, which will predispose to passive regurgitation of gastric contents. In addition, intraabdominal pressure > 15 mmHg → ↓venous return + ↑SVR → ↓CO. Controlled ventilation will minimize the possibility of hypercarbia from absorbed CO_2.

Emergence Given the high incidence of N/V (~50%), prophylactic antiemetics (e.g., metoclopramide 10 mg iv) are recommended and should be given 30-60 min before the end of the case.

Blood and fluid requirements	IV: 16-18 ga × 1 NS/LR @ 8-12 ml/kg/h Fluid warmer	Blood loss should be minimal, although assessment may be difficult 2° concealed bleeding.
Monitoring	Standard monitors (see p. B-1). Urinary catheter NG tube	Others as clinically indicated. Prevent hypothermia (forced air warmer, heated and humidified gases, warming blanket, warm OR, etc.).
Positioning	✓ and pad pressure points. ✓ eyes.	Initially in Trendelenburg position (↑venous return, ↓lung volumes, potential for mainstem intubation) for trocar placement; then reverse Trendelenburg (↓venous return, ↑lung volumes) during subsequent portions of the surgical procedure .
Complications	Respiratory: Pneumoperitoneum Hypercarbia/hypoxemia Pneumothorax, pneumomediastinum Endobronchial intubation	Pneumoperitoneum with CO_2 allows the surgeon to operate laparoscopically. This creates cephalad displacement of the diaphragm with ↓FRC, ↓pulmonary compliance and atelectasis. This can manifest as ↑PIP, ↓PO_2 and ↑PCO_2. Ventilation should be controlled during the operation to minimize the effects of pneumoperitoneum and hypercarbia. An increase in MV is appropriate. Pneumothorax can occur 2° retroperitoneal dissection of insufflated CO_2. Pneumothorax will manifest as ↓PO_2, ↑PIP, hemodynamic instability (↑HR, ↓BP), and possibly subcutaneous emphysema. The position of the ETT may change with altered patient position → endobronchial intubation.
	Cardiovascular: Hypotension Hemorrhage Dysrhythmias	↓BP can occur 2° patient positioning (reverse Trendelenburg) and from ↓venous return 2° pneumoperitoneum (↑intraabdominal pressure > 15 mmHg). Hemorrhage can result from inadvertent injury to blood vessels (during

Complications, cont.		trocar placement). Vascular injection of CO_2 (air embolism) can cause ↓BP, dysrhythmias and even cardiovascular collapse. If cardiopulmonary compromise occurs, the pneumoperitoneum can be released to allow for differential diagnosis and treatment.
	Visceral injury	Injury to the viscera may necessitate an open procedure or may go undiagnosed and → other postop complications, depending on the organ that is injured.
	Hypothermia	2° dry gas insufflation
	Subcutaneous emphysema	Dx: Sudden ↑$ETCO_2$ + subcutaneous crepitation (abdomen/chest wall). Rx: Stop insufflation of CO_2, D/C N_2O, ↑ventilation. Prevention: Keep CO_2 insufflation pressure < 12 mmHg.

POSTOPERATIVE

Complications	N/V (common)	Metoclopramide (10 mg iv), ondansetron (4 mg iv).
	Shoulder pain	From pneumoperitoneum; usually self-limited.
	Respiratory	Respiratory complications can be seen in the postop period as well. See list in Intraop Complications, above.
Pain management	PCA (see p. C-3). Percocet 2 tabs po q 6 h	
Tests	As indicated from H&P.	

References

1. Alponat A: Predictive factors for conversion of laparoscopic cholecystectomy. *World J Surg* 1997; 21(6):629-33.
2. Callery MP, Strasberg SM, Soper NJ: Complications of laparoscopic general surgery. *Gastrointest Endosc Clin N Am* 1996; 6(2):423-44.
3. Cervantes J: Changes in gallbladder surgery: comparative study 4 years before and 4 years after laparoscopic cholecystectomy. *World* J *Surg* 1997; 21(2):201-4.
4. Cunningham AJ, Brull SJ: Laparoscopic cholecystectomy: anesthetic implications. *Anesth Analg* 1993; 76: 1120-33.
5. Gurbuz AT, Peetz ME: The acute abdomen in the pregnant patient. Is there a role for laparoscopy? *Surg Endosc* 1997; 11(2):98-102.
6. Hein HA: Hemodynamic changes during laparoscopic cholecystectomy in patients with severe cardiac disease. *J Clin Anesth* 1997; 9(4):261-65.
7. Joris JL: Anesthetic management of laparoscopy. In *Anesthesia.* Miller RD, ed. Churchill Livingstone, New York: 1994, 2011-29.
8. Karim SK, Panton ON, Finley RJ, et al: Comparison of total versus partial laparoscopic fundoplication in the management of gastroesophageal reflux disease. *Am J Surg* 1997; 172:375-78.
9. Lew JKL, Gin T, Oh TE: Anaesthetic problems during laparoscopic cholecystectomy. *Anaesthes Intens Care* 1992; 20:91-2.
10. Millat B, Atger J, Deleuze A, Briandet H, Fingerhut A, Guillon F, Marrel E, De Seguin C, Soulier P: Laparoscopic treatment for choledocholithiasis: a prospective evaluation in 247 consecutive unselected *patients. Hepatogastroenterology* 1997; 44(13):28-34.
11. Mjaland O: Outpatient laparoscopic cholecystectomy. *Br J Surg* 1997; 84(7):958-61.
12. Safran DB: Cholecystectomy following the introduction of laparoscopy; more, but for the same indication. *Am Surg* 1997; 63(6):506-11.
13. Savader SJ, Lillemoe KD, Prescott CA, Winick AB, Venbrux AC, Lund GB, Mitchell SE, Cameron JL, Osterman FA Jr: Laparoscopic cholecystectomy-related bile duct injuries: a health and financial disaster. *Ann Surg* 1997; 225(3):268-74.
14. Zucker KA, ed: *Surgical Laparoscopy Update*. Quality Medical Publishing, St Louis: 1993.

LAPAROSCOPIC SPLENECTOMY

SURGICAL CONSIDERATIONS

Description: Laparoscopic splenectomy may be performed for most conditions in which splenectomy is indicated, and when the spleen is of normal size or only modestly enlarged. Although it may be possible to isolate larger spleens within the abdomen, it is difficult to place them in a bag large enough to permit morcellation (piecemeal removal of tissue). There are no absolute size criteria, however, and we have laparoscopically removed spleens that are several times normal size.

The patient is placed on a bean bag in the lateral decubitus position with the left side elevated. The kidney rest is elevated and the OR table is flexed to open up the space between the lower ribs and the hips. Care is taken to pad all pressure points.

The abdomen is entered with a Veress needle, either at the umbilicus or along the left costal margin, and insufflated to 15 mmHg. A total of 3-5 ports are placed along the left costal margin. The posterior attachments of the spleen are divided and the short gastric vessels are severed. Bleeding from the hilum of the spleen is controlled with serial firings of the vascular stapler. The spleen is placed in an endoscopic bag, morcellated and removed. The 10- and 12-mm port sites are closed after perfect hemostasis is ensured.

Variant procedure or approaches: Some surgeons perform the procedure with the patient supine or only partially rotated. The most important alternative approach is by laparotomy.

Usual preop diagnosis: Most common – idiopathic thrombocytopenic purpura (ITP); less common – hemolytic anemia, thrombotic thrombocytopenic purpura (TTP), hypersplenism

SUMMARY OF PROCEDURE

Position	Decubitus, flexed
Incision	3-5 trocar ports
Special instrumentation	Vascular staplers; consider Harmonic Scalpel; bipolar instruments
Antibiotics	Cefazolin 1 g
Surgical time	1-3 h
Closing considerations	Rapid closure not requiring muscle relaxation
EBL	Generally minimal; if significant enough to require transfusion, may require conversion to laparotomy.
Postop care	Minimal. Generally begin liquids POD 1 and discharge POD 2.
Mortality	Rare: Predominately related to underlying disease
Morbidity	Minimal Hemorrhage Conversion to laparotomy Injury to pancreas, stomach or splenic flexure of colon
Pain score	4

PATIENT POPULATION CHARACTERISTICS

Age range	All ages; more common, adults
Male:Female	1:1
Incidence	Uncommon
Etiology	Hematologic disorders (e.g., ITP, TTP); tumor of the spleen (e.g., Hodgkin's disease); hypersplenism
Associated conditions	Steroid dependence; neutropenia; thrombocytopenia

ANESTHETIC CONSIDERATIONS

PREOPERATIVE

Patients will present for laparoscopic splenectomy with a variety of diseases, including ITP, lymphomatous disease (Hodgkin's and non-Hodgkin's), autoimmune hemolytic anemia, TTP, hereditary spherocytosis, Evans's syndrome, hairy-cell leukemia, hypersplenism 2° portal HTN, sarcoidosis, polycythemia vera and myelofibrosis. Open splenectomy is usually reserved for traumatic laceration of the spleen. Previous upper abdominal surgery does not absolutely mitigate against the laparoscopic procedure. Laparoscopic cases tend to take longer than open splenectomies. Patients who have been treated with chemotherapeutic drugs will require careful preop exam to evaluate for potentially toxic side effects. (See Anesthetic Considerations for Splenectomy, p. 449.) Patients should receive antipneumococcal, meningococcal and Haemophilus influenzae vaccinations at least 1 wk preop.

Respiratory — Patients who present with splenomegaly may have a degree of left lower-lobe atelectasis, which should be evaluated by physical exam. Intraabdominal CO_2 insufflation → further atelectasis, ↓FRC, ↑PIP, ↑$PaCO_2$ and ↓PaO_2; therefore, laparoscopic procedures may be contraindicated in patients with severe respiratory disease.
Tests: Consider P/A & lateral CXR; ABG; PFTs, if clinically indicated.

Hematologic — Cytopenias are very common.
Tests: CBC & Plt count

Laboratory — As indicated from H&P.

Premedication — Standard premedication (see p. B-2).

INTRAOPERATIVE

Anesthetic technique: GETA

Induction — Standard induction (see p. B-2).

Maintenance — Standard maintenance (see p. B-3) without N_2O, to prevent distension of bowel.

Emergence — No special considerations. Prophylactic antiemetics (e.g., metoclopramide 10 mg) are appropriate.

Blood and fluid requirements	IV: 16-18 ga × 1 NS/LR @ 8-12 ml/kg/h Fluid warmer	Blood loss should be < 1 U. If Plt transfusion is necessary, it should be given after ligation of splenic vessels (↓sequestration).
Monitoring	Standard monitors (see p. B-1). Urinary catheter NG tube	Others as indicated by patient status. Prevent hypothermia (forced air warmer, heated and humidified inspired gases, warming blanket, warm OR, etc.).
Positioning	✓ and pad pressure points. ✓ eyes.	Careful positioning and padding of patient is essential.
Complications	Respiratory: Pneumoperitoneum Hypercarbia/hypoxemia Pneumothorax, pneumomediastinum Endobronchial intubation Cardiovascular: Hypotension Hemorrhage Dysrhythmias Visceral injury Hypothermia Subcutaneous emphysema	The complications of laparoscopy are discussed in Anesthetic Considerations for Laparoscopic Cholecystectomy, p. 420.
	Bleeding	Typically, when blood loss > 750-1000 ml, convert to open splenectomy. Plt transfusion may be necessary.

POSTOPERATIVE

Complications	N/V	Metoclopramide (10 mg iv), ondansetron (4 mg iv)
	Shoulder pain	2° pneumoperitoneum; usually self-limited. Ketorolac (30 mg iv).
	Atelectasis	Usually left lower lobe
Pain management	PCA (see p. C-3).	
Tests	As indicated by patient status.	

References

1. Diaz J, Eisenstat M, Chung R: A case-controlled study of laparoscopic splenectomy. Am J *Surg* 1997; 173:348-50.
2. Farab RR: Comparison of laparoscopic and open splenectomy in children with hematologic disorders. *J Pediatr* 1997; 131(1):41-6.
3. Flowers JL: Laparoscopic splenectomy in patients with hematologic diseases. *Ann Surg 1996;* 224(1):19-28.
4. Hicks BA: Laparoscopic splenectomy in childhood hematologic disorders. *J Laparoendosc Surg* 1996; 6:S31-S34.
5. Leggett PL: Laparoscopic splenectomy. *Ann Surg* 1997; 226(1), 111-12.
6. Park A, Gagner M, Pomp A: The lateral approach to laparoscopic splenectomy. *Am J Surg* 1997; 173:126-30.
7. Tsiotos G: Laparoscopic splenectomy for immune thrombocytopenic purpura. *Arch Surg* 1997; 132(6):642-46.
8. Zucker KA ed: *Surgical Laparoscopy Update*. Quality Medical Publishing, Inc., St. Louis: 1993.

LAPAROSCOPIC ADRENALECTOMY

SURGICAL CONSIDERATIONS

Description: Adrenalectomies are relatively uncommon procedures, and **laparoscopic adrenalectomies** are presently carried out at only a small number of centers. They are performed for a variety of benign conditions or for indeterminate adrenal masses, depending on their size. A laparoscopic approach generally would not be used for a known carcinoma and, similarly, a laparoscopic approach for removal of a pheochromocytoma is controversial.

Generally, laparoscopic adrenalectomies are performed with the patient on a bean bag in the lateral decubitus position, with the side to be operated on up and the OR table flexed to open up the distance between the costal margin and the iliac crest. The adrenal may be approached transperitoneally or preperitoneally. On the left, the spleen and tail of pancreas must be dissected away from the adrenal; on the right, the liver must be mobilized. Vessels to the adrenal are divided, and the tumor is placed into an endoscopic bag and removed by extending one of the port sites. The port sites are closed and the procedure is completed.

Variant procedure or approaches: Laparotomy

Usual preop diagnosis: Indeterminate adrenal mass (nonfunctional adenoma); also can be performed for functional adenomas, rarely for pheochromocytoma. Contraindicated for known carcinoma.

SUMMARY OF PROCEDURE

Position	Decubitus with arms extended out from the table.
Incision	4-5 ports
Special instrumentation	Balloon dissector can be used for preperitoneal approach.
Antibiotics	At surgeon's discretion; cefazolin 1 g iv
Surgical time	1-4 h
Closing considerations	Brief closure; muscle relaxation helpful.
EBL	< 150 ml, although occasionally significant blood loss may occur.
Postop care	Begin diet POD 1, usually discharged POD 2-3
Mortality	Rare
Morbidity	Hemorrhage/hematoma Conversion to laparotomy Injury to pancreas or kidney
Pain score	4

PATIENT POPULATION CHARACTERISTICS

Age range	Adults, all ages
Male:Female	Equal
Incidence	Uncommon
Etiology	Adrenal tumors
Associated conditions	Depending on function of tumor (e.g., HTN for aldosteronoma, Cushing's disease)

ANESTHETIC CONSIDERATIONS

PREOPERATIVE

The preop evaluation of patients undergoing laparoscopic adrenalectomy is discussed under Anesthetic Considerations for (open) Adrenalectomy, p. 482.

INTRAOPERATIVE

Anesthetic technique: GETA. An epidural should not be necessary for postop analgesia if the procedure is performed laparoscopically. If the surgical team feels that there is a high likelihood of conversion to an open procedure, consider placement of an epidural catheter for postop analgesia.

Induction	See induction under (open) Adrenalectomy, p. 483.
Maintenance	See maintenance under (open) Adrenalectomy, p. 483.
Emergence	See emergence under (open) Adrenalectomy, p. 484. Case is likely to take longer if performed laparoscopically but usually has a less painful postop course. Prophylactic antiemetics (e.g., metoclopramide 10 mg) are appropriate.

Blood and fluid requirements	IV: 14-16 ga × 1 NS/LR @10-15 ml/kg/h	Warming techniques important (forced air warmers, fluid warmers, humidified inspired gases, etc.).
Monitoring	Standard monitors (see p. B-1). UO Arterial line	
	± PA catheter	A PA catheter is useful in the management of patients with pheochromocytoma.
	TEE	TEE may be needed to evaluate cardiac function and filling.
Positioning	✓ and pad pressure points. ✓ eyes.	Careful support and padding of extremities and torso is very important.
Complications: laparoscopic	Respiratory: Pneumoperitoneum Hypercarbia/hypoxemia Pneumothorax, pneumomediastinum Endobronchial intubation Cardiovascular: Hypotension Hemorrhage Dysrhythmias Visceral injury Subcutaneous emphysema Hypothermia	The complications of laparoscopy are discussed in Anesthetic Considerations for Laparoscopic Cholecystectomy, p. 420.
Complications: endocrine	Pheochromocytoma: BP lability Myocardial dysfunction	Rx: intraop HTN with SNP or phentolamine (2.5-5 mg q 5 min); ↑HR with esmolol; ↓BP with phenylephrine or dopamine. (See Anesthetic Considerations for Adrenalectomy, p. 482.)
	Conn's syndrome: CHF 2° hypervolemia	See Anesthetic Considerations for Adrenalectomy, p. 484.

Complications: endocrine, cont.	↑BP Electrolyte disturbances Hyperglycemia	
	Cushing's syndrome: ↑BP/↑BP Acute adrenal insufficiency	Continue replacement steroids. (See Anesthetic Considerations for Adrenalectomy, p. 482.)

POSTOPERATIVE

Complications	N/V Shoulder pain Other	Metoclopramide (10 mg iv), ondansetron (4 mg iv). 2° pneumoperitoneum; usually self-limited. Ketorolac (30 mg iv).
Pain management	PCA (see p. C-3).	See Anesthetic Considerations for Adrenalectomy, p. 484.
Tests	As indicated	

References

1. Chapuis Y: Bilateral laparoscopic adrenalectomy for Cushing's disease. *Br J Surg* 1997; 84(7):1009.
2. Duy QY: Laparoscopic adrenalectomy. Comparison of the lateral and posterior approaches. *Arch Surg* 1996; 131(8):870-75.
3. Fernandez-Cruz L: Technical aspects of adrenalectomy via operative laparoscopy. *Surg Endosc* 1994; 8(11)1348-51.
4. Horgan S, Sinan M, Helton WS, Pellegrini CA: Use of laparoscopic techniques improves outcome from adrenalectomy. *Am J Surg* 1997; 173:371-74.
5. Linos DA, Stylopoulos N, Boukis M, et al: Anterior, posterior, or laparoscopic approach for the management of adrenal diseases. *Am J Surg* 1997; 173-120-25.
6. Naito S: Laparoscopic adrenalectomy: comparison with open adrenalectomy. *Eur Urol* 1994; 26(3):253-57.
7. Staren ED: Adrenalectomy in the era of laparoscopy. *Surgery* 1996; 120(4):706-9.
8. Terai A: Laparoscopic adrenalectomy for bilateral pheochromocytoma: a case report. *Int J Urol* 1997; 4(3):300-3.
9. Vargas HI, Kavoussi LR, Bartlett DL, et al: Laparoscopic adrenalectomy: A new standard of care. *Urology* 1997; 49:673-78.
10. Winfield HN, Hamilton BD, Bravo EL: Technique of laparoscopic adrenalectomy. *Urol Clin N Am* 1997; 24(2):459-65.
11. Zucker KA, ed: *Surgical Laparoscopy Update*. Quality Medical Publishing, St. Louis: 1993.

LAPAROSCOPIC BOWEL RESECTION

SURGICAL CONSIDERATIONS

Description: Intestinal resection by laparoscopy remains an advanced procedure performed by relatively few surgeons, and the techniques are not yet standardized. Most of these resections are of the large intestine, typically performed for intestinal obstructions or inflammatory conditions. Laparoscopic procedures for cancer are still controversial, and at least 2 large, multicenter trials are presently under way to examine the safety of these procedures.

Most **laparoscopic bowel resections** will require 4 or more ports, and insufflation is routine. The patient is usually placed in the low lithotomy position, and the surgeon may have to move to all sides of the patient to complete the procedure. For this reason, it is important that the arms be tucked in at the patient's sides. Often it is preferable to let the drape fall over the patient's face, which optimizes surgical access.

Unipolar and bipolar cautery, the Harmonic Scalpel and many different surgical staplers may be used during these procedures. These generally require longer operative times than the corresponding open procedures but, typically, they are associated with shorter hospitalization stays and earlier return to work than traditional laparotomy.

Variant Procedure or approaches: Laparotomy or **laparoscopic-assisted** procedures. Many variations of laparoscopic (versus open) procedures may be performed. In some—such as the creation of an end sigmoid colostomy—the entire procedure may be performed intracorporeally. Sometimes the specimen is removed via the anus or through a vaginotomy. In other cases, the procedure is "laparoscopic-assisted." In these, the mobilization is performed intracorporeally and the specimen is exteriorized and resected, and the anastomosis is performed through a small, strategically placed laparotomy incision. An example of this is a right colectomy, in which an incision is needed to remove the specimen, making it logical to perform the anastomosis through the same incision.

Usual preop diagnosis: Intestinal obstruction; inflammatory conditions (e.g., diverticulitis, bleeding, neoplasms); cancer (controversial). Laparoscopic intestinal procedures may be performed for intestinal obstruction and inflammatory conditions.

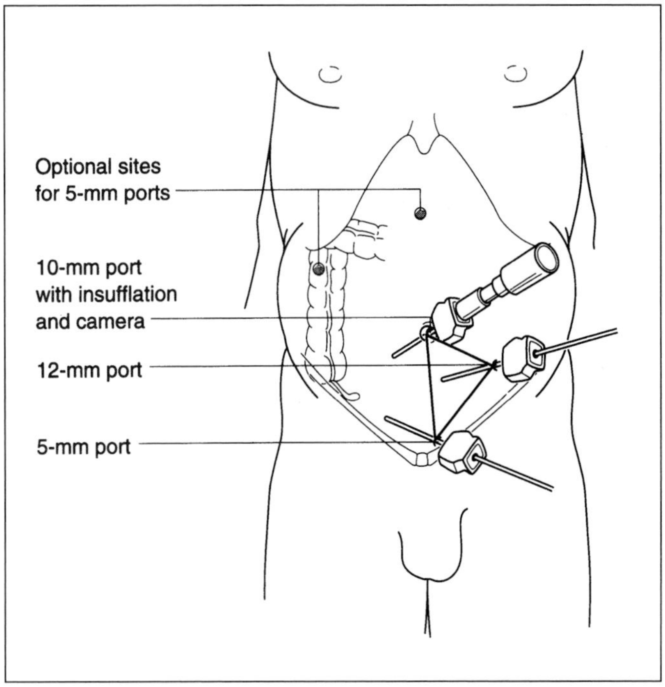

Figure 7.7-2. Trocar placement for a right colectomy. The general principle is to place the camera port so that the surgeon's visual axis is parallel to the telescope, and to place the working ports so that the operative site is at the apex of an isosceles triangle. (Reproduced with permission from Greenfield LJ, et al, eds: *Surgery: Scientific Principles and Practice*, 2nd edition. Lippincott-Raven Publishers, Philadelphia: 1997, 738.)

SUMMARY OF PROCEDURE

Position	Supine, usually lithotomy
Incision	4 or more trocar ports (Fig 7.7-2), sometimes with a small laparotomy incision for specimen removal and anastomosis.
Special instrumentation	May require Harmonic Scalpel, various laparoscopic stapling instruments.
Antibiotics	Cefazolin 1 g
Surgical time	1.5-5 h
Closing considerations	< laparotomy, but usually requires closure of several port sites.
EBL	Variable, but transfusion should be exceedingly rare.
Postop care	NG tube seldom used. Most patients begin regular diet within 48 h; discharge, generally 3-5 d.
Mortality	Minimal
Morbidity	Generally uncommon; similar in magnitude to those seen with open operations. Complications include: Hemorrhage Infection Anastomotic leak Intestinal obstruction
Pain score	3-7

PATIENT POPULATION CHARACTERISTICS

Age range	Adult
Male:Female	1:1. Endometriosis only in females; other pathology slightly more common in men.
Incidence	Laparoscopic bowel procedures still relatively uncommon
Etiology	Tumor; inflammatory process
Associated conditions	Bowel obstruction; hemorrhage

ANESTHETIC CONSIDERATIONS

PREOPERATIVE

For respiratory, cardiovascular, musculoskeletal, gastrointestinal and renal considerations, see Anesthetic Considerations for Intestinal and Peritoneal Procedures, p. 370.

Premedication Standard premedication (see p. B-2). If patient is at risk for a full stomach, administration of metoclopramide (10 mg iv) and H_2 blocker (ranitidine 50 mg iv), as well as Na citrate 0.3 M 30 ml po. Metoclopramide should not be used in patients with bowel obstructions or perforations.

INTRAOPERATIVE

Anesthetic technique: GETA

Induction Standard induction (see p. B-2). Standard rapid-sequence induction if at risk for aspiration (see p. B-5).

Maintenance Standard maintenance (see p. B-3) without N_2O, to prevent distension of the bowel.

Emergence No special considerations unless the patient is at risk for aspiration; extubation should then occur after the patient is fully awake and has protective airway reflexes.

Blood and fluid requirements	IV: 16-18 ga × 1 NS/LR @ 8-12 ml/kg/h Fluid warmer	Blood loss should be < 1 U.
Monitoring	Standard monitors (see p. B-1). Urinary catheter NG tube to decompress the stomach	Others as indicated by patient status. Prevent hypothermia (forced air warmer, heated humidified gases, warming blanket, warm room, etc).
Positioning	✓ and pad pressure points. ✓ eyes.	
Complications	Respiratory: Pneumoperitoneum Hypercarbia/hypoxemia Pneumothorax, pneumomediastinum Endobronchial intubation Cardiovascular: Hypotension Hemorrhage Dysrhythmias Visceral injury Hypothermia Subcutaneous emphysema	These complications (associated with the preperitoneal approach), as well as the general complications of laparoscopy, are discussed in Anesthetic Considerations for Laparoscopic Cholecystectomy, p. 420.

POSTOPERATIVE

Complications	N/V Shoulder pain	Metoclopramide (10 mg iv), ondansetron (4 mg iv) 2° pneumoperitoneum. Usually self-limited. Ketorolac (30 mg iv).
Pain management	PCA (see p. C-3).	
Tests	As indicated by patient status.	

References

1. Bessler M, Whelan RL, Halverson A, Treat MR, Nowygrod R: Is immune function better preserved after laparoscopic versus open colon resection? *Surg Endosc* 1994; 8:881-83.
2. Bohm B, Milsom JW, Fazio VW: Postoperative intestinal motility following conventional and laparoscopic intestinal surgery. *Arch Surg* 1995; 130:415-19.
3. Bokey EL: Morbidity and mortality following laparoscopic-assisted right hemicolectomy for cancer. *Dis Colon Rectum* 1996; 39(10): S24-S28.
4. Callery MP, Strasberg SM, Soper NJ: Complications of laparoscopic general surgery. *Gastrointest Endosc Clin N Am* 1996; 6:423-44.

5. Darzi A: Laparoscopic sigmoid colectomy: total laparoscopic approach. *Dis Colon Rectum* 1994; 37(3): 268-71.
6. Ehrmantraut W, Sardi A: Laparoscopy-assisted small bowel resection. *Am Surg* 1997; 63:996-1001.
7. Fleshman JW, Nelson H, Peters WR, Kim HC, Larach S, Boorse RR, Ambroze W, Leggett P, Bleday R, Stryker S, Christenson B, Wexner S, Senagore A, Rattner D, Sutton J, Fine AP: Early results of laparoscopic surgery for colorectal cancer. Retrospective analysis of 372 patients treated by Clinical Outcomes of Surgical Therapy (COST) Study Group. *Dis Colon Rectum* 1996; 39(10 Suppl): S53-S58.
8. Goh YC: Early postoperative results of a prospective series of laparoscopic vs. open anterior resections for rectosigmoid cancers. *Dis Colon Rectum* 1997; 40(7):776-80.
9. Jacobs M, Plasencia G, Caushaj P: *Atlas of Laparoscopic Colon Surgery*. Williams & Wilkins, Baltimore: 1996.
10. Milsom JW: Use of laparoscopic techniques in colorectal surgery. Preliminary study. *Dis Colon Rectum* 1994; 37(3):215-18.
11. Nezhat CR, Nezhat FR, Luciano AA, Siegler AM, Metzger DA, Nezhat CH: *Operative Gynecologic Laparoscopy: Principles and Techniques*. McGraw-Hill, New York: 1995.
12. Paik PS: Laparoscopic colectomy. *Surg Clin North Am* 1997; 77(1):1-13.
13. Reissman P: Laparoscopic colorectal surgery: ascending the learning curve. *World J Surg* 1996; 20(3):277-81.
14. Van Ye TM: Laparoscopically assisted colon resections compare favorably with open technique. *Surg Laparosc Endosc* 1994; 4(1):25-31.
15. Zucker KA, ed: *Surgical Laparoscopy Update*. Quality Medical Publishing, St. Louis: 1993.

LAPAROSCOPIC APPENDECTOMY

SURGICAL CONSIDERATIONS

Description: The indications for **laparoscopic appendectomy** are not well defined. In women of childbearing age, the negative appendectomy rate approaches 40%; most negative explorations will involve pelvic pathology that cannot always be seen well through a right lower quadrant (RLQ) incision. Some surgeons restrict laparoscopy to these cases; others prefer to perform most or all of their appendectomies by laparotomy.

Generally, 3-4 trocar sites are necessary, with the initial trocar usually placed at the umbilicus and subsequent trocars placed in the lower abdomen, according to surgeon's preference. Women are often placed in low lithotomy position, and some surgeons prefer this position in men as well. Generally, the surgeon stands at the patient's left, and an assistant stand's either beside the surgeon or between the patient's legs. The Trendelenburg position with elevation of the right side of the abdomen facilitates exposure of the appendix. Under direct vision, using monopolar cautery, the peritoneal attachments of the cecum and appendix are divided. The appendiceal vessels are clipped or cauterized and the appendix amputated, using an endoscopic stapler or between laparoscopic ties. The appendix may be placed in a specimen bag for removal or retracted into one of the ports and removed in this fashion. The umbilical fascia is closed and the skin is loosely approximated. When unexpected pathology is identified, it can be dealt with by laparoscopy or by laparotomy, with incision placement dependent on findings.

Variant Procedure or approaches: Open appendectomy via RLQ or midline incision

Usual preop diagnosis: Acute abdomen; possible acute appendicitis

SUMMARY OF PROCEDURE

Position	Supine: possible lithotomy
Incision	3-4 ports
Antibiotics	Cefazolin 1 g
Surgical time	30-60 min
Closing considerations	Muscular relaxation helpful for umbilical closure.
EBL	Minimal
Postop care	Usual discharge POD 1
Mortality	Minimal
Morbidity	Minimal Risk of intraabdominal abscess, mostly dependent on pathology (e.g., early acute inflammation vs perforation) Hemorrhage Infection Stump leak: exceedingly rare Conversion to open procedure: dependent on pathology and experience of surgeon
Pain score	3

PATIENT POPULATION CHARACTERISTICS

Age range	All ages
Male:Female	1:1
Incidence	Common
Etiology	Acute appendicitis
Associated conditions	Consider other pelvic pathology in women of childbearing age.

ANESTHETIC CONSIDERATIONS

PREOPERATIVE

This patient population is generally fit and healthy apart from their acutely presenting illness. Full-stomach precautions are appropriate in these patients (see p. B-5).

Respiratory Respiratory impairment can occur 2° acute abdominal pain and splinting. Tachypnea and hyperpnea can be heralding Sx of appendiceal perforation and sepsis. Patients with acute abdomen should be treated as if they have full stomachs.
Tests: As indicated from H&P.

Cardiovascular May be dehydrated from fever, emesis and decreased oral intake. Assess volume status with vital signs in the supine and standing positions (if possible) and hydrate adequately prior to proceeding with anesthetic induction.
Tests: ECG, if indicated from H&P.

Gastrointestinal Patient typically has abdominal pain with N/V. Muscular resistance to palpation of abdominal wall frequently parallels the severity of the inflammatory process. With spreading peritoneal irritation (as with perforation), patient will develop abdominal distension and paralytic ileus.
Tests: Electrolytes

Hematologic Moderate leukocytosis (10,000-18,000) with moderate left shift. Hemoconcentration is probable, if patient is dehydrated.
Tests: CBC

Laboratory Others as indicated from H&P.

Premedication Patients with acute appendicitis should be treated as if they have full stomachs. Consider administration of metoclopramide (10 mg iv) and H_2 blocker (ranitidine 50 mg iv), as well as Na citrate 0.3 M 30 ml po. Opiate premedication (morphine 0.08-0.15 mg/kg im) is indicated after patient is scheduled for surgery. If surgical intervention is still in question, administration of opiates may mask Sx of appendicitis.

INTRAOPERATIVE

Anesthetic technique: GETA, with rapid-sequence iv induction.

Induction	Preoxygenate patient and have an assistant apply cricoid pressure. Etomidate 0.1-0.4 mg/kg, STP 3-5 mg/kg + succinylcholine 1.5 mg/kg, for intubation.
Maintenance	Standard maintenance (see p. B-3), without N_2O.
Emergence	Extubate when the patient is awake and with active laryngeal protective reflexes.
Blood and fluid requirements	IV: 16-18 ga × 1 NS/LR @ 5-8 ml/kg/h

Monitoring	Standard monitors (see p. B-1). Urinary catheter NG tube	Others as indicated by patient status. Prevent hypothermia (forced air warmer, heated humidified gases, warming blanket, warm room, etc.)
Positioning	✓ and pad pressure points. ✓ eyes. Secure or tuck arms.	Trendelenburg position with elevation of the right side of the abdomen improves surgical exposure.
Complications	Respiratory: Pneumoperitoneum Hypercarbia/hypoxemia Pneumothorax, pneumomediastinum Endobronchial intubation Cardiovascular: Hypotension Hemorrhage Dysrhythmias Visceral injury Hypothermia Subcutaneous emphysema	These complications (associated with the preperitoneal approach), as well as the general complications of laparoscopy, are discussed in Anesthetic Considerations for Laparoscopic Cholecystectomy, p. 420.

POSTOPERATIVE

Complications	N/V Urinary retention	Metoclopramide (10 mg iv), ondansetron (4 mg iv) Straight catheterization of the bladder
Pain management	PCA (see p. C-3). Oral opiates Ketorolac	Tylenol #3 – 2 tabs po q 6 hr (weak) or Percocet – 2 tabs po q 6 hr. 30 mg iv
Tests	As indicated by patient status.	

References

1. Amos JD, Schorr SJ, Norman PF, et al: Laparoscopic surgery during pregnancy. *Am J Surg* 1996; 171:425-37.
2. Apelgren KN: Laparoscopic appendectomy and the management of gynecologic pathologic conditions found at laparoscopy for presumed appendicitis. *Surg Clin North Am* 1996; 76(3):469-82.
3. Callery MP, Strasberg SM, Soper NJ: Complications of laparoscopic general surgery. *Gastrointest Endosc Clin N Am* 1996; 6:423-44.
4. Chiarugi M: Laparoscopic compared with open appendicectomy for acute appendicitis: a prospective study. *Eur J Surg* 162(5), 385-90, 1996.
5. Cox MR: Prospective randomized comparison of open versus laparoscopic appendectomy in men. *World J Surg* 1996; 20(3):263-66.
6. Kaplan A, Dorman BH, Harvey SC: Laparoscopic versus conventional appendectomy. *Ann Surg* 1995; 221:119-21.
7. Kluiber RM: Laparoscopic appendectomy. A comparison with open appendectomy. *Dis Colon Rectum* 1996; 39(9):1008-11.
8. Laine S: Laparoscopic appendectomy—is it worthwhile? A prospective, randomized study in young women. *Surg Endosc* 1997; 11(2):95-7.
9. Lueken RP, Moeller CP, Heeckt B, Schaefer C: Review of 47 laparoscopic appendectomies. *J Am Assoc Gynecol Laparosc* 1995; 2:269-72.
10. McCahill LE: A clinical outcome and cost analysis of laparoscopic versus open appendectomy. *Am J Surg* 1996; 171(5):533-37.
11. Reiertsen O: Randomized controlled trial with sequential design of laparoscopic versus conventional appendectomy. *Br J Surg* 1997; 84(6):842-47.
12. Zucker KA, ed: *Surgical Laparoscopy Update*. Quality Medical Publishing, St Louis: 1993.

LAPAROSCOPIC INGUINAL HERNIA REPAIR

SURGICAL CONSIDERATIONS

Description: A variety of different techniques have evolved for the performance of **laparoscopic hernia repairs,** but all require GA or at least extensive regional anesthesia such as a spinal or epidural anesthetic.

The **preperitoneal approach** is the most commonly performed since it offers the advantages of shortened operative time and decreased morbidity. The hernia is approached at the umbilicus with a cutdown into the preperitoneal space. The balloon dissector is introduced into this extraperitoneal space and gently advanced toward the groin, establishing an area between the abdominal and peritoneal walls within which to work. This space is continuous with the subcutaneous space. The insufflation pressures for the preperitoneal procedures are generally less than for the transperitoneal procedures (9 versus 15 mmHg), although CO_2 absorption may be greater with the preperitoneal approach. Two additional ports are placed in the lower abdomen. Once the dissection has been completed, the defect is bridged with a sheet of prosthetic mesh that is stapled in place. The ports are withdrawn, and port sites are closed.

In the **transperitoneal approach**, the abdomen is entered with a Veress needle as for a laparoscopy and the laparoscope is placed through the umbilical port. Two additional ports are then placed, the peritoneum overlying the hernial orifices is dissected off, and the hernial orifices are covered with a sheet of prosthetic mesh that is stapled in place. The peritoneum is then approximated over the mesh, the trocars are withdrawn and the trocar sites are closed.

There is still considerable controversy surrounding techniques of hernia repair. Fewer than 20% of hernia repairs in the U.S. are presently performed laparoscopically; however, for patients with recurrent hernias and bilateral hernias there may be advantages to the laparoscopic approach.

Variant Procedure or approaches: Open hernia repair (see Inguinal Herniorrhaphy, p. 455).

Usual preop diagnosis: Inguinal hernia

SUMMARY OF PROCEDURE

Position	Supine
Incision	Umbilical port with 2 additional lower abdominal ports
Special instrumentation	May require balloon dissector.
Antibiotics	Cefazolin 1 g
Surgical time	1-2 h
Closing considerations	Minimal time; no muscular relaxation
EBL	Minimal
Postop care	1-2 h in PACU/holding area → home
Mortality	Rare
Morbidity	Generally minimal Orchialgia, neuralgia Conversion to open procedure Recurrence of hernia: Rare in experienced hands Bowel obstruction Bladder injury: Rarely reported
Pain score	3

PATIENT POPULATION CHARACTERISTICS

Age range	Mostly adults
Male:Female	Male > Female
Incidence	Common
Etiology	Most hernias congenital; chronically increased intraabdominal pressure (e.g., chronic cough, obesity)
Associated conditions	None important

ANESTHETIC CONSIDERATIONS

PREOPERATIVE

The preop evaluation of patients undergoing laparoscopic hernia repair is discussed under Anesthetic Considerations for Inguinal Hernia, p. 462. Patients presenting for this procedure are generally healthy. Laparoscopic repair of inguinal hernia is usually associated with less pain and earlier return to preop function when compared to the open procedure. Patients with strangulated or incarcerated hernias usually require open procedures.

Laboratory	Hb/Hct (healthy patients); otherwise, as indicated from H&P.
Premedication	Standard premedication (see p. B-2).

INTRAOPERATIVE

Anesthetic technique: GETA (or LMA). Spinal or epidural anesthetics may be appropriate in patients where the abdomen is not insufflated.

Induction	Standard induction (see p. B-2).	
Maintenance	Standard maintenance (see p. B-3) without N_2O, to prevent distension of the bowel.	
Emergence	No special considerations except to minimize coughing on emergence. Consider 1 mg/kg iv lidocaine.	
Blood and fluid requirements	IV: 18 ga × 1 NS/LR @ 5-8 ml/kg/h Fluid warmer	Blood loss should be minimal.
Monitoring	Standard monitors (see p. B-1). Urinary catheter NG tube	Others as indicated by patient status. Prevent hypothermia (forced air warmer, heated and humidified gases, warming blanket, warm OR, etc.).
Positioning	✓ and pad pressure points. ✓ eyes.	Careful positioning and padding of the patient is essential.
Complications	Hemorrhage from trocar insertion. Subcutaneous reverse	These complications (associated with the preperitoneal approach), as well as the general complications of laparoscopy, are discussed in Anesthetic Considerations for Laparoscopic Cholecystectomy, p. 420.

POSTOPERATIVE

Complications	N/V Urinary retention	Metoclopramide (10 mg iv), ondansetron (4 mg iv) Straight catheterization of the bladder
Pain management	Oral opiates	Tylenol #3 – 2 tabs po q 6 h (weak) or Percocet – 2 tabs po q 6 h.
	Ketorolac	30 mg iv
Tests	As indicated by patient status.	

References

1. Arregui ME, Navarrete J, Davis C, et al: Laparoscopic inguinal herniorrhaphy. *Surg Clin North Am* 1993; 73(3):513-27.
2. Atabek U: A survey of preferred approach to inguinal hernia repair: laparoscopic or inguinal incision? *Am Surg* 1994; 60(4):255-58.
3. Cooper SS: Laparoscopic inguinal hernia repair: is the enthusiasm justified? *Am Surg* 1997; 63(1):103-6.
4. Cunningham AJ: Laparoscopic surgery—anesthetic implications. *Surg Endosc* 1994; 8(11):1272-84.
5. Kozal R, Lange PM, Kosir M, et al: A prospective, randomized study of open vs laparoscopic inguinal hernia repair. *Arch Surg* 1997;132:292-95.
6. Liem MS: Comparison of conventional anterior surgery and laparoscopic surgery for inguinal-hernia repair. *N Engl J Med* 1997; 336(22):1541-47.
7. Notaras MJ: Laparoscopic inguinal hernia repair. *Br J Surg* 1997; 84:579-80.
8. Schrenk P: Prospective randomized trial comparing postoperative pain and return to physical activity after transabdominal preperitoneal, total preperitoneal or Shouldice technique for inguinal hernia repair. *Br J Surg* 1996; 83(11):1563-66.
9. Stoker DL: Laparoscopic versus open inguinal hernia repair: randomised prospective trial. *Lancet* 1994; 343(8908): 1243-45.

10. Tschudi J: Controlled multicenter trial of laparoscopic transabdominal preperitoneal hernioplasty vs Shouldice herniorrhaphy. Early results. *Surg Endosc* 1996; 10(8):845-47.
11. Wilson MS: Prospective trial comparing Lichtenstein with laparoscopic tension-free mesh repair of inguinal hernia. *Br J Surg* 1995; 82(2):274-77.
12. Zucker KA, ed: *Surgical Laparoscopy Update*. Quality Medical Publishing, St Louis: 1993.

Surgeon

Harry A. Oberhelman, MD, FACS

7.8 PANCREATIC SURGERY

Anesthesiologist

Steven K. Howard, MD

OPERATIVE DRAINAGE FOR PANCREATITIS

SURGICAL CONSIDERATIONS

Description: Operative drainage for pancreatitis is usually indicated when a peripancreatic collection of fluid becomes infected. Pancreatic abscesses often develop in the lesser sac or, less often, adjacent to and along the pancreas. The infection may subsequently spread to the subphrenic spaces or into the pericolic gutters. Fistulization into adjacent organs, particularly the transverse colon, is common. Severe intraabdominal hemorrhage from erosion into major arteries lying adjacent to the pancreas may also occur.[1] Exploration of the peritoneal cavity is performed before opening the lesser sac. Fluid or abscess collection lateral to the left and right sides of the colon should be palpated, as should the base of the transverse mesocolon and its subhepatic areas. The gastrocolic ligament is incised to approach the pancreas. There are different operative approaches, depending on location of involvement and surgeon's preference. Upper midline or transverse abdominal incisions are used most often. Posterior drainage through the bed of the 12th rib or retroperitoneal lateral approaches may be used (Fig 7.8-1).

Usual preop diagnosis: Pancreatitis 2° to biliary tract disease, alcoholism, idiopathic

SUMMARY OF PROCEDURE

Position	Supine
Incision	Midline, transverse, synchronous anterior and posterior
Unique considerations	Must perform adequate debridement of necrotic tissue and provide adequate drainage of abdomen; NG tube
Antibiotics	Cefotetan 1-2 g 30 min preop
Surgical time	1-2 h
Closing considerations	Adequate drainage of pancreatic bed and fluid resuscitation of patient
EBL	300-750 ml
Postop care	Routine wound and drain care; PACU → room (occasionally ICU)
Mortality	8-30%
Morbidity	Fistulae formation: 18-55% Delayed gastric emptying: 50% Unremitting sepsis: 10-30% Atelectasis: 5-10% Respiratory deterioration: 5% Hemorrhage Bowel perforations
Pain score	7-9

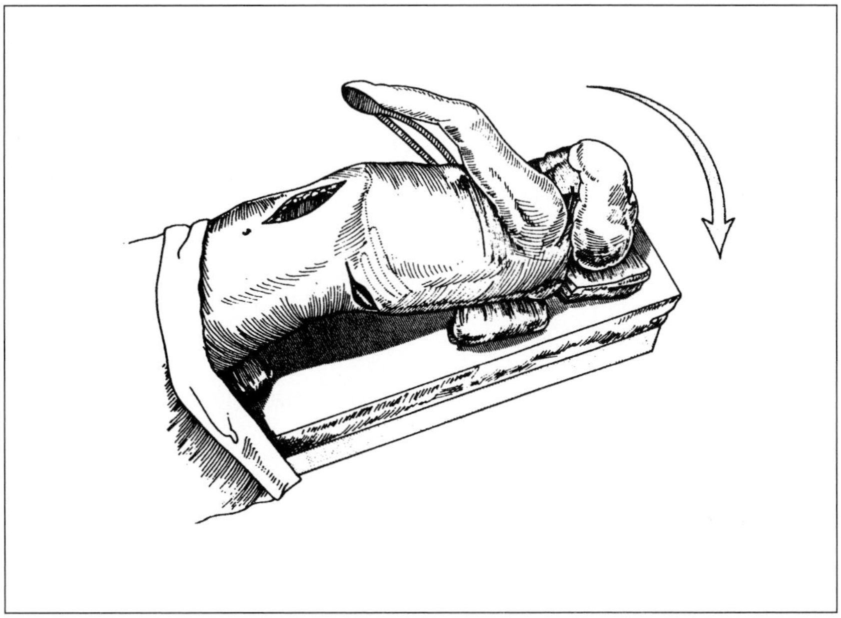

Figure 7.8-1. Incision for anterior and posterior drainage in pancreatitis. Note that bed or table is rotated until patient is almost supine. (Reproduced with permission from Berne TV, Donovan AJ: Synchronous anterior and posterior drainage of pancreatic abscess. *Arch Surg* 1981; 116: 527-33. Copyright 1981, American Medical Association.)

PATIENT POPULATION CHARACTERISTICS

Age range	30-60 yr
Male:Female	1:1
Incidence	10-40% of patients with pancreatitis
Etiology	Alcoholism (30-50%); postop pancreatitis (15-40%); biliary tract disease (20-30%); idiopathic pancreatitis (15-20%)
Associated conditions	See Etiology, above.

ANESTHETIC CONSIDERATIONS

See Anesthetic Considerations for Pancreatic Surgery, p. 443.

Reference

1. Berne TV: Pancreatic abscesses. *Probl Gen Surg* 1984; 1:569-82.

DRAINAGE OF PANCREATIC PSEUDOCYST

SURGICAL CONSIDERATIONS

Description: Internal drainage of a pancreatic pseudocyst may be accomplished by anastomosing the cyst to the stomach, duodenum or other small bowel via a Roux-en-Y loop of jejunum. The procedure of choice for internal decompression depends on the location of the pseudocyst in relation to the portion of the GI tract that will provide maximal dependent drainage of the cyst. Operation is best delayed for a period of 4-6 weeks to permit maturation of the cyst wall.[3] If operation is indicated, the abdomen is entered via a midline incision. If the pseudocyst lies behind the stomach (or duodenum), it is approached anteriorly, through the posterior wall of the stomach (or duodenum). A circular portion of the posterior wall is excised, allowing entry into the cyst cavity, which is then drained. An anastomosis is created between the cyst and stomach (or duodenum) by using interrupted sutures. The anterior wall of the stomach (or duodenum) is then closed. If the cyst presents inferior to the stomach, it is anastomosed in a similar fashion to a Roux-en-Y loop of jejunum. Drains are placed appropriately. External drainage may suffice, if it is not possible to provide internal drainage. Spontaneous resolution of pancreatic pseudocyst may be expected in 20% or more of patients.[1] If infection of the pseudocyst occurs with clinical signs of sepsis, **external drainage** percutaneously under CT guidance or operative **internal drainage** is indicated.

Usual preop diagnosis: Pseudocyst of pancreas 2° to acute pancreatitis

SUMMARY OF PROCEDURE

	Internal Drainage	External Drainage
Position	Supine	⇐
Incision	Midline abdominal	⇐
Unique considerations	Location of pseudocyst in relation to GI tract; NG tube	Accessibility for percutaneous decompression; NG tube
Antibiotics	Cefotetan 1-2 g 30 min preop	⇐
Surgical time	1-2 h	1 h
Closing considerations	Adequate drainage	⇐
EBL	100-300 ml	⇐
Postop care	NG decompression	⇐
Mortality[3]	10-12%	3-4%

	Internal Drainage	External Drainage
Morbidity[3]	Bleeding: 5-7%	< 2%
	Recurrence: 2-3%	2-5%
	Sepsis: < 5%	⇐
Pain score	6-8	5-7

PATIENT POPULATION CHARACTERISTICS

Age range	15-80 yr
Male:Female	1:1
Incidence	Rare
Etiology	Acute pancreatitis; trauma; malignancy
Associated conditions	Acute pancreatitis: 90%

ANESTHETIC CONSIDERATIONS

See Anesthetic Considerations for Pancreatic Surgery, p. 443.

References

1. Bradley EL, Clements JL Jr, Gonzalez AC: The natural history of pancreatic pseudocysts: a unified concept of management. *Am J Surg* 1979; 137(1):135-41.
2. Criad E, Destefano AA, et al: Long-term results of percutaneous catheter drainage of pancreatic pseudocysts. *Surg Gynecol Obstet* 1992; 175:293.
3. Grace RR, Jordan PH Jr: Unresolved problems of pancreatic pseudocysts. *Ann Surg* 1976; 184(1):16-21.
4. Warshaw AL, Rattner DW: Timing of surgical drainage for pancreatic pseudocyst: clinical and chemical criteria. *Ann Surg* 1985; 202(6):720-24.

PANCREATICOJEJUNOSTOMY

SURGICAL CONSIDERATIONS

Description: **Pancreaticojejunostomy,** as advocated by **Puestow,**[3] consists of a longitudinal opening of the pancreatic duct, from the site of transection of the tail of the pancreas to a point just to the right of the mesenteric vessels. The widely opened duct is then anastomosed to a Roux-en-Y loop of jejunum (Fig 7.8-2A). This is necessary because of the multiple strictures and dilatations that occur along the duct system. Resection of the pancreatic tail and spleen are optional. Through a midline or transverse abdominal incision, the pancreas is exposed by mobilizing the duodenum (**Kocher maneuver**), exposing the head of the pancreas, and opening the lesser sac to visualize the body and tail. The pancreas is mobilized by dissecting it away from portal vein, celiac plexus and splenic vessels. Hemorrhage may complicate this stage of the surgery. The pancreatic duct may be aspirated to identify its location. A Roux-en-Y loop of jejunum is then brought up to the pancreas and anastomosed to the opened duct or pancreatic capsule. A drain is left along the anastomosis. The wound is closed in the usual fashion.

Variant procedure or approaches: If the obstruction of the pancreatic duct is limited to the head of the pancreas, one may merely perform a retrograde drainage; that is, anastomosing the distal transected pancreas to a Roux-en-Y loop of the jejunum (**Duval procedure** [Fig 7.8-2B]).[1] A Whipple resection (pancreatoduodenectomy) is an alternative surgical treatment for chronic pancreatitis confined to the head of the gland.

Usual preop diagnosis: Chronic pancreatitis

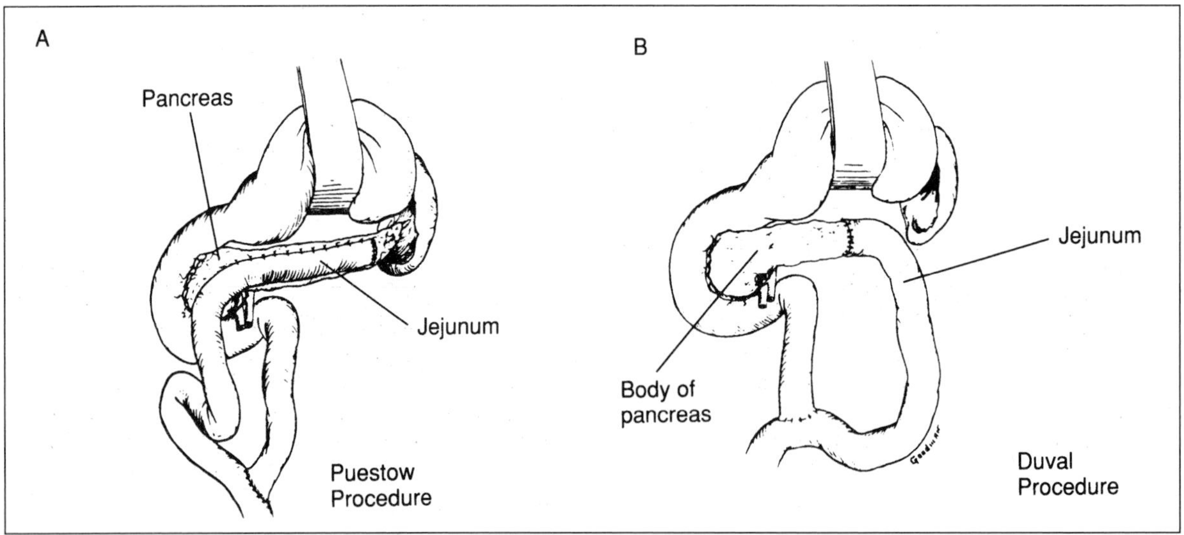

Figure 7.8-2. Operative management of chronic pancreatitis: (A) onlay Roux-en-Y pancreaticojejunostomy (Puestow); (B) distal Roux-en-Y pancreaticojejunostomy (Duval). (Reproduced with permission from Hardy JD: *Hardy's Textbook of Surgery*. JB Lippincott: 1988.)

SUMMARY OF PROCEDURE

	Longitudinal Pancreaticojejunostomy (Puestow)	**Caudal Pancreaticojejunostomy (Duval)**
Position	Supine	⇐
Incision	Midline abdominal or transverse	⇐
Antibiotics	Cefotetan 1-2 g 30 min preop	⇐
Surgical time	2-3 h	1-2 h
Closing considerations	NG tube; adequate drainage	⇐
EBL	300-400 ml	100-200 ml
Postop care	NG decompression	⇐
Mortality	1-4%	2-3%
Morbidity	Failure to relieve pain: 25-50%	25-60%
	Pancreatic leak: 5-10%	5%
	Wound infection: 5%	⇐
Pain score	6-8	6-8

PATIENT POPULATION CHARACTERISTICS

Age range	17-72 yr
Male:Female	2.5:1
Etiology	Alcoholism; biliary tract disease; idiopathic; traumatic; familial
Associated conditions	Biliary tract disease (25-50%); hyperparathyroidism (< 5%)

ANESTHETIC CONSIDERATIONS

See Anesthetic Considerations for Pancreatic Surgery, p. 443.

References

1. Duval MK Jr: Caudal pancreatico-jejunostomy for chronic relapsing pancreatitis. *Ann Surg* 1954; 140(6):775-85.
2. Howard VM, Zhaug Z: Pancreaticodenectomy (Whipple resection) in the treatment of chronic pancreatitis. *World J Surg* 1990; 14:77-82.
3. Morrow CE, Cohen JI, Sutherland DE, Najarian JS: Chronic pancreatitis: long-term surgical results of pancreatic duct drainage, pancreatic resection, and near total pancreatectomy and islet autotransplantation. *Surgery* 1984; 96(4):608-16.
4. Puestow CB, Gillesby WJ: Retrograde surgical drainage of the pancreas for chronic relapsing pancreatitis. *Arch Surg* 1958; 76:898-907.

PANCREATECTOMY

SURGICAL CONSIDERATIONS

Description: **Distal pancreatectomy** is performed for tumors in the distal half of the pancreas. The peritoneum is incised along the inferior surface of the pancreas, with care being taken to avoid tearing the middle colic vessels. Following mobilization of the spleen, the splenic artery is ligated near its origin. The gastrosplenic ligament is divided, ligating the short gastric vessels and the left gastroepiploic vessel. The inferior mesenteric vein is ligated at the inferior border of the pancreas, and the splenic vein is ligated at the proposed point of transection. The transected pancreas (Fig 7.8-3) is usually stapled and drained, although some surgeons suture the cut end and ligate the duct. The spleen may be preserved when operating for benign disease, provided the splenic vessels are ligated proximal to the splenic hilum in order to preserve collateral blood flow.

Variant procedure or approaches: **Subtotal pancreatectomy** usually implies resecting the pancreas from the mesenteric vessels distally, leaving the head and uncinate process intact. This procedure may be performed for tumor or chronic pancreatitis. **Child's procedure** consists of removing all of the pancreas except a rim of tissue along the lesser curvature of the duodenum; preserving the duodenum makes it unnecessary to reconstruct the bile duct. This procedure is usually reserved for patients with chronic pancreatitis.

Usual preop diagnosis: Carcinoma of pancreas; islet cell tumors; chronic pancreatitis

SUMMARY OF PROCEDURE

	Distal Pancreatectomy	Subtotal Pancreatectomy	Child's Procedure
Position	Supine	⇐	⇐
Incision	Midline abdominal or chevron	⇐	⇐
Special instrumentation	Denier retractor	⇐	⇐
Unique considerations	NG tube	⇐	Preservation of vasculature of duodenum
Antibiotics	Cefotetan 1-2 g 30 min preop	⇐	⇐
Surgical time	2-3 h	⇐	3-4 h
Closing considerations	Adequate drainage	⇐	⇐
EBL	300-500 ml	500-750 ml	500-1000 ml
Postop care	NG decompression; PACU	⇐	⇐
Mortality	< 5%	⇐	⇐
Morbidity	Diabetes: 5%	⇐	⇐
	Wound infection: 5%	⇐	⇐
	Pancreatic fistula: < 5%	⇐	90%
	Common bile duct injury	⇐	⇐
	Hemorrhage	⇐	⇐
	Duodenal necrosis	⇐	⇐
	Pancreatic leakage	⇐	⇐
	Pancreatic insufficiency	⇐	⇐
Pain score	6-8	6-8	6-8

PATIENT POPULATION CHARACTERISTICS

Age range	30-60 yr
Male:Female	1:1
Incidence	~ 26,000/yr in U.S.
Etiology	Adenocarcinoma; chronic pancreatitis; islet cell tumors
Associated conditions	Alcoholism and biliary tract disease with chronic pancreatitis (90%); other endocrine disorders (3-5%)

ANESTHETIC CONSIDERATIONS

See Anesthetic Considerations for Pancreatic Surgery, p. 443.

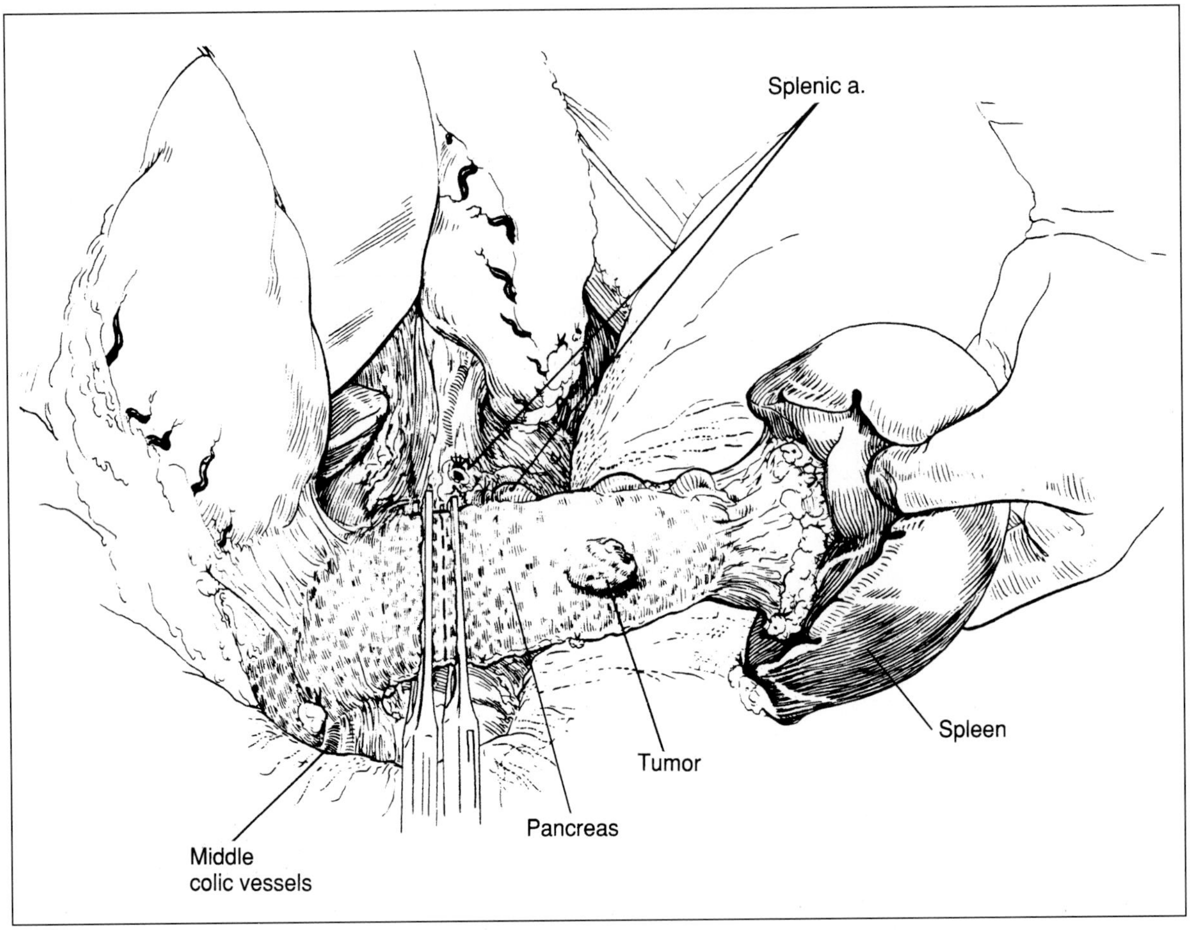

Figure 7.8-3. Resection of pancreatic tumor. (Reproduced with permission from Zollinger RM Jr, Zollinger RM: *Atlas of Surgical Operations*, 6th edition. MacMillan: 1988.)

Reference

1. Mulholland MW: Chronic pancreatitis. In *Surgery: Scientific Principles and Practice*, 2nd edition. Greenfield LJ, et al, eds. Lippincott-Raven Publishers, Philadelphia: 1997, 889-900.

WHIPPLE RESECTION

SURGICAL CONSIDERATIONS

Description: A **Whipple resection** consists of a **pancreatoduodenectomy**, followed by an **anastomosis** of the distal pancreatic stump into the jejunum, a **choledochojejunostomy** and a **gastrojejunostomy** (Fig 7.8-4). On entering the peritoneal cavity, one determines the resectability of the pancreatic lesion. Contraindications to resection include: involvement of the superior mesenteric vessels; infiltration by tumor into root of the mesentery; extension into the porta hepatis, with involvement of the hepatic artery; and liver metastases. If the tumor is deemed resectable, further mobilization of the head of the pancreas is performed. The common duct is transected above the cystic duct entry and the gall bladder is removed. Once the superior mesenteric vein is freed from the pancreas, the latter is transected, with care being taken not to injure the splenic vein. The stomach is transected at the antral-body junction or beyond the pylorus if uninvolved by tumor. The jejunum is transected beyond the ligament of Treitz and the specimen removed by severing the vascular connections with the mesenteric vessels. Reconstitution is achieved by anastomosing the distal pancreatic stump, bile duct and stomach into the jejunum. Drains are placed adjacent to the pancreatic anastomosis. Some surgeons stent the latter until healing has occurred.

Variant procedure or approaches: There are several variants that consist of an extension of the Whipple procedure: **total pancreatectomy**; **regional pancreatectomy**, involving resection and reconstruction of the retropancreatic superior mesenteric vein and/or artery; and the pylorus-preserving anastomosed **pancreatic resection**. In addition, the distal pancreatic stump may be anastomosed to the posterior wall of the stomach.

Usual preop diagnosis: Carcinoma of the pancreas; malignant cystadenomas; chronic pancreatitis

SUMMARY OF PROCEDURE

	Whipple[2]	Total Pancreatectomy[4]	Regional Pancreatectomy[4]
Position	Supine	⇐	⇐
Incision	Midline abdominal or generous oblique	Midline abdominal or chevron	Midline abdominal or generous oblique
Special instrumentation	Denier retractor	⇐	⇐
Unique considerations	Stenting of pancreatic duct	None	Stenting of pancreatic duct
Antibiotics	Cefotetan 2 g preop	⇐	⇐
Surgical time	4-5 h	4-6 h	5-6 h
Closing considerations	Securing pancreatic stent, if used	None	Securing pancreatic stent, if used
EBL	500-750 ml	750-1000 ml	750-1500 ml
Postop care	NG decompression; pancreatic decompression; PACU/ICU	NG decompression; diabetes management	⇐
Mortality	8-12%	12%	15%
Morbidity	Delayed gastric emptying: 25%	⇐	< 2%
	Sepsis: 5-15%	5%	25%
	Hemorrhage: 5%	< 5%	5%
	MI: 1-3%	⇐	< 5%
	Biliary fistula: < 2%	< 1%	< 2%
	Pancreatic fistula: 3-5%	NA	3-5%
Pain score	7-9	7-9	7-9

PATIENT POPULATION CHARACTERISTICS (for cancer of pancreas[1])

Age range	50-80 yr
Male:Female	1:1
Incidence	10th most common cancer in U.S. – 28,000/yr
Etiology	Familial and genetic factors (probably most important); diabetes; alcohol, tobacco, coffee intake; diet; pancreatitis
Associated conditions	See Etiology, above.

ANESTHETIC CONSIDERATIONS FOR PANCREATIC SURGERY

(Procedures covered: drainage for pancreatitis; drainage of pancreatic pseudocyst; pancreaticojejunostomy; pancreatectomy; Whipple resection)

PREOPERATIVE

Patients presenting for pancreatic surgery typically can be divided into three groups: (1) those with acute pancreatitis who have failed medical treatment in the past and who may be extremely ill, presenting for surgery during an exacerbation of pancreatitis or when the diagnosis is in doubt; (2) patients with carcinoma of the pancreas, including hormone-

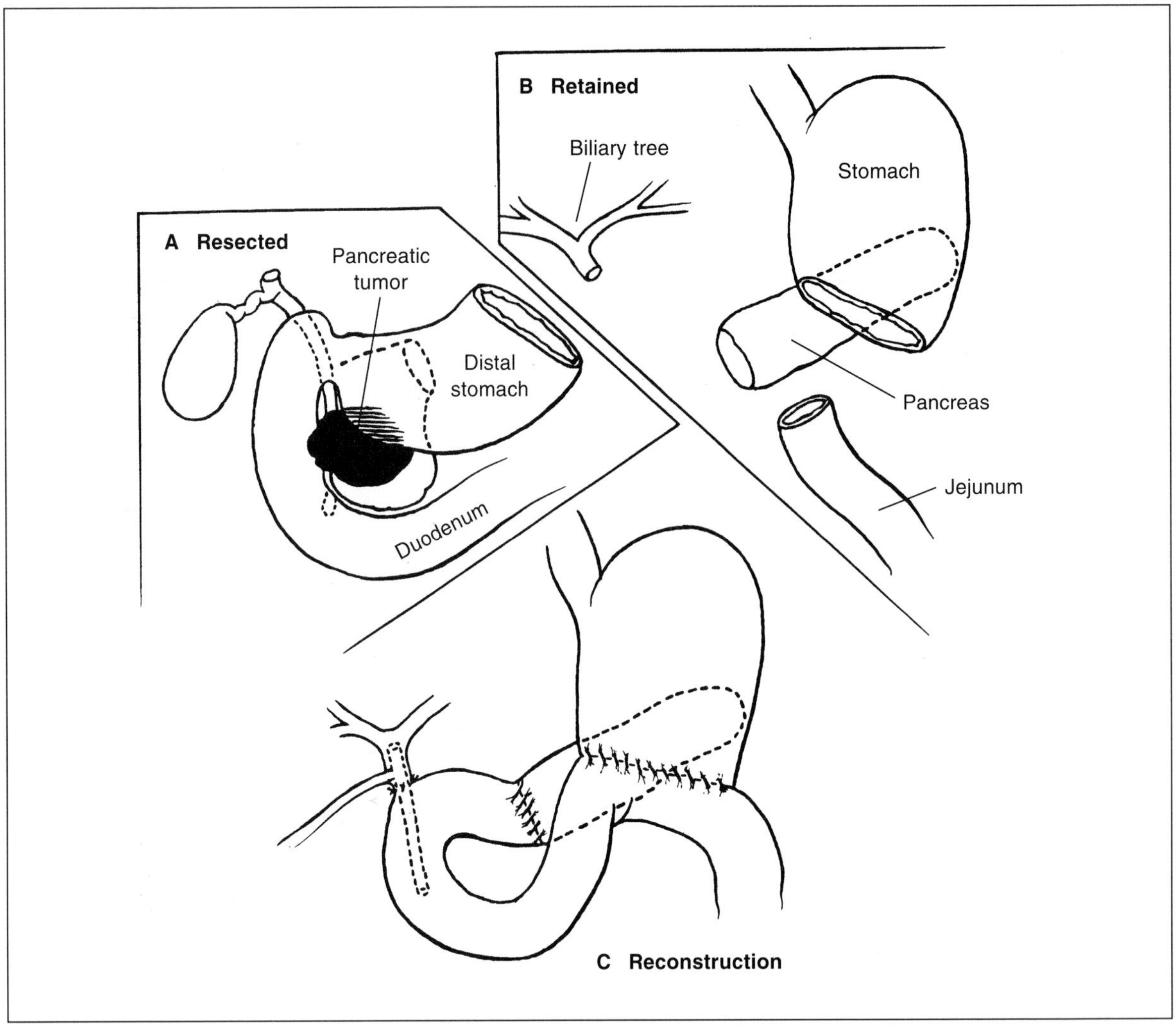

Figure 7.8-4. Standard pancreaticoduodenectomy. **(A)** Structures resected, including distal stomach, entire duodenum, head and neck of pancreas with tumor, gallbladder, and distal extrahepatic biliary tree. **(B)** Structures retained, including proximal stomach, body and tail of pancreas, proximal biliary tree, and jejunum distal to ligament of Treitz. **(C)** Reconstruction: proximal pancreaticojejunostomy, hepaticojejunostomy over T tube, and distal gastrojejunostomy. (Reproduced with permission from Hardy JD: *Hardy's Textbook of Surgery*, 2nd edition. JB Lippincott, Philadelphia: 1988, 718.)

secreting tumors such as insulinoma and gastrinoma (Zollinger-Ellison syndrome); and (3) patients suffering from the sequelae of chronic pancreatitis, e.g., pseudocyst or abscess.

Respiratory Respiratory compromise—such as pleural effusions, atelectasis and ARDS, progressing to respiratory failure—may occur in up to 50% of patients with acute pancreatitis. Postop mechanical ventilation may be needed for these patients.
Tests: Consider CXR; ABG; as indicated from H&P.

Cardiovascular Patients with acute pancreatitis may be hypotensive and may require aggressive volume resuscitation with crystalloid and even blood prior to surgery. ECG change simulating myocardial ischemia may be seen in patients with acute pancreatitis. Severe electrolyte disturbances may be associated with acute pancreatitis and some hormone-secreting tumors of the pancreas. ↓K^+ may be severe and should be corrected preop (correction of ↓Mg^{++} may improve ↓K^+.)
Tests: ECG; electrolytes; others as indicated from H&P.

Gastrointestinal Jaundice and abdominal pain are common presenting Sx in this group of patients. The presence of ileus or intestinal obstruction should mandate full-stomach precautions and rapid-sequence induction. Electrolyte disturbances are common with acute pancreatitis and may include hypochloremic metabolic alkalosis, ↓Ca^{++}, ↓Mg^{++} and ↑glucose. These abnormalities should be

Gastrointestinal, cont. corrected preop. Zollinger-Ellison syndrome is associated with diarrhea and severe peptic ulcer disease which may be complicated by perforation and bleeding. Vipomas are associated with massive watery diarrhea and electrolyte disturbances.
Tests: Electrolytes; glucose; LFTs; CA^{++}; amylase; others as indicated from H&P.

Renal Patients should be evaluated for renal insufficiency and anesthetic plan adjusted accordingly.
Tests: BUN; creatinine; others as indicated from H&P.

Endocrine Many patients with acute pancreatitis may have diabetes 2° loss of pancreatic tissue. Hormone-secreting tumors of the pancreas are occasionally associated with multiple endocrine neoplasia syndromes (MEN-I, parathyroid, pancreas, pituitary and pheochromocytomas). Insulinoma is the most common hormone-secreting tumor of the pancreas and can result in hypoglycemia. Perioperative blood glucose measurements are essential.
Tests: Electrolytes; glucose; others as indicated from H&P (e.g., urinary VMA if pheochromocytoma suspected).

Hematologic Hct may be falsely elevated, due to hemoconcentration, or low, 2° hemorrhage. Coagulopathy may be present.
Tests: CBC with differential; Plt; consider PT, PTT.

Laboratory Other tests as indicated from H&P.

Premedication Standard premedication (see p. B-2). Note: full-stomach precautions in patients with intestinal obstruction (see p. B-5): ranitidine 50 mg iv and 0.3 M Na citrate (30 ml po 10 min preop).

INTRAOPERATIVE

Anesthetic technique: GETA ± epidural for postop analgesia. If postop epidural analgesia is planned, insertion of the catheter prior to anesthetic induction is helpful to establish correct placement in the epidural space (accomplished by injecting 5-7 ml of 1% lidocaine in order to elicit a segmental block).

Induction The patient with bowel obstruction or ileus is at risk for pulmonary aspiration, and rapid-sequence induction with cricoid pressure is indicated (see p. B-5). If the patient is clinically hypovolemic, restore intravascular volume (colloid, crystalloid or blood) prior to induction and titrate induction dose of sedative/hypnotic agents. Etomidate (0.2-0.4 mg/kg iv) or ketamine (1-3 mg/kg iv) may provide less hemodynamic depression on induction of anesthesia.

Maintenance Standard maintenance (see p. B-3). Avoid N_2O to minimize bowel distension. **Combined epidural/GA:** A local aesthetic (2% lidocaine with 1:200,000 epinephrine) can be injected into a thoracic (3-5 ml) or lumbar (5-10 ml) epidural catheter (q 60 min) to provide both anesthesia and optimal surgical exposure (contracted bowel and profound muscle relaxation). A continuous infusion of local anesthetic (e.g., 2% lidocaine or 0.25% bupivacaine at 5-10 ml/h [lumbar], or 5 ml/h [thoracic]) may enhance hemodynamic stability. Be prepared to treat hypotension with fluid and vasopressors (e.g., ephedrine 5-10 mg iv). If epidural opiates are used for postop analgesia, a loading dose (e.g., hydromorphone 1.0 mg) should be administered 1-2 h before conclusion of surgery. Systemic sedatives (droperidol, opiates, benzodiazepines, etc.) should be minimized during this type of anesthesia as they increase the likelihood of postop respiratory depression.

Emergence The decision to extubate at the end of surgery depends on the patient's underlying cardiopulmonary status and extent of the surgical procedure. Patients should be hemodynamically stable, warm, alert, cooperative, and fully reversed from any muscle relaxants prior to extubation.

Blood and fluid requirements

Anticipate large fluid loss.
IV: 14-16 ga × 2
NS/LR @ 10-20 ml/kg/h
Warm all fluids.
Humidify inhaled gases.

Blood loss can be significant, and blood should be immediately available. Procedures tend to be long and extensive, leading to hypothermia and large 3rd-space fluid loss. If procedure does not involve cancer or infection, cell-saving devices can be utilized. Guide fluid management by UO, filling pressures, CO.

Monitoring

Standard monitors (see p. B-1).
UO
Arterial line
± CVP or PA catheter

Most pancreatic surgery is associated with major fluid shifts and fluid loss. Invasive monitoring is usually required. In patients with cardiopulmonary compromise, a PA catheter may prove helpful for intraop fluid management. Use forced-air warmer to maintain normothermia.

Positioning	✓ and pad pressure points. ✓ eyes.	
Complications	Hypocalcemia Hypovolemia	Release of pancreatic lipase → omental fat saponification → ↓Ca^{++}. Significant 3rd-space and evaporative losses contribute to hypovolemia. Major hemorrhage can occur during dissection of the pancreas from the mesenteric and portal vessels.

POSTOPERATIVE

Complications	Hyperglycemia Electrolyte imbalance Hypovolemia Hypothermia Hypocalcemia	Total pancreatectomy is associated with a brittle diabetes that can be very difficult to control. Subtotal resections lead to variable hyperglycemia.
Pain management	Continuous epidural analgesia (see p. C-1). PCA (see p. C-3).	Patient should be recovered in an ICU or hospital ward that is accustomed to treating the side effects of epidural opiates (e.g., respiratory depression, breakthrough pain, nausea, pruritus).
Tests	CXR (if CVP placed); ABG; Hct	Electrolytes; calcium; glucose; platelets—as indicated for postop management.

References

1. Bell RH Jr: Neoplasms of the exocrine pancreas. In *Surgery: Scientific Principles and Practice*, 2nd edition. Greenfield LJ, et al, eds. Lippincott-Raven Publishers, Philadelphia: 1997, 901-17.
2. Longmire WP Jr: Cancer of the pancreas: palliative operation, Whipple procedure, or total pancreatectomy. *World J Surg* 1984; 8(6):872-79.
3. Merritt WT: Anesthesia for gastrointestinal surgery. In *Principles and Practice of Anesthesiology*. Longnecker DE, Tinker JH, Morgan GE, eds. Mosby-Year Book Inc, St Louis: 1998, 1881-1903.
4. Moossa AR, Scott MH, Lavelle-Jones M: The place of total and extended total pancreatectomy in pancreatic cancer. *World J Surg* 1984; 8(6):895-99.
5. Yeo CY: Neoplasms of the endocrine pancreas. In *Surgery: Scientific Principles and Practice*, 2nd edition. Greenfield LJ, et al, eds. Lippincott-Raven Publishers, Philadelphia: 1997, 918-30.

Surgeon

Harry A. Oberhelman, MD, FACS

7.9 PERITONEAL SURGERY

Anesthesiologist

Steven K. Howard, MD

EXPLORATORY OR STAGING LAPAROTOMY

SURGICAL CONSIDERATIONS

Description: Exploratory laparotomy is indicated primarily in patients suffering penetrating or severe abdominal blunt trauma. It is important that a thorough and systematic intraabdominal examination be carried out to prevent missing significant injuries (e.g., ruptured duodenum or transected pancreas). Any active bleeding should be controlled prior to a systematic examination. Other indications for laparotomy include certain patients with fever of undetermined origin or those in whom a specific diagnosis cannot be made, or for staging of selected patients with Hodgkin's disease. A **staging laparotomy** consists of **splenectomy**, **wedge** and **needle biopsies** of both lobes of the liver, and biopsies of the periaortic, celiac, mesenteric and portahepatic lymph nodes. In young women, suturing (pexing) the ovaries in the midline protects them from radiation. Indications for staging in Hodgkin's disease and lymphomas vary from institution to institution.

Basically, the procedure begins with a midline abdominal incision; then the abdomen is explored, and both needle and wedge biopsies of the liver are performed. The spleen is removed by incising the lateral peritoneal attachment and delivering the spleen into the wound. The short gastric vessels are cut and ligated and the splenic vessels exposed. These are cut individually and ligated, and the spleen is removed. Paraaortic nodes are exposed through a left paraaortic incision in the retroperitoneum, and removed for biopsy. Lymph channels are clipped to prevent lymphatic leakage. The nodes dissected extend to the inferior margin of the duodenum. It may be necessary to cross the aorta and biopsy the enlarged nodes on the right side.

Usual preop diagnosis: Abdominal trauma; Hodgkin's disease or other lymphomas

SUMMARY OF PROCEDURE

	Staging Laparotomy	Exploratory Laparotomy
Position	Supine	⇐
Incision	Midline abdominal	⇐ + Transverse
Special instrumentation	Abdominal retractor	⇐
Unique considerations	Ovarian pexy	Careful monitoring of BP in trauma patients
Antibiotics	Cefazolin iv 1 g preop	Cefazolin 1-2 g iv in trauma patients
Surgical time	1.5-2 h	Variable, 1-2 h+
Closing considerations	Splenic bed hemostasis	Hemostasis
EBL	100-200 ml	Variable, 200-500 ml
Postop care	NG decompression; PACU → room	ICU for trauma patients
Mortality	< 1%	2-5%
Morbidity	Prolonged ileus: 10-15%	⇐ + In trauma patients:
	Pulmonary complications: 5-10%	Atelectasis: 5-10%
	Wound infection: 2-3%	Wound infection: 5-10%
	Small bowel obstruction: 1%	Hemorrhage: 1-3%
	Intraperitoneal bleeding: < 1%	Pneumonia: < 1%
Pain score	6-8	6-8

PATIENT POPULATION CHARACTERISTICS

Age range	15-60 yr	15-75 yr
Male:Female	1:1.5	1:1
Incidence	Common	⇐
Etiology	Unknown	Trauma
Associated conditions	Hodgkin's disease (95%); lymphoma (5%)	Other visceral or vascular injuries in trauma

ANESTHETIC CONSIDERATIONS

(Procedures covered: exploratory/staging laparotomy; splenectomy)

PREOPERATIVE

Typically, patients presenting for **staging laparotomy** (which usually includes splenectomy) have Hodgkin's disease or some other lymphomatous disorder. Apart from the primary disease, these patients are in reasonably good health and will not have undergone radiation or chemotherapy prior to the staging laparotomy. Patients presenting for **splenectomy** may be divided into two less healthy groups: (1) trauma patients (whose management is described in Chapter 7.13, Trauma Surgery) and (2) a more complex group that includes myeloproliferative disorders and other varieties of hypersplenism. These two groups may present complex perioperative management problems.

Respiratory Patients who have splenomegaly may have a degree of left lower lobe atelectasis which should be evaluated by physical exam. Some may have been treated with bleomycin, a chemotherapeutic drug that causes pulmonary fibrosis at total doses > 200 mg/m^2. Methotrexate and cytarabine may also cause pulmonary fibrosis. Toxic drug effects are potentiated by smoking, XRT and high FiO_2.
Tests: CXR; others as clinically indicated.

Cardiovascular Patients with systemic disease requiring splenectomy may be chronically ill and have decreased cardiovascular reserve. Patients who have received doxorubicin (Adriamycin) at doses > 550 mg/m^2, may have a dose-dependent cardiotoxicity that can be worsened by XRT. Manifestations include ↓QRS amplitude, CHF, pleural effusions and dysrhythmias.
Tests: ECG; consider ECHO or MUGA scan to determine LV function, if indicated.

Neurological Patients may have neurological deficits from receiving chemotherapeutic agents (e.g., vinblastine and cisplatin can cause peripheral neuropathies). Any evidence of neurologic dysfunction should be documented in the preop evaluation.

Hematologic Patients are likely to present with splenomegaly 2° hematologic disease (Hodgkin's disease, non-Hodgkin's lymphoma, reticulum cell sarcoma, chronic leukemia, Felty's syndrome, myeloid metaplasia, thrombotic thrombocytopenic purpura, idiopathic thrombocytopenic purpura, idiopathic autoimmune hemolytic anemia, sickle cell disease, thalassemia, hereditary elliptocytosis, hereditary spherocytosis). Cytopenia is very common.
Tests: CBC with differential; Plt count

Hepatic Some chemotherapeutic agents (e.g., methotrexate) may be hepatotoxic. Evaluation of LFTs should be considered in patients deemed to be at risk.
Tests: LFTs, if indicated from H&P.

Renal Some chemotherapeutic drugs (e.g., methotrexate, cisplatin) are nephrotoxic; therefore, patients exposed to such agents can present with renal insufficiency.
Tests: Consider UA, electrolytes, BUN, creatinine, others as indicated from H&P.

Laboratory Other tests as indicated from H&P.

Premedication Standard premedication (see p. B-2). Administer stress dose of steroids (e.g., 100 mg hydrocortisone q 8 h on day of surgery) if patient has received them as part of chemotherapeutic regimen.

INTRAOPERATIVE

Anesthetic technique: GETA ± epidural for postop analgesia. If postop epidural analgesia is planned, placement of catheter prior to anesthetic induction is helpful to establish correct placement in the epidural space (accomplished by injecting 5-7 ml of 1% lidocaine via the epidural catheter, eliciting a segmental block).

Induction Standard induction (see p. B-2).

Maintenance Standard maintenance (see p. B-3). **Combined epidural/GA:** Local anesthetic (2% lidocaine with 1:200,000 epinephrine (5-10 ml q 60 min) can be injected incrementally into the epidural catheter to provide both anesthesia and optimal surgical exposure (contracted bowel and profound muscle relaxation). Be prepared to treat hypotension with fluids and vasopressors (e.g., ephedrine 5-10 mg iv). A continuous infusion of local anesthesia (e.g., 2% lidocaine or 0.25% bupivacaine) at 5-10 ml/h may enhance hemodynamic stability. If epidural opiates are used for postop analgesia, a loading dose (e.g., hydromorphone 1.0 mg) should be administered 1-2 h before conclusion of surgery. Systemic sedatives (droperidol, opiates, benzodiazepines, etc.) should be minimized as they increase the likelihood of postop respiratory depression.

Emergence No special considerations.

Blood and fluid requirements
IV: 14-16 ga × 1
NS/LR @ 10-15 ml/kg/h
Fluid warmer
Airway humidifier

Potential for major blood loss. In splenectomy patients, Plt transfusions should be given after ligation of splenic vessels (↓sequestration).

Monitoring	Standard monitors (see p. B-1).	Others as indicated by patient's status. Try to prevent hypothermia during long operations. Consider heated humidifier, warming blanket, warming room temperature, keeping patient covered until ready for prep, etc.
Positioning	✓ and pad pressure points. ✓ eyes.	
Complications	Unexpected bleeding	Plt transfusion may be necessary.

POSTOPERATIVE

Complications	Bleeding Atelectasis (usually left lower lobe)	Patient should be recovered in ICU or hospital ward that is accustomed to treating side effects of epidural opiates (e.g., respiratory depression, breakthrough pain, nausea, pruritus).
Pain management	Epidural analgesia PCA (see p. C-3).	
Tests	CXR, if CVP placed perioperatively; CBC and Plt count.	

References

1. Fitch JCK, Rinder CS: Cancer therapy and its anesthetic implications. In *Clinical Anesthesia*, 2nd edition. Barash PG, Cullen BF, Stoelting RK, eds. Lippincott-Raven Publishers, Philadelphia: 1997, 1219-36.
2. Merritt WT: Anesthesia for gastrointestinal surgery. In *Principles and Practice of Anesthesiology,* 2nd edition. Longnecker DE, Tinker JH, Morgan GE, eds. Mosby-Year Book, St Louis: 1998, 1881-1903.
3. Rutledge R, Sheldon GF: Abdominal Trauma. In *Operative Surgery*, 3rd edition. Nora PF, ed. WB Saunders Co., Philadelphia: 1990.
4. Taylor MA, Kaplan HS, Nelsen TS: Staging laparotomy with splenectomy for Hodgkin's disease: The Stanford experience. *World J Surg* 1985; 9(3):449-60.

SPLENECTOMY

SURGICAL CONSIDERATIONS

Description: Through a midline abdominal or left subcostal incision, the spleen is mobilized by dividing the lateral peritoneal attachments while the spleen is retracted medially. (Relevant anatomy is shown in Fig 7.9-1.) Once delivered into the operative wound, the short gastric vessels are clamped, cut and ligated. The splenic artery and vein are then exposed, with care being taken not to injure the tail of the pancreas. By keeping the splenic hilum between the operator's fingers and thumb, inadvertent bleeding can be controlled easily. Accessory spleens (incidence, 15-30%) should also be looked for if the splenectomy is being done for a hematologic disorder. They are found along the cephalad and caudad edges of the pancreas behind the stomach and in the area of the gastrohepatic ligament, greater omentum and the splenic hilum. All patients undergoing splenectomy should receive polyvalent pneumococcal vaccine either prior to operation or following surgery.

Variant procedure or approaches: Following trauma, efforts at splenic salvage (**splenorrhaphy**) should be made, if possible, to preserve all or part of the spleen. This may be accomplished by the use of local hemostatic techniques (electrocoagulation, argon beam coagulator, Surgicel or Gelfoam soaked in thrombin, microfibrillar collagen, and the use of fine sutures or mattress sutures with Teflon felt pledgets). Recently, splenectomy has been performed laparoscopically if the spleen is near normal size (see Laparoscopic Splenectomy, p. 422).

Usual preop diagnosis: Staging laparotomy; trauma; immune thrombocytopenic purpura; hereditary spherocytosis; other hereditary hemolytic anemia types; or a variety of myeloproliferative disorders

SUMMARY OF PROCEDURE

	Splenectomy	Splenorrhaphy
Position	Supine	⇐
Incision	Midline or left subcostal	⇐
Special instrumentation	Suitable abdominal retractors	⇐
Unique considerations	Potential for major blood loss during procedure; avoid splenic laceration and damage to tail of pancreas.	⇐
Antibiotics	Cefotetan 1 g preop	⇐
Surgical time	1-1.5 h	1-2 h
Closing considerations	Adequate hemostasis	⇐
EBL	50-100 ml	200-500 ml
Postop care	NG decompression; PACU (nontrauma)	⇐
Mortality	0-3%	⇐
Morbidity[2]	Thrombocytosis: 50-75% → DVT Pulmonary complications: 3-23% Pancreatitis and/or pancreatic fistula: 1.5-7.7% Subphrenic abscess: 0-6% Bleeding: 1-5% Overwhelming sepsis:[3] Adults – 0.3-1.8% Children – ≤ 4%	⇐ (Overall complication rate: 11.8%[1])
Pain score	5-7	5-7

PATIENT POPULATION CHARACTERISTICS

Age range	Any age
Male:Female	1:1
Incidence	Common
Etiology	See Usual preop diagnosis, above.
Associated conditions	Blood dyscrasia (30-50%); abdominal or thoracic trauma (25%); Hodgkin's disease (5-10%); tumors (5%)

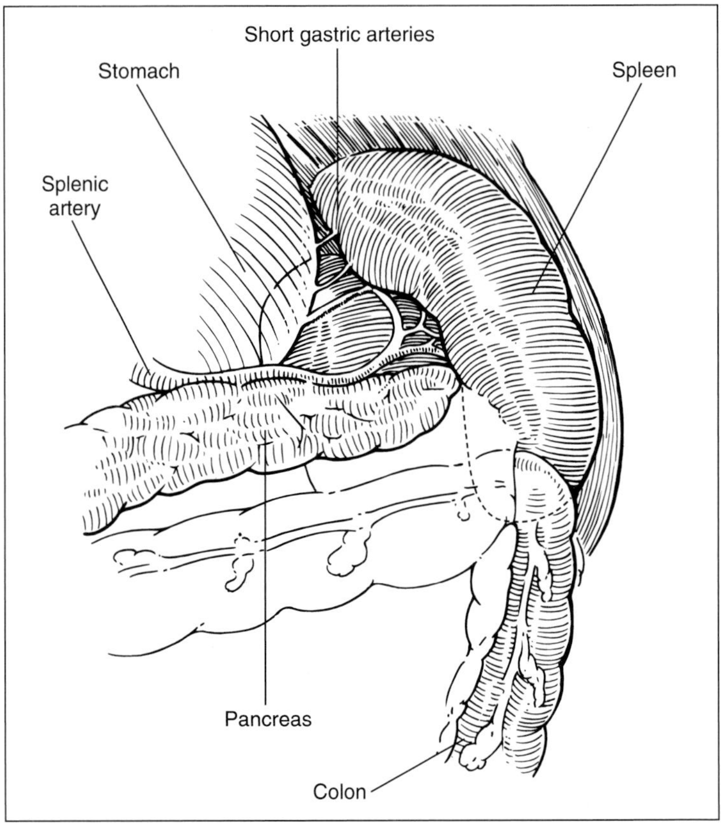

Figure 7.9-1. Relevant anatomy for splenectomy. (Reproduced with permission from Calne S, Pollard SG: *Operative Surgery*. Gower Medical Pub: 1992.)

ANESTHETIC CONSIDERATIONS

See Anesthetic Considerations following Exploratory or Staging Laparotomy, p. 449.

References

1. Feliciano DV et al: A four-year experience with splenectomy versus splenorrhaphy. *Ann Surg* 1985; 201(5):568-75.
2. Meyer, AA: Spleen. In *Surgery: Scientific Principles and Practice*, 2nd edition. Greenfield LJ, et al, eds. Lippincott-Raven Publishers, Philadelpha: 1997, 1262-82.
3. Pate JW, Peters TG, Andrews CR: Postsplenectomy complications. *Am Surg* 1985; 51(8):437-41.
4. Schwartz PE, et al: Postsplenectomy sepsis and mortality in adults. *JAMA* 1982; 248(18):2279-83.

EXCISION OF INTRAABDOMINAL, RETROPERITONEAL TUMORS

SURGICAL CONSIDERATIONS

Description: Intraabdominal and retroperitoneal tumors, other than those of visceral origin, consist primarily of sarcomas (liposarcoma, fibrous histiocytomas, mesenteric fibromas). They are usually approached through a long, midline incision for adequate exposure and to assess their resectability. Resection of such lesions may require excision of adjacent or involved small bowel or large intestine or other involved abdominal viscera. Care must be taken not to injure the ureters or major vessels, particularly at the root of the mesentery to the small bowel. If residual tumor remains, IORT may be indicated. In certain tumors the patient may still benefit from "tumor debulking" (removing as much tumor as possible and treating the remaining tumor with radiation and/or chemotherapy). Operative approaches are dictated by location of tumor. Although most operative approaches are transabdominal, some retroperitoneal tumors may be approached retroperitoneally via oblique incision on either side of the abdomen.

Usual preop diagnosis: Intraabdominal or peritoneal tumor

SUMMARY OF PROCEDURE

Position	Supine
Incision	Midline abdominal
Unique considerations	Availability of blood
Antibiotics	Cefazolin 1-2 g iv preop
Surgical time	3-4 h
Closing considerations	Hemostasis
EBL	300-1000 ml
Mortality	1-3%
Morbidity	Respiratory problems: 5-10% Wound infection: 2-4% Hemorrhage: 1-3%
Pain score	8-10

PATIENT POPULATION CHARACTERISTICS

Age range	Variable, 20-75 yr
Male:Female	1:1
Incidence	Common
Etiology	Unknown
Associated conditions	Partial bowel obstruction (15-20%); hydronephrosis (10-15%)

ANESTHETIC CONSIDERATIONS

See Anesthetic Considerations for Intestinal and Peritoneal Procedures, p. 370.

Reference

1. *Color Atlas of Demonstrations in Surgical Pathology*, Vol 1. Royal College of Surgeons of Edinburgh. Williams & Wilkins: 1983, 530-43.

DRAINAGE OF SUBPHRENIC ABSCESS

SURGICAL CONSIDERATIONS

Description: Abscesses may occur in subphrenic spaces, including the right subphrenic, right subhepatic, left subphrenic, lesser sac, or bare area of the liver, following peritonitis (Fig 7.9-2), abdominal surgery or trauma. It is important to know the anatomy of these spaces for making a correct diagnosis and for treatment.

Drainage is accomplished by a posterior or anterior extraperitoneal approach or by a transpleural approach, depending on the location of the abscess. Lesser sac abscesses are best approached by an anterior transperitoneal route. Abscesses in the bare area of the liver are drained posteriorly. Once the abscess has been localized, the cavity is entered by finger dissection and drained. Loculations are broken up and the cavity thoroughly irrigated with NS or a suitable antibiotic solution. Appropriate drains are placed and the wound is closed in a conventional manner. Cultures are routinely obtained.

Variant procedure or approaches: Percutaneous approaches are becoming more popular as experience is gained by interventional radiologists. This technique should be reserved for unilocular collections, where sterile cavities are not penetrated, and a safe route is available.

Usual preop diagnosis: Subphrenic abscess

SUMMARY OF PROCEDURE

	Subphrenic Abscess Drainage	Percutaneous Approach
Position	Supine or lateral decubitus, right or left	⇐
Incision	Subcostal or oblique abdominal	None
Special instrumentation	Drainage tubes	Special catheters; CT guidance
Antibiotics	Cefotetan 1-2 g preop	⇐
Surgical time	1 h	⇐
EBL	50-100 ml	10-25 ml
Postop care	Maintain patency of the drainage tubes	⇐
Mortality	< 5%	⇐
Morbidity	Inadequate drainage: 5-10% Pulmonary complications: 5-10% Bowel perforation: < 2%	⇐
Pain score	7-9	4-5

PATIENT POPULATION CHARACTERISTICS

Age range	Variable, 15-80 yr
Male:Female	1:1
Incidence	Common
Etiology	Postop (70-80%); peritonitis (25-30%); trauma (5-10%)
Associated conditions	See Etiology, above.

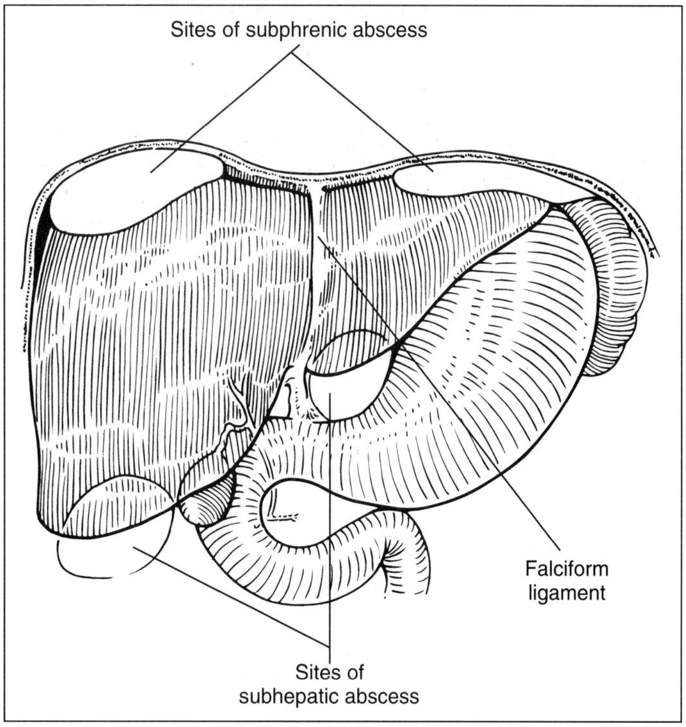

Figure 7.9-2. Anatomy of subphrenic abscess. (Reproduced with permission from Calne S, Pollard SG: *Operative Surgery*. Gower Medical Pub: 1992.)

ANESTHETIC CONSIDERATIONS

See Anesthetic Considerations for Intestinal and Peritoneal Procedures, p. 370.

Reference

1. Nora PF: *Operative Surgery: Principles and Techniques*. WB Saunders Co, Philadelphia: 1990, 466-73.

INGUINAL HERNIORRHAPHY

SURGICAL CONSIDERATIONS

Description: Groin hernias are defects in the transverse abdominis layer, where a direct hernia comes through the posterior wall of the inguinal canal and an indirect hernia comes through the internal inguinal ring. Surgical approach can be either anterior or posterior. In general, an **anterior approach** (Bassini, McVay's, Shouldice, or mesh repair) is used for primary repair of an indirect or direct inguinal hernia. The **Bassini repair** consists of ligation of the hernia sac and suturing the conjoint tendon to the shelving edge of Poupart's ligament. **McVay's repair** sutures the conjoint tendon to Cooper's ligament and is usually reserved for direct inguinal hernias. **Shouldice** emphasizes the closing of the transverse fascia and transversus abdominal muscle layers. More recently, the interposing of Marlex mesh between the conjoint tendon, the internal oblique muscle and the inguinal ligament is widely used. Other modifications are indicated in special situations.

A **posterior approach** is used by some surgeons for the repair of femoral hernias and recurrent inguinal hernias[3] and for treating incarcerated and strangulated hernias. The **posterior preperitoneal approach** is normally performed by suturing the transversus abdominis arch on the superior aspect of the hernia defect to Cooper's ligament and the iliopubic tract on the inferior aspect of the defect. This approach also may be utilized laparoscopically with the insertion of mesh to repair the defect.

The **laparoscopic approach** to hernia repair commonly utilizes a **preperitoneal patch repair** and results in less postop pain and an earlier return to normal physical activity (see Laparoscopic Inguinal Hernia Repair, p. 432).

Usual preop diagnosis: Groin pain or lump

SUMMARY OF PROCEDURE

Position	Supine
Incision	Oblique or transverse
Unique considerations	Avoid damage to nerve structure and spermatic cord. Avoid interfering with blood supply to testes.
Antibiotics	None
Surgical time	1-1.5 h
Postop care	PACU → room
EBL	25-50 ml
Mortality	< 0.3%
Morbidity	Wound abscess: < 3% Wound hematoma: < 2%
Pain score	4-5

PATIENT POPULATION CHARACTERISTICS

Age range	1-90 yr
Male:Female	85:15
Incidence	15/1000
Etiology	Congenital variants; reduced collagen synthesis in adults
Associated conditions	Chronic cough; urinary retention; chronic constipation

ANESTHETIC CONSIDERATIONS

See Anesthetic Considerations following Repair of Abdominal Dehiscence, p.460.

References

1. Abrahamson J: Hernias. In *Maingot's Abdominal Operations*, 10th edition. Zinner MJ, Schwartz SI, Ellis H, eds. Appleton & Lange, Stanford CT: 1997, 479-580.
2. Barbier J, Carretier M, Richer JP: Cooper ligament repair: an update. *World J Surg* 1989; 13(5):499-505.
3. Read RC: Preperitoneal herniorrhaphy: a historical review. *World J Surg* 1989; 13(5):532-40.
4. Wantz GE: The Canadian repair: Personal observation. *World J Surg* 1989; 13(5):516-21.

FEMORAL HERNIORRHAPHY

SURGICAL CONSIDERATIONS

Description: The hernia sac is exposed as it exits the preperitoneal space through the femoral canal (Fig 7.9-3). If the hernia cannot be reduced, the possibility of strangulation needs to be kept in mind. The peritoneal sac in most cases should be opened proximal to the femoral canal in order to gain control of the intestine before it reduces itself into the peritoneal cavity. If the bowel is ischemic, it may require resection. The repair consists of suturing the iliopubic tract to Cooper's ligament, taking care not to compromise the femoral vein.[2]

Usual preop diagnosis: Bulging of tissues over femoral canal

SUMMARY OF PROCEDURE

Position	Supine
Incision	Oblique
Antibiotics	Cefazolin 1 g iv
Surgical time	1-1.5 h
EBL	25-50 ml
Postop care	PACU → room
Mortality	< 1% (6-20%, if strangulated)
Morbidity	Recurrence: 6%
Pain score	5-6

PATIENT POPULATION CHARACTERISTICS

Age range	Adults; rare in children
Male:Female	1:4
Incidence	1.5% of all groin hernias
Etiology	Failure of preformed peritoneal sac to obliterate; muscle atrophy in older age group

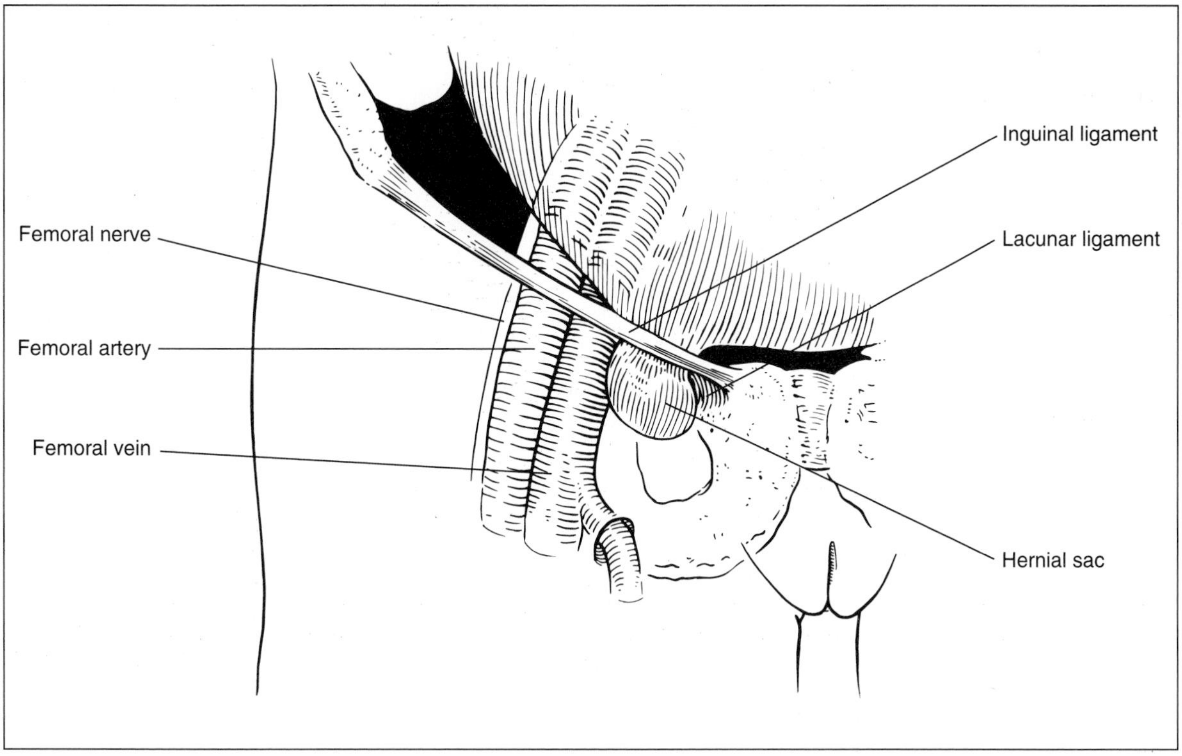

Figure 7.9-3. Anatomy of a femoral hernia. (Reproduced with permission from Calne R, Pollard SG: *Operative Surgery*. Gower Medical Pub: 1992.)

ANESTHETIC CONSIDERATIONS

See Anesthetic Considerations following Repair of Abdominal Dehiscence, p. 460.

References

1. Abrahamson J: Hernias. In *Maingot's Abdominal Operations*, 10th edition. Zinner MJ, Schwartz SI, Ellis H, eds. Appleton & Lange, Stanford CT: 1997, 479-580.
2. Bendavid R: New techniques in hernia repair. *World J Surg* 1989; 13(5):522-31.

REPAIR OF INCISIONAL HERNIA

SURGICAL CONSIDERATIONS

Description: Incisional hernias can occur after any abdominal incision, but are most common following midline incisions. Factors leading to herniation are: wound infection, trauma, inadequate suturing and weak tissues. Following skin incision, the skin edges and subcutaneous fat are retracted and the dissection carried down to the hernia defect. The redundant hernia sac is excised and the fascia freed up on both sides of the wound. Primary closure is preferred, if possible.

Variant procedure or approaches: In addition to primary repair, the latter may be reinforced by an onlay mesh prosthesis, or the prosthesis may be used to fill the hernial defect or placed behind the muscle layer.

Usual preop diagnosis: Incisional hernia

SUMMARY OF PROCEDURE

Position	Supine
Incision	Vertical or transverse
Special instrumentation	Mesh prosthesis (when indicated)
Antibiotics	Cefazolin 1 g iv preop
Surgical time	1-2 h
Closing considerations	Retention sutures
EBL	100-200 ml
Postop care	NG decompression; abdominal binder; PACU → room
Mortality	< 1%
Morbidity	Ileus: 5-10%
	Respiratory complications: 5-10%
	Wound infection: 1-2%
Pain score	5-6

PATIENT POPULATION CHARACTERISTICS

Age range	20-70 yr
Male:Female	1:1
Incidence	3-5% of midline abdominal incision
Etiology	Wound infection; trauma; inadequate suturing; weak tissues
Associated conditions	Obesity; malnutrition

ANESTHETIC CONSIDERATIONS

See Anesthetic Considerations following Repair of Abdominal Dehiscence, p. 460.

Reference

1. Condon RE, Telford G: Anterior Abdominal Wall Hernia. In *Operative Surgery Principles and Techniques*, 3rd edition. Nora PF, ed. WB Saunders Co, Philadelphia: 1990, Ch 33.

REPAIR OF ABDOMINAL DEHISCENCE

SURGICAL CONSIDERATIONS

Description: Dehiscence implies a "splitting apart" or "bursting open" of a wound. A complete dehiscence is a separation of all layers of the abdominal wall and is often associated with an extrusion of abdominal viscera. If incomplete, the separation of fascial and muscular layers results in an incisional hernia or an obstruction of a herniated loop of intestine. The earliest sign of a wound dehiscence is the presence of a serosanguineous drainage from the wound. Minimal disruptions may be treated conservatively with occlusive dressings and an abdominal binder. Major dehiscence requires operative repair using retention sutures.

Variant procedure or approaches: Variations in the type of closure depend on surgeon's preference. Interrupted, nonabsorbable sutures and skin bridges are often used.

Usual preop diagnosis: Wound dehiscence

SUMMARY OF PROCEDURE

Position	Supine
Incision	Closure of previous incision
Unique considerations	Adequate muscle relaxation essential
Antibiotics	Cefotetan 1-2 g preop
Surgical time	1-1.5 h
EBL	50-100 ml
Postop care	Abdominal binder to relieve tension on suture line; PACU → room
Mortality	5-10%
Morbidity	Incisional hernia: 5-10% Wound infection: < 5% Wound ischemia: 1-2%
Pain score	4-5

PATIENT POPULATION CHARACTERISTICS

Age range	25-90 yr
Male:Female	1:1
Incidence	1.3% in patients < 45 yr 5.4% in patients > 45 yr
Etiology	Wound infection; excessive coughing or sneezing; excessive abdominal distention; weak tissue; poor nutrition; hematoma formation; poor surgical technique
Associated conditions	Malnutrition (25-30%); ascites (20-25%); hypoproteinemia (20%); chronic anemia (5-10%) vitamin C deficiency (< 5%)

ANESTHETIC CONSIDERATIONS

Procedures covered: inguinal herniorrhaphy; femoral herniorrhaphy; incisional hernia repair; repair of abdominal dehiscence)

PREOPERATIVE

Predisposing factors for hernia often include increased abdominal pressure 2° chronic cough, bladder outlet obstruction, constipation, pregnancy, vomiting and acute or chronic muscular effort. These factors should be controlled preop to avoid postop recurrence. The patient population may range from premature infants to the elderly with the potential for having multiple medical problems.

Musculoskeletal Pain is likely to be present in area of hernia; evaluate bony landmarks if regional anesthetic is planned.

Gastrointestinal Hernias may become incarcerated, obstructed or strangulated, requiring emergency surgery. Fluid and electrolyte imbalance is likely.
Tests: Electrolytes, if indicated from H&P.

Hematologic For regional anesthesia, check patient's coagulation status, if indicated from H & P.
Tests: As indicated from H&P.

Laboratory Other tests as indicated from H&P.

Premedication If necessary, standard premedication (see p. B-2).

INTRAOPERATIVE

Anesthetic technique: GA, regional or local anesthesia ± sedation (MAC) are all appropriate anesthetic techniques. Choice depends on factors such as site of incision, patient physical status and preference of both patient and surgeon. GA may be preferred for incisions made above T8. Profound muscle relaxation may be necessary to facilitate exploration and repair.

Regional anesthesia:

Spinal Single-shot vs continuous: Patient in sitting or lateral decubitus position (operative site down) for placement of hyperbaric subarachnoid block. Doses of local anesthetics are as follows for T4-T6 level: 5% lidocaine in 7.5% dextrose (75-100 mg); 0.75% bupivacaine in 8.25% dextrose (10-15 mg); 0.5% tetracaine in 5% dextrose (12-18 mg). For continuous spinal, titrate local anesthetic to desired surgical level (T6). Large doses of hyperbaric local anesthetic should be avoided as they can cause postop cauda equina syndrome.

Epidural Patient in sitting or lateral decubitus position for placement of epidural catheter. After locating the epidural space, administer a test dose (e.g., 3 ml of 1.5% lidocaine with 1:200,000 epinephrine) to elucidate whether the catheter is subarachnoid or intravascular. Titrate local anesthetic until desired surgical level is obtained (3-5 ml at a time) usually less than 20 ml.

Local Requires gentle surgical technique. Surgical field block, plus ilioinguinal and iliohypogastric nerve blocks using 0.5% bupivacaine with 1:200,000 epinephrine. Usually done by surgeon.

General anesthesia:

Induction LMA vs ETT: Standard induction (see p. B-2). Mask may be suitable for the patient who presents with a simple chronic hernia. If there is obstruction, incarceration or strangulation, however, a rapid-sequence induction (see p. B-5) with ET intubation is indicated. GETA also may be indicated in the patient with wound dehiscence.

Maintenance Standard maintenance (see p. B-3). Muscle relaxants may be necessary to facilitate surgical repair.

Emergence Consider extubating the trachea while patient is still anesthetized to prevent coughing and straining. Patients who are at risk for pulmonary aspiration and require awake intubation or rapid-sequence induction are not candidates for deep extubation.

Blood and fluid requirements Minimal blood loss
IV: 16-18 ga × 1
NS/LR @ 5-8 ml/kg/h

Monitoring	Standard monitoring (see p. B-1).	
Positioning	✓ and pad pressure points. ✓ eyes.	
Complications	↓↓HR + ↓BP	Vagal reflex evoked by bowel traction.

POSTOPERATIVE

Complications	Cauda equina syndrome	The diagnosis of cauda equina syndrome (urinary and fecal incontinence, paresis of lower extremities, perineal hyperesthesia) should be sought in the postop period in patients who have received large doses of intrathecal local anesthetic during continuous spinal techniques. ✓ patients for bowel or bladder dysfunction and perineal sensory deficits. If present, consider a neurology consultation and continue followup of the patient's neurologic dysfunction.
	Urinary retention, common with regional anesthesia	Patients with urinary retention may require intermittent catheterization until urinary function resumes.
	Wound dehiscence with coughing/straining	
Pain management	PO analgesics: Acetaminophen and codeine (Tylenol #3 1-2 tab q 4-6 h) or oxycodone and acetaminophen (Percocet 1 tab q 6 h)	Surgical field block or regional anesthesia should provide sufficient analgesia postop.

References

1. Cousins MJ, Bridenbaugh PO, eds: *Neural Blockade Pain Management*, 3nd edition. Lippincott-Raven Publishers, Philadelphia: 1998.
2. Hardy JD: *Critical Surgical Illness*, 2nd edition. WB Saunders Co, Philadelphia: 1980, 203-9.
3. Horlocker TT, McGregor DG, Matsushige DK, Chantigian RC, Schroeder DR, Besse JA: Neurologic complications of 603 consecutive continuous spinal anesthetics using macrocatheter and microcatheter techniques. Perioperative Outcomes Group. *Anesth Analg* 1997; 84(5):1063-70.
4. Horlocker TT, McGregor DG, Matsushige Dk, Schroeder DR, Besse JA: A retrospective review of 4767 consecutive spinal anesthetics: central nervous system complications. Perioperative Outcomes Group. *Anesth Analg* 1997; 84(3):578-84.

Surgeon

Stefanie S. Jeffrey, MD, FACS

7.10 BREAST SURGERY

Anesthesiologist

Steven K. Howard, MD

BREAST BIOPSY

SURGICAL CONSIDERATIONS

Description: Breast biopsy is the surgical removal of breast tissue for pathologic examination. Breast biopsies are done for palpable abnormalities, such as breast masses or asymmetric breast thickenings, or for nonpalpable abnormalities that are seen only on mammogram. Mammographic abnormalities include microcalcifications, mammographic masses (densities) and areas of architectural distortion. With mammographic abnormalities, the breast tissue may look and feel normal at surgery and the abnormality may only be appreciated by x-ray or by microscopic examination; therefore, the surgeon requires accurate preop localization of the abnormality to be removed. This is done under local anesthesia following placement of a percutaneous hook-wire by the radiologist using mammographic or sonographic guidance. The patient goes directly to the OR, where the surgeon dissects along the wire and excises the abnormality nearby its hooked tip. The tissue specimen is sent for a radiograph to confirm whether the abnormality has been adequately excised. This is known as **wire localization**, **needle localization**, or **hook-wire localization breast biopsy**.

Breast biopsies generally are done under local anesthesia; however, the patient may require monitoring by an anesthesiologist if large amounts of intravenous sedation are anticipated or if the patient has any medical problems. Some surgeons prefer to do breast biopsies under GA if the biopsy is particularly deep in the breast, the patient is very anxious and prefers not to be awake, or the patient has submammary breast implants that may be punctured accidentally by needle injection of local anesthetic.

Usual preop diagnosis: Breast mass or mammographic abnormality

SUMMARY OF PROCEDURE

	Breast Biopsy	Wire Localization Breast Biopsy
Position	Supine, with ipsilateral arm abducted. Table may be banked to center breast.	⇐
Incision	Overbreast mass or circumareolar	⇐ + Incision may or may not incorporate skin entry site of wire.
Special instrumentation	None	Wire placed immediately preop in mammography suite.
Antibiotics	Cefazolin 1 g iv (optional)	⇐
Surgical time	0.5-1 h	1-1.5 h, depending on time needed to get results of specimen radiograph.
Closing considerations	Gauze bandage over wound. Some surgeons prefer patient to sit upright so breast can resume normal shape before bandaging.	⇐ + Specimen radiograph result must be obtained prior to completion of operation.
EBL	< 25 ml	⇐
Postop care	PACU → home	⇐
Mortality	Minimal	⇐
Morbidity	Hematoma: < 10%	⇐
	Infection: 2-5%	⇐
		Inability to excise mammographic abnormality: Infrequent (due to inaccurate wire placement in radiology or wire movement during patient transport or surgical prepping)
		Placement or migration of the wire into the thorax or mediastinum: Very rare
Pain score	2-5	2-5

PATIENT POPULATION CHARACTERISTICS

Age range	6-90 (usually >30 yr)	35-80 yr
Male:Female	Mainly female	Only female
Incidence	Common	⇐
Etiology	Unknown	⇐

ANESTHETIC CONSIDERATIONS

See Anesthetic Considerations for Breast Biopsy and Sentinel Lymph Node Biopsy, p. 467.

SENTINEL LYMPH NODE BIOPSY

SURGICAL CONSIDERATIONS

Description: Sentinel lymph node biopsy is a technique applied to patients with small, invasive breast cancers who do not have clinically pathologic lymph nodes. The sentinel lymph node is the first lymph node to drain afferent lymphatics from the particular region of the breast where the cancer is located. The sentinel node is not necessarily the lowest lymph node in the axilla. It is usually located somewhere in the axilla but may be situated in the internal mammary chain for some medial, midline or lower outer-quadrant breast tumors. Because the sentinel lymph node is the first node to drain a breast cancer, it is the most likely lymph node to harbor any metastatic tumor cells that may have traveled via lymphatic pathways. Early studies suggest that if, on careful histologic examination, the sentinel lymph node is negative for tumor metastases, this is highly predictive for the absence of metastatic disease. Larger clinical trials are under way to determine whether sentinel lymph node biopsy will eventually replace standard axillary lymph node dissection in the surgical treatment of breast cancer when the sentinel node is tumor-negative.

One method for identification of the sentinel node is by injection of isosulfan blue vital dye (Lymphazurin 1%) around the periphery of the breast tumor or the previous biopsy site and then visually identifying the blue lymphatic tract and blue sentinel lymph node within the axilla. The blue vital dye is injected intraop within 10 min of performing the axillary incision, since the blue dye may pass beyond the sentinel node after 30 min following injection. Another method of sentinel node identification is through the use of technetium-99m-labeled sulfur colloid, which is injected around the periphery of the breast tumor or biopsy cavity. Two to 6 h later, the patient is brought to surgery and the sentinel lymph node, now radioactive, is identified intraop using a special handheld gamma-detection probe (similar to a pencil-sized Geiger counter). Frequently, isosulfan blue vital dye is used in conjunction with the technetium-99m sulfur colloid so that the sentinel node may be identified both visually and with the handheld gamma-detection probe.

Usual preop diagnosis: Breast cancer

SUMMARY OF PROCEDURE

Position	Supine
Incision	Small axillary incision
Special instrumentation	Handheld gamma-detection probe
Unique considerations	Radiation exposure negligible. Avoid BP cuff or iv in ipsilateral arm. Possible need to avoid muscle relaxants. Isosulfan blue vital dye → allergic reaction (1-2:100).
Antibiotics	Cefazolin 1 g iv (optional)
Surgical time	10-30 min up to 1.5 h for axillary lymph node dissections
EBL	Minimal
Postop care	PACU → home
Mortality	Rare
Morbidity	Allergic dye reaction: 1.5% Anaphylaxis 1:2000
Pain score	2-5

PATIENT POPULATION CHARACTERISTICS

Age range	20-90 yr; typically > 40 yr
Incidence	Approximately 1 in 8 American women will develop breast cancer
Etiology	Unknown; possible familial predisposition

ANESTHETIC CONSIDERATIONS FOR BREAST BIOPSY AND SENTINEL LYMPH NODE BIOPSY

PREOPERATIVE

Breast masses may vary in size and depth, which will, in part, determine what type of anesthetic is most suitable for the procedure in these otherwise healthy patients. Typically, these excisional biopsies can be accomplished with MAC/ sedation and local anesthesia; however, patient wishes must be considered in the anesthetic plan. The suitability of local vs GA may be best addressed by preop discussion with the surgical team.

Psychosocial Patients are likely to be very anxious concerning the possibility of breast malignancy, and should be counseled and premedicated appropriately.

Laboratory CBC; other tests as indicated from H&P.

Premedication Standard premedication (see p. B-2).

INTRAOPERATIVE

Anesthetic technique: GA or local anesthesia ± sedation are both appropriate techniques. Choice of anesthetic technique depends on the size and depth of lesion and the wishes of the patient. Often done on an outpatient basis.

MAC Propofol infusion (25-100 μg/kg/min) combination of analgesics (e.g., fentanyl/remifentanil) and anxiolytics (e.g., midazolam), titrated to effect, are most commonly used. The surgeon may choose to add Na bicarbonate to 1% lidocaine (1:10) to reduce injection pain. The anesthesiologist may give remifentanil 0.5-1 μg/kg 90 sec before the initial injection of local anesthetic in the skin.

Induction Standard induction (see p. B-2). Mask or LMA anesthetic may be appropriate.

Maintenance Standard maintenance (see p. B-3). Muscle relaxants are not necessary for surgical procedure.

Emergence No special considerations

Blood and fluid requirements
Minimal blood loss
IV: 18-20 ga × 1
NS/LR @ 3-5 ml/kg/h

Monitoring Standard monitors (see p. B-1). Maintain verbal contact with patient if MAC. Other monitors as clinically indicated. Isosulfan blue vital dye → artifactual ↓O_2 sat as low as 92-94%.

Positioning
✓ and pad pressure points.
✓ eyes.

Complications
Inadequate analgesia — May have to supplement surgical field block with local anesthetic or convert to GA.
Isosulfan dye reaction — Pruritus, localized swelling, blue hives. Rx: diphenhydramine (10-50 mg iv). ↓BP may require epinephrine.

POSTOPERATIVE

Complications No specific complications anticipated. Inform patients that urine, vomit, or stool may be blue for 24-48 h.

Pain management PO analgesics (see p. C-1).

Tests As clinically indicated.

References

1. Albertini JJ, Lyyman GH, Cox C, et al: Lymphatic mapping and sentinel node biopsy in the patient with breast cancer. *JAMA* 1996; 276:1818-22.
2. Alex JC, Krag DN: The gamma-probe guided resection of radiolabeled primary lymph nodes. *Surg Oncol Clin N Am* 1996; 5:33-41.
3. Bland KI, Copeland EM III, eds: *The Breast: Comprehensive Management of Benign and Malignant Diseases*. WB Saunders Co, Philadelphia: 1991.
4. Giuliano AE, Jones RC, Brennan M, Statman R: Sentinel lymphadenectomy in breast cancer. *J Clin Oncol* 1997; 15:2345-50.

5. Harris JR, Lippman ME, Morrow M, Hellman S, eds: *Diseases of the Breast.* Lippincott-Raven Publishers, Philadelphia, 1996.
6. Hietala S-O, Hirsch JI, Faunce HF: Allergic reaction to Patent Blue Violet during lymphography. *Lymphology* 1977; 10:158-60.
7. Hirsch JI, Tisnado J, Cho S-R, Beachley MC: Use of isosulfan blue for identification of lymphatic vessels: experimental and clinical evaluation. *AJR Am J Roentgenol* 1982; 139:1061-64.
8. Larsen VH, Freudendal-Pedersen, Fogh-Andersen. The influence of Patent Blue V on pulse oximetry and haemoximetry. *Acta Anaesthesiol Scand* 1995; 39(suppl 107):53-5.
9. Longnecker SM, Gussardo MM, Van Voris LP: Life-threatening anaphylaxis following subcutaneous administration of isosulfan blue 1%. *Clin Pharm* 1985; 4:219-21. (Case Report)
10. Saito S, Fukura H, Shimada H, Fijita T: Prolonged interference of blue dye "patent blue" with pulse oximetry readings. *Acta Anaesthesiol Scand* 1995; 39:268-69.
11. Zelcer J, White PF: Monitored anesthesia care. In *Anesthesia*, 4th edition. Miller RD, ed. Churchill Livingstone, New York: 1994, 1465-80.

MASTECTOMY ± RECONSTRUCTION

SURGICAL CONSIDERATIONS

Description: The treatment of breast cancer has evolved greatly in the last 30 years. The **radical mastectomy**, which removes the breast, the underlying pectoral muscles and the axillary lymph nodes, is no longer the mainstay of treatment. The two major treatment alternatives now are the **modified radical mastectomy** and **wide local excision** of the tumor (**partial mastectomy** or **lumpectomy**) with **axillary dissection**, followed by postop radiation therapy to the remaining breast tissue (breast conservation therapy). Modified radical mastectomy entails removal of the breast and axillary lymph nodes, while the pectoral muscles remain in place (except in unusual cases when surgeons perform the **Patey procedure**, in which the pectoralis minor muscle is removed to allow a more complete dissection of the axillary lymph nodes). When a wide local excision is performed, it removes the tumor with a rim of normal surrounding tissue (i.e., surgical margins free of tumor). When a wide local excision and axillary dissection are performed at the same time, separate incisions normally are performed and separate instruments may be used so that there is no cross-contamination of cancer cells between the wounds.

The axillary dissection generally removes levels I and II axillary lymph nodes: those lymph nodes that lie lateral to the edge of the pectoralis minor muscle and those that lie posterior to the pectoralis minor muscle. The level III, or highest group of axillary lymph nodes, are medial to the pectoralis minor muscle. For prognostic and treatment purposes, no survival advantage can be shown in removing level III axillary lymph nodes. The disadvantages include a significant increase in postop lymphedema of the arm when these high lymph nodes are excised. As part of the axillary dissection, the surgeon preserves the thoracodorsal nerve to the latissimus dorsi muscle and the long thoracic nerve to the serratus anterior muscle, as well as the blood and nerve supply to the pectoral muscles. Preservation of the intercostobrachial nerve (sensory to the upper arm), which courses through the axillary fat pad, is optional.

A **total mastectomy** (also known as a **simple** or **complete mastectomy**) removes only the breast. There is no formal axillary dissection involved and it is done mainly for treatment of extensive duct carcinoma *in situ*.

Immediate breast reconstruction may be planned for patients who will not require radiotherapy. Two approaches are commonly used: (1) prosthetic reconstruction, in which a saline-filled implant or tissue expander is placed in a subpectoral pocket; and (2) TRAM or latissimus dorsi myocutaneous flap (see p. 832) either rotated into position as a vasicular pedicle or as a free flap.

Usual preop diagnosis: Breast cancer; *in situ* breast cancer

SUMMARY OF PROCEDURE

	Modified Radical Mastectomy	Total Mastectomy (Simple Mastectomy)	Lumpectomy, Axillary Lymph Node Dissection
Position	Supine, with ipsilateral arm abducted. Some surgeons prep arm. May require repositioning (latissimus dorsi).	⇐	⇐
Incision	Elliptical oblique or elliptical transverse to include nipple/areola and previous biopsy incision.	⇐	Incision over breast mass or previous biopsy site. Separate transverse incision in axilla (sometimes using different instruments).
Special instrumentation	Pectoral, axillary drains usually placed prior to closure.	Pectoral drain usually placed prior to closure.	Axillary drain may be placed prior to closure.
Unique considerations	Avoid iv and BP cuff on ipsilateral arm.	⇐	⇐
Antibiotics	Cefazolin 1 g iv	⇐	⇐
Surgical time	1.5-3 h (+ 1-7 h if immediate breast reconstruction performed)	1-2 h (+ 1-7 h if immediate breast reconstruction performed)	2-3 h
Closing considerations	Gauze bandage over incision site	⇐	⇐
EBL	150-500 ml, depending on whether scalpel or electrocautery is used.	⇐	25-100 ml
Postop care	PACU → room × 2 d	PACU → hospital × 1-2 d or occasionally → home	⇐
Mortality	Rare	⇐	⇐
Morbidity	Lymphedema: 5-30% (depending on extent of axillary dissection)	–	Lymphedema: 5-30% (depending on extent of axillary dissection)
	Seroma: 25%	⇐	⇐
	Infection: 2-10%	⇐	⇐
	Flap necrosis: < 5%	⇐	–
	Hematoma: < 5%	⇐	< 10%
	Injury to axillary neurovascular structures: Rare	–	⇐
	Pneumothorax: Rare (may occur with attempts to obtain hemostasis of intercostal perforating vessels)	⇐	–
Pain score	4-8	4-6	4-8

PATIENT POPULATION CHARACTERISTICS

Age range	20-90 yr (generally > 40 yr)
Incidence	Over their lifetime, approximately 1/8 of American women develop breast cancer; in 1997, 182,200 new cases of female breast cancer were diagnosed. The incidence has been increasing at a rate of 3%/yr since 1980.
Etiology	Unknown; possible familial predisposition (BRCA genes)

ANESTHETIC CONSIDERATIONS

PREOPERATIVE

Patients often have no other underlying medical problems. Some consideration, however, should be given to the anesthetic implications of metastatic spread to bone, brain, liver, lung, etc.

Respiratory	Respiratory compromise can be present if patient has received XRT to the thorax as part of treatment. **Tests:** CXR (✓ for pleural effusion and rib or vertebral lesions). If patient shows any signs of respiratory compromise, obtain room air ABG. Consider PFTs (FVC, FEV_1, $MMEF_{25-75}$) if CXR or ABG abnormal. This will help predict pulmonary reserve and patient tolerance to GA. Patients who show signs of impaired pulmonary function might require postop care in an ICU for various reasons (e.g., mechanical ventilation, aggressive pulmonary toilet, close observation, etc.).	
Cardiovascular	Chemotherapeutic agents (e.g., doxorubicin at doses > 550 mg/m^2) also cause severe cardiomyopathies. If patient was exposed to this type of drug, cardiac dysfunction may be present, and a cardiac consultation to evaluate ventricular function may be necessary. **Tests:** Consider ECHO or MUGA scan; ECG.	
Neurological	Breast cancer often metastasizes to the CNS and can present with focal neurologic deficits, ↑ICP or altered mental status. If patient has altered mental status, full workup should proceed without delay; postpone surgery until cause is found. **Tests:** CT/MRI scan should be recommended, if indicated from H&P.	
Hematologic	Patient may be anemic 2° chronic disease or chemotherapeutic agents. **Tests:** CBC, with differential and Plt count	
Laboratory	Routine lab exam; other tests as indicated from H&P.	
Premedication	Standard premedication (see p. B-2).	

INTRAOPERATIVE

Anesthetic technique: GETA

Induction	Standard induction (see p. B-2).	
Maintenance	Standard maintenance (see p. B-3). The use of muscle relaxants during axillary dissection should be avoided to permit surgical identification of nerves by nerve stimulator or if electrocautery is used in the axilla.	
Emergence	Pressure dressings may be applied with the patient anesthetized and "sitting up" at the end of the procedure. Discuss with surgeons whether or not they intend to apply this type of dressing to enable emergence to be timed appropriately.	
Blood and fluid requirements	Minimal-to-moderate blood loss IV: 16-18 ga × 1 (avoid operative side) NS/LR @ 3-5 ml/kg/h	
Monitoring	Standard monitors (see p. B-1).	Others as indicated by patient status. BP cuff on arm opposite surgical site.
Positioning	✓ and pad pressure points. ✓ eyes.	
Complications	Pneumothorax	Deep surgical exploration may cause inadvertent pneumothorax; monitor patient for Sx (e.g., ↑PIP, ↓$PaCO_2$, asymmetric breath sounds, hyperresonance to percussion over the affected side, hemodynamic instability). Dx: CXR. Rx: Chest tube, 100% O_2.

POSTOPERATIVE

Complications	Pneumothorax Psychological trauma	Pneumothorax: If index of suspicion is high, maintain oxygenation (100% FiO_2) and ventilation; inform surgeons of the likelihood of the Dx. If patient is hemodynamically unstable (suggesting a tension pneumothorax), place a 14-ga iv catheter in the 2nd intercostal space while the surgeons set up for placement of a chest tube. If patient is hemodynamically stable and not hypoxemic, a portable CXR may aid in diagnosis.
Pain management	PCA (see p. C-3). PO analgesics (see p. C-1).	
Tests	Postop portable CXR, if pneumothorax is a consideration.	

Surgeons

Ronald J. Weigel, MD, PhD
Harry A. Oberhelman, MD, FACS

7.11 ENDOCRINE SURGERY

Anesthesiologist

Steven K. Howard, MD

EXCISION OF THYROGLOSSAL DUCT CYST

SURGICAL CONSIDERATIONS

Description: The majority of patients with thyroglossal duct cysts are diagnosed before the age of 20 yr. The usual presentation is a superficial midline/neck mass near hyoid bone. Following incision of the deep cervical fascia, the cyst is freed from secondary structures (Fig 7.11-1). Since the duct is in close association with the hyoid bone, the mid-portion of the bone should be excised with the cyst. The dissection is continued superiorly and posteriorly to the foramen cecum. If the duct is not entirely removed, recurrence is very likely.

Usual preop diagnosis: Thyroglossal duct cyst

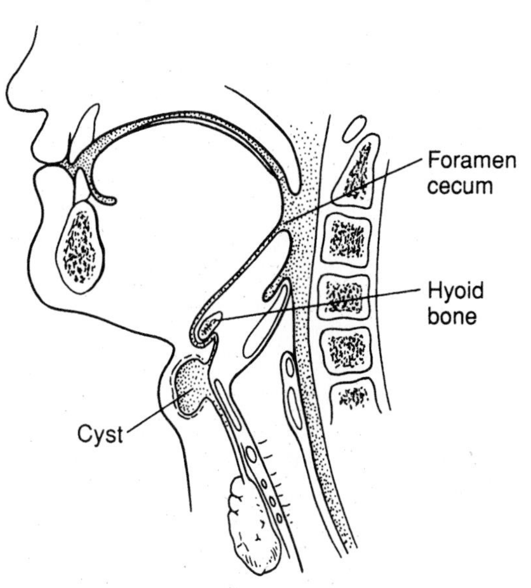

Figure 7.11-1. Course of thyroglossal duct, with cyst. (Reproduced with permission from Healey JE Jr: *Surgical Anatomy*, 2nd edition. BC Decker: 1990.)

SUMMARY OF PROCEDURE

Position	Supine, with neck in hyperextended position
Incision	Transverse skin incision
Antibiotics	None routinely used
Surgical time	1-1.5 h
Closing considerations	Careful hemostasis
EBL	25-50 ml
Mortality	< 0.1%
Morbidity	Bleeding: < 5%
	Infection: < 5%
Pain score	5-7

PATIENT POPULATION CHARACTERISTICS

Age range	10-20 yr
Male:Female	1:1
Incidence	Not uncommon
Etiology	Persistence of undifferentiated epithelial cells in area of hyoid bone that later became squamous-cell epithelium or glandular tissue

ANESTHETIC CONSIDERATIONS

See Anesthetic Considerations following Thyroidectomy, p. 475.

Reference

1. Nora PF, ed: *Operative Surgery*, 3rd edition. WB Saunders Co, Philadelphia: 1990, Ch 7.

THYROIDECTOMY

SURGICAL CONSIDERATIONS

Description: Thyroidectomy, partial or total, is performed for benign and malignant conditions. Through a transverse Kocher collar incision, the thyroid gland is exposed by dividing the strap muscles in the neck. The thyroid lobe is freed from the strap muscles by sharp/blunt dissection, which exposes the superior thyroid vessels (Fig 7.11-2). The latter are clamped, cut and ligated, with care being taken not to injure the superior laryngeal nerves. Following division of the middle thyroid vein and inferior thyroid vessels, the thyroid gland is retracted medially and its remaining attachments severed. Again, care is taken not to injure the recurrent laryngeal nerve or the parathyroid glands. Any enlarged or suspicious lymph nodes should be excised for biopsy. If a **total thyroidectomy** is to be performed, the isthmus and opposite lobe are removed as described above. Again, it is important to preserve the parathyroid glands. Careful hemostasis is achieved prior to suturing the strap muscles of the neck and wound closure. Drains are optional, but not commonly used. When a **subtotal thyroidectomy** is performed, a rim of the posteriorly located thyroid gland is preserved. Clamps are placed across the gland at a safe distance from the region of the recurrent laryngeal nerve. The superior thyroid vessels are mobilized and ligated, with care being taken not to injure the superior laryngeal nerves. Following division of the middle thyroid vein and inferior thyroid vessels, the thyroid gland is removed subtotally or totally, again with care being taken not to injure the recurrent laryngeal nerves or parathyroid glands. Careful hemostasis is achieved prior to suturing the strap muscles of the neck and wound closure.

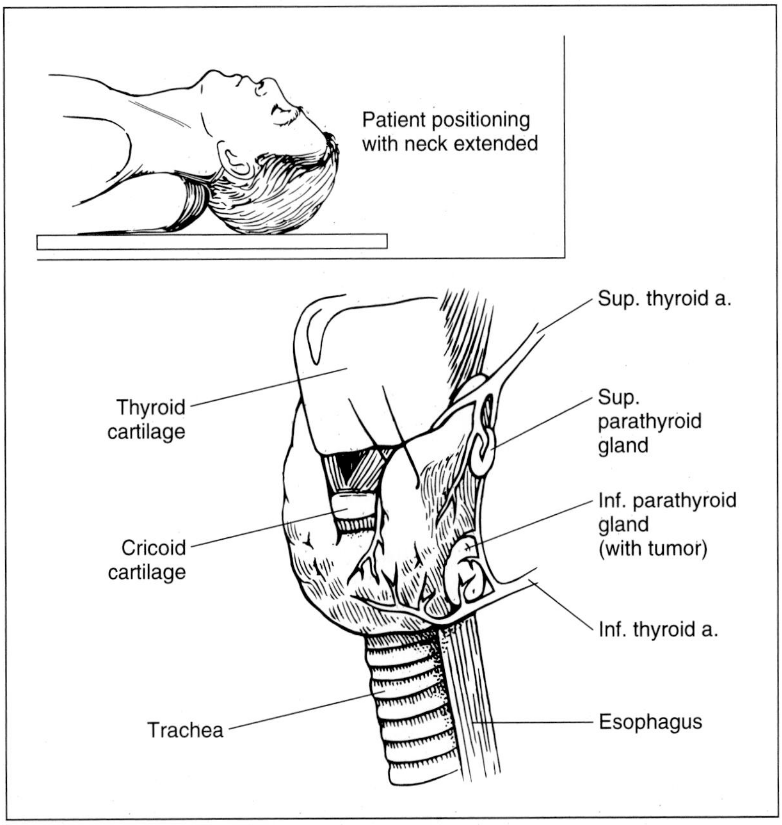

Figure 7.11-2. Blood supply to the thyroid gland. (Reproduced with permission from Healey JE Jr: *Surgical Anatomy*, 2nd edition. BC Decker: 1990.) Inset shows patient positioning with neck extended.

Usual preop diagnosis: Goiter; thyroid cancer; thyroid nodule; hyperthyroidism

SUMMARY OF PROCEDURE

Position	Supine with head elevated to 30°
Incision	Transverse collar
Antibiotics	None routinely used.
Surgical time	1-2 h
Closing considerations	Adequate hemostasis
EBL	50-75 ml
Postop care	Observe for postop respiratory problems, hypocalcemia, bleeding
Mortality	< 0.5%
Morbidity	Hypoparathyroidism: 2-3% Bleeding: 0.3-1% Respiratory obstruction

Morbidity, cont.	Thyroid storm (usually in association with Graves' disease) Wound infection Recurrent laryngeal nerve damage: 0.2% Superior laryngeal nerve damage Hoarseness
Pain score	5-7

PATIENT POPULATION CHARACTERISTICS

Age range	15-80 yr
Male:Female	1:6 for hyperthyroidism 5:8 for thyroid cancer
Incidence	Common
Etiology	Thyroid cancer or suspicion of malignancy (50%); benign thyroid lesion (50%)
Associated conditions	Other endocrine disorders (e.g., pheochromocytoma in association with medullary thyroid carcinoma in patients with MEN 2A and 2B)

ANESTHETIC CONSIDERATIONS

PREOPERATIVE

Hyperthyroidism may be 2° Graves' disease, toxic multinodular goiter, thyroid adenomas, TSH-secreting tumor (rare), thyroiditis or overdosage of thyroid hormone. Common Sx are sweating, intolerance to heat, increased appetite, ↑HR, weight loss or gain, thyroid goiter, exophthalmos. Hypothyroidism may be iatrogenic or 2° autoimmune thyroiditis. Common Sx are intolerance to cold, anorexia, fatigue, weight gain or loss, constipation, ↓HR. Patients presenting for thyroidectomy are usually made euthyroid prior to surgery and may be taking one or more of the following medications: propylthiouracil, methimazole, potassium iodide, glucocorticoids or β-blockers. An important aspect of the preop visit is to assure that the patient is in a physiologically euthyroid state.

Respiratory

Beware of tracheal compression with large goiters → tracheal deviation, stridor.
Hyperthyroid: ↑BMR → ↑VO_2 → rapid desaturation on induction.
Hypothyroid: ↓ventilatory response to ↑CO_2 and ↓O_2 (beware of opioids and sedatives).
Tests: CXR; consider preop CT scan of neck to evaluate possible tracheal involvement, especially in patients with large goiters.

Cardiovascular

Hyperthyroid: Tachycardia, atrial fibrillation, palpitations, CHF. A normal resting HR is helpful in determining whether or not the patient is ready for surgery. If the situation calls for it (e.g., emergency surgery), the patient can be treated with β-blockers to blunt the sympathomimetic effects of the hyperthyroid state. β-blocker therapy can be problematic in patients with CHF (titrate while monitoring filling pressures and CO).
Hypothyroid: Bradydysrythmias, diastolic HTN, pericardial effusions, ↓voltage of ECG. Thyroid replacement must be weighed against the risk of precipitating myocardial ischemia. Addison's disease is more common in patients with hypothyroidism; some patients may receive a "stress dose" of steroids (hydrocortisone 100 mg iv q 8 h × 3) in the perioperative period.
Tests: ECG; consider ECHO for evaluation of LV function.

Endocrine	T4	T3ru	T3	TSH
Hyperthyroid	↑	↑	↑	Normal or ↓
1° hypothyroid	↓	↓	↓ or normal	↑
2° hypothyroid	↓	↓	↓	↓

Tests: Thyroid function, Ca^{++}, Mg, phosphate, alkaline phosphatase, glucose

Thyroid storm

A life-threatening exacerbation of hyperthyroidism occurring during periods of stress, which is manifested by hyperthermia, cardiac instability, anxiety, altered mental state and tachycardia (and

Thyroid storm, cont.	has been mistaken intraop for malignant hyperthermia [MH]). Rx: ↑FiO_2, sodium iodide (1-2.5 g iv) + hydrocortisone (100 mg iv) + β-blockers q s; maintain fluids, electrolytes. This is a condition most often associated with Graves' disease that has been incompletely treated prior to surgery.
Myxedema coma	Severe hypothyroidism constituting a medical emergency, with mortality of > 50%. Manifestations include stupor or coma, hypothermia, hypoventilation with hypoxemia, bradycardia, hypotension, apathy, hoarseness and hyponatremia. Rx: T4 (400-500 μg loading dose; 50-200 μg maintenance dose q d); hydrocortisone (100-300 mg iv q d).
Neurological	Hyperthyroid: warm, moist skin, nervousness, anxiety (may require generous sedation), tremor. Hypothyroid: ↓BMR → slow mentation and movement, cold intolerance.
Musculoskeletal	Hyperthyroid: higher incidence of myasthenia gravis (↑sensitivity to muscle relaxants), skeletal muscle weakness (↑sensitivity to muscle relaxants), clubbing of the fingers, weight loss Hypothyroid: arthralgias and myalgias
Renal	Hypothyroid: impaired renal function 2° amyloidosis, urinary retention, oliguria **Tests:** Consider BUN; creatinine
Hematologic	Hyperthyroid: mild anemia, thrombocytopenia Hypothyroid: coagulation abnormalities, anemia **Tests:** CBC
Gastrointestinal	Hyperthyroid: weight loss and diarrhea Hypothyroid: GI bleeding, constipation, ileus **Tests:** As indicated from H&P.
Laboratory	Other tests as indicated from H&P.
Premedication	Midazolam 0.025-0.05 mg/kg iv. Continue antithyroid medications preop. Hyperthyroid patients must be made euthyroid prior to elective surgery and may be on the following drugs: propylthiouracil, methimazole, potassium iodide, β-blockers and glucocorticoids. Hypothyroid patients can undergo surgery if they have mild-to-moderate disease. Severely hypothyroid patients should be given thyroid replacement prior to elective surgery.

INTRAOPERATIVE

Anesthetic technique: Normally, GETA; infrequently, under local anesthesia. For inadequately treated hyperthyroid patients, it is important to establish an adequate depth of anesthesia to prevent an exaggerated sympathetic response to surgical stimulation. Avoid agents that stimulate the sympathetic nervous system (e.g., ketamine, pancuronium, meperidine). Hypothyroidism may be associated with ↑sensitivity to anesthetic agents and muscle relaxants.

Induction	Standard induction for euthyroid patients (p. B-2). If the patient has airway compromise 2° a large thyroid goiter, consider an awake fiber optic intubation (p. B-7).
Maintenance	Standard maintenance (p. B-3). Maintain muscle relaxation.
Emergence	Airway obstruction 2° recurrent laryngeal nerve damage, tracheomalacia or hematoma can occur. Consider visualizing vocal cord function prior to extubation.

Blood and fluid requirements	Minimal blood loss IV: 18 ga × 1 NS/LR @ 5-8 ml/kg/h Head-up position	Slight head-up position can help make for a bloodless surgical field without substantially increasing the risk of VAE.
Monitoring	Standard monitors (see p. B-1).	+ Others as indicated by patient's status. Maintain temperature, especially in hypothyroid patients.
Positioning	✓ and pad pressure points. ✓ eyes.	Supine, with head slightly hyperextended, allows for surgical exploration of the neck.
Complications	Cardiorespiratory depression	In hypothyroid patients, marked ↓BP and ↓RR may occur with minimal anesthetic doses.

POSTOPERATIVE

Complications	Recurrent laryngeal nerve damage	Bilateral: patient will be unable to speak and will require reintubation. Unilateral: characterized by hoarseness.

Complications, cont.	Tracheomalacia or hematoma with airway compromise	Acute airway obstruction may occur immediately postop, and rapid reintubation may be life-saving. If airway compromise is 2° hematoma, reopen incision and drain remaining blood; if patient still requires artificial airway, consider awake reintubation.
	Acute hypoparathyroid state (hypocalcemia)	Acute hypocalcemia can present as laryngeal stridor (24-48 h postop), although it most often presents with tingling in the fingertips and in the lips. If untreated and severe, this can progress to tetany and seizures. Administering 1 amp Ca^{++} gluconate given iv over 20 min usually alleviates symptoms. Rx: measure Ca^{++}; replace if necessary.
	Thyroid storm	Can mimic MH (see Rx above).
Pain management	PCA morphine (see p. C-3).	
Tests	Vocal cord function	Ability to phonate "e" implies continued vocal cord function.

References

1. Brown BR: Anesthetic management of endocrine emergencies. *ASA Annual Refresher Course Lectures* 1992; 224:1-7.
2. Roizen MF: Diseases of the endocrine system. In *Anesthesia and Uncommon Diseases.* Katz J, Benumof JL, Kadis LB, eds. WB Saunders Co, Philadelphia: 1990, 254-62.
3. Schwartz JJ, Rosenbaum SH, Graf GJ: Anesthesia and the endocrine system. In *Clinical Anesthesia*, 3rd edition. Barash PG, Cullen BF, Stoelting RK, eds. Lippincott-Raven Publishers, Philadelphia: 1997, 1039-60.
4. Sieber FE: Evaluation of the patient with endocrine disease and diabetes mellitus. In *Principles and Practice of Anesthesiology.* Rogers MC, Tinker JH, Covino BG, Longnecker DE, eds. Mosby-Year Book Inc., St. Louis: 1993, 278-84.
5. Thompson NW: Thyroid gland. In *Surgery: Scientific Principles and Practice*, 2nd edition. Greenfield LJ, et al, eds. Lippincott-Raven Publishers, 1997, 1283-1307.

PARATHYROIDECTOMY

SURGICAL CONSIDERATIONS

Description: Through a transverse cervical incision, the thyroid gland is exposed and the strap muscles dissected to increase the exposure of the parathyroid glands. It is necessary to divide the superior thyroid vessels to free the upper lobe for visualization of the superior parathyroid glands. The inferior glands are located near the junction of the inferior thyroid artery and the recurrent laryngeal nerve (Fig 7.11-3). Hemostasis is required in order to visualize the parathyroid glands easily. The classic operation involves identification of all four parathyroid glands with removal of the enlarged gland(s). Current techniques of localization (e.g., high-resolution ultrasound), possibly in combination with intraop PTH monitoring, have gained acceptance for performing localized operations. When one or more adenomas are present, they are excised, along with one normal gland or part of a normal gland. If the adenoma cannot be found in the neck, the thymus should be resected to identify parathyroid adenomas in the superior mediastinum. If one parathyroid cannot be identified on a side, **thyroid lobectomy** should be performed, since the adenoma may be located within the thyroid substance. If the operation is performed for hyperplasia, all glands are removed except for one-half of one gland. Some surgeons preserve parathyroid tissue by freezing it in case subsequent hypoparathyroidism develops. The preserved tissue may be transplanted into various muscles.

Usual preop diagnosis: Parathyroid adenoma; hyperparathyroidism (primary, secondary or tertiary); parathyroid carcinoma

SUMMARY OF PROCEDURE

Position	Supine; roll beneath thoracic spine
Incision	Transverse cervical
Special instrumentation	Thyroid retractor
Antibiotics	Cefotetan 1 g iv preop
Surgical time	1-2 h
EBL	25-50 ml
Postop care	Monitor serum Ca^{++} (Normal = 8.5-10.5 mg% total Ca; 1-1.3 mM ionized Ca^{++})
Mortality	< 0.5%
Morbidity	Hypocalcemia: < 15% Hypoparathyroidism: < 5% Recurrent laryngeal paralysis: < 1%
Pain score	5-6

PATIENT POPULATION CHARACTERISTICS

Age range	Increases with age
Male:Female	1:2
Incidence	50-100/100,000
Etiology	Hyperplasia (10-15%); cancer (1%)
Associated conditions	Bone disease (5-15%); duodenal ulcer (5-10%); peptic ulcer; renal calculi (60-70%); MEN-1 association (parathyroid + pituitary + pancreatic tumors); HTN (20-50%)

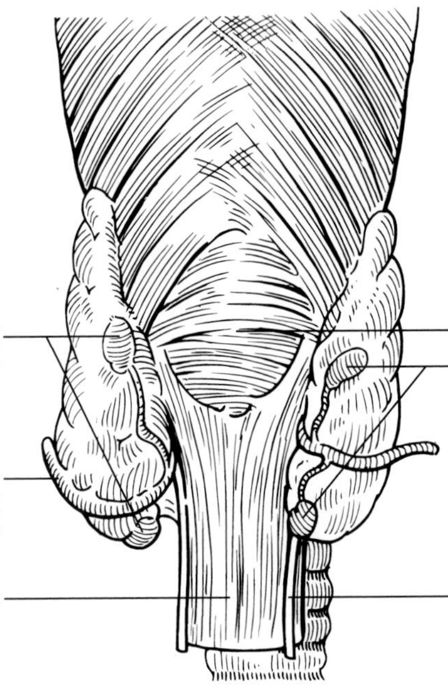

Figure 7.11-3. Common position of parathyroid glands (posterior view). (Reproduced with permission from Calne R, Pollard SG: *Operative Surgery*. Gower Medical Pub: 1992)

ANESTHETIC CONSIDERATIONS

PREOPERATIVE

These patients typically present with hypercalcemia (hyperparathyroidism), which must be controlled prior to surgery. Although 25-50% of cases are asymptomatic, many will present with a variety of Sx, including fatigue, muscle weakness, depression, anorexia, nausea, constipation, abdominal and bone pain, HTN, renal stones and polydipsia. Differential diagnosis for the hypercalcemic patient includes: metastatic disease, multiple myeloma, milk-alkali syndrome, vitamin D intoxication, sarcoidosis, hyperthyroidism, thiazide diuretics, adrenal insufficiency, Paget's disease, immobilization or an exogenous parathyroid hormone-producing tumor.

Respiratory — Hyperparathyroidism is associated with decreased clearance of secretions from the tracheobronchial tree → postop atelectasis. Avoid respiratory or metabolic acidosis, which will increase the free fraction of Ca → hypercalcemia (↑BP, ↑muscle weakness, ↑HR).
Tests: As indicated from H&P.

Cardiovascular — HTN (usually resolves with treatment); ECG may show tachycardia with ↓PR and ↓QT intervals. Patients may be hypovolemic (2° anorexia, nausea, vomiting and polyuria) and have increased

Cardiovascular, cont.	sensitivity to digitalis, resistance to catecholamines. Preop management includes correction of intravascular volume and electrolyte abnormalities. Preop treatment of hypercalcemia may include expansion of intravascular volume and diuresis in order to increase renal calcium excretion, usually accomplished with iv NS and furosemide. Hypophosphatemia can impair myocardial contractility and should be corrected; hemodialysis or peritoneal dialysis can be used to lower dangerously elevated serum calcium levels. Mithramycin is not useful for acute Rx of ↑Ca^{++}. **Tests:** ECG; electrolytes; others as indicated from H&P.
Neurological	Patient may present with seizures, hyporeflexia, mental status changes (somnolence, depression, memory loss, psychosis, coma) or peripheral neuropathy. Significant improvement may follow correction of hypercalcemia.
Musculoskeletal	These patients may have muscle atrophy and weakness, osteopenia, arthralgia, pathologic fractures (careful laryngoscopy and positioning), osteitis fibrosa cystica. Response to neuromuscular blockers may be enhanced 2° ↑Ca^{++} → muscle weakness.
Hematologic	Patients also tend to be hypophosphatemic and may show signs of hemolysis, Plt dysfunction, impaired ventricular contractility and leukocyte dysfunction. **Tests:** CBC with Plt count
Endocrine	Primary hyperparathyroidism is most commonly due to benign parathyroid adenoma (90%), or hyperplasia (9%) and rarely to carcinoma. It may be associated with multiple endocrine adenopathy (MEA) syndrome. MEA-1 consists of tumors of the parathyroid, pancreatic islets and pituitary. MEA-2 consists of pheochromocytoma, mucosal neuromas, parathyroid tumors and medullary thyroid carcinoma. **Tests:** As indicated from H&P.
Renal	Patients may have renal dysfunction 2° nephrolithiasis, nephrocalcinosis, renal tubular disorders and glomerular disorders. Polyuria 2° ↑Ca^{++} → electrolyte disturbances. **Tests:** Creatinine
Laboratory	Serum calcium (< 12 mg/dL likely asymptomatic; 12-14 mg/dL, mild symptoms; >16 mg/dL, life-threatening); albumin (increase in albumin by 1 g/dL will increase total serum calcium by 0.8 mg/dL); electrolytes; Mg; phosphate (usually low).
Premedication	All medications to lower hypercalcemia should be continued unless calcium levels have normalized. If patient has been treated with steroids in the preop period, administer a stress dose (hydrocortisone 100 mg iv q 8 h × 24 h) prior to induction of anesthesia and continue into the early postop period. Standard premedications (p. B-2) are usually appropriate in this patient group.

INTRAOPERATIVE

Anesthetic technique: GETA, with head slightly hyperextended, allows for surgical exploration of the neck.

Induction	Standard induction (p. B-2). If patient is clinically hypovolemic, restore intravascular volume prior to induction and titrate induction dose of sedative/hypnotic agents.	
Maintenance	Standard maintenance (p. B-3), with muscle relaxant titrated to effect, using peripheral nerve stimulator. Avoid hyperventilation or hypoventilation (acidosis will increase calcium levels, while alkalosis will lower calcium levels). Maintain adequate hydration and UO throughout the procedure.	
Emergence	No special considerations (see postop complications, below).	
Blood and fluid requirements	Minimal blood loss IV: 18 ga × 1 NS @ 5-8 ml/kg/h	Avoid calcium-containing iv solution (e.g., LR).
Monitoring	Standard monitors (p. B-1)	Others as indicated by patient status.
Positioning	✓ and pad all pressure points. ✓ eyes.	Patients should be carefully positioned as they tend to be osteopenic and are prone to pathologic bone fractures. Slight head-up position may ↓ blood loss and improve surgical visibility without significantly ↑ risk of VAE.
Complications	Hypocalcemia	See postop complications (below).

POSTOPERATIVE

Complications	Hypocalcemia Hypophosphatemia Hypocalcemic tetany Seizures Laryngospasm	Hypocalcemia may occur in the immediate postop period. Sx include parathesias, muscle spasm and tetany, as well as laryngospasm, bronchospasm and apnea. Rx: includes 10-20 ml calcium gluconate 10% over 10 min. Follow levels and repeat therapy until the clinical signs of hypocalcemia are controlled.
	Recurrent laryngeal nerve injury Laryngeal edema 2° surgical manipulation Stridor Hematoma with airway compromise	Recurrent laryngeal nerve dysfunction can be monitored by having the patient vocalize the letter "e." Unilateral vocal cord dysfunction results in hoarseness, while bilateral vocal cord dysfunction results in aphonia.
	Pneumothorax	Dx: pleuritic chest pain, dyspnea, ↑RR, ↓breath sounds, hypoxemia; ✓ CXR. Rx: O_2; chest tube and reintubation as necessary.
Pain management	PCA (p. C-3)	
Tests	Serial measurements of: Ca^{++} Phosphate Mg Others as clinically indicated CXR to rule out pneumothorax	The lowest Ca^{++} level is usually seen after 4-5 d postop. Follow clinical signs of hypocalcemia: Trousseau's sign (carpopedal spasm in response to application of a BP cuff at a level above SBP for 3 min); Chvostek's sign (contracture of the facial muscles produced by tapping on the facial nerve).

References

1. Roizen MF: Diseases of the endocrine system. In *Anesthesia and Uncommon Diseases*, 3rd edition. Katz J, Benumof JL, Kadis LB, eds. W.B. Saunders Co, Philadelphia: 1990, 245-55.
2. Schwartz JJ, Rosenbaum SH, Graf GJ: Anesthesia and the endocrine system. In *Clinical Anesthesia*, 3rd edition. Barash PG, Cullen BF, Stoelting RK, eds. Lippincott-Raven Publishers, Philadelphia: 1997, 1039-60.
3. Wang C: The anatomic basis of parathyroid surgery. *Ann Surg* 1976; 183(3):271-75.

ADRENALECTOMY

SURGICAL CONSIDERATIONS

Description: Adrenalectomy is performed for cortical and medullary tumors or hyperplasia (Fig 7.11-4). The glands are removed by sharp/blunt dissection, with care being taken not to injure the adrenal vein. The latter should be exposed and ligated, avoiding damage to the vena cavae on the right side and the renal vein on the left side. Through a midline or subcostal incision (**transabdominal approach**), the left adrenal gland is exposed by incising the lateral peritoneal attachment of the spleen, allowing it to be mobilized and retracted medially along with the tail of the pancreas. Gerota's fascia is then incised at the upper pole of the left kidney, exposing the adrenal gland. The gland is mobilized by sharp/blunt dissection until the prominent adrenal vein is exposed. It is then carefully transected between ligatures and the adrenal gland is removed. On the right side, the adrenal gland is exposed by retracting the right lobe of the liver cephalad and depressing the hepatic flexure inferiorly. After the peritoneum is incised lateral to the duodenum, and the latter mobilized, the IVC is exposed. The right kidney is pulled downward and the adrenal gland is visualized, along with the right adrenal vein entering the vena cava. On occasion, there may be two adrenal veins that require ligating. Once the adrenal vein has been secured, the adrenal gland is removed easily by blunt dissection and any significant vascular attachments are ligated.

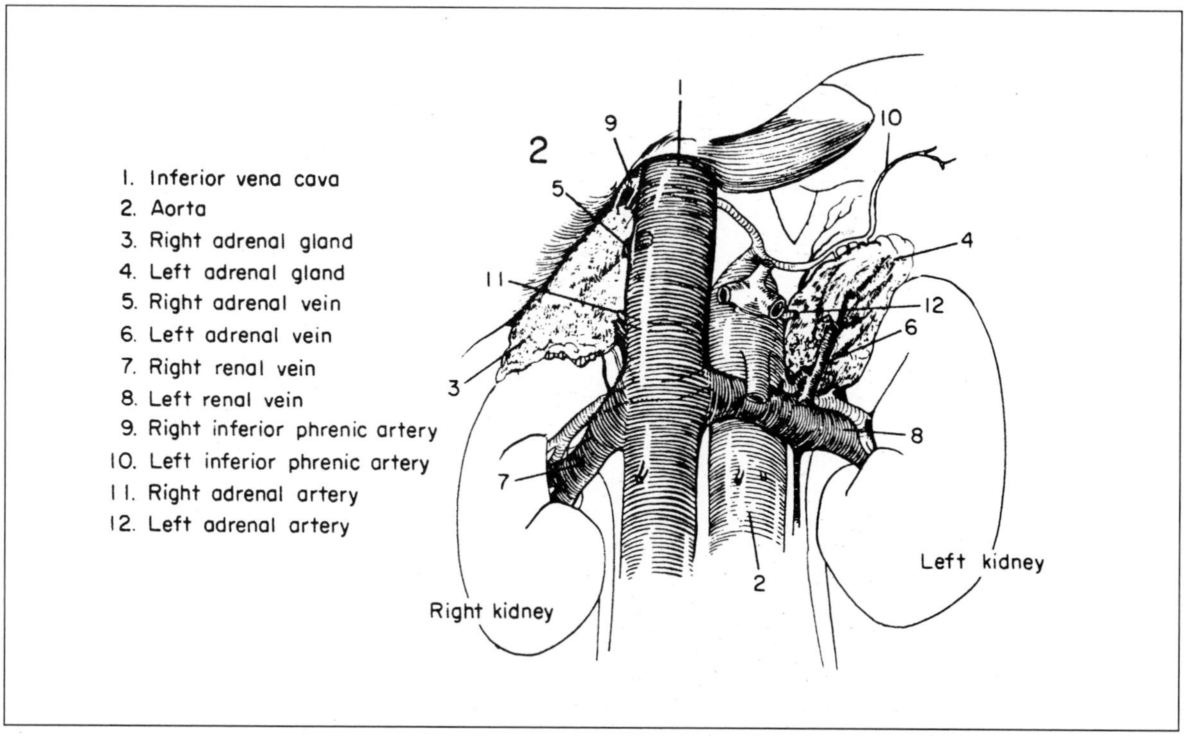

Figure 7.11-4. Surgical anatomy for an adrenalectomy. (Reproduced from: Zollinger RM Jr., Zollinger RM. *Atlas of Surgical Operations*, 6th edition. Macmillan: 1988.)

Variant procedure or approaches: The **flank, or posterior approach** (Fig 7.11-5) is preferred for unilateral adrenalectomy; e.g., a portion of the 12th rib is resected, exposing Gerota's fascia. After incising the fascia, the adrenal gland is exposed, mobilized and resected, following ligation of the adrenal vein. Laparoscopic adrenalectomy is being performed with greater frequency (see p. 424).

Usual preop diagnosis: Cushing's syndrome; aldosteronism; pheochromocytoma; other adrenal tumors

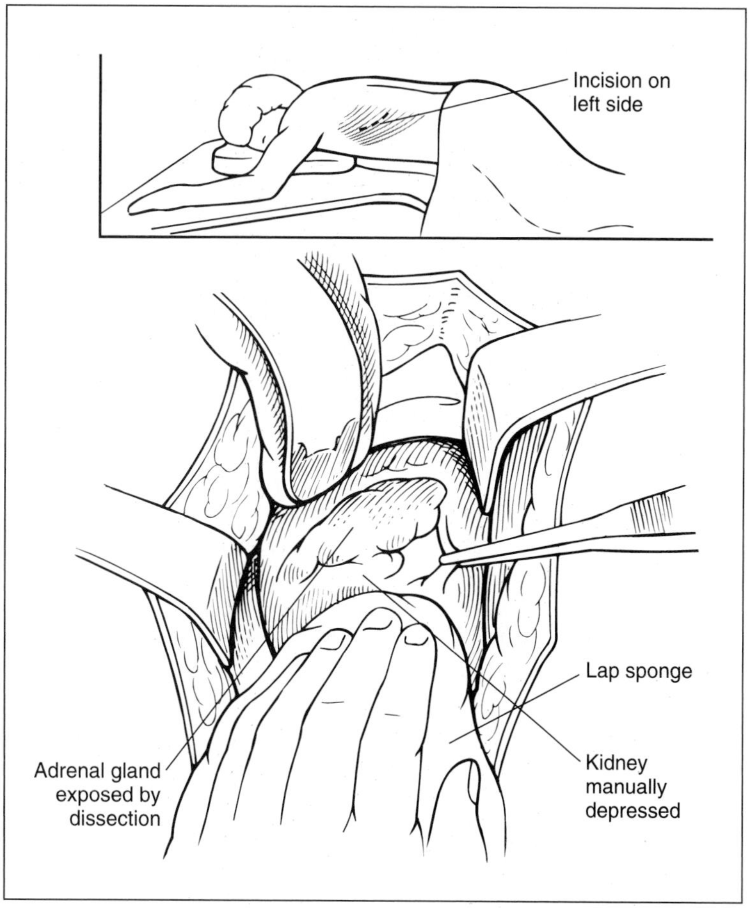

Figure 7.11-5. Flank exposure of adrenal gland. The diaphragm has been transected and Gerota's fascia opened to expose the adrenal gland. (Redrawn with permission from Macdonald J, Haller D, Weigel RJ: Endocrine System. In *Clinical Oncology.* Abeloff MD, et al, eds. Churchill Livingstone, New York: 1995.

SUMMARY OF PROCEDURE

	Transabdominal	Flank or Posterior
Position	Supine	Nephrectomy or prone jackknife
Incision	Midline abdominal or bilateral subcostal	Dorsal flank oblique or curved posterior
Special instrumentation	Denier retractor	None
Unique considerations	BP monitoring essential for pheochromocytoma patients	⇐
Antibiotics	None	⇐
Surgical time	1-2 h	⇐
Closing considerations	Hemostasis	⇐
EBL	200-300 ml	⇐
Postop care	Continue monitoring BP; PACU → room; ± ICU	⇐
Mortality	5.6% (Cushing's)	⇐
Morbidity	Respiratory difficulties: 26%	⇐
	Wound problems: 9%	⇐
	Hemorrhage: 3%	
	Venous thrombosis with embolism (Cushing's): 2%	⇐
Pain score	6-8	7-9

PATIENT POPULATION CHARACTERISTICS

Age range	13-75 yr
Male:Female	1:2.8
Incidence	Pheochromocytoma: 0.4-2% of all hypertensive patients Primary hyperaldosteronism: ~4% of all hypertensive patients Cushing's syndrome: 6/1 million
Etiology	Adenoma or adenocarcinoma (90%); Ectopic ACTH (15% of patients with Cushing's); Cushing's syndrome (hyperadrenocorticism) (10-15%); Conn's syndrome (hyperaldosteronism). Idiopathic hyperplasia is usually treated medically.
Associated conditions	HTN (75-80%); diabetes mellitus (10-15%)

ANESTHETIC CONSIDERATIONS

PREOPERATIVE

Cushing's syndrome: Hyperadrenocorticism can be due to adrenal hyperplasia, adrenal carcinoma, pituitary hypersecretion (Cushing's disease), hypersecretion from exogenous tumor or exogenous steroid administration (most common). Adrenalectomy is the traditional treatment for hyperadrenocorticism due to adrenal carcinoma. These typically moon-faced patients present with one or more of the following: HTN (2° glucocorticoids, renin), renal calculi, osteoporosis, glucose intolerance, personality changes and myopathy. In addition, a fragile vasculature predisposes these patients to easy bruising and difficult vascular access.

Pheochromocytoma: Tumors of chromaffin tissue origin release massive amounts of catecholamines (norepinephrine > epinephrine) and are responsible for the patient's clinical presentation. The tumor is usually found unilaterally in one of the adrenal glands, but also can be found anywhere in the body that chromaffin tissue arises (e.g., urinary bladder, sympathetic chain). These patients require extensive preop preparation, consisting of α-blockade (phenoxybenzamine 40-100 mg/d × 1-2 wk) and concomitant volume expansion. Patients with tachydysrhythmias may require β-blockade only after institution of the α-blockers to prevent serious hypertensive sequelae. Adrenergic blockade and volume expansion may take up to 2 wk prior to surgical removal of the tumor. Inadequate preop preparation will increase the perioperative morbidity of patients with pheochromocytomas. The adequacy of medical therapy is assessed by the absence of symptoms of catecholamine excess, BP of ≤ 160/90 on 2 measurements in the 36 hours preceding surgery, SBP dropping by ≥ 15% on standing, but not less than an absolute BP of 80/45; no ST-T wave changes for 2 wk prior to surgery. There is an increased incidence of pheochromocytoma in certain diseases (multiple-endocrine neoplasia II, neurofibromatosis, tuberous sclerosis, Sturge-Weber syndrome, von Hippel-Lindau disease).

Conn's syndrome: Hyperaldosteronism can be primary (Conn's syndrome–adrenal adenoma or hyperplasia) or secondary (caused by excess renin secretion related to renal dysfunction). These patients are typically hypokalemic and alkalotic →

muscle weakness, parathesias, tetany and polyuria. They may also be hypervolemic (→ CHF), hypernatremic and hypertensive (diastolic).

Respiratory Cushing's syndrome: Patient may be obese with all attendant problems of morbid obesity (see Preoperative Considerations in Operations for Morbid Obesity, p. 354).
Conn's syndrome: respiratory muscle weakness
Tests: As indicated from H&P.

Cardiovascular Cushing's syndrome: HTN, hypervolemia, dysrhythmias 2° hypokalemia
Pheochromocytoma: Paroxysmal HTN, tachydysrhythmias, orthostatic hypotension, hypovolemia, myocardial dysfunction, cardiomyopathy, ventricular ectopy, ↓intravascular volume, ↓sensitivity of α-receptors to normal levels of catecholamines, CHF
Conn's syndrome: HTN, dysrhythmias, ↓T wave, + U wave
Tests: ECG; orthostatic vital signs; consider ECHO or MUGA scan, to evaluate LV function, if indicated from H&P.

Renal Cushing's syndrome: Excess steroid production → Na^+ retention, K^+ excretion and glucose intolerance (hyperglycemia).
Conn's syndrome: renal HTN, polyuria, polydipsia, ↓K^+, ↑Na^+. Correction of hypokalemia requires > 24 h supplemental K^+ infusion (e.g., 5-20 mEq/h).
Pheochromocytoma: HTN from excess catecholamine state may damage kidneys; hyperglycemia.
Tests: UA; creatinine; glucose; urine concentrations of catecholamine metabolites; others as appropriate

Neurological Cushing's syndrome: Psychiatric changes, headache
Pheochromocytoma: Tremulousness, headache, anxiety, nervousness, paresthesia in arms, hypertensive retinopathy, dilated pupils

Musculoskeletal Cushing's syndrome: Striae, muscular wasting, buffalo hump, truncal obesity, thin skin, easy bruisability, osteopenia (compression fractures), weakness
Pheochromocytoma: Weight loss, weakness, fatigue
Conn's syndrome: muscle weakness, tetany, ↑sensitivity to muscle relaxants, osteoporosis

Hematologic Cushing's syndrome: Polycythemia
Pheochromocytoma: Polycythemia (due to hemoconcentration)

Laboratory Tests as indicated from H&P.

Premedication Conn's syndrome: Spironolactone often given to inhibit excess aldosterone effects. Midazolam (0.025-0.05 mg/kg); hydrocortisone 100 mg q 8 h.
Pheochromocytoma: Midazolam (0.025-0.05 mg/kg iv). Preop steroid replacement if bilateral adrenalectomy is contemplated.

INTRAOPERATIVE

Anesthetic technique: GETA (± epidural for postop analgesia). If postop epidural analgesia is planned, placement of catheter prior to anesthetic induction is helpful in establishing correct placement in the epidural space and assuring a bilateral block (accomplished by placing 5-7 ml of 1% lidocaine via the epidural and eliciting a segmental block). Epidurals cannot be used for a posterior approach since they are in the operative field.

Induction Gentle iv induction (titration to effect with STP or etomidate) and muscle relaxation (vecuronium 0.1 mg/kg). Patient should be adequately anesthetized prior to any stimulation. Unopposed parasympathetic response can occur to laryngoscopy, with resultant bradycardia/asystole.

Maintenance Volatile anesthetic (isoflurane), opiate, muscle relaxant. N_2O can cause bowel distention and is best avoided. Local anesthetic (2% lidocaine **without** epinephrine [pheochromocytoma] [5-10 ml q 60 min]) can be injected into the epidural catheter to provide both anesthesia and optimal surgical exposure (contracted bowel and profound muscle relaxation). A continuous infusion of local anesthetic (e.g., 2% lidocaine or 0.25% bupivacaine) at 5-10 ml may enhance hemodynamic stability. Some anesthesiologists will not use the epidural catheter intraop because chemical "sympathectomy" is more difficult to reverse. If epidural opiates are used for postop analgesia, a loading dose (e.g., hydromorphone 1.0 mg) should be administered at least 1 h before the conclusion of surgery. Systemic sedatives (droperidol, opiates, benzodiazepines, etc.) should be minimized during this type of anesthetic as they increase the likelihood of postop respiratory depression. Intraop HTN in pheochromocytomic patients is best treated with SNP, tachycardia with esmolol, and hypotension

Maintenance, cont.	with phenylephrine or dopamine. Good communication with surgical team is very important, especially when the adrenal gland is being mobilized.	
Emergence	Depends on ease of the surgical procedure and the hemodynamic stability of the patient intraop. If patient is hemodynamically unstable, hypothermic, or has a large 3rd-space fluid requirement, consider postop ventilation.	
Blood and fluid requirements	Anticipate large fluid loss. IV: 14-16 ga × 2 NS/LR @ 10-15 ml/kg/h Warm all fluids. Humidify inhaled gases. Cell Saver	As blood loss can be significant, blood should be immediately available. If procedure does not involve cancer, cell-saving devices can be utilized. Guide fluid management by UO, filling pressures, CO.
Monitoring	Standard monitors (p. B-1) UO Arterial line CVP/PA catheter ± TEE	Others as clinically indicated (e.g., PA catheter for patients with pheochromocytoma). Forced air warmer useful for maintaining body temperature. The use of TEE may be helpful in establishing fluid status and other hemodynamic parameters.
Complications	Labile HTN Dysrhythmias	Surgical manipulation of the adrenal may cause ↑↑BP and dysrhythmias. Rx: Alert surgeon and control BP with esmolol/SNP.
	↓BP (postexcision)	↓BP not uncommon after removal of tumor. Rx: phenylephrine/dopamine infusions.
Positioning	✓ and pad pressure points. ✓ eyes.	Strict attention to patient positioning, padding and taping are important in patients with glucocorticoid excess because of osteopenia and thin, easily traumatized skin.

POSTOPERATIVE

Complications	Pneumothorax (incidence approaches 20%)	Dx: pleuritic chest pain, dyspnea, ↑RR, ↓breath sounds, hypoxemia. ✓ CXR. Rx: O_2; chest tube and reintubation as necessary.
	Hypoglycemia	
	Hypoadrenocorticism after tumor resection	Consider glucocorticoid and mineralocorticoid replacement—hydrocortisone 100 mg q 8 h.
	Cushing's syndrome: Hypoventilation 2° to obesity (hypoxemia, hypercarbia) HTN Pheochromocytoma: BP lability Myocardial dysfunction	
Pain management	Epidural analgesia (p. C-1) PCA (p. C-3)	Patient should be recovered in an ICU or ward accustomed to treating the side effects of epidural opiates (e.g., respiratory depression, breakthrough pain, nausea, pruritus).
Tests	CXR; ECG; electrolytes; glucose	

References

1. Christopherson R, Parris WCV: Anesthesia for endocrine surgery. In *Principles and Practice of Anesthesiology*, 2nd edition. Longnecker DE, Tinker JH, Morgan GE Jr, eds. Mosby-Year Book, Inc, St. Louis: 1998, 1948.
2. Cousins MJ, Rubin RB: The intraoperative management of pheochromocytoma with total epidural sympathetic blockade. *Br J Anaesth* 1974; 46(1):78-81.
3. Roizen MF, Horrigan RW, Koike M, et al: A perspective randomized trial of four anesthetic techniques for resection of pheochromocytoma. *Anesthesiology* 1982; 57:A43.
4. Roizen MF, Hunt TK, Beaupre PN, et al: The effect of alpha-adrenergic blockade on cardiac performance and tissue oxygen delivery during excision of pheochromocytoma. *Surgery* 1983; 94(6):941-45.
5. Roizen MF, Schreider BD, Hassan SZ: Anesthesia for patients with pheochromocytoma. *Anesthesiol Clin North Am* 1987; 5:269.
6. Sieber FE: Evaluation of the patient with endocrine disease and diabetes mellitus. In *Principles and Practice of Anesthesiology*, 2nd edition. Longnecker DE, Tinker JH, Morgan GE Jr, eds. Mosby-Year Book, Inc, St Louis: 1998, 303-22.

Surgeons

Edward J. Alfrey, MD (*Kidney transplantation*)
Donald C. Dafoe, MD (*Kidney transplantation*)
Carlos O. Esquivel, MD, PhD (*Liver transplantation*)

7.12 LIVER/KIDNEY TRANSPLANTATION

Anesthesiologists

Gordon R. Haddow, MB, ChB, FFA(SA) (*Liver/kidney transplantation*)
E. Price Stover, MD (*Multiorgan procurement*)

KIDNEY TRANSPLANTATION—CADAVERIC AND LIVE DONOR

SURGICAL CONSIDERATIONS

Description: Kidney transplantation offers patients with end-stage renal disease freedom from dialysis. The source of the renal graft may be a cadaveric donor, a relative (e.g., parent, sibling) or a genetically unrelated, but emotionally related individual (e.g., spouse).

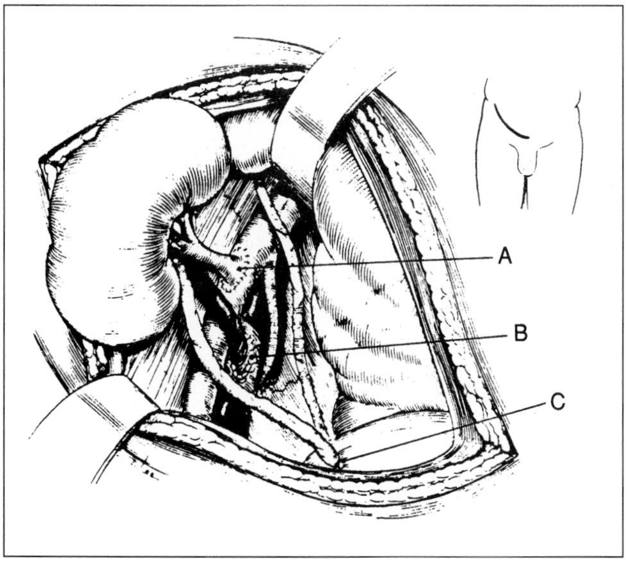

Figure 7.12-1. Kidney transplantation, showing anastomoses of: (A) renal artery to external iliac artery; (B) renal vein to iliac vein; and (C) ureter to bladder. To increase exposure of bladder for a ureteroneocystostomy, antibiotic solution is used to fill the bladder. Lower quadrant curvilinear incision is shown in inset. (Reproduced with permission from Hardy JD: *Hardy's Textbook of Surgery*, 2nd edition. JB Lippincott: 1988.)

After induction of anesthesia, a 3-way Foley catheter is placed into the bladder, and the kidney allograft is placed in the extraperitoneal iliac fossa. A curvilinear incision is made in the right or left lower quadrant. The dissection is maintained in the extraperitoneal space by retracting the peritoneum medial and cephalad, and a self-retaining retractor is usually placed. The external iliac artery and vein are identified, surrounding lymphatics are divided after ligation, and the vessels are mobilized for several centimeters. The external iliac vein is clamped first and the renal-vein-to-iliac-vein anastomosis is performed. Then the external iliac-artery-to-renal-artery anastomosis is performed, and the clamps are released (Fig 7.12-1). The patient should be euvolemic at this point; mannitol and/or furosemide can be given. The bladder is filled with an antibiotic irrigation solution to allow reimplantation of the ureter, which is performed after the detrusor muscle of the bladder has been dissected away from the mucosa. The wound is closed, normally leaving native kidneys intact.

Variant procedure or approaches: Cadaveric or live-donor transplantation

Usual preop diagnosis: End-stage renal disease (ESRD)

SUMMARY OF PROCEDURE

	Cadaveric	Live Donor
Position	Supine	⇐
Incision	Lower quadrant curvilinear (Fig 7.12-1 inset)	⇐
Special instrumentation	Self-retaining retractor; vascular instruments; CVP; Foley catheter (3-way)	⇐
Unique considerations	Adequate hydration, CVP 10-12 mmHg; mannitol 12.5-25 g; intraop immunosuppression prior to reperfusion (steroids, azathioprine 10 mg/kg); potassium-free iv fluid; protection of shunt or fistula important.	⇐
Antibiotics	Gentamicin 1.7 mg/kg; cefazolin 1 g, 1 h preop	Cefazolin 1 g, 1 h preop
Surgical time	2.5-3 h	3 h
EBL	500 ml	⇐
Postop care	Replace UO ml/ml; may have delayed graft function 2°prolonged cold storage and ↓UO or clearance; ICU selectively.	Fluid replacement; delayed graft function unlikely; ICU
Mortality	1%	1-3%
Morbidity	Lymph or serous leak: 3-5%	⇐
	Postop bleeding: 3-5%	1-2%
	MI: 2-3%	⇐
	Ureteral leak: 2-3%	⇐

	Cadaveric	Live Donor
Morbidity, cont.	Wound infection: 2-3%	⇐
	Arterial thrombosis: 1-2%	⇐
	Venous thrombosis: 1-2%	⇐
	Wound hematoma: 1-2%	⇐
	Other infectious complications: 15-40%	⇐
Pain score	5	6

PATIENT POPULATION CHARACTERISTICS

Age range	3-70 yr
Male:Female	1:1
Incidence	60/1,000,000
Etiology	Glomerulonephritis (25%); HTN (25%); diabetes mellitus (25%); polycystic disease and others (25%)
Associated conditions	CAD (40%); HTN (25%); uremic and/or diabetic neuropathy (25%); hyperparathyroidism (15-20%)

ANESTHETIC CONSIDERATIONS

See Anesthetic Considerations following Cadaveric Kidney/Pancreas Transplant, p. 490.

Reference

1. Morris PJ: Renal transplantation: a quarter century. *Semin Nephrol* 1997; 17:188-95.

CADAVERIC KIDNEY/PANCREAS TRANSPLANTATION

SURGICAL CONSIDERATIONS

Description: Pancreas transplantation: Patients near end-stage renal disease 2° diabetes mellitus (DM) can maintain relative normoglycemia with a successful pancreas transplant. The immunosuppressive requirements differ from a kidney transplant alone in the use of an anti-T cell preparation, beginning in the OR. The kidney transplant is placed in the iliac fossa on one side (see Kidney Transplantation, p. 487) and the pancreas transplant is placed in the opposite iliac fossa, with the pancreas normally transplanted first (Fig 7.12-2). The graft is prepared first, on the back table. For the arterial in-flow, either a patch of aorta, including the superior mesenteric and celiac artery trunks, is utilized; or a Y-graft is fashioned, using the donor iliac artery bifurcation anastomosed to the graft splenic and superior mesenteric arteries. The graft duodenal segment, which includes most of the C-loop of the duodenum, is shortened on the back table. The arterial anastomosis is accomplished by anastomosing either the aortic patch or the iliac extension to the donor external iliac artery. The portal vein is anastomosed to the external iliac vein. The exocrine secretions of the pancreas graft may be drained via a segment of donor duodenum into either the urinary bladder (as depicted in Figure 7.12-2) or bowel. The bladder should be filled after revascularization of the pancreas to allow good visualization of it while the duodenal segment is sewn to the bladder. Pancreas transplantations can have significant blood loss if the graft mesenteric vessels are not occluded properly. Once the pancreas is transplanted, the kidney transplant is placed into the opposite iliac fossa (as described in the preceding section).

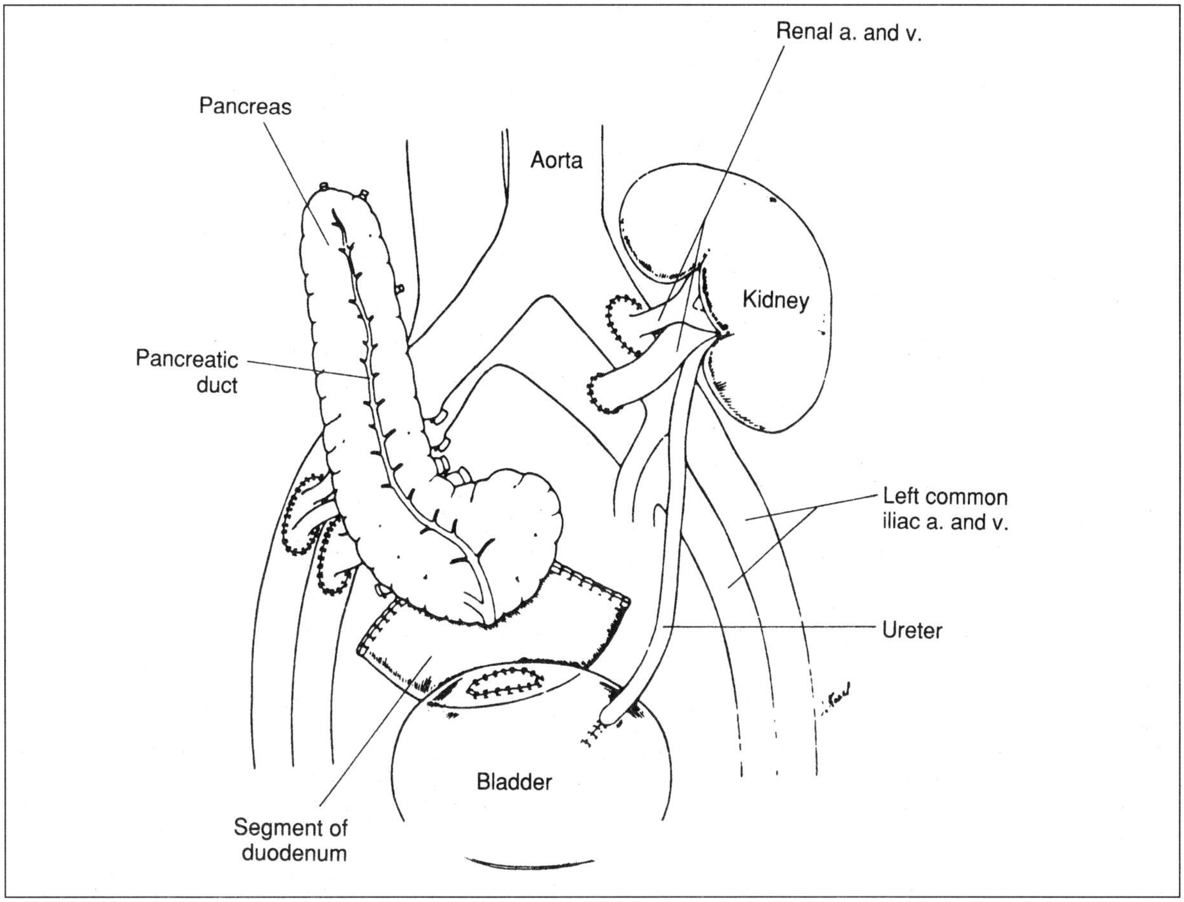

Figure 7.12-2. Transplantation of pancreas with bladder drainage through a pancreaticoduodenocystostomy. Renal transplant also shown. (Modified with permission from Moody FG, ed: *Surgical Treatment of Digestive Disease*, 2nd edition. Mosby-Year Book: 1990.)

Variant procedure or approaches: Isolated islet cells have been transplanted beneath the renal capsule of a renal allograft or into native portal vein; however, the success rate has been limited.

Usual preop diagnosis: End-stage renal disease (ESDR) 2° diabetes mellitus (DM)

SUMMARY OF PROCEDURE

Position	Supine; cushion heels
Incision	Midline or bilateral lower quadrant
Special instrumentation	Bookwalter retractor; vascular instruments; Foley catheter; NG tube; CVP; arterial line
Unique considerations	Do not correct hyperglycemia < 300 mg/dL. Maintain adequate hydration, CVP 10-12 mmHg; mannitol 0.25-0.5 g/kg on unclamping; intraop immunosuppression prior to reperfusion (1 g methylprednisolone, 10 mg/kg azathioprine after incision); potassium-free iv fluid; protection of shunt or fistula important.
Antibiotics	Gentamicin (1.7 mg/kg iv slowly), cefazolin (1 g q 6 h for 5 d)
Surgical time	5-6 h
EBL	750 ml
Postop care	ICU × 1-2 d, hourly monitoring of glucose; serum glucose should decline by 50 mg/dL each h and remain < 200 mg/dL.
Mortality	2%
Morbidity	Thrombosis of graft: 10% Wound infection: 2-6% Postop bleeding: 3-5% Pancreatitis: 2-4% Anastomotic leak: 1%
Pain score	6

PATIENT POPULATION CHARACTERISTICS

Age range	15-45 yr
Male:Female	1:1
Incidence	15-20% of all patients with ESRD
Etiology	Autoimmune (pancreas); glomerulonephritis (25%); HTN (25%); diabetes mellitus (25%); polycystic disease and others (25%)
Associated conditions	Retinopathy (100%); CAD (50-70%); uremic and/or diabetic neuropathy (50%); gastropathy (25%); hyperparathyroidism (15-20%)

ANESTHETIC CONSIDERATIONS FOR KIDNEY AND KIDNEY/PANCREAS TRANSPLANTATION

PREOPERATIVE

Typically, patients presenting for renal transplantation fall into two patient populations: (1) the young and relatively healthy (following dialysis), or (2) an older, more chronically ill group. Rarely, patients will present for transplant surgery without adequate preparation (e.g., ↑K^+, ↓pH). Patients presenting for pancreas transplantation are usually severe diabetics with many of the associated problems, such as CAD, autonomic neuropathy, gastroparesis and stiff-joint syndrome (difficult intubation).

Respiratory Pleuritis and pleural effusions may occur in this patient population. Increased susceptibility to infection is common in the patient with chronic uremia.

Cardiovascular Pericarditis (acute or constrictive), HTN, CHF, dysrhythmias, pericardial effusion are common, especially in the undialized patient. Diabetes, a common cause of ESRD, is often associated with PVD, CAD and autonomic neuropathy.
Tests: ECG (rhythm, electrolyte abnormalities, pericarditis, LVH). Other tests (ECHO, stress, etc.) as indicated from H&P.

Gastrointestinal Gastroparesis may occur, especially in diabetic patients with autonomic neuropathy. It is safer to assume that these patients will require full-stomach precautions. Ranitidine (50 mg iv) and metoclopramide (10 mg iv) should be given 60 min preop to aid gastric emptying and ↓acidity. Na citrate (30 ml, 0.3 M po) should be given immediately before induction.

Renal Patients are usually on dialysis. Postdialysis goals include: K^+ = 4-5 mEq/L, BUN < 60 mg%, creatinine < 10 mg%. Metabolic acidosis, hypocalcemia and hypermagnesemia may be present, and require correction preop. Patient may be hypovolemic following dialysis; ✓ pre- and post-dialysis weight (> 2 kg loss is significant). Rapid correction of severe hyperkalemia can be achieved by giving iv 50 ml of 50% glucose, together with 12 U regular insulin and 50 mEq $NaHCO_3$.
Tests: Creatinine; BUN; creatine clearance; electrolytes

Hematologic These patients are typically anemic (Hct = 18-24%). Usually it is not necessary to correct this anemia (unless < 18%). A coagulation disorder may be present with abnormal Plt function (improved by dialysis) and possibly thrombocytopenia, resulting in a prolonged bleeding time. There is a high incidence of post transfusion hepatitis in this patient population.
Tests: Hct; PT; PTT; Plt count; bleeding time; hepatic screen

Neurologic Peripheral neuropathy may occur and specific deficits should be documented. Autonomic neuropathy can → cardiac problems (e.g., orthostatic hypotension, ↑HR or ↓HR), silent MI, and gastrointestinal problems.

Premedication Patients should continue their routine medications up to the time of surgery. A small dose of midazolam is usually a safe premedication for Rx anxiety. Consider the possibility of a full stomach and use full-stomach precautions (see p. B-5).

INTRAOPERATIVE

Anesthetic technique: GETA. Epidural anesthesia may be considered for some cases of renal transplantation.

Induction Rapid-sequence induction (see p. B-5). ET intubation is aided by succinylcholine (1 mg/kg) if K^+

Induction, cont.	< 5.5 mEq/L; otherwise, use cisatracurium (0.2-0.5 mg/kg) or vecuronium (0.2 mg/kg). Fentanyl (2-5 μg/kg) may be used to suppress the cardiovascular response to intubation.	
Maintenance	Standard maintenance (see p. B-3). Maintain muscle relaxation with cisatracurium or vecuronium, titrated to effect using a nerve stimulator. Avoid meperidine (accumulation of normeperidine may cause CNS toxicity). Anticipate prolonged drug effects, and avoid agents that are primarily excreted by the kidney.	
Emergence	Usually extubated in the OR after protective laryngeal reflexes have returned. Pancreatic transplant patients (e.g., brittle diabetics, hemodynamically unstable) are sent to the ICU.	
Blood and fluid requirements	IV: 14 ga × 1 NS q s CVP = 10-15 mmHg Warm fluids. Humidify gases.	Preop fluid status is highly variable. Fluids should be given to maintain CVP 10-15 mmHg. It is important to maintain adequate vascular volume and BP. Mannitol (0.25-1 g/kg), furosemide (5-20 mg) and low-dose dopamine are often given with reperfusion of the kidney.
Monitoring	Standard monitors (see p. B-1). Arterial line CVP/PA line	Arterial pressure is often monitored. Avoid the side of A-V fistulae. Axillary artery is a useful alternative. CVP is essential and occasionally a PA line is needed (severe cardiac disease). CVP is kept at 10-15 mmHg, especially after the new kidney is reperfused, to ensure adequate renal blood flow.
	Hct, K^+ and glucose	In pancreatic transplant patients, glucose should be checked q 30 min and q 10 min for the first h following reperfusion. Keep glucose < 300 mg % prior to reperfusion.
	Neuromuscular	Monitor neuromuscular block to avoid excessive use of neuromuscular relaxants.
Positioning	✓ and pad pressure points. ✓ eyes.	
Complications	Hemorrhage Low UO	

POSTOPERATIVE

Complications	Respiratory depression Femoral neuropathy Hemorrhage Electrolyte abnormalities	Monitor UO. Dialysis may be needed until renal function returns. Sudden cardiac arrest can complicate pancreatic transplantation (due to autonomic neuropathy).
Pain management	PCA (see p. C-3).	
Tests	Hct Electrolytes Creatinine, BUN Amylase Glucose	A rise in amylase and blood glucose may indicate failure of the pancreatic transplant.

References

1. Graybar GB, Deierhoi MH: Anesthesia and pancreatic transplantation. *Anesth Clin North Am* 1989; 7(3)515-49.
2. Moote CA: Anesthesia for renal transplantation. In *Organ Transplantation*. Benumof JL, ed. Anesthesiology Clinics of North America. WB Saunders, Philadelphia: 1994; 12(4) 691-716.
3. Sutherland DER: State of the art in pancreas transplantation. *Transplant Proc* 1994; 26:316.

LIVE-DONOR NEPHRECTOMY

SURGICAL CONSIDERATIONS

Description: Use of a kidney donated by a healthy relative or emotionally related donor greatly increases the number and quality of available kidneys for transplantation. The better the histocompatibility, the lesser the chance of rejection, lower immunosuppression, lesser the risk of infectious complications and better long term graft survival. The donor/patient is placed in a lateral decubitus position on a flexible OR table with a "kidney rest." (A bean bag or sand bags are also helpful for positioning.) An incision is made from the rectus muscle, angling slightly cephalad to cross into the flank just below the tip of the 12th rib and then past it posteriorly to the paraspinous muscles. The retroperitoneum is exposed using a sternal retractor. The kidney is then mobilized, which takes about 1.5 h. A clamp is placed across the renal artery at the aorta and the renal vein at the IVC; the renal artery is doubly ligated distally and divided. Just prior to clamping the renal artery, furosemide and/or mannitol may be given to stimulate a diuresis. It is important to keep the vascular volume expanded in these patients prior to removal of the kidney. The ureter is transected and the kidney is removed and taken to the back table where it is flushed with a cold preservation solution. It is then transported into the recipient room for reimplantation.

Variant approach: A transperitoneal laparoscopic approach to donor nephrectomy is gaining acceptance. Port incisions are made in the flank; then, a midline infraumbilical incision is made to deliver the kidney graft. Postop pain is significantly reduced with this approach.

Usual preop diagnosis: Donor nephrectomy

SUMMARY OF PROCEDURE

Position	Lateral decubitus (supine at some centers, where a midline incision is used).
Incision	Flank; may require 12th rib resection. (Midline in some centers.)
Special instrumentation	Foley catheter; chest retractor; flexible OR table with "kidney rest"; bean bag or sand bags; SCDs for DVT prophylaxis
Unique considerations	Possible pneumothorax; avoid ETT dislodgement when turning patient from supine to flank position. Vigorous hydration to encourage urine production.
Antibiotics	Cefazolin 1 g, 1 h preop
Surgical time	2-2.5 h
Closing considerations	Deflex table to facilitate closure
EBL	100 ml
Postop care	CXR to rule out pneumothorax. Epidural or PCA (morphine) is helpful for pain management. PACU → room.
Mortality	< 0.1%
Morbidity	Ileus: 5-10% Urinary retention: 5-10% Wound infection: 1-3% Pneumothorax: 1% Bleeding: 0.1-0.5%
Pain score	7

PATIENT POPULATION CHARACTERISTICS

Age range	18-70 yr
Male:Female	1:1
Incidence	Up to 20% of all kidney transplants at some centers
Etiology	Kindness
Associated conditions	Good health is mandatory for renal donation.

ANESTHETIC CONSIDERATIONS

PREOPERATIVE

In order to be a live donor, one must be in good health with bilaterally functional kidneys. Diabetes, HIV infection, liver disease and malignancy are all contraindications to kidney donations.

Cardiovascular	R/O HTN, CAD.	
Renal	Normal bilateral renal function is required. **Tests:** IVP; creatinine, creatinine clearance	
Fluid status	Adequate hydration is important and UO should be >1.5 ml/kg/h. Various regimes are used to ensure adequate hydration, usually with iv fluid starting the night before.	
Premedication	Adequate anxiolysis is beneficial. These patients are making a great sacrifice and should be treated with special care. Standard premedication (see p. B-2).	

INTRAOPERATIVE

Anesthetic technique: GETA ± epidural for postop pain management

Induction	Standard induction (see p. B-2).	
Maintenance	Standard maintenance (see p. B-3). Avoid long-acting, renally excreted drugs. Ventilate to maintain eucapnia to avoid possible renal artery vasoconstriction. Use of an epidural with local anesthetic and/or narcotic may aid both intraop and postop pain relief, but hypotension should be avoided.	
Emergence	Routine extubation in OR	
Blood and fluid requirements	IV: 14 ga × 2 NS/LR @ 6-8 ml/h Warm all fluids. Humidify gases. UO 1.5 ml/kg/h	Aim for a minimum of 1.5 ml/kg/h UO. Mannitol (0.25-1 g/kg) given iv once kidney is being manipulated, and if UO decreases.
Monitoring	Standard monitors (see p. B-1).	CVP or invasive arterial monitoring are rarely required.
Positioning	✓ and pad pressure points. ✓ eyes.	Positioning may impair venous return → ↓BP. Ensure that the head is properly padded and that the cervical spine is in line with thoracic spine.
Complications	Hemorrhage	Because the vessels are tied close to the aorta and IVC, the possibility of severe hemorrhage exists.
	Pneumothorax	Pneumothorax is always possible, especially when the 12th rib is resected.

POSTOPERATIVE

Complications	Pneumothorax Hemorrhage Infection Pulmonary problems Hypokalemia (diuretics) Ileus	
Pain management	Epidural narcotics (see p. C-1). PCA (see p. C-3).	Epidural analgesia is recommended.
Tests	CXR Hct	

References

1. Moote CA: Anesthesia for renal transplantation. In *Organ Transplantation*. Benumof JL, ed. Anesthesiology Clinics of North America. WB Saunders, Philadelphia: 1994; 12(4) 691-716.
2. Simmons RL, Finch ME, Ascher NL, Najarian JS, eds: *Manual of Vascular Access, Organ Donation and Transplantation*. Springer-Verlag, New York: 1984.

LIVER TRANSPLANTATION

SURGICAL CONSIDERATIONS

Description: Liver transplantation is the treatment of choice for patients with acute and chronic end-stage liver disease (ESLD). The liver transplant operation can be divided into three stages: (1) hepatectomy; (2) anhepatic phase, which involves the implantation of the liver; and (3) postrevascularization, which includes hemostasis and reconstruction of the hepatic artery and common bile duct.[13] There are many variations in the technical aspects of the liver transplant operation that may result in physiologic changes during anesthesia. The anesthesiologist must be aware of these technical variations to optimize the intraop management of the liver transplant recipient. Examples of these variations include: cross-clamping of the vena cava during the implantation of the liver, which results in impairment of the systemic venous return with subsequent profound hypotension; utilization of the venovenous bypass, which may be associated with thrombus, air embolism and/or fibrinolysis; and the use of a "cutdown liver," which may result in significant bleeding from the raw surface following revascularization.

The **hepatectomy** may be a formidable task in patients with severe portal HTN, coagulopathy and previous surgery in the upper abdomen. In such circumstances, blood loss is significant and may be minimized by placing the patient on venovenous bypass or by creating a temporary portocaval shunt to relieve the portal HTN. Table 7.12-1 lists factors that may be associated with significant blood loss during the transplant operation. The hepatectomy is usually much easier in patients with acute fulminant hepatitis or primary biliary cirrhosis than in patients with shrunken cirrhotic livers, such as in postnecrotic cirrhosis from hepatitis B or C, alpha-1 antitrypsin deficiency or Wilson's disease, among others.

Table 7.12-1. Contributing Factors Associated With Increased Blood Loss in Liver Transplantation

1. Severe coagulopathy
2. Severe portal HTN
3. Previous surgery in the right upper quadrant
4. Renal failure
5. Uncontrolled sepsis
6. Retransplantation
7. Transfusion reaction
8. Venous bypass-induced fibrinolysis
9. Primary graft nonfunction
10. Intraop vascular complications

The **anhepatic phase** may be associated with significant hemodynamic changes, depending on the technique used for vascular control. This stage of the operation consists of implantation of the liver allograft, with or without venovenous bypass. The use of the venovenous bypass is particularly helpful in coagulopathic patients with severe portal HTN. In these high-risk patients, the goal of the venovenous bypass system is to relieve the portal HTN by "bypassing" the liver.[10] Cannulas, placed in the portal and femoral veins, draw the blood out of the systemic and splanchnic venous systems into a Biomedicus pump that delivers the blood into the axillary vein, maintaining the venous return (Fig 7.12-3). This system allows the interruption of the vena cava with mild-to-moderate hemodynamic changes, depending on the blood flow rate through the system. The benefits and potential complications of the venovenous bypass system are listed in Table 7.12-2.[10] Wound complications and nerve injuries may be prevented by introducing the bypass cannulas percutaneously rather than approaching the vessels through a surgical incision.

Because of these complications, several transplant teams have opted not to use the venovenous bypass. Vascular control is obtained by placing vascular clamps across the supra- and infrahepatic vena cava and the portal vein. The systemic and splanchnic venous return is interrupted during the anhepatic phase, leading to significant hypotension unless preventive measures, as reviewed in Anesthetic Considerations (p. 499), are taken (Fig 7.12-4).

Table 7.12-2. Benefits and Potential Complications of the Venovenous Bypass System

Benefits	Complications
Improved hemodynamics during anhepatic phase	PE
↓blood loss	Air embolism
May improve perioperative renal function.*	Brachial plexus injury
	Wound seroma/infection

* In a prospective randomized trial comparing venovenous bypass with no bypass, no difference was found in the perioperative renal function between the two groups.[4]

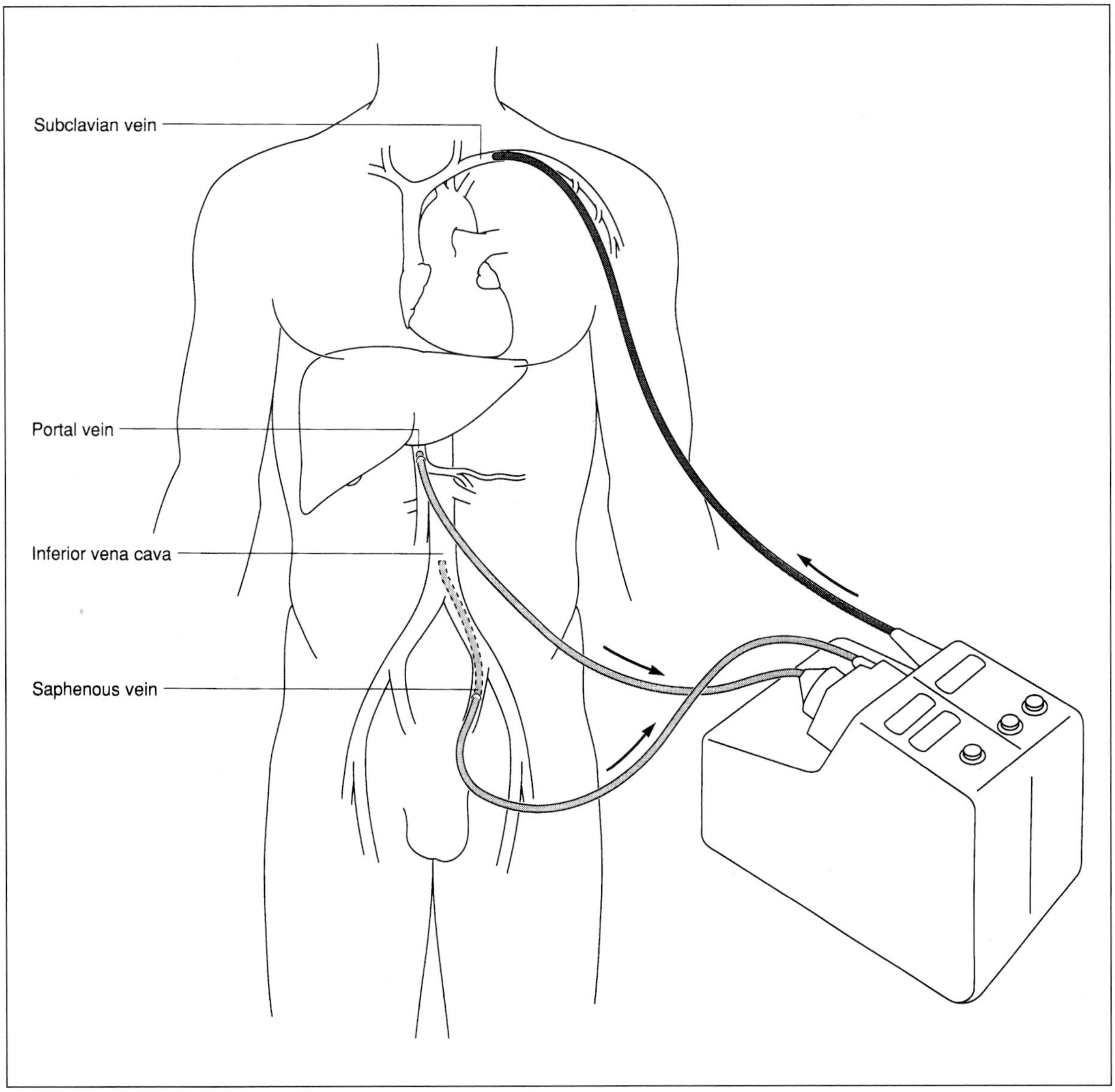

Figure 7.12-3. Setup for venovenous bypass during hepatic transplantation. Cannulas are placed into the portal vein to decompress the splanchnic bed and inferior vena cava (through the greater saphenous vein) to decompress the lower extremities and kidneys during the anhepatic phase of the transplant. A centrifugal pump is used to deliver bypassed blood to the central circulation by means of a cannula passed into the axillary vein. (Reproduced with permission from Greenfield LJ, et al, eds: *Surgery: Scientific Principles and Practice*, 2nd edition. Lippincott-Raven Publishers, Philadelphia: 1997.)

In a standard orthotopic liver transplantation, with or without venovenous bypass, the recipient's vena cava is removed, leaving two cuffs—one just below the diaphragm and the other above the entry of the renal veins. A cadaveric donor liver comes with a segment of the vena cava that is used for restoring the continuity of the recipient's vena cava. The first vascular anastomosis consists of an end-to-end anastomosis of the allograft suprahepatic vena cava and the cuff of the recipient's infradiaphragmatic vena cava. This is followed by the reconstruction of the infrahepatic vena cava with an end-to-end anastomosis. Lastly, the portal vein reconstruction is completed with an end-to-end anastomosis. At this point, the clamps are removed, ending the anhepatic phase of the operation.

Before **revascularization** (i.e., before removing the vascular clamps), the liver must be flushed with a cold solution (e.g., albumin 5%) through the portal vein and out the infrahepatic vena cava. This replaces the preservation solution, which has a very high content of K^+ (~145 mEq/L) and air. Hyperkalemia could be troublesome following revascularization, particularly from livers that sustained significant preservation (cold-storage) injury. Massive air embolism may lead to cardiac arrest following revascularization.

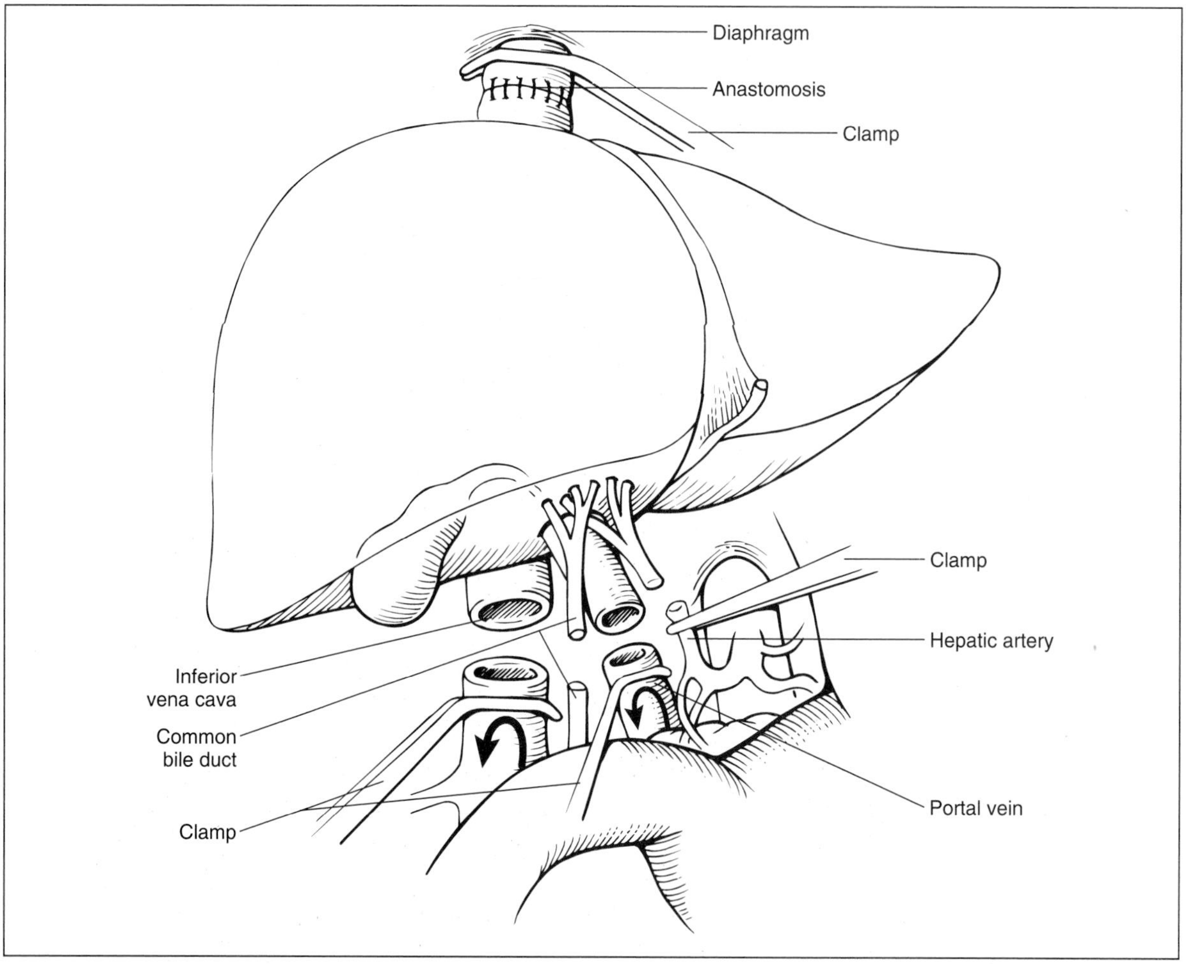

Figure 7.12-4. Standard liver transplantation without venovenous bypass. Venous return is significantly impaired.

Venovenous bypass is not necessary in **piggyback liver transplantation** since the diseased liver is separated from the vena cava (systemic venous return remains unimpaired), and vascular control is obtained by placing a clamp across the confluence of the hepatic veins as they join the vena cava (Fig 7.12-5). A temporary portocaval shunt may be created to minimize bleeding in cases with severe portal HTN. The first anastomosis is between the suprahepatic vena cava of the liver allograft and the cuff created from the hepatic veins. The infrahepatic vena cava of the liver allograft is ligated, and the portal vein reconstruction is completed. The clamps are then removed and the liver is revascularized.

Postrevascularization begins with the removal of the vascular clamps. The reperfusion of the liver may be the most critical part of the operation. It is during this stage that patients may experience pulmonary HTN, followed by RV failure and profound hypotension. This must be treated aggressively; otherwise, the liver is subjected to high outflow resistance leading to congestion and worsening of the preservation injury. The cause of this phenomenon is not well understood; fortunately, it is seen in very few patients.

The hepatic artery reconstruction is performed after stabilization of the patient following revascularization of the liver. The last part of the procedure involves hemostasis, removal of the gallbladder and reconstruction of the bile duct (Fig 7.12-6). There are two basic methods for the bile duct reconstruction: an end-to-end anastomosis, with or without a T tube (in patients with normal common bile ducts); or a choledochojejunostomy to a Roux-en-Y (in patients with biliary atresia, primary sclerosing cholangitis or diseased common bile ducts, or when there is a size discrepancy between the donor and recipient common bile duct). In cadaveric or live-donor segmental transplantation, the technique for the recipient's hepatectomy and the implantation of the allograft is not different from that of full-size liver transplantation; however, the technique of piggyback liver transplantation must be used with live donors since the allograft segment does not include the vena cava. The anesthesiologist must be alert during the reperfusion of a segmental graft since significant bleeding may ensue from the raw surface of the liver (Fig 7.12-7).

Usual preop diagnosis: End-stage liver disease (ESLD)

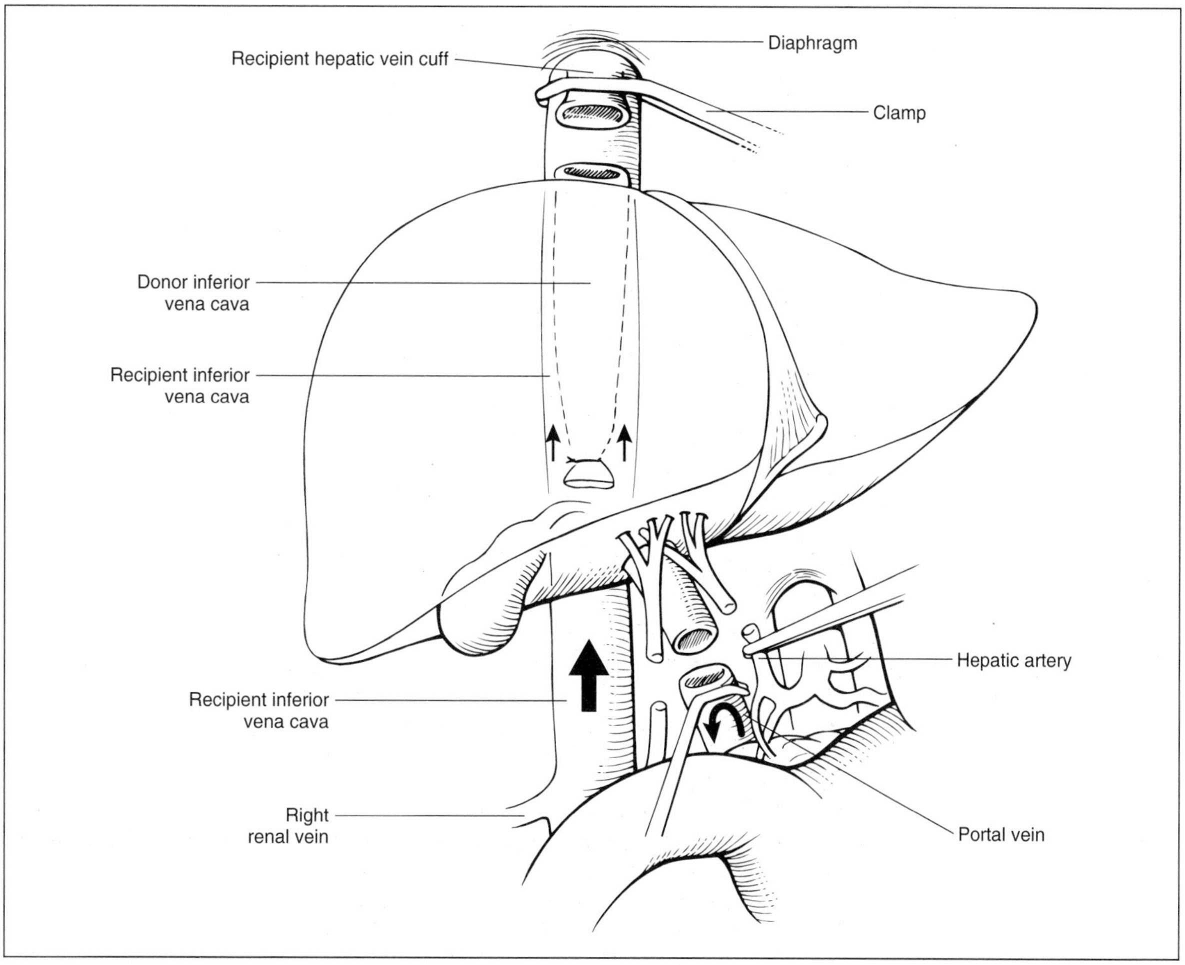

Figure 7.12-5. Piggyback liver transplantation. Note that the recipient's vena cava is left intact and systemic venous return is unimpaired.

SUMMARY OF PROCEDURE

Position	Supine; arms tucked. Left arm and left groin area out for access to the axillary and femoral veins if venous bypass is used.
Incision	Bilateral subcostal, in children; in adults, incision must extend cephalad to the xiphoid process.
Special instrumentation	Upper hand retractor, venous bypass pump; rapid-infusion system; Cell Saver; argon beam coagulator.
Unique considerations	Thrombus or VAE may occur during removal of clamps from vena cava. RV failure, ↓BP and ↓SVR may be observed after revascularization. Continuous arteriovenous hemofiltration may be required if renal failure is present. Head and extremities should be covered with plastic to maintain body temperature, particularly in children.
Antibiotics	Ampicillin (1 g q 8 h) and ceftriaxone (1 g q 24 h) prior to making incision
Surgical time	4-12 h
EBL	6 U average blood loss (range 0-100 U)
Postop care	ICU: 1-2 d. HTN commonly seen.
Mortality	10% at 1 yr
Rejection	35-70% during first yr
Morbidity	Infectious complications: 20-50% Biliary stenosis or leaks: 6-15% Retransplantation: 6-14% Primary graft nonfunction: 2-6% Hepatic artery thrombosis: 0-6% Portal vein thrombosis: 1-4%
Pain score	7-8

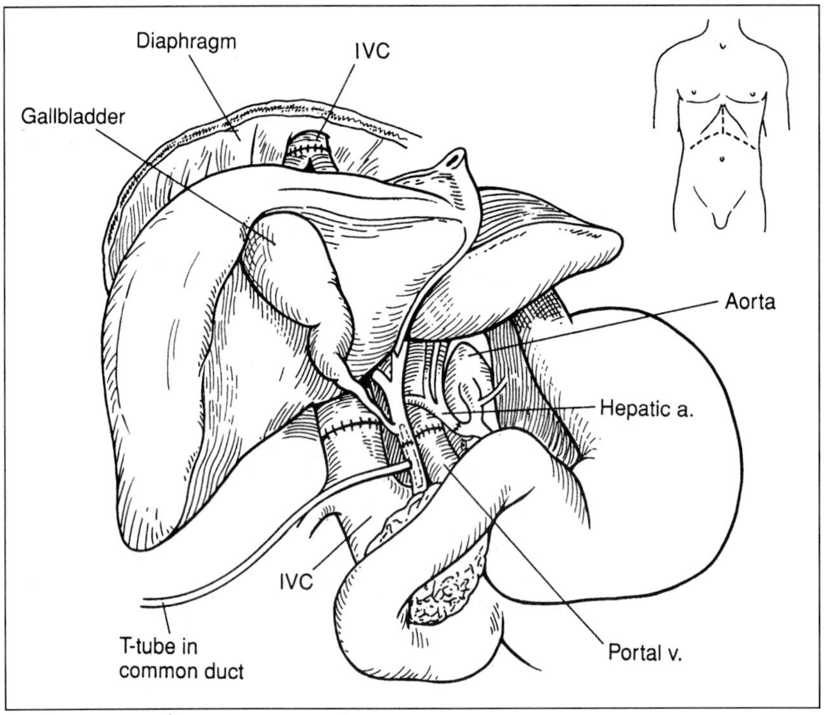

Figure 7.12-6. Liver transplantation. Anastomoses – including suprahepatic and infrahepatic IVC, portal vein, hepatic artery and common bile duct – are complete as shown here. Roux-en-Y loop of small intestine is an alternative biliary drainage conduit. Inset shows a chevron incision with midline extension. (Reproduced with permission from Hardy JD: *Hardy's Textbook of Surgery*, 2nd edition. JB Lippincott: 1988.)

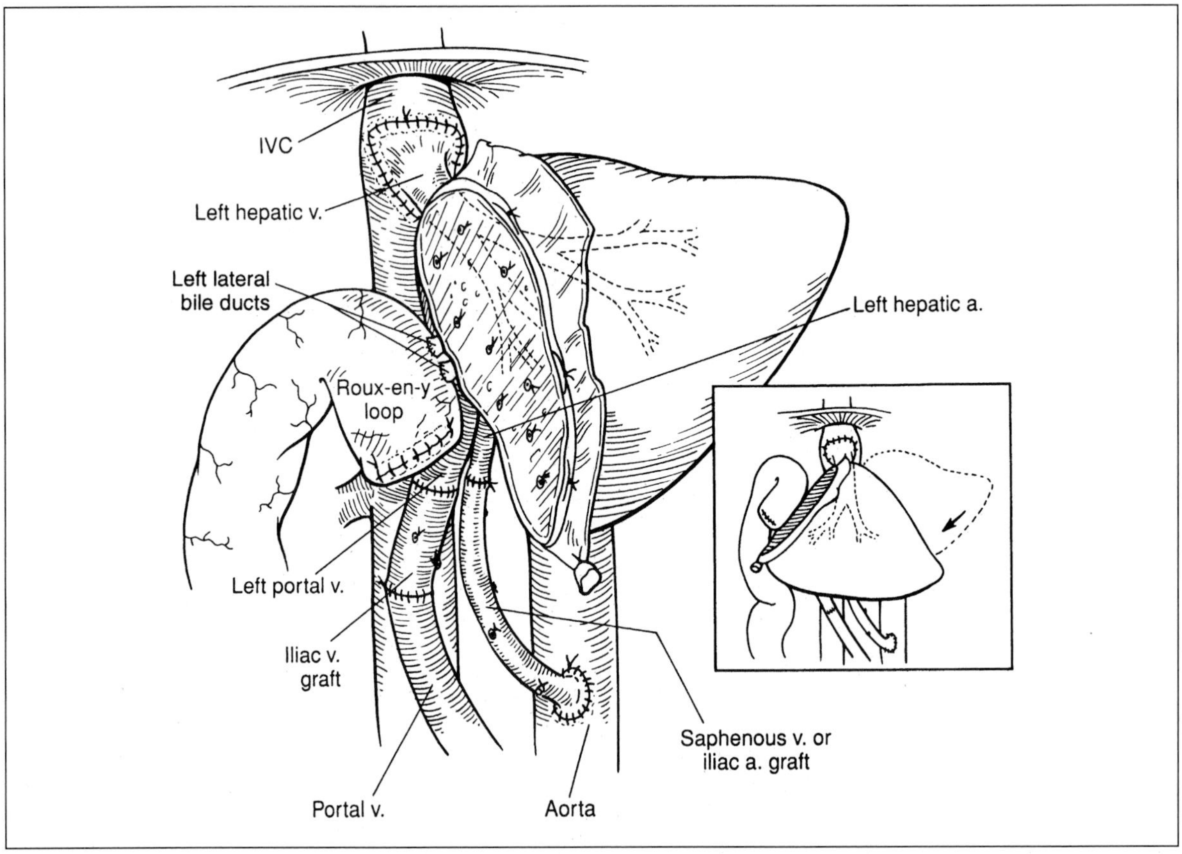

Figure 7.12-7. Liver transplantation (child) using left lateral segment from an adult liver. The hepatic artery and portal vein are extended with donor iliac artery and vein, respectively. The final position of the graft is shown (inset). A Roux-en-Y loop of small intestine is used to drain the bile duct(s). The IVC is left intact. The cut surface of the liver can bleed excessively if CVP is too high. (Reproduced with permission from Broelsch CE, et al: Liver transplantation in children from living related donors: surgical techniques and results. *Ann Surg* 1991; 214(4):432.)

PATIENT POPULATION CHARACTERISTICS

Age range Neonate-70 yr
Male:Female 1:1
Incidence 10/million/yr (15% pediatrics)
Etiology Adult: hepatitis C cirrhosis; alcoholic cirrhosis; primary biliary cirrhosis; primary sclerosing cholangitis; hepatitis B cirrhosis; hepatocellular carcinoma
Pediatric: biliary atresia; inborn errors of the metabolism

Associated conditions Coagulopathy; hypoalbuminemia; ascites; cardiomyopathy (in alcoholic patients); hepatorenal syndrome; hypoglycemia in acute fulminant hepatitis

ANESTHETIC CONSIDERATIONS

PREOPERATIVE

Patients presenting for liver transplantation represent a formidable challenge to the anesthesiologist. Frequently, these patients present for surgery with multiorgan system failure. Due to the emergent nature of the surgery, there may be insufficient time available for the customary evaluation and correction of abnormalities in this patient population.

Respiratory These patients are often hypoxic because of ascites, pleural effusions, atelectasis, V/Q mismatch and pulmonary AV shunting. As a result, they are usually tachypneic and have a respiratory alkalosis. Evidence of pulmonary infection is usually a contraindication to surgery, but ARDS that may occur with hepatic failure is not.
Tests: ABG; PFT, as indicated. CXR: ✓ infection, effusions, atelectasis.

Cardiovascular These patients demonstrate a hyperdynamic state with ↑CO and ↓SVR (probably 2° AV fistulae and endogenous vasodilators). This inefficient circulatory state is manifested by a high SO_2. The SVR usually is not responsive to α-agents. AV fistulae also occur across the pulmonary circulation, so that precautions to prevent air embolism are important. Ejection fraction (EF) is usually high (> 60%). Pericardial effusions may be present, and should be drained at surgery. Many of these patients will have dysrhythmias, HTN, pulmonary HTN (very high risk), valvular disease, cardiomyopathy (alcoholic disease, hemochromatosis, Wilson's disease) and CAD. These patients will require appropriate preop consultation and workup.
Tests: ECG; ECHO: ✓ EF, contractility, pulmonary HTN, wall motion abnormalities, valve problems. If abnormal, consider a MUGA scan and/or right- and left-heart catheterization with coronary artery angiography.

Neurological Patients are often encephalopathic and may be in hepatic coma; however, other organic causes of coma should be ruled out. In fulminant hepatic failure, ↑ICP is common, accounting for 40% of mortality (herniation), and may require prompt treatment (mannitol, hyperventilation, etc.).
Tests: Continuous ICP monitoring in fulminant hepatic failure

Hepatic Hepatitis serology and the cause of hepatic failure should be determined. Vascular abnormalities, previous RUQ surgery or portal-vein decompressive surgery places the patient in a high-risk group. Albumin usually low, with consequent low plasma oncotic pressure → edema, ascites. The magnitude and duration of drug effects may be unpredictable but, generally, these patients have ↑sensitivity to all drugs and their actions are prolonged.
Tests: Bilirubin; PT; ammonia level; SGOT; SGPT; albumin

Gastrointestinal Portal HTN, esophageal varices and coagulopathies ↑ risk of GI hemorrhage. Gastric emptying is often slow and, together with the emergent nature of this surgery, warrants rapid-sequence induction. H_2-antagonists are indicated preop.

Renal ↓Renal function, especially in fulminant hepatic failure (hepatorenal syndrome). The kidneys often recover after transplantation, but simultaneous kidney transplantation may be justified. These patients are often hypervolemic, hyponatremic and possibly hypokalemic. Ca^{++} is usually normal. Metabolic alkalosis may be present. Consider preop dialysis and intraop continuous AV hemofiltration. Low-dose dopamine (2-4 μg/kg/min) and/or mannitol (0.5-1 g/kg) are often used intraop to maintain renal function.
Tests: BUN; creatinine, creatinine clearance; electrolytes; ABG

Endocrine Patients often glucose-intolerant or frankly diabetic, although acute hypoglycemia may be seen in acute hepatic failure. Hyperaldosteronism may be present.
Tests: Glucose; electrolytes

Hematologic These patients are often anemic 2° either blood loss or malabsorption. Coagulation is impaired because of ↓hepatic synthetic function (all factors except VIII and fibrinogen are ↓), abnormal fibrinogen production, ↓/impaired Plt, fibrinolysis, and low-grade DIC.
Tests: PT; PTT; Plt count; bleeding time; fibrinogen; fibrin split products (FSP); TEG

Premedication Low doses of benzodiazepines may be used judiciously, but often nothing is given prior to surgery. Usually good preop evaluation and discussion suffice. Intramuscular injection should be avoided. Full-stomach precautions are justified. Metoclopramide 10 mg iv, ranitidine 50 mg iv and Na citrate 0.3 M 30 ml po should be given prior to surgery.

INTRAOPERATIVE

Anesthetic technique: GETA. These patients are extremely complex to manage because of the hemodynamic variability, massive blood loss, coagulopathy and metabolic problems. It is convenient to divide the operation into three stages: preanhepatic, anhepatic and neohepatic (discussed below).

Induction Often, a narcotic (e.g., fentanyl 2-5 μg/kg) is given just prior to induction; and rapid-sequence induction is preferred. STP (3-5 mg/kg) or etomidate (0.3 mg/kg) with succinylcholine (1-2 mg/kg), together with cricoid pressure.

Maintenance Standard maintenance (see p. B-3) with fentanyl 10-50 μg/kg. A benzodiazepine (e.g., midazolam 0.1-0.3 μg/kg) often is given to ensure amnesia during periods of hemodynamic instability when the volatile agent may need to be off. N_2O is avoided because of bowel distention and possible air embolism. Ventilation with $FiO_2 > 0.5$ and $PaCO_2 = \sim 35$ mmHg. Occasionally, PEEP (5 cm H_2O) is added. Antibiotics and immunosuppressants should be given per surgeon's direction. Muscle relaxation is usually maintained with pancuronium.

Preanhepatic phase The **preanhepatic phase** starts at skin incision and ends with removal of the recipient liver. Pleural and pericardial effusions are drained, which may improve oxygenation. Hyperglycemia is common during this period. ↓filling pressures 2° hemorrhage or vascular compression. Hemorrhage can be severe 2° portal HTN. Coagulation problems usually increase during this period, although fibrinolysis is not usually a problem. Blood loss replacement is accomplished with blood (PRBC) and FFP. Cryoprecipitate and Plts are given as needed, but a hypercoaguable state should be avoided, particularly if venovenous bypass is contemplated. Hemodynamic instability is not uncommon during the hepatic vascular dissection 2° manipulation of the liver and ↓venous return.

Venovenous bypass relieves most of the complications of portal and IVC cross-clamping (↓venous return, low CO, tachycardia, acidosis, ↓renal function, intestinal swelling.) Blood is pumped from the femoral vein and the portal system (either portal vein or inferior mesenteric) via a centrifugal pump to the left axillary vein. Generally, no heparin is used, but heparin-bonded cannulas and tubing are used. Bypass flows need to be at least 1 L/min to avoid possible thromboembolism. Bypass flow depends on venous inflow and is drawn into the pump by negative pressure. Low flows may be caused by hypovolemia or obstructed cannulae. Complications include: unexpected decannulation, thromboembolism and air embolism, all of which may need rapid termination of bypass and treatment of hypotension. Venovenous bypass is not always used.

Massive blood transfusion is associated with $\downarrow Ca^{++}$ and replacement is usually needed (± 500 mg/1000 ml of blood/FFP/plasmalyte mixture). If hyperkalemia occurs, it should be treated aggressively. Metabolic acidosis > 5 mEq/L should be treated with bicarbonate. Occasionally, inotropic support is needed, but α-adregenic agents should be avoided because of ↓renal and peripheral perfusion. UO needs to be maintained by ensuring adequate intravascular volume; occasionally, low-dose dopamine and/or mannitol may be needed.

Anhepatic phase The **anhepatic stage** begins with clamping of the hepatic vessels and vena cava and removal of the liver; it ends with the reperfusion of the donor liver. Problems during this period include: hemorrhage, increasing coagulopathy and fibrinolysis, acidosis, hypothermia and ↓renal function. The hemodynamic instability associated with clamping of the hepatic vessels and the congestion of the bowel that occurs can be decreased by venovenous bypass (see above). Care should be taken to maintain intravascular volume, while avoiding volume overload, since this will worsen fluid

Anhepatic phase, cont.

overloading on reperfusion. At the completion of vena caval anastomoses, the liver is flushed via the portal vein to remove air, preservation fluid and metabolites. Reperfusion may take place after completion of the portal vein anastomosis or after both portal vein and hepatic artery anastomoses are completed. As in the preanhepatic phase, acidosis, ↓Ca^{++}, glucose, coagulation and other electrolyte abnormalities should be treated. Fibrinolysis usually starts in this period, but is not usually treated unless severe because of the potential for embolism during venovenous bypass.

Neohepatic phase

The **neohepatic phase** begins with the unclamping of the portal vein, hepatic artery and vena cava and reperfusion of the donor liver. Preparation for this phase is important because this may be a period of great hemodynamic instability. Before removal of the clamps, acidosis should be corrected, ionized Ca^{++} should be normal and K^+ should be < 4.5 mEq/L. $CaCl_2$, $NaHCO_3$ and epinephrine should be readily available. Fluid overload prior to declamping should be avoided. High venous filling pressures decrease hepatic perfusion, especially prior to hepatic artery anastomosis. Declamping can be attended by ↓BP, ↓HR, dysrhythmias, hypothermia, lactic acidosis, coagulopathy and hyperglycemia.

Reperfusion syndrome

The "reperfusion syndrome" (which can occur in this phase) is characterized by ↓HR, ↓BP (30% develop MAP < 70% of baseline), conduction defects and ↓SVR in the face of acutely ↑RV filling pressures. Cause unknown. CO is often maintained. A rapid ↑K^+ can lead to cardiac arrest. (Rx: ensure normal pH and electrolytes prior to unclamping, rapid therapy when it occurs.) ↓BP and ↓HR are treated with epinephrine (10 μg increments), while $CaCl_2$ and $NaHCO_3$ are used to correct hyperkalemia and acidosis. Pulmonary edema may occur as a result of fluid overload and can be treated with diuretics, inotropes and phlebotomy. A high venous pressure will cause graft congestion and should be avoided. Reperfusion is associated with severe coagulopathy due to fibrinolysis (usually primary), release of heparin and hypothermia. As liver function returns, there should be an improvement in coagulation, acid-base status (metabolic alkalosis may occur), ↓lactic acidosis, return of glucose to normal and bile production. Hypokalemia may occur 2° uptake by the liver. HTN may be a problem. (Rx: SNP infusion.) Graft failure is associated with coagulopathy, ↑lactic acid, citrate intoxication, hyperglycemia and ↓bile formation.

Emergence

Extubation is deferred to ICU, with patient intubated and ventilated. These patients are generally ventilated postop until they are stable and able to be weaned from ventilatory support. Apart from the usual tests, hepatic function needs to be monitored, immunosuppression provided, infection controlled, analgesia ensured (usually morphine) and peptic ulcer prophylaxis given (ranitidine preferred).

Blood and fluid requirements

Massive blood loss
IV: 10 Fr × 2

Plasmalyte A or Normasol
UO >1 ml/kg/h
Warm all fluids.
Humidify gases.
Rapid-infusion system
Cell Saver
20 U PRBC
20 U FFP
20 U PLT

Generally, ivs are placed in the right antecubital fossa, left or right IJ or EJ. The left arm is avoided because the axillary vein is used for venovenous bypass.
Plasmalyte A or Normasol are preferred (absence of glucose, Ca^{++} and lower Na^+ content) over NS/LR. Hypernatremia can be a problem due to administration of $NaHCO_3$. The ability to give up to 1.5 L/min of blood should be available. Usually a mixture of Normasol (250 ml), PRBC (1 U) and FFP (1 U) is used, yielding Hct = 26-30%. Actual blood loss estimation is extremely difficult, and usually replacement is judged by hemodynamic status, UO and S_vO_2. Cell Savers are used to conserve blood. Anticoagulation is with a citrate solution to avoid heparin contamination and cells are washed with Normasol/Plasmalyte A. D/C use before biliary reconstruction (infection) or in neoplasms, hepatitis B or spontaneous bacterial peritonitis.

Monitoring

Standard monitors (see p. B-1).
ECG (5-lead)
Temp-bladder
ETN_2

Include 5-lead ECG and bladder temperature. (These patients sustain significant temperature loss.)
A full-time anesthesia technologist and lab/blood bank runner are useful. Lab and blood bank should be notified of the expected transplant. An automated data acquisition system also is useful, since there are times during the case when the record may be neglected in favor of working with the patient.

Monitoring, cont.	Arterial line(s)	One or two arterial lines are placed at the outset – one in the right radial, for ongoing lab and blood gas sampling, with 1 port being designated as heparin-free; another line, in the right femoral artery is utilized for continuous pressure measurement. All flush solutions contain citrate for anticoagulation in order to avoid heparin contamination.
	PA catheter/S_vO_2/CO	A PA catheter is essential for management of hemodynamics in these patients because of the rapid changes in vital signs. A catheter capable of measuring mixed-venous O_2 sat is very useful, as it gives early clues to impending decompensation. Coagulopathy complicates the placement of central lines, and the use of ECHO or ultrasound-guided needles is useful.
	TEE	TEE is useful to monitor cardiac filling and function and to diagnose problems such as PE or air embolism. Care needs to be taken in placing the TEE, since many of these patients have esophageal varices.
	ICP	ICP should be measured in patients with fulminant hepatic failure if ↑ICP is a concern. ABG, acid base status, electrolyte, lactate, osmolality, Ca^{++}, PT, PTT < Plt, Hct – all should be monitored on a regular basis (hourly or half-hourly and, occasionally, more frequently).
	TEG	The thromboelastograph (TEG) is useful for monitoring coagulation (see discussion of coagulation management, below).
Coagulation management	TEG PT PTT Plt counts Fibrinogen FSP	Patients are prone to a variety of coagulopathies (↓Plt, ↓coagulation factors, DIC, fibrinolysis, etc.) because of preop factors, massive hemorrhage, anhepatic period and reperfusion of the new liver; therefore, monitoring and treatment are necessary. Also, states of hypercoagulopathy need to be avoided because of unheparinized venovenous bypass. While PT, PTT, Plt counts, fibrinogen and FSP may provide relevant information, they may not reflect the true coagulability of patient's blood and tend to take considerable time to perform. Thus, in some centers, TEG has gained in popularity. It measures whole blood coagulability, not specific factors. TEG works by measuring viscoelastic properties of blood as it forms clot (fibrin connections) between a rotating cuvette and a spindle. Characteristic patterns are formed by the various coagulopathies with the common types shown in Fig 7.12-8. Evaluation of the TEG leads to more rational transfusion therapy, reducing the number of U of blood/blood products used. Comparing specimens of native whole blood vs blood mixed with EACA or protamine can guide pharmacologic therapy of coagulopathies. Table 7.12-3 gives specific recommendations.
Positioning	✓ and pad pressure points. ✓ eyes.	Table and arm boards should be very well padded. Head should be placed on a foam rest. Particular care should be taken to pad the retractor supports where they may impinge on the arms and on the radial nerve as it curls around the humerus.
Temperature control	Warming blanket Humidifier	Patient's arms, head and legs should be wrapped in plastic to protect against heat loss. Plastic drapes and the use of a cesarian section-type drape to protect the ECG electrodes

Table 7.12-3. Coagulation Therapy Guided by TEG Monitoring

1. Maintenance fluid
   RBC: FFP: Plasmalyte A = 300:200:250 ml
2. Replacement therapy
   a. FFP (2 U) for prolonged reaction time (R > 15 min)
   b. Plt (10 U) for small MA (MA < 40 mm)
   c. Cryoprecipitate (6-12 U) for persistent slow-clot formation rate ($\alpha < 40°$) with normal MA
3. Pharmacologic therapy
   a. Compare coagulability of whole blood, blood treated with protamine sulfate, and blood treated with epsilon aminocaproic acid.
   b. Epsilon aminocaproic acid (1 g) for severe fibrinolysis (F < 60 min)
   c. Protamine sulfate (50 mg) for severe heparin effect
   d. Heparin (1000-2000 U) for hypercoagulable state

(Used with permission from Kang YG: Anesthesia for liver transplantation. *Anes Clin North Am* 1989; 7(3): 507.)

Temperature control, cont.

and direct fluid flow off the table are useful to prevent the patient from lying in a pool of fluid. A warming blanket under the patient and over the lower legs is very useful.

Complications

Coagulopathy
Hemorrhage
Air embolism
RV failure
Metabolic acidosis

POSTOPERATIVE

Monitoring of hepatic function

Serial LFTs
PT, PTT
Ammonia level
Lactate
TEG
Bile output

Initial LFTs often show very high liver enzymes, which subside over a period of days. PT generally improves to normal levels, while lactic acidosis usually corrects quickly. Often a metabolic alkalosis follows and may need treatment with HCl.

Complications

Bleeding
Partial vein thrombosis
Hepatic artery thrombosis
Biliary tract leaks
Primary nonfunction
Rejection
Infection
Pulmonary complication
HTN
Electrolyte abnormalities (hypokalemia, ↓Ca^{++}, ↑Na)
Alkalosis
Renal failure
Peptic ulceration
Neurologic

This is not a complete list. Feared complications which may result in graft loss include portal vein thrombosis, hepatic artery thrombosis, bile leaks and rejection. These are attended by ↑LFTs, lactic acidosis, coagulopathy, hypoglycemia, ↓renal function and poor bile formation. The reader is referred to Reference 5, below, for a more complete discussion.

References

1. Carmicheal FJ, Lindop MJ, Farman JV: Anesthesia for hepatic transplantation: cardiovascular and metabolic alterations and their management. *Anesth Analg* 1985; 64(2):108-16.
2. Carton EG, Rettke SR, Plevak, et al: Perioperative care of the liver transplant patient. Parts I & II. *Anesth Analg* 1994; 78:120-33, 382-99.
3. Gelman S, Kang YG, Pearson JD: Anesthetic consideration in liver transplantation. In *Anesthesia for Organ Transplantation*. Fabian JA, ed. JB Lippincott Co, Philadelphia: 1992, Ch 7, 115-39.

4. Grande L, Rimola A, Cugat E, Alvarez L, Garcia-Valdecasas JC, Taura P, et al: Effect of venovenous bypass on perioperative renal function in liver transplantation: results of a randomized controlled trial. *Hepatology* 1996; 23:1418-28.
5. Kang YG, Lewis JH, Navalgund A, Russell MW, Bontempo FA, Niren LS, Starzl TE: Epsilon-aminocaproic acid for treatment of fibrinolysis during liver transplantation. *Anesthesiology* 1987; 66(6):766-73.
6. Kang YG, Martin DJ, Marguez J, Lewis JH, Bontempo FA, Shaw BW Jr, Starzl TE, Winter PM: Intraoperative changes in blood coagulation and thromboelastic monitoring in liver transplantation. *Anesth Analg* 1985; 64(9):888-96.
7. Kutt JL, Mezon BR: Anesthesia and liver transplantation. In *Organ Transplantation.* Benumof JL, ed. Anesthesiology Clinics of North America. WB Saunders, Philadelphia: 1994; 12(4):717-28.
8. Jawan B, Cheung HK, Lee JH: Anesthesia for living related donor liver transplantation. *Transplant Proc* 1996; 28(4):2409-11.
9. Nakazato PZ, Concepcion W, Bry W, Limm W, Tokunaga Y, Itasaka H, et al: Total abdominal evisceration: an en-bloc technique for abdominal organ harvesting. *Surgery* 1992; 111:37-47.
10. Paulsen AW, Whitten CW, Ramsay MA, Klintmalm GB: Considerations for anesthetic management during veno-venous bypass in adult hepatic transplantation. *Anesth Analg* 1989; 68(4):489-96.
11. Ramsey MAE: Anesthesia for liver transplantation. In *Transplantation of the Liver.* Busuttil RW, Klintmalm GB, eds. WB Saunders, Philadelphia: 1996, 419-33.
12. Shaw BW, Martin DJ, Marquez JM, Kang YG, Bugbee AC, Iwatsuki S, et al: Venous bypass in clinical liver transplantation. *Ann Surg* 1984; 200:524.
13. Starzl TE, Demetris AJ: Liver transplantation: a 31-year perspective. In *Current Problems in Surgery.* Wells SA Jr, ed. 1990 XXVII: 2-4.
14. Starzl TE, Iwatsuki S, Esquivel CO, Todo S, Kam I, Lynch S, et al: Refinements in the surgical technique of liver transplantation. *Semin Liver Dis* 1985; 5:349-59.

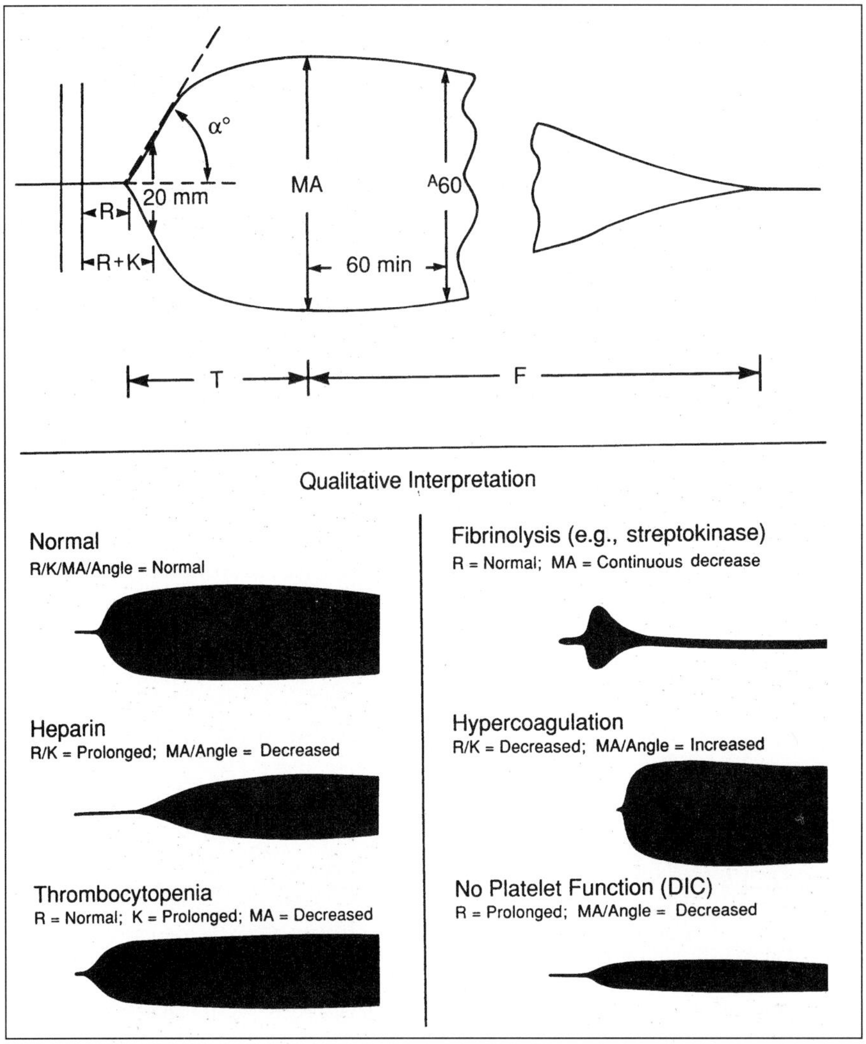

Figure 7.12-8. Variables and normal values measured by TEG:

R – reaction time, 6-8 min

R + k – coagulation time, 10-12 min

α – clot formation rate, >50°

MA – maximum amplitude, 50-70 mm

A_{60} – amplitude 60 min after MA

A_{60}/MA-100 – whole blood clot lysis index, >85%

F – whole blood clot lysis time, > 300 min

(Reproduced with permission from Kang YG, et al: Intraoperative changes in blood coagulation and thromboelastographic monitoring in liver transplantation. *Anesth Analg* 1985; 64:891.)

MULTIORGAN PROCUREMENT

SURGICAL CONSIDERATIONS

Description: The families of brain-dead patients may allow donation of the patient's other functioning organs, and this act of altruism can save or enhance the lives of as many as 10 others. Multiorgan procurement begins with an *in situ* flush used to exsanguinate and cool organs. The donor patient's chest and abdomen are opened from pubis to sternal notch. The chest is opened with a sternal saw, and, generally, an extra-large Balfour retractor is used to widely retract the abdomen. The aorta and IVC are dissected first to allow rapid placement of a flush line in the event that the patient decompensates. Following this, the liver vasculature is identified in the hepatoduodenal ligament below the liver and dissected out. This part of the procedure generally takes about 1.5 h. In cases where the pancreas is procured, an additional 45 min-1 h is required for mobilization of the pancreas. During pancreas procurement, Betadine is placed through an NG tube into the stomach and duodenum. A total of about 100-200 ml of Betadine should be passed. Once the heart, liver, pancreas and kidneys have been mobilized, heparin must be given. For an average-size adult, 30,000 U of heparin is given prior to clamping. The organs are then perfused with Viaspan. At this point, the ventilator can be turned off and the aorta cross-clamped below the diaphragm. The heart is the first organ to be removed. If the lungs are removed, an extra 20-30 min of perfusion time is required. After removal of the heart and/or lungs, the liver can be removed, followed by the pancreas and kidneys. Total time for multiorgan harvest, including heart, lungs, liver, pancreas and kidneys, is approximately 4 h, although anesthesia time typically ends with aortic cross-clamping.

Variant procedure: During the **"rapid-flush" technique** used by some procurement teams, the dissection of individual abdominal organs is minimized and an *en bloc* resection is done after clamping the aorta below the diaphragm and flushing preservation solution through the distal aorta. The *en bloc* organs are then dissected *ex vivo*, often at the transplant center, in preparation for transplantation. This technique is more rapid, requiring only about 1.5 h.

Usual preop diagnosis: Brain death

SUMMARY OF PROCEDURE

Position	Supine
Incision	Midline only, neck to pubis, ± bilateral transverse extensions
Special instrumentation	Chest and abdominal retractors
Unique considerations	Maintain oxygenation and BP as if live patient. May require pressors and/or blood transfusion. Temporarily deflate lungs for sternal sawing.
Antibiotics	Ampicillin (1 g iv), ceftriaxone (1 g iv); Betadine via NG tube for pancreas (with duodenal segment) procurement
Surgical time	4 h; rapid-flush technique: 1.5 h
EBL	200 ml

PATIENT POPULATION CHARACTERISTICS

Age range	3-60 yr
Male:Female	N/A
Incidence	Approximately 5000/yr in U.S.
Etiology	Usually head trauma (e.g., motor vehicle accidents, gunshot wounds to the head) or intracranial bleeding
Associated conditions	Vasomotor instability; diabetes insipidus (DI); intracranial HTN

ANESTHETIC CONSIDERATIONS

PREOPERATIVE

In general, organ donors are previously healthy individuals who have suffered catastrophic, irreversible brain injury of known etiology, most commonly due to blunt head trauma, penetrating head injury, or intracranial hemorrhage. A declaration of brain death by physicians not participating in the organ procurement must be documented. This documentation, together with certification of death and familial consent, should be verified by the anesthesiologist prior to organ procurement. There should be no evidence of disease or trauma involving the organs targeted for donation and, in general, the patient should be hemodynamically stable with minimal inotropic requirements. Once brain death has been declared, it is important to shift the emphasis away from cerebral resuscitation efforts and to focus instead on the maintenance of adequate tissue perfusion and oxygenation. Brain death is frequently followed by a series of pathophysiological events that may complicate the management of these patients.

Respiratory

Pulmonary dysfunction following brain death has many possible etiologies: aspiration, atelectasis, pneumonia and pulmonary edema. In addition, trauma may cause pulmonary dysfunction related to contusion, pneumothorax or hemothorax. Meticulous pulmonary toilet is essential to prevent atelectasis and pneumonia. Maintenance of adequate oxygenation is requisite to insure preservation of other organs for transplantation. Use mechanical ventilation with TVs of 10-12 ml/kg and a minute ventilation that maintains $PaCO_2$ 35-45 mmHg and pH 7.35-7.45. The FiO_2 should insure a PaO_2 75-150 mmHg and arterial saturation > 95%. PEEP is usually applied at 3-5 cmH_2O and should not exceed 7.5 cmH_2O because of the deleterious effects on CO and regional blood flow, and possible barotrauma. The FiO_2 generally should be increased to 100% prior to transport to the OR. An important exception is in the case of heart-lung or lung retrieval where it is important to maintain FiO_2 < 40% to minimize possible effects of O_2 toxicity. Ideally, PIP should be < 30 cmH_2O to minimize possible barotrauma to the lungs.

Tests: Frequent ABGs, including immediate preop period. Proper position of the ETT should be confirmed preop.

Cardiovascular

Hypotension should be anticipated in all organ donors. This results most commonly from neurogenic shock (derangement of descending vasomotor control → progressive ↓SVR and venous pooling) and hypovolemia. Hypovolemia is usually the result of dehydration therapy for cerebral edema, hemorrhage, DI or osmotic diuresis due to hyperglycemia. Hypothermia, LV dysfunction and endocrine abnormalities also can contribute to ↓BP. Fluid resuscitation with crystalloid, colloid and PRBCs to maintain Hct > 30% should be initiated preop. Hemodynamic goals are: (1) CVP 10-12 cmH_2O (6-8 cmH_2O if lungs are to be procured), MAP between 60-100 mmHg, SBP > 100 mmHg, and UO > 1 ml/kg/h. Donors are often placed on inotropic therapy to maintain these parameters; however, following adequate volume resuscitation, preop inotropic therapy often may be gradually decreased or discontinued. If inotropic therapy remains necessary, typically it would consist of dopamine (2-10 μg/kg/min), followed by dobutamine (3-15 μg/kg/min) or epinephrine (0.1-1.0 μg/kg/min), then norepinephrine. The latter 3 agents may be combined with dopamine (2-3 μg/kg/min) in an attempt to augment or preserve renal, mesenteric and coronary arterial blood flow. It should be noted that brain death may be accompanied initially by a transient hypertensive crisis which may require short-term treatment with SNP and/or esmolol.

ECG abnormalities are common in patients with intracranial injury and are of no pathologic consequence. Atrial and ventricular dysrhythmias and various degrees of conduction block occur frequently in organ donors; the etiology may be electrolyte imbalance, ABG disturbance, ↑ICP, loss of the vagal motor nucleus, inotropic therapy, hypothermia or myocardial contusions or ischemia. Antidysrhythmic therapy should follow the usual guidelines except for ↓HR, which is resistant to atropine in this setting. Bradycardia, if accompanied by ↓BP, should be treated with isoproterenol, dopamine, epinephrine or temporary cardiac pacing.

Tests: ECG; ECHO (to assess wall motion abnormalities) and possibly coronary angiography (if CAD is suspected).

Neurological

DI frequently occurs in brain-dead donors; it is likely the result of destruction of the hypothalamic-pituitary axis. Untreated, it may cause marked hypovolemia and electrolyte disturbances (↑Na, ↑Mg, ↓K, ↓PO_4, ↓Ca). Therapy with iv vasopressin (titrated from 2 μg/kg/min) or desmopressin acetate (DDAVP) (titrated from 0.3 μg/kg/min) is often initiated to maintain UO < 1.5-3 ml/kg/h. Many believe the benefits of minimizing electrolyte imbalance, fluid shifts and reduction of core temperature outweigh the risks of vasopressin or desmopressin therapy, including coronary and renal vasoconstriction and possible organ ischemia or uneven distribution of the preservation solutions during flushing. It may be prudent, however, to D/C vasopressin or DDAVP infusions for at least 1 h prior to aortic cross-clamping and infusion of preservation solutions. Thermoregulation is abnormal in brain-dead donors due to hypothalamic dysfunction; and core temperature should be monitored (bladder, esophageal or rectal). Aggressive warming techniques may have to be employed early to maintain a core temperature > 34-35°C as there are numerous undesirable consequences of significant hypothermia (< 32°C) in the organ donor – e.g., cardiac dysrhythmia, cardiac instability, ↓GFR and cold diuresis, a left shift in the oxyhemoglobin dissociation curve

Neurological, cont. and pancreatitis. While other endocrine or metabolic disturbances may exist as a result of destruction of the hypothalamic-pituitary axis, currently there is no consistent recommendation for any other hormonal replacement therapy.
Tests: Serum electrolytes and osmolality every 4-6 h

Hematologic Donors may be anemic from hemodilution and/or hemorrhage. In order to ensure adequate tissue O_2 delivery, PRBCs are transfused to maintain Hct > 30. Some donors may exhibit a coagulopathy; clinically significant bleeding should be treated with clotting factors and Plts. Persistent or severe primary fibrinolysis or DIC may require rapid transfer of the donor to the OR for organ retrieval. Administration of epsilon-aminocaproic acid to treat fibrinolysis is avoided for fear of microvascular thrombosis in the donor organs.
Tests: Hb/Hct; PT; PTT; Plt count; DIC screen as clinically indicated.

Other The role of oxygen-free radicals, with regard to reperfusion injury, has prompted the suggested use of mannitol and steroids (and other compounds) as scavengers.

INTRAOPERATIVE

Anesthetic technique: Although anesthesia is unnecessary in brain-dead organ donors, both visceral and somatic reflexes can lead to physiologic responses during the procedure. The goals of intraop management with regard to respiratory, cardiovascular, hematologic and neurologic status are identical to those discussed under preop considerations.

Induction Settings for mechanical ventilation parallel those of the ICU, although it may be advisable to begin with an FiO_2 of 100% until the first ABG result is obtained. The exception is when procurement of the lungs or heart-lungs is anticipated; then FiO_2 should not exceed 40%. To eliminate reflex neuromuscular activity and to facilitate surgical retraction, a long-acting neuromuscular blocking agent such as pancuronium or pipecuronium (0.15 mg/kg) should be given at the beginning of the procedure and supplemented as necessary.

Maintenance Reflex hypertensive responses to surgical stimulation occur frequently and may lead to excessive intraop blood loss and damage to donor kidneys; management should include the weaning of vasopressors and the initiation of vasodilator therapy with isoflurane, SNP or NTG.
Anesthetic care continues until the proximal aortic cross-clamp is applied. D/C all monitoring and supportive therapy at this point. The notable exception is the case of heart-lung or lung procurement; in this situation, all monitoring except FiO_2 should cease with proximal aortic cross-clamping. All supportive care is terminated, with the exception of mechanical ventilation of the lungs at 4 breaths/min or as directed by the transplant team, and suctioning of the ETT after cessation of mechanical ventilation just prior to removal of the tube. Extubation marks the termination of anesthetic care of the heart-lung or lung donor.

Blood and fluid requirements	IV: 14-16 ga × 1-2 NS/LR @ 2-4 ml/kg/h	Significant 3rd-space losses; may need to administer large volumes of crystalloid, colloid (up to 1 L) and PRBCs (not uncommon to transfuse 2 or more U to maintain Hct >30). Central venous access is necessary for monitoring and for vasoactive drug delivery.
Monitoring	Standard monitors (see p. B-1). Intraarterial BP CVP line UO	If a PA catheter is in place, it may be used or removed based on concerns of catheter-related, right-side endocardial lesions. Rarely is insertion of a PA catheter warranted in these operations. ABG, Hb/Hct, serum electrolytes and glucose should be monitored hourly; for operations involving procurement of lungs or heart-lungs, ABGs should be obtained at least every 30 min.
Complications	Hypotension	Most commonly 2° hypovolemia and neurogenic shock (loss of descending vasomotor control). Ensure adequate volume repletion as described above, then institute or increase inotropic/vasopressor therapy as previously outlined.
	Dysrhythmias	Multiple possible etiologies as described above. Standard treatment and diagnosis should be employed, with the exception of bradycardia, which is atropine-resistant and should be treated with isoproterenol, dopamine, epinephrine or transvenous pacing.

Complications, cont.	Cardiac arrest	CPR should be instituted in an effort to maintain the viability of the liver, kidneys and other abdominal viscera intended for transplantation. Procurement of the liver and kidneys should proceed rapidly to aortic cross-clamping at the diaphragm and administration of cold preservation fluid into the aorta and portal vein. This series of events will undoubtedly preclude use of the heart and lungs for transplantation.
	Oliguria	Ensure adequate volume replacement and BP as outlined, then add dopamine (2-3 μg/kg/min), if not previously instituted to promote renal vasodilation and to increase renal blood flow, glomerular filtration rate and UO. If these measures are ineffective at restoring adequate UO (> 1 ml/kg/h), then furosemide or mannitol may be used after consultation with the transplant team.
	DI	Fluid and electrolyte therapy as determined by filling pressures and hourly serum electrolyte values. Adjustment of vasopressin or DDAVP infusion to maintain UO < 1.5-3.0 ml/kg/h; initiation of this infusion should be done in consultation with the transplant team. As previously discussed, it may be advisable to D/C vasopressin or DDAVP at least 1 h prior to aortic cross-clamping.
	Coagulopathy	Transfuse Plt, FFP and cryoprecipitate as necessary for clinical bleeding in the setting of abnormal coagulation studies. Avoid EACA due to risk of microvascular thrombosis in the donor organs.
	Hyperglycemia	Avoid dextrose-containing solutions which may aggravate existing hyperglycemia and contribute to osmotic diuresis and electrolyte abnormalities.
	Hypothermia	Early aggressive attempts to minimize intraop heat loss are essential and include warming the OR, use of a warming blanket, insulating exposed areas (head, neck, shoulders), warming all fluids, and using heated, humidified inspired gases.
Special considerations	Heart-lung procurement	Division of the mediastinal pleura and tracheal dissection with manipulation of each lung outside the mediastinum may result in profound hypotension and may cause problems with oxygenation and ventilation. Adequate intravascular volume is essential, and inotropic therapy may be required during this period. Problems with ventilation and oxygenation must be communicated immediately to the transplant team. Following aortic cross-clamping and infusion of cardioplegia solution, the lung preservation fluid will be infused via the right and left PAs. During this period, the lungs should be ventilated manually with 4 bpm, or as otherwise directed by the transplant team. It is prudent early on in the procurement procedure to verify the position of the ETT with the transplant surgeon to insure that the tube does not contribute to mucosal injury at the site of the anticipated suture line.
	Organ preservation	Therapy aimed at improving organ preservation may require several pharmacologic manipulations as directed by the transplant team. Agents commonly used during organ procurement include dopamine (2-3 μg/kg/min), furosemide, mannitol, allopurinol (free-radical scavenger), chlorpromazine and phentolamine (vasodilators), heparin (prevents microvascular thrombosis and promotes

Special considerations, cont.

reperfusion), and PGE_1 (vasodilator, membrane stabilizer, antiplatelet effect). Systemic infusion of PGE_1 prior to aortic cross-clamping (commonly used in heart-lung or lung procurement) will lead to predictable and profound hypotension; efforts at volume resuscitation toward optimal CVP should continue until the aortic cross-clamp is applied. If heparin is to be administered iv, a catheter should be used after verifying the ability to freely aspirate blood. Methylprednisolone (30 mg/kg) is commonly administered at least 2 h before organ retrieval in an effort to protect the heart and kidneys from ischemic injury.

General Liver/Kidney Transplantation References

1. Firestone L, Firestone S: Anesthesia for organ transplantation. In *Clinical Anesthesia*, 2nd edition. Barash PG, Cullen BF, Stoelting RK, eds. Lippincott-Raven Publishers, Philadelphia: 1997, 1249-78.
2. Flye MW, ed: *Principles of Organ Transplantation*. WB Saunders Co, Philadelphia: 1989.
3. Gelb AW, Robertson KM: Anaesthetic management for the brain dead for organ donation. *Can J Anaesth* 1990; 37:(7)806-12.
4. Phillips MG, ed: *Organ Procurement, Preservation and Distribution in Transplantation*. William Byrd Press, Richmond, VA: 1991.
5. Robertson KM, Cook DR: Perioperative management of the multiorgan donor. *Anesth Analg* 1990; 70(5):546-56.
6. Salter DR, Dyke CM: Cardiopulmonary dysfunction after brain death. In *Anesthesia for Organ Transplantation*. Fabian JA, ed. JB Lippincott Co, Philadelphia: 1992, 81-94.
7. Simmons RL, Finch ME, Ascher NL, Najarian JS, eds: *Manual of Vascular Access, Organ Donation and Transplantation*. Springer-Verlag, New York: 1984.
8. Sutherland DER, et al: Results of pancreas transplantation in the United States for 1987-90. *Clin Transplantation* 1991; 5:330-41.
9. Terasaki PI, ed: *Clinical Transplants*. UCLA Tissue Typing Laboratory, Los Angeles: 1990.

Surgeons

Aleksander R. Komar, MD
J. Augusto Bastidas, MD

7.13 TRAUMA SURGERY

Anesthesiologist

Linda E. Foppiano, MD

INITIAL ASSESSMENT AND AIRWAY MANAGEMENT

The Advanced Trauma Life-Support System (ATLS), developed by the American College of Surgeons' Committee on Trauma, represents the best current approach to the severely injured patient. The sequence of management includes: 1) primary survey and initial resuscitation, 2) evaluation with continuation of resuscitation, and 3) secondary survey with definitive management.

The primary survey attempts to identify and treat immediate life-threatening conditions. This is accomplished by following the ABCs: **airway control,** with cervical spine precautions; assisted **breathing** or mechanical ventilation; and support of the **circulation** via volume resuscitation and tamponade of external bleeding. Once alveolar ventilation is ensured, the next priority is to optimize O_2 delivery by maximizing cardiovascular performance. Hypovolemia is the most likely etiology of postinjury shock; therefore, fluid resuscitation should be initiated via two large-bore iv cannulas placed in the antecubital veins. Any external source of bleeding should be controlled with manual compression. When vascular collapse precludes peripheral percutaneous access, saphenous vein cutdown at the ankle is preferred. ECG monitoring, serial vital signs, rapid physical examination, rectal temperature reading and initiation of flow sheet complete the primary survey. Response of the patient to fluid resuscitation is then evaluated and, if crystalloid volume exceeds 50 ml/kg, type-specific or O(-) blood should be given. If shock persists despite fluid resuscitation, cardiogenic shock, tension pneumothorax or ongoing hemorrhage should be considered. Cardiogenic shock may require ER thoracotomy; tension pneumothorax should be vented immediately with chest tube placement. Ongoing hemorrhage should be treated surgically, without an attempt to normalize vital signs with fluid administration.

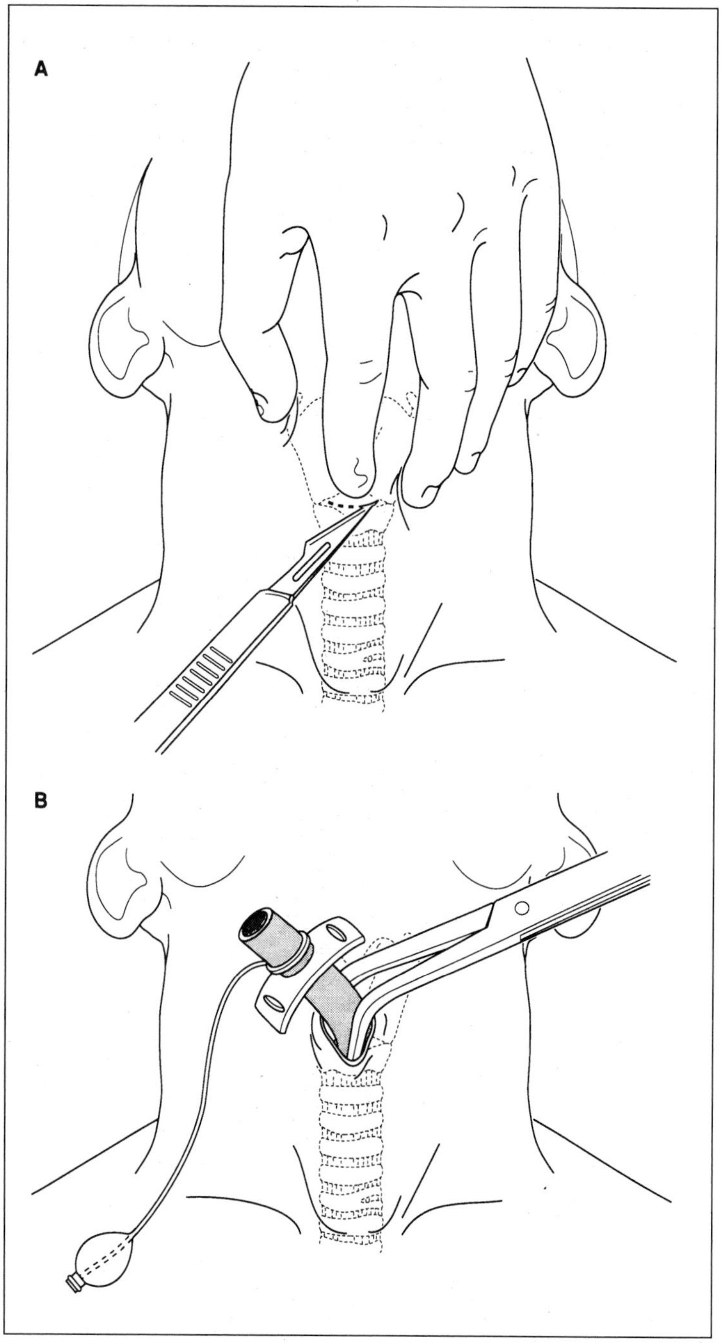

Figure 7.13-1. Cricothyroidotomy. **(A)** Identification of the cricothyroid membrane by palpation and incising the membrane transversely. **(B)** Insertion of a tracheostomy tube through the cricothyroid membrane, which is spread with a tracheal dilator. (Reproduced with permission from Greenfield LJ, et al, eds: *Surgery: Scientific Principles and Practice, 2nd edition.* Lippincott-Raven, Philadelphia: 1997, 1479.)

MANAGEMENT OF AIRWAY

Airway obstruction, inadequate ventilation, hypoxemia, abnormal mental status and cardiovascular instability are the usual indications for airway intervention. The three commonly accepted methods of airway control are: **blind nasotracheal intubation, orotracheal intubation** and **cricothyroidotomy.**

Nasotracheal intubation, recommended for spontaneously breathing trauma patients, can be performed without the use of pharmacologic agents or special equipment. It is, however, associated with higher incidence of vomiting and aspiration and, in the intoxicated patient with a depressed level of consciousness, the success rate may be as low as 65%.

Oral intubation, with the use of appropriate neuromuscular blockade and the Sellick maneuver, is the preferred choice in many trauma centers. The approach is rapid but at least three people are required to perform it safely in the patient with suspected cervical spine injury. In-line stabilization of the neck has replaced in-line traction as the protective measure. Because muscle paralysis may force operative airway intubation, equipment for cricothyrotomy should be immediately accessible.

Patients in respiratory distress with severe facial trauma or unstable cervical spine injury require a surgical airway.

Cricothyrotomy (Fig 7.13-1) is the preferred surgical airway in adults and has virtually replaced tracheostomy in the emergency department. The important anatomic landmarks of the superior and inferior borders of the thyroid and cricoid cartilages are palpated. The thyroid cartilage is then stabilized with the left hand of the surgeon, a longitudinal incision is made and rapidly advanced through subcutaneous tissue. The cricothyroid membrane lies very superficially, being covered by only the skin and platysma muscle. The cricothyroid membrane is incised transversely with a scalpel (blade No. 11), and an ETT or tracheostomy tube should be inserted (Fig 7.13-1B). Only after the airway is secured should bleeding from transsected vessels be controlled. Cricothyrotomies should be converted to tracheotomies within 72 h after the initial injury, provided the patient's condition permits.

Tracheostomy is indicated for patients requiring surgical airway in less dramatic situations or if cricothyroidotomy cannot be performed due to direct laryngeal injury. It can be accomplished through the same incision, extended caudally, if laryngeal injury is found.

On rare occasion, the injury is in the distal cervical or proximal intrathoracic trachea. In such cases, median sternotomy and lateral retraction of the innominate artery is required for exposure of the trachea. Right thoracotomy provides access to the more distal intrathoracic trachea (see Chest Trauma, p. 521).

Usual preop diagnosis: Airway compromise

SUMMARY OF PROCEDURE

Position	Supine
Incision	Midline longitudinal incision in the neck
Unique considerations	The large number of legal claims involving failed intubation suggests that surgical cricothyroidotomy remains an underutilized technique.
Antibiotics	Usually not given until clear indications related to the primary injury are apparent.
Surgical time	2 min
EBL	Minimal
Postop care	Mechanical ventilation
Mortality	Related to the primary injury
Morbidity	Cricothyrotomy is more likely to result in airway stricture or damage to more proximal structures in the larynx. On the basis of this rationale, cricothyrotomies are converted to tracheostomies within 48-72 h of admission if patient's general condition permits.
Pain score	3

EMERGENCY TUBE THORACOSTOMY

SURGICAL CONSIDERATIONS

Description: In the United States, trauma is the most common cause of death in young people; 25% of these deaths (approximately 16,000 per year) are due to thoracic trauma. Proper management of thoracic trauma is extremely important since 75% of these deaths occur after the patient reaches the hospital. Early deaths are commonly due to airway obstruction, flail chest, open pneumothorax, massive hemothorax, tension pneumothorax and cardiac tamponade. Later deaths are due to respiratory failure, sepsis and unrecognized injuries.

Eighty percent of blunt thoracic injuries are caused by motor vehicle accidents (MVAs). Penetrating injuries to the chest are almost as common as blunt trauma. The death rate in hospitalized patients with isolated chest injury is 4-8%; this increases to 10-15% when one other organ system is involved and to 35% if multiple additional organs are injured. Eighty-five percent of chest injuries do not require thoracotomy, and the patient can be managed with relatively simple measures, such as airway control and tube thoracostomy.

Blunt trauma can induce injury by three distinctive mechanisms: direct blow, deceleration injury and compression injury. Rib fracture is the most common sign of blunt thoracic trauma. Fracture of the upper ribs (1st-3rd), clavicle or scapula implies high-energy impact and is associated with major vascular injury.

Life-threatening injuries caused by penetrating trauma are distinctly different from those caused by blunt trauma. In penetrating chest injuries, pneumothorax is almost always present and hemothorax is present in 80% of cases. Hypovolemia from intrathoracic hemorrhage is second only to rib fractures as a sequela of thoracic trauma.

Uncomplicated or **tension pneumothorax** may be caused by blunt or penetrating trauma. Positive intrathoracic pressure interferes with venous return to the heart and adequate ventilation. Since sequela of thoracic injuries interfere with air exchange, treatment must take high priority, just after securing the airway, obtaining iv access and beginning fluid resuscitation. In the hemodynamically stable patient, suspicion of a pneumothorax should be confirmed by x-ray. On the CXR, a 20% loss of lung dimension corresponds to approximately 50% loss of lung volume. Any tendency to observe a "small" pneumothorax should be resisted since delayed recognition of progression of the pneumothorax may occur and become life-threatening at any time (for example, after intubation, during transport to another, less well monitored area [e.g., radiology]). Release of a major hemothorax or pneumothorax in a patient with chest trauma is essential to establish adequate ventilation and cannot wait for radiologic diagnosis. The presence of subcutaneous emphysema, absent breath sounds and acute respiratory distress warrants chest tube thoracostomy without delay. After the placement of the chest tube, a CXR helps to evaluate decompression.

As much as 40% of the circulating blood volume can accumulate in a hemothorax. The most frequent sources of bleeding are the intercostal and internal mammary vessels. Some degree of hemothorax is present in almost every patient with chest injury. A supine CXR may miss up to 1 liter of blood; therefore, an upright chest film should be performed whenever possible. Following chest tube placement, blood loss > 1500 ml or an ongoing loss of 250 ml for 3 consecutive h suggests the need for surgical intervention.

Simple pneumothorax without associated hemothorax can be treated with a 20-22 Fr chest tube placed in the 3rd intercostal space in the midclavicular line or in the 5th intercostal space in the anterior axillary line. Hemothorax and tension pneumothorax requires a large-bore, 38-40 Fr chest tube placed in the midaxillary line through the 5th or 6th intercostal space (Fig 7.13-2). A 20 ml syringe with 1% lidocaine can be used not only to provide local anesthesia, but also to locate the upper edge of the rib in the obese patient. A generous, 3 cm incision should be made one interspace below the targeted level. The subcutaneous tissues are dissected bluntly, creating a tunnel that is directed upwards. The pleural space should be entered just above the upper edge of the rib to avoid injury to the intercostal neurovascular bundle, located just below the lower edge of the rib. After the pleural space has been entered bluntly, it should be explored with the operator's finger swept around to ensure proper location and to free potential adhesions. The chest tube should be inserted and advanced in the posterior and superior direction. The tube then should be connected to a suction/collection system under 20 cm of water negative pressure, preferably

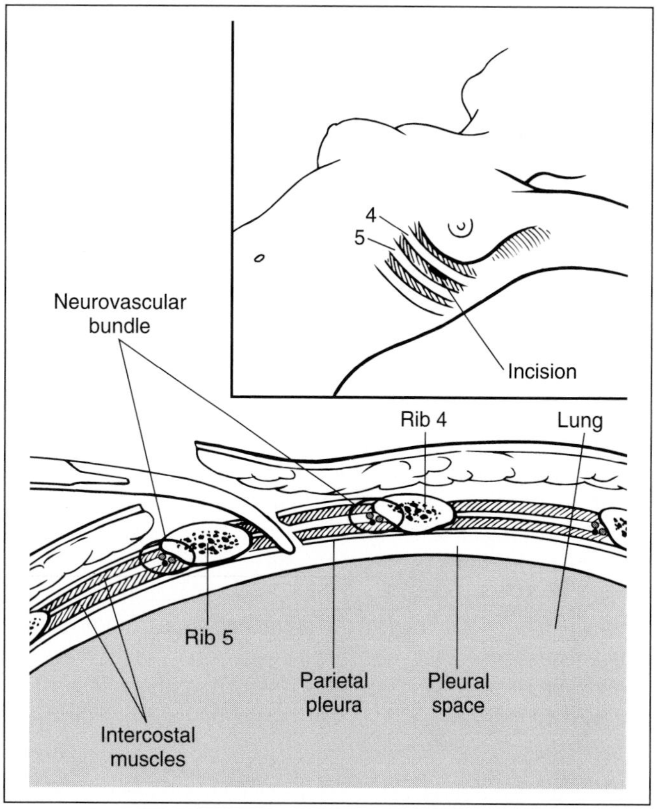

Figure 7.13-2. Tube thoracostomy. Incision through 4th or 5th interspace at anterior axillary line. Forceps are used to tunnel over the superior edge of the rib and to bluntly enter the pleural space.

through an autotransfusion device. CXR should immediately follow chest tube placement. If the pleural space still contains blood, another chest tube should be inserted.

Usual preop diagnosis: Tension pneumothorax; pneumothorax; hemothorax

SUMMARY OF PROCEDURE

Position	Supine, with arm extended overhead
Incision	3 cm in interspace below 5th intercostal space in anterior axillary line.
Special instrumentation	38-40 Fr chest tube should be used in most patients. Small, 20-22 Fr tube reserved for simple pneumothorax in stable patients. Autotransfusion device should be available in ER.
Unique considerations	In tension pneumothorax, a large-bore needle inserted in the midclavicular line in the 2nd intercostal space can relieve a tension pneumothorax and save a patient's life until a chest tube is available.
Antibiotics	No clear benefit in simple stab wound or low-velocity gunshot wound. In immunocompromised patients and patients with associated injuries and high-velocity gunshot wounds, use cefazolin 1 g iv.
Surgical time	5 min
EBL	Minimal, from tube placement. Variable amounts drained out, depending on extent of hemothorax and associated injuries.
Postop care	Chest tube may be removed after at least 48 h, when there is no air leak from lung and < 100-150 ml of fluid drainage per 24 h.
Mortality	In isolated chest injury: 4-8% When one other organ system is involved: 0-15% If multiple additional organs injured: 35%
Morbidity	Clotted hemothorax Empyema Lung abscess Lung contusion
Pain score	5

EMERGENCY ROOM THORACOTOMY

SURGICAL CONSIDERATIONS

Description: Emergency department thoracotomy may offer the only chance of survival for the trauma patient arriving *in extremis*. Various conditions may warrant such a dramatic procedure: 1) **Intrathoracic vascular or cardiac bleeding** requires immediate control of exsanguinating hemorrhage to offer any chance for survival. 2) **Pericardial tamponade** initially is a protective mechanism, but ultimately results in cardiac arrest unless there is immediate evacuation of blood from the pericardium and repair of the cardiac laceration. 3) **Air embolism** often presents as a profound hypotensive shock after PPV is initiated. Air embolism to the coronary vessels causes myocardial ischemia. This condition requires immediate cross-clamping of the hilum and aspiration of the air from the ventricles. 4) **Open cardiac massage** in a hypovolemic patient may provide better coronary and systemic perfusion than external chest compressions. 5) **Aortic cross-clamping** at the level of the descending thoracic aorta enhances coronary and cerebral perfusion and can be tolerated up to 30 min without detrimental peripheral acidosis. As an additional benefit, it may restrict intraabdominal blood loss.

The probability of survival following emergency thoracotomy depends on the mechanism of injury as well as the patient's condition at the time of thoracotomy. In patients with isolated cardiac injury presenting with signs of life, a survival rate approaches 50% but drops to 1% if there are no signs of life on presentation. For blunt trauma patients requiring ER thoracotomy, survival rate does not exceed 2%, regardless of their initial condition.

A **left anterolateral thoracotomy** is the incision of choice, since pericardiotomy, open cardiac massage and aortic occlusion are best achieved through this approach. This incision can be extended easily across the sternum and into the right chest to improve exposure and to control massive blood loss and/or air embolism from the right lung. The entire chest is prepped liberally, and left anterolateral thoracotomy is performed rapidly in the 5th intercostal space using a large-blade scalpel. Heavy scissors can be used to quickly divide the intercostal muscles and to cut across the sternum. If pericardial tamponade is encountered, the pericardium is opened anteriorly to the phrenic nerve. Blood and clot are evacuated and bleeding sites controlled with pressure on the ventricles and vascular clamps on the atrium or blood vessels. Attempts to repair cardiac lacerations should be delayed until resuscitative measures have been completed. In the nonbeating heart, suturing is performed prior to defibrillation. If coronary or systemic air embolism is present, the appropriate hilum is cross-clamped and air is aspirated from the left ventricle through the elevated apex. Cardiac arrest is an indication for immediate internal massage. The two-hand method is preferred and internal defibrillation should be instituted. If internal defibrillation does not restore proper cardiac activity, cross-clamping of the aorta will improve coronary perfusion. To cross-clamp the aorta, the left lung is retracted anteriorly and superiorly and the posterior pleura is dissected under direct vision. With proper exposure and an NG tube in the esophagus, the aorta can be identified and a vascular clamp applied.

Usual preop diagnosis: Penetrating chest trauma with cardiac arrest and recent recorded signs of life.

SUMMARY OF PROCEDURE

Position	Supine
Incision	Left anterolateral thoracotomy. Extension of incision across sternum should be considered routinely for improved exposure.
Special instrumentation	Emergency department thoracotomy tray; internal defibrillator paddles; suction device; rapid-infusion device; O(-) blood
Unique considerations	Airway should be secured first. NG tube should be placed if possible. Typically, patients are not anesthetized for this procedure.
Antibiotics	Cefazolin, 1 g iv
Surgical time	10 min
EBL	1-2 L
Postop care	ICU
Mortality	Blunt trauma: 98% All penetrating chest injuries requiring ER thoracotomy: 85% Penetrating cardiac injury: 50%
Morbidity	ARDS Arrhythmias
Pain score	10

EXPLORATORY SURGERY FOR NECK TRAUMA

SURGICAL CONSIDERATIONS

Description: The cervical region contains a greater variety of vital structures than any other region of the body (Fig 7.13-3). The cardiovascular, respiratory, digestive, endocrine and CNS systems are all represented in the neck; injury to any of these can be fatal.

Injury to the neck can result from blunt or penetrating trauma. Most blunt injuries to the neck are managed nonoperatively. Blunt airway injury is rarely a surgical emergency; in this instance, it is managed similarly to penetrating neck injuries. Cervical spine injury is present in fewer than 5% of cases of blunt trauma; however, all patients should be screened for cervical spine injury (PE, x-ray, CT) and full spinal precautions should be maintained until the cervical spine is cleared.

The neck is usually divided into three horizontally oriented zones (Fig 7.13-3, inset). Zone I extends from the sternal notch to the cricoid cartilage. Penetrating injuries in this area are associated with a high mortality. Zone II extends from the cricoid cartilage to the angle of the mandible. Because this is the most exposed region of the neck, injuries can be evaluated and explored relatively easily. Zone III extends from the angle of the mandible to the base of the skull. Because of anatomic constraints, injuries to Zones I and III can be difficult to identify and repair. In patients with a Zone I injury, iv access should be established in the contralateral upper extremity because of possible injury to ipsilateral IJ vein or subclavian vein.

Until recently, evaluation and management of stable patients with neck injuries that penetrated the platysma depended on location of injury. Injuries to Zones I and III were evaluated radiographically, whereas injuries to Zone II were indications for mandatory exploration. With the increased availability and improved safety of arteriography, however, a selective exploration strategy is now favored.

Management of hemodynamically unstable or symptomatic patients with penetrating neck injuries should be limited to applying direct pressure, protecting the airway, establishing iv access and obtaining CXR. Exploration and definitive management of the injury in the OR should follow as soon as possible. In all stable patients with an injury penetrating the platysma where surgical exploration is not planned, angiographic evaluation of the carotid artery is mandatory as carotid artery injuries are present in ~10% of patients.

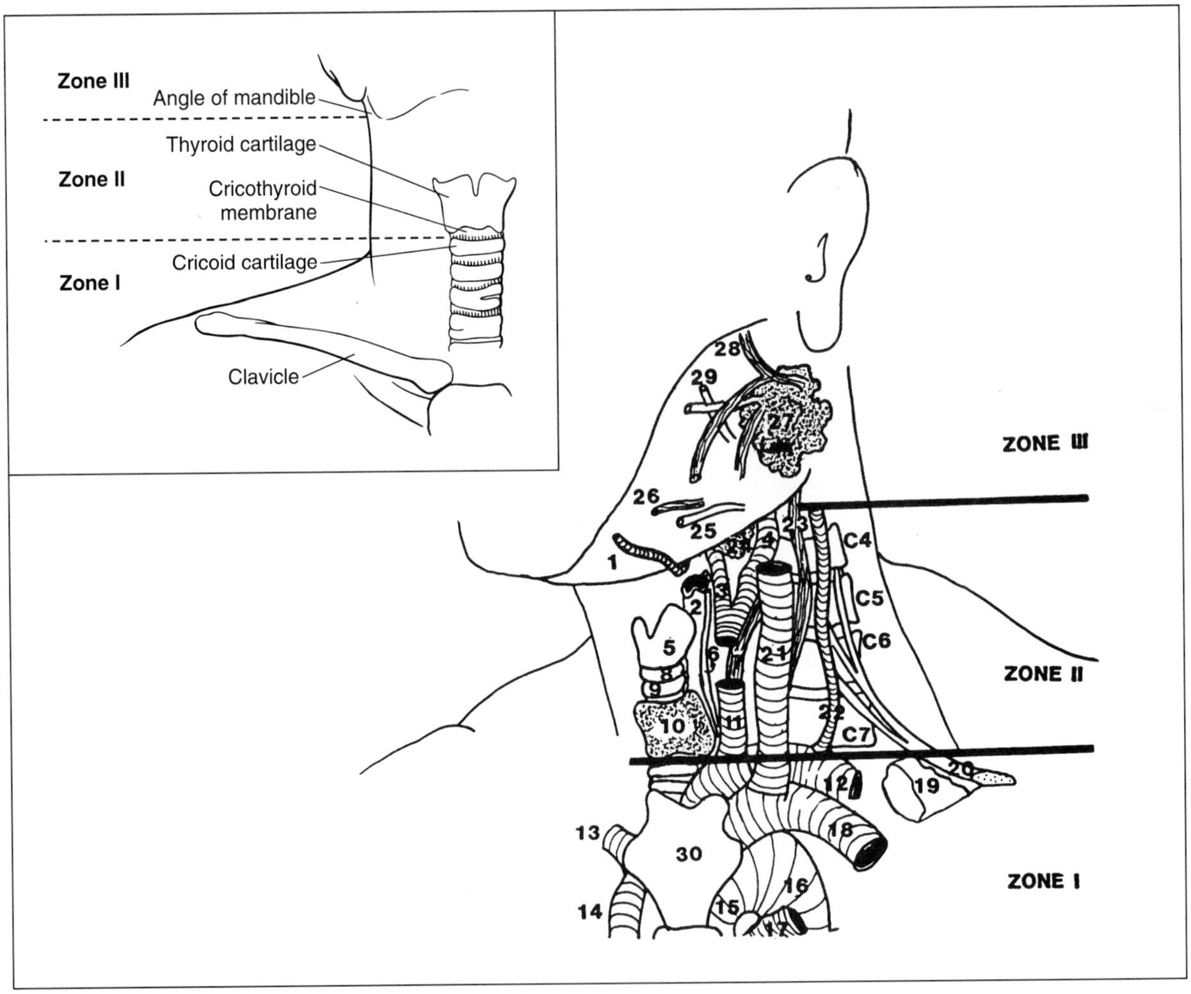

Figure 7.13-3. Cervical structures contained in zones I, II and III. (1) facial artery; (2) esophagus; (3) internal carotid artery; (4) external carotid artery; (5) thyroid cartilage; (6) sympathetic trunk; (7) vagus nerve; (8) cricothyroid membrane; (9) cricoid cartilage; (10) thyroid cartilage; (11) common carotid artery; (12) subclavian artery; (13) right innominate vein; (14) SVC; (15) ascending aorta; (16) descending aorta; (17) PA; (18) subclavian vein; (19) clavicle; (20) brachial plexus; (21) IJ vein; (22) vertebral artery; (23) phrenic nerve; (24) submandibular gland; (25) lingual artery; (26) hypoglossal nerve; (27) parotid gland and duct; (28) facial nerve and its branches; (29) maxillary artery; (30) sternal manubrium. The thoracic duct is not shown in this figure. (Adapted with permission from Ordog GJ, et al. *J Trauma* 1985; 25:238). (Inset redrawn with permission from Epstein M, Chan D, eds: *Emerg Med Clin North Am,* Vol. 16, No. 1, Feb. 1998, 87.)

Evaluation of the larynx, pharynx, trachea and esophagus should be performed if Sx are present. A penetrating neck wound should never be probed or explored locally, as this may dislodge a clot and precipitate a significant hemorrhage or air embolus.

Possible **median sternotomy incision** is used for patients with right-neck Zone I injury or if injuries to mediastinum involving innominate artery or right subclavian artery are suspected. Exposure of injuries to the proximal left subclavian artery is extremely difficult via median sternotomy. In this case, a left anterior thoracotomy is necessary. The chest and left arm should be prepped and draped so as to allow arm manipulation.

Usual preop diagnosis: Penetrating neck injury

SUMMARY OF PROCEDURE

Position	Supine with head turned away from side of exploration and neck extended. If both sides of neck require exploration, head should be in midposition. It is helpful to clear the cervical spine before exploration.
Incision	Sternocleidomastoid
Unique considerations	Monitor BP and HR carefully during carotid sinus manipulation.
Antibiotics	Cefazolin 1 g iv for 1-2 d postop. If pharyngoesophageal injury: ampicillin 1 g + gentamicin 80 mg iv.
Surgical time	1 h
Closing considerations	Wound requires drainage, especially in Zone I exploration and if esophagus or airways were violated.
EBL	Variable
Postop care	ICU 12-24 h for neurologic and airway monitoring. After carotid injury repair, angiography should be considered.
Mortality	1%
Morbidity	Hemorrhage Airway injury Damage to neural or vascular structures Esophageal fistula
Pain score	4

PATIENT POPULATION CHARACTERISTICS

Age range	Typically young adult
Etiology	Typically male
Incidence	5-10% of all trauma involves neck structures.
Associated conditions	Intrathoracic injuries; spinal cord injuries; recurrent laryngeal nerve injury; phrenic nerve injuries; thoracic duct injury

ANESTHETIC CONSIDERATIONS

PREOPERATIVE

Patients with neck injuries often present unique challenges for ET intubation. Extensive internal damage may be present despite minimal external signs. High-velocity deceleration events, or "clothesline" injuries, are often associated with airway compromise. Vascular injuries, particularly involving the carotid artery, can markedly distort internal anatomy and prevent visualization of laryngeal structures or passage of an ET tube. Known or suspected cervical spine injuries will restrict optimal positioning of the head and neck for laryngoscopy. Facial or dental injuries may impede access for laryngoscopy because of limited mouth opening or the presence of blood in the oropharynx. The use of alternative methods to secure the airway (e.g., fiber optic bronchoscopy) or a surgical approach may be the safest option.

Airway Preop assessment of the airway and nature and extent of the cervical injury is crucial. Stridor and hoarseness may be present with laryngeal injury or compression of the trachea. Assess patient's ability to talk as a part of the airway evaluation. C-spine injury (though not common with penetrating neck injuries) should be evaluated by x-ray or CT scan. Airway injury can be associated with subcutaneous emphysema or pneumothorax. The extent of mouth opening, dental injuries and any distortion of internal and external structures due to tissue swelling or hematoma should be

Airway, cont.	determined before induction. The CXR should be carefully examined for evidence of tracheal deviation compression or pneumothorax. **Tests:** X-ray; CT scan; ABG	
Cardiovascular	The patient should be evaluated for the extent of blood loss (BP, HR, capillary refill, peripheral pulse, skin condition). In addition to vascular injuries, associated facial and dental injuries may result in significant occult blood loss accumulated in the stomach. Venous lacerations can allow VAE.	
Neurological	Deficits associated with acute compromise of cerebral arterial blood flow should be evaluated on physical exam. Damage to the recurrent laryngeal nerve can occur, resulting in changes in voice and ↑aspiration risk. Cervical spine injuries should be assessed by physical exam (neck pain, neurologic examination) and radiologic studies (lateral cervical spine x-rays [including C-7], CT scan, MRI).	
Premedication	Full-stomach precautions (see p. B-5).	

INTRAOPERATIVE

Anesthetic technique: GETA

Induction	The induction technique will depend on the associated injuries and physical exam. In the hypovolemic patient, induction doses of STP or propofol should be reduced by 50-75% to minimize ↓↓BP. Consider etomidate (0.2-0.3 mg/kg) as alternative induction agent. A rapid-sequence iv induction with cricoid pressure is usually required. In the presence of a vascular injury, the cough reflex and the BP response to intubation should be suppressed (e.g., remifentanil 1 μg/kg iv), in addition to induction agents to prevent expansion of the hematoma. A wide range of ETT sizes (5.0-8.0 mm) should be available. If cervical spine injury is suspected, in-line stabilization of the patient's head and neck should be provided by an assistant. In the presence of an unstable c-spine, cricoid pressure should be avoided to prevent further injury. If a difficult intubation is anticipated, fiber optic intubation (see p. B-6) or an awake surgical airway (cricothyrotomy or tracheotomy) should be considered.	
Maintenance	Standard maintenance (p. B-3) is usually appropriate for the normotensive neck-trauma patient. In cases of vascular injury, careful control of BP in the low normal range is advantageous. When nerve testing is anticipated, no muscle relaxation or a short-acting agent (e.g., mivacurium) should be used.	
Emergence	Awake extubation is the goal in patients with minimal distortion of the airway at the conclusion of the procedure. Postop intubation and mechanical ventilation is prudent in patients with residual neurological deficits or oropharyngeal swelling. BP control at low normal levels and slight elevation of the head of the bed (10-20°) will help to resolve tissue edema.	
Blood and fluid requirements	IV: 14-16 ga × 1 NS/LR @ 4-6 ml/kg/h	Blood transfusion may be necessary with vascular injuries.
Monitoring	Standard monitors (see B-1). ± Arterial line	Invasive monitoring may be indicated for patients with major vascular injuries; however, the placement should not delay the start of emergency surgery.
Positioning	✓ and pad pressure points. ✓ eyes.	With suspected or known cervical spine injuries, stabilization of the head and neck in the neutral position is required.
Complications	Awareness Hypothermia	

POSTOPERATIVE

Complications	Hemorrhage Hematoma Airway compromise	BP control at low normal levels (SNP infusion, labetalol, NTG) and elevation of the head of the bed (10-20°) will help minimize tissue edema and hematoma formation, which could lead to airway compromise.
Pain management	See p. C-1+.	
Tests	As indicated	

References:

1. Kendall JL, Anglin D, Demetriades D: Penetrating neck trauma. In *Emerg Med Clin North Am: Contemporary Issues in Trauma*. Eckstein M, Chan D, eds. WB Saunders, Philadelphia: 1998, 16(1), 85-106.
2. Wisner D, Blaisdell FW: Neck injuries. In *Scientific American Surgery*, Vol 1. Scientific American, New York: 1998.

CHEST TRAUMA: PERICARDIAL WINDOW, RELEASE OF TAMPONADE, REPAIR OF CARDIAC LACERATION

SURGICAL CONSIDERATIONS

Description: Cardiac contusions occur in 20% of patients with blunt chest trauma, most often 2° compression by a steering wheel. The degree of injury varies from localized contusion to cardiac rupture. Autopsy studies of victims of immediately fatal accidents show that as many as 65% have rupture of one or more cardiac chambers and 45% have pericardial lacerations. Most of the patients with cardiac rupture die at the scene; however, survivors are reported if vital signs are present during transport. Early clinical findings include friction rub, chest pain, ↑HR, murmurs, dysrhythmias or signs of ↓CO. ECGs show nonspecific ST-T wave changes. Serial tracings should be obtained, since abnormalities may not appear for 24 h. Serum enzymes are not valuable; elevation is usually masked by enzymes released from injured muscles. ICU monitoring for 24 h is indicated when ECG abnormalities are present or major contusion is suspected. Management of myocardial contusion should be the same as for acute MI. Pericardial lacerations from stab wounds tend to seal and cause tamponade, present in 80-90% of patients with stab wounds to the heart. Accumulation of 150 ml of blood in the pericardium may impair preload and cause shock. **Beck's triad** of distended neck veins, muffled heart sounds, and ↓BP is present in only 30% of the patients with tamponade. Pulsus paradoxus is even less reliable.

Treatment of penetrating cardiac injuries has gradually changed from initial management by **pericardiocentesis** to prompt **thoracotomy** and **pericardial decompression**. Pericardiocentesis, falsely negative in approximately 15% of cases, is reserved for selected cases when the diagnosis is uncertain or in preparation for thoracotomy. A subxiphoid pericardial window is an option, but is best performed in the OR.

Gunshot wounds produce more extensive myocardial damage, multiple perforations and massive bleeding into the pleural space. Hemothorax, shock and exsanguination occur in nearly all cases of cardiac gunshot wounds. Pericardial tamponade is often absent. Hemodynamically stable patients with penetrating injuries close to the heart should have ECG evaluation in the ER only if equipment is immediately available. The presence of pericardial fluid should be further evaluated with a pericardial window. If a hemopericardium is confirmed, blood should be evacuated and injury treated in the OR.

Patients who are stable enough to be transported to the OR have excellent prognosis, with reported survival of 97% for stab wounds and 71% for gunshot wounds. In contrast, patients who require emergency department thoracotomy have only a 25% survival rate for penetrating injuries.

Subxiphoid pericardial window under local or GA: The entire chest is prepped for potential sternotomy. A vertical midline incision is made over the xiphoid process and upper epigastrium. The xiphoid is elevated or excised, allowing access to the pericardiophrenic membrane and anterior mediastinum. Pericardium is opened between two stay sutures and inspected for the presence of blood. If blood is found, definitive repair should follow without delay.

Median sternotomy can be performed easily as an extension of a pericardial window, and provides excellent exposure to the heart, great vessels and pulmonary hila. This approach is ideal for anterior injuries and for the unstable patient, but is less well suited for posterior injuries and left subclavian injuries.

Left anterior/anterolateral thoracotomy in the 5th intercostal space is the incision of choice for a stable patient. The pericardium is opened anterior to the phrenic nerve and tamponade is relieved. The bleeding heart is controlled with digital occlusion and the laceration is closed with mattress sutures, with care being taken not to occlude coronary flow. Small coronary branches can be ligated, while others should be repaired and may even require CPB.

Usual preop diagnosis: Cardiac laceration

SUMMARY OF PROCEDURE

Position	Supine, L arm extended overhead
Incision	Median sternotomy or left anterior or anterolateral thoracotomy in 5th intercostal space. Further exposure may be obtained by transsternal extension into the R chest.
Special instrumentation	Rapid-infusion device; active rewarming system
Unique considerations	Massive blood loss is expected upon opening pericardium and during repair of laceration. Large-bore peripheral lower extremity iv and central venous access recommended for monitoring of volume replacement.
Antibiotics	Cefazolin 1 g iv
Surgical time	45 min
Closing considerations	Hypothermia and coagulopathy contribute to mortality.
EBL	1-2 L
Postop care	ICU
Mortality	With tamponade: ~30% Without tamponade: ~90%
Morbidity	Overall: 50% Intracardiac shunts Valvular lesions Ventricular aneurysms Retained foreign bodies
Pain score	8

PATIENT POPULATION CHARACTERISTICS

Age range	Usually young adult
Etiology	Blunt trauma 2° MVA, penetrating trauma 2° stab or gunshot wounds
Associated conditions	Hemothorax; pneumothorax; great vessels injury; lung contusion

ANESTHETIC CONSIDERATIONS

See Anesthetic Considerations for Chest Trauma, p. 525.

CHEST TRAUMA: REPAIR OF GREAT VESSELS

SURGICAL CONSIDERATIONS

Description: Thoracic great vessel injury accounts for 8-9% of all vascular injuries seen in the trauma center. The subclavian artery and descending thoracic aorta are the vessels injured most often (21% of cases) followed by PA (16%), subclavian vein (13%), vena cava (11%), innominate artery and pulmonary veins (9%).

Rupture of the thoracic aorta is the most lethal injury following blunt chest trauma and causes up to 50% of fatalities in MVA. Proposed mechanism of injury is a deceleration force causing flexion or torsion of the aortic arch and subsequent disruption of the aortic wall at the ligamentum arteriosum immediately distal to the left subclavian artery. Survival of the patient depends on retention of the hematoma by the adventitial layer of the aorta. This protective mechanism is only temporary and, of those who survive the first h after the accident, 15% will die within the next 6 h and another 25% will die within 24 h. Arteriography is the standard for evaluating aortic injuries and may reveal pseudoaneurysms, arteriovenous fistulas (AFs) or intimal flaps. The mechanism of injury and the mediastinal silhouette are the two most sensitive markers for an injured thoracic aorta. Depressed left mainstem bronchus, apical capping, deviated trachea or deviated NG tube in the esophagus seen on CXR may be suggestive of aortic injury.

Ascending aorta: Rupture requires median sternotomy, CPB and repair with a Dacron graft. Penetrating injury to the anterior aspect of the aorta can be repaired primarily, if there is additional posterior injury, CPB is required for successful repair.

Aortic arch: Complete exposure of great vessels is required, median sternotomy with extension to the neck and division of the innominate vein may be utilized. Complex injuries may require CPB.

Innominate artery, right carotid artery: Approach is via a median sternotomy with right cervical extension and division of the innominate vein, if necessary. Blunt trauma typically involves the proximal innominate artery, in contrast to penetrating trauma, which usually involves the distal portion of the artery near the carotid or subclavian bifurcation. Injuries are repaired using the **bypass exclusion technique** in which a Dacron tube graft is placed between ascending aorta and distal innominate artery; then the injury site is repaired after bypass is completed. Since cerebral perfusion is maintained through the L carotid and subclavian arteries, shunting is not necessary.

Descending thoracic aorta: 97% of patients who arrive alive at the hospital will have an injury at the isthmus. Clamping and direct reconstruction are required under temporary bypass shunt or pump-assisted shunt. Posterolateral thoracotomy via the 4th intercostal space is the preferred access. Distal control of the descending aorta is obtained first; then the transverse aortic arch is exposed and umbilical tape is applied between L carotid and L subclavian arteries. Vascular clamps are applied at the proximal aorta, distal aorta and subclavian artery. Graft interposition is utilized in 85% of cases. An aortic cross-clamp time < 30 min decreases the incidence of paraplegia.

Subclavian artery or vein: Approach is via a cervical extension of the median sternotomy for right-sided injuries. Exposure of injuries to the proximal, left, subclavian artery via median sternotomy is usually inadequate. In patients with such injuries, a left thoracotomy is needed. Graft interposition is often necessary.

Pulmonary artery and veins: In major hilar injury, a pneumonectomy may be necessary despite high mortality. Cross-clamping of the hilum prevents air embolus and hemorrhage.

Thoracic vena cava: Intrathoracic IVC injury causes hemopericardium and tamponade. Repair requires total CPB and is often performed through the R atrium. SVC repair is often performed via a lateral venorrhaphy.

Usual preop diagnosis: Thoracic great vessel injury

SUMMARY OF PROCEDURE

Position	Supine
Incision	Anterolateral thoracotomy is preferred as it provides access to the descending aorta for cross-clamping, good access to heart and may be extended across sternum into right chest.
Special instrumentation	Intraop blood recovery device; rapid-infusion device; graft materials for any vessels larger than 5 mm. CPB often necessary.
Unique considerations	Use of vasodilators (SNP) prevents cardiac strain during cross-clamping of the aorta. Large amount of fluid is required to prevent hypotension after clamp removal.
Antibiotics	Cefazolin 1 g iv
Surgical time	1-3 h
EBL	≥ 1-2 L
Postop care	ICU. Careful hemodynamic monitoring is critical since underlying pulmonary contusion may be worsened by inappropriate fluid administration. PA catheter may be necessary to optimize hemodynamic parameters, particularly in older patients. Coagulation studies must be carefully monitored and corrected with appropriate blood products.
Mortality	Subclavian artery injury: 5% Blunt injury to the descending thoracic aorta: 5-25% Ascending thoracic aorta, aortic arch (in patients with stable vital signs on arrival), 50%; pulmonary artery or vein, suprahepatic IVC or SVC: > 70% In general, mortality is associated with multisystem trauma and usually 2° concomitant head injury, infection, respiratory insufficiency and renal insufficiency.
Morbidity	Paraplegia: ~8% (with descending aortic injuries)
Pain score	10

PATIENT POPULATION CHARACTERISTICS

Age range	Typically young adult
Incidence	Thoracic great vessel injury accounts for 8-9% of all vascular injuries seen in the trauma center.
Etiology	Blunt trauma from MVA; penetrating trauma from stab or gunshot wounds
Associated conditions	Pneumothorax; hemothorax, head injury

ANESTHETIC CONSIDERATIONS

See Anesthetic Considerations for Chest Trauma, p. 525.

CHEST TRAUMA: PNEUMONECTOMY, LOBECTOMY, REPAIR OF TRACHEOBRONCHIAL INJURY

SURGICAL CONSIDERATIONS

Description: Penetrating injuries to the chest can be divided into high- and low-velocity injuries. All stab wounds are classified as low-velocity injuries. Gunshot wounds may be considered low- or high-velocity injuries, depending on energy of the bullet. The majority of gunshot wounds seen in the ER are low velocity, however, higher velocity injuries are being seen with increased frequency. The extent of tissue destruction in high-velocity injuries is related to blast effect, tumbling and fragmentation of the missile and secondary missiles such as bone fragments. Patients with such injuries are more likely to require thoracotomy and pulmonary resection. In general, pulmonary resection is required in 1% of stab wounds and 2% of gunshot wounds. The indications for early operation are continued shock, prolonged bleeding, a larger air leak with inability to oxygenate or ventilate the patient and suspected concomitant injuries to the vital intrathoracic structures. In most patients with stab wounds or low-velocity gunshot wounds, bleeding from the lung tissue stops spontaneously after evacuation of the hemothorax and reexpansion of the lung. Only 5-10% of such patients will require thoracotomy to control bleeding, compared to a thoracotomy rate of 70% for high-velocity injuries. Pulmonary contusion is a frequent sequela of gunshot injuries or blunt trauma to the chest. Pulmonary contusion occurs in 75% of patients with flail chest but also can occur following blunt trauma without rib fracture. Alveolar rupture with fluid transudation and extravasation of blood are early findings.

The incidence of tracheobronchial injuries reported in the autopsy series from MVA is 1%. Mechanisms of injury include rapid deceleration, direct blow or sudden increase of intratracheal pressure against a closed glottis. The most common injury is transverse rupture, occurring in 74%, followed by longitudinal rupture, in 18%, and complex, comprising the remaining 8%. Approximately 80% of cases with tracheal rupture occur within 2.5 cm of the carina. Patients with injury to the airway may present in severe dyspnea and with massive subcutaneous emphysema. About 90% of these patients will have an abnormal CXR, showing pneumothorax, pneumomediastinum, subcutaneous emphysema or pleural effusion.

Tracheobronchoscopy should be performed in all patients with suspected tracheobronchial injuries to establish the diagnosis and plan operative treatment.

Parenchymal lacerations are repaired by the simplest method available to stop bleeding or air leak. If pulmonary resection is required, formal segmental resection is not necessary. A stapling device should be used to preserve as much lung tissue as possible.

Anatomic pulmonary resections are indicated when bronchial injury repair is not feasible or may lead to complete lobar collapse. **Pneumonectomy** may be required for major hilar injuries but is associated with a mortality rate of 75%. **Primary repair of tracheobronchial injuries** should be performed as soon as possible. Transverse rupture may require the placement of a sterile tracheal tube into the distal trachea through the operative field. After posterior sutures are placed, an orotracheal tube is advanced beyond the area of injury. **Main-stem bronchial repair** is performed under one-lung ventilation. High-frequency jet ventilation may be required to maintain oxygenation. Occasionally, total CPB is necessary for repair of complex airway injuries. Before closing, the suture line is pressure-tested and evaluated by fiber optic bronchoscopy.

Usual preop diagnosis: Tracheobronchial injury; penetrating/blunt chest trauma

SUMMARY OF PROCEDURE

Position	Supine, with neck extended for proximal tracheal injury, or lateral decubitus
Incision	Transverse cervical for almost all proximal tracheal injuries Right posterolateral thoracotomy in 5th intercostal space for thoracic trachea and right bronchial wounds Left posterolateral thoracotomy for L bronchial injury
Special instrumentation	Fiber optic bronchoscope, intrabronchial tube, jet ventilator/oscillator
Unique considerations	In patients with lobar resection or after pneumonectomy, PEEP may result in bronchopleural fistula
Antibiotics	Cefazolin 1 g iv
Surgical time	2-3 h
EBL	Variable
Postop care	ICU (typically)
Mortality	Penetrating tracheobronchial injuries: ~15% Pneumonectomy for trauma: 75%
Morbidity	Broncheopleural fistula Pneumothorax Hemothorax ARDS
Pain score	Cervical approach: 5-7 Thoracic approach: 8-10

ANESTHETIC CONSIDERATIONS FOR CHEST TRAUMA

Hemopericardium may rapidly progress to pericardial tamponade requiring immediate pericardiocentesis or pericardial window, followed by surgical exploration and repair of the cardiac or vascular laceration. These patients typically present in shock (↓↓BP) with distended neck veins (↑↑venous pressure) and distant heart sounds (Beck's triad) without evidence of tension pneumothorax. Preop, and particularly during the induction of GA, the patient's intravascular volume must be expanded and myocardial contractility, HR and SVR maintained. Inotropes and antiarrhythmic drugs may be required if hemodynamic instability occurs and does not respond to iv fluid administration. CPB is usually not required.

PREOPERATIVE

Respiratory Associated injuries such as hemothorax and/or pneumothorax may be present, requiring thoracostomy tube placement. A widened mediastinum, apical pleural capping or fracture of the first or second rib often occurs with injury to the great vessels. Multiple rib fractures are often associated with pulmonary contusions, which may not be apparent on the initial CXR, but can progressively impair oxygenation. With tamponade, spontaneous respiration is preferred over PPV (→ ↓ venous return + ↓ CO).

Tests: CXR (PA + lateral views). Upright inspiratory films best delineate chest structures; expiratory films enhance visualization of pneumothorax. ABG.

Cardiovascular BP and HR should be followed and responses to fluid resuscitation noted. With adequate resuscitation, the EJ veins should appear full. CO can be significantly reduced despite normal BP measurements. Pulsus paradoxus may be present, with decreases in SBP of 10-12 mmHg during inspiration. Preop, intravascular volume should be restored, and myocardial contractility supported with inotropes (e.g., dopamine 5-10 μg/kg/min) as necessary. Correction of metabolic acidosis with iv bicarbonate is indicated (e.g., 1 mEq/kg, then ✓ ABG). Myocardial contusion also can occur and can be associated with ventricular arrhythmias, RBBB and RV failure, since the right heart is substernal and most directly involved in blunt trauma to the sternum. Supportive therapy with antiarrhythmics (e.g., lidocaine 1-2 mg/min) and inotropes (dopamine or epinephrine) may be required.

Cardiovascular, cont.	**Tests:** ABG, serial ECGs with myocardial contusion. ECHO may show pericardial effusion, though clotted blood can be interpreted as myocardium.
Neurological	Hypotension and ↓CO may compromise cerebral perfusion. Associated head injury also can contribute to alterations in mental status. Pupil size and reactivity should be noted. Glasgow Coma Scale score ≤ 8 indicates significant brain injury.
Musculoskeletal	Known or suspected cervical spine fractures require intubation precautions, with laryngoscopy performed while an assistant provides in-line stabilization of the patient's head in the neutral position. **Tests:** Lateral cervical spine x-rays, including C-7

INTRAOPERATIVE

★ **Anesthetic technique:** GETA with full-stomach precautions (see p. B-5). **NB:** In the patient with an unstable C-spine, cricoid pressure (nl ≈ 10 lbs) may cause spinal cord injury, and consideration should be given to the establishment of a surgical airway under local anesthesia.

Induction	A pericardial window through a subxiphoid incision can be performed with local anesthesia. More often, GETA is required for exploration through a median sternotomy or left thoracotomy. In the latter case, a DLT or BB is desirable. Rapid-sequence induction with ketamine (0.5-1 mg/kg) and succinylcholine is attractive since ketamine is usually associated with ↑HR, ↑BP and ↑CO. Etomidate (0.2-0.6 mg/kg) is a useful alternative for patients with head injuries. Inotropic agents (ephedrine, dopamine, epinephrine) should be immediately available to treat hypotension. Agents which tend to decrease SVR, such as inhalational anesthetics and narcotics, should be introduced with caution. The potential for sudden and substantial blood loss exists and PRBCs (cross-matched, type-specific or O[-]) should be available in the OR prior to induction.
Maintenance	Initially, low-dose inhalational agents and low-dose narcotics may be used, as tolerated. Hypotension may require dopamine infusion (1-50 μg/kg/min). Muscle relaxation and PPV are used. NO should be avoided if laceration of the heart or great vessel is suspected. If the patient is hypotensive and acidotic, scopolamine (0.2-0.4 mg iv) will provide amnesia. As cardiac and vascular injuries are repaired, BP and CO will often improve, permitting increased depth of anesthesia and decreased inotropic support.
Emergence	Trauma patients often require prolonged intubation; however, hemodynamically stable patients with limited injuries may be extubated awake. Patients who received significant blood replacement (> 50% of blood volume), those requiring inotropic support, and patients with head injuries should remain intubated and mechanically ventilated postop.

Blood and fluid requirements	Be prepared for blood loss. IV: 14 ga × 2 Fluid warmer Rapid-infusion device Airway humidifier T&C PRBCs.	Large blood losses occur occasionally, depending on the severity of the injury. Crystalloid and/or blood products should be infused to maintain BP and CVP (full jugular veins).
Monitoring	Standard monitors (see p. B-1). Arterial line CVP ± PA catheter ± TEE	ECG should be observed for changes associated with myocardial contusion (ventricular arrhythmias, RBBB, ST-T wave changes). CVP monitoring is very useful in guiding fluid management. With release of tamponade, CVP rapidly drops toward normal.
Positioning	✓ and pad pressure points. ✓ eyes.	Axillary roll, if lateral decubitus position, chest roll if median sternotomy.
Complications	Hypothermia	Hypothermia → dysrhythmias + ↓CO → acidosis. Rx: warm OR, warm iv fluids, humidify gases and use patient warming devices.
	Awareness	May be unavoidable in unstable patients. Rx: Consider scopolamine 0.2-0.4 mg iv.
	Renal failure	Usually 2° ↓renal perfusion (prerenal). Rx: Restore BP and circulating volume.

Complications, cont.	Coagulopathy	Most commonly 2° dilutional thrombocytopenia. DIC may require replacement therapy with Plts, FFP and cryoprecipitate.

POSTOPERATIVE

Complications	Hypotension Arrhythmias	Cardiogenic shock may be 2° prolonged hypotension or cardiac contusion. Hemodynamic instability with ventricular arrhythmias may occur. Treatment with inotropic infusions (dopamine 5-10 μg/kg/min or epinephrine 50-200 ng/kg/min) and antiarrhythmics.
	Hypothermia	Active warming of iv fluids and warming blankets should be continued in ICU or PACU if hypothermia persists.
	ARDS	Interstitial and alveolar edema → progressively worsening pulmonary function requiring prolonged mechanical ventilation.
	Coagulopathy Renal failure	Based on clinical assessment and laboratory data (PT, Plt count, fibrinogen); transfusion of Plts, FFP and/or cryoprecipitate may be indicated.
Pain management	PCA or parenteral narcotics Epidural	Epidural infusions of narcotic and/or low-dose local anesthetics can be effective in patients without coagulopathy.

ABDOMINAL TRAUMA: DAMAGE CONTROL

SURGICAL CONSIDERATIONS

Description: The incidence of abdominal injuries requiring laparotomy approaches 25% for penetrating and 5% for blunt abdominal trauma. In blunt trauma, liver and spleen injuries occur with an incidence of ~50%. In penetrating trauma, the most common injuries are small bowel (29%), liver (28%), colon (23%) and stomach (13%). Ninety percent of preventable deaths in trauma patients are related to shock from unrecognized intraabdominal hemorrhage caused by solid viscus injury.

Victims of severe multisystem trauma are particularly susceptible to development of a fatal coagulopathic state 2° hypothermia, acidosis, dilution and consumption. Replacement of two or more blood volumes with NS or PRBCs will decrease the level of coagulation factors to 15%. Because of delays in obtaining coagulation profile results, coagulation factors should be replaced empirically in the setting of a large transfusion requirement (e.g., 1 U FFP/4 U PRBC). Metabolic acidosis affects both the circulatory system and coagulation, → ↓ CO and triggering DIC. Chances of salvaging a patient with pH < 7.0 are close to zero. To stop this self-perpetuating downward cycle, the concept of "Damage Control" has evolved. This involves rapid laparotomy to control major injuries, followed by temporary closure of the abdomen and another exploration after the patient is rewarmed and stabilized. With the use of this technique, approximately 40% of critically injured patients can be saved from otherwise fatal injuries.

With the patient on a heated operating table, the abdomen and chest are prepped from the thighs to the neck and draped, and the abdomen is entered through a midline incision. This critical moment can be associated with significant blood loss and may require rapid blood transfusion. Four-quadrant packing with laparotomy pads is performed in the abdominal cavity, and manual compression of the subdiaphragmatic aorta may be instituted if packing alone does not control the hemorrhage. If necessary, the operation is stopped and blood/fluid resuscitation is performed. After consultation with the anesthesiologist, the surgeon proceeds with the sequential unpacking of each of the four quadrants and identifying injuries. Vascular injuries are controlled with clamping and ligation, bowel injuries are stapled across, but no attempt is made for primary repair. Liver and retroperitoneal injuries are controlled with packing alone. When damage control is performed, the abdomen is closed rapidly either with towel clips or running suture. The patient is then transported to

ICU and actively rewarmed and resuscitated. Reoperation should be performed at 24-48 h and definitive repair of the injured organs should be completed.

Usual preop diagnosis: Intraabdominal trauma and hemorrhage

SUMMARY OF PROCEDURE

Position	Supine
Incision	Midline abdominal
Special instrumentation	Fluid-warming, rapid-infusion device
Unique considerations	Autotransfusion device may be of use if no contamination of abdominal cavity (e.g., Cell Saver).
Antibiotics	Cefotetan 1 g iv
Surgical time	45 min
Closing considerations	Even temporary closure may not be possible because of severe bowel edema. A silo made from a plastic iv bag may be used to cover the bowel.
EBL	Average transfusion requirement: 12 L crystalloids, 20 U PRBCs, 5 U FFP, 6 U Plts
Postop care	ICU; patient remains intubated. Active rewarming is of primary importance.
Mortality	70%
Morbidity	Intraabdominal abscesses: 30% Fistulas: 10%
Pain score	10

PATIENT POPULATION CHARACTERISTICS

Age range	Typically young adult
Male:Female	9:1
Incidence	25% for penetrating and 5% for blunt abdominal trauma
Etiology	MVA; penetrating injury (e.g., GSW or stab wound)
Associated conditions	Chest trauma; closed head trauma; pelvic fracture

ABDOMINAL TRAUMA: HEPATIC AND SPLENIC INJURIES

SURGICAL CONSIDERATIONS

Description: The liver is the most commonly injured organ with penetrating trauma, while the spleen is the most commonly injured organ with blunt trauma. Approximately 30% of all patients requiring laparotomy for trauma will have hepatic injuries. Minor hepatic injuries (grades I and II) constitute the majority of cases, require simple repairs and are associated with minimal mortality. Twenty percent of patients will have complex injuries (grades III-V) with mortality up to 30%.

Several maneuvers can be used to facilitate **repair of liver injuries: Manual compression** temporarily controls bleeding and allows time for volume resuscitation. **Portal triad occlusion (Pringle maneuver)** (Fig. 7.13-4B) decreases blood loss and identifies the patient who would benefit from left or right hepatic artery ligation. **Intrahepatic omental packing** is superior to gauze packing for controlling bleeding and obliterating the space resulting from parenchymal debridement. More extensive liver injuries may require rapid and extensive **finger fracture technique (blunt parenchymal dissection)** for vascular control. Wide mobilization of hepatic attachments with medial rotation of the liver exposes the supra- and infrahepatic portions of the vena cava. Placement of an atriocaval shunt may be used to control retrohepatic caval hemorrhage. **Perihepatic packing and planned reexploration** is a life-saving procedure for coagulopathic, acidotic or hypothermic patients (damage control surgery). Continuous arterial bleeding after packing can be managed with **selective hepatic embolization**. All liver injuries should be drained to control potential bile leaks. Closed suction drains have the lowest septic complication rate.

Portal triad (portal vein, hepatic artery, common bile duct) injuries, although rare, are associated with extremely high mortality. Isolated portal vein injuries are associated with a 70% mortality. The portal vein should be repaired if possible; however, ligation can be tolerated. Careful volume resuscitation should follow portal vein ligation to avoid ↓BP 2° fluid sequestration in the splanchnic bed. Simple ligation of the hepatic artery, preferably proximal to the gastroduodenal artery, is recommended for most major hepatic artery injuries. Shock and transfusion-related coagulopathy occurring in the immediate postop period are responsible for 80% of the deaths in liver injury patients. Control of hemorrhage remains the critical component in the successful management of liver injuries.

The treatment of **splenic injuries** has changed over the past 2 decades from prompt **splenectomy** in all cases to **splenic salvage** whenever possible. More than 90% of splenic injuries are caused by blunt trauma. Approximately 25% of these patients can be managed nonoperatively. Of the 75% who require laparotomy, only 1/3 (25% of all splenic injuries) require splenectomy. The remainder (50% of all splenic injuries) can be managed by techniques that preserve the spleen. The splenic salvage rate in the pediatric population approaches 90%.

In a patient with massive **intraabdominal hemorrhage**, sudden cardiovascular collapse is predictable when the abdomen is opened. To prevent this, a left thoracotomy with temporary thoracic aortic occlusion may be indicated. For the exsanguinating patient with detectable BP and suspected abdominal source of bleeding, laparotomy with manual compression of the aorta at the aortic hiatus is recommended. Similarly, if the patient becomes unexpectedly hypotensive when the abdominal cavity is entered, a medium-sized Richardson retractor, wrapped in a laparotomy pad, can be used to compress the abdominal aorta against the spinal column just under the diaphragm. Access for aortic clamping is rapidly obtained by blunt finger dissection of the lesser sac. After removing all clots and free blood, four-quadrant packing is used to control bleeding. If, during subsequent packing removal, a significant liver injury is encountered, lateral extension of the incision may be required. If atriocaval shunt is preferred over finger-fracture technique to control a retrohepatic vascular injury, extension of the midline incision through a median sternotomy is performed. A modified chest tube (36 Fr) or 9 mm ETT is commonly used as a vascular shunt. The tube is inserted through the right atrial appendage and secured at the intrapericardial vena cava and suprarenal vena cava with vascular snares (Fig 7.13-4).

Massive bleeding from the LUQ is probably caused by splenic injury. Hilar vascular injury, extensive fragmentation, total avulsion or associated severe injuries are indications for splenectomy. The tail of the pancreas should be palpated and vascular control of the splenic vessels obtained. In case of a life-threatening emergency, the spleen is delivered into the wound in blunt fashion, LUQ tightly repacked and control of short gastric vessels delayed until better resuscitation can be obtained.

Usual preop diagnosis: Hepatic injury; splenic injury

SUMMARY OF PROCEDURE

Position	Supine
Incision	Midline abdominal; possible extension into thorax via median sternotomy and L or R subcostal extensions.
Special instrumentation	Chest tube or ETT as an atriocaval shunt; active rewarming device; Cell Saver
Unique considerations	Most emergency laparotomies require close cooperation between anesthesiologist and surgeon. The procedure may need to be interrupted for fluid or blood resuscitation if patient becomes hypotensive. The entire chest and abdomen, including both groins, need to be accessible to the surgeon; ECG electrodes preferably are placed on the patient's back.
Antibiotics	Cefazolin 1 g iv
Surgical time	1-2 h
Closing considerations	After massive fluid resuscitation, interstitial edema may preclude primary fascial closure. Absorbable mesh or nonabsorbable synthetics may be necessary to close the abdomen.
EBL	2-10 L (transfusion requirement 6-20 U)
Postop care	ICU—shock and coagulopathy management. Monitoring for possible rebleeding and abdominal compartment syndrome.
Mortality	Liver: 10% Spleen: 10%
Morbidity	Liver – perihepatic abscess: 10% Spleen – septic complications: 7%
Pain score	8-10

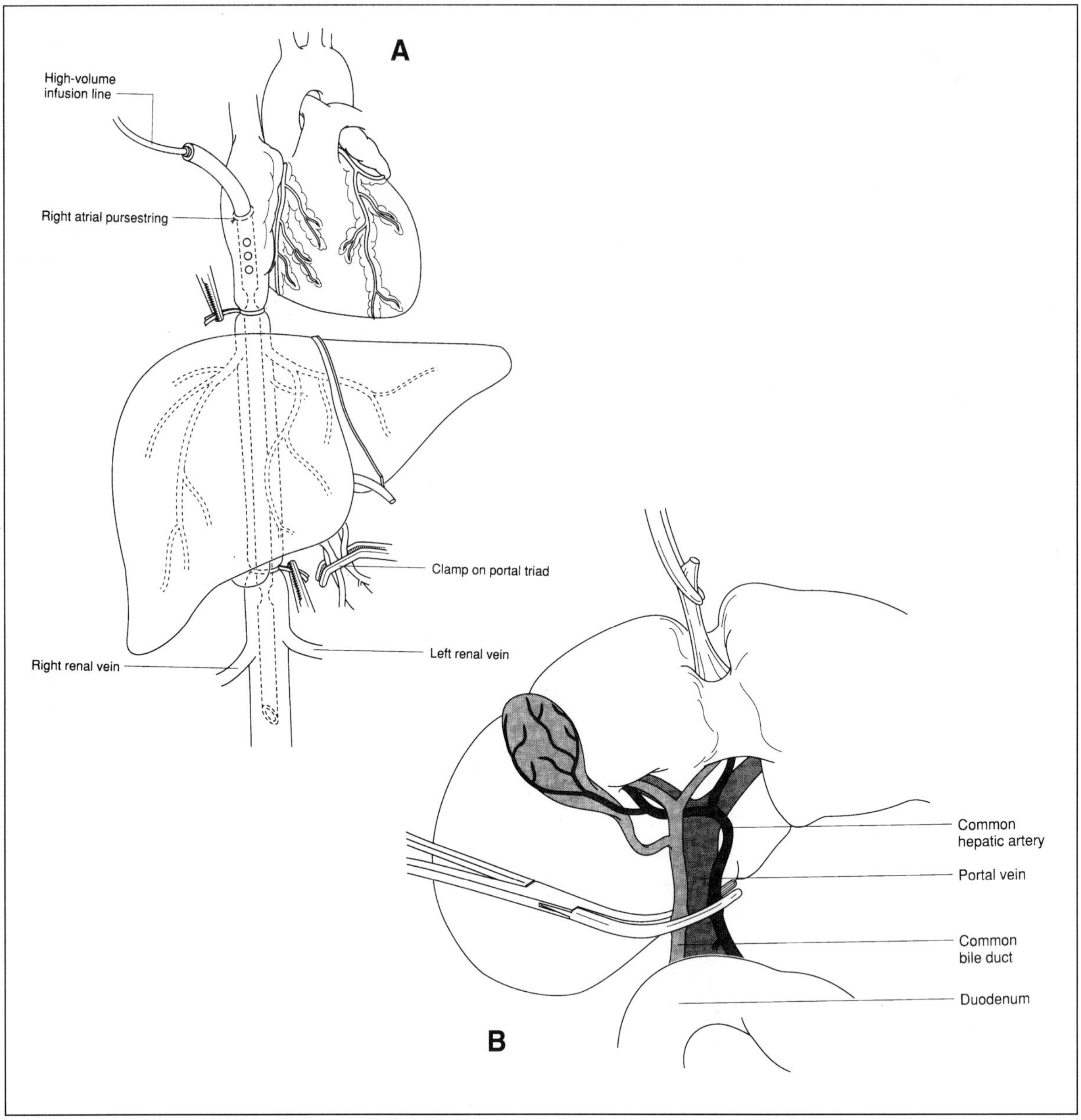

Figure 7.13-4. (A) Intracaval shunt used for retrohepatic venous injuries, combined with a Pringle maneuver for isolation of the retrohepatic vena cava for operative repair. (B) Pringle maneuver compression of the portal triad structures with a noncrushing vascular clamp for hepatic inflow control. (Reproduced with permission from Greenfield LJ, et al, eds: *Surgery: Scientific Principles and Practice*, 2nd edition. Lippincott-Raven Publishers, Philadelphia: 1997, 340, 276).

PATIENT POPULATION CHARACTERISTICS

Age range	Any age
Male:Female	3:1
Incidence	Liver: 30% of patients requiring laparotomy for trauma Spleen: 10% of patients requiring laparotomy for trauma
Etiology	Liver: penetrating wound (80%) with gunshot wounds responsible for 60% and stab wounds for 40% Spleen: blunt trauma (90%), mostly due to MVA
Associated conditions	Liver: isolated hepatic injury (30%); injury to one or two other organs: 50%, with diaphragm, major vascular structures, stomach, lung and colon being most common.

TRAUMA SURGERY FOR ABDOMINAL VASCULAR INJURIES

SURGICAL CONSIDERATIONS

Description: Penetrating trauma is the most common cause of abdominal vascular injuries — IVC/hepatic veins: 36%; celiac/mesenteric vessels: 30%; iliac vessels: 11%; and aorta, portal/splenic and renal vessels: each 5%. Patients with gunshot wounds to the abdomen have ~25% incidence of major vascular injury; however, only ~10% of patients with penetrating stab wounds will have vascular injuries. Patients sustaining blunt abdominal trauma have a 5-10% incidence of vascular injury.

Initial resuscitation of the patient with abdominal vascular injuries depends on the patient's condition at arrival. Multiple large-bore catheters should be inserted in the upper extremities or, if necessary, central venous access should be obtained. Because of the probable intraabdominal venous injury, lower-extremity venous access is not indicated. In the agonal patient with a distended abdomen (indicating major intraperitoneal bleeding), emergency-department thoracotomy with cross-clamping of the descending aorta may be necessary. Blood replacement during resuscitation is done preferably with type-specific blood. It is a good practice to have two U of O(-) blood available immediately in the ER in case there is no time even for limited cross-match. Efforts to limit hypothermia should start as soon as patient arrives (use of prewarmed fluids and high-flow blood warmers and covering the patient with prewarmed blankets).

Injuries to the abdominal vessels can be grouped into four regions, which require different surgical approaches:

Midline supramesocolic hemorrhage or hematoma (superior to the transverse mesocolon) is usually 2° injury to the suprarenal aorta, celiac axis, proximal superior mesenteric artery or proximal renal artery. Proximal aortic control should be obtained at the hiatus by either aortic compression or manually by entering the lesser sack and digitally splitting the muscle fibers of the crura. Once this is done, direct access to the vessels is achieved through retroperitoneal mobilization of all left-sided abdominal viscera or extensive **Kocher's maneuver** (duodenal mobilization to expose the IVC and aorta on the right side). Injuries to the aorta are then repaired directly or with the appropriate graft. An injured celiac axis probably can be safely ligated. Access to the superior mesenteric artery and vein may require transection of the pancreas, and ligation of the superior mesenteric vein may be a better option than repair.

Midline inframesocolic hemorrhage or hematoma results from infrarenal aorta or IVC injury. Exposure is obtained by incising posterior peritoneum in the midline after displacement of the small bowel and cephalic retraction of the transverse mesocolon. A proximal aortic clamp is then placed just below the left renal vein, and a distal clamp near the aortic bifurcation. The defect is repaired primarily, using patch aortoplasty, end-to-end anastomosis or a graft. If the aorta is intact and an inframesocolic hematoma seems to be more extensive on the right side, or if there is active bleeding coming through the base of the mesentery, then injury to the IVC should be suspected. Access to the infrahepatic IVC is preferably obtained by mobilization of the R colon, and duodenum. Repair will require proximal and distal control of the IVC and application of a clamp to the injury, or Fogarty balloon tamponade of the laceration. In young patients with exsanguinating hemorrhage, the infrarenal IVC can be ligated, providing time for appropriate fluid management.

Lateral perirenal hematoma or hemorrhage suggests injury to the renal vessels or kidney. In patients with blunt abdominal trauma who have a negative abdominal CT, IVP or arteriogram, surgery is not required. A penetrating injury usually requires surgical exploration. Vascular control of the ipsilateral renal artery is obtained before the hematoma is entered. If there is active bleeding from the kidney or overlying retroperitoneum, then the kidney is exposed via a lateral incision, and a vascular clamp is applied to the renal vessels. This is usually followed by nephrectomy after palpation to verify the existence of a normal contralateral kidney. Only 30-40% of kidneys with arterial injuries can be salvaged.

Lateral pelvic hematoma or hemorrhage indicates injury to the iliac vessels. Vascular control is obtained at the aortic bifurcation proximally and close to the inguinal ligament distally. An injury to the right common iliac vein may require division of the overlying right common iliac artery. The internal iliac artery is best visualized by elevating common and external iliac arteries on vascular tapes. The iliac artery can be repaired primarily or by using a graft. If fecal contamination is severe, an extraanatomic crossover femorofemoral graft may be required. Injuries to the iliac veins are treated with lateral venorrhaphy or ligation.

Usual preop diagnosis: Abdominal vascular injury

SUMMARY OF PROCEDURE

Position	Supine, with left arm extended overhead
Incision	Midline abdominal
Special instrumentation	Autotransfusion device (e.g., Cell Saver); thoracotomy tray; aortic compressor
Unique considerations	Prevent heat loss and warm all infusions and irrigation solutions. For the patient requiring massive transfusion, 1 U FFP/4 U PRBCs. After prolonged aortic cross-clamp, prophylactic administration of $NaHCO_3$ (1-2 mEq/kg) may be indicated to prevent "washout" acidosis. Patients after infrarenal vena cava ligation require volume expansion and prevention of lower extremity venous pooling. Elastic wraps and lower-extremity elevation should be maintained for at least 1 wk. Similarly, after superior mesenteric vein ligation, splanchnic hypervolemia requires vigorous fluid resuscitation and lasts approximately 3 d.
Antibiotics	Cefazolin 1 g iv
Surgical time	Variable
Closing considerations	Once vascular injuries are repaired, hepatic injuries are controlled with packing, bowel injuries are closed with staplers and the skin is rapidly closed with towel clips.
EBL	5-10 L
Postop care	ICU
Mortality	Aorta: 60% Superior mesenteric artery: 40-80% Superior mesenteric vein: 20% Combined injury to the suprarenal aorta and IVC: 100% Infrarenal abdominal aorta: 50% Infrarenal vena cava: 30% Renal artery: 15% Iliac artery: 40% Iliac vein: 30%
Morbidity	Abscess Fistula Sepsis Shock Coagulopathy
Pain score	8-10

PATIENT POPULATION CHARACTERISTICS

Age range	Typically young adult
Male:Female	Male > female
Incidence	15% of patients with abdominal trauma
Etiology	10% of penetrating stab wounds and 25% of gunshot wounds to the abdomen will cause a major vascular injury
Associated conditions	Multiple vascular injuries; hollow viscus perforation; fecal contamination

ANESTHETIC CONSIDERATIONS

Abdominal injuries range from relatively simple penetrating injuries (e.g., a stab wound) to severe blunt trauma (e.g., liver lacerations and pelvic fractures) and are often associated with massive hemorrhage. Head injuries and spinal fractures may complicate management plans. The ability to provide rapid, aggressive volume replacement is often the key to survival. Coagulopathy (DIC) and hypothermia present additional challenges.

PREOPERATIVE

Respiratory Associated injuries such as hemothorax and/or pneumothorax may be present, requiring thoracostomy tube placement. A widened mediastinum, apical pleural capping or fracture of the 1st or 2nd rib often occur with serious vascular injuries. Multiple rib fractures suggest possible pulmonary contusions, which may not be evident on initial CXR but can progressively impair oxygenation and ventilation with time and fluid resuscitation.

Respiratory, cont.

Tests: CXR (PA + lateral views). Upright inspiratory films best delineate chest structures; expiratory films enhance detection of pneumothorax; ABG.

Cardiovascular

BP and HR should be followed and responses to fluid resuscitation noted. Tachycardia can maintain an adequate BP with reduced pulse pressure, despite 25-30% loss of blood volume. Attempt to quantify overt blood loss (e.g., scalp lacerations, open fracture sites). Blunt chest trauma (e.g., steering wheel contact) may result in myocardial contusion with various dysrhythmias, most often premature ventricular or atrial complexes.

Tests: Serial Hct; ECG in patients > 50 yrs of age or with blunt chest trauma

Neurological

Seek physical evidence of open or closed head injuries, such as palpable depressions of the skull or scalp lacerations, abrasions or contusions. Pupil size and reactivity should be noted. Intubation in the ER is necessary for patients who are unable to protect their airway, require hyperventilation, or are combative and unable to cooperate with medical staff for exam and treatment. In general, any patient with a Glasgow Coma Scale (GCS) ≤ 8 (no spontaneous eye opening, inappropriate or incomprehensible speech and only reflexive motor responses) requires intubation. Motor and/or sensory deficits may reflect spinal cord injury and may be associated with neurogenic ("spinal") shock, particularly with upper thoracic or cervical cord injuries.

Tests: Cervical spine x-rays – lateral view, including C7, is a good screening exam; ✓ for altered vertical alignment and unequal disk interspaces. CT scan or MRI of head, ✓ for gross asymmetry, hemorrhage or obliterated ventricles.

Musculoskeletal

Known or suspected cervical spine injuries require intubation precautions. In urgent cases, intubation without neck extension is achieved with an assistant providing in-line stabilization of the head in the neutral position. If time permits, awake, blind or fiber optic intubation may be attempted. Basilar skull fractures contraindicate passage of nasal ET or OG tubes. Pelvic and femur fractures may represent sources of significant (>1000 ml) occult blood loss.

Tests: Radiographs of cervical spine (see above), skull, extremities

Hematologic

Depending on estimations of prior, ongoing and anticipated surgical blood losses, preop blood T&C may be desired. O(-) or type-specific blood should be available until the T&C is complete.

Tests: Serial Hct; T&C

Laboratory

Other tests, as indicated from H&P or suspected injuries, including: electrolytes; liver panel; toxicology screen; blood alcohol level.

Premedication

Premedication is rarely useful due to the urgency of the procedures and the need to have an alert, responsive patient for serial evaluations of mental status or abdominal pain. Sedative premedication should be avoided in patients who are hemodynamically unstable and those with probable head injuries. Virtually all patients are considered to have full stomachs, and any compromise of the ability to protect the airway is inappropriate. While Na citrate (30 ml po) may be administered to patients at risk for aspiration, ranitidine and metoclopramide may not reach effective levels in the short interval before induction.

INTRAOPERATIVE

Anesthetic technique: GETA with full-stomach precautions

Induction

Before induction, a variety of laryngoscope blades (e.g., Miller 1 and 2, Mac 3 and 4) and ETTs with stylets (6.0, 7.0 and 8.0 mm) should be ready. LMA may be useful for providing temporary airway control without cervical spine manipulation if direct laryngoscopy is difficult. LMA may be used as a conduit for fiber optic endotracheal intubation. A size 7.0 mm JD ETT will pass through a #4 LMA. Equipment for emergent cricothyrotomy (a 14 ga iv catheter + adapter) and jet ventilation should be in OR.

Most often, preoxygenation is followed by a rapid-sequence iv induction with cricoid pressure (Sellick's maneuver) using STP (3-5 mg/kg) and succinylcholine (1.0-1.5 mg/kg). If hypotension is present or a concern, alternate induction agents (e.g., ketamine 0.5-1.0 mg/kg iv or etomidate 0.1-0.3 mg/kg iv) may be used. Axial head and neck stabilization is necessary if cervical spine injury is present or suspected.

Some trauma patients will have been intubated in the ER. Induction consists of verifying ETT placement by auscultation and $ETCO_2$ monitoring. Very low $ETCO_2$ values may be obtained in patients with markedly reduced CO_2. Ventilation with 100% O_2 and muscle relaxation with

Induction, cont. pancuronium or vecuronium (0.1 mg/kg iv) is appropriate. Ongoing fluid resuscitation should be continued during this time.

Maintenance O_2/air, muscle relaxants, narcotics and volatile agents are titrated as tolerated. Avoid N_2O in the presence of pneumothorax, pneumocephalus, bowel distention, or prolonged procedures. Shorter-acting agents (e.g., volatile agents, fentanyl, vecuronium), carefully titrated, may be preferred in patients with head injuries to facilitate early postop assessment of neurologic status. If hypotension precludes use of volatile agents, low-dose scopolamine (0.1-0.2 mg iv) or ketamine (0.25 mg/kg/15-30 min) can provide amnesia. Heated or passive humidifiers should be used, particularly in prolonged cases. Forced air warming blankets, elevated OR temperatures and warmed irrigation fluids (surgical field, bladder) also may be necessary if hypothermia becomes problematic.

Emergence Prior to extubation, patient should be awake and able to protect his/her airway, and should be hemodynamically stable and spontaneously ventilating with ease through the ETT. Patients who should not be extubated at the end of the case include elderly patients with rib fractures, hemodynamically unstable patients, those who have received massive fluid and blood product transfusion (e.g., with evidence of intestinal edema), or those with coagulopathy.

Blood and fluid requirements	Anticipate large blood loss. IV: 14-16 ga × 2 or 7-9 Fr × 2 NS/LR @ 8-10 ml/kg/h Fluid warmers Rapid-infusion device Airway humidifier ± T&C PRBCs.	Large blood losses may be anticipated, depending on the mechanism of injury (e.g., liver lacerations, major vascular injury, pelvic fractures). Crystalloid, colloid and PRBCs should be given to preserve blood volume as estimated by blood losses, systemic BP, CVP/PCWP and Hct. With massive transfusion, Plts and FFP will also be needed. In general, 2 U FFP and 6-10 U of Plts should be transfused after approximately 10 U of PRBCs (1 blood volume in a 70-kg person) have been given. Postop hypothermia is best minimized by warming all iv and irrigating fluids, maintaining OR temperature @ 78-80°F, warming and humidifying inspired gases, and using warming blankets.
Monitoring	Standard monitors (see B-1). Urinary catheter ± Arterial line	Standard monitoring should be applied as soon as the patient enters the OR. Arterial lines may be useful in unstable patients or those in whom frequent blood samples are anticipated.
	± CVP line ± PA catheter ± TEE	CVP line or PA catheter may be useful if vasoactive drips are needed or if ventricular dysfunction is apparent. In truly emergent cases, the placement of additional monitoring should be accomplished without delaying the surgical control of hemorrhage or without interrupting aggressive volume resuscitation.
Positioning	✓ and pad pressure points. ✓ eyes.	If C-spine has not been cleared by radiographs, the neck should remain immobilized intraop and postop.
Complications	Hypothermia	Hypothermia → dysrhythmias + ↓CO → acidosis. Rx: warm OR, warm iv fluids, humidify gases and use patient warming devices.
	Awareness	May be unavoidable in unstable patients. Rx: Consider scopolamine 0.2-0.4 mg iv.
	Renal failure	Usually 2° dilutional thrombocytopenia. DIC may require replacement therapy with Plts, FFP and cryoprecipitate.

POSTOPERATIVE

Complications	Hypothermia	Active warming of blood products and forced air warming blankets (Bair-Hugger) and warm room temperatures should be continued in PACU if hypothermia persists.
	Atelectasis, V/Q mismatch	Pulmonary compliance is often increased with large volumes of fluid replacement. Pulmonary contusions may

Complications, cont.		aggravate this problem and severely compromise oxygenation and ventilation, requiring high inspired O_2 concentration, high PIP and PEEP.
	Coagulopathy	Coagulation products may be necessary, based on Plt counts, PT/PTT, and ongoing RBC transfusion requirements.
Pain management	PCA or parenteral narcotics (see p. C-3, C-1), epidural narcotic.	Patients with rib fractures benefit from epidural narcotic and/or low-dose local anesthetic infusions.
Tests	Hb/Hct CXR, if postop intubation or intraop central line or thoracostomy tubes were placed.	PT/PTT, Plt counts, if unexplained bleeding postop. Fibrinogen, fibrin split products, if DIC is suspected.

PEDIATRIC TRAUMA: AIRWAY AND VASCULAR ACCESS

SURGICAL CONSIDERATIONS

Description: Children younger than 15 yr are victims in about 25% of all trauma occurring in the U.S. This incidence translates to approximately 200,000 hospitalizations and 10,000 deaths. Another 10,000-12,000 children sustain permanent impairment as a result of their injuries. According to the National Pediatric Trauma Registry, 40% of all pediatric injuries occur as a result of MVA and 35% are injuries sustained at home. Falls remain the most common cause of severe injury in infants and toddlers, while bicycle accidents cause most of the injuries in older pediatric groups. The majority of pediatric injuries occur 2° blunt trauma, and infants < 2 yr of age are known to have higher mortality rates for the same level of injury compared to older children.

The sequence of primary survey, resuscitation, secondary survey and definitive care should be followed. Confirmation of a patent airway is the essential first step. The best method for restoring airway patency is the **jaw thrust maneuver** and removal of any debris from the mouth. The most common reason for intubation in the pediatric trauma patient is loss of consciousness or as part of resuscitation from shock. Only 2% of children sustaining trauma will present with complete mechanical obstruction to the airway. In the rare child who presents with acute airway obstruction, **needle cricothyroidostomy** is the preferred method of securing the airway until definitive airway control can be achieved. This technique of ventilation uses the principle of jet insufflation as defined in the adult. Surgical cricothyrotomy in children results in a high incidence of subglottic stenosis, but it is still a viable option if needle cricothyroidostomy fails to be effective.

Because infants are obligatory nasal and diaphragmatic breathers, fractures and soft-tissue injuries that occlude the nostrils may actually obstruct the airway. Since air swallowed by the infant or insufflated into the stomach may cause acute gastric distention and restrict diaphragmatic excursion, the stomach should be decompressed with an OG tube.

Once the airway is secured and breathing assured, attention should be given to the circulation. In the noncrying child, the SBP should be approximately 80+ their age in years × 2. Children may compensate for as much as 25% of circulating volume blood loss without a change in BP. Poor peripheral perfusion, decreased level of consciousness and decreased UO are suggestive of hypovolemia. IV access must be obtained rapidly to begin crystalloid resuscitation in any child with impending signs of shock. If the peripheral iv access is difficult to obtain, as is often the case, saphenous vein cutdown at the saphenofemoral junction should be performed. In infants, if iv access cannot be obtained within 2 min, intraosseous access should be attempted (Fig 7.13-5). Once iv access has been obtained, as many as 3 boluses of crystalloid, using a volume of 20 ml/kg, can be given. If the hypovolemic shock state has not been reversed after the third bolus, and other causes of shock such as spinal injury, cardiac tamponade or pneumothorax were excluded, blood should be administered without delay.

Another important problem in the management of pediatric trauma is related to high ratio of body surface area to body mass and lack of substantial subcutaneous tissue. The small infant who is hypothermic may be refractory to therapy; therefore, every attempt should be made to prevent heat loss and all iv fluids should be warmed.

Needle cricothyrostomy: With the head in neutral position (which may require placement of towels under the shoulders), the neck should be prepped from the jaw to the chest. The neck is protected by in-line immobilization. The cricothyroid membrane should be identified, and the thyroid cartilage is immobilized with the surgeon's left hand. The cricothyroid membrane is punctured perpendicularly with a 14-16 ga iv catheter over a needle. The needle is then redirected caudally, the catheter slid off into the trachea and jet insufflation initiated. Placement of a permanent airway should follow.

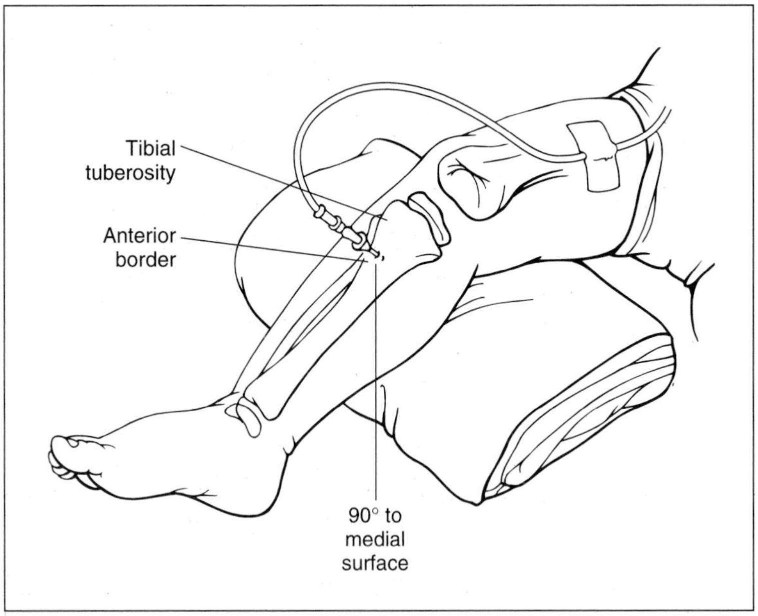

Figure 7.13-5. Intraosseous infusion. (Reproduced with permission from *Textbook of Pediatric Life Support*. American Heart Association, 1994.)

Saphenous cutdown: The groin should be prepped and draped and a curvilinear incision made 1-2 cm below and parallel to the inguinal ligament. The saphenous vein is identified at the saphenofemoral junction medially to the femoral artery, and two ligatures are passed underneath if the distal ligature is tied and used to apply tension to the vein. The vein is punctured with a scalpel blade (No. 11) and cut, creating a small flap. Tension applied to the proximal ligature reduces backbleeding during cannulation. A catheter is then introduced, the proximal ligature is tied and the distal ligature is used to secure the catheter in place.

Intraosseous infusion: After skin preparation, an incision is made 2 cm distal to the tibial tuberosity on the flattened medial aspect of the tibia. An 18-20 ga spinal needle (with obturator) can be used in children < 18 mo of age. Older patients may require use of a 13-16 bone marrow biopsy needle. Pressure and rotatory motion are applied in a direction perpendicular to the bone until a decrease in resistance is felt. Position of the needle can be confirmed by bone marrow or blood aspiration. This route can be used for rapid fluid infusion and most resuscitation medications can be given this way. Interosseus infusion, however, is only an emergency maneuver and should be used to restore circulating volume to the level that enables more permanent iv access.

Usual preop diagnosis: Airway obstruction; hypovolemic shock; hypovolemic shock with difficult iv access

General Trauma Surgery References

1. Hirshberg A, Mattox KL: Damage control surgery. *Surg Clin North Am* 1997; 77(4):909-20.
2. Karlin A, Anesthesia for Trauma. In *Reference Courses in Anesthesiology*. American Society of Anesthesiologists, Lippincott-Raven Publishers, Philadelphia: 1997; Vol 25, 107-16.
3. Stere JK, Carbonde: Anesthesia for trauma. In *Anesthesia*. Miller RD, ed. Churchill-Livingstone, New York: 1994, 2157-73.

8.0 OBSTETRIC/GYNECOLOGIC SURGERY

Surgeons

Babak Edraki, MD
Nelson N. Teng, MD, PhD
Daniel S. Kapp, MD

8.1 GYNECOLOGIC ONCOLOGY

Anesthesiologists

Jon W. Propst, MD, PhD
Myer H. Rosenthal, MD, FACCP

STAGING LAPAROTOMY FOR OVARIAN CANCER

SURGICAL CONSIDERATIONS

Description: Ovarian carcinoma has the highest mortality rate of all gynecologic malignancies because it is usually discovered in advanced stages, with pelvic mass and ascites being common findings at presentation. Surgery is used for staging as well as therapy. Studies have demonstrated an inverse relationship between postop residual tumor mass and survival; therefore, the goals of surgery are accurate staging and optimal tumor debulking (< 1 cm residual disease). The standard procedure consists of meticulous exploration of the abdominopelvic cavity, abdominopelvic cytology, multiple random and targeted biopsies, **total abdominal hysterectomy (TAH)**, **bilateral salpingo-oophorectomy (BSO)**, **pelvic** and **paraaortic lymph node dissection**, **infracolic omentectomy** and **appendectomy**. After access to the abdomen is obtained through a midline or paramedian abdominal incision, cytologic washings of the pelvis, pericolic gutters, lesser sac and hemidiaphragms are done. The peritoneal cavity is carefully explored. A TAH/BSO is then performed by ligating and transecting the round, infundibulopelvic, broad, cardinal and uterosacral ligaments on both sides. The specimen is cut away from the vagina and the cuff closed. The pelvic and paraaortic lymph nodes are dissected in a manner similar to that described under Radical Hysterectomy, p. 566. All residual tumor is removed, using sharp dissection and/or CUSA and/or Argon beam coagulator (ABC), and then an appendectomy is usually performed. The omentum is clamped, transected and ligated along its attachment to the transverse colon. A bowel resection with possible colostomy formation may be necessary to achieve optimal cytoreductive surgery (see Pelvic Exenteration, p. 559). Next, the peritoneal cavity is copiously irrigated with warm water. Targeted and random biopsies of bladder, cul-de-sac of Douglas, pericolic gutters, hemidiaphragms, small bowel, large bowel and anterior abdominal wall are performed. A permanent peritoneal port may be placed subcutaneously for use in future dose-intensive intraperitoneal chemotherapy. A less extensive surgical procedure may be appropriate if a large volume of unresectable tumor is discovered. Surgery in these cases must be individualized.

In some Stage I lesions, a **unilateral salpingo-oophorectomy** is sufficient therapy. The decision to use this approach depends on cell type, age, reproductive status and extent of disease. Generally, a retroperitoneal **lymph node dissection**, **omentectomy** and **appendectomy** are also performed. Approximately 25% of patients undergoing **cytoreductive surgery** for advanced stages of ovarian carcinoma require bowel resection with either primary reanastomosis or colostomy. A splenectomy is not routinely done unless the spleen is involved with tumor. A permanent central venous infusion port may be placed for convenient venous access. This is usually done at the completion of the abdominal surgery following skin closure. Some patients with unresectable disease and bowel obstruction will require a gastrostomy tube placement at this time.

Usual preop diagnosis: Ovarian cancer/pelvic mass

SUMMARY OF PROCEDURE

Position	Supine
Incision	Midline or paramedian abdominal
Special instrumentation	CUSA, Vital View (suction-irrigation device combined with light source) helpful; laparoscopic biopsy forceps (laparoscope, laparoscopic instruments for evaluation of upper abdomen through lower vertical abdominal incision); ABC; TA, GIA, EEA stapling devices.
Unique considerations	Removal of large amounts of ascites may result in fluid shifts and intravascular volume depletion intraop and postop.
Antibiotics	Cefotetan 2 g iv on call to OR; then q 12 h × 2 doses
Surgical time	1-4 h; 4-5 h, including splenectomy and bowel surgery for more advanced stages.
Closing considerations	NG tube placement by anesthesiologist; permanent peritoneal or central venous access for subsequent chemotherapy
EBL	500-1000 ml; 250-500 ml for Stage I lesions; 1300 ml for more advanced stages
Postop care	Extensive peritoneal raw surfaces lead to intraperitoneal fluid 3rd-spacing. Patients require good hydration to maintain intravascular volume. Central hemodynamic monitoring and ICU admission are useful in selected patients. Use SCDs and mini-dose heparin for DVT prophylaxis.
Mortality	1-2/1000
Morbidity	Postop fever: 14-19% Wound infection: < 5% Wound dehiscence: 0.3-3% PE: 1-2% Ureteral injury: < 1% Vaginal vault prolapse: Rare
Pain score	7-8

PATIENT POPULATION CHARACTERISTICS

Age range	All age groups; most common, 50-59 yr.
Incidence	15/100,000 (26,700+ new cases/yr); 1.4% lifetime risk of ovarian cancer
Etiology	Unknown
Predisposing factors	Family Hx of ovarian carcinoma; personal or family Hx of breast cancer (BRCA gene mutations); ↑age at first pregnancy; gonadal dysgenesis; exposure to radiation; environmental factors
Associated conditions	Familial cancer syndromes (e.g., endometrial, colon, breast); Peutz-Jeghers syndrome—5% of cases develop gonadal stromal tumor; XY gonadal dysgenesis—gonadoblastomas; multiple nevoid basal cell carcinoma (Gorlin's syndrome); ataxia telangiectasia (hereditary, progressive cerebellar lack of muscular coordination associated with recurrent pulmonary infections and ocular and cutaneous telangiectasias)

ANESTHETIC CONSIDERATIONS

PREOPERATIVE

Ovarian carcinoma is usually diagnosed at a relatively late stage and, therefore, the patient may have significant ascites and a fairly large tumor mass. Surgery is indicated for cure of localized tumor and for staging of distant and local metastases. Additional procedures, such as bowel resection or lymph node dissection, occasionally are performed at the same time.

Respiratory Significant ascites may distend the abdomen and produce respiratory compromise. The presence of orthopnea, tachypnea or other signs of impaired ventilation need to be investigated. Underlying lung diseases such as asthma also may be exacerbated by the abdominal distension.
Tests: Consider CXR; others as indicated from H&P.

Cardiovascular An ECHO, MUGA scan or other studies may be requested to evaluate cardiac function. Exercise tolerance should be evaluated in every patient and any preexisting cardiac disease explored in the preop visit.
Tests: Consider ECG, as indicated from H&P.

Gastrointestinal Patient should have adequate preop iv hydration if given a bowel prep overnight.

Neurological Not usually significant. Taxol and cisplatin can produce peripheral neuropathy.

Hematologic Bone marrow suppression common following chemotherapy
Tests: Hct; WBC; Plt

Laboratory LFT; CT scan of abdomen and pelvis

Premedication Anxiolytic such as midazolam 1-2 mg iv on the morning of surgery

INTRAOPERATIVE

Anesthetic technique: GETA ± epidural analgesia. Typically, a balanced anesthetic with inhalational agents or **propofol** infusion (100-200 μg/kg/min) and narcotics. An epidural catheter may be placed for postop pain management and also may be used intraop to decrease anesthetic requirements.

Induction Standard induction (see p. B-2).

Maintenance Standard maintenance (p. B-3). Continue muscle relaxant based on nerve stimulator response. Epidural 2% lidocaine with epinephrine 1:200,000 (~10 ml/h) if catheter is placed preop. A NG tube should be placed after induction and kept on low suction to help prevent postop N/V. Patients with combined regional/general anesthetic may require increased fluids due to vasodilation.

Emergence The patient may be extubated at the conclusion of surgery unless hemodynamically unstable or requiring continued vigorous fluid resuscitation. Reverse muscle relaxant with neostigmine 0.07 mg/kg and glycopyrrolate 0.01 mg/kg, and give supplemental O_2 after extubation. It is reasonable to schedule a postop ICU bed for unstable patients or those who require invasive monitoring for fluid management.

Blood and fluid requirements	± Significant blood loss IV: 16 ga × 2	Blood loss may be 1-2 L. Give PRBCs to keep Hct ~27%. 5% albumin or 6% hetastarch are useful for rapid volume

Blood and fluid, cont.	NS/LR @ 4-6 ml/kg/h 5% albumin 6% hetastarch	replacement if the Hct is acceptable. If large volumes of ascites are removed, significant hypotension can develop from fluid shifts. Third-space losses, therefore, may be 10-15 ml/kg/h. Alternating NS and LR is recommended to avoid development of a nonanion gap hyperchloremic acidosis 2° excessive NS.
Monitoring	Standard monitors (p. B-1). ± Arterial catheter ± CVP/PA catheter Foley catheter NG tube	Arterial and PA catheters are indicated for extensive surgery and/or patients with underlying medical conditions (e.g., CAD, COPD). The measurements of cardiac filling pressures and CO help to guide fluid replacement when surgery is extensive.
Positioning	✓ and pad pressure points. ✓ eyes. Antiembolism stockings and SCD	
Complications	Hypothermia	These patients tend to become hypothermic, so it is important to warm all iv fluids and inspired gasses. A heating blanket on the bed is helpful, as is wrapping the head with towel or plastic. Keep the OR as warm as practical. Central temperature should be monitored in the bladder or esophagus during surgery.
	Renal failure	Renal dose dopamine (1-3 μg/kg/min) with adequate preload may be indicated to maintain UO > 0.5 ml/kg/h in patients with borderline renal function; however, adequate levels of preload are essential to maintain renal perfusion.

POSTOPERATIVE

Complications	Excess fluid requirement	If patient required large volumes of fluid, extubation may need to be delayed until a diuresis can be started. IPPV with PEEP may be beneficial in maintaining lung volumes and decreasing lung-water accumulation. Measurement of cardiac filling pressures is helpful in guiding therapy. Pulmonary edema may develop 3-5 d postop.
Pain management	PCA Epidural spinal narcotics	See PCA and epidural narcotic recommendations on pages C-1 and C-3.

References

1. Burghardt E, et al: Pelvic lymphadenectomy in operative treatment of ovarian cancer. *Am J Obstet Gynecol* 1986; 155(2):315-19.
2. Cruikshank DP, Buchsbaum HJ: Effects of rapid paracentesis. Cardiovascular dynamics and body fluid composition. *JAMA* 1973; 225(11):1361-62.
3. DiSaia PJ, Creasman WT: Advanced epithelial ovarian cancer. In *Clinical Gynecologic Oncology*. DiSaia PJ, Creasman WT, eds. CV Mosby, St Louis: 1989, 325-416.
4. Halpin TF, McCann TO: Dynamics of body fluids following the rapid removal of large volumes of ascites. *Am J Obstet Gynecol* 1971; 110(1):103-6.
5. Morrow CP: Malignant and borderline epithelial tumors of the ovary: clinical features, staging, diagnosis, operative assessment and review of management. In *Gynecologic Oncology: Fundamental Principles and Clinical Practice*. Coppleson M, ed. Churchill-Livingstone, New York: 1981, 655-79.
6. Ozols RF, Rubin SC, Thomas G, Robboy S: Epithelial ovarian cancer. In *Principles and Practice of Gynecologic Oncology, 2nd edition.* Hoskins WJ, Perez CA, Young RC, eds: Lippincott-Raven Publishers, Philadelphia: 1996, 919-86.
7. Roizen MF: Anesthetic implications of concurrent diseases. In *Anesthesia*, 4th edition. Miller RD, ed. Churchill Livingstone, New York: 1994; 903-1014.
8. Wheeless CR Jr: Staging of gynecologic oncology patients with exploratory laparotomy. In *Atlas of Pelvic Surgery*, 2nd edition. Lea & Febiger, Philadelphia: 1988, 378-79.
9. Wu PC, Lang JH, Huang RL, et al: Lymph node metastasis and retroperitoneal lymphadenectomy in ovarian cancer. *Bailliere's Clin Obstet Gynaecol* 1989; 3:143.

SECOND-LOOK/REASSESSMENT LAPAROTOMY FOR OVARIAN CANCER

SURGICAL CONSIDERATIONS

Description: The clinical evaluation of an ovarian cancer patient's response to chemotherapy may be unreliable because tumor that may defy detection by noninvasive methods can be present in the abdominopelvic cavity. Surgery in the form of **"second-look" laparotomy** is the most accurate method of evaluation of ovarian cancer patients' response to chemotherapy. It is usually undertaken to determine whether the patient is surgically and pathologically free of disease, after an appropriate number of treatment cycles with platinum-based (CDDP or carboplatin) chemotherapy. In addition, in cases where optimal debulking could not be performed, a second-look debulking laparotomy is done to achieve optimal cytoreduction. The surgery involves methodical and meticulous exploration of all of the abdomen and pelvis, multiple cytologies and biopsies, lysis of adhesions, resection of the residual tumor, as well as the pelvic and periaortic lymph nodes (if not done at time of first surgery).

Usual preop diagnosis: Ovarian carcinoma

SUMMARY OF PROCEDURE

Position	Supine
Incision	Midline or paramedian vertical abdominal
Antibiotics	Cefotetan 2 g preop; then q 12 h × 2 doses
Surgical time	2-3 h
Closing considerations	Placement of permanent central venous or intraperitoneal access
EBL	350-700 ml
Postop care	PACU → room
Mortality	1-2/1000
Morbidity	Postop fever: 14-19% Wound infection: < 5% Wound dehiscence: 0.3-3% PE: 1-2% Incisional hernia: 0.5-1% Ureteral injury: 0.5-1% Necrotizing fasciitis: Rare Posthysterectomy prolapse of vaginal vault: Rare
Pain score	7-8

PATIENT POPULATION CHARACTERISTICS

Age range	All ages; most common, 50-59 yr
Incidence	15/100,000; 26,700+ new cases/yr; 1.4% lifetime risk of ovarian cancer
Etiology	Risk factors include: positive family Hx; nulliparity; ↑age at first pregnancy; gonadal dysgenesis; exposure to radiation; environmental factors
Associated conditions	Familial cancer syndromes (e.g., endometrial, colon, breast); Peutz-Jeghers syndrome (5% of cases develop gonadal stromal tumor); XY gonadal dysgenesis (gonadoblastomas); multiple, nevoid basal-cell carcinoma (Gorlin's syndrome); ataxia telangiectasia

ANESTHETIC CONSIDERATIONS

PREOPERATIVE

Patients having a second-look laparotomy have undergone surgical resection of a tumor with lymph node biopsy, usually followed by chemotherapy and/or radiation therapy. Depending on the type of adjunctive treatment given, the patient may come to surgery in poor physical condition from malnutrition, or toxicity from chemotherapy (see Table 8.1-1). Vascular access may be difficult to obtain due to sclerosis or thrombosis of peripheral veins.

Respiratory Pulmonary function may be impaired by several chemotherapeutic drugs, most commonly bleomycin. Patients often have a Hickman catheter or other central line already in place which can

Respiratory, cont.

be used for induction of anesthesia. A preop CXR is mandatory to assess the presence of lung injury. Patients who have dyspnea at rest or with mild exertion, or who have known pulmonary fibrosis, should be evaluated by PFTs, including FVC, FEV_1, $MMEF_{25\text{-}75}$, and ABGs. Patients who have received bleomycin should not receive O_2 > 39% intraop, but arterial O_2 saturation ideally should be kept ≥ 93%[5]. The pulmonary toxicity of bleomycin is dose-related, with a much higher incidence occurring if over 200 mg/m^2. Combination chemotherapy with vincristine or cisplatin also increases pulmonary toxicity. Severe lung disease is an indication for the use of spinal or epidural anesthesia whenever possible; otherwise, postop mechanical ventilation may be necessary.
Tests: Consider CXR; others as indicated from H&P.

Cardiovascular

Cardiotoxicity is seen with several anti-neoplastic agents, especially daunorubicin and doxorubicin. The cardiomyopathy produced by these drugs occurs in two forms: (1) acute – ST-T wave changes and dysrhythmias, which are transient and usually not a serious problem; and (2) chronic – a dose-related toxicity manifested by CHF. Total doses of doxorubicin as low as 250 U can cause myocardial damage, but is more common at doses > 400 units. Cardiac irradiation, or combination chemotherapy with cyclophosphamide, increases the risk of cardiac toxicity. Patients who have received cardiotoxic drugs are usually followed by serial ECHOs or MUGA scans, and the results of these tests should be reviewed preop. Patients with CHF or ECG changes should have a cardiology consultation to optimize their medical condition preop.
Tests: ECG; others as indicated from H&P.

Neurological

Peripheral neuropathies are produced by vincristine, cyclophosphamide, Taxol (paclitaxel), 5-fluorouracil and several other drugs. Vincristine can also produce SIADH. Other CNS effects include N/V, seizures and cerebellar dysfunction. A preop neurologic exam is required for those patients with evidence of neurotoxicity. It is important to document the presence of neurologic deficits preop for subsequent comparisons.

Endocrine

Steroids such as prednisone are commonly used together with chemotherapeutic agents, as treatment for pulmonary fibrosis and other complications of chemotherapy. The use of steroids for several wk suppresses the endogenous secretion of the adrenal cortex, which may take up to 6 mo to recover fully. Hydrocortisone 100 mg iv, therefore, is given perioperatively every 8 h to cover the stress associated with surgery. The dose is tapered rapidly over 2 or 3 d postop. If the patient is receiving hormone replacement for hypothyroidism, it may be continued as scheduled perioperatively. Diabetics should be managed to keep blood sugar at 150-250 mg/dL. A glucose and insulin infusion (100 U regular insulin/L D5W) is useful for maintaining proper blood glucose levels intraop. Infuse at 10-20 ml/h, based on the results of hourly blood glucose determinations during surgery; 20 mEq KCl/L may be added in patients with normal renal function to prevent hypokalemia. Oral hypoglycemic agents should be withheld on the day of surgery.
Tests: Fasting blood sugar (if diabetic)

Renal

Many chemotherapeutic drugs have renal toxicity; therefore, a preop set of renal function tests is mandatory. Patients with impaired renal function should be given appropriate dosages of medications (e.g., antibiotics) which depend on renal excretion.
Tests: Renal function tests

Musculoskeletal

Vincristine produces a neurotoxicity manifested by numbness and tingling in the extremities, weakness, foot drop, loss of reflexes, ataxia and muscle pains. Muscle weakness in the arms and legs indicates that the drug should be discontinued. Muscle weakness also may involve the larynx and extraocular muscles of the eye. Reduced amounts of neuromuscular blocking drugs should be used intraop and a nerve stimulator used to follow twitches.

Gastrointestinal

Consider hydration overnight if given a bowel prep or if there is significant N/V.
Tests: Consider serum electrolytes, if indicated from H&P.

Hematologic

Bone marrow suppression is a very common side effect of antineoplastic drugs. The toxicity usually produces a reversible drop in leukocytes, erythrocytes and Plt with a nadir 10-14 d posttreatment. Patients with a total neutrophil count of < 1,000 should be kept in isolation until counts improve. A low Plt count (< 75,000) is an indication for Plt transfusion preop. Regional anesthesia in patients with thrombocytopenia needs to be carefully considered due to the increased risk of bleeding complications. It is useful to check PT/PTT preop when in doubt about the coagulation status of a patient. A preop transfusion of Plts and/or RBCs is recommended if lab values are below acceptable limits (Plt < 75,000, Hct < 25).
Tests: Hb/Hct; WBC; Plt; PT; PTT

Laboratory	Liver function tests if indicated by H&P.	
Premedication	Anxiolytic such as midazolam 1-5 mg im or iv. Stress-dose hydrocortisone (100 mg) if indicated.	

INTRAOPERATIVE

Anesthetic technique: GETA usually indicated. Combined GETA/epidural or spinal are also excellent choices; however, surgery should be done under regional anesthesia in patients with severe bleomycin pulmonary toxicity.

General anesthesia:

Induction Standard induction (p. B-2 and Anesthetic Considerations for Staging Laparotomy for Ovarian Cancer, p. 542). Consider renal function and surgery duration when deciding on agent.

Maintenance Standard maintenance: see Anesthetic Considerations for Staging Laparotomy, p. 542. An epidural may be used to reduce GA requirements (p. B-3).

Emergence Extubate when patient is responsive and neuromuscular block is fully reversed. In patients with borderline pulmonary function, extubation may be delayed until patient is in the PACU or ICU, and after ABG is checked while the patient breathes spontaneously.

Regional anesthesia:

Epidural 2% lidocaine ± epinephrine 1:200,000 (10-15 ml) or 0.5% bupivacaine (10-15 ml) are used; then at ~10 ml/h. Narcotics such as morphine (2-4 mg) or hydromorphone (0.3-0.5 mg) may be given in the epidural for postop pain control.

Blood and fluid requirements	IV: 16-18 ga × 1-2 NS/LR @ 7-10 ml/kg/h Keep UO > 0.5 ml/kg/h. PRBC for Hct < 30%	Excessive use of NS can lead to hyperchloremic metabolic acidosis; therefore, alternating NS and LR solutions makes sense when giving large volumes of iv fluids.
	5% albumin 6% hetastarch	5% albumin or 6% hetastarch may be used as volume replacement when Hct > 30%, although they have no proven advantages over crystalloid solutions.
	FFP/Plt	FFP and Plt are used if there is evidence of coagulopathy (↑PT, ↑PTT, ↓Plt).
Monitoring	Standard monitors (see p. B-1). ± Arterial line ± CVP/PA catheter Foley catheter NG tube	Arterial and CVP catheters are indicated for patients with compromised cardiac or pulmonary function or patients having extensive surgical procedures.
Positioning	✓ and pad pressure points. ✓ eyes. Anti-embolism stockings and SCD	It is useful to maintain access to at least one arm for blood drawing and additional iv access.
Complications	Hypothermia	Warm all fluids and humidify inspired gasses. Heating pad on the bed. Wrap head in plastic or towels.
	Bleeding	✓ PT; PTT, Plts periodically for large blood loss.

POSTOPERATIVE

Complications	Bleeding Nausea Infection Respiratory insufficiency	Antiemetics (i.e., metoclopramide 10 mg iv) should be given for nausea. Supplemental O_2 should be given in PACU.
Pain management	PCA (see p. C-3). Epidural/spinal narcotics (see p. C-1).	Surgeons may infiltrate wound edges with 0.25% bupivacaine in those patients without epidurals.
	CXR; ABG	As indicated by postop clinical findings.

References

1. Calabresi P, Chabner BA: Antineoplastic agents. In *Goodman and Gilman's: The Pharmacologic Basis of Therapeutics*, 8th edition. Gilman AG, Rall TW, Nies AS, Taylor P, eds. Pergamon Press, New York: 1990, 1209-63.

2. Copeland LJ, Gershenson DM, Wharton JT, Atkinson EN, Sneige N, Edwards CL, Rutledge FN: Microscopic disease at second-look laparotomy in advanced ovarian cancer. *Cancer* 1985; 55(2):472-78.
3. Creasman WT: Second look laparotomy in ovarian cancer. *Gynecol Oncol* 1994; 55:S122-S127.
4. DiSaia PJ, Creasman WT: Advanced epithelial ovarian cancer. In *Clinical Gynecologic Oncology*. DiSaia PJ, Creasman WT, eds. CV Mosby, St. Louis: 1989, 325-416.
5. Manufacturer's drug information from Bristol-Myers, Squibb Oncology/Immunology Division. In *Physicians Desk Reference*, 51st edition. Medical Economics Co., Montvale, New Jersey: 1997: 696-734.
6. Ozols RF, Rubin SC, Thomas G, Robboy S: Epithelial ovarian cancer. In *Principles and Practice of Gynecologic Oncology, 2nd edition.* Hoskins WJ, Perez CA, Young RC, eds. Lippincott-Raven Publishers, Philadelphia: 1996, 919-86.
7. Podratz KC, Cliby WA: Second look surgery in the management of epithelial ovarian carcinoma. *Gynecol Oncol* 1994: 55:S128-S133.
8. Speyer J: Second-look laparotomy in an ovarian cancer patient responding to chemotherapy. In *Expert Consultations in Gynecological Cancers.* Markman M, Belinson JL, eds. Marcel Dekker, Inc. New York: 1997, 285-87.

Table 8.1-1. Toxicities of Selected Antineoplastic Chemotherapeutic Agents

Agent	Site of Toxicity
Vincristine, vinblastine	Neuropathies, SIADH, myelosuppression
Cyclophosphamide	Prolonged neuromuscular block
Mechlorethamine	Prolonged neuromuscular block
Bleomycin	Pulmonary fibrosis
Doxorubicin, daunorubicin	Cardiotoxicity, GI upset, myelosuppression
Methotrexate	Myelosuppression, GI upset, stomatitis, pulmonary infiltrates
Fluorouracil	Myelosuppression, hepatic and GI alterations, nervous system dysfunction
Mercaptopurine	Myelosuppression
Thioguanine	Myelosuppression
Actinomycin D	Myelosuppression, GI upset, stomatitis
Mitomycin	Myelosuppression, GI upset
Cisplatin, carboplatin	Peripheral neuropathy, GI upset, electrolyte disturbances, nephrotoxicity, myelosuppression
Paclitaxel	Myelosuppression, peripheral neuropathy, GI upset, arthralgia/myalgias, mucositis

RADICAL VULVECTOMY

SURGICAL CONSIDERATIONS

Description: ***En bloc* dissection** of the inguinal-femoral region and the vulva is the time-honored treatment for invasive vulvar carcinoma. The surgery involves bilateral excision of lymphatic and areolar tissue in the inguinal and femoral regions, combined with removal of the entire vulva between the labia-crural folds, from the perineal body to the upper margin of mons pubis (Fig 8.1-1). A large surgical wound is created and, if 1° closure without tension is not possible, a skin or myocutaneous graft may be necessary. Deep pelvic nodes are almost never involved with metastases when the superficial and deep groin nodes are free of disease; therefore, a **pelvic lymphadenectomy** is no longer routinely performed. If presence of tumor is documented in the groin nodes, particularly in Cloquet's sentinel nodes (the most cephalad, deep inguinal nodes), a **deep pelvic lymphadenectomy** may be performed. **Postop radiation therapy**, however, is widely used instead of a pelvic lymph node dissection to minimize operative morbidity and confer a survival advantage.

A skin incision in the shape of a bull's head (Fig 8.1-1) allows access to the inguinal-femoral region. (The incision ideally should extend 2+ cm beyond the tumor margin.) The inguinal ligament and rectus fascia should be cleared bilaterally of all nodal tissues, and the fossae ovalis on both sides identified. The lateral aspect of the femoral sheath is incised along the sartorius muscle, with care being taken not to injure the femoral nerve or vessels and the cribriform fascia is cleaned off the femoral artery. The external pudendal artery, which marks the entrance of the saphenous vein into the fossa ovalis, should be identified and ligated. The proximal and distal segments of the saphenous vein should be ligated and excised as the fibrofatty, lymph-bearing tissue of the femoral sheath is resected. Cloquet's nodes at the femoral ring beneath the inguinal ligaments on both sides should be resected and submitted for frozen-section pathology evaluation. The deep inguinal lymphatic chain is removed on both sides by opening the inguinal canal from the external inguinal ring. The vulvar incision is carried down through the labia-crural folds. The internal pudendal vessels at the posterior lateral margin of the vulvar incision are identified as they emerge from Alcock's canal, then are ligated and incised.

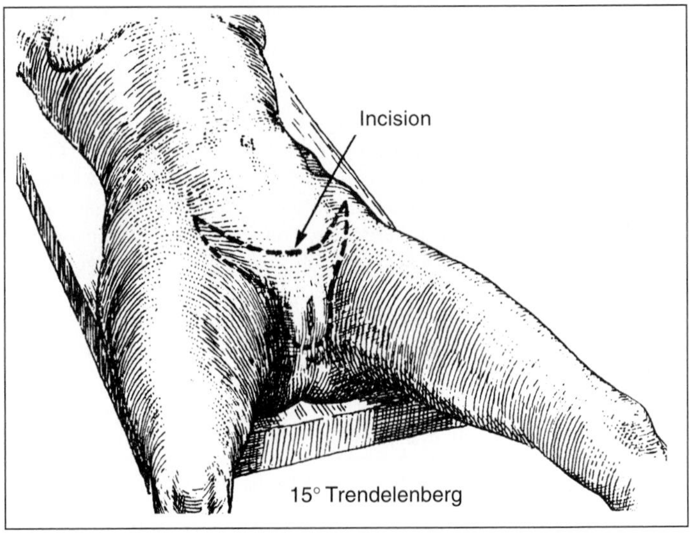

Figure 8.1-1. *En bloc* radical vulvectomy and bilateral groin lymph node dissection; with bull's head incision. (Reproduced with permission from Wheeless CR Jr: *Atlas of Pelvic Surgery*. Lea & Febiger: 1988.)

Use of electrocautery in this portion of the procedure usually tends to decrease operative blood loss. The dissection is continued along the periosteum of the symphysis at the level of the fascia of the deep muscles of the urogenital diaphragm. The bulbocavernosus, ischiocavernosus and superficial transverse perinei muscles are removed. A circumferential vaginal incision, excluding the urethral meatus, is then performed and the vulva is removed. The incisions overlying the groin node dissections should be closed with minimal tension after placement of closed-suction Jackson-Pratt drains. The vulvar surgical wound is closed by slightly undermining the skin of the edges of the incision and suturing them to the vaginal mucosa. A **vulvar reconstruction**, using myocutaneous flaps, also can be performed at this time (see Pelvic Exenteration, p. 559).

Variant procedure or approaches: In 1962, Byran and associates popularized a **3-incision technique** first described by Kehrer in 1918. Separate incisions are made in each groin and the vulva (Fig 8.1-2). This operative approach has led to a significant decrease in wound infection and breakdown, apparently without increasing tumor recurrence in the inguinal dermal bridge above the symphysis pubis. Another variant is the **hemivulvectomy** (Fig 8.1-3), in which unilateral radical hemivulvectomy and groin node dissection are performed in selected stage I, nonmidline, unifocal vulvar cancer patients. This procedure will minimize morbidity, disfigurement and sexual dysfunction. The observation that almost no contralateral groin metastases occur in the absence of positive ipsilateral groin nodes allows the surgeon to perform only a **unilateral groin node dissection**.

Usual preop diagnosis: Invasive vulvar cancer

SUMMARY OF PROCEDURE

	***En Bloc* Dissection**	**3-Incision**	**Hemivulvectomy**
Position	Modified dorsolithotomy in Allen universal stirrups	⇐	⇐
Incision	Bull's head, from iliac crest to iliac crest and along labia-crural folds (Fig 8.1-1)	2 separate groin incisions from iliac crest to pubic tubercle, 1 vulvar incision (Fig 8.1-2)	1 or 2 separate groin incisions from iliac crest to pubic tubercle; vulvar incision (Fig 8.1-3)
Special instrumentation	Argon beam coagulator (ABC)	⇐	⇐
Unique considerations	Two-team approach to minimize surgical time. Preop bowel prep and constipating medications (e.g., Lomotil) to decrease postop bowel movements.	⇐	⇐
Antibiotics	Cefotetan 2 g iv on call to OR; then 2 g iv q 12 h × 72 h.	⇐	⇐
Surgical time	3-4 h	⇐	2-3 h

	En Bloc Dissection	3-Incision	Hemivulvectomy
Closing considerations	Possible skin graft; vulvar and groin suction drains	⇐	⇐
EBL	500-1000 ml	⇐	250-1000 ml
Postop care	PACU or ICU, if necessary. SCDs and mini-dose heparin ★ for DVT prophylaxis. (**NB:** trauma to femoral vessels at time of groin lymph node dissection increases risk of thrombophlebitis and PE. Aggressive local wound care.)	⇐	⇐
Mortality	1-2%	⇐	⇐
Morbidity	Wound infection and breakdown: 40-80%	15%	< 15%
	Introital stenosis and dyspareunia: 50%	⇐	⇐
	Lymphedema of lower extremities: 25-30%	⇐	< 25% (if deep groin nodes not dissected)
	Lymphocysts: 10%	⇐	⇐
	Genital prolapse: 7%	⇐	1-2%
	Stress incontinence: 5%	⇐	1-2%
	Thrombophlebitis: 3-5%	⇐	1-2%
	Hernia: 1-2%	⇐	⇐
	PE: 1-2%	⇐	⇐
Pain score	8	8	7

PATIENT POPULATION CHARACTERISTICS

Age range Median 70 yr

Incidence 2.5/100,000; 3-5% of female genital malignancies

Etiology Exact etiology unknown; risk factors include: vulvar dystrophies; granulomatous disease of vulva; Bowen's disease; condyloma acuminata

Associated conditions Diabetes; obesity; HTN; arteriosclerosis; nulliparity; positive serology for syphilis; cervical malignancy; human papilloma virus infection

---

ANESTHETIC CONSIDERATIONS

PREOPERATIVE

Patients with vulvar carcinoma are typically in the 6th or 7th decade of life and, hence, have a high incidence of concurrent medical problems, such as HTN, CAD and diabetes. Radical vulvectomy is performed for invasive tumor which has not metastasized to distant sites. An ICU bed should be reserved for patients with a significant medical Hx.

Respiratory The presence of lung disease and smoking Hx should be discussed with the patient preop. CXR or PFTs are indicated for patients with significant respiratory disease. The response to bronchodilators should be tested in patients with bronchospastic disease or COPD.
Tests: Consider CXR; others as indicated from H&P.

Cardiovascular There is an increased incidence of HTN and atherosclerosis in these patients. A cardiology consultation is indicated for angina, recent MI, CHF or heart murmurs. An ECG should be ordered for all patients > 50 yr old.
Tests: ECG; others as indicated from H&P.

Renal In old age, creatinine clearance is decreased due to decreased renal mass, but serum creatinine remains unchanged because of decreased muscle mass. A preop creatinine clearance, therefore, should be checked in patients > 70 yr old or with known renal dysfunction to assess the degree of impairment.
Tests: As indicated from H&P.

Gastrointestinal Patients should have iv hydration preop if given bowel prep overnight.

Neurological Document a neurological exam if Hx of stroke, seizures or other neurologic disease. Hx of peripheral neuropathy or autonomic dysfunction should be assessed in diabetic patients.
Tests: As indicated from H&P.

Musculoskeletal Elderly patients are prone to arthritis and osteoporosis. Inquire about NSAID usage in the last 4 wk preop.

Endocrine Diabetes, obesity and hypothyroidism are common in this patient population.
Tests: Fasting blood sugar; thyroid function; others as indicated from H&P.

Hematologic Chronic anemia may be present. Encourage autologous blood donation if Hct is adequate.
Tests: Hb/Hct; Plt count

Laboratory LFTs, if indicated.

Premedication Usually no premedication is needed, but occasionally small doses of midazolam (1-3 mg iv) are useful for anxiety.

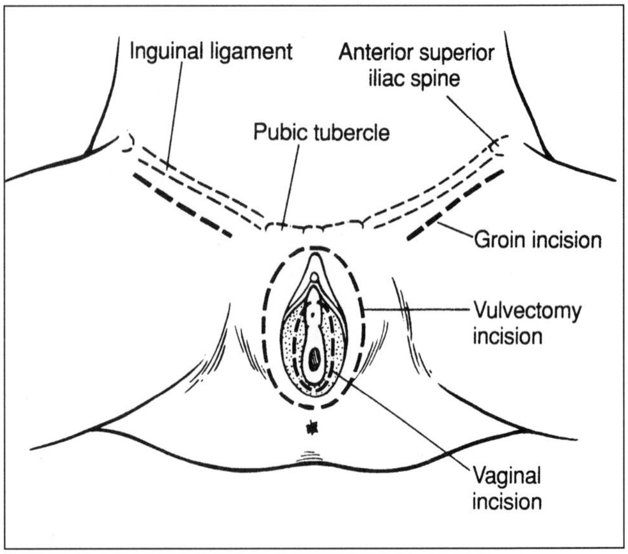

Figure 8.1-2. 3-incision radical vulvectomy and bilateral groin lymph node dissection. (Produced with permission from Mattingly RF, Woodruff JD, eds: *TeLinde's Operative Gynecology*. JB Lippincott: 1985.)

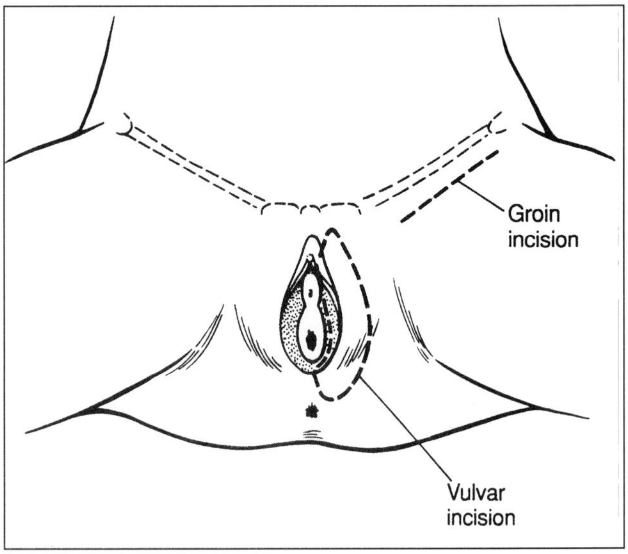

Figure 8.1-3. Radical hemivulvectomy with unilateral groin lymph node dissection through a separate incision. (Produced with permission from Mattingly RF, Woodruff JD, eds: *TeLinde's Operative Gynecology*. JB Lippincott: 1985.)

INTRAOPERATIVE

Anesthetic technique: GETA or regional anesthesia, alone or in combination. Regional techniques may be supplemented by the use of a propofol infusion (25-100 μg/kg/h).

General anesthesia:

Induction Standard induction (see p. B-2). Elderly patients usually require reduced dosages of medications. Titration to effect is advised when using any induction agent.

Maintenance Standard maintenance (see p. B-3).

Emergence No special considerations

Regional anesthesia:

Epidural 2% lidocaine ± epinephrine 1:200,000 (10-20 ml) or 0.5% bupivacaine (10-20 ml) are used; then @ ~10 ml/h. Narcotics such as morphine (2-4 mg) in the epidural for postop pain control.

Spinal Tetracaine (12 mg) or bupivacaine (13-15 mg), preservative-free morphine (0.3-0.5 mg) → T8 sensory level.

Blood and fluid requirements IV: 8-16 ga × 2
NS/LR @ 6-8 ml/kg/h

Occasionally, femoral vessels may be injured, requiring rapid blood replacement. Controlled hypotension to MAP =

Blood and fluid, cont.	Warm iv fluids. UO > 0.5 ml/kg/h PRBCs for Hct < 25% in healthy patients and < 30% in patients with cardiac or pulmonary disease	60-70 mmHg may be helpful in minimizing blood loss (in patients without cardiac or cerebrovascular disease).
Monitoring	Standard monitors (p. B-1) ± Arterial line ± CVP line Foley catheter	Invasive monitors indicated for patients in poor condition or with cardiovascular or respiratory disease. An arterial catheter is useful for drawing labs in surgery to check Hct, glucose or ABGs.
Positioning	✓ and pad pressure points. ✓ eyes. Antiembolism stockings and SCD	

POSTOPERATIVE

Complications	Hypothermia Nerve injury Bleeding Atelectasis	 Diagnosis of nerve injury may be delayed by epidural anesthesia. Give supplemental O_2 postop.
Pain management	PCA (p. C-3) Epidural or spinal narcotics (p. C-1)	Incisions may be left open to granulate in or be covered with skin grafts. Epidural analgesia allows earlier ambulation with less sedation in elderly patients.
Tests	Tests as indicated	From postop clinical findings

References

1. Burke TW, Eifel P, McGuire W, Wilkinson EJ: Vulva. In *Principles and Practice of Gynecologic Oncology, 2nd edition.* Hoskins WJ, Perez CA, Young RC, eds. Lippincott-Raven Publishers, Philadelphia: 1996, 717-51.
2. Burke TW, Levenback C, Coleman RC, et al: Surgical therapy of T1 and T2 vulvar carcinoma: further experience with radical wide excision and selective inguinal lymphadenectomy. *Gynecol Oncol* 1995; 57:215.
3. DiSaia PJ, Creasman WT: Invasive cancer of the vulva. In *Clinical Gynecologic Oncology.* DiSaia PJ, Creasman WT, eds. CV Mosby, St. Louis: 1989, 241-72.
4. DiSaia PJ, Creasman WT, Rich WM: An alternate approach to early cancer of the vulva. *Am J Obstet Gynecol* 1979; 133(7):825-32.
5. Mattingly RF, Woodruff JD: Invasive carcinoma of the vulva. In *TeLinde's Operative Gynecology.* Mattingly RF, Thompson JD, eds. JB Lippincott, Philadelphia: 1985, 715-41.
6. Stehman FB, Bundy BN, Dvoretsky PM, Creasman WT: Early stage I carcinoma of the vulva treated with ipsilateral superficial inguinal lymphadenectomy and modified radical hemivulvectomy: a prospective study of the Gynecologic Oncology Group. *Obstet Gynecol* 1992a; 79:490.
7. Wheeless CR Jr: Radical vulvectomy with bilateral inguinal lymph node dissection. In *Atlas of Pelvic Surgery.* Lea & Febiger, Philadelphia: 1988, 405-11.

CONIZATION OF THE CERVIX

SURGICAL CONSIDERATIONS

Description: Conization of the cervix can be used for both diagnostic and therapeutic purposes. It is performed in cases of biopsy-proven dysplasia with unsatisfactory colposcopy (inadequate visualization of the endocervical canal) or following endocervical curettage showing dysplasia or atypical glandular epithelial cells. Persistent abnormal cytology associated with normal colposcopy, colposcopic suspicion of invasion and/or cervical biopsy showing microinvasive cancer are also indications for this procedure. The surgery consists of the annular removal of a cone-shaped wedge of tissue from the cervix with a scalpel. With the advent of the LEEP (loop electrosurgical excision procedure), most cone biopsies are done under local paracervical/intracervical block in an office setting and do not require the services of an anesthesiologist.

Variant procedure or approaches: In selected patients, a **laser** is used in place of the scalpel. This procedure can be performed under local anesthesia with less blood loss, but operative time is usually longer. The thermal effect of the laser at the cone margins, although usually minimal, may interfere with pathologic interpretation. In pregnant patients, a **shallower cone** is done to minimize complications. Approximately 1% of women with cervical carcinoma are pregnant at the time of diagnosis, and 1/1240 pregnancies is complicated by cervical cancer. Recognition and therapy of preinvasive cervical lesions during pregnancy, therefore, are of paramount importance. Because of the increased vascularity of the pregnant uterus and cervix, conization is usually associated with increased blood loss and morbidity.

Usual preop diagnosis: Cervical dysplasia

SUMMARY OF PROCEDURE

	Conization	Laser Conization	Shallow Cone In Pregnancy
Position	Lithotomy	⇐	Lithotomy; with left lateral tilt in 3rd trimester
Incision	Cervical	⇐	⇐
Special instrumentation	Colposcope	CO_2 laser; protective eye wear; colposcope	Colposcope
Unique considerations	Infiltration of cervix with dilute vasopressin or phenylephrine solution. A solution of 1:200,000 epinephrine also can be used. Vaginal pack necessary in selected patients.	⇐	Phenylephrine, vasopressin or epinephrine should not be used during pregnancy. Liberal use of hemostatic sutures should be made.
Antibiotics	None	⇐	⇐
Surgical time	30-60 min	30-90 min	⇐
EBL	50-200 ml	50 ml	100-350 ml
Postop care	Be aware of postop bleeding.	⇐	⇐
Mortality	< 0.01%	⇐	⇐
Morbidity	Hemorrhage: 5-10%	⇐	10-15%
	Cervical incompetence: 2-3%	⇐	⇐
	Cervical stenosis: 2-3%	⇐	⇐
	Dysmenorrhea: Rare	⇐	⇐
	Infertility: Rare	⇐	⇐
	Injury to rectum and bladder: Rare	⇐	⇐
	Pelvic cellulitis: Rare	⇐	–
	Uterine perforation: Rare	⇐	–
			Fetal loss: 10-15% (up to 30% in 1st trimester)*
			Premature labor: 5-10% (controversial)
			Rupture of membrane: 2-5%
Pain score	3	3	3

* The naturally higher incidence of spontaneous miscarriages in the 1st trimester contributes to this figure.

PATIENT POPULATION CHARACTERISTICS

Age range	Reproductive and postreproductive years
Incidence	~5% of Pap smears (+ for dysplasia); 10-17% of patients who undergo colposcopic exams
Etiology and predisposing factors	Smoking; human papilloma virus (HPV); herpes simplex virus (HSV); multiple sexual partners; early age of onset of coitus; multiparity; lower socioeconomic status; human immunodeficiency virus (HIV); immunocompromised hosts

ANESTHETIC CONSIDERATIONS

PREOPERATIVE

Conization is done for diagnosis and treatment of cervical lesions. Occasionally it is necessary to perform the procedure during pregnancy, which increases the risk of bleeding complications. The effect of anesthetic agents on the fetus (especially 1st trimester) also needs to be considered when choosing anesthetic technique (see p. 616).

Respiratory	Not usually a problem, unless there is Hx of lung disease or smoking.
Cardiovascular	These patients are generally young and, therefore, less likely to have significant heart disease.
Neurological	Usually not significant, unless there is Hx of seizure disorder or other neurologic illness.
Hematologic	**Tests**: Hct
Laboratory	Consider pregnancy test.
Premedication	Usually none, although an anxiolytic may be given if not pregnant. Na citrate (0.3 M) 30 ml po should be given 30 min prior to induction in all pregnant patients.

INTRAOPERATIVE

Anesthetic technique: Usually a local or MAC anesthetic; occasionally, GETA or spinal. Pregnancy makes it desirable to perform the procedure under local or regional anesthesia if possible. The minimalist approach to pharmacologic intervention is appropriate in a pregnant patient.

General anesthesia:

Induction	Standard induction (p. B-2). In pregnant patients, rapid-sequence induction (p. B-5) with cricoid pressure is appropriate. If patient is to be intubated, use either succinylcholine 1 mg/kg iv or vecuronium 0.1 mg/kg iv for muscle relaxation; otherwise, in nonpregnant patients, mask or LMA ventilation may suffice.
Maintenance	Standard maintenance (p. B-3). It is not necessary to maintain muscle relaxation throughout the case; and either controlled or spontaneous ventilation can be used.
Emergence	Reverse muscle relaxants with neostigmine or edrophonium and insure that the patient is awake and able to protect her airway prior to extubation. It may be prudent to give an antiemetic, such as metoclopramide 10 mg iv or droperidol 0.5-1 mg iv, 30 min prior to emergence in nonpregnant patients.

Regional anesthesia: Both spinal and epidural techniques are acceptable, and may be preferred for pregnant patients who cannot tolerate local anesthesia. Prehydration with 1000 ml LR prior to the block is recommended. Treat hypotension with ephedrine 5-10 mg iv, titrated to effect.

Blood and fluid requirements	Minimal blood loss IV: 18 ga × 1 NS/LR @ 2-4 ml/kg/h	
Monitoring	Standard monitors (see p. B-1). Fetal monitoring may be indicated for pregnancies > 16 wk.	A labor and delivery nurse should accompany patients. Monitor for Sx of fetal distress or onset of labor. Magnesium or terbutaline may be necessary to suppress the sudden onset of premature labor. Consult with obstetrician on the need for these tocolytic agents. Any evidence of fetal distress should be communicated to the surgeon immediately.
Positioning	✓ and pad pressure points. ✓ eyes. Left uterine displacement	★ **NB**: peroneal nerve compression at lateral fibular head → foot drop. Left uterine displacement with a wedge under mattress should be used for pregnant patients (after ~20 wk).
Complications	Laser eye damage Fire Premature labor	If a laser is used, eye protection is required for the patient and all OR personnel; be alert for fire hazards when using a laser.

POSTOPERATIVE

Complications	Peroneal nerve injury (2° lithotomy position)	Nerve injury manifested as foot drop and loss of sensation over dorsum of foot.
	N/V	Rx: metoclopramide 10 mg iv
	Premature labor	Tocolytic agents (e.g., terbutaline, magnesium) may be needed, administered in consultation with obstetrician.
	Bleeding	
	PDPH	May require epidural blood patch.
Pain management	Oral analgesic	Acetaminophen (325-360 mg po)

References

1. Averette HE, Nasser N, Yankow SL, Little WA: Cervical conization in pregnancy. Analysis of 180 operations. *Am J Obstet Gynecol* 1970; 106(4):543-49.
2. Delmore J, Horbelt DV, Kallail KJ: Cervical conization: cold knife and laser excision in residency training. *Obstet Gynecol* 1992; 79(6):1016-19.
3. DiSaia PJ, Creasman WT: Cancer in pregnancy. In *Clinical Gynecologic Oncology*. DiSaia PJ, Creasman WT, eds. CV Mosby, St. Louis: 1989, 511-22.
4. Jones HW III: Cone biopsy in the management of cervical intra-epithelial neoplasia. In *Clinical Obstetrics and Gynecology*. Pitkin RM, Scott JR, Weingold AB, Stafl A, eds. Harper & Row, Philadelphia: 1983, 26(4):968-79.
5. Kristensen GB, Jensen LK, Holund B: A randomized trial comparing two methods of cold knife conization with laser conization. *Obstet Gynecol* 1990; 76(6):1009-13.
6. Mazze RI, Kallen B. Reproductive outcome after anesthesia and operation during pregnancy: a registry study of 5405 cases. *Am J Obstet Gynecol* 1989; 161:(5) 1178-85.
7. Samuels F, Landon MB: Medical complications. In *Obstetrics. Normal and Problem Pregnancies*. Gabbe SG, Niebyl JR, Simpson JL, eds. Churchill Livingstone, New York: 1986, 855-57.
8. Tabor A, Berget A: Cold knife and laser conization for cervical intra-epithelial neoplasia. *Obstet Gynecol* 1990; 76(4):633-35.

ANESTHETIC CONSIDERATIONS FOR LASER THERAPY TO VULVA, VAGINA, CERVIX

PREOPERATIVE

Laser therapy is indicated for preinvasive lesions of the vulva, vagina or cervix. It destroys tissues by the selective application of light energy focused into a beam. Vaporized tissues tend to heal without scarring, and blood loss is minimal due to the cauterizing effect of the laser.[1] Most gynecological laser procedures are done with local anesthesia in the clinic setting and do not require the services of an anesthesiologist.

Respiratory	Not significant unless there is underlying lung disease.
Cardiovascular	In elderly patients, exercise tolerance should be assessed. **Tests:** ECG if > 50 yr.
Hematologic	**Tests:** Hct
Laboratory	Consider pregnancy test in young women.
Premedication	Anxiolytic such as midazolam 1-2 mg iv, if needed.

INTRAOPERATIVE

Anesthetic technique: Usually MAC; occasionally, GETA/LMA or regional technique may be used. Sedation with propofol, midazolam and fentanyl in small doses usually is adequate.

General anesthesia:

Induction	Standard induction (p. B-2)
Maintenance	Standard maintenance (see p. B-3). Muscle relaxation not necessary. A technique with relatively rapid emergence (e.g., propofol or sevoflurane/desflurane) is useful for outpatient surgery.
Emergence	No special considerations

Regional anesthesia: Spinal or epidural anesthesia may be used with a sensory level to T10. Either lidocaine, tetracaine or bupivacaine is acceptable, depending on anticipated length of surgery. Provide supplemental O_2 if sedation given.

Spinal	A T10 sensory level is desirable; and lidocaine 75 mg, tetracaine 10 mg or bupivacaine 12 mg can be used. Small-diameter spinal needles (e.g., 26 ga Quincke or 25 ga Sprotte needles) minimize chance of postdural puncture headache (PDPH).	
Epidural	2% lidocaine, ± epinephrine 1:200,000 (10-15 ml) or 0.5% bupivacaine (10-15 ml) are used; then @ ~10 ml/h. Narcotics such as morphine (4 mg) or hydromorphone (0.5 mg) may be given in the epidural for postop pain control.	
Blood and fluid requirements	Minimal blood loss IV: 18 ga × 1 NS/LR @ 2-4 ml/kg/h	Give 1000 ml LR prior to regional block to compensate for vasodilatation.
Monitoring	Standard monitors (see p. B-1).	
Positioning	✓ and pad pressure points. ✓ eyes.	
Complications	Eye injury OR fires Aerosolization of viral particles	Goggles should be worn by both patient and all OR personnel during laser use to prevent injury to eyes from light. If the patient is asleep, cover eyes with saline-soaked gauze. Whenever laser is in use, be prepared for fires: know where fire extinguisher is located, and watch for improper handling of lasers. Vaporization of condyloma may produce aerosolization of viral particles; therefore, appropriate ventilation is suggested to disperse smoke.

POSTOPERATIVE

Complications	N/V PDPH	N/V may respond well to 10 mg iv metoclopramide. PDPH may require epidural blood patch for treatment.
Pain management	Oral analgesics	E.g., acetaminophen 325-650 mg po

Reference

1. McKenzie AL, Carruth JA: Lasers in surgery and medicine. *Phys Med Biol* 1984; 29(6):619-41.

SUCTION CURETTAGE FOR GESTATIONAL TROPHOBLASTIC DISEASE

SURGICAL CONSIDERATIONS

Description: Suction curettage is the most efficient method of evacuating a gestational trophoblastic neoplasm (mole). The procedure involves dilation of the cervix by instruments or by laminaria tents, followed by insertion of suction cannula of appropriate diameter into the uterine cavity. Standard negative pressures used are in the range of 30-70 mmHg. Intravenous oxytocin to maintain uterine contraction and minimize blood loss is started after a moderate amount of tissue has been removed. This procedure is followed by gentle, sharp curettage of the uterus. Paracervical injection of dilute vasopressin solution or 1% xylocaine with 1:200,000 epinephrine may decrease operative blood loss (in cases not complicated by thyrotoxicosis or HTN).

Variant procedure or approaches: Evacuation of a mole > 16 wk gestation size is associated with a significant risk of trophoblastic embolization and cardiorespiratory embarrassment (2° pulmonary HTN/edema, cyanosis, ↓CO, ↓BP, right heart failure). Central hemodynamic monitoring using a PA catheter is useful in the management of cardiovascular changes associated with trophoblastic embolization and to prevent inadvertent fluid overload.

Usual preop diagnosis: Gestational trophoblastic disease (GTD)

SUMMARY OF PROCEDURE

	Small Mole < 16 Weeks Size	Large Mole > 16 Weeks Size
Position	Lithotomy	⇐
Incision	None	⇐
Special instrumentation	Suction evacuation kit	⇐
Unique considerations	If mole > 12 wk size, laparotomy setup should be readily available. Oxytocin drip. In some cases, thyrotoxicosis may be present, requiring control with β-blockers.	⇐ + Central hemodynamic monitoring with PA catheter; avoid overzealous use of crystalloids and blood transfusions. Preop ABG.
Antibiotics	Cefotetan 2 g iv on call to OR	⇐
Surgical time	30-60 min	⇐
EBL	200-400 ml	⇐
Postop care	Outpatient (usually)	ICU admission in selected cases
Mortality	Rare	⇐
Morbidity	Trophoblastic embolization: 2.6%	11-27%
	Excessive bleeding: 2%	10%
	Infection: < 2%	⇐
	Uterine perforation: < 1%	1-2%
		Acute pulmonary edema: 2-11%
Pain score	3	3

PATIENT POPULATION CHARACTERISTICS

Age range	Reproductive age group
Incidence	1/1200 deliveries in U.S.
Etiology	Genetics, androgenous (all chromosomes in true moles are paternal in origin); nutritional deficiency: protein, folic acid, carotene (vitamin A)
Associated conditions	Lower socioeconomic status; Asian, Hispanic populations; hyperemesis gravidarum (due to ↑levels of HCG); preeclampsia in first trimester; thyrotoxicosis (because of its analogy to TSH molecule, ↑levels of HCG can bind TSH receptors and cause thyrotoxicosis); prior GTD (incidence ↑ to 0.6-2.0%)

ANESTHETIC CONSIDERATIONS

PREOPERATIVE

Some 80% of cases are diagnosed at the 12th-18th wk of development.[1] Most patients have an unusually large uterus for the length of the pregnancy and vaginal bleeding is common. Trophoblastic disease is classified by the degree of invasiveness: retained mole is the most common type and the least invasive. Invasive mole involves the wall of the uterus, and metastatic mole involves more distant sites. Chemotherapy with methotrexate and actinomycin D usually is given postop for invasive or metastatic disease.[2] (See Table 8.1-1, p. 547 for toxicities of chemotherapeutic agents.)

Respiratory Pulmonary edema may complicate preeclampsia, which occurs in 25% of patients with GTD. If respiratory distress is present, it also may be due to embolization of tumor to lungs.[7] Avoid overhydration → pulmonary complications in patients with large moles.

Tests: ABGs should be obtained preop if there is a question about the pulmonary function of the patient or in patients at high risk of developing trophoblastic embolization. Others as indicated by H&P.

Cardiovascular Blood volume is often depleted due to hyperemesis and vaginal bleeding. Patients may be dehydrated 2° hyperemesis gravidarum preop, and adequate hydration should be given preop if patient shows signs of hypovolemia (e.g., tachycardia, orthostatic hypotension, low UO). Preeclampsia may also complicate this disease and can be diagnosed by HTN, proteinuria and edema. If the patient has preeclampsia, invasive monitoring of BP may be advisable. Also, if patient is receiving magnesium therapy, a serum level should be checked preop. Magnesium therapy may inhibit myocardial

Cardiovascular, cont.	contractility in high doses. Ca is the preferred antidote for myocardial depression. $MgSO_4$ → uterine atony → ↑blood loss.
Neurological	Seizure prophylaxis with Mg^{++} is indicated for women with severe preeclampsia. If seizures occur, a small dose of STP (50-100 mg) or diazepam (2.5-5 mg) should be given iv and respiration assisted with supplemental O_2 by mask. The trachea should be intubated for airway protection in patients with full stomachs and in those who are difficult to ventilate by mask.
Musculoskeletal	✓ reflexes if patient has received Mg^{++}. Reduce amount of nondepolarizing muscle relaxant to compensate for the effects of Mg^{++} on muscle strength.
Hematologic	Anemia may be masked by hypovolemia. Rh– patients with Rh+ partners should receive 300 μg of Rh immune globulin (RhoGAM) within 72 h postop to ↓ possibility of Rh isoimmunization in future pregnancies. **Tests:** CBC; ✓ Plt in preeclamptics. If patient has received chemotherapy recently, ✓ HCT; complete blood count (WBC, Plt). Plt count should also be checked in women who have preeclampsia.
Endocrine	Hyperthyroidism occurs in 5% of women with hydatidiform moles[2] and is due to the thyroid-stimulating effects of HCG. **Tests:** Thyroid function tests should be checked preop in women with Sx of hyperthyroidism, and corrected prior to surgery.
Laboratory	Serum HCG level; consider thyroid function tests; LFTs; PT; PTT; Plt count; Mg^{++} level; UA; as indicated from H&P.
Premedication	Usually an anxiolytic such as midazolam 1-2 mg iv. A nonparticulate antacid (Na citrate 30 ml 0.3 M) should be given po just before induction.

INTRAOPERATIVE

Anesthetic technique: Usually GETA, although may be carried out under spinal or epidural anesthesia. Chemical sympathectomy in regional anesthesia may ↑ blood loss.

General anesthesia:

Induction	A rapid-sequence induction (p. B-5) with cricoid pressure should be used; STP 5 mg/kg iv or propofol 2-3 mg/kg iv is usually recommended. Analgesia is provided by fentanyl 1-3 μg/kg iv or sufentanil 0.1-0.3 μg/kg iv. Succinylcholine (1 mg/kg iv) or rocuronium (0.5 mg/kg iv) provides muscle relaxation for intubation.
Maintenance	Standard maintenance (p. B-3). Prophylaxis for N/V (e.g., metoclopramide 10 mg iv or droperidol 0.5-1.25 mg iv) is recommended. Control BP, if preeclamptic, with labetalol, hydralazine or SNP. Try to keep DBP at 90-100 mmHg.
Emergence	Extubate when fully awake and protective airway reflexes have returned. Watch for emesis after extubation. Give supplemental O_2.

Regional anesthesia:

Spinal	A T8 sensory level is desirable; and lidocaine (75 mg), tetracaine (10-12 mg) or bupivacaine (10-12 mg) can be used. Small-diameter spinal needles (e.g., 26-ga Quincke or 25-ga Sprotte needles) will minimize the chances of postdural puncture headache (PDPH).
Epidural	Use 2% lidocaine ± epinephrine 1:200,000 (10-15 ml) or 0.5% bupivacaine (10-15 ml).

Blood and fluid requirements	Possible large blood loss IV: 18-16 ga × 1 NS/LR @ 2-4 ml/kg/h	One large-volume iv line should be placed and blood readily available. The usual causes of bleeding are uterine perforation, cervical laceration or uterine atony.
Control of bleeding	Oxytocin (30 U/L) infusion Isoflurane < 1%	Oxytocin is begun about halfway through procedure at 30-60 drops/min (consult obstetrician). Try to keep isoflurane < 1% to prevent uterine relaxation.
	Ergonovine maleate 0.2 mg im	Ergonovine may be given for severe bleeding. Since this drug can cause HTN, it is contraindicated in cases of pre-eclampsia with elevated BP.

Monitoring	Standard monitors (p. B-1). ± Arterial catheter ± CVP/PA catheter Foley catheter	An arterial catheter and CVP are indicated in cases of thyrotoxicosis, preeclampsia or significant hemorrhage. The use of vasodilators such as SNP is also an indication for invasive monitors.
Positioning	✓ and pad pressure points. ✓ eyes.	★ **NB**: peroneal nerve compression at lateral fibular head → foot drop. Lifting the legs may cause the level of spinal or epidural anesthesia to move cranially if performed too quickly after the block.
Complications	Embolization of trophoblastic material	Embolization may occur, especially if > 16 wk gestation. Significant respiratory compromise can occur, requiring postop ventilation and PEEP.

POSTOPERATIVE

Complications	Bleeding N/V HTN Hypotension	Continue oxytocin infusion. Significant hemorrhage should be evaluated by surgeons for possible perforation, laceration or atony. Antiemetics such as droperidol (0.6 mg), Compazine (5-10 mg) or metoclopramide (10 mg) may be useful. BP should be monitored closely in preeclamptics. Consider ICU admission if unstable.
	Peroneal nerve injury (2° to lithotomy position)	Nerve injury manifested as foot drop and loss of sensation over dorsum of foot.
Pain management	Oral analgesics	Acetaminophen (325-650 mg po)

References

1. Bruun T, Kristoffersen K: Thyroid function during pregnancy with special reference to hydatidiform mole and hyperemesis. *Acta Endocrinol* 1978; 88(2)383-89.
2. Curry SL, Hammond CB, Tyrey L, Creasman WT, Parker RT: Hydatiform mole: Diagnosis, management and long-term followup of 347 patients. *Obstet Gynecol* 1975; 45(1):1-8.
3. DiSaia PJ, Creasman WT: Gestational trophoblastic neoplasia. In *Clinical Gynecologic Oncology*. DiSaia PJ, Creasman WT, eds. CV Mosby, St. Louis: 1989, 214-40.
4. Edraki B, Chambers JT: Gestational trophoblastic disease: persistent mole. In *Expert Consultations in Gynecological Cancers*. Markman M, Belinson JL, eds. Marcel Dekker, New York: 1997, 124-26.
5. Goldstein DP, Berkowitz RS. Current management of complete and partial molar pregnancy. *J Reprod Med* 1994; 39:139.
6. Hammond CB, Weed JC Jr, Currie JL: The role of operation in the current therapy of gestational trophoblastic disease. *Am J Obstet Gynecol* 1980; 136(7):844-58.
7. Kohorn EI: Clinical management and the neoplastic sequelae of trophoblastic embolization associated with hydatiform mole. In *Obstet Gynecol Surv*, Vol 42(8). Williams & Wilkins, Baltimore: 1987, 484-88.
8. Lipp RG, Kindrchi JD, Selmitz R: Death from pulmonary embolism associated with hydatiform mole. *Am J Obstet Gynecol* 1962; 83(12):1644-47.
9. Soper JT, Lewis JL Jr., Hammond CB: Gestational trophoblastic disease. In *Principles and Practice of Gynecologic Oncology, 2nd edition*. Hoskins WJ, Perez CA, Young RC, eds. Lippincott-Raven Publishers, Philadelphia: 1996, 1039-77.
10. Wheeless CR Jr: Suction curettage for abortion. In *Atlas of Pelvic Surgery*. Lea & Febiger, Philadelphia: 1988, 208-9.

PELVIC EXENTERATION

SURGICAL CONSIDERATIONS

Description: Pelvic exenteration was introduced by Brunschwig as an ultraradical surgical approach for advanced and radioresistant cervical cancer. Although advanced vaginal and vulvar carcinoma have occasionally been treated with this procedure, its most important role is in the management of centrally recurrent, surgically resectable, radioresistant cervical carcinoma. Pelvic exenteration involves ***en bloc* resection** of all pelvic tissues, including uterus, cervix, vagina, bladder and rectum. Involvement of distal vagina may require resection of vulva and groin nodes. The goal of this procedure is curative, with removal of all cancer tissue and reconstruction of appropriate diversions for the urine and stool if the colon cannot be reanastomosed to the rectum. It is rare for cervical and vaginal cancer to involve the lower 5 cm of the rectum and anus. It is, therefore, possible to mobilize the descending colon and anastomose it primarily to the distal rectum. A continent or incontinent urinary diversion, **omental pelvic carpet** or **sling** and **gracilis myocutaneous flaps** for vaginal and perineal reconstruction are then performed. A rectus abdominis muscle flap also can be used for vaginal reconstruction. This type of flap yields excellent aesthetic and functional results. In cases where an omental sling (shown in Fig 8.1-4) cannot be developed, an absorbable synthetic mesh is sutured to the pelvic peritoneum to create a pelvic lid (like a hammock) to keep the small bowel off the denuded pelvic peritoneum, thus decreasing the possibility of small-bowel obstruction. In general, an additional 2-3 h of surgical time and an additional 300 ml of EBL are expected when a vaginal reconstruction is undertaken. An exploratory laparotomy is needed prior to initiation of the exenterative procedure to rule out spread of disease outside the pelvis and/or extension to pelvic sidewalls and pelvic lymph nodes, all of which are absolute contraindications to this procedure.

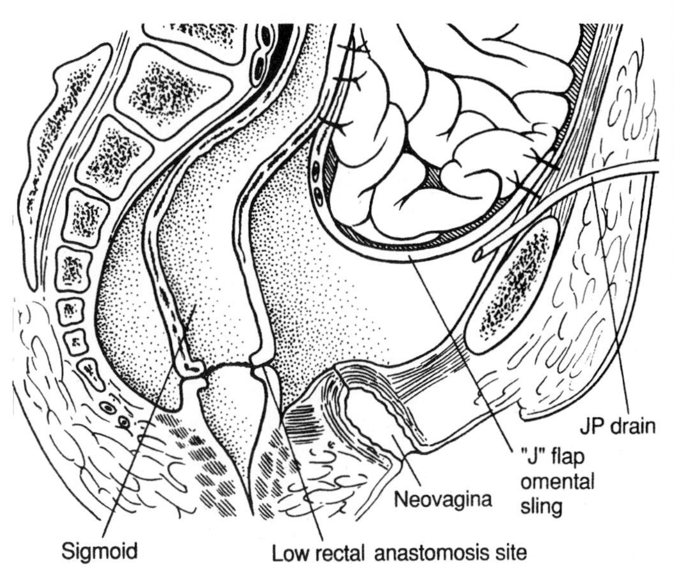

Figure 8.1-4. Sagittal section of the pelvis after a total pelvic exenteration. Note that all the reproductive organs, along with their supporting structures, the rectum and the bladder, have been resected. Drains can be placed through separate stab incisions in the abdomen. The small bowel is kept away from the operative site by a pelvic lid. The urinary and fecal diversions are not diagrammed. (Reproduced with permission from Wheeless CR: *Atlas of Pelvic Surgery*. Lea & Febiger: 1988.)

Resectability is evaluated by palpation of pelvic and paraaortic lymph nodes, liver, hemidiaphragms and peritoneal surfaces of the upper abdomen and pelvis. Washings should be obtained for cytology. A thorough lymph node dissection should then be performed and all suspicious nodes should be submitted for frozen-section pathologic examination. The pararectal, paravesical and presacral spaces should then be developed. If the patient is found to be inoperable, CUSA can be used to decrease the tumor burden. Consideration also should be given to IORT. If the patient is deemed operable, the space of Retzius is developed. The round ligaments are then transected close to the pelvic sidewall bilaterally; and the infundibulopelvic ligaments are also ligated and transected. The ureters are divided as close to the bladder as possible. The superior hemorrhoidal vessel is ligated and transected; and the colon is transected at the appropriate level. The anterior divisions of the internal iliac artery on both sides are ligated and divided; and the web of tissue is clamped close to the pelvic sidewall, transected and suture-ligated. Following this, sharp dissection can be done to free up the specimen from the low attachments to the levator muscles. In larger tumors, the levator muscle is partially removed with the specimen to provide adequate margins. From a combined perineal and abdominal approach, the distal vagina, urethra and perineum (± rectum) can be resected. The specimen is handed off the field, hemostasis is achieved, an ileal loop or other urinary conduit is performed, low rectal anastomosis is done, vaginal reconstruction is undertaken, and the pelvic floor is covered. (Figs 8.1-4 and 8.1-5 show the completed exenteration.)

Variant procedure or approaches: Anterior pelvic exenteration involves preservation of rectosigmoid, while **posterior pelvic exenteration** involves preservation of bladder. Posterior exenteration has proved more useful in cancer of vulva or vagina than in cervical cancer. Anterior and posterior exenterations are used in selective cases because of the increased risk of an incomplete tumor resection and multiple complications and malfunctioning of the preserved organ.

Usual preop diagnosis: Recurrent cervical carcinoma following radiotherapy

SUMMARY OF PROCEDURE

Position	Modified dorsolithotomy with Allen stirrups
Incision	Midline longitudinal, perineal
Special instrumentation	Vital View and argon beam coagulator (may be helpful); EEA, GIA, TA staplers; Robo-retractor or similar devices
Unique considerations	Full and thorough mechanical and antibiotic intestinal prep. NG tube placement intraop. SCD and minidose heparin intraop for DVT prophylaxis. Preop PFTs. Consider preop Greenfield IVC filter placement to avoid PE for high-risk patients. Consider intraop radiation of tumor bed and/or of resection margins. Abort case if extrapelvic metastases and/or tumor extension to pelvic sidewalls noted.
Antibiotics	Cefotetan 2 g iv q 12 h to begin, 12 h preop, and continue 72 h postop. Alternatively, a combination of ampicillin (1 g), gentamicin (80 mg) and metronidazole (500 mg).
Surgical time	8-12 h (2-team approach); 5-10 h (for anterior and posterior exenteration)
Closing considerations	Abdominal drains; colostomy; ureteral stents; urostomy; intraop radiation therapy. Triple-lumen central line placement. Copious irrigation of the operative sites.
EBL	1200-4000 ml
Postop care	ICU: 2-3 d. Correction of electrolyte imbalance. Extensive peritoneal raw surfaces lead to intraperitoneal fluid 3rd-spacing. Patients require good hydration to maintain intravascular volume. SCDs and minidose heparin for DVT prophylaxis. Consider concentrated albumin infusion to maintain intravascular volume. Early and aggressive use of TPN is important. Maintain Hct in the low 30s as concentrated blood may lead to sludging and contribute to flap necrosis and wound breakdown. Remove ureteral stents 1-2 wk postop, when the edema at the ureterointestinal site has subsided.
Mortality	5-11%
Morbidity	Intraop hemorrhage requiring a median of 5 U PRBC transfusion Infectious: Nonspecific: 25% Flap necrosis: 20% Pelvic cellulitis: 19% Pyelonephritis: 17% Wound infection: 6% Sepsis: 3% Psychiatric: Confusion: 24% Intestinal: Ileus: 18% GI fistula: 13% Stoma breakdown: 3% Small bowel obstruction: 5% Renal: Ureteral fistulae: 14% Failure: 5% Cardiovascular: CHF: 8% Venous thrombosis: 3-7% DIC: 3% Dysrhythmia: 3% MI: 3% Pulmonary: Pneumonia: 3% PE: 2% Neurologic: CVA: 2% Spinal cord infarction: < 2%
Pain score	7-8

PATIENT POPULATION CHARACTERISTICS

Age range	All age groups
Incidence	1.5-17% of cervical cancers treated with radiation therapy (depending on stage and cell type)
Associated conditions	Advanced or recurrent gynecologic malignancies; radiation injury

ANESTHETIC CONSIDERATIONS

PREOPERATIVE

This procedure is performed for recurrent central cervical or other gynecologic carcinomas and involves removal of all pelvic tissues. Occasionally, the bladder or rectum is preserved, if not involved with tumor. Most patients have undergone preop radiation or chemotherapy.

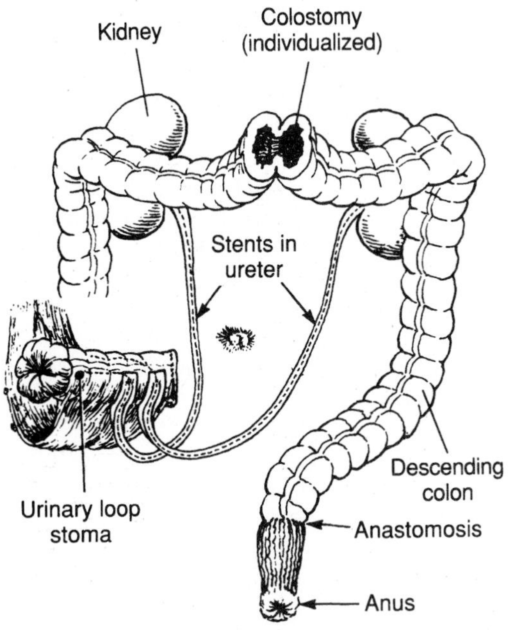

Figure 8.1-5. Conceptual drawing shows the urinary and fecal diversions after a total pelvic exenteration. (Reproduced with permission from Wheeless CR: *Atlas of Pelvic Surgery*. Lea & Febiger: 1988.)

Respiratory Usually not significant unless there is Hx of smoking or lung disease. Ask about prior chemotherapy. (See Anesthetic Considerations for Second-Look/Reassessment Laparotomy for Ovarian Cancer, p. 544.)
Tests: Consider CXR; others as indicated from H&P.

Cardiovascular Exercise tolerance should be assessed. Underlying CAD or CHF should be medically optimized preop in consultation with a cardiologist. Any exposure to cardiotoxic chemotherapy should be investigated and may require further tests, such as an ECHO.
Tests: Consider ECG; others as indicated from H&P.

Neurological Any Hx of stroke, seizure, carotid artery disease or other neurologic disease should be evaluated and documented.

Endocrine Any endocrine disease, such as diabetes, should be optimized in consultation with the patient's primary care physician or endocrinologist. Ask about recent corticosteroid use.
Tests: Fasting blood sugar in the diabetic; others as indicated from H&P.

Gastrointestinal Patients should have iv hydration if given a bowel prep. A long intestinal tube (Miller-Abbot or Cantor tube) should be placed preop for bowel decompression.

Hematologic Many patients will be anemic from chronic disease and malnutrition. Preop transfusion of packed cells to increase Hct > 30% is indicated. Ask about recent NSAID usage.
Tests: CBC, PT, PTT, if indicated.

Laboratory LFTs; CT scan of pelvis and abdomen

Premedication Anxiolytic such as midazolam (1-2 mg iv) or diazepam, 10 mg po. Careful explanation about the procedure and the potential for postop intubation and mechanical ventilation is beneficial.

INTRAOPERATIVE

Anesthetic technique: GETA ± supplemental epidural anesthesia. Inhalation anesthetics or propofol infusion may be used in relatively healthy patients. A high-dose narcotic technique should be used for patients with significant CAD or in poor overall physical condition.

General anesthesia:

Induction Standard induction (p. B-2), unless otherwise indicated by patient condition. Long-acting muscle relaxants (e.g., pancuronium [0.1 mg/kg] or pipecuronium [0.08 mg/kg]) should be used unless patient has significant renal dysfunction, in which case cisatracurium (0.2 mg/kg) should be used.

Maintenance Isoflurane, propofol (100-200 μg/kg/min) or high-dose fentanyl (50-75 μg/kg) combined with midazolam[1] (0.1-0.5 mg/kg). Epidural anesthetic or epidural narcotic (morphine or hydromorphone)

Maintenance, cont. can be given to reduce anesthetic requirements when using inhalation agents. Atracurium or cisatracurium infusion (1-2 mg/kg/min) should be used to maintain muscle relaxation in patients with renal dysfunction.

Emergence If patient is hemodynamically stable, warm and responsive at the end of surgery, extubation may be appropriate. Any patient who is unstable, hypothermic, has had a high-dose narcotic, has significant edema of the face or airway, or who has ongoing excessive fluid requirements should be ventilated overnight in the ICU prior to an attempt at extubation. Due to the large fluid shifts that can occur, all patients need to be monitored in an ICU postop.

Regional anesthesia:

Epidural 2% lidocaine (10-15 ml), with or without epinephrine 1:200,000 or 0.5% bupivacaine (10-15 ml) are used; then at ~10 ml/h. Narcotics such as morphine (2-4 mg) or hydromorphone (0.3-0.5 mg) may be given in the epidural for postop pain control.

Ventilation	5 cm H_2O PEEP may help prevent atelectasis.	✓ ABGs during surgery. Adjust ventilation accordingly to keep normocarbic. HCO_3 is given for metabolic acidosis when pH < 7.20.
Blood and fluid requirements	Possible large blood loss IV: 14-16 ga × 2 NS/LR @ 10-15 ml/kg/h Colloid solutions Hetastarch PRBCs when Hct < 30% Keep PAWP < 20 mmHg.[12] Maintain UO of 0.5-1 ml/kg/h. Ionized Ca^{++} FFP/PLT	Renal ultrafiltration is improved by NS/LR, but bowel edema is also increased. LR is useful when acidosis is present and NS is better when giving blood products or when metabolic alkalosis is present. Rapid infuser device should be available. Colloid solutions are superior in restoring hemodynamic stability when large fluid volumes are required. The use of 6% hetastarch should be limited to 1,000 ml due to potential coagulopathy with larger volumes. UO should guide fluid therapy, in addition to PA pressures and CO. Dopamine 2-3 μg/kg/min also may be used to maintain UO. Use of furosemide or mannitol is controversial and probably a last resort to prevent anuric renal failure. Controlled hypotension to a MAP of 60-70 mmHg is useful in healthy patients to reduce blood loss. Measure ionized calcium and potassium after rapid administration of blood products; replace calcium as necessary. Plt or FFP may be given for coagulation abnormalities studies as necessary to treat significant bleeding.
Monitoring	Standard monitors (see p. B-1). ± Arterial line Foley catheter ± PA catheters ± TEE	Invasive hemodynamic monitoring with arterial and PA catheters usually is required. TEE allows intraop assessment of myocardial function and may be appropriate in selected patients.
Positioning	✓ and pad pressure points. ✓ eyes. Antiembolism stockings and SCD	★ **NB:** peroneal nerve compression at lateral fibular head → foot drop.
Complications	Hypothermia Bleeding Coagulopathy Trauma to kidney	Warm OR. Humidify gases. Wrap head in towels. Use warm saline lavage of abdomen. Rapid infuser device is helpful for giving large volumes of iv fluids. Watch for hematuria or ↓UO.

POSTOPERATIVE

Complications	Bleeding Fluid overload	✓ Hct and coags periodically. Be prepared for continued increased fluid requirements for 24 h postop. It is essential to maintain optimal cardiac filling pressures. After 24 h, fluid mobilization will begin, usually requiring diuretic therapy.
	Peroneal nerve injury 2° lithotomy position	Nerve injury manifested as foot drop and loss of sensation over dorsum of foot.

Pain management	Epidural or iv opiates	See p. C-1.
Tests	Hct	Others as indicated from H&P.

References

1. Anthopoulos AP, Manetta A, Larson JE, Podczaski ES, Bartholomew MJ, Mortel R: Pelvic exenteration: a morbidity and mortality analysis of a seven year experience. *Gynecol Oncol* 1989; 35(2):219-23.
2. Counts RB, Haisch C, Simon TL, Maxwell NG, Heimbach DM, Carrico CJ: Hemostasis in massively transfused trauma patients. *Ann Surg* 1979; 190(1):91-9.
3. Craig RL, Poole GV: Resuscitation in uncontrolled hemorrhage. *Am Surg* 1994: 60:59.
4. DiSaia PJ, Creasman WT: Invasive cervical cancer. In *Clinical Gynecologic Oncology*. DiSaia PJ, Creasman WT, eds. CV Mosby, St. Louis: 1989, 67-132.
5. Eisenkop SM, Nalick RH, Teng NH: Modified posterior exenteration for ovarian cancer. *Obstet Gynecol* 1991; 78(5P+1): 879-85.
6. Fiorica JV, Roberts WS, Hoffman MS, Barton DP, Finan MA, Lyman G, Cavanagh D: Concentrated albumin infusion as an aid to postoperative recovery after pelvic exenteration. *Gynecol Oncol* 1991; 43(3):265-69.
7. Hatch KD, Gelder MS, Soong SJ, Baker VV, Shingleton HM: Pelvic exenteration with low rectal anastomosis: survival, complications, and prognostic factors. *Gynecol Oncol* 1990; 38(3):462-67.
8. Jackowatz JG, Porudominsky D, Riihimaki DU, Kemeny M, Kokal WA, Braly PS, Terz JJ, Beatty DJ: Complications of pelvic exenteration. *Arch Surg* 1985; 120:(11)1261-65.
9. Martino M, Houvenaeghel G, Hardwigsen J, Moutardier V, et al: Pelvic recurrence of cancers of the uterine cervix. A study of a series of 49 cases. *Ann Chir* 1997; 51:36-45.
10. Matthews CM, Morris M, Burke TW, Gershenson DM, Wharton TJ, Rutledge FN: Pelvic exenteration in the elderly patient. *Obstet Gynecol* 1992; 79(5):773-77.
11. Morley GW, Lindenauer SM: Pelvic exenterative therapy for gynecologic malignancy: an analysis of 70 cases. *Cancer* 1976; 38(1 Suppl):581-86.
12. Numa F, Ogata H. Suminami Y, Tsunaga N, et al: Pelvic exenteration for the treatment of gynecological malignancies. *Arch Gynecol Obstet* 1997; 259:133-38.
13. Penalver MA, Benjany DE, Averette HE, et al: Continent urinary diversion in gynecologic oncology. *Gynecol Oncol* 1989; 34:274.
14. Rutledge FN, Smith JP, Wharton JT, O'Quinn AG: Pelvic exenteration: Analysis of 296 patients. *Am J Obstet Gynecol* 1977; 129(8):881-92.
15. Shires GT III, Peitzman AB, Albert SA, Illner H, Silane MF, Perry MO, Shires GT: Response of extravascular lung water to intraoperative fluids. *Ann Surg* 1983; 197(5):515-19.
16. Skillman JJ, Restall S, Salzman EW: Randomized trial of albumin vs. electrolyte solutions during abdominal aortic operations. *Surgery* 1975; 78(3):291-303.
17. Stanhope CR, Webb MJ, Podratz KC: Pelvic exenteration for recurrent cervical cancer. *Clin Obstet Gynecol* 1990; 33(4): 897-909.
18. Stehman FB, Perez CA, Kurman RJ, Thigpen JT: Uterine cervix. In *Principles and Practice of Gynecologic Oncology, 2nd edition*. Hoskins WJ, Perez CA, Young RC, eds. Lippincott-Raven Publishers, Philadelphia: 1996, 785-858.
19. Symmonds RE, Pratt JH, Webb MJ: Exenterative operations: experience with 198 patients. *Am J Obstet Gynecol* 1975; 121(7):907-18.
20. Wheeless CR Jr: Total pelvic exenteration. In *Atlas of Pelvic Surgery*. Lea & Febiger, Philadelphia: 1988, 445-55.

EXPLORATORY LAPAROTOMY, HYSTERECTOMY/BSO FOR UTERINE CANCER

SURGICAL CONSIDERATIONS

Description: Currently, endometrial cancer is the most common gynecologic malignancy in the U.S. The first step in the management of this cancer is an **exploratory laparotomy**, concurrent with a **hysterectomy**. The objective, aside from 1° therapy, is to obtain as much surgical and pathological staging data as feasible for determination of adjuvant postop therapy. Careful exploration is carried out for evidence of omental, liver, peritoneal and adnexal metastases. Aortic and pelvic areas are palpated for metastases and suspicious nodes are removed. If no suspicious nodes are present, some pelvic and periaortic lymph nodes are sampled. Note that this is less extensive than the more complete lymph node dissection of a radical hysterectomy. The lymph node sampling may be omitted in the treatment of some uterine sarcomas. A **total hysterectomy** with **BSO** is then performed in the usual manner (see discussion of TAH/BSO in Staging Laparotomy for Ovarian Cancer, p. 541).

Variant procedure or approaches: A combined laparoscopically assisted vaginal hysterectomy and BSO as well as laparoscopic pelvic and paraaortic node sampling is appropriate in selected patients and is being performed with increasing frequency. The benefits of this approach are shorter hospital stay and convalescence, as well as decreased postop pain. Adhesions of variable severity may be present from prior surgery or radiation. Care should be taken to avoid possible bowel injury at time of trocar insertion. Patient needs to be in steep Trendelenburg position for duration of the procedure. Both arms should be tucked in at the patient's side. Since argon is a heavy gas, prolonged use of the endoscopic argon beam coagulator (ABC) in a patient in steep Trendelenburg can cause significant facial and neck subcutaneous emphysema. As with the open technique, the lymph nodes being removed are in immediate proximity of the great pelvic vessels. The surgeon and anesthesiologist should be mindful of the potential for severe hemorrhage if these vessels are injured.

Usual preop diagnosis: Endometrial carcinoma

SUMMARY OF PROCEDURE

	Open Technique	Laparoscopic Technique
Position	Supine	Modified dorsolithotomy in Allen stirrups
Incision	Midline longitudinal abdominal	Vertical infraumbilical and multiple small transverse incisions
Special instrumentation	None	Videolaparoscopy equipment. Endoscopic GIA staplers, endoscopic ABC, endoscopic vascular clips and CO_2 laser.
Unique considerations	None	Mechanical bowel preop; steep Trendelenburg
Antibiotics	Cefotetan 2 g iv on call to OR; then 2 g iv q 12 h × 2 doses	⇐
Surgical time	2-4 h	2-3 h
Closing considerations	NG tube placement	Release the pneumoperitoneum completely. Closure of fascia at trocar sites ≥ 10 mm in diameter
EBL	400-750 ml	100-500 ml
Postop care	Consider using SCDs and minidose heparin for DVT prophylaxis.	Begin early ambulation and feeding. Patients generally can be discharged on POD 1 or 2.
Mortality	0.1%	⇐
Morbidity	Hemorrhage requiring transfusion: 15%	0.3-3%
	Thrombophlebitis: 7%	⇐
	UTI: 7%	⇐
	Paralytic ileus: 2-5%	1-2%
	Wound infection: 3%	Rare
	PE: 1-2%	⇐
	Pelvic infection: 1.5%	⇐
	Wound dehiscence: 1%	N/A
	Bowel injuries: < 1%	1.1%
	Urinary tract injuries: < 1%	0.3-3%
		Trocar site herniation: 0.5-2%
		Trocar site tumor: 1.6% (estimated)
Pain score	7	2-3

PATIENT POPULATION CHARACTERISTICS

Age range	Reproductive and postreproductive ages (average = 61 yr)
Incidence	70-80/100,000
Etiology	Exposure to unopposed endogenous or exogenous estrogen; increased extraglandular conversion of androstenedione to estrone; sequential oral contraceptive pills; exposure to radiation (sarcomas)
Associated conditions	Obesity; diabetes; HTN; nulliparity; late menopause; early menarche; family Hx; Stein Leventhal syndrome; chronic anovulation; ovarian and colon cancer; granulosa cell ovarian tumors; arthritis; hypothyroidism

ANESTHETIC CONSIDERATIONS

PREOPERATIVE

Endometrial cancer is usually diagnosed in postmenopausal women who present with vaginal bleeding. Exploratory laparotomy and TAH/BSO are commonly performed for removal of the primary tumor as well as staging of metastatic disease. Occasionally, preop radiation therapy may be in progress, with consequent systemic effects.

Respiratory Check for Hx of lung disease or smoking.
Tests: Others as indicated from H&P.

Cardiovascular Hx of CAD, HTN or CHF Sx (e.g., angina, dyspnea or peripheral edema) should be investigated. Assess patient's exercise tolerance and current medications. Tests such as an exercise treadmill or ECHO may be indicated if patient has significant angina or CHF.
Tests: All patients > 50 yr should have a preop ECG.

Neurological Seldom a significant problem unless there is Hx of cerebrovascular disease, seizures or other neurologic disease.

Endocrine Inquire about the presence of endocrine diseases, such as diabetes and hypothyroidism, which have been associated with this tumor. If the patient has received corticosteroids within the previous 6 mo, a supplemental dose of hydrocortisone (100 mg iv q 12 h × 2 d) should be given for surgery.
Tests: Consider tests if indicated from H&P.

Neuromuscular Osteoarthritis and osteoporosis common in this patient population. Ask about NSAID usage.
Tests: Bleeding time is indicated if considering regional anesthesia.

Hematologic If vaginal bleeding has been profuse or of long duration, significant anemia may occur. Consider preop iron supplements if there are several days until surgery.
Tests: CBC

Laboratory LFTs; CT scan of abdomen and pelvis

Premedication Anxiolytic, such as midazolam 1-5 mg iv, if necessary. Discuss anesthetic plan and options for postop pain management with patient.

INTRAOPERATIVE

Anesthetic technique: GETA ± epidural or spinal analgesia/anesthesia. In unusual circumstances (e.g., severe lung disease) surgery may be done under spinal or epidural anesthesia only.

General anesthesia:

Induction Standard induction (p. B-2)

Maintenance Standard maintenance (p. B-3). Continued muscle relaxation is usually required to facilitate surgery. Epidural 2% lidocaine with epinephrine 1:200,000 at 10 ml/h may be given to reduce anesthetic requirements.

Emergence Reverse muscle relaxant with neostigmine (0.07 mg/kg with glycopyrrolate 0.01 mg/kg). Patient should awaken at the end of surgery and be extubated in the OR; provide supplemental O_2 until patient is fully recovered from anesthesia.

Regional anesthesia:

Epidural 2% lidocaine (10-20 ml) ± epinephrine 1:200,000 or 0.5% bupivacaine (10-20 ml) are used; then @ ~10 ml/h. Narcotics such as morphine (2-4 mg) or hydromorphone (0.3-0.5 mg) may be given in the epidural for postop pain control.

Spinal Tetracaine (12-14 mg) ± preservative-free morphine (0.3-0.5 mg). Sensory level ~T5.

Blood and fluid requirements	IV: 18-16 ga × 1 NS/LR @ 4-6 ml/kg/h PRBC for Hct < 25%	Crystalloid is used for volume replacement. If anemia is present preop, it may be necessary to give PRBCs to keep Hct > 25%.
Monitoring	Standard monitors (p. B-1). Foley catheter ± Arterial line, CVP NG tube	Direct monitoring of arterial pressure is indicated in patients with CAD, severe HTN or lung disease. CVP or PA catheters may be appropriate in selected patients.

Positioning	✓ and pad pressure points. ✓ eyes. Antiembolism stockings and SCD	
Complications	Hypothermia (mild)	Warm iv fluids and inspired gasses. Heating pad on OR table. Wrap head in towels or plastic.
	Trauma or obstruction of ureter	Watch for hematuria or decreased urine flow.

POSTOPERATIVE

Pain management	PCA (p. C-3) Epidural/spinal narcotics (p. C-1)	Ketorolac (30 mg im/iv) is useful for breakthrough pain.

References

1. Barakat RR, Park RC, Grigsby PW, Muss HD, Norris HJ: Corpus: epithelial tumors. In *Principles and Practice of Gynecologic Oncology, 2nd edition.* Hoskins WJ, Perez CA, Young RC, eds. Lippincott-Raven Publishers, Philadelphia: 1996, 859-96.
2. Berman ML, Ballon SC, Lagasse LD, Watring WG: Prognosis and treatment of endometrial cancer. *Am J Obstet Gynecol* 1980; 136(5):679-88.
3. Dicker RC, Greenspan JR, Straus LT, et al: Complication of abdominal and vaginal hysterectomy among women of reproductive age in the United States. The Collaborative Review of Sterilization. *Am J Obstet Gynecol* 1982; 144(7):841-48.
4. DiSaia PJ, Creasman WT: Adenocarcinoma of the uterus. In *Clinical Gynecologic Oncology.* DiSaia PJ, Creasman WT, eds. CV Mosby, St. Louis: 1989, 161-97.
5. Edraki B, Schwartz PE. Operative laparoscopy and the gynecologic oncologist. Commentary and review. *Cancer* 1995; 76:1987-91
6. Liu CY: Complications of laparoscopic hysterectomy: prevention, recognition and management. In *Laparoscopic Hysterectomy and Pelvic Floor Reconstruction.* Liu CY, ed. Blackwell Science, Cambridge: 1996; 277-96.

RADICAL HYSTERECTOMY

SURGICAL CONSIDERATIONS

Description: **Radical hysterectomy** is the preferred mode of therapy for young women with Stage IA, IB, or nonbulky IIA cervical carcinoma who want to preserve ovarian function. It is also appropriate with Stage II endometrial and Stage I vaginal carcinoma. The operation involves the removal of the uterus, along with the upper vagina and all the parametrial tissues to the pelvic sidewall. A pelvic and paraaortic **lymph node dissection** is usually performed at the beginning of the procedure. Suspicious nodes are submitted for pathological frozen-section evaluation. The paravesical and pararectal spaces are then developed, with the "web" of tissue between these two spaces being palpated carefully (Fig 8.1-6). If parametrial tumor extension is noted and/or the lymph nodes are positive on frozen section, the hysterectomy may be aborted. The radical hysterectomy is performed after the pararectal and paravesical spaces have been developed. The uterine arteries are divided at their origin from the anterior division of the internal iliac artery. The ureters are dissected free of the parametrial tissues, which are then transected close to the pelvic sidewall. Next, the rectovaginal space is developed (Fig 8.1-7). The uterosacral ligaments

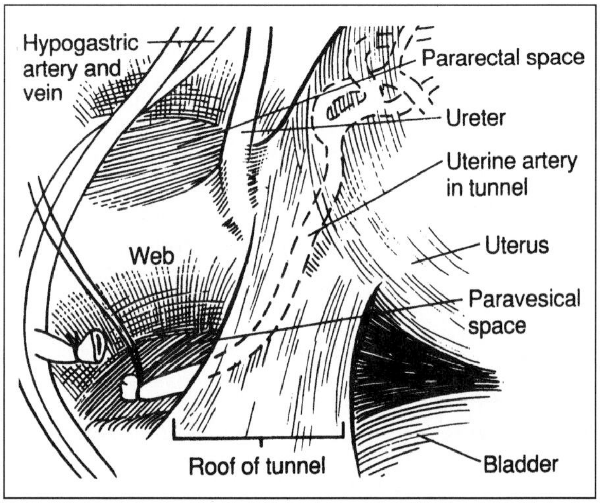

Figure 8.1-6. View of parametrial area, showing positions of ureter and uterine artery to web, hypergastric vessels, paravesical and pararectal spaces. (Reproduced with permission from Wheeless CR: *Atlas of Pelvic Surgery*. Lea & Febiger: 1988.)

are transected between their uterine and sacral attachments. The upper third of the vagina is cross-clamped and divided in such a manner as to provide a 3 cm margin, and the specimen is delivered *en bloc*. Note that, during this procedure, the ureters and bladder are dissected free and left intact.

In selected women younger than 45 yr who may require postop radiotherapy, ovarian function is preserved by performing an **oophoropexy**. This is accomplished by severing the uteroovarian ligament and mobilizing the ovarian vessels as they course through the infundibulopelvic ligament. The ovaries are then sutured outside the radiation therapy field and marked with metal clips for future identification.

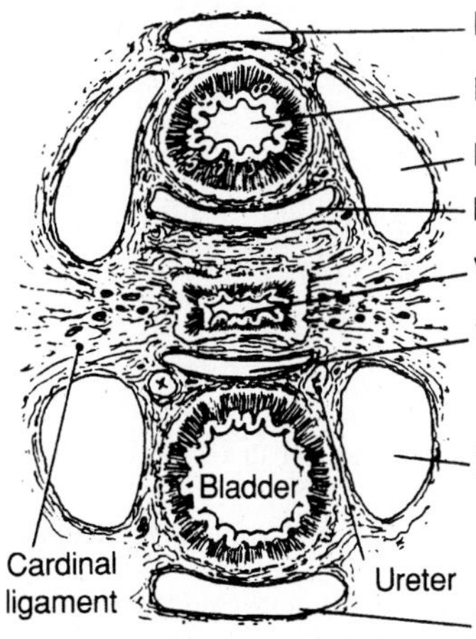

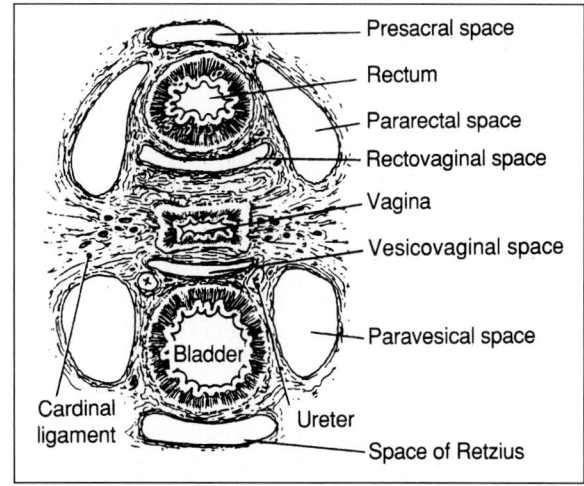

Figure 8.1-7. Schematic diagram of a cut in the anteroposterior plane with positions of all spaces in relation to pelvic organs. (Reproduced with permission from Wheeless CR: *Atlas of Pelvic Surgery*. Lea & Febiger: 1988.)

Variant procedure or approaches: **Stallworthy**, **Dolstad**, **Novak**, **Rutledge**, **Wertheim,** and other surgeons have proposed several modifications in an effort to reduce the incidence of ureteral and bladder fistulae. These approaches include preservation of blood supply to the terminal 2 cm of the pelvic ureter by widely displacing ureters (not dissecting them from their fascial beds) and limiting parametrial dissection to the proximal 1/3 or 1/2.

Usual preop diagnosis: Stage IA, IB, or nonbulky IIA cervical carcinoma; Stage II endometrial or Stage I vaginal carcinoma (less common)

SUMMARY OF PROCEDURE

Position	Supine
Incision	Midline longitudinal or low transverse abdominal (Maylard)
Special instrumentation	Argon beam coagulator, Vital View (suction, irrigation and light source combined in 1 instrument) helpful
Unique considerations	Abort case if positive paraaortic lymph nodes found on frozen section, or if obvious parametrial involvement noted. Consider intraop radiation therapy (investigational), if patient is inoperable.
Antibiotics	Cefotetan 2 g iv on call to OR; then q 12 h × 2 doses
Surgical time	3-6 h
Closing considerations	Vaginal and abdominal drains; NG tube placement; suprapubic bladder catheter placement; oophoropexy; copious irrigation
EBL	500-1500 ml
Postop care	Transient ileus very common. Advance diet slowly. Transient bladder dysfunction very common; therefore, continued bladder drainage for 1+ wk may be necessary. Consider using SCDs and minidose heparin for DVT prophylaxis.
Mortality	0.3-2.0%
Morbidity	Paralytic ileus: 3-11% Pelvic lymphocyst: 6.4% Intraop hemorrhage: 5.6% Thrombophlebitis: 5% Pneumonia: 1.5-4% Wound infection: 3.5% Pelvic infection: 2.2% PE: 2.2% Vesical injury: 2-3.5% Vesical fistulae: 1.8% Small bowel obstruction: 1.5% Ureteral fistulae: 1.1% Ureteral injury: 1.1% Wound dehiscence: 1% Postop lymphedema: < 1% Rectal injury: < 1% Pelvic urinoma: Rare
Pain score	8

PATIENT POPULATION CHARACTERISTICS

Age range	Reproductive and postreproductive yr
Incidence	10/100,000
Etiology	Human papilloma virus (HPV), subtypes 16, 18 (most common) and others
Associated conditions	Smoking; venereal warts; genital herpes; multiple sexual partners; early-age onset of coitus; multiparity; lower socioeconomic status; HIV infection

---

ANESTHETIC CONSIDERATIONS

PREOPERATIVE

This surgery usually is performed for cervical carcinoma in young women who wish to preserve ovarian function, and whose tumor has not spread beyond local invasion. Lymph nodes are removed to confer a therapeutic advantage and to plan postop adjuvant therapy, if any.

Respiratory	These tumors have been associated with cigarette smoking. ✓ for preexisting lung disease. **Tests:** As indicated from H&P.
Cardiovascular	Patients > 50 yr need a preop ECG. **Tests:** As indicated from H&P.
Neurological	Not usually significant unless Hx of neurologic disease.
Musculoskeletal	Question patient about any joint or muscle disease and their exercise tolerance.
Gastrointestinal	Consider supplemental iv hydration in patients given a bowel prep.
Endocrine	Not usually important unless preexisting disease. ✓ for corticosteroid use in the previous 6 mo.
Hematologic	✓ NSAID usage in the previous week. Encourage autologous blood donation. **Tests:** Consider coags if regional anesthetic planned; Hb/Hct; Plt count.
Laboratory	Electrolytes; renal panel; UA; CT scan of pelvis and abdomen (helpful but not necessary)
Premedication	Anxiolytic such as midazolam (1-2 mg iv)

INTRAOPERATIVE

Anesthetic technique: GETA ± epidural or spinal analgesia for postop pain control. (Surgery may be performed in patient with respiratory compromise under epidural or spinal anesthesia).

Induction	Standard induction (p. B-2)	
Maintenance	Standard maintenance (p. B-3). Muscle relaxation usually required to assist with surgical exposure. Prophylactic antiemetic (e.g., metochlopramide 10 mg iv) should be given before the end of surgery.	
Emergence	No special considerations	
Blood and fluid requirements	Occasional blood loss >1500 ml IV: 16-18 ga × 1-2 NS/LR @ 6-8 ml/kg/h Maintain UO > 0.5 ml/kg/h. Warm iv fluids. Humidify inspired gases.	Good iv access is necessary to deal with potential for bleeding. Controlled hypotension to a MAP of 60-70 mmHg may help reduce blood loss. A lymph node dissection will increase 3rd-space losses and should be accounted for in fluid management. Fluid requirements generally are increased by a functioning epidural catheter due to vasodilation. Controversy exists with regard to recurrence of cancer in patients who have received nonautologous blood transfusions.
Monitoring	Standard monitors (p. B-1) Foley catheter CVP catheter ± Arterial catheter	Invasive monitoring is indicated for patients with underlying cardiopulmonary disease, advanced age, or where controlled hypotension is planned.

Positioning	✓ and pad pressure points. ✓ eyes. Antiembolism stockings and SCD	Heating pad on table
Complications	Injury to ureters Hypothermia	Watch for hematuria or decreased urine flow. Warm iv fluids and humidify gases.

POSTOPERATIVE

Complications	Atelectasis Hypothermia Bleeding	Give supplemental O_2 postop. Encourage use of incentive spirometer.
Pain management	PCA (p. C-3) Epidural or spinal narcotics (p. C-1)	Add ketorolac 30 mg im/iv q 8 h for breakthrough pain.

References

1. Ayhan A, Tuncer ZS: Radical hysterectomy with lymphadenectomy for treatment of early stage cervical cancer: clinical experience of 278 cases. *J Surg Oncol* 1991; 47(3):175-77.
2. Ayhan A, Tuncer ZS, Yarali H: Complications of radical hysterectomy in women with early stage cervical cancer: clinical analysis of 270 cases. *Eur J Surg Oncol* 1991; 17(5):492-94.
3. DiSaia PJ, Creasman WT: Invasive cervical cancer. In *Clinical Gynecologic Oncology*. DiSaia PJ, Creasman WT, eds. CV Mosby, St. Louis: 1989, 67-132.
4. Hoskins WJ, Ford JH Jr, Lutz MH, Averette HE: Radical hysterectomy and pelvic lymphadenectomy for the management of early invasive cancer of the cervix. *Gynecol Oncol* 1976; 4(3):278-90.
5. Kindermann G, Debus-Thiede G: Postoperative urological complication after radical surgery for cervical cancer. In *Baillière's Clinical Obstetrics and Gynaecology, Operative Treatment of Cervical Cancer*. Baird DT, et al, eds. Baillière Tindall/WB Saunders Co, London: 1988; 2(4):933-41.
6. Lee YN, Wang KL, Lin MH, Liu CH, Wang KG, Lan CC, Chuang JT, Chen AC, Wu CC: Radical hysterectomy with pelvic lymph node dissection for treatment of cervical cancer: a clinical review of 954 cases. *Gynecol Oncol* 1989; 32:135-42.
7. Meigs JV: Radical hysterectomy with bilateral pelvic lymph node dissections. A report of 100 patients operated on five or more years ago. *Am J Obstet Gynecol* 1951; 62:854-70.
8. Stehman FB, Perez CA, Kurman RJ, Thigpen JT: Uterine cervix. In *Principles and Practice of Gynecologic Oncology, 2nd edition*. Hoskins WJ, Perez CA, Young RC, eds. Lippincott-Raven Publishers, Philadelphia: 1996, 785-858.
9. Symmonds RE, Pratt JH: Prevention of fistulas and lymphocysts in radical hysterectomy. *Obstet Gynecol* 1961; 17:57-64.
10. Webb MJ: Radical hysterectomy. *Baillieres Clin Obstet Gynaecol* 1997; 11(1):149-66.

INTERSTITIAL PERINEAL IMPLANTS

SURGICAL CONSIDERATIONS

Description: Radiotherapy is the treatment modality of choice for International Federation of Gynecology and Obstetrics (FIGO) Stage IIB-IVA carcinoma of the cervix; Stage I, II, III and IVA vaginal cancers; selected vulvar cancers; and pelvic recurrences of gynecologic cancers. Often, **external-beam therapy** is combined with **brachytherapy**, either in the form of **intracavitary insertion** or as an **interstitial perineal template implant**. Intracavitary radiotherapy utilizes devices such as Fletcher-Suit or cylinders that are fitted into the vagina and provide a therapeutic boost to the vaginal apex region after external beam irradiation. In general, these devices do not require a laparotomy or laparoscopy for guidance. For selected patients with distorted anatomy and/or bulky tumors, interstitial implants provide superior dose distribution and better local tumor control. The two most widely used systems are the **Martinez Universal Perineal Interstitial Template (MUPIT)** and the **Syed-Neblett applicator**. These systems have similar efficacy and both are performed in the OR with the patient under local or GA. A **laparotomy** is frequently performed at the time of interstitial implant placement to accurately guide the needles into their target tissues and to avoid radiation injury to bowel and/or other pelvic organs not involved with tumor. To minimize postop patient discomfort, some centers use **laparoscopy** instead of laparotomy for needle guidance. A two-team approach is used: gynecologic/oncology team performs the laparotomy or laparoscopy and guides the needles from above; radiation/oncology team inserts the implants from below. The implants are afterloaded with the appropriate radiation source when the patient has returned to her shielded room. If a hysterectomy has been done before, an omental pelvic carpet, or a pelvic lid made of delayed, absorbable mesh, is performed to provide additional space between the radiation source and bowel.

SUMMARY OF PROCEDURE

	Laparotomy-Guided	Laparoscopy-Guided
Position	Modified dorsolithotomy; Allen stirrups	⇐
Incision	Midline longitudinal abdominal	Vertical infraumbilical and multiple small transverse incisions at the pubic hairline
Special instrumentation	Syed-Neblett or MUPIT systems, or modifications thereof	⇐ + Videolaparoscopy equipment, preferably with a 3-chip camera
Unique considerations	MRI and/or CT scans + information from physical exam are used to pre plan implant with a computer dosimetry program. Patients require thorough preop mechanical and antibiotic bowel prep. Preop epidural placement or postop PCA (see pp. C-1-3) may prove helpful for pain control. Foley catheter needs to be inserted through an opening at the top of the clear plastic template prior to implant positioning.	⇐ + Adhesions of variable severity may be present from prior surgery or radiation. Care should be taken to avoid possible bowel injury at time of trocar insertion. Patient needs to be in steep Trendelenburg position for duration of procedure.
Antibiotics	Cefotetan 2 g iv on call to OR; then q 12 h × 3 doses	⇐
Surgical time	1.5-3 h	⇐
EBL	150-350 ml	Minimal
Closing considerations	Suture template to perineum. Perform rectal exam and adjust any needles that are too close to, or have protruded through, the rectal mucosa. Pack any space between template and perineum with Vaseline gauze. Obtain A-P and lateral orthogonal localization films with the patient in the supine bed rest position. Insert Hypaque dye into bladder (via Foley catheter) prior to localization films. Consider insertion of a large Foley into the rectum and attach to a drainage bag. Consider NG tube placement.	⇐ + Release the pneumoperitoneum completely. Consider insertion of 1 L heparinized LR to cause the bowel to float and remain mobile, thus minimizing the risk of radiation injury.
Postop care	Patient is confined to bed while interstitial implants are in place. SCDs and minidose heparin for DVT prophylaxis. Vigorous use of incentive spirometry. Consider constipating medications (e.g., Lomotil). Patient must be placed in a shielded room. Visitors and medical personnel should interact with patient from behind a lead shield until radiation sources have been removed.	⇐
Mortality	0.1-0.3%	⇐
Morbidity	Rectovaginal fistula: 10-20%	⇐
	Vesicovaginal fistula: 6-20%	⇐
	Hemorrhagic proctitis with diarrhea and tenesmus: 7-18%	⇐
	Radiation cystitis: 7-10%	⇐
	Cervical necrosis: 5-6%	⇐
	Vaginal vault necrosis: 3-5%	⇐
	Rectal fibrosis: 2-5%	⇐
	Pelvic infection: 2-3%	⇐
Pain score	8-9	8-9

PATIENT POPULATION CHARACTERISTICS

Age range	Reproductive and postreproductive yr; childhood, rare
Etiology	Cervical, vaginal or vulvar carcinomas; pelvic recurrence of gynecologic malignancies

ANESTHETIC CONSIDERATIONS

PREOPERATIVE

Radiation implants are used for palliation or cure in cervical, endometrial and ovarian carcinoma. The implants concentrate the radiation close to the site of the tumor and may be supplemented by external beam radiation as well. The unusual tolerance of the uterus and vagina to radiation permit large doses to be given, and accounts for the success in treating cervical lesions.[11] The sigmoid, rectum and large bowel are much more sensitive to radiation injury and limit the dose of radiation that may be given to the pelvis.

Respiratory Usually not significant unless underlying lung disease is present.

Cardiovascular Many patients with pelvic tumors are elderly and prone to cardiovascular disease. There are no specific recommendations except to check a preop ECG in all patients > 50 yr who are otherwise asymptomatic.
Tests: ECG; others as indicated from H&P.

Neurological Usually not significant unless there is Hx of neurologic disease.

Musculoskeletal Inquire about any Hx of arthritis or osteoporosis. ✓ NSAID usage.

Hematologic **Tests:** CBC; PT; PTT

Laboratory UA; electrolytes; renal panel

Premedication An anxiolytic such as midazolam (1-3 mg iv) may be used if necessary.

INTRAOPERATIVE

Anesthetic technique: Regional or GA, depending on site involved. A postop epidural is useful for pain management.

Induction Standard induction (see p. B-2).

Maintenance Standard maintenance (see p. B-3). It is not necessary to maintain neuromuscular blockade after intubation.

Emergence Metoclopramide (10 mg iv) or droperidol (0.5-1 mg iv) can be given for prophylaxis against nausea 30 min before emergence.

Blood and fluid requirements Small blood loss
IV: 18-20 ga × 1
NS/LR @ 2-4 ml/kg/h

Monitoring Standard monitors (see p. B-1).

Positioning ✓ and pad pressure points.
✓ eyes.
Antiembolism stockings and SCD

POSTOPERATIVE

Pain management Epidural narcotics (see p. C-1).
PCA (see p. C-3).

Ketorolac 30-60 mg im/iv q 6 h is useful for breakthrough pain, unless the patient has peptic ulcer disease or renal insufficiency.

References

1. Ampuero F, Doss LL, Khan M, Skipper B, Hilgers RD: The Syed-Neblett interstitial template in locally advanced gynecological malignancies. *Int J Radiat Oncol Biol Phys* 1983; 9(12):1897-1903.
2. Aristizabal SA, Surwit EA, Hevezi JM, Heusinkveld RS: Treatment of advanced cancer of the cervix with transperineal interstitial irradiation. *Int J Radiat Oncol Biol Phys* 1983; 9(7):1013-17.

3. DiSaia PJ, Nolan JF, Arneson AN: Radiation therapy in gynecology. In *Obstetrics and Gynecology*, 4th edition. Danforth DN, ed. Harper and Row, Philadelphia: 1982, 1214-30.
4. Edraki B, Teng NNH, Kapp DS, O'Hanlan KA: Laparoscopically assisted interstitial perineal implantation and pelvic lid construction: description of an effective and minimally invasive method (abstract). *Gynecol Oncol* 1995; 56:133.
5. Feder BH, Syed AM, Neblett D: Treatment of extensive carcinoma of the cervix with the "transperineal parametrial butterfly," a preliminary report on the revival of Waterman's approach. *Int J Radiat Oncol Biol Phys* 1978; 4(7-8):735-42.
6. Fu KK, Snead PK, Leibel SA, Nori D, Peschel RE: Carcinoma of the cervix. In *Interstitial Brachytherapy: Physical, Biological, and Clinical Considerations*. Anderson LL, Nath R, Weaver KA, Nori D, Phillips TL, Son YU, Chin-Tsao ST, Meigooni AS, Meli JA, Smith V, eds. Interstitial Collaborative Working Group. Raven Press, New York: 1990, 179-88.
7. Hockel M, Knapstein PG: The combined operative and radiotherapeutic treatment (CORT) of recurrent tumors infiltrating the pelvic wall: first experience with 18 patients. *Gynecol Oncol* 1992; 46(1):20-8.
8. Hughes-Davies L, Silver B, Kapp DS: Parametrial interstitial brachytherapy for advanced or recurrent pelvic malignancy: the Harvard/Stanford experience. *Gynecol Oncol* 1995; 58:24-7.
9. Martinez A, Edmundson GK, Cox RS, Gunderson LL, Howes AE: Combination of external beam irradiation and multiple-site perineal application (MUPIT) for treatment of locally advanced or recurrent prostatic, anorectal, and gynecologic malignancies. *Int J Radiat Oncol Biol Phys* 1985; 11(2):391-98.
10. Monk BJ, Walker JL, Tewari K, Ramsinghani NS, Nisar Syed AM, DiSaia PJ: Open interstitial brachytherapy for the treatment of local-regional recurrences of uterine corpus and cervix cancer after primary surgery. *Gynecol Oncol* 1994; 52:222-28.
11. Montana GS, Fowler WC, Varia MA, Walton LA, Mack Y, Shemanski L: Carcinoma of the cervix, Stage III. Results of radiation therapy. *Cancer* 1986; 57(1):148-54.
12. Perez CA, Hall EJ, Purdy JA, Williamson J: Biologic and physical aspects of radiation oncology. In *Principles and Practice of Gynecologic Oncology, 2nd edition.* Hoskins WJ, Perez CA, Young RC, eds. Lippincott-Raven Publishers, Philadelphia: 1996, 305-80.
13. Phillips TL, Nori D, Peschel RE: Carcinoma of the vagina and vulva. In *Interstitial Brachytherapy: Physical, Biological, and Clinical Considerations*. Anderson LL, Nath R, Weaver KA, Nori D, Phillips TL, Son YU, Chin-Tsao ST, Meigooni AS, Meli JA, Smith V, eds. Interstitial Collaborative Working Group. Raven Press, New York: 1990, 189-97.
14. Rotman M, Aziz H: Techniques in the radiation treatment of carcinoma of the uterine cervix. *Int J Radiat Oncol Biol Phys* 1991; 20(1):173-75.

Surgeons

M. Thomas Margolis, MD
W. LeRoy Heinrichs, MD, PhD

8.2 GYNECOLOGY/INFERTILITY SURGERY

Anesthesiologist

Emily F. Ratner, MD

DILATATION AND CURETTAGE

SURGICAL CONSIDERATIONS

Description: During dilatation and curettage (D&C), the endometrial lining of the uterus and coexisting lesions (myoma, polyp) are removed. This procedure is performed to diagnose and treat bleeding from uterine and cervical lesions, to complete an incomplete or missed spontaneous abortion (SAB), or to treat cervical stenosis. It is used infrequently as a primary method for pregnancy termination. A D&C is performed less frequently with the advent of the office endometrial biopsy and medical management of bleeding problems.

With the patient in the dorsal lithotomy position, the surgeon initially performs a bimanual examination under anesthesia to obtain information about both the presence of adnexal pathology and anatomic detail of the uterus. A speculum is inserted into the vagina, and the cervix is grasped with a clamp. The cervix is pulled gently toward the operator, who then uses a uterine probe to delineate the length of the uterus and the angulation between the cervical canal and uterus. The uterine cavity is reached by dilating the cervical canal with progressively larger dilators (Hegar's or Pratt) to an 8-9 mm diameter. A ureteral stone forceps is often used at this stage to remove existing polyps; and a curette is used to systematically remove the endometrial lining (Fig 8.2-1).

Usual preop diagnosis: Uncontrolled uterine bleeding refractory to hormonal treatment in young women; abnormal uterine bleeding in perimenopausal/postmenopausal women; incomplete, missed or induced abortion; cervical stenosis causing dysmenorrhea or infertility

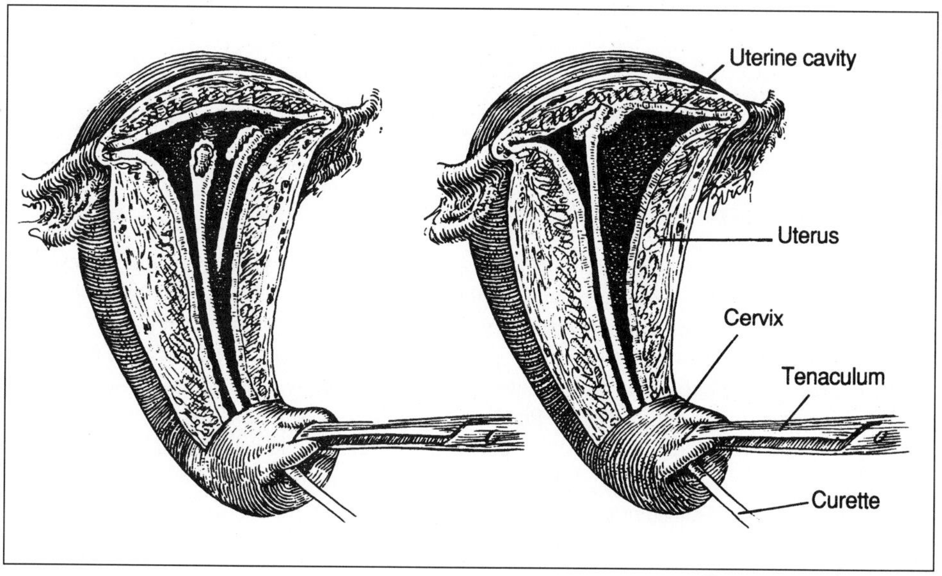

Figure 8.2-1. Curettage of endometrial lining. (Reproduced with permission from Thompson JD, Rock JA, eds: *TeLinde's Operative Gynecology*, 7th edition. JB Lippincott: 1992.)

SUMMARY OF PROCEDURE

Position	Dorsal lithotomy with stirrups
Incision	None
Special instrumentation	To prevent peroneal nerve injury, the area of the leg leaning against the stirrup should be well cushioned. Following induction, perineum is positioned at the very end of the table to ensure optimum exposure. During the cervical dilatation, a vasovagal response can occur, with subsequent bradycardia and hypotension. Uterine perforations will often cause severe postop pain.
Antibiotics	None
Surgical time	5-15 min
EBL	50-100 ml
Mortality	Minimal
Morbidity	Postop fever: 1.7% Uterine perforation: 0.63% Severe immediate postop bleeding (caused by either uterine artery perforation or cervical injury): < 1%
Pain score	3-5

PATIENT POPULATION CHARACTERISTICS

Age range	20-80 yr
Incidence	> 1/50 females
Etiology	Dysfunctional uterine bleeding
Associated conditions	Obesity; HTN

ANESTHETIC CONSIDERATIONS

See Anesthetic Considerations following Therapeutic Abortion, Dilatation and Evacuation, p. 578.

References

1. Mackenzie IZ, Bibby JG: Critical assessment of dilatation and curettage in 1029 women. *Lancet* 1978; 2(8089):566-68.
2. Rock JA, Thompson JD, eds: *TeLinde's Operative Gynecology*, 8th edition. Lippincott-Raven Publishers, Philadelphia: 1997.

THERAPEUTIC ABORTION, DILATATION AND EVACUATION

SURGICAL CONSIDERATIONS

Description: **Therapeutic abortion (TAB)** is the elective termination of a pregnancy prior to viability (usually considered to be 24 wk). In 1982, 1,574,000 legal abortions were performed in the U.S., a ratio of 426 abortions per 1,000 live births. **Suction curettage** is the most efficient method to terminate pregnancies during the first trimester (< 12 wk), and the great majority of abortions are performed this way. Few (< 5%) of first trimester abortions in the U.S. are performed with a sharp curette. Increased operative time and blood loss is seen with this method, resulting in its being practiced mainly in locations where a suction apparatus is not available. Suction curettage for a spontaneous abortion (SAB) is performed in a manner identical to a regular TAB, except that a cervical dilatation might not be needed and the blood loss is usually 2-3 times greater. Very early termination (< 4 wk following LMP) can be performed without anesthesia, using a method called "menstrual regulation."

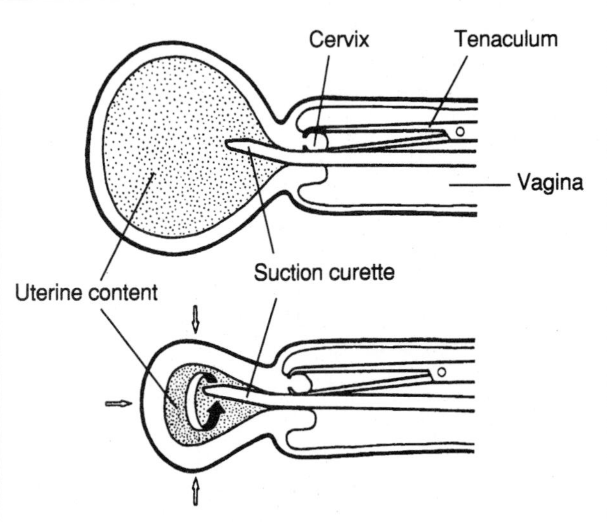

Figure 8.2-2. Uterine aspiration. Top—uterus at beginning of procedure; bottom—at conclusion of procedure. (Reproduced with permission from Thompson JD, Rock JA, eds: *TeLinde's Operative Gynecology*, 7th edition. JB Lippincott: 1992.)

The **TAB procedure** consists of a standard cervical dilatation (required for gestations > 6 wk), followed by vacuum aspiration of the uterine contents, using a plastic suction curette (Fig 8.2-2). Alternatively, the cervical canal can be dilated > 6 hr prior to the operation with laminaria or synthetic osmotic dilators which, after insertion, swell to provide dilatation. A sharp curette is often used at the very end to gently verify the emptiness of the cavity, followed by reaspiration. Due to the risk of missing the pregnancy, most physicians wait until 7-8 wk following the LMP before performing the operation. Ergonovine maleate (0.4 mg im) and oxytocin (Pitocin) 20-30 U/1000 ml iv is often used during the procedure to reduce bleeding, although the efficacy of oxytocin has been questioned. The procedure is performed under either local or GA; it is generally felt that local is safer. Regardless of the method used, the obtained product of conception (POC) is sent for histological examination to exclude the presence of trophoblastic tissue or ectopic pregnancy.

Variant procedure: Dilatation and evacuation (D&E) remains the safest method for mid-trimester pregnancy termination.[2] It is performed similarly to first-trimester suction curettage, with the addition of using large-ring forceps to grasp and remove fetal parts intermittently. This procedure is often performed under paracervical block.

Usual preop diagnosis: Pregnancy (viable or nonviable): 52% within 8 wk estimated gestational age; 90% within 12 wk estimated gestational age

SUMMARY OF PROCEDURE

	1st-Trimester Suction Curettage		2nd-Trimester D&E	
Position	Dorsal lithotomy with patient in Allen stirrups. Following induction, perineum positioned at end of table to ensure optimum exposure.		⇐	
Incision	None		⇐	
Special instrumentation	Suction		⇐ + Large-ring forceps	
Unique considerations	To prevent peroneal nerve injury, the area of the leg leaning against stirrup should be well cushioned. During cervical dilatation, a vasovagal reaction can occur → ↓HR + ↓BP. During injection of lidocaine for paracervical block, seizures may occur if > 12 ml of 1% solution are injected. Uterine perforations will often cause excessive postop pain.		⇐	
Antibiotics	Doxycycline 100 mg iv		⇐	
Surgical time	5-15 min		15-45 min	
EBL[6]	No. wk gestation:		300-500 ml	
	1-4	10 ml		
	5-8	10-30 ml		
	9-10	30-80 ml		
	11-12	80-200 ml		
	13-14	200-400 ml		
Postop care	PACU		⇐	
Mortality	0-3.1/100,000[3,4]		13/100,000[2]	
Morbidity	Mild infection	1/216	T > 38° for > 1 d	13.4/1,000
	Resuctioned day of surgery	1/553	Cervical injury	11.6/1,000
	Resuctioned subsequently	1/596	Cervical tear	10/1,000
	Cervical stenosis causing amenorrhea	1/6,071	Retained POC	9/1,000
	Cervical incompetence	1/9,444	Hemorrhage	7.1/1,000
	Underestimation of gestational age	1/15,454	UTI	1.8/1,000
	Convulsive seizure (after local anesthesia)	1/25,086		
	Total	1/118		
Complications requiring hospitalization	Incomplete abortion	1/3,617	Endometritis	8.5/1,000
	Sepsis	1/4,722	Uterine perforation	3.2/1,000
	Uterine perforation	1/10,625	Need for laparotomy	2.1/1,000
	Vaginal bleeding	1/14,166	Need for blood transfusion	1.9/1,000
	Inability to complete	1/28,333		
	Coexisting tubal pregnancy	1/42,500		
	Total	1/1,405		
Pain score	5		5	

PATIENT POPULATION CHARACTERISTICS

Age range	15-45 yr
Incidence	> 1/5 females
Etiology	Wishing pregnancy termination

ANESTHETIC CONSIDERATIONS

(Procedures covered: dilatation and curettage [D&C]; therapeutic abortion [TAB], dilatation and evacuation [D&E])

PREOPERATIVE

These are among the most common procedures performed in gynecology. Patients presenting for these procedures are generally healthy; however, bleeding and sepsis may alter ASA status.

Cardiovascular Hemodynamic status may be impaired 2° preop uterine bleeding, and patient may be septic from retained uterine products. ✓ BP, HR, orthostatic vital signs.
Tests: As indicated from H&P.

Laboratory Hb/Hct; other tests as indicated from H&P.

Premedication Anxiolytic (e.g., midazolam 1-2 mg iv) as needed.

INTRAOPERATIVE

Anesthetic technique: Local, regional or GA all may be appropriate. In the younger patient population, spinal anesthesia may be less desirable because of increased incidence of postdural puncture headache (PDPH).

Local anesthesia: Some obstetricians/gynecologists perform these procedures under local anesthesia. Paracervical block has the potential for inadvertent iv administration with consequent toxic reaction.

Regional anesthesia: A T10 sensory level is sufficient to provide anesthesia for procedures on the uterus.

Spinal 5% lidocaine 75-100 mg (controversial); 0.75% bupivacaine 10-15 mg in 7.5% dextrose. (See Anesthetic Considerations for Cesarean Section, p. 602.) If spinal anesthesia is indicated, a pencil-point spinal needle (e.g., Whitacre or Sprotte) should be used to decrease the incidence of PDPH.[9]

Epidural 1.5-2.0% lidocaine with epinephrine 5 μg/ml, 15-25 ml; supplement with 5-10 ml as needed. Supplemental iv sedation. (See Anesthetic Considerations for Cesarean Section, p. 602.)

General anesthesia:

Induction Standard induction (see p. B-2).

Maintenance Standard maintenance (see p. B-3) used commonly, although frequently done by mask with O_2/N_2O + volatile anesthetic and spontaneous respiration. May also use propofol infusion (100-250 μg/kg/min), with N_2O, without volatile anesthetic. A small amount of opiate may be used. High incidence of postop N/V warrant prophylactic treatment with metoclopramide (5-10 mg iv). Ondansetron (4 mg iv) may prove useful in these patients.

Emergence Be ready with suction in the event of vomiting on emergence.

Blood and fluid requirements	Minimal blood loss IV: 18 ga × 1 (unless hypovolemic) NS/LR @ 2 ml/kg/h	Usual replacement of maintenance fluids and overnight deficit with crystalloid. Blood replacement rarely indicated.
Control of blood loss	Oxytocin (Pitocin) 20-30 U Ergonovine maleate (0.2 mg)	Oxytocin causes uterine contraction, with a consequent decrease in blood loss. Rapid iv bolus may lead to hypotension. Oxytocin is usually diluted in 1 L of crystalloid and then infused. Ergonovine maleate also causes uterine contraction and is usually given im. Side effects include HTN, myocardial ischemia and dysrhythmias, especially if given iv.[7]
Monitoring	Standard monitors (p. B-1)	
Positioning	✓ hip, leg, hand position. ✓ and pad pressure points. ✓ eyes. Shoulder abducted < 90°	Lithotomy position can be deleterious to pulmonary function, as it may impair respiratory mechanics. Rarely, hemodynamic changes can occur on elevation of the legs into the stirrups, as this increases venous return to the heart. Problems with hypotension on lowering legs postop are more common.
Vagal stimulation	Bradycardia	When cervix is grasped and dilated, patient may have excessive vagal stimulation, which can be treated by

Vagal stimulation, cont.		prompt cessation of stimulation and with atropine (0.4 mg iv), if indicated.
Complications	Nerve injury	Be sure that no peripheral nerve injury (e.g., foot drop) occurs. Common peroneal nerve palsy is possible if pressure on the nerve over fibula is not prevented by adequate padding or positioning. Hyperflexion of the hip joint can cause femoral and lateral femoral cutaneous nerve palsy. Obturator and saphenous nerve injury are also complications of the lithotomy position.[1]
	Finger trauma	Take care to insure safety of patient's fingers when manipulating foot of the bed. Avoid finger injury by placing patient's arms on arm boards or by wrapping her hands.[6]

POSTOPERATIVE

Complications	High incidence of N/V Uterine rupture with severe abdominal pain (rare) Severe hemorrhage, necessitating blood transfusion (rare)	Antiemetics, including metoclopramide 10 mg iv, droperidol 1 mg iv and ondansetron 4 mg iv, can be useful in this setting. Severe immediate postop bleeding caused by uterine atony, retained POCs, uterine artery perforation, or cervical injury.[2]
Pain management	IV opiate	Oral pain medications may be satisfactory. Extreme pain may be caused by uterine perforation.
Tests	Hb/Hct, if hemorrhage	

References

1. Courtney, MA: Neurologic sequelae of childbirth and regional anesthesia. In *Manual of Obstetric Anesthesia.* Churchill Livingstone, New York: 1992.
2. Grimes DA et al: Mid-trimester abortion by dilatation and evacuation. *N Engl J Med* 1977; 296(20):1141-45.
3. Grimes DA, Cates W Jr: Complications from legally-induced abortion: a review. *Obstet Gynecol Surg* 1979; 34(3):177-91.
4. Hakim-Elahi E: Complications of first-trimester abortion: a report of 170,000 cases. *Obstet Gynecol* 1990; 76(1):129-35.
5. Nakata DA, Stoelting RK: Positioning. *In Patient Safety in Anesthetic Practice.* Morell RC, Eichhorn JH, eds. Churchill Livingstone, New York: 1997, 293-318.
6. Pernoll ML, ed: *Current Obstetrics and Gynecologic Diagnosis and Treatment.* Appleton & Lange, Norwalk, CT: 1991, 686-91.
7. *Physician's Desk Reference*, 52nd edition. Medical Economics Data, Inc, Montvale NJ: 1998.
8. Rock JA, Thompson JD, eds: *TeLinde's Operative Gynecology*, 8th edition. Lippincott-Raven Publishers, Philadelphia: 1997.
9. Ross BK, Chadwick HS, Mancuso JS, Benedetti C: Sprotte needle for obstetric anesthesia: Decreased incidence of post dural puncture headache. *Reg Anesth* 1992; 17:29-33.

HYSTEROSCOPY

SURGICAL CONSIDERATIONS

Description: Hysteroscopy is a procedure in which the endometrial cavity can be examined, allowing for direct visualization of lesions. The procedure is used primarily to investigate abnormal uterine bleeding, often caused by intrauterine submucous myoma and polyps. After the diagnosis, these lesions can be removed using a variety of techniques. For example, ablation of the endometrial lining may be carried out with a rollerball, resectoscope or Nd:YAG laser.

Variant procedure or approaches: Diagnostic hysteroscopies can be performed under both GA and local anesthesia, while **operative hysteroscopies** are usually performed under GA. An examination under anesthesia is performed, followed by the insertion of open speculum and the attachment of a tenaculum to the cervix. The cervical canal is dilated until the hysteroscope with its sheath can be introduced (Fig 8.2-3). A distention medium is then used to provide adequate visualization (Table 8.2-1). Several different distention media are used (e.g., CO_2 is frequently used for diagnostic cases). The flow is limited to 1200 ml/min and the intrauterine pressure is kept < 200 mmHg in order to prevent cardiac dysrhythmias.

For optimum operative hysteroscopy in the presence of bleeding, dextran 70 (Hyskon) is the most frequently used medium. It is highly viscous and not miscible with blood; thus, it provides superb visibility. Although fatal anaphylaxis has been noted only rarely, an attempt should be made to keep the amount used to < 50 ml. Dextrose, 4-6% dextran and 3% sorbitol in water also have been used; but due to their miscibility with blood, fewer operative cases are performed with this media. A view camera can be attached to the hysteroscope to allow for easier visualization. During operative cases, an accompanying laparoscope is often introduced from above to evaluate the progress of the hysteroscopy and to safeguard against uterine perforation and potential bowel injury.

Usual preop diagnosis: Abnormal uterine bleeding; infertility; recurrent pregnancy loss

Table 8.2-1: Choice of Distention Media (++ = preferred; + = satisfactory; – = not used)

	CO_2	Hyskon	Low-viscosity fluid
Office use	++	–	+
OR use	++	++	++
Diagnostic	++	++	+
Operative	–	++	–

SUMMARY OF PROCEDURE

Position	Dorsal lithotomy (Allen stirrups)
Incision	None
Special instrumentation	CO_2 insufflator; Hyskon or fluid pump; laser; electrocautery equipment
Unique considerations	Accelerated fluid absorption with prolonged procedures or with resections may lead to pulmonary edema. Laparoscopy often accompanies this procedure.
Surgical time	15 min-2 h
Antibiotics	Cefazolin 1 g iv
EBL	0-100 ml
Postop care	Excessive postop bleeding can be controlled by using a 5 ml Foley balloon catheter in the uterus for several h.[5]
Mortality	1/10,000 anaphylaxis to Hyskon[2]
Morbidity	Shoulder pain can occur from CO_2 used as a distention medium. Pleural effusion can be seen with use of low-viscosity medium.[1]
Pain score	3-5

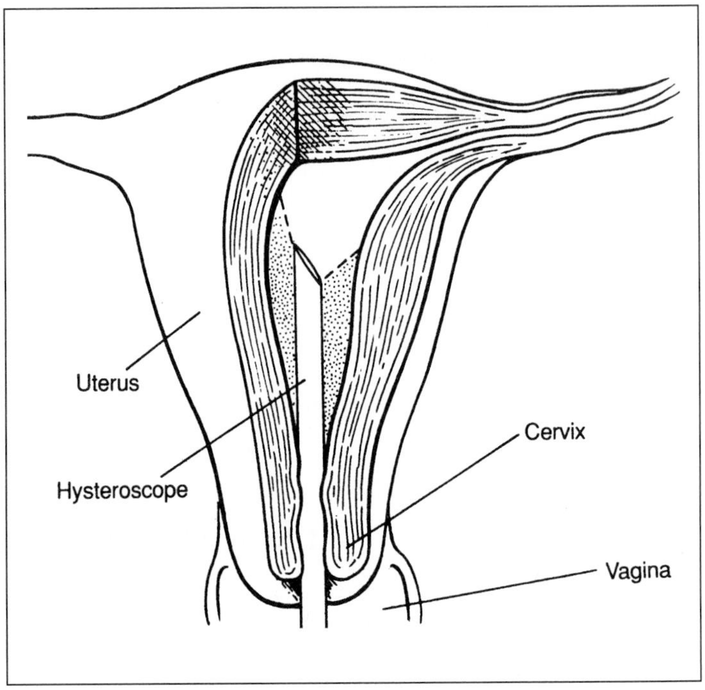

Figure 8.2-3. Hysteroscopy. (Reproduced with permission from Baggish MS, Barbot S, Valle RF: *Diagnostic & Operative Hysteroscopy*. Year Book Medical Pub: 1989.)

PATIENT POPULATION CHARACTERISTICS

Age range	20-80 yr
Incidence	> 1/50
Etiology	Unexplained uterine bleeding; infertility
Associated conditions	Obesity

ANESTHETIC CONSIDERATIONS

PREOPERATIVE

Hysteroscopy may be performed for diagnostics or treatment of intrauterine pathology. Patients presenting for this procedure are generally healthy.

Cardiovascular As patient may be undergoing hysteroscopy for uterine bleeding, BP, HR and orthostatic vital signs should be noted.
Tests: As indicated from H&P.

Laboratory Hb/Hct if bleeding Hx. Other tests as indicated from H&P.

Premedication Anxiolytic (e.g., midazolam 1-2 mg iv) as needed.

INTRAOPERATIVE

Anesthetic technique: Local, regional or GA may be used. In the younger patient population, spinal anesthesia may be less desirable because of increased incidence of postdural puncture headache (PDPH). If spinal anesthesia is indicated, pencil point spinal needles (e.g., Sprotte or Whitacre) should be used to decrease the incidence of PDPH.[9]

Local anesthesia: Some procedures may be done under local, especially if they are diagnostic. Paracervical block has the potential for an inadvertent intravenous administration, with consequent toxic reaction.

Regional anesthesia: A T10 sensory level is sufficient to provide anesthesia for these procedures.

Spinal 5% lidocaine 75-100 mg (controversial); 0.75% bupivacaine 10-15 mg in 7.5% dextrose. (See Anesthetic Considerations for Cesarean Section, p. 602.)

Epidural 1.5-2.0% lidocaine with epinephrine 5 μg/ml, 15-25 ml; supplement with 5-10 ml as needed. Supplemental iv sedation. (See Anesthetic Considerations for Cesarean Section, p. 602.)

General anesthesia:

Induction Standard induction (see p. B-2).

Maintenance Standard maintenance (see p. B-3). Patients have a high incidence of vomiting, so prophylaxis (e.g., metoclopramide 10 mg iv), as in patients for D&C, is warranted.

Emergence Be ready with suction in the event of vomiting on emergence.

Blood and fluid requirements Minimal blood loss
IV: 18 ga × 1 (unless hypovolemic)
NS\LR @ 2 ml/kg/h

Usual replacement of maintenance fluids and overnight deficit in the form of crystalloid. Blood replacement is almost never indicated.

Positioning ✓ hip, leg and hand positions.
✓ and pad pressure points.
✓ eyes.
Shoulder abduction < 90°

Lithotomy position can be deleterious to pulmonary function, as it may impair respiratory mechanics. Rarely, hemodynamic changes occur on elevation of legs into the stirrups, as this increases venous return to the heart. Problems with hypotension on lowering legs postop are common. Take care to insure that no peripheral nerve injury occurs. Common peroneal nerve palsy is possible if pressure on the nerve over the fibula is not prevented by adequate padding or positioning. Hyperflexion of hip joint can cause femoral and lateral femoral cutaneous nerve palsy. Obturator and saphenous nerve injury are also complications of the lithotomy position.[3] Take care to ensure safety of patient's fingers when manipulating the foot of the bed. Avoid finger injury by placing patient's arms on arm boards or by wrapping her hands.

Monitoring Standard monitors (see p. B-1).

Surgical stimulation When cervix is grasped and dilated, patient may have excessive vagal nerve stimulation.

RX: prompt cessation of stimulation by surgeons and treatment with atropine, if indicated.

Complications	Pulmonary edema Coagulopathy Anaphylactoid reactions Finger injury	Dextran 70 (Hyskon) and dextran 40 are frequently infused into the uterus during hysteroscopy to facilitate visualization of intrauterine structures. Case reports of ARDS, pulmonary edema, DIC, as well as Plt dysfunction, have been reported when large volumes have been used.[4,5,11] It has been recommended that no more than 300 ml of this solution be infused to avoid these potentially serious complications. Anaphylactoid reactions have also occurred after exposure to Hyskon.

POSTOPERATIVE

Complications	High incidence of N/V Respiratory compromise from excessive Hyskon absorption	Antiemetics, including metoclopramide 10 mg iv, droperidol 1 mg iv and ondansetron 4 mg iv, can be useful in this setting.
Pain management	Small dose of titrated opiate	Patients usually tolerate oral pain medications.
Tests	Consider CXR and ABG.	If respiratory compromise

References

1. Adoni A, et al: Postoperative pleural effusion caused by dextran. *Int J Gynaecol Obstet* 1980; 18(4):243-44.
2. Borten M, Seibert CP, Taymor ML: Recurrent anaphylactic reaction to intraperitoneal dextran 75 used for prevention of postsurgical adhesions. *Obstet Gynecol* 1983; 61(6):755-57.
3. Courtney MA: Neurologic sequelae of childbirth and regional anesthesia. In *Manual of Obstetric Anesthesia*. Churchill Livingstone, New York: 1992.
4. Jedeikin R, Olsfanger D, Kessler I: Disseminated intravascular coagulopathy and adult respiratory distress syndrome: life-threatening complications of hysteroscopy. *Am J Obstet Gynecol* 1990; 162(1):44-5.
5. Leake JF, Murphy AA, Zacur HA: Noncardiogenic pulmonary edema: a complication of operative hysteroscopy. *Fertil Steril* 1987; 48(3):497-99.
6. Nakata DA, Stoelting RK: Positioning. In *Patient Safety in Anesthetic Practice*. Morell RC, Eichhorn JH, eds. Churchill Livingstone, New York: 1997, 293-318.
7. Pellicer A, Diamond MP: Distending media for hysteroscopy. *Obstet Gynecol Clin North Am* 1988; 15:23-8.
8. Rock, JA, Thompson JD, eds: *TeLinde's Operative Gynecology*, 8th edition. Lippincott-Raven Publishers, Philadelphia: 1997.
9. Ross BK, Chaduck HS, Mancuso JJ, Benedelti C. Sprotte needle for obstetric anesthesia: Decreased incidence of post dural puncture headache. *Reg Anesth* 1992; 17:29-33.
10. Soderstrom RM, ed: *Operative Laparoscopy*, 2nd edition. Lippincott-Raven Publishers, Philadelphia: 1998.
11. Vercellini P, Rossi R, Pagnoni B, Fedele L: Hypervolemic pulmonary edema and severe coagulopathy after intrauterine dextran instillation. *Obstet Gynecol* 1992; 79(5[P + 2]):838-39.

PELVIC LAPAROTOMY

SURGICAL CONSIDERATIONS

Description: These are all common gynecological procedures. **Laparotomy** is most frequently performed via a Pfannenstiel's incision, which permits good pelvic exposure. A vertical incision is used in oncological surgery or in the presence of a large uterus. A knife or Bovie is used to cut through the skin and underlying tissue until the rectus fascia is reached. The fascia is nicked, and then sharply incised bilaterally 2-4" with scissors or electrocautery (Bovie). The rectus muscle is separated sharply in the midline down to the pubis and the peritoneum is entered. The peritoneal incision is then extended vertically or transversely. The pelvis and entire abdominal cavity are first explored by palpation. Then the bowels usually are packed in a cephalad direction with surgical laparotomy sponges (laps) to prevent them from falling back into the pelvis. Good muscle relaxation is important during this stage to ensure optimum packing. A self-retaining retractor is frequently used to keep the laps in place and to enhance exposure. After the desired operation has been performed, the retractor and packs are removed. During the peritoneal closure, abdominal muscle relaxation is again critical in order to minimize tension on this layer and risk of bowel injury with the needle. The rectus fascia, the subcutaneous tissue and, finally, the skin are closed in succession.

Variant procedures: Myomectomies are performed to remove myomata that are causing pain, abnormal bleeding or infertility. Myomata are heavily vascularized at the base, and the surgeon has several ways to minimize this bleeding. A clamp can be placed across the uterine vasculature to minimize blood flow to the uterus. A common alternative is the use of a vasoconstrictor such as diluted epinephrine (1:200,000) or vasopressin solution (1-5 U/10 ml NS). The solution (2-10 ml) is injected around the myoma prior to incising the uterus, which invariably → ↑HR and ↑BP. Gonadotropin releasing hormone (GNRH) agonists may be used for a few months prior to the operation in order to render the patient hypoestrogenic and thus decrease the vascularity of the myomata. After the myomata have been removed, the uterine defects are closed with several layers of suture, and the uterine serosa is closed.

Ovarian cystectomies are performed to alleviate related pain and to diagnose the identity of asymptomatic cysts. Small, single-functional ovarian cysts are found at different stages in a woman's menstrual cycle. At times, due to hormonal imbalance, these cysts can increase in size and quantity, which may cause severe pain. The ovary also can contain various nonfunctional cysts (e.g., tumors) which have to be removed, even if asymptomatic, to rule out malignancy. After the pelvic structures are well visualized, the cystic ovary is stabilized with instruments or surgical laps. Sharp or blunt dissection is used to shell out the cyst intact. If there is any suspicion about the nature of the cyst, an intraop frozen section is obtained. The ovary is then reapproximated and the abdomen closed. If the cyst is large and little healthy ovarian stroma remains, an **oophorectomy** is performed.

Ectopic pregnancies are usually medical emergencies. Increasingly, **laparoscopy** is being used to treat this condition (see p. 628), although laparotomies for ectopic pregnancies are still widely performed. The abdomen is entered, and the pregnancy located quickly. An attempt is made to control the bleeding with the surgeon's hand, a clamp or suture. Frequently, large amounts of blood in the pelvis are suctioned and the ectopic pregnancy is removed via a partial **tubal resection, salpingostomy** or **salpingectomy**; then the abdomen is closed. A **D&C** is often performed at the end to prevent late bleeding from the pregnancy-induced endometrial proliferation (see D&C, p. 575).

In **abdominal colpopexy** (fixation of vagina), the patient is initially placed in the lithotomy position in order to perform an examination under anesthesia, as well as to insert a vaginal pack needed to identify the vaginal apex. A urethral catheter is inserted prior to staging the laparotomy. A rectus fascia graft is obtained during the opening of the abdomen (a synthetic graft can be used instead). The bowel is packed and the defect is examined from the abdominal perspective. Frequently there is an accompanying enterocele which must be closed initially (see **Moschowitz procedure,** below). The peritoneum over the vaginal apex is then entered and the neighboring rectum and bladder are dissected a distance away from the vaginal apex. The peritoneum over the sacrum is incised and the cephalad end of the graft is sutured to the anterior sacral ligament of the third vertebrae. The caudal end of the graft is attached to the vaginal apex, with the surgeon frequently using a vaginal hand to place these last sutures. The peritoneum and abdomen are closed, and the patient is placed back in the dorsal lithotomy position for a high posterior **colporrhaphy** (repair of vagina).

The **Moschowitz procedure** is used to reduce enteroceles via an abdominal approach. The abdomen is entered in the usual fashion, the uterus held up with a traction suture, the bowel packed, and the patient placed in the Trendelenburg position. Multiple concentric purse-string sutures close the defect in the pouch of Douglas; and the abdomen is closed.

The **presacral neurectomy** is an operation performed for women with severe chronic midline pelvic pain. Usually the patient has a history of prior surgeries to diagnose and treat the problem. A laparotomy is initially performed with packing of the bowels. The rectosigmoid is brought over to the left in order to make a vertical, posterior, parietal, peritoneal incision over the sacral area. The anatomy is examined closely and the presacral nerves are ligated; then the peritoneum and abdomen are closed. Severe bleeding can be seen intraop from the hemorrhoidal and sacral veins, but usually can be controlled with pressure.

Usual preop diagnosis: Myomata (pelvic pain, hypermenorrhea, infertility); ovarian cysts and oophorectomy (pelvic pain, undiagnosed ovarian mass); ectopic pregnancy; vaginal vault prolapse; enterocele; presacral neurectomy (chronic pelvic pain)

SUMMARY OF PROCEDURE

Position	Supine or lithotomy
Incision	Pfannenstiel's or low midline abdominal
Unique considerations	Muscle relaxation is important during bowel packing and abdominal closure. Vasoconstrictor substances for controlling myomata bleeding (1:200,000 epinephrine and 1-5 U vasopressin/10 ml NS) are often used and can alter BP and HR.
Antibiotics	1-2 g iv cefoxitin or cefotetan

Surgical time	45 min-4 h Abdominal colpopexy: 4-5 h
EBL	150-1000 ml (maximum related to procedure)
Postop care	PACU
Mortality	Minimal
Morbidity[2]	Gastric dilatation: 3% Thrombophlebitis: 3% PE: 2% Ureteral stenosis: 1%
Pain score	8

PATIENT POPULATION CHARACTERISTICS

	Myomectomy	Ovarian Cystectomy, Oophorectomy	Ectopic Pregnancy	Abdominal Colpopexy, Moschowitz	Presacral Neurectomy
Age range	20-45 yr	20-85 yr	15-45 yr	40-80 yr	20-50 yr
Incidence	> 1/5 females	⇐	1/100 females	1/500 females	⇐
Etiology	Congenital	Endometriosis Anovulation Adenoma	Preexisting tubal disease	Multiparous obesity Chronic cough	Endometriosis
Associated conditions	Menorrhagia	Endometriosis	Pelvic adhesions	Pelvic relaxation	Endometriosis

ANESTHETIC CONSIDERATIONS

See Anesthetic Considerations following Infertility Operations, p. 585.

References

1. Rock JA, Thompson JD, eds: *TeLinde's Operative Gynecology*, 8th edition. Lippincott-Raven Publishers, Philadelphia: 1997.
2. Uyttenbroeck F: *Gynecologic Surgery - Treatment of Complications and Prevention of Injuries*. Masson Publishing, New York: 1980.

INFERTILITY OPERATIONS/*IN VITRO* FERTILIZATION

SURGICAL CONSIDERATIONS

Description: These operations all deal with reproductive problems. The general trend is to avoid laparotomies and to perform operations using outpatient laparoscopy and hysteroscopy techniques whenever possible.

Fimbrioplasty is used to repair distal fallopian tubal occlusion—a common cause for infertility—which is usually a consequence of pelvic inflammatory disease. The operation is performed most often via a **pelvic laparotomy** (see p. 582). A urethral catheter is inserted to empty the bladder, followed by the insertion of a transcervical uterine catheter for chromopertubation (dye injection). The abdomen is opened and the pelvic structures are exposed. During the operation microsurgical techniques are followed closely to minimize trauma. Meticulous hemostasis is important. A wound protector is often used instead of self-retaining retractors. The peritoneum and pelvic structures are kept moist with intermittent irrigation. An overhead salpingolysis and ovariolysis are performed microsurgically. Once the adnexae have been freed, they are elevated by loosely packing the pouch of Douglas with insulated pads (plastic sheathed covered laps). Chromopertubation is then performed and, if occlusion is present, a new stoma is created using microsurgical instruments and sutures. The abdomen is then closed.

Tubal reanastomosis, performed to restore fertility, is very similar to fimbrioplasty, with microsurgical techniques followed diligently. After the tubal segments have been freed slightly from their underlying mesosalpinx, the occluded ends are cut and chromopertubation is performed to ensure patency. After patency has been established, anastomosis is performed in two layers. The mesosalpinx is reapproximated to the tubal serosa and the abdomen closed.

The uterus is embryologically formed by the fusion of two paramesonephric tubes. At times, the fusion is incomplete and a septated uterus or bicornuate uterus is formed. The malformed uterus is associated with an increased risk for miscarriages and preterm labor. **Metroplasty** is used to correct this condition. The **Strassmann procedure** for bicornuate uteri uses a standard pelvic laparotomy. Following uterine exposure, an incision is made on the medial side of each hemicorpus and carried down until the uterine cavity is entered. The edges are reapproximated to form a single uterus. The **Tompkins procedure** for septated uteri also uses the standard pelvic laparotomy approach. A uterine wedge containing the septum is removed, followed by closure of the uterus. More recently, septated uteri have been repaired via a hysteroscopic approach (see Hysteroscopy, p. 579) with scissors or laser.

Proximal tubal cannulation is a relatively new technique with great promise, in which proximal tubal occlusion can be repaired through either a fluoroscopic or a hysteroscopic approach. The hysteroscopic approach, usually performed under GA, allows the surgeon to insert a small cannula to restore tube patency. This procedure is often done with laparoscopy in order to follow the progress of the cannulization and to visualize the chromopertubation (see Hysteroscopy, p. 579, and Laparoscopy).[1]

Gamete intrafallopian transfer[7] (GIFT) and **tubal embryo transfer** (TET) are methods of **advanced reproductive technology.** Couples who have undergone extensive infertility workups and treatment without success eventually become candidates for GIFT and TET procedures. Ovarian follicles are stimulated to grow with the help of gonadotropins. These follicles are then punctured with a needle transvaginally to "harvest" the eggs. These eggs can be mixed with semen and placed directly into the distal end of the fallopian tube using laparoscopic techniques and a small tubal catheter (see Laparoscopy). In the TET procedure, the semen and eggs are allowed to incubate a few days *in vitro;* embryos form and are transferred to the fallopian tubes in a manner similar to the GIFT procedure.

Usual preop diagnosis: Infertility; history of multiple spontaneous abortion and preterm labor (see Pelvic Laparotomy, p. 582, Laparoscopy and Hysteroscopy)

SUMMARY OF PROCEDURE

(For summaries of specific procedures, see Laparoscopy, Hysteroscopy, p. 579 or Pelvic Laparotomy, p 582.)

PATIENT POPULATION CHARACTERISTICS

Age range	20-40 yr
Incidence	1/20 (female)
Etiology	PID; endometriosis; idiopathic
Associated conditions	Obesity

ANESTHETIC CONSIDERATIONS

(Procedures covered: pelvic laparotomy for myomectomy; ovarian cystectomy; oophorectomy; ectopic pregnancy removal; abdominal colpopexy; Moschowitz enterocele repair; presacral neurectomy; infertility operations)

PREOPERATIVE

This is generally a healthy patient population; however, this procedure can be performed for a wide variety of pathologic conditions.

Cardiovascular Patients undergoing myomectomy and, especially, ectopic pregnancy removal, may have had a significant amount of preop bleeding; therefore, BP, HR and orthostatic vital signs should be noted.

Tests: As indicated from H&P.

Laboratory	Hb/Hct. Patients with ectopic pregnancy may have urine/serum pregnancy tests, as well as pelvic ultrasound.	
Premedication	Patients with ruptured ectopic pregnancies may come to the OR urgently, and should be treated as for full stomach. This includes premedication with a nonparticulate antacid, Na citrate 30 ml po, metoclopramide 10 mg iv, and ranitidine 50 mg iv.	

INTRAOPERATIVE

Anesthetic technique: GETA is preferred in patients undergoing laparoscopic surgery and in patients presenting for emergency surgery. Regional anesthesia is best avoided in hemodynamically unstable patients (i.e., ectopic pregnancies), and for laparoscopy where breathing difficulty may develop 2° to pneumoperitoneum and Trendelenburg position. GA may be suitable for simple laparotomies. In the younger patient population, spinal anesthesia is less desirable because of increased incidence of postdural puncture headache (PDPH). If spinal anesthesia is indicated, a pencil-point needle (e.g., Whitacre, Sprotte) should be used in order to decrease the incidence of PDPH.[6]

General anesthesia:

Induction	Standard induction (see p. B-2). A patient with an intact ectopic pregnancy undergoing laparoscopy should have an ETT placed and be mechanically ventilated to assure adequate oxygenation, ventilation and acid-base balance.[3] In a patient with a ruptured ectopic pregnancy, ketamine 1-2 mg/kg or etomidate 0.1-0.4 mg/kg may be preferable if a large blood loss has occurred. These patients may also have full stomachs; and, in this case, they require a rapid-sequence induction with cricoid pressure and immediate ET intubation (succinylcholine 1.5 mg/kg).
Maintenance	Standard maintenance (see p. B-3). A high incidence of N/V warrants prophylaxis with metoclopramide 10 mg iv, droperidol 1 mg iv, or ondansetron 4 mg iv.
Emergence	Be ready with suction in the event of vomiting on emergence.

Regional anesthesia: A T4-6 sensory level is recommended for pelvic/lower abdominal surgery.

Spinal	5% lidocaine 75-100 mg (controversial); 0.75% bupivacaine 10-15 mg in 7.5% dextrose. (See Anesthetic Considerations for Cesarean Section, p. 602.)
Epidural	1.5-2.0% lidocaine with epinephrine 5 μg/ml, 15-25 ml; supplement with 5-10 ml as needed. Supplemental iv sedation. (See Anesthetic Considerations for Cesarean Section, p. 602.)

Blood and fluid requirements	Possible heavy blood loss IV: 16-18 ga × 1-2 NS/LR @ 5-7 ml/kg/h	Patients with ectopic pregnancies may have large blood loss both preop and intraop. Adequate iv access is imperative in these patients, as is the availability of blood.
Control of blood loss	Epinephrine Vasopressin	During myomectomies, surgeons may inject vasopressors into the area surrounding myomata prior to excision. This can cause HTN and cardiac dysrhythmias.
Monitoring	Standard monitors (p. B-1) ± Foley catheter	
	Ectopic pregnancy: ± Arterial catheter	Patients with ectopic pregnancies may need intraarterial monitoring if major hemorrhage occurs.
Positioning	✓ and pad pressure points. ✓ eyes.	During abdominal colpopexy, patient is placed intermittently in both the lithotomy and supine positions. (See p. 578 for concerns regarding the lithotomy position.)
Complications	Respiratory: Pneumoperitoneum ↑$PaCO_2$, ↓PaO_2 ETT migration	Pneumoperitoneum with CO_2 and steep Trendelenburg position cause cephalad displacement of diaphragm with ↓FRC, ↓pulmonary compliance, and ↑airway closure/atelectasis. Hypercarbia and hypoxia, due to respiratory compromise, can result unless ventilation is controlled during GA. Check for endobronchial migration of ETT upon assumption of Trendelenburg position.
	Pneumothorax	Pneumothorax due to retroperitoneal dissection of insufflated gas into the mediastinum can cause hypoxemia, ↑airway pressure, subcutaneous emphysema and hypotension.

Complications, cont.	Cardiovascular:		
	↓BP	↓BP can result from ↓venous return caused by pneumoperitoneum.	
	Hemorrhage	Hemorrhage can result from blood vessel injury or rapid reversal of head-down position. Unintended intravascular injection of CO_2 gas can lead to hypotension and dysrhythmias.	
	Dysrhythmias		
	Neurological:	Use of Trendelenburg position incurs risk of nerve injury. Hyperextension of arm may result in brachial plexus injury and careful padding of vulnerable points is necessary. Shoulder brace can compress nerve roots in retroclavicular region.	
	Nerve injury		
	Brachial plexus injury		
	Nerve root compression		

POSTOPERATIVE

Complications	N/V	Rx: metoclopramide 10 mg iv, droperidol 1 mg iv, or ondansetron 4 mg iv.
	Anemia	
	Shoulder pain	Postop pain may be referred to the shoulder, due to irritation of diaphragm by residual pneumoperitoneum or bleeding.
Pain Management	PCA (p. C-3)	
Tests	Hb/Hct, if hemorrhage occurs.	

ANESTHETIC CONSIDERATIONS FOR *IN VITRO* FERTILIZATION

PREOPERATIVE

This is generally a fit, healthy patient population. Little is required beyond routine tests, unless otherwise indicated.

Laboratory Hct; other tests as indicated from H&P.

Premedication Standard premedication (see p. B-1).

INTRAOPERATIVE

Anesthetic technique: Conscious sedation, local anesthesia, regional (e.g., spinal and epidural) and GA all have been employed for *in vitro* fertilization. If the *in vitro* fertilization technique consists of transvaginal egg retrieval and embryo transfer (not laparoscopic technique), one study suggests higher pregnancy and delivery rates if conscious sedation or epidural anesthesia is used as opposed to GA.[2] However, if laparoscopy is performed, local anesthesia may result in inadequate pain relief and require heavy iv sedation. Regional anesthesia provides better pain relief, but breathing difficulty can develop due to pneumoperitoneum and Trendelenburg position. Therefore, GETA with controlled ventilation is most commonly used. If GA is used, an isoflurane-N_2O technique has a higher reproductive success rate than propofol-N_2O.[8]

Induction Standard induction (see p. B-2). Avoidance of succinylcholine may decrease postop myalgia.

Maintenance Standard maintenance (see p. B-3). N_2O does not appear to adversely affect success of fertilization.[4]

Emergence No special considerations

Blood and fluid requirements	Minimal blood loss	Blood loss minimal, unless trauma to vasculature. Rarely, trauma to blood vessels or organs following laparoscopy may necessitate laparotomy.
	IV: 18 ga × 1	
	NS/LR @ 2 ml/kg/h	
Monitoring	Standard monitors (p. B-1)	
Positioning	✓ and pad pressure points.	
	✓ eyes.	
Complications	Respiratory:	Pneumoperitoneum with CO_2 and steep Trendelenburg position cause cephalad displacement of diaphragm with ↓FRC, ↓pulmonary compliance, and ↑airway closure/atelectasis. Hypercarbia and hypoxia, due to respiratory compromise, can result unless ventilation is controlled dur-
	Pneumoperitoneum:	
	↑$PaCO_2$, ↓PaO_2	
	ETT migration	

Complications, cont.		ing GA. Check for endobronchial migration of ETT upon assumption of Trendelenburg position.
	Pneumothorax	Pneumothorax due to retroperitoneal dissection of insufflated gas into the mediastinum can cause hypoxemia, ↑airway pressure, subcutaneous emphysema and hypotension.
	Cardiovascular: ↓BP Hemorrhage VAE (CO_2) Dysrhythmias	↓BP can result from ↓venous return caused by pneumoperitoneum. Hemorrhage can result from blood vessel injury or rapid reversal of head-down position. Unintended intravascular injection of CO_2 gas (VAE) can lead to ↓BP and dysrhythmias.
	Neurological: Nerve injury Brachial plexus injury Nerve root compression Bowel injury	Use of Trendelenburg position incurs risk of nerve injury. Hyperextension of arm may result in brachial plexus injury and careful padding of vulnerable points is necessary. Shoulder brace can compress nerve roots in retroclavicular region.

POSTOPERATIVE

Complications	Shoulder pain	Postop pain may be referred to the shoulder, due to irritation of diaphragm by residual pneumoperitoneum or bleeding.
Pain management	Oral analgesics are usually sufficient.	

References

1. Confino ET: Transcervical balloon tuboplasty: a multicenter study. *JAMA* 1990; 264:2079-82.
2. Gonen O, Shulman A, Ghetler Y, Shapiro A, Judekin R, Beyth Y, Ben-Nun I. The impact of different types of anesthesia or *in vitro* fertilization-embryo transfer treatment outcome. *J Assist Reprod Genet* 1995 Nov.; 12(10): 678-82.
3. Resiner, LS. The pregnant patient and the disorders of pregnancy. In *Anesthesia and Uncommon Diseases*. WB Saunders Co, Philadelphia: 1990, 165-66.
4. Rosen MA, Roizen MF, Eger EI II, Glass RH, Martin M, Dandekar PV, Dailey PA, Litt L: The effect of nitrous oxide on *in vitro* fertilization success rate. *Anesthesiology* 1987; 67(1):42-4.
5. Rock JA, Thompson JD, eds: *TeLinde's Operative Gynecology*, 8th edition. Lippincott-Raven Publishers, Philadelphia: 1997.
6. Ross BK, Chaduck HS, Mancuso JJ, Benedelti C. Sprotte needle for obstetric anesthesia: Decreased incidence of post dural puncture headache. *Reg Anesth* 1992; 17:29-33.
7. Tanbo T: Assisted fertilization in infertile women with patient tubes: a comparison of *in vitro* fertilization, gamete intrafallopian transfer and tubal embryo stage transfer. *Hum Reprod* 1990; 5:266-70.
8. Vincent RD, Syrop CH, Van Voorhis BJ, Chestnut DH, Sparks AE, McGrath JM, Choi WW, Bates JN, Penning DH. An evaluation of the effect of anesthetic technique on reproductive success after laparoscopic pronuclear stage transfer. Propofol/nitrous oxide versus isoflurane/nitrous oxide. *Anesthesiology* 1995 Feb.; 82(2): 352-8.

HYSTERECTOMY—VAGINAL OR TOTAL ABDOMINAL

SURGICAL CONSIDERATIONS

Description: After cesarean section (C-section), **hysterectomy** is the most commonly performed operation in the U.S. (650,000/year). Two approaches are possible: vaginal and abdominal. The **vaginal approach**, performed with the patient in a dorsal lithotomy position, is preferred since it offers significantly less morbidity and mortality. Its use is limited by situations in which pelvic bony architecture, uterine size, pelvic adhesions, or the presence of gynecological cancers require an **abdominal approach**. Often the approach is decided upon in the OR, where a pelvic examination under anesthesia will determine the true uterine size, degree of prolapse and the presence of pelvic pathology. A laparoscopy may very well be performed at the outset of surgery in order to evaluate the pelvis and free up adhesions which would have made a vaginal approach initially unsafe. In patients ≥ 45 years, **bilateral salpingo-oophorectomy** (BSO) is often performed in addition to the hysterectomy to provide ovarian cancer prophylaxis. Pelvic relaxation syndrome is the most frequent preop diagnosis in patients having a vaginal hysterectomy. Pelvic relaxation includes one or more of the following: prolapse of the uterus; intestine into the pouch of Douglas (enterocele); bladder into the anterior vaginal wall (cystocele); urethra into the anterior vaginal wall (urethrocele); and rectum into the posterior vaginal wall (rectocele). In these cases, the hysterectomy is often accompanied by an anterior/posterior colporrhaphy, bladder neck suspension, and perineoplasty.

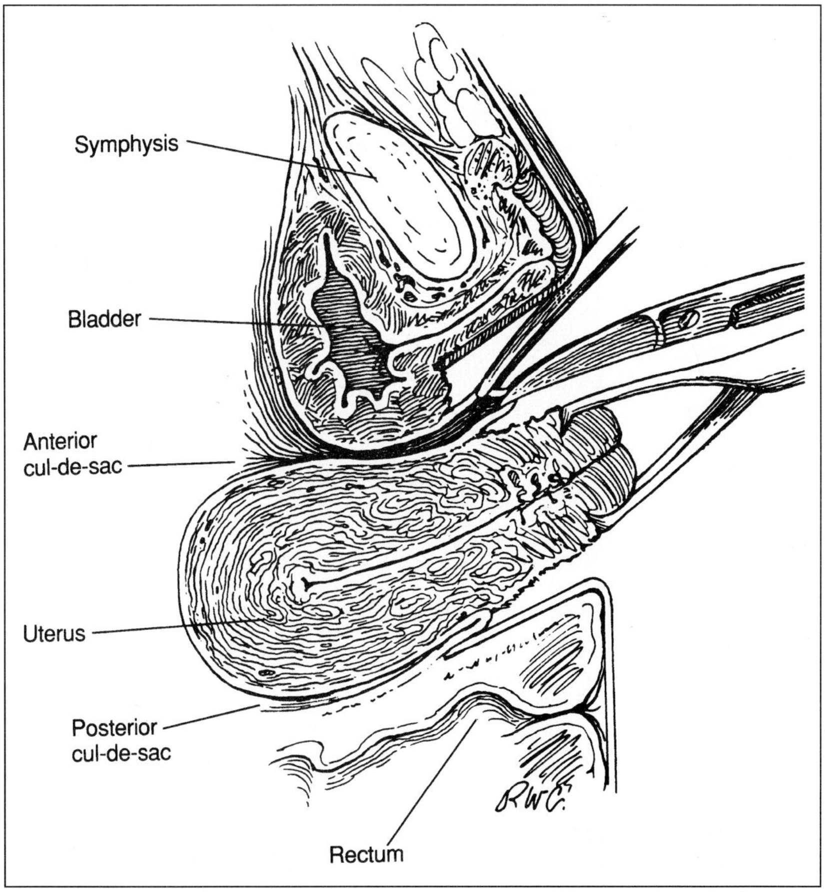

Figure 8.2-4. Surgical anatomy for vaginal hysterectomy. (Reproduced with permission from Thompson JD, Rock JA, eds: *TeLinde's Operative Gynecology*, 7th edition. JB Lippincott: 1992.)

Variant approaches: Abdominal hysterectomy is performed through a Pfannenstiel's or midline incision, depending on the uterine size and the need to perform a lymph node dissection for cancer. A Pfannenstiel's incision often can be improved with two types of muscle-splitting steps: the **Maylard**, in which the rectus muscles are cut, or a **Cherney rectus muscle detachment** performed at the pubic insertion. After entering the abdomen, a self-retaining retractor is placed and the round, ovarian and broad ligaments clamped, cut and tied, in that order. The uterine vessels are identified and ligated, followed by the creation of a bladder flap and, finally, the cutting and ligation of the uterosacral and cardinal ligaments. The vagina is entered and the cervix removed. Then the vaginal cuff is closed in a way to incorporate the uterosacral ligaments for support. The visceral peritoneum is reapproximated, the retractor removed, and the abdominal layers closed.

In a **vaginal hysterectomy**, the cervix is retracted, a paracervical incision is made, and the anterior and posterior cul de sacs are entered (Fig 8.2-4). The uterosacral and cardinal ligaments and the uterine vessels are cut and ligated. With steady downward traction, the broad ligament is ligated in a step-wise manner until either the ovarian or infundibulopelvic ligament is reached, and one of the two is ligated, depending on whether the ovaries are to be removed or not. After the uterus has been removed, the peritoneum is reapproximated, followed by the closing of the vaginal cuff, which often includes the uterosacral and cardinal ligaments for support. A vaginal pack is often left in place. Frequently, laparoscopy is being combined with vaginal hysterectomy to evaluate the pelvis for unrecognized disease and to ensure prophylactic adnexectomy in women ages ≥ 40-45 yr.

Usual preop diagnosis: Uterine myoma; pelvic relaxation syndrome; pelvic pain 2° endometriosis or adhesions; uncontrolled uterine bleeding/dysmenorrhea; endometrial hyperplasia; gynecological cancers

SUMMARY OF PROCEDURE

	Abdominal Approach	Vaginal Approach
Position	Supine	Lithotomy. Following induction, position patient so that the perineum is at the end of operating table to ensure optimum surgical exposure.

	Abdominal Approach		Vaginal Approach
Incision	Pfannenstiel's or low midline. The Pfannenstiel's incision can be extended with a Maylard muscle-splitting procedure or a Cherney rectus muscle detachment at pubic insertion.		Pericervical vaginal
Special instrumentation	None		Stirrups
Unique considerations	None		To prevent peroneal nerve injury, the area of leg leaning against stirrup should be well cushioned. Often, vasoconstriction agents (1:200,000 epinephrine and vasopressin) are used to cut down perioperative vaginal cuff bleeding.[3]
Antibiotics	1-2 g cefoxitin or cefotetan		⇐
Surgical time	1-2 h		45 min-1.5 h
EBL	1500 ml		750-1000 ml
Postop care	PACU		⇐
Mortality[2]	Overall 14.6/10,000		0.2%[2]
	< 25 yr	8.9/10,000	0/10,000
	25-34	4.7	0.9
	35-44	3.8	0.5
	45-54	6.5	2.7
	55-64	41.3	1.9
	65-74	93.0	18.3
	> 75	255.8	56.8
Morbidity[1,2,4,5]	Febrile morbidity	32.3/100	15.3/100
	Hemorrhage requiring transfusion	15.4/100	8.3/100
	Femoral nerve injury	11.6/100	–
	Wound infection	7/100	–
	Unintended major surgical procedure	1.7/100	5.1/100
	Vaginal cuff infection	3.1/100	2.1/100
	Rehospitalization	2.8/100	1.8/100
	Bladder injury	2.5/100	
	Ureter injury	2.0/100	
	Life-threatening event	0.4/100	
Pain score	5-8		4-6

PATIENT POPULATION CHARACTERISTICS

Age range	30-80 yr
Incidence	> 1/5 females; 650,000/yr in U.S.
Etiology	Uterine myomata; endometriosis; uterine prolapse; uterine cancer
Associated conditions	Stress urinary incontinence; obesity

ANESTHETIC CONSIDERATIONS

PREOPERATIVE

Although many patients presenting for this procedure are otherwise healthy, others may have metastatic cancer.

Respiratory CXR may be indicated to rule out pleural effusion or other lung pathology in cancer patients. Additionally, ABGs, ± PFTs, may be indicated preop in patients with significant pulmonary involvement.
Tests: As indicated from H&P.

Cardiovascular Patient may have blood loss from the primary problem. Additionally, she may have undergone bowel prep, which can cause dehydration and electrolyte abnormalities. Assessment of volume status, using BP and orthostatic vital signs, is important.
Tests: As indicated from H&P.

Hematologic	Hb/Hct. Patients with Hx of easy bruising or bleeding should have coagulation parameters evaluated (PT, PTT, Plt).
Laboratory	Other tests as indicated from H&P.
Premedication	Anxiolytic (e.g., midazolam 1-2 mg iv) as needed.

INTRAOPERATIVE

Anesthetic technique: GA is commonly used; however, either spinal or epidural anesthesia is appropriate for adequately hydrated patients who are undergoing simple hysterectomy through a Pfannenstiel's incision, or vaginal hysterectomy. In the younger patient population, spinal anesthesia may be less desirable because of the increased incidence of post-dural puncture headache (PDPH) in using this technique. If spinal anesthetic is indicated, a pencil-point needle (e.g., Sprotte or Whitacre) should be used to decrease the incidence of PDPH.[9] Patients with extensive cancer who undergo exploratory laparotomy with lymph node dissection may benefit from combined epidural/GA with decreased postop pulmonary complications and early ambulation. Some studies advocate the use of epidural anesthesia in order to decrease intraop blood loss.[6]

General anesthesia:

Induction	Standard induction (see p. B-2).
Maintenance	Standard maintenance (see p. B-3). Muscle relaxation is necessary if the procedure is performed abdominally. These patients have a high incidence of N/V, and prophylaxis with metoclopramide 10 mg iv, droperidol 1 mg iv or ondansetron 4 mg iv is indicated.
Emergence	Be ready with suction in the event the patient vomits on emergence.

Regional anesthesia: A T4-6 sensory level is sufficient to provide anesthesia for procedures on the uterus.

Spinal	5% lidocaine 75-100 mg (controversial); 0.75% bupivacaine 10-15 mg in 7.5% dextrose. (See Anesthetic Considerations for Cesarean Section, p. 602)
Epidural	1.5-2.0% lidocaine with epinephrine 5 μg/ml, 15-25 ml; supplement with 5-10 ml as needed. Supplemental iv sedation. (See Anesthetic Considerations for Cesarean Section, p. 602.)

Blood and fluid requirements	Possible heavy blood loss IV: 16-18 ga × 2 Warm all fluids. Heat, humidify gases. Autologous blood donation	Preop autologous blood transfusion may not be possible in patients who are already anemic. Blood and evaporative losses are usually greater in patients undergoing abdominal, rather than vaginal, hysterectomy. Patients having a Pfannenstiel's incision should also have smaller fluid requirements than those having a larger midline incision.
Control of blood loss	**Vaginal hysterectomy:** Moderate blood loss NS/LR @ 4-5 ml/kg/h.	In order to avoid blood transfusion, consider colloid infusion in patients who have a good cardiac function and can tolerate a low Hct. May need blood transfusion.
	Abdominal hysterectomy: Moderate-to-heavy blood loss NS/LR @ 6-10 ml/kg/h	
Monitoring	**Vaginal hysterectomy:** Standard monitors (p. B-1) ± Foley catheter	A Foley catheter may be helpful (to monitor fluid status) during vaginal hysterectomy if the procedure is expected to be longer than usual.
	Abdominal hysterectomy: Standard monitors (p. B-1) Foley catheter ± Arterial line ± CVP line	During abdominal hysterectomy, a Foley catheter is useful, since this procedure is longer, involves more fluid shifts and may involve a significant blood loss. Intra-arterial and CVP monitoring are useful in patients undergoing large tumor resections and in whom large blood losses are anticipated.
Positioning	✓ and pad pressure points. Shoulder abduction < 90°	The lithotomy position has several considerations for safety. (See p. 578 for details.)
Complications	**Vaginal hysterectomy:** Cervical stimulation	Vagal stimulation may occur when the surgeons grasp the cervix; subsequent bradycardia may ensue. This can be

Complications, cont.	Epinephrine/vasopressin injection → HTN or cardiac dysrhythmias **Abdominal hysterectomy:** Cervical stimulation Epinephrine/vasopressin injection **Abdominal hysterectomy:** Blood loss	treated by cessation of the surgical stimulus and treatment with atropine if indicated. The surgeons may use epinephrine or vasopressin to decrease local bleeding. Either of these agents may cause HTN or cardiac dysrhythmias.[8] Hemorrhage is possible with large tumor resections, and must be treated with adequate fluid and blood replacement. Attention must be given to associated problems such as hypothermia, hypocalcemia and dilutional coagulopathy.

POSTOPERATIVE

Complications	N/V Anemia	Rx with metoclopramide 10 mg, droperidol 1 mg iv, or ondansetron 4 mg iv.
Pain management	Epidural opiates (p. C-1) PCA (p. C-3)	If catheter to be used postop
Tests	Hct; CXR (if CVP catheter placed intraop)	CXR to evaluate central line placement and rule out pneumothorax.

References

1. Daly JW, Higgins KA: Injury to the ureter during gynecological surgical procedures. *Surg Gynecol Obstet* 1988; 167(1):19-22.
2. Dicker RC, Greenspan Jr, Strauss LT et al: Complications of abdominal and vaginal hysterectomy among women of reproductive age in the United States. The Collaborative Review of Sterilization. *Am J Obstet Gynecol* 1982; 144(7):841-48.
3. England GT, Randall HW, Graves WL: Impairment of tissue defenses by vasoconstrictors in vaginal hysterectomies. *Obstet Gynecol* 1983; 61(3):271-74.
4. Georgy FM: Femoral neuropathy following abdominal hysterectomy. *Am J Obstet Gynecol* 1975; 123(8):819-22.
5. Kvist-Poulsen H, Borel J: Iatrogenic femoral neuropathy subsequent to abdominal hysterectomy: incidence and prevention. *Obstet Gynecol* 1982; 60(4):516-20.
6. Modig, J: Regional anaesthesia and blood loss. *Acta Anaesthesiol Scand Suppl*: 1988, 89; 44-8.
7. *Physician's Desk Reference*, 52nd edition. Medical Economics Data, Inc, Montvale, NJ: 1998.
8. Rock JA, Thompson JD, eds: *TeLinde's Operative Gynecology*, 8th edition. Lippincott-Raven Publishers, Philadelphia: 1997.
9. Ross BK, Chaduck HS, Mancuso JS, Benedetti C: Sprotte needle for obstetric anesthesia: Decreased incidence of post dural puncture headache. *Reg Anesth* 1992; 17:29-33.
10. Wingo PA, et al: The mortality risk associated with hysterectomy. *Am J Obstet Gynecol* 1984; 152(7):803-8.

ANTERIOR AND POSTERIOR COLPORRHAPHY, ENTEROCELE REPAIR, VAGINAL SACROSPINOUS SUSPENSION

SURGICAL CONSIDERATIONS

Description: Cystocele (Fig 8.2-5A) and rectocele (Fig 8.2-5B) are prolapses (relaxation) of the anterior and posterior vaginal wall, respectively. They occur 2° multiparity and congenital weakening of pelvic tissue. The term "pelvic relaxation syndrome" includes the often coexisting anatomical "relaxations" (e.g., enterocele [Fig 8.2-5C] and uterine prolapse). Cystoceles are often symptomatic due to bladder protrusion past the introitus during straining. Often this relaxation will allow the bladder neck to lose its important anatomical relationship to the urethra and the rest of the bladder. The result can be bothersome stress urinary incontinence for the patient (see Operations for Stress Urinary Incontinence, p. 595). The rectocele is often experienced as a vaginal bulge during straining, and tends to cause severe constipation. Enterocele herniation of the small bowel into the rectovaginal septum is often experienced as pelvic pain. The goal of the colporrhaphy is to restore the original anatomy. Due to the frequent coexisting relaxations, a posterior colporrhaphy (vaginal repair), enterocele repair and vaginal hysterectomy are frequently performed at the same time.

In an **anterior colporrhaphy**, the patient is placed in a high dorsal lithotomy position with the perineum at the end of the operating table for surgical access. The bladder is emptied and a weighted speculum is inserted into the vagina. A **vaginal hysterectomy** is performed at this point, if indicated (see Vaginal Hysterectomy, p. 588). The extent of the urethrocystocele is determined manually and the vaginal mucosa is grasped at its cephalic border with two clamps. From this point to the external urethral meatus, the mucosa is undermined with a vasoconstrictive solution (epinephrine 5-10 ml, 1:200,000), phenylephrine (1:200,000) or vasopressin (1-5 U/10 ml NS). This decreases blood loss significantly and helps to determine the depth of the vaginal mucosa. The mucosa is cut over this undermined area and, with the help of sharp and blunt dissection, the mucosa is dissected laterally from its underlying fascia. A series of fascial plication sutures are placed to reduce the cystourethrocele. The redundant mucosa is excised and the edges are reapproximated. A suprapubic catheter is most often inserted at the end to prevent bladder over-distention. If necessary, a **posterior colporrhaphy** may be performed. A small portion of perineum posterior to the introitus is removed initially. The vaginal mucosa over the rectocele is undermined with vasoconstrictor fluid prior to incision, followed by dissection of the overlying mucosa in a manner nearly identical to anterior colporrhaphy. One or several layers of stitches are placed to plicate the pararectal fascia, allowing for reduction of the rectocele. Sometimes, part of the levator ani muscle is included to provide better support. Redundant mucosa is excised and the edges reapproximated. A vaginal pack is usually placed in order to minimize bleeding.

An **enterocele** often is first noticed during a posterior colporrhaphy procedure, and is repaired prior to finishing the posterior repair. The enterocele is well identified and dissected away from the surrounding tissue. Two or more parallel purse-string stitches are used to close the enterocele. The enterocele tissue distal to the purse-string closure is excised. In order to reduce the enterocele in an optimum fashion, intraabdominal pressure has to be at a minimum.

Variant procedure or approaches: Vaginal sacrospinous suspension with the Miya hook is an elegant alternative to the abdominal colpopexy procedure for women with severe uterine and/or vaginal vault prolapse. The patient is placed in a dorsal lithotomy position and an examination under anesthesia is performed. A vasoconstrictive solution is injected (usually 1:200,000 epinephrine 3-5 ml) in the posterior vaginal wall. A vertical incision is made and the mucosa is bluntly dissected off the rectum in an anterolateral direction. An enterocele, if found, is repaired at this time. The pararectal tissue is then bluntly pierced to enter the pararectal space. The anatomy surrounding the sacrospinous ligament is well palpated and, with the help of the special Miya hook, a large suture is placed into the sacrospinous ligament. The other end of the suture is placed at the apex of the vagina which, after tying, is pulled in a lateral cephalad direction. The mucosa is finally closed.

The **Le Fort procedure** is now a rare operation and is performed in very elderly women with complete prolapse of the uterus and/or vagina who do not desire to remain

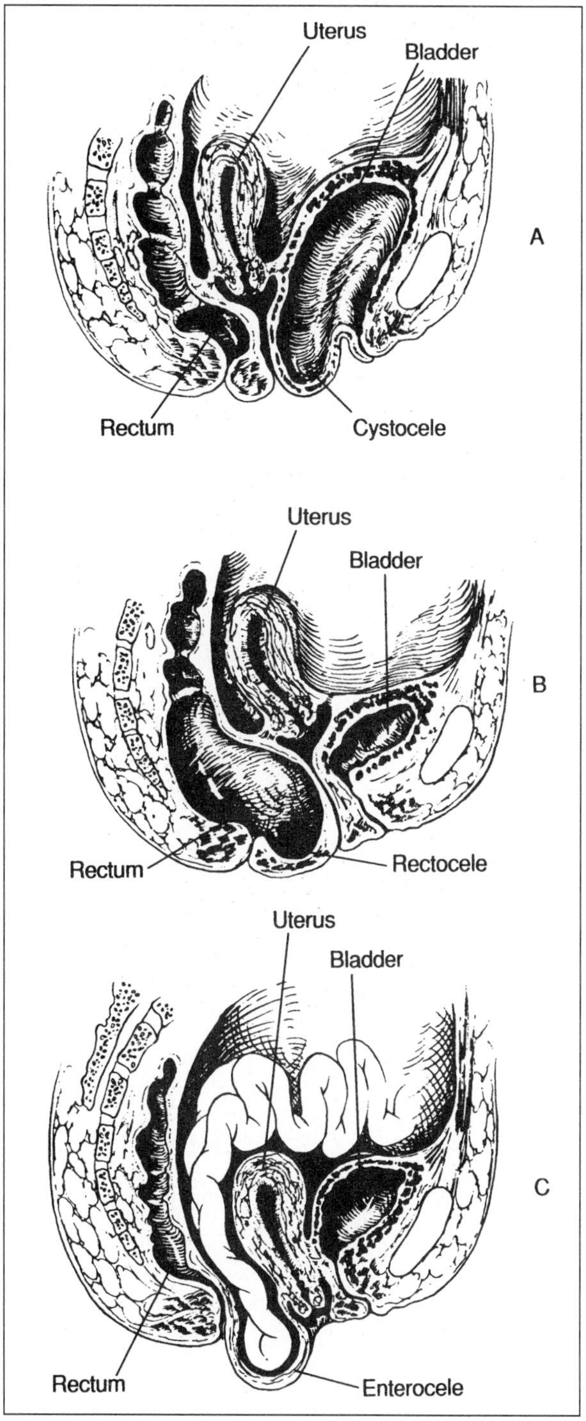

Figure 8.2-5. (A) Anatomy of cystocele. (B) Anatomy of rectocele. (C) Anatomy of enterocele. (Reproduced with permission from Pernoll ML, ed: *Current Obstetrics and Gynecological Diagnosis and Treatment*. Appleton & Lange: 1991.)

sexually active. With the patient in a dorsal lithotomy position, a rectangular strip from the anterior and posterior vaginal wall is removed initially, followed by closure of the margins each to the other. The result is a near-complete closure of the vagina.

Usual preop diagnosis: Symptomatic cystocele or stress urinary incontinence; symptomatic uterine prolapse; enterocele; rectocele causing severe constipation; dyspareunia

SUMMARY OF PROCEDURE

Position	Dorsal lithotomy	
Incision	Vaginal mucosal; peritoneum for enterocele repair	
Unique considerations	To prevent peroneal nerve injury, the area of the leg leaning against the stirrup should be well cushioned. Putting the legs in a high position increases venous return to the heart. Infiltration with epinephrine and vasopressin are often used to reduce intraop bleeding. This causes changes in CO, HR and BP. Low intraabdominal pressure (good muscle relaxation) is needed during the enterocele reduction. A urethral catheter is not used intraop.	
Antibiotics	1-2 g iv cefoxitin/cefotetan	
Surgical time	45 min (anterior colporrhaphy) 30 min (posterior colporrhaphy/enterocele repair)	
Closing considerations	Suprapubic catheter (anterior colporrhaphy); vaginal pack (enterocele repair)	
EBL	20-500 ml	
Postop care	PACU	
Mortality	1%	
Morbidity	Anterior colporrhaphy[1]	Vaginal sacrospinous suspension (Miya hook)
	Delayed voiding 1-7 d: 30%	Bleeding in gluteal and pudendal vessels
	Foul vaginal discharge: 14%	Pararectal burning pain ≥ 2 mo
	Bacteriuria: 13%	Sciatic pain (indicating misplaced sutures which must be removed)
	Pyrexia (>100.4F): 11%	Peritoneal tear (during Miya hook insertion)
	Atelectasis: 3%	
	Delayed voiding > 7 d: 0.6%	
	Need for blood transfusion: 0.6%	
	Urethrovaginal fistula: 0.4%	
	Acute gastric dilatation: 0.2%	
Pain score	5-8	

PATIENT POPULATION CHARACTERISTICS

Age range	40-80 yr
Incidence	> 1/5
Etiology	Multiparous state; obesity; chronic cough
Associated conditions	Pelvic relaxation syndrome

ANESTHETIC CONSIDERATIONS

See Anesthetic Considerations following Operations for Stress Urinary Incontinence, p. 596.

References

1. Beck RP, et al: A 25-year experience with 519 anterior colporrhaphy procedures. *Obstet Gynecol* 1991; 78(6):1011-18.
2. DeCherney AH, Pernoll ML, eds: *Current Obstetrics and Gynecologic Diagnosis and Treatment.* Appleton & Lange, Norwalk, Ct: 1994.
3. Miyazaki F: Miya hook ligature carrier for sacrospinous ligament suspension. *Obstet Gynecol* 1987; 70(2):286-88.
4. Rock JA, Thompson JD, eds: *TeLinde's Operative Gynecology*, 8th edition. Lippincott-Raven Publishers, Philadelphia: 1997.

OPERATIONS FOR STRESS URINARY INCONTINENCE

SURGICAL CONSIDERATIONS

Description: Stress urinary incontinence is a common condition affecting mostly older and multiparous women. It is a disorder of the musculofascial support to the bladder neck and pelvic floor. These patients usually have extensive preop workup to exclude urge incontinence and almost all have been treated with pelvic floor exercises (Kegel) and estrogen prior to surgery. Two surgical approaches exist: **abdominal suspension** procedures and **suspension by the vaginal route**. Ongoing controversy exists concerning which approach is best. Patient position is crucial for all vaginal surgery.

Vaginal approaches: The **Kelly urethral plication** is often the primary surgical treatment, especially when other vaginal surgery needs to be performed. The patient initially is placed in a high dorsal lithotomy position with the perineum at the end of the operating table for surgical exposure. The bladder is emptied and a weighted speculum is inserted into the vagina. The extent of the cystourethrocele is determined and the vaginal mucosa is grasped at its cephalic border with two clamps. From this point to the external urethral meatus, the mucosa is usually undermined with 5-10 ml of a vasoconstrictive solution (epinephrine 1:200,000), phenylephrine (1:200,000) or vasopressin (1-5 U/10 ml NS). This decreases blood loss significantly and helps to determine the depth of the mucosa. With the help of sharp and blunt dissection, the mucosa is freed laterally from its underlying adherent fascia. A series of vertical mattress sutures are placed in the mobilized paraurethral and paravesicle fascia in order to reduce the cystourethrocele and elevate the posterior urethra to a high retropubic position. The redundant mucosa is excised and the edges are reapproximated. A suprapubic catheter is often inserted at the end of the surgery to prevent bladder overdistention.

Anterior vesicle neck suspension (**Stamey** and modified **Pereyra**) are two very similar procedures wherein the vaginal mucosa is incised and dissected off the underlying paravesicle and paraurethral fascia much the same way as in the Kelly plication. Instead of using a layer of mattress sutures, both suspension methods use two lateral sutures that suspend the vesicle neck on each side (Fig 8.2-6A). The ends of the sutures are tied over the rectus fascia to provide support. The Stamey method uses a small Dacron cuff to prevent the suture from tearing through the paravesicle fascia, while in the modified Pereyra method, the posterior loop is firmly attached to the pubourethral ligament. One or two small suprapubic abdominal incisions must be made to allow for the tying of the sutures. Specialized long needles are used to help the placement of these sutures, and a cystoscope is often used to verify their placement. Perforation of the bladder is a common complication found upon cystoscopy. Finally, a suprapubic catheter is placed at the end of the operation. (See Urology, p. 668.)

Abdominal approaches: The **Marshall-Marchetti-Krantz (M-M-K)** and **Burch** are probably the most common abdominal suspension procedures. The patient is placed in the frog-leg position with a urethral catheter in place. A Pfannenstiel's incision is used to enter the space of Retzius, which lies between the parietal peritoneum and the rectus fascia under the pubic bone. Blunt dissection is used to open and extend this space. The surgeon then inserts two fingers into the vagina to raise the anterior vagina and bladder neck. This enables the surgeon to place two or more sutures in the tissue just lateral to the urethra and attach them to the pubic fibrocartilage or Cooper's ligament (Burch).

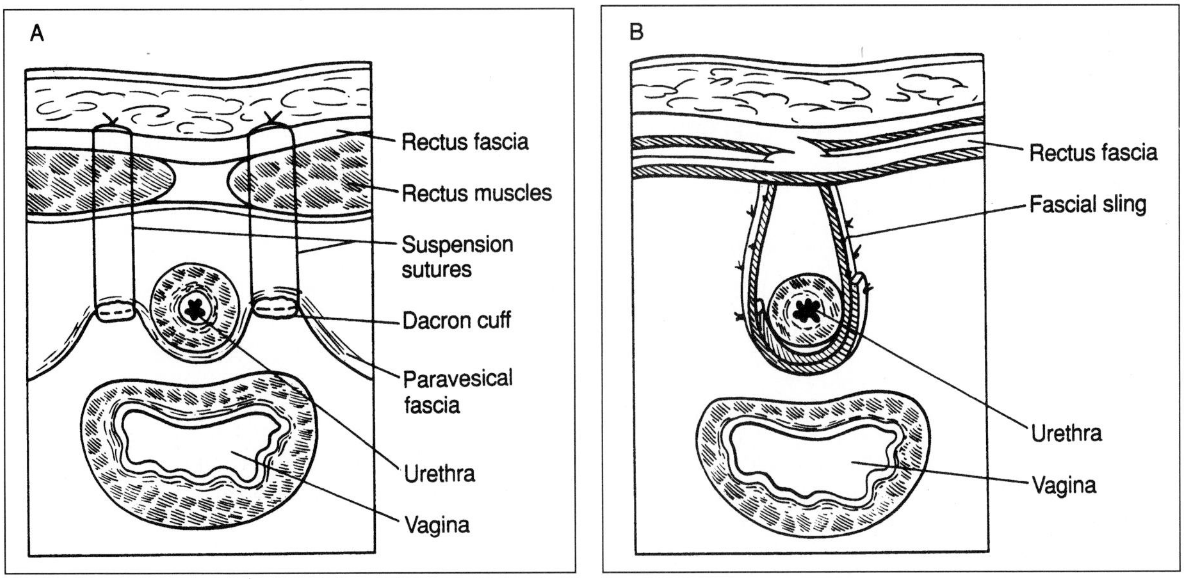

Figure 8.2-6. (A) Stamey procedure. (B) Urethral sling procedure. (Reproduced with permission from Varner RE, Sparks JM: Surgery for Stress Urinary Incontinence. *Surg Clin North Am* 1991; 71(5):1124, 1128.)

The **urethral sling procedure** is reserved for women with low urethral pressure and/or for whom other incontinence operations have failed. The goal of the sling procedure is to produce extrinsic compression of the urethrovesical junction with the help of a strip anchored to the rectus fascia (Fig 8.2-6B). With the patient in the dorsal lithotomy position, a urethral catheter is placed and the vaginal mucosa incised and dissected off the underlying paravesicle and paraurethral fascia similar to the Kelly plication. The retropubic space is entered through a Pfannenstiel's incision and a strip of rectus fascia is obtained. The strip is then brought through the vagina, around the urethra and back to the abdomen, where it is fastened to the rectus fascia, creating a sling under the urethra at the junction of the bladder neck. The vaginal and abdominal incisions are closed, and a suprapubic catheter is placed.

Usual preop diagnosis: Stress urinary incontinence

SUMMARY OF PROCEDURE

	Kelly Plication	M-M-K/Burch
Position	Dorsal lithotomy	Frog leg
Incision	Vaginal mucosa	Pfannenstiel's
Unique considerations	Cushion area of leg against stirrup to prevent peroneal injury. Epinephrine (1:200,000) or vasopressin are often infiltrated to reduce intraop bleeding for vaginal approaches. This causes changes in CO, bleeding, HR and rhythm. The urethral catheter is frequently removed and reinserted during surgery.	⇐
Antibiotics	Cefoxitin 1-2 g iv	⇐
Surgical time	1 h	⇐
Closing considerations	Suprapubic catheter	⇐
EBL	50 ml	100-200 ml
Postop care	Inpatient	⇐
Mortality	Minimal	⇐
Morbidity	Prolonged catheter time: 54%	Rare
	Bladder perforation: 1%	Rare
	Outlet obstruction: 2%	Rare
	Urethral perforation: 1%	Rare
	Detrusor instability: Rare (due to vaginal approach)	14%
	Enterocele: Rare	15%
	Incisional hernia: Rare	0.09%
	Osteitis pubis: Rare	Rare
	Uterine prolapse: Rare	4%
	UTI: Rare	10.4%
	Voiding difficulties: Rare	2%
	Wound infection: Rare	8.7%
Pain score	4-6	6-8

PATIENT POPULATION CHARACTERISTICS

Age range	40-80 yr
Incidence	>1/5 females
Etiology	Multiparous state; obesity; chronic cough
Associated conditions	Other components of pelvic relaxation syndrome (rectocele, uterine prolapse, enterocele)

ANESTHETIC CONSIDERATIONS

(Procedures covered: anterior and posterior colporrhaphy; enterocele repair; vaginal sacrospinous suspension; operations for stress urinary incontinence)

PREOPERATIVE

This is usually an older patient population, past child-bearing age. Patient may be relatively healthy otherwise. ✓ for concurrent disease.

Laboratory	Hb/Hct, as indicated from H&P.	
Premedication	Anxiolytic (e.g., midazolam 1-2 mg iv) as needed.	

INTRAOPERATIVE

Anesthetic technique: Regional or GA may be used. In the younger patient population, spinal anesthesia may be less desirable because of increased incidence of postdural puncture headache (PDPH). If spinal anesthesia is indicated, a pencil-point needle (e.g., Sprotte or Whitacre) should be used to decrease the incidence of PDPH.[7]

Regional anesthesia: A T10 sensory level is sufficient to provide anesthesia for procedures on the uterus and bladder, but a T4 level is recommended if the peritoneum is opened.

Spinal	5% lidocaine 75-100 mg (controversial); 0.75% bupivacaine 10-15 mg in 7.5% dextrose. (See Anesthetic Considerations for Cesarean Section, p. 602.)	
Epidural	1.5-2.0% lidocaine with epinephrine 5 μg/ml, 15-25 ml; supplement with 5-10 ml as needed. Supplemental iv sedation. (See Anesthetic Considerations for Cesarean Section, p. 602.)	
General anesthesia:		
Induction	Standard induction (see p. B-2).	
Maintenance	Standard maintenance (see p. B-3).	
Emergence	No special considerations	
Blood and fluid requirements	Normally minimal blood loss IV: 16-18 ga × 1 NS/LR @ 2-4 ml/kg/h	Only 1 iv is normally necessary for adequate intraop hydration.
Control of blood loss	Epinephrine, vasopressin, phenylephrine used by surgeons.	Surgeons may inject vasopressors into the submucosa to minimize blood loss. This may cause intraop and cardiac dysrhythmias.[5]
Monitoring	Standard monitors (p. B-1)	Although bladder catheterization prior to incision is normal, the catheter is not left in place throughout surgery in those patients undergoing anterior and posterior colporrhaphy, enterocele repair and Kelly urethral plication. Suprapubic bladder catheters are placed toward the end of surgery in these procedures, as well as in the Stamey, Pereyra and urethral sling procedures.
Positioning	✓ and pad pressure points. ✓ eyes.	See p. 578 for concerns regarding the lithotomy position.

POSTOPERATIVE

Complications	N/V	Rx: metoclopramide 10 mg iv, droperidol 1 mg iv or ondansetron 4 mg iv.
Pain management	IV opiates Usually rapid conversion to po pain medications	
Tests	None indicated.	

References

1. Blaivas JG, et al: Pubovaginal fascial sling for the treatment of complicated stress urinary incontinence. *J Urol* 1991; 145(6):1214-18.
2. Galloway NT, et al: The complications of colposuspension. *Br J Urol* 1987; 60(2):122-24.
3. Lee RA, et al: Surgical complications and results of modified Marshall-Marchetti-Krantz procedure for urinary incontinence. *Obstet Gynecol* 1979; 53(4):447-450.
4. Pereyra AJ, et al: Pubourethral supports in perspective: modified Pereyra procedure for urinary incontinence. *Obstet Gynecol* 1982; 59(5):643-48.
5. *Physician's Desk Reference*, 52nd edition. Medical Economics Data, Inc, Montvale, NJ: 1998.

6. Rock JA, Thompson JD, eds: *TeLinde's Operative Gynecology*, 8th edition. Lippincott-Raven Publishers, Philadelphia: 1997.
7. Ross BK, Chaduck HS, Mancuso JS, Benedetti C: Sprotte needle for obstetric anesthesia: Decreased incidence of post dural puncture headache. *Reg Anesth* 1992; 17:29-33.
8. Stamey TA: Endoscopic suspension of the vesical neck for urinary incontinence in females. *Ann Surg* 1980; 192(4):465-71.
9. Varner RE, Sparks JM: Surgery for stress urinary incontinence. *Surg Clin North Am* 1991; 71(5):1111-34.

Surgeons

Yasser El-Sayed, MD
Ronald N. Gibson, MD
Babak Edraki, MD
R. Harold Holbrook Jr, MD

8.3 OBSTETRIC SURGERY

Anesthesiologist

Sheila E. Cohen, MB, ChB, FRCA

CESAREAN SECTION—LOWER SEGMENT AND CLASSICAL

SURGICAL CONSIDERATIONS

R. Harold Holbrook, Jr

Description: Cesarean section (C-section) is the delivery of the fetus through a horizontal or vertical incision into the **lower uterine segment**. The skin incision is made either as a Pfannenstiel's (transverse in the crease above the pubis) or vertical midline from umbilicus to pubis. The peritoneal cavity is entered as in any laparotomy. A retractor is placed inferiorly and the reflection of visceral peritoneum from the bladder dome to the anterior lower segment of the uterus (bladder flap) is incised and displaced inferiorly, along with the bladder. The uterus is entered sharply and the incision extended with digital pressure and/or bandage scissors. The fetal head is elevated out of the pelvis and delivered through the uterine incision. In cases of nonvertex lie, the infant's breech is grasped and brought out of the incision. After the delivery of the fetus, the cord is double-clamped and cut, and cord blood is obtained for analysis. The placenta is removed manually and the uterine cavity cleared of all debris and clots. The uterine incision is closed with a running, interlocking stitch, followed by a 2nd imbricating layer. The bladder flap and parietal peritoneum do not require closure. Finally, the fascia is closed and the skin reapproximated with staples. **Classical C-section** usually involves a vertical skin incision and fundal vertical uterine incision (Fig 8.3-1). Patients with a history of prior classical C-section should be delivered abdominally via a repeat C-section, since the risk of uterine rupture with labor of vaginal delivery is 2%.

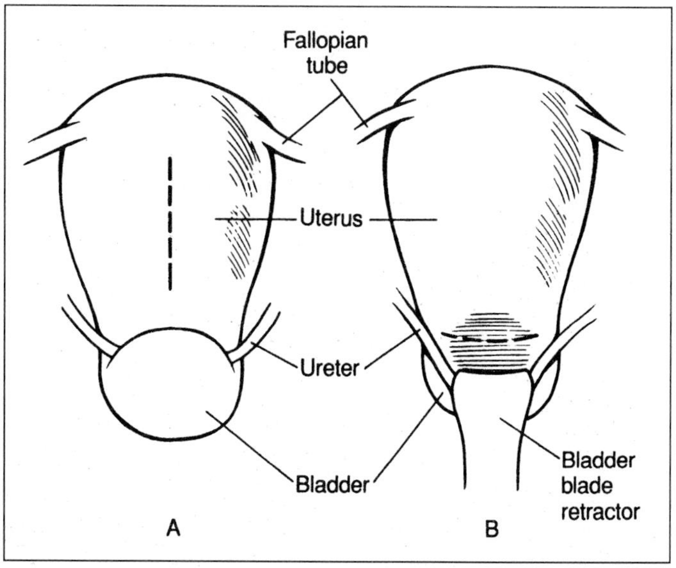

Figure 8.3-1. Typical C-section incisions. (A) Classic incision, in upper uterine segment. (B) Low transverse incision.

Usual preop diagnosis: Failure to progress in labor; elective repeat C-section; fetal distress

SUMMARY OF PROCEDURE

	Lower-Segment C-Section	Classical C-Section
Position	Supine with left lateral tilt. (In obese patients, the pannus may be lifted superiorly by tape or towel clips.)	⇐
Incision	Skin: transverse low abdominal (Pfannenstiel's) or repeat vertical. Uterus: transverse (Kerr) or low vertical (for premature infants or nonvertex lie)	Skin: Pfannenstiel's or, more commonly, vertical midline. Uterus: vertical fundal
Special instrumentation	Bladder blade retractor; small ring forceps; bandage scissors; suction bulb; DeLee suction trap (if meconium)	⇐
Unique considerations	✓ fetal heart tones before procedure. If for CPD: cervical exam within last 15 min before procedure. If for fetal distress: continuous monitoring until skin incision.	⇐
Antibiotics	If in labor or membranes ruptured: cefazolin 2 g iv, immediately after cord clamping.	⇐
Surgical time	20-90 min	40-90 min
Closing considerations	Low transverse: closed in 2 layers. Low vertical: 2 layers; may require additional opera-	3-layer closure requires additional time.

	Lower-Segment C-Section	Classical C-Section
Closing considerations, cont.	tive time for repair of incision if extension into cervix or fundus.	
EBL	750-1000 ml	1000-2000 ml
Postop care	Observation for bleeding and hypotension	Special attention to vital signs needed due to additional blood loss.
Mortality	< 0.1%	⇐
Morbidity	Infection:	
	Not in labor: < 5%	⇐
	In labor/ruptured membranes: ≤ 50% (antibiotics reduce to 15%)	⇐
	Small-bowel obstruction (SBO): Rare	⇐
Pain Score	4	7

PATIENT POPULATION CHARACTERISTICS

Age range 14-40+ yr

Incidence[8] 10-25%

Etiology[7] Failure to progress (30%); repeat C-section (30%); fetal anomaly/other (20%); abnormal presentation (10%); fetal distress (10%)

Associated conditions Preeclampsia/eclampsia; DIC; hemolysis, elevated liver enzyme, low Plt count (HELLP) syndrome; obstetrical hemorrhage/ shock; chorioamnionitis

---

ANESTHETIC CONSIDERATIONS

(Procedures covered: cesarean section; emergent obstetrical hysterectomy; repair of uterine rupture)

PREOPERATIVE

In general, these patients are young and healthy, although the pregnant patient has undergone profound physiologic changes which affect the conduct of anesthesia. Patients present for emergency C-section for fetal distress and hemorrhage (placenta previa, abruptio placenta and, rarely, uterine rupture).

Respiratory The pregnant patient has a compensated respiratory alkalosis (PCO_2 = 32-34), ↑minute ventilation (MV) (↑50%), and ↓FRC (↓20%). ↑O_2 consumption (↑20%) with ↓FRC results in rapid onset of hypoxemia if ventilation is compromised. Small airway closure due to elevation of diaphragm (exaggerated by obesity and supine position) can result in shunting and ↓PaO_2. ↑MV and ↓FRC enhance uptake of inhalational anesthetics. Mucosal capillary engorgement in upper airways may necessitate a smaller ETT and mandates careful airway suctioning to avoid bleeding.
Tests: As indicated from H&P.

Cardiovascular Typically, there is a ↓SVR (↓15%), ↓diastolic pressure and ↓MAP (↓15%) with ↑HR (↑30%) and ↑CO (↑30%). To minimize aortocaval compression and hypotension, the supine position should be avoided by the use of left lateral tilt. Immediately postpartum, 600-800 ml blood enters the central circulation, due to placental transfusion, with further increase in CO.
Tests: As indicated from H&P.

Hematologic These patients have ↑blood volume (↑35%), ↑plasma volume (↑45%), ↑red cell mass (↑20%). WBC count may increase to 15,000/mm^2. Iron deficiency anemia often is superimposed on the dilutional anemia of pregnancy (Hct 33%). The typical blood loss of 500-800 ml is usually well tolerated. Excessive blood loss is possible with multiple gestation, previous C-section, PIH, placenta previa, abruptio placenta and uterine atony. Repeat C-section associated with placenta previa poses high risk for hemorrhage because of placenta accreta.
Tests: Hb/Hct

Gastrointestinal Abnormalities, including ↓gastric motility (after onset of labor), gastroesophageal reflux, raised intragastric pressure and gastric hyperacidity, predisposes to aspiration pneumonitis. All parturients

Gastrointestinal, cont.

should be considered to have full stomachs and should receive clear antacid (e.g., 0.3 M Na citrate 30 ml) immediately prior to GA or regional anesthesia. Administer iv metoclopramide 10 mg and ranitidine 50 mg before emergent C-section. Before elective C-section, parturients at high risk for aspiration (e.g., planned or potential GA, difficult airway, or any patient with esophageal reflux, or obesity) should receive an H_2-blocker (e.g., ranitidine 150 mg po) the night before and the morning of surgery.

Hepatic

Liver enzymes can be mildly elevated and plasma protein concentration is diminished (↑unbound drug levels); however, liver function is usually normal.
Tests: As indicated from H&P.

Renal

These patients have ↑renal blood flow (↑50%), ↑glomerular filtration rate and ↑creatinine clearance, and ↓serum creatinine and ↓blood urea N_2. Dependent edema results from increased water and sodium retention 2° resetting of the osmotic threshold for thirst and vasopressin secretions.
Tests: As indicated from H&P.

Laboratory

T&S maternal blood if risk factors for blood loss are present (e.g., third c-section). Cross-match unnecessary unless significant blood loss is anticipated. Routine autologous blood donation is not recommended. Coagulation studies and Plt count recommended with pregnancy-induced hypertension (PIH), abruptio placenta, heavy maternal bleeding. BUN; creatinine; UA; fasting blood glucose; others as indicated from H&P.

Premedication

Agents to decrease risk of aspiration pneumonitis are discussed on p. B-5. Sedatives are not routinely administered. In extremely anxious patients, however, 0.5-1.0 mg midazolam iv is an excellent anxiolytic without apparent affect on maternal memory or alertness or neonatal condition.

SPECIAL CONSIDERATIONS

Pregnancy-induced hypertension (PIH)

PIH is characterized by generalized vasoconstriction with relative intravascular volume depletion and, occasionally, diffuse capillary leak. There may be an increased risk of hypotension with regional anesthesia. Cautious hydration prior to regional anesthesia is necessary to prevent hypotension or pulmonary edema. Hepatic dysfunction may be present (HELLP syndrome: hemolysis, elevated liver enzymes and low Plt count). Epidural anesthesia is preferred over spinal by some, because of lower risk of hypotension. Cardiovascular stability is better with regional than GA, provided intravascular volume is adequate. Abnormal coagulation (↓Plt count or dysfunctional Plt) contraindicates regional anesthesia. If GA is necessary, control BP with small doses of labetalol (5-20 mg iv over 3-5 min) and/or low doses of a short-acting opioid (e.g., fentanyl 50-100 μg) prior to induction to blunt hypertensive response to laryngoscopy. There is a potential for difficult intubation in PIH due to airway edema; therefore, a small ETT (6.0 mm) should be available. $MgSO_4$ potentiates neuromuscular blocking agents; avoid defasiculating dose of muscle relaxant prior to induction, use smaller than normal doses of nondepolarizing agents and monitor neuromuscular function.
Tests: PT; PTT; Plt; TEG or bleeding time; LFTs

Eclampsia

Treat eclamptic seizures with adequate oxygenation and a small dose of STP (50-100 mg) or diazepam (5 mg). Intubate if necessary to protect airway. Initiate Mg sulfate therapy (loading dose: 1-4 g iv over 20-30 min, then infuse @ 1-2 g/h).

Massive maternal hemorrhage:
- **Placenta previa**
- **Abruptio placenta**
- **Ruptured uterus**

Insert 2 large-bore iv catheters (14-16 ga). Assure immediate availability of cross-matched blood. Rapidly restore intravascular volume with crystalloid, colloid or both. Induction of GA with ketamine (1-1.5 mg/kg) is preferred in hypovolemic patients. DIC can follow abruptio placenta or amniotic fluid embolism. Dilutional thrombocytopenia following massive blood loss might require Plt transfusion. Uterine atony is treated with oxytocin 20-40 U/L, NS @ rate sufficient to control atony (risk of hypotension with boluses); methylergonovine, 0.2 mg im (risk of HTN); or 15-methylprostaglandin F_2-alpha, 0.25 mg im or intramyometrially (risk of pulmonary HTN, bronchospasm). Emergency hysterectomy following cesarean delivery may be the only solution to continued bleeding. Induction of GA may be necessary if massive bleeding occurs during regional anesthesia.

Diabetes

Diabetic patients have an increased propensity to hypotension following regional anesthesia, with the fetus becoming more acidotic than normal as a result. Determine blood glucose hourly and maintain at 80-100 mg/dL. Insulin requirements decrease drastically after delivery, and insulin dosage must be reduced to prevent maternal hypoglycemia.
Tests: Fasting blood glucose; UA

Response to anesthetic drugs In pregnant patients, MAC is ↓ ≤ 40% for inhaled agents; combined with more rapid uptake, this predisposes to anesthetic overdose. Sensitivity to local anesthetics also increased. Epidural space capacity decreased, due to engorgement of epidural veins; this decreases requirements for local anesthetics and increases possibility of intravascular injection of drugs. Increased sensitivity to nondepolarizing muscle relaxants (especially in patients receiving $MgSO_4$) mandates careful monitoring and use of reduced doses. Decreased protein binding may increase toxicity of highly protein-bound drugs such as bupivacaine.

INTRAOPERATIVE

Anesthetic technique: General considerations involve primarily the choice of anesthetic. Compared with regional anesthesia, the risks of aspiration and difficult intubation with GA significantly increase maternal morbidity and mortality.[3] Anesthetic choice in specific circumstances depends on maternal and fetal conditions and degree of urgency. Properly conducted GA or regional anesthesia probably are equally safe for the fetus.

Epidural or spinal anesthesia is preferred for elective or semielective C-section when no contraindications to regional anesthesia exist (e.g., patient refusal, coagulopathy, active neurological disease, hypovolemia, sepsis). Spinal anesthesia is increasingly popular in obstetrics coincident with the use of pencil-point needles (e.g., Sprotte, Whitacre). Risk of headache with these needles is low (1-2%). Advantages of spinal over epidural anesthesia include: technical ease, more rapid onset of block, more solid anesthesia and less shivering. Hypotension, however, is more common with spinal anesthesia. Fluid loading (e.g., 1000-1500 ml LR with or without colloid) helps to minimize the risk of hypotension, and pressors (e.g., ephedrine [5-10 mg] or phenylephrine [50-100 μg]) are often required.

General anesthesia normally is used when regional anesthesia is contraindicated or when there is inadequate time to institute regional blockade. Obstetric emergencies for which rapid induction of GA may be indicated include: severe maternal hemorrhage, prolapsed umbilical cord, severe fetal bradycardia, severe persistent fetal decelerations, or the need for intrauterine manipulations. Less dire situations often permit the performance of a "quick spinal" or extension of a functioning epidural block with an agent having a rapid onset (e.g., 15-20 ml 3% 2-chloroprocaine or 2% lidocaine with epinephrine). Continuous monitoring of the fetal heart rate (FHR) in the OR may allow use of regional anesthesia if the FHR tracing is reassuring. Constant communication with the obstetrician regarding maternal and fetal condition is essential. Although situations exist in which a GA is preferable to regional, the risks must be weighed against the benefits for patients with greater potential for complications. If difficult intubation is anticipated, rapid-sequence induction of GA should not be undertaken. Alternative approaches include awake intubation, spinal anesthesia or local infiltration by the obstetrician. Sometimes, a nonreassuring FHR pattern is diagnosed as "fetal distress" and the patient is delivered immediately. Fetal distress is an imprecise and nonspecific term with little positive predictive value. The severity of any FHR abnormality should be considered when the urgency of delivery and type of anesthesia are determined. C-section performed for a nonreassuring FHR pattern does not necessarily preclude the use of regional anesthesia.[6]

Regional anesthesia:

Epidural Apply monitors, fluid load and place the patient in the sitting or lateral decubitus position. A 3 ml test dose of 1.5-2% lidocaine (45-60 mg) with 1:200,000 epinephrine (15-20 μg) is given through the epidural needle or catheter to exclude intravascular injection (Sx: tachycardia palpitations, dizziness, tinnitus, new taste in mouth) or subarachnoid placement (motor/sensory block in lower extremities). After 3-5 min, inject 15-20 ml 2% (300-400 mg) lidocaine with 1:200,000 epinephrine (75-100 μg) incrementally over 5 min. Sodium bicarbonate, 1 mEq/10 ml lidocaine, hastens onset of block, but increases risk of hypotension. Bupivacaine or ropivacaine 0.5%, 15-20 ml (75-100 mg), with or without epinephrine 1:200,000 and/or fentanyl (50-75 μg), or 3% 2-chloroprocaine, 15-20 ml (450-600 mg) also can be used. To ensure a T4 level of anesthesia throughout surgery, additional local anesthetic is often needed. If a functioning epidural catheter is in place and an urgent C-section becomes necessary, 15-20 ml 3% 2-chloroprocaine (450-600 mg) or 2% lidocaine with epinephrine should produce adequate surgical anesthesia within 5-10 min.

Tilt table or use left hip elevation. Administer O_2 by mask or nasal cannula, and check FHR prior to abdominal prep. Monitor BP every min until stable, then every 3-5 min. Treat ↓20% in BP or SBP < 95-100 mmHg with further uterine displacement, additional fluids, and ephedrine 5-10 mg iv. For inadequate anesthesia, give additional epidural local anesthetic, 50-100 μg fentanyl iv or epidurally, 50% N_2O/O_2, ketamine 5-10 mg iv and/or infiltrate with local anesthetic. The patient must remain conscious to avoid risk of aspiration. If anesthesia is still inadequate, induce GA (see below). After delivery of infant and placenta, rapidly infuse oxytocin 20-30 U/L. Antibiotics given at surgeon's request. Observe for excessive blood loss. Chest pain, mild oxyhemoglobin desaturation

Epidural, cont.	and SOB after delivery may be due to irritation of diaphragm by blood or packs, too high or inadequate level of anesthesia, or venous air or amniotic fluid embolization. S-T segment changes on ECG occur, but do not usually signify myocardial ischemia.[8]
Spinal	Apply monitors, administer fluid, and position as for epidural anesthesia. Metoclopramide 10 mg iv, 5-10 min prior to block decreases intraop N/V. Insert 24-25 ga pencil-point needle (or small diamond-tip needle) and verify free flow of CSF. In urgent situations, a larger pencil-point needle (e.g., 22 ga Sprotte) is easier and faster to place with minimal increase in headache. Inject hyperbaric 0.75% spinal bupivacaine, 11.25-12.0 mg (1.5-1.6 ml) ± fentanyl 10-15 μg or preservative-free MS 0.1-0.25 mg, and position the patient with left uterine displacement. Prophylactic ephedrine, 5-10 mg iv, at time of spinal injection decreases the incidence of hypotension. Monitor and treat BP as for epidural. Adjust operating table position to insure a T4 level of anesthesia. If anesthesia is inadequate and time permits, consider repeating spinal block or placement of an epidural catheter. Treat persistent inadequate anesthesia as for epidural. Induce GA if other measures fail.

General anesthesia:

Induction	Tilt table or use left hip displacement and administer 500-750 ml dextrose-free crystalloid prior to induction. Preoxygenation for 3 min is optimal; however, 4 maximal inspiratory breaths in 30 sec is a satisfactory substitute in an emergency. Place patient in maximal "sniff" position with elevation of shoulders, if necessary, to optimize position for intubation. After patient is prepped and draped and obstetric team is ready to begin, perform rapid-sequence induction with cricoid pressure. Administer STP, 4-5 mg/kg (or ketamine, 1-1.5 mg/kg, in hypovolemic patients) and succinylcholine 1-1.5 mg/kg to induce GA and facilitate intubation. Inflate cuff of ETT and verify tracheal placement by $ETCO_2$ waveform and auscultation of bilateral breath sounds.
Failed intubation[1,2]	If tracheal intubation is unsuccessful, monitor O_2 saturation and mask ventilate, maintaining cricoid pressure. Summon experienced help and quickly decide whether surgery must proceed. The risks of continuing with mask GA and cricoid pressure must be weighed against the risk of allowing the mother to awaken. If mask ventilation is impossible, quickly attempt ventilation with an LMA. If this succeeds, either continue to use throughout the case or place special, long ETT (MLT) through LMA blindly or with fiber optic laryngoscopy. If LMA fails to allow ventilation, attempt emergency transtracheal ventilation using a 12-14-ga iv catheter and appropriate tubing to connect to a high-pressure O_2 source (e.g. jet ventilator). If these measures are unsuccessful, an emergency cricothyrotomy or tracheostomy should be performed by experienced personnel. **Planning for a failed intubation must occur before it actually happens.** A difficult intubation tray, including equipment for emergency jet ventilation, must be immediately accessible in the delivery room.
Maintenance	50% N_2O/O_2 with 0.7-1.0% isoflurane or sevoflurane, or 0.5% halothane. Control ventilation, avoiding extreme hypocapnia ($PCO_2 < 30$ mmHg) which decreases umbilical blood flow. After delivery, substitute an opioid (e.g., fentanyl 50-100 μg) for volatile agent and increase concentration of N_2O to 70%. Administer small doses of muscle relaxants (e.g., vecuronium 2-3 mg) as needed. Reverse with neostigmine 0.05 mg/kg and glycopyrrolate 0.01 mg/kg or atropine 0.02 mg/kg. Midazolam (1-2 mg) given after delivery helps avoid maternal awareness, which occasionally occurs with this anesthetic technique.
Emergence	Delay extubation until patient is fully awake and muscle strength has returned to normal.

Blood and fluid requirements	Moderate blood loss IV: 16-18 ga × 1 NS/LR 1-3 L typical replacement	Infuse 1-2 L dextrose-free crystalloid immediately prior to regional anesthesia. Typical blood loss = 500-800 ml. A rapid-fluid infuser and blood warmer should be available in the event that large-volume blood transfusion is required.
Monitoring	Standard monitors (p. B-1). FHR monitor ± CVP or PA catheter	Arterial BP monitoring via automated BP device or arterial line for severe or labile HTN. CVP or PA catheter useful in PIH for oliguric patients unresponsive to fluid challenges. PA catheter indicated for pulmonary edema.
Positioning	Left uterine displacement (blanket under right hip and/or table tilt)	Minimizes aortocaval compression.

Complications	Amniotic fluid embolism	Rare cause of hemodynamic instability, hypoxemia and DIC. Often fatal. Rx: supportive – 100% O_2, PEEP and vasopressors.

POSTOPERATIVE

Complications	PE	DX: pleuritic chest pain, hypoxemia, ↑RR, ↑HR, ↑A-a gradient. Rx: supportive – 100% O_2, volume expansion and vasopressors.
	Postpartum hemorrhage	See Anesthetic Considerations for Removal of Retained Placenta, p. 618.
Pain management	**Epidural:** 4-5 mg preservative-free morphine in 10 ml after delivery. **Intrathecal:** morphine 0.1-0.25 mg given with spinal local anesthetic. Chloroprocaine interferes with analgesia from epidural opioids.	Common side effects include: pruritus 70%, nausea 30-40% and, rarely, respiratory depression. Nalbuphine (5-10 mg) and naloxone (0.1-0.4 mg) are used for reversal of these side effects. Metoclopramide (10 mg iv) and/or ondansetron (4 mg iv) may be needed for persistent nausea. Risk of delayed respiratory depression in healthy patients is small; however, adequately trained nursing staff and a protocol for treatment of complications are mandatory if intraspinal opioids are used. These patients should not routinely receive sedatives or other systemic opioids for 12 h, and close monitoring of RR and level of consciousness is necessary. Pulse oximetry is recommended in high-risk patients.
	Parenteral opioids: iv or im opioids or PCA instituted in recovery room.	
Tests	As indicated.	

References

1. Benumof JL: Laryngeal mask airway and the ASA difficult airway algorithm. *Anesthesiology* 1996; 84:686-99.
2. Benumof JL: Management of the difficult adult airway: With special emphasis on awake tracheal intubation. *Anesthesiology* 1991; 75(6):1087-1110.
3. Chadwick HS, Posner K, Caplan RA, Ward RJ, Cheney FW: A comparison of obstetric and nonobstetric anesthesia malpractice claims. *Anesthesiology* 1991; 74(2):242-49.
4. Cunningham FG, MacDonald PC, Gant NF, Leveno KJ, Gilstrap LC, Hankins GDV, Clark SL: Cesarean delivery and cesarean hysterectomy. In *Williams Obstetrics*, 20th edition. Appleton & Lange, Stamford, CT: 1997, 509-32.
5. Hawkins JL, Koonin LM, Palmer SK, Gibbs CP: Anesthesia-related deaths during obstetric delivery in the United States, 1979-1990. *Anesthesiology* 1997; 86:277-84.
6. Marx GF, Luykx WM, Cohen S: Fetal-neonatal status following caesarean section for fetal distress. *Br J Anaesth* 1984; 56(9):1009-13.
7. McLintic AJ, Pringle SD, Lilley S, Houston AB, Thorburn J: Electrocardiographic changes during cesarean section under regional anesthesia. *Anesth Analg* 1992; 74(1):51-6.
8. O'Driscoll K, Foley M: Correlation of decrease in perinatal mortality and increase in cesarian section rates. *Obstet Gynecol* 1983; 61(1):1-5.

EMERGENT OBSTETRICAL HYSTERECTOMY

SURGICAL CONSIDERATIONS

Yasser El-Sayed

Description: The most common indications for emergency obstetrical hysterectomy are intractable postpartum bleeding and rupture of the gravid uterus. Causes of intractable postpartum bleeding include uterine rupture after a vaginal delivery, placenta accreta or previa, and postpartum uterine atony nonresponsive to other interventions, either medical (oxytocin, methylergonovine, prostaglandins) or surgical (ligation of uterine or internal iliac arteries). Causes of uterine rupture include breakdown of a previous uterine scar, obstructed labor or trauma. The emergent nature of these conditions requires rapid intervention by the anesthesiologist, including iv fluid resuscitation, as well as blood and blood product administration, if necessary. The patient's oxygenation and coagulation parameters must be monitored closely, given the risk of hypoxia and DIC 2° massive blood loss. Prompt transfer to a well equipped OR should be undertaken.

The technique for an emergent obstetrical hysterectomy is largely similar to a hysterectomy for other indications. Of note is the engorged and prominent nature of the vessels supplying the gravid uterus. The edematous tissues surrounding the uterus are very friable and may bleed profusely if improperly manipulated. A **supracervical** or **total hysterectomy** may be performed. Through a midline or Pfannenstiel's incision, the uterus is elevated out of the abdominal cavity. The round ligaments are clamped, transected and ligated; and the anterior leaf of the broad ligament is incised bilaterally from the transected round ligaments to the vesicouterine reflection. The posterior leaf of the broad ligament adjacent to the uterus is entered at a level just below that of the fallopian tubes and uteroovarian ligaments. These are then clamped, transected and ligated. Next, incision of the posterior leaf of the broad ligament toward the cardinal ligaments is performed. With gentle blunt dissection, the bladder and attached vesicouterine peritoneal flap are dissected off the lower uterine segment. The ascending uterine arteries and veins are identified bilaterally, then clamped, transected and ligated. If a subtotal hysterectomy is planned, the body of the uterus is amputated at this level, and the cervical stump is closed with interrupted sutures. If a total hysterectomy is planned, dissection of the bladder off the cervix is continued until the cervicovaginal margin is identified. The cardinal and uterosacral ligaments are clamped, transected and ligated, with clamps placed as close to the cervix as possible without including cervical tissue. Once the level of the lateral vaginal fornix is reached, a clamp is swung below the cervix, across the lateral vaginal fornix. The cervix is then amputated off the vaginal cuff. Throughout the procedure, it is vital to clamp and ligate any bleeding vessels, and to take extra care to avoid damage to the ureter or bladder. Following removal of the uterus and cervix, the vaginal cuff angles are sutured to the ipsilateral cardinal ligament stumps, and the vaginal cuff is closed with a running locked stitch. The abdominal wall is closed in layers.

Usual preop diagnosis: Intractable postpartum bleeding; rupture of gravid uterus

SUMMARY OF PROCEDURE

Position	Supine, with left lateral tilt
Incision	Pfannenstiel's or midline longitudinal
Unique considerations	Monitoring of coagulation parameters and correction of DIC. Consider central venous hemodynamic monitoring. Pediatrics team present, if indicated.
Antibiotics	Cefotetan 2 g iv q 12 h; total 3 doses
Surgical time	2-3 h
Closing considerations	Subcutaneous intraperitoneal drains, if indicated.
EBL	3000-4000 ml
Postop care	ICU if blood loss severe; patient may require continued intubation and mechanical ventilatory support. Monitor for infectious morbidity and acute renal failure.
Mortality	< 1%
Morbidity	Hemorrhage Postop febrile morbidity DIC Wound infection Sheehan's syndrome Bladder injury Intraperitoneal bleeding requiring reoperation Vesicovaginal fistula Ureterovaginal fistula Transfusion-related complications
Pain score	7

PATIENT POPULATION CHARACTERISTICS

Age range	Reproductive age
Incidence	0.11% of obstetric patients
Etiology	Unknown
Associated conditions	Placenta accreta; uterine atony nonresponsive to medical or other surgical intervention; extension of cervical tear to lower uterine segment; placenta previa; uterine rupture; uterine inversion

ANESTHETIC CONSIDERATIONS

See Anesthetic Considerations following Cesarean Section, p. 602.

References

1. Al-Sibai MH, Rahman J, Rahman MS, Butalack F: Emergency hysterectomy in obstetrics—a review of 117 cases. *Aust NZ J Obstet Gynaecol* 1987; 27(3):180-84.
2. Chestnut DH, Dewan DM, Redick LF, Caton D, Spielman FJ: Anesthetic management for obstetric hysterectomy: a multi-institutional study. *Anesthesiology* 1989; 70(4):607-10.
3. Chestnut DH, Eden RD, Gall SA, Parker RT: Peripartum hysterectomy: a review of cesarean and postpartum hysterectomy. *Obstet Gynecol* 1985; 65(3):365-70.
4. Clark SL, Yeh SY, Phelan JP, Bruce S, Paul RH: Emergency hysterectomy for obstetric hemorrhage. *Obstet Gynecol* 1984; 64(3):376-80.
5. Creasy RK, Resnik R, eds: *Maternal-Fetal Medicine: Principles and Practice*, 3rd edition. WB Saunders, Philadelphia: 1994, 602-19.
6. Cunningham FG, MacDonald PC, Gant NF, Leveno KJ, Gilstrap LC, Hankins GDV, Clark SL: Cesarean delivery and cesarean hysterectomy. In *Williams Obstetrics*, 20th edition. Appleton & Lange, Stamford, CT: 1997, 509-32.
7. O'Grady JP, Gimovsky ML, McIlhargie, eds: *Operative Obstetrics*. Williams & Wilkins, Baltimore: 1995, 264-67.
8. Plauche WC: Peripartum hysterectomy. *Obstet Gynecol Clin North Am* 1988; 15(4):783-95.

REPAIR OF UTERINE RUPTURE

SURGICAL CONSIDERATIONS

Babak Edraki

Description: Rupture of the gravid uterus is considered a true obstetric emergency and can be catastrophic, with significant maternal and fetal mortality. The classic symptoms are "shearing" pain, cessation of uterine contractions, loss of fetal heart tones and the onset of vaginal bleeding. Unfortunately, these warning symptoms occur only in a minority of uterine rupture cases. Extrusion of the placenta through the uterine rupture may result in late decelerations due to uteroplacental insufficiency. Extrusion of the umbilical cord may be manifested by recurrent variable decelerations. Suprapubic pain as the only symptom has not been associated with uterine rupture. In cases where the uterine rupture occurs at the site of a prior uterine scar, the clinical course is usually less severe and the blood loss less than in cases of primary rupture of an intact uterus. The incidence of uterine rupture at the site of the old scar is 0.5% for lower-uterine transverse cesarean sections, and 2% for classic cesarean sections. Uterine rupture mimics abruptio placenta in its presentations; however, once the diagnosis is made, prompt surgical intervention is mandated. **Total abdominal hysterectomy** (see p. 588), or **supracervical hysterectomy** (p. 607), is the definitive therapy; however, depending on the clinical situation and patient's wishes for future fertility, a **uterine repair** may be undertaken. This consists of a 2-3-layered closure of the defect, using synthetic absorbable sutures. A transverse abdominal incision is made approximately 3 cm above the symphysis pubis and carried to the anterior rectus fascia. The fascia is incised and the muscles of the anterior abdominal wall separated from the midline sharply and bluntly. The peritoneum is elevated and entered sharply. Because of the emergent nature of this condition and the possible massive blood loss associated with rupture of a gravid uterus, the anesthesiologist must act quickly. Prompt O_2 administration, together with aggressive iv fluid resuscitation, is indicated. Serious consideration should be given to the use of unmatched O-negative or type-specific blood until cross-matched blood becomes available. Intraop hypogastric or uterine artery ligation may help minimize blood loss. Patient's coagulation parameters must be monitored, since hypoxia and massive blood loss are associated with DIC.

Usual preop diagnosis: Uterine rupture

SUMMARY OF PROCEDURE

Position	Supine with left-lateral tilt
Incision	Pfannenstiel's (low, transverse abdominal) or midline longitudinal
Unique considerations	Pediatrics team present for infant resuscitation, if necessary. Thorough surgical exploration of the urinary tract (bladder and ureters) since ~10% of cases are associated with bladder lacerations. Cell Saver may be helpful.
Antibiotics	Cefotetan 2 g iv q 12 h × 3 doses
Surgical time	1-2 h
EBL	500-3000 ml
Postop care	ICU if blood loss severe; continued intubation and mechanical ventilatory support if aggressive fluid resuscitation results in pulmonary edema. Acute renal failure may occur 2° hypoxic and hypovolemic renal injury at time of acute uterine rupture with massive bleeding; monitor UO and serial renal function tests.
Mortality	Fetal: 35-45% Maternal: 5%
Morbidity	Blood transfusion > 5 U: 58.3% Postop wound infection: 33% Pelvic abscess: 8.3% Repeat uterine rupture with subsequent pregnancies: 5%
Pain score	6

PATIENT POPULATION CHARACTERISTICS

Age range	Reproductive age
Incidence	1/1400 deliveries
Etiology	Prior uterine surgery; grand multiparity; obesity; manual removal of placenta; injury from tools of abortion; direct or indirect violence; oxytocin use; intraamniotic or vaginal prostaglandins; breech extractions; internal or external version; forceps rotation; shoulder dystocia; fundal pressure; neglect (cephalopelvic disproportion, etc.); congenital uterine anomaly; cornual pregnancy; gestational trophoblastic neoplasia; placenta percreta; abruptio placenta

ANESTHETIC CONSIDERATIONS

See Anesthetic Considerations following Cesarean Section. p. 602.

References

1. Akasheh F: Rupture of the uterus. Analysis of 104 cases of rupture. *Am J Obstet Gynecol* 1968; 101(3):406-8.
2. Chazotte C, Cohen WR: Catastrophic complications of previous cesarean section. *Am J Obstet Gynecol* 1990; 163(3):738-42.
3. Claman P, Carpenter RJ, Reiter A: Uterine rupture with the use of vaginal prostaglandin E_2 for induction of labor. *Am J Obstet Gynecol* 1984; 150(7):889-90.
4. Cunningham FG, MacDonald PC, Gant NF, Leveno KJ, Gilstrap LC, Hankins GDV, Clark SL: Surgical contraception. In *Williams Obstetrics*, 20th edition. Appleton & Lange, Stamford, CT: 1997, 137-8.
5. Eden RD, Parker RT, Gall SA: Rupture of the pregnant uterus: a 53-year review. *Obstet Gynecol* 1986; 68(5):671-74.
6. Golan A, Sandbank O, Rubin A: Rupture of the pregnant uterus. *Obstet Gynecol* 1980; 56(5):549-54.
7. Plauche WC, VonAlmen W, Muller R: Catastrophic uterine rupture. *Obstet Gynecol* 1984; 64(6):792-97.
8. Reyes-Ceja L, Cabrera R, Insfran E, Herrera-Lasso F: Pregnancy following previous uterine rupture. Study of 19 patients. *Obstet Gynecol* 1969; 34(3):387-89.
9. Sawyer MM, Lipshitz J, Anderson GD, Dilts PV Jr: Third-trimester uterine rupture associated with vaginal prostaglandin E_2. *Am J Obstet Gynecol* 1981; 140(6):710-11.-9
10. Yussman MA, Haynes DM: Rupture of the gravid uterus. A 12-year study. *Obstet Gynecol* 1970; 36(1):115-20.

POSTPARTUM TUBAL LIGATION

SURGICAL CONSIDERATIONS

Ronald N. Gibson

Description: Postpartum tubal ligation (PPTL) is female surgical sterilization performed at the time of cesarean section (C-section) after delivery of the infant and repair of the uterine incision or within the first several days after a vaginal delivery. Although PPTL can be performed immediately postpartum, problems in the neonate may not be immediately evident, and a delay in surgery may be appropriate. If performed after a vaginal delivery, a small infraumbilical incision is made in the skin and carried down through the parietal peritoneum. The fallopian tubes are identified and brought out of the incision. It is important to identify the fimbriated end of the tube to ensure that the structure ligated is not the round ligament. A midsegment portion of the tube over an avascular portion of mesosalpinx is selected and tubal patency is disrupted by a variety of methods (**Pomeroy, Parkland, Irving, Uchida,** etc.). The Pomeroy, or a modification of it, is the most common technique used. The segment of tube grasped is ligated with absorbable suture and the knuckle of tube formed is excised. The cut ends of the tubes should be hemostatic before replacing the tubes into the abdomen. The wound is closed in layers in the usual fashion.

The consent for sterilization requires special consideration. The procedure is strictly elective and voluntary and must be considered permanent, even though reversal may be possible. Some patients will eventually regret their decision to undergo permanent sterilization. The risk of sterilization failure and an increased risk of ectopic pregnancy in case of failure must be reviewed. The full range of alternatives to PPTL, including an interval sterilization procedure (sterilization performed remote from pregnancy) must also be considered.

Usual preop diagnosis: Desire for permanent sterilization

SUMMARY OF PROCEDURE

Position	Supine; steep Trendelenburg often required to allow bowel to fall away for exposure.
Incision	Infraumbilical
Special instrumentation	Small Richardson and Army/Navy retractors; Babcock clamps; vein retractor
Unique considerations	A special consent form for sterilization must be signed by the patient in advance of the surgery. The bladder must be drained prior to the procedure.
Antibiotics	None recommended
Surgical time	15-25 min (Uchida technique may ↑ operative time)
EBL	10 ml
Postop care	Routine postpartum care after recovery from anesthesia
Mortality	3/100,000
Morbidity	Hemorrhage Infection Incidental damage to bowel or bladder
Pain score	3

PATIENT POPULATION CHARACTERISTICS

Age range	Reproductive age
Incidence	The most common contraceptive procedure in the U.S.

ANESTHETIC CONSIDERATIONS

PREOPERATIVE

Optimal timing of tubal ligation is controversial. The patient with a functioning epidural catheter may benefit from having surgery immediately after delivery. Many surgeons, however, favor waiting 8-24 h, when adequate assessment of the neonate should be complete and risk of maternal hemorrhage lessened. Alternatively, the epidural catheter can be left in place and reinjected later. Because pulmonary aspiration remains a theoretical risk, initiation of GA or spinal anesthesia often is delayed 8-24 h until the acute GI changes of pregnancy have regressed. There is no benefit to delaying surgery beyond this time. Shorter hospital stays after vaginal delivery are encouraging more tubal ligations during the first 12 h after delivery. It is unknown whether this will affect morbidity or mortality.

Respiratory	FRC returns to normal almost immediately after delivery. **Tests:** As indicated from H&P.
Cardiovascular	The physiologic changes of pregnancy return to normal at varying intervals after delivery. For example, risk of aortocaval compression disappears immediately. Blood volume returns to prepregnant values over several days. Postpartum hemorrhage can occur without warning. **Tests:** As indicated from H&P.
Gastrointestinal	Postpartum patients continue to be at risk for acid aspiration, although it is not known exactly when normal GI function returns. Precautions for prevention of acid aspiration should be followed as discussed in Cesarean Section, p. 602.
Neurological	Local anesthetic requirements for spinal anesthesia remain decreased after delivery but are greater than for pregnant patients.
Laboratory	Hct; other tests as indicated from H&P.
Premedication	Precautions should be taken to decrease risk of aspiration pneumonitis, as discussed under Cesarean Section, p. 603.

INTRAOPERATIVE

Anesthetic technique: Spinal anesthesia is preferred if a functioning epidural catheter is not in place. Epidural catheters frequently become dislodged after patient becomes ambulatory. GA is acceptable if patient has a strong preference or if contraindications to regional anesthesia exist. These patients may be at risk for aspiration of gastric contents at least 8-24 h postdelivery.

Regional anesthesia:

Spinal	For technique and monitoring for spinal anesthesia, see Cesarean Section, p. 605. Hyperbaric 5% lidocaine was the drug of choice for this procedure, but concerns about transient radicular irritation after spinal lidocaine have led some to abandon its use.[6] Most procedures for PPTL last 20-40 min, but some (e.g., Uchida, Irving) may last ~1 h. If more prolonged surgery is likely (e.g., obese patient, or patient with adhesions) or for routine use, bupivacaine (7.5-12 mg) ± fentanyl (10-25 μg) may be preferable. With the patient supine, adjust position of the operating table to obtain a T6 level of anesthesia. Sedate patient as necessary with small doses of iv midazolam 0.5-1.0 mg, or opioid.
Epidural	A 3 ml epidural test dose, followed after 3-5 min by 15-20 ml 3% 2-chloroprocaine or 1.5-2% lidocaine with 1:200,000 epinephrine injected incrementally. Additional local anesthetic as needed to ensure adequate level of anesthesia.

General anesthesia:

Induction	Rapid-sequence induction with STP (4-5 mg/kg) or propofol (1-2 mg/kg) and succinylcholine (1 mg/kg) for ET intubation.
Maintenance	Standard maintenance (p. B-3)
Emergence	Extubation should be delayed until patient is fully awake and protective airway reflexes have returned.

Blood and fluid requirements	Minimal blood loss IV: 18 ga × 1 NS/LR @ 2-4 ml/kg/h	1-1.5 L dextrose-free crystalloid immediately prior to regional anesthesia
Monitoring	Standard monitors (p. B-1)	
Positioning	✓ and pad pressure points. ✓ eyes.	
Complications	None specific	

POSTOPERATIVE

Complications	Minimal bleeding	
Pain management	**Intraspinal opioids**: 10-25 μg fentanyl **Parenteral opioids**: IV or im opioids (e.g., meperidine 10-20 mg iv q 10-15 min titrated to RR and patient's level of pain) instituted in recovery room.	Intrathecal fentanyl 10-25 μg, given with spinal local anesthetic, enhances intraop anesthesia, particularly with low doses of bupivacaine, and provides several h postop analgesia.
Tests	None routinely indicated.	

References

1. Abouleish EI: Postpartum tubal ligation requires more bupivacaine for spinal anesthesia than does cesarean section. *Anesth Analg* 1986; 65(8):897-900.
2 American College of Obstetricians and Gynecologists: Ethical considerations in sterilization. ACOG Committee Opinion 73. Washington, DC: 1989.
3. American College of Obstetricians and Gynecologists: Female sterilization by tubal interruption. ACOG Criteria, Set 9. Washington, DC: 1995.
4. American College of Obstetricians and Gynecologists: Postpartum tubal sterilization. ACOG Committee Opinion 105. Washington, DC: 1992.
5. Cunningham FG, MacDonald PC, Grant NF, et al, eds: *Williams Obstetrics*, 20th edition. Appleton & Lange, Stamford, CT: 1997, 1375-81.
6. Hampl KF, Schneider MC, Pargger H, Gut J, Drewe J, Drasner K: A similar incidence of transient neurologic symptoms after spinal anesthesia with 2 percent and 5 percent lidocaine. *Anesth Analg* 1996; 83:1051-54.
7. Hatcher RA, Stewart F, Trussell J, et al: *Contraceptive Technology*, 15th revised edition. Irvinton Publishers, New York: 1990, 387-421.
8. Wheeless CR Jr: *Atlas of Pelvic Surgery*, 2nd edition. Lea & Febiger, Philadelphia: 1988, 282-88.

REPAIR OF VAGINAL/CERVICAL LACERATIONS

SURGICAL CONSIDERATIONS

Ronald N. Gibson

Description: Vaginal and cervical lacerations may occur 2° trauma of spontaneous and operative vaginal delivery. Adequate repair requires optimal surgical assistance, exposure and patient comfort. Repair may be performed in a birthing bed, or may require patient positioning, lighting, anesthesia or monitoring capabilities available only in an OR. Vaginal and cervical lacerations can extend into the perineum, rectum, urethra, bladder, lower uterine segment, broad ligament or peritoneal cavity.

Lacerations of the lower vagina are generally easy to identify and repair. Small superficial lacerations that do not bleed often do not need repair, while larger ones should be approximated. Deep lacerations may cause profuse bleeding; if it persists despite placement of multiple stitches, brief tamponade may be adequate to achieve hemostasis, or vaginal packing may be required. Lacerations involving the perineum are classified as follows. First degree: involves break in mucosa and skin. Second degree: involves deeper tissue (bulbocavernosus and levator ani fascia and muscle). Third degree: involves anal sphincter. Fourth degree: extends into rectal mucosa. First- and second-degree lacerations are repaired in layers with continuous or interrupted stitches. The skin is usually closed with a subcuticular stitch. When the anal sphincter is lacerated, it often retracts. The ends are grasped with Allis clamps and approximated with multiple figure-of-eight stitches. When the laceration extends into the rectum, the rectal mucosa usually is closed in two layers, with the second layer imbricating the first. With periurethral lacerations, a catheter may need to be placed in the urethra to prevent passing a stitch through it. A laceration involving the urethra or bladder should be closed in multiple layers, followed by bladder drainage for several days.

Lacerations of the upper vagina are often difficult to visualize. Uterine bleeding and the umbilical cord of an undelivered placenta can obscure the field, and it can be difficult to determine if bleeding is vaginal or uterine. It is helpful to deliver the placenta and control uterine bleeding before proceeding. Once visualization is adequate, it is important to place the first stitch above the apex of the laceration to control bleeding from vessels that may have retracted. Again, vaginal packing may be required if oozing of blood persists.

Superficial **lacerations of the cervix** occur with most deliveries but usually require no treatment. Deep lacerations can cause significant blood loss, especially when they involve larger branches from the uterine artery or extend into the lower uterine segment. Again, the first stitch must be placed above the apex of the laceration to control bleeding from vessels that may have retracted. A **laparotomy** may be necessary if a laceration extends into the lower uterine segment or broad ligament and is causing significant bleeding that cannot be controlled otherwise.

Usual preop diagnosis: Vaginal or cervical laceration

SUMMARY OF PROCEDURE

Position	Dorsal lithotomy
Incision	None (unless exploratory laparotomy is performed)
Special instrumentation	Right-angle retractors; ring forceps; Allis clamps; Gelpi retractor; vaginal packing
Antibiotics	May be used for lacerations involving entry into the peritoneal cavity or the rectal mucosa.
Surgical time	10-45 min (possibly longer if exploratory laparotomy is performed)
EBL	Variable. Possible need for transfusion. Areas that persistently ooze after repeated placement of suture may be managed with vaginal packing.
Postop care	PACU → ward
Mortality	Rare
Morbidity	Hemorrhage Hematoma Infection Rectovaginal fistula Vesicovaginal fistula
Pain score	3

PATIENT POPULATION CHARACTERISTICS

Age range	Reproductive age
Incidence	Not uncommon
Etiology	Trauma 2° spontaneous or operative vaginal delivery (98%); other vaginal/pelvic trauma (2%)
Associated conditions	Major blood loss possible; with nonobstetric etiology, the possibility of sexual assault needs to be explored.

ANESTHETIC CONSIDERATIONS

PREOPERATIVE

Vaginal and cervical lacerations may go undetected until a considerable loss of blood has occurred. Patients should be examined carefully for Sx of hypovolemia with appropriate volume resuscitation prior to anesthesia.

Respiratory	FRC returns to normal almost immediately after delivery. **Tests:** As indicated from H&P.
Cardiovascular	The physiologic changes of pregnancy return to normal at varying intervals after delivery. For example, risk of aortocaval compression disappears immediately. Blood volume returns to prepregnant values over several days. Postpartum hemorrhage can occur without warning. Ensure adequate fluid resuscitation prior to induction of GA or regional anesthesia. **Tests:** As indicated from H&P.
Gastrointestinal	Postpartum patients continue to be at risk for acid aspiration, although it is not known exactly when normal GI function returns. Precautions for prevention of acid aspiration should be followed as discussed in Cesarean Section, p. 602.
Neurological	Local anesthetic requirements for spinal anesthesia remain decreased after delivery.
Laboratory	Hct; other tests as indicated from H&P.
Premedication	Precautions should be taken to decrease risk of aspiration pneumonitis, as discussed under Cesarean Section, p. 603.

INTRAOPERATIVE

Anesthetic technique: In many patients, a functioning epidural catheter will be in place, and supplemental doses of anesthetic may be given to provide adequate analgesia for the surgery. If no epidural is placed and the patient is hemodynamically stable, a spinal anesthetic may be satisfactory. Occasionally GA may be required.

Regional anesthesia:

Epidural	Supplemental doses of local anesthetic (2-chloroprocaine or 1.5-2% lidocaine 10-15 ml) injected incrementally with patient in sitting position (if tolerated) to promote perineal anesthesia.
Spinal	Hyperbaric lidocaine 5% 50-70 mg (see comments regarding transient radicular irritation on p. 611) or hyperbaric bupivacaine 0.75% 7.5-10 mg with patient in sitting position, if tolerated. 24-25 ga pencil-point needle (Sprotte or Whitacre) to decrease incidence of spinal headache. Anesthesia to T10 is usually adequate. Repair of more extensive lacerations may require a higher level and, consequently, a higher dose of anesthetic.

General anesthesia:

Induction	Rapid-sequence induction with STP (4-5 mg/kg) and succinylcholine (1 mg/kg) for ET intubation. If significant blood loss, ketamine 1.5 mg/kg is preferred for induction.
Maintenance	Standard maintenance (p. B-3). If significant blood loss, ketamine 1.5 mg/kg is preferred for induction.
Emergence	Extubation should be delayed until patient is fully awake and protective airway reflexes have returned.

Blood and fluid requirements	IV: 16-18 ga × 1 NS/LR @ 2-4 ml/kg/h	1-1.5 L dextrose-free crystalloid immediately prior to regional anesthesia. Blood loss may be extensive until laceration is repaired.
Monitoring	Standard monitors (p. B-1)	
Complications	Bleeding	
Positioning	✓ and pad pressure points. ✓ eyes.	★ **NB:** peroneal nerve compression at lateral fibular head → foot drop.

POSTOPERATIVE

Complications	Bleeding Peroneal nerve injury (2° lithotomy position)	Nerve injury manifested as foot drop and loss of sensation over dorsum of foot.
Pain management	**Intraspinal opioids**: 10 μg fentanyl **Parenteral opioids**: iv or im opioids (e.g., meperidine 10-20 mg iv q 10-15 min up to 50 mg instituted in recovery room.	Intrathecal fentanyl 10 μg given with spinal local anesthetic – enhances intraop anesthesia and provides several h postop analgesia.
Tests	Hct	

References

1. Cunningham FG, MacDonald PC, Grant NF, et al, eds: *Williams Obstetrics*, 20th edition. Appleton & Lange, Stamford, CT: 1997, 327-46, 745-82.
2. Golan A, David MP: Repair of birth injuries. In *Operative Perinatology: Invasive Obstetric Techniques*. Iffy L, Charles D, eds. MacMillan, New York: 1984, 730-50.
3. Zuspan P, Quilligan EJ, eds: *Douglas-Stromme: Operative Obstetrics*, 5th edition. Appleton & Lange, New York: 1988.

CERVICAL CERCLAGE—ELECTIVE AND EMERGENT

SURGICAL CONSIDERATIONS

Ronald N. Gibson

Description: Cervical cerclage is the reinforcement of the cervix to prevent premature cervical dilation in a patient with an incompetent cervix. With cervical incompetence there is painless dilation of the cervix in the midtrimester of pregnancy. The membranes bulge through the cervix and rupture, followed by delivery of a severely premature infant.

An **elective cerclage** is performed prophylactically before pregnancy or usually after the first trimester of pregnancy on a patient with a past history of cervical incompetence. If cerclage is performed before pregnancy, it may need to be removed because of spontaneous abortion or fetal anomalies. It generally is performed between 14-16 wk gestation, but may be performed as early as 10 wk gestation. An **emergent cerclage** is performed in a patient who presents in the second trimester with painless cervical dilation and/or effacement. Ultrasound is performed before the procedure to confirm viability and to rule out major congenital anomalies. An emergent cerclage should not be performed if there is advanced cervical dilation or any evidence of infection, contractions or uterine bleeding.

There are two types of cerclage procedures generally performed: the McDonald and the Shirodkar. The **McDonald cerclage** is technically easier, and the one most commonly performed. A purse-string stitch with nonabsorbable monofilament suture is placed high around the cervix near the level of the internal os and tied at the twelve o'clock position. The end of the suture is cut long to facilitate removal. The cerclage is removed electively at term or earlier if there is rupture of membranes, persistent contractions, bleeding or evidence of infection. The **Shirodkar cerclage** involves incising the cervix transversely, anteriorly and posteriorly, and advancing the bladder off the cervix. A nonabsorbable monofilament suture is placed submucosally between the incisions, and the mucosa is closed, burying the stitch. A Shirodkar cerclage may be left for future pregnancies if abdominal delivery is performed.

Usual preop diagnosis: Cervical incompetence

SUMMARY OF PROCEDURE

Position	Dorsal lithotomy, with use of cane stirrups. Left lateral pelvic tilt (if performed during pregnancy); Trendelenburg.
Incision	None with McDonald cerclage; transverse cervical with Shirodkar cerclage
Special instrumentation	Right-angle retractors; monofilament, nonabsorbable stitch
Unique considerations	For emergent cerclage, when prolapsing membranes are present, they may be reduced by filling the bladder and/or possibly removing amniotic fluid transabdominally.
Antibiotics	None recommended.
Surgical time	30 min-1 h (May be longer for Shirodkar cerclage.)
EBL	25-50 ml (May be higher with the Shirodkar cerclage.)
Postop care	PACU → ward; tocolysis with indomethacin or other agent can be considered.
Mortality	Rare
Morbidity	Morbidity is increased for emergent cerclage, especially when performed later in 2nd trimester. The McDonald cerclage is associated with less trauma and bleeding than the Shirodkar cerclage. Cervical trauma Rupture of membranes Chorioamnionitis Preterm labor Spontaneous abortion
Pain score	McDonald—2; Shirodkar—3

PATIENT POPULATION CHARACTERISTICS

Age range	Reproductive age
Incidence	Not uncommon
Etiology	Cervical trauma from previous vaginal delivery; cervical trauma at time of previous D&C; previous treatment for cervical dysplasia (laser therapy, cryotherapy, LEEP/large loop excision of transitional zone [LLETZ], cone biopsy); congenital anomalies; idiopathic

ANESTHETIC CONSIDERATIONS

PREOPERATIVE

This is a generally fit and healthy patient population. Little will need to be done other than routine tests, unless otherwise indicated. Cerclage is usually performed between 14-24 wk of pregnancy. When performed after 20 wk, relevant physiologic changes are as discussed under Cesarean Section, p. 602. Patient may receive drugs such as ß-sympathomimetics (e.g., terbutaline), nifedipine or indomethacin to decrease uterine irritability.

Laboratory Hct; other tests as indicated from H&P.

Premedication None usually. If > 18 wk gestation, precautions should be taken to decrease risk of aspiration pneumonitis, as discussed under Cesarean Section, p. 603.

INTRAOPERATIVE

Anesthetic technique: Drug exposure during the critical period of organogenesis (15-56 d) should be minimized, although no particular anesthetic techniques or agents have proven teratogenic in humans. Through an action on vitamin B_{12}, N_2O inhibits methionine synthetase, which is involved in thymidine and methionine synthesis. This may explain why N_2O is teratogenic in rodents. There is no evidence, however, that N_2O is teratogenic when used for cervical cerclage or other operations in humans. Avoid diazepam during the period of organogenesis (cleft lip). Ensure adequate uteroplacental perfusion and fetal oxygenation by maintaining normal maternal BP and oxyhemoglobin saturation. Use left uterine displacement after 20 wk gestation. Maternal hyperventilation and IPPV may diminish uteroplacental and umbilical blood flow. Monitoring FHR may permit optimization of fetal well being by adjustment of anesthetic technique or patient position. Spinal anesthesia is ideal as it minimizes fetal drug exposure and provides good operating conditions. Risk of headache is low with the use of pencil-point needles (e.g., Sprotte, Whitacre). Epidural anesthesia is an appropriate alternative for this procedure. GA may be used if regional anesthesia is contraindicated.

Regional anesthesia:

Spinal Hyperbaric 5% spinal lidocaine 70-80 mg (see comments regarding transient radicular irritation, p. 611) or bupivacaine 7-10 mg ± fentanyl 10-15 µg. Position patient to obtain T8 block. Monitor BP every min until stable, then every 3-5 min. Treat > 20% decrease in BP or SBP < 95-100 mmHg with additional fluids and ephedrine 5-10 mg iv.

General anesthesia:

Induction Standard induction (p. B-2). If > 18 wk gestation, rapid-sequence induction is indicated (p. B-5).

Maintenance Standard maintenance (p. B-3). If < 15-18 wk gestation, use of LMA or mask anesthesia with O_2/N_2O/volatile agent/opioid is appropriate. If > 18 wk gestation, ET intubation will be necessary.

Emergence If > 18 wk gestation, extubate patient when fully awake and protective airway reflexes have returned.

Blood and fluid requirements	Minimal blood loss IV: 18 ga × 1 NS/LR @ 4 mg/kg/h	1-1.5 L dextrose-free crystalloid immediately prior to regional anesthesia
Monitoring	Standard monitors (p. B-1)	
Positioning	Left uterine displacement, if > 20 wk gestation ✓ and pad pressure points. ✓ eyes.	Left uterine displacement with a wedge under mattress should be used for pregnant patients (after ~ 20 wk). ★ **NB:** peroneal nerve compression at lateral fibular head → foot drop.

POSTOPERATIVE

Complications	Preterm labor Maternal dysrhythmias Hypotension Peroneal nerve injury	Observe for preterm labor in recovery area. Tocolytic agents (β-adrenergic agents) given to inhibit uterine contractions can cause maternal dysrhythmias or hypotension. Nerve injury manifested as foot drop and loss of sensation over dorsum of foot.
Pain management	**Intraspinal opioids**: 10-15 µg fentanyl **Parenteral opioids**: iv or im opioids (e.g., meperidine 10-20 mg q 15 min up to 50 mg) instituted in recovery room.	Intrathecal fentanyl given with spinal improves intraop analgesia and provides short-period postop analgesia. Risk of delayed respiration depression minimal in healthy patients.

References

1. Aldridge LM, Tunstall ME: Nitrous oxide and the fetus. A review and the results of a retrospective study of 175 cases of anaesthesia for insertion of a Shirodkar suture. *Br J Anaesth* 1986; 58(12):1348-56.
2. American College of Obstetricians and Gynecologists: Cervical cerclage, prophylactic. ACOG Criteria, Set 17. Washington, DC: ACOG, 1996.
3. American College of Obstetricians and Gynecologists: Cervical cerclage, therapeutic. ACOG Criteria, Set 18. Washington, DC: ACOG, 1996.
4. Crawford JS, Lewis M: Nitrous oxide in early human pregnancy. *Anaesthesia* 1986; 41(9):900-5.
5. O'Grady JP, Gimovsky ML, McIlhargie, eds: *Operative Obstetrics.* Williams & Wilkins, Baltimore: 1995, 44-51.
6. Mazze RI, Kallen B: Reproductive outcome after anesthesia and operation during pregnancy: a registry study of 5405 cases. *Am J Obstet Gynecol* 1989; 161(5):1178-85.
7. Parisi VM: Cervical incompetence. In *Maternal–Fetal Medicine: Principles and Practice*, 3rd edition. Creasy RK, Resnik R, eds. WB Saunders Co, Philadelphia: 1994, 453-66.
8. Safra MJ, Oakley GP Jr: Association between cleft lip with or without cleft palate and prenatal exposure to diazepam. *Lancet* 1975; 2(7933):478-84.

REMOVAL OF RETAINED PLACENTA

SURGICAL CONSIDERATIONS

Yasser El-Sayed

Description: In most deliveries, the placenta is easily removed with gentle cord traction and uterine massage. If, after 30 min, the placenta remains undelivered, **manual removal**, following either parenteral analgesia or GA, must be initiated. NTG (100-200 μg iv or 0.4 mg sublingually) may induce uterine relaxation during manual removal. A possible alternative to manual removal involves injection of 10 ml of oxytocin (10 U/ml) into the umbilical vein; however, the success of this procedure is unpredictable. A retained placental fragment may cause immediate or late postpartum hemorrhage. An ultrasound evaluation of the uterus may help in the detection of a retained fragment. If retained products are found, **curettage** is recommended. Frequently, the retained product will already have been flushed out of the uterus by brisk bleeding. In such cases, iv oxytocin, im prostaglandins or methylergonovine may be administered to contract the uterus prior to curettage.

Bleeding from a retained placenta or fragment is frequently brisk, so the anesthesiologist must be ready to administer iv fluids and O_2, and to correct any coagulopathy. Cross-matched blood must be available. Placenta accreta, if extensive, can cause profuse bleeding at delivery, and a hysterectomy is often necessary.

Oxytocin 20-40 U in 1000 ml of LR should be administered at a rate sufficient to maintain uterine tone after manual removal of the placenta or after sharp/suction curettage of a retained placental fragment.

Usual preop diagnosis: Retained placenta

SUMMARY OF PROCEDURE

Position	Dorsal lithotomy
Incision	None
Special instrumentation	Banjo curette/suction cannula
Unique considerations	IV fluids; use of blood and blood products, as needed; monitoring of vital signs
Antibiotics	Cefotetan 2 g iv q 12 h; 3 total doses
Surgical time	30 min
EBL	Variable—300-900 ml
Postop care	PACU → ward. Monitor for infection and further bleeding.
Mortality	Rare

Morbidity	Hemorrhage Endometritis Uterine perforation 2° curettage Asherman's syndrome Transfusion-related morbidity (hepatitis, HIV, transfusion reactions)
Pain score	5

PATIENT POPULATION CHARACTERISTICS

Age range	Reproductive age
Incidence	0.25-0.8% of vaginal deliveries
Etiology	Unknown
Associated conditions	Placenta accreta; avulsed cotyledon; succenturiate lobe

ANESTHETIC CONSIDERATIONS

PREOPERATIVE

The degree of urgency associated with these patients may vary dramatically. Some patients may be hemodynamically unstable as a result of continued bleeding in the postpartum period; others may have a retained placenta with minimal bleeding. Patient's volume status should be carefully assessed.

Respiratory FRC returns to normal almost immediately after delivery.
Tests: As indicated from H&P.

Cardiovascular Restore intravascular volume prior to institution of analgesia or anesthesia. Extension of existing lumbar epidural blockade may aggravate hypovolemia and should proceed with caution. Consider possibility of placenta accreta (placental villi are attached to myometrium).

Gastrointestinal Postpartum patients continue to be at risk for acid aspiration, although it is not known exactly when normal GI function returns. Precautions for prevention of acid aspiration should be followed as discussed in Cesarean Section, p. 602.

Neurological Local anesthetic requirements for spinal anesthesia remain decreased after delivery.

Hematologic Coagulopathy can develop with retained placenta if bleeding is severe and persistent.
Tests: Hct, PT; PTT; Plt; FSP, as indicated.

Laboratory Other tests as indicated from H&P. T&C for 2 U+ if time permits. Emergency transfusion with Type O(-) or type-specific blood may be necessary.

Premedication Precaution should be taken to decrease risk of aspiration, as discussed in Cesarean Section, p. 603.

INTRAOPERATIVE

Anesthetic technique: Anesthesia for the removal of a retained placenta may vary from MAC to GA performed as an emergency. In the multiparous patient, MAC may be sufficient to enable the obstetrician to empty the uterus. If better analgesia and additional uterine relaxation are needed, however, then GA may be required. The incidence of retained placenta is about 1%. If intravascular volume has been restored and an existing epidural catheter is in place, the block can be extended to provide adequate anesthesia. Initiating spinal anesthesia is also an option if: intravascular volume status is adequate, there is no active bleeding, and uterine relaxation is not required. Small doses of opioids and midazolam sometimes provide sufficient analgesia and sedation to allow removal of a retained placenta without compromising maternal safety. If this proves inadequate or hemorrhage is severe, however, GA with ET intubation is required. Anecdotal experience indicates that NTG in 100-200 μg iv boluses or sublingual NTG 400 μg provides uterine relaxation and delivery of retained placenta in normovolemic patients receiving iv analgesia.[3]

Regional anesthesia:

Spinal For technique and monitoring of spinal anesthesia, see Cesarean Section, p. 602. Hyperbaric 5% spinal lidocaine 50-75 mg (controversial, see comments on pg. 611) or bupivacaine 8-10 mg; adjust the position of operating table to obtain T8 level of anesthesia.

Epidural	For technique and monitoring, see Cesarean Section, p. 604. Administer increments of 3% 2-chloroprocaine or 2% lidocaine with 1:200,000 epinephrine until block level adequate. Additional local anesthetic as needed to ensure adequate level of anesthesia.	
MAC	Titrate small doses opioid (e.g., fentanyl 25-50 μg) and midazolam 0.5-1.0 mg. Ensure patient is awake and responsive throughout. Consider NTG 100-200 μg iv for uterine relaxation repeated as necessary to obtain the desired effect. Transient hypotension may follow vasodilation due to NTG, and should be treated with volume and pressors if necessary.	
General anesthesia:		
Induction	Preoxygenation, rapid-sequence induction with cricoid pressure, and hydration, as discussed in Cesarean Section (p. 605). Ketamine (1 mg/kg) preferred for induction of hypotensive patient, but in larger doses (> 1.5 mg/kg) theoretically may increase uterine tone and make removal of placenta more difficult. Anesthesia with N_2O/O_2 + opioid (but no volatile agent) often permits delivery of the placenta.	
Maintenance	If uterine relaxation is necessary, administer volatile agent (> 1 MAC) or NTG (see above) until uterine tone decreases.	
Emergence	Extubation should be delayed until patient is fully awake and protective airway reflexes have returned.	
Blood and fluid requirements	Anticipate large blood loss IV: 16-18 ga × 1-2 NS/LR @ 6-8 ml/kg/h	Infuse crystalloid solution to maintain BP (1-1.5 L iv) prior to regional anesthesia. Treat hypotension with fluids and ephedrine, and by decreasing concentration of volatile agent. Surgery is usually brief in duration; additional muscle relaxation not usually necessary.
Monitoring	Standard monitors (p. B-1)	
Complications	Bleeding	
Positioning	✓ and pad pressure points. ✓ eyes.	★ **NB:** peroneal nerve compression at lateral fibular head → foot drop.

POSTOPERATIVE

Complications	Peroneal nerve injury (2° lithotomy position) Bleeding	Nerve injury manifested as foot drop and loss of sensation over dorsum of foot.
Pain management	IV or im opioids, titrated to effect, as usual, instituted in recovery room.	
Tests	Hct	

References

1. Creasy RK, Resnik R, eds: *Maternal-Fetal Medicine: Principles and Practice*, 3rd edition. WB Saunders, Philadelphia: 1994.
2. Cunningham FG, MacDonald PC, Gant NF, eds: *Williams Obstetrics*, 20th edition. Appleton & Lange, Norwalk CT: 1997.
3. Desimone CA, Norris MC, Leighton BL: Intravenous nitroglycerin aids manual extraction of a retained placenta. [Letter] *Anesthesiology* 1990; 73(4):787.
4. Huber MG, Wildschut HI, Boer K, Kleiverda G, Hoek FJ: Umbilical vein administration of oxytocin for the management of retained placenta: is it effective? *Am J Obstet Gynecol* 1991; 164(5 P+1):1216-19.
5. Lee CY, Madrazo B, Drukker BH: Ultrasonic evaluation of the postpartum uterus in the management of postpartum bleeding. *Obstet Gynecol* 1981; 58(2):227-32.
6. O'Grady JP, Gimovsky ML, McIlhargie, eds: *Operative Obstetrics.* Williams & Wilkins, Baltimore: 1995, 503-4.
7. Pernoll LM, ed: *Current Obstetric and Gynecologic Diagnosis and Treatment*, 8th edition. Appleton & Lange, Norwalk CT: 1994, 575-79.
8. Riley ET, Flanagan B, Cohen SE, Chitkara U: Intravenous nitroglycerin: a potent uterine relaxant for emergency obstetrical procedures. Report of 3 cases and review of literature. *Int J Obstet Anesth* 1996; 5:264-68.
9. Robinson HP: Sonar in the puerperium. A means of diagnosing retained products of conception. *Scott Med J* 1972; 17(11):364-66.
10. Schenker JG, Margalroth EJ: Intrauterine adhesions: an updated appraisal. *Fertil Steril* 1982; 37(5):593-610.
11. Wilken-Jensen C, Strom V, Nielsen MD, Rosenkilde-Gram B: Removing a retained placenta by oxytocin — a controlled study. *Am J Obstet Gynecol* 1989; 161(1):155-56.

MANAGEMENT OF UTERINE INVERSION

SURGICAL CONSIDERATIONS

Yasser El-Sayed

Description: Uterine inversion is associated with fundal implantation of the placenta whereby a thinning of the uterine wall, together with placental separation, causes an invagination of the myometrium, resulting in inversion. Vigorous fundal pressure or cord traction also can contribute to uterine inversion, which can be complete or incomplete. Complete inversion results in the inverted fundus extending beyond the cervix and appearing at the vaginal introitus, whereas in an incompletely inverted uterus, the fundus does not extend beyond the external cervical os. Uterine inversion can cause hemorrhage and shock out of proportion to observed bleeding, and must be managed as an obstetrical emergency. An anesthesiologist must be called to the delivery room as soon as a diagnosis of uterine inversion is made. The ready availability of GA is paramount. Intravenous access with two infusion systems and appropriate fluid resuscitation must be initiated emergently. Blood and blood products should be available for administration as indicated.

Frequently, reinversion can be accomplished with iv tocolytics, such as terbutaline, magnesium sulfate and, more recently, NTG; however, GA with a volatile agent may be necessary. Three primary methods for uterine reinversion are the Johnson, Huntington and Haultain procedures. Normally, the **Johnson method** is attempted first. Persistent pressure applied to the fundus is used to elevate the uterus into the vagina. The placenta, if attached, is not removed until iv resuscitation has been initiated, and iv tocolytics (or anesthesia) have been administered. Oxytocin is given when the uterus has been reinverted. **Laparotomy** must be performed if reinversion with the Johnson method is unsuccessful. The **Huntington procedure** involves grasping the round ligaments and applying upward traction on them, while an assistant exerts upward pressure on the uterus via a hand in the vagina. If the inverted uterus is trapped below the cervical ring, the **Haultain procedure** is used. This procedure involves making a longitudinal fundal incision posteriorly to allow easier reinversion of the fundus.

Usual preop diagnosis: Uterine inversion

SUMMARY OF PROCEDURE

	Manual Reinversion	Huntington/Haultain
Position	Dorsal lithotomy	Supine
Incision	None	Pfannenstiel's or midline longitudinal
Unique considerations	Prompt O_2 and iv fluid resuscitation; use of blood and blood products as necessary.	⇐
Antibiotics	Cefotetan 2 g iv q 12 h; total 3 doses	⇐
Surgical time	30 min	1-2 h
EBL	150-4000 ml	⇐
Postop care	± ICU. ARDS may necessitate mechanical ventilation. Monitor for acute renal failure 2° hypoxia and hypovolemia.	⇐
Mortality	Rare	⇐
Morbidity	Febrile morbidity	⇐
	Clinical shock	⇐
	Infectious morbidity from blood transfusion	⇐
Pain score	5	7

PATIENT POPULATION CHARACTERISTICS

Age range	Reproductive age
Incidence	1/2000-6000 deliveries
Etiology	Unknown
Associated conditions	Fundal implantation of the placenta; primiparity; intrapartum oxytocin; placenta accreta; therapy of preeclampsia with magnesium sulfate; macrosomic fetus

ANESTHETIC CONSIDERATIONS

PREOPERATIVE

These patients often present in shock out of proportion to blood loss; immediate resuscitation may be necessary. Since patient condition will improve as soon as the uterus is replaced, however, surgical treatment should not be delayed.

Respiratory	FRC returns to normal almost immediately after delivery. **Tests:** As indicated from H&P.	
Cardiovascular	Massive hemorrhage and pain usual with complete inversion. Prior to induction, insert large-bore iv and rapidly infuse fluids, including colloid to treat hypotension. Blood transfusion may be necessary, although is seldom available until after surgery.	
Gastrointestinal	Postpartum patients continue to be at risk for acid aspiration, although it is not known exactly when normal GI function returns. Precautions for prevention of acid aspiration should be followed as discussed in Cesarean Section, p. 602.	
Neurological	Local anesthetic requirements for spinal anesthesia remain decreased after delivery.[3]	
Laboratory	Hct; Plt; other tests as indicated from H&P. T&C for 2 U; keep 2 U ahead.	
Premedication	Na citrate 30 ml po within 30 min of induction. If time permits, other agents to decrease risk of aspiration pneumonitis, as discussed in Cesarean Section, p. 603.	

INTRAOPERATIVE

Anesthetic technique: Attempted uterine replacement and induction of anesthesia should not await intravascular volume replacement. Bleeding usually stops when uterus is replaced. NTG may provide adequate uterine relaxation, and can be given in the patient's room. (See p. 618 for dosages.) Sometimes, however, GETA is required, often with increasing concentrations of volatile agents to facilitate uterine replacement. If regional anesthesia (e.g., epidural or spinal) was used for delivery, replacement of uterus may be accomplished with little further anesthetic intervention, with or without NTG. If regional anesthesia was not used for delivery, iv analgesia with small doses of fentanyl (25-50 μg iv) occasionally allows reduction.

Induction	Rapid-sequence induction with ketamine (1.0 mg/kg) preferred. Higher dose may adversely increase uterine tone.	
Maintenance	Halothane, isoflurane (and probably sevoflurane), are all effective uterine relaxants, but sevoflurane is most rapidly eliminated. Hypotension should be treated with fluids + vasopressors.	
Emergence	Extubation should be delayed until patient is fully awake and protective airway reflexes have returned.	
Blood and fluid requirements	Significant blood loss IV: 16-18 ga × 1 or 2	Possible continued blood loss after reduction of uterus, due to uterine atony.
Monitoring	Standard monitors (p. B-1)	Arterial line may be useful if time allows.
Positioning	✓ and pad pressure points. ✓ eyes.	
Complications	Uterine atony Massive blood loss	Rx: ↓volatile anesthetic concentrations. Oxytocin infusion, uterine massage, ± methylergonovine (0.2 mg iv/im → ↑BP.

POSTOPERATIVE

Complications	Bleeding
Pain management	Parenteral opiates
Tests	Hct

References

1. Brar HS, Greenspoon JS, Platt LD, Paul RH: Acute puerperal uterine inversion. New approaches to management. *J Reprod Med* 1989; 34:(2)173-77.
2. Creasy RK, Resnik R, eds: *Maternal-Fetal Medicine: Principles and Practice*, 2nd edition. Saunders, Philadelphia: 1989, 519-20.
3. Cunningham FG, MacDonald PC, Gant NF, eds: *Williams Obstetrics*, 18th edition. Appleton & Lange, Norwalk: 1989, 422-23.
4. Kitchin J, Thiagarajah S, May HV Jr, Thornton WN Jr: Puerperal inversion of the uterus. *Am J Obstet Gynecol* 1975; 123:51-8.
5. Riley ET, Flanagan B, Cohen SE, Chitkara J: Intravenous nitroglycerin: a potent relaxant for emergency obstetrical procedures. Review of literature and reports of 3 cases. *Int J Obstet Anesth* 1996; 5:264-68.
6. Shah-Hosseini R, Evrard JR: Puerperal uterine inversion. *Obstet Gynecol* 1989; 73(4):567-70.

Surgeons

B. Hannah Ortiz, MD
Camran R. Nezhat, MD

8.4 LAPAROSCOPIC PROCEDURES FOR GYNECOLOGIC SURGERY

Anesthesiologist

Edward T. Riley, MD

LAPAROSCOPIC SURGERY FOR ENDOMETRIOSIS

SURGICAL CONSIDERATIONS

Description: There are numerous theories about the etiology of endometriosis, including: (1) The peritoneal cavity is seeded with endometrial cells via the fallopian tubes during menses;[7] (2) totipotential cells in the peritoneal cavity are transformed by hormonal exposure into endometrial cells; (3) endometrial cells are transported intravascularly or via lymphatics to ectopic sites where they respond to hormonal stimuli (this theory has been used to explain the presence of endometriosis in the brain and pleura); (4) decreased cytotoxic response of the immune system suggests that it is a failure of natural killer-cell activity to eliminate ectopic endometrial cells; and (5) it is an inherited disorder, since the incidence of endometriosis is higher in first-degree relatives. Intervention is usually indicated for intractable pain, infertility or impaired function of the gastrointestinal (GI) or genitourinary (GU) tracts. GU endometriosis may range from superficial involvement of peritoneum overlying the ureters and bladder to frankly invasive endometriosis penetrating through to bladder mucosa. Scarring and fibrosis can result in ureteral obstruction and hydronephrosis with renal insufficiency. Patients with GI endometriosis may have thickening of the rectovaginal septum, suggesting obliteration of the posterior cul-de-sac or rectosigmoid involvement. Adhesions may make rectovaginal examination difficult or painful. Pelvic structures may be immobile, suggesting adhesions fixing bowel or bladder to the uterus. Sigmoidoscopy should be performed to rule out malignancy and to determine whether endometriosis has penetrated through to the bowel mucosa.

Two treatment approaches can be taken. **Hysterectomy** and **bilateral salpingo-oophorectomy** (BSO) may be indicated for patients with severe symptoms who have not responded to medical or conservative surgical treatment and who do not desire fertility (see Laparoscopic Hysterectomy, p. 631). **Bilateral oophorectomy** might be necessary to eliminate the estrogen that sustains and stimulates the ectopic endometrium.[4] Conservative surgery is indicated for women who desire pregnancy and whose disease is responsible for their symptoms of pain or infertility. Though seldom curative, surgery improves fertility and offers at least temporary pain relief. **Laparoscopy** (Fig 8.4-1) is the most appropriate surgical technique for the diagnosis and treatment of endometriosis. Data from animal and clinical studies suggest that laparoscopic surgery is more effective for adhesiolysis, causes fewer de novo adhesions than laparotomy and reduces impairment of tuboovarian function.[8] Special consideration must be given to the patient's past history of abdominal or pelvic surgery, pelvic inflammatory disease and endometriosis as this will affect the choice of surgical approach. Ovarian endometriosis is common and can be challenging to diagnose and treat. Ovarian endometriosis can be divided into Type I (primary endometriomas or small cysts measuring > 3 cm on the ovarian surface) or Type II (secondary endometriomas, usually functional [e.g., follicular] in origin which become enlarged to > 3 cm). Regardless of classification, it is critical to remove all endometriotic lesions to prevent exacerbation and recurrence.

Bladder endometriosis: If the lesions are superficial, hydrodissection and vaporization are adequate for removal. Using hydrodissection, the areolar tissue between the serosa and muscularis beneath the implants is dissected. The lesion is circumscribed with a laser and fluid is injected into the resulting defect. The lesion is grasped with forceps and dissected with the laser. Traction allows the small blood vessels supplying the surrounding tissue to be coagulated as the lesion is resected. Frequent irrigation is necessary to remove char, ascertain the depth of vaporization and ensure that the lesion does not involve the muscularis and mucosa. Endometriosis extending to the muscularis but without mucosal involvement can be treated laparoscopically, and any residual or deeper lesions may be treated successfully with hormonal therapy. When endometriosis involves full bladder-wall thickness, the lesion is excised and the bladder reconstructed in one layer.[2] Simultaneous cystoscopy is performed and bilateral ureteral catheters are inserted. The bladder dome is held near the midline with the grasping forceps and the endometriotic nodule is excised 5 mm beyond the lesions. An incision is made with the CO_2 laser using the suction-irrigating probe as a backstop. The specimen is removed from the abdominal cavity with a long grasping forceps. The lesion is regrasped and removed with the laparoscope as one unit. CO_2 distends the bladder cavity, allowing excellent observation of its interior. After again identifying the ureters and examining the bladder mucosa, the bladder is closed. Cystoscopy is performed to identify possible leaks. The duration of laparoscopic segmental cystectomy is approximately 35 min. Patients are discharged the following day and instructed to take trimethoprim and sulfamethoxazole for 2 wk. The Foley catheter is removed 7-14 d later, and cystograms are made.

GI/GU endometriosis: In a patient with no Hx of pelvic surgery, the **direct-trocar insertion method** may be used with an intraumbilical incision. The incision is made within the umbilicus because this is the anatomical area closest to the fascia and peritoneum and involves the least risk of injury to retroperitoneal structures.[5] Once the incision is made, the trocar is placed through the skin incision. Using an intraumbilical incision and inserting the trocar at 90 degrees facilitates access to the abdominal cavity and decreases the risk of aortocaval injury. This technique of direct-trocar insertion may not be recommended for patients who have had prior laparotomy or laparoscopy that revealed adhesive disease. After insufflation of the abdomen with CO_2, assessment of intraabdominal and pelvic structures is made. A second skin incision

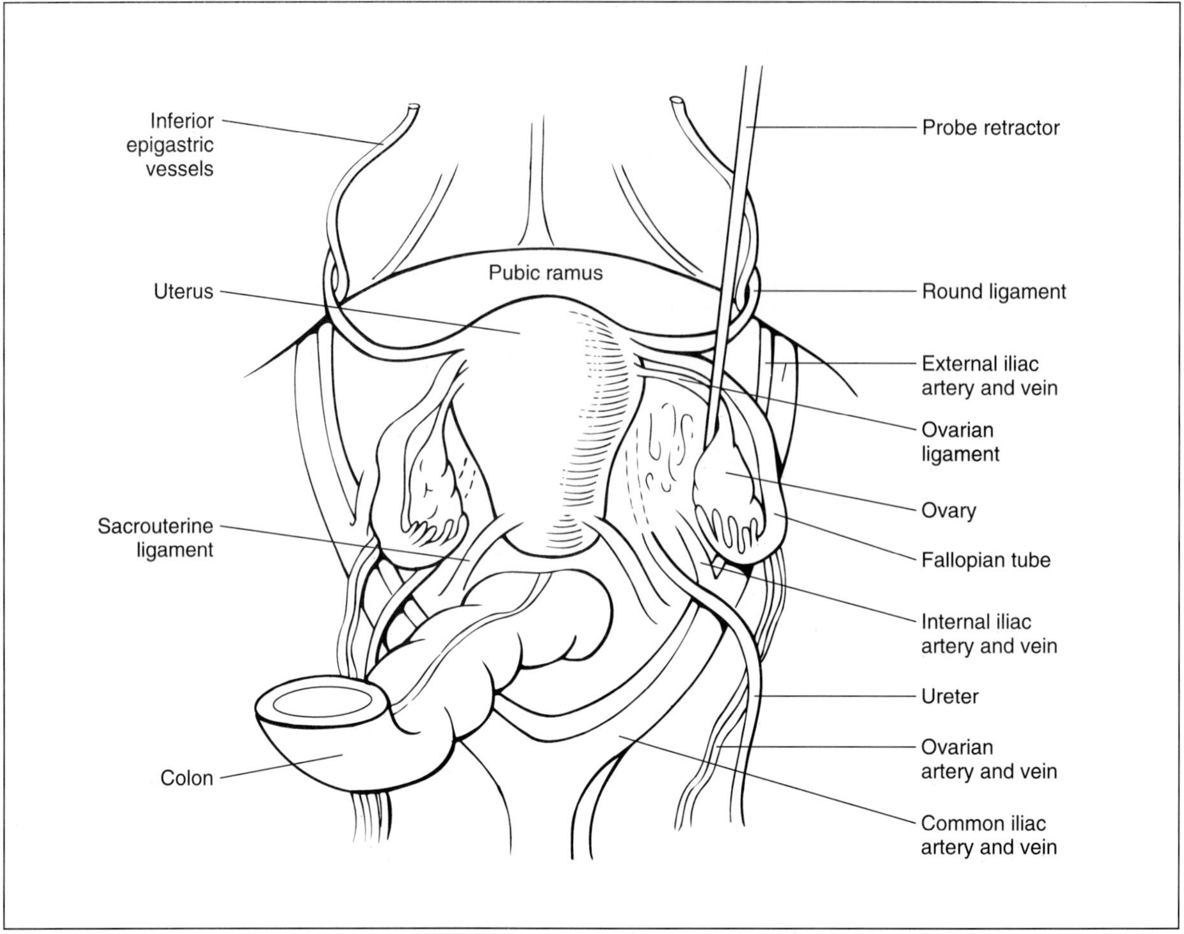

Figure 8.4-1. Laparoscopic view of the female pelvis.

is made 2-3 cm above the symphysis. A Foley catheter should be in place throughout the procedure to allow continuous drainage of the bladder, thereby reducing the likelihood of trocar injury to the bladder. A 5 mm trocar is placed under direct visualization with attention to peritoneal vessels and bladder. Two lateral ports are placed in a similar fashion, taking care to avoid the inferior epigastric vessels. The suction irrigator, a blunt grasper and the bipolar cautery are placed into the trocars. Filmy adhesions of the bowel or omentum to the anterior abdominal wall or uterus are lysed using CO_2 laser, bipolar cautery, monopolar scissors or hydrodissection. Treatment of peritoneal endometriosis ranges from laser ablation of superficial peritoneal implants to excision and dissection of deeply embedded, fibrotic areas. Scarring from endometriosis which has penetrated the peritoneum to involve deeper structures destroys normal surgical planes and distorts anatomical relationships. Identification of structures and landmarks is critical before attempting to treat the peritoneal disease. At laparoscopy, normal anatomic relationships along the pelvic sidewall may appear distorted. Because scarring from endometriosis may change these relationships, patients are at risk for accidental ureteral or vascular injury at the time of surgery. Identification of ureters and blood vessels is critical prior to treatment of pelvic sidewall disease. Although different modalities have been used, hydrodissection and high-power superpulse or ultrapulse CO_2 laser are the best options for endometriosis treatment.[2] Because the CO_2 laser does not penetrate water, this fluid backstop allows the surgeon to work on selected tissue with a greater safety margin.

Ovarian endometriosis: A Type I endometrioma of < 2 cm is vaporized using laser or bipolar coagulation. Larger Type I lesions may require excision using scissors or biopsy forceps. For Type IIA endometriomas, the procedure begins with lysis of periovarian adhesions using laser or monopolar scissors. The ovarian cortex is evaluated, the endometrioma cyst is identified, the cyst wall is perforated (using laser or scissors), and an irrigation device is inserted to assess cyst contents and wall. Suspicious areas are biopsied and sent for frozen-section analysis. A plane is developed between the cyst wall and ovary by grasping the wall and separating it from ovarian stroma, using traction and countertraction. Difficult areas where endometriosis has embedded through the cyst wall, disrupting the planes, require hydrodissection and bipolar cautery to control bleeding vessels in the ovarian bed. In some cases it is necessary to remove a portion of the ovary attached to the cyst wall until a plane can be found. Redundant ovarian tissue is approximated with low-power laser or electrosurgery to avoid adhesions. Suturing should be avoided; but, if necessary, 4-0 polydioxanone sutures can be placed to close the defect.

Usual preop diagnosis: Endometriosis

SUMMARY OF PROCEDURE

	Ovarian Endometriosis Procedure	GI/GU Endometriosis Procedure
Position	Dorsal lithotomy, legs in stirrups ± steep Trendelenburg	⇐
Incision	Intraumbilical; lateral suprapubic; or midline suprapubic	⇐
Special instrumentation	CO_2 laser or other cutting instrument; bipolar Kleppinger forceps; suction irrigator	⇐ ± Ureteral stenting, cystoscope, sigmoidoscope
Antibiotics	Cefotetan 1 g iv	⇐
Surgical time	45 min–3 h, depending on extent of disease	1-4 h
Closing considerations	Close fascia of all 10-12 mm ports; subcuticular closure for 5 mm trocar sites	⇐
EBL	Minimal	⇐
Postop care	Mild disease: PACU → home; otherwise, discharge on POD 1 (peritoneal disease).	Ambulate POD 0; Foley catheter.
Mortality	0.08-0.2/1000[5]	⇐
Morbidity	Overall complication rate: 2.5%[5] Conversion to laparoscopy: 0.42% VAE (CO_2 embolism) Peroneal nerve damage Vascular damage Bowel injury: Rare Urinary tract injury: Rare	Urinary tract injury
Pain score	4-8	4-8

PATIENT POPULATION CHARACTERISTICS

Age range	Reproductive age	20s–40s
Incidence	10-15% of all reproductive age women/ 25% of all gynecologic laparotomies	1-11% of women with known endometriosis
Etiology	Numerous theories (see above).	Extensive disseminated endometriosis
Associated conditions	Infertility; pelvic pain; bladder or bowel symptoms; HTN (2° to urinary tract involvement); GI tract involvement (3-7%)	Pelvic pain; GI or GU symptoms

ANESTHETIC CONSIDERATIONS

See Anesthetic Considerations following Laparoscopic Hysterectomy, p. 633.

References

1. Chantigian RC, Chantigian PDM: Anesthesia for laparoscopy. In *Complications of Laparoscopy and Hysteroscopy*. Corfman RS, Diamond MP, DeCherney A, eds. Blackwell Scientific Publications, Cambridge: 1993, 11.
2. Nezhat C, et al: *Operative Gynecologic Laparoscopy: Principles and Techniques.* McGraw Hill, New York: 1995, 122.
3. Nezhat C, Nezhat F: Laparoscopic segmental bladder resection for endometriosis: a report of two cases. *Obstet Gynecol* 1993; 81:886.
4. Nezhat F, et al: Videolaseroscopy for oophorectomy. *Am J Obstet Gynecol* 1991; 165:1323-30.
5. Querleu D, Chapron C: Complications of gynecologic laparoscopic surgery. *Curr Opin Obstet Gynecol* 1995; 7:257-61.
6. Samper ER, et al: Colonic endometriosis, its clinical spectrum. *South Med J* 1984; 77:912.
7. Samson JA: Peritoneal endometriosis due to menstrual dissemination of endometrial tissue into the pelvic cavity. *Am J Obstet Gynecol* 1927; 14:422.
8. Schenken SR, et al: Reoperation after initial treatment of endometriosis with conservative surgery. *Am J Obstet Gynecol* 1978; 131:416.

LAPAROSCOPIC SURGERY FOR ECTOPIC PREGNANCY

SURGICAL CONSIDERATIONS

Description: Ectopic pregnancy is defined as a pregnancy occurring outside the uterus. The majority of ectopic pregnancies occur in the fallopian tubes (95-97%); the remainder occur in the cornua (2-4%), ovary (0.1%), cervix (0.1%) or abdomen (0.03%). Ectopic pregnancy remains a leading cause of maternal morbidity and mortality. Predisposing factors include history of tubal ligation or other tubal surgery, pelvic inflammatory disease (PID), IUD use and a history of *in vitro* fertilization (IVF) or other treatments for infertility. Other associations include developmental anomalies of the Müllerian system, intrauterine polyps or myomas.

Patients present with lower quadrant pain, vaginal bleeding and an elevated β-hCG. Shoulder pain from subdiaphragmatic intraperitoneal blood is a less frequent finding. Treatment options for an asymptomatic ectopic gestation include operative laparoscopy or a trial of medical management with intramuscular methotrexate. In cases where the size of the ectopic pregnancy is too large for conservative medical management (> 3.5 cm), and the patient is hemodynamically stable, operative management is essential.[3] Hypotension or an acute abdomen in the presence of a positive β-hCG value are strongly suggestive of rupture and require expeditious surgical intervention.

Access to the abdomen is obtained in the usual fashion (e.g., through a Veress needle or direct-trocar insertion, followed by insufflation and insertion of accessory trocars). Ruptured tubal pregnancies can be treated endoscopically if the bleeding has ceased or can be controlled. Actively bleeding vessels are identified and cauterized, and forced irrigation is used to dislodge clots and trophoblastic tissue. Depending on their size, the products of conception (POCs) are removed through either a 5 or 10 mm trocar sleeve or placed into an endoscopic bag for removal; or a minilaparotomy can be performed. Copious irrigation should follow to ensure hemostasis and identify and remove any remaining trophoblastic tissue. Trophoblast is invasive, and residual tissue may implant into bowel, bladder, peritoneum or other abdominal structures and cause significant future morbidity.

For an unruptured ectopic pregnancy, the tube is identified and stabilized using laparoscopic forceps. To minimize bleeding, 5-7 ml of a solution of 50 U vasopressin in 100 ml NS is injected into the mesosalpinx just below the ectopic pregnancy and over the antimesenteric surface of the tubal segment containing the gestation. Intravascular injection of vasopressin solution can precipitate acute arterial HTN, bradycardia or even death; therefore, care must be taken to avoid such injection. A linear incision is made over the thinnest portion of the tube. The pregnancy usually protrudes through the incision, and forceful irrigation will dislodge the gestation from its implantation site. Oozing from the tube is common, but usually ceases spontaneously.

In a ruptured tubal or isthmic pregnancy, resection of the tubal segment containing the gestation is preferable to salpingostomy. **Segmental tubal resection** is performed with bipolar electrosurgery, laser (KTP, argon, Nd:YAG or CO_2), sutures or stapling devices. Similarly, **total salpingectomy** can be performed by progressive coagulation and cutting the mesosalpinx, which is separated from the uterus using bipolar coagulation and scissors or laser. The isolated tube segment containing the ectopic pregnancy is removed intact or in sectioned parts through the 10 mm trocar sleeve. At the completion of the procedure, the abdomen is irrigated and inspected and incisions are closed in the usual fashion.

Usual preop diagnosis: Ectopic pregnancy

SUMMARY OF PROCEDURE

Position	Dorsal lithotomy, legs in Allen universal stirrups, steep Trendelenburg
Incision	Intraumbilical, lateral suprapubic, midline suprapubic
Special instrumentation	CO_2 laser; laparoscopic instrumentation
Unique considerations	Intraperitoneal hemorrhage and hemodynamic instability are potential risks. Patient should be cross-matched for 2 U PRBCs.
Antibiotics	Cefotetan 1 g iv
Surgical time	45 min-2 h
Closing considerations	Fascia of 10-12 mm trocar sites closed in layers. Smaller 5 mm ports closed in a subcuticular fashion.
EBL	100 ml – severe hemorrhage, if ruptured.
Postop care	The patient may be admitted overnight for observation. Quantitative β-hCG should be followed until undetectable, to rule out the possibility of retained trophoblastic tissue.
Mortality	5/1000. For any laparoscopy: 0.08 to 0.2/1000.[4]
Morbidity	Overall complication rate: 2.5%[4] Hemorrhage and need for transfusion

Morbidity, cont.	Conversion to laparotomy: 4.2/1000[3]
	Air embolism: Rare
	Unintended puncture of a viscus: Rare
	Puncture of a major vessel: Rare
	Insufflation of incorrect site: Rare
Pain score	3-5

PATIENT POPULATION CHARACTERISTICS

Age range	Reproductive-age females
Incidence	1/100 pregnancies
Etiology	Distorted tubal or uterine anatomy
Associated conditions	Hx of PID; endometriosis; tubal damage; IUD; IVF

ANESTHETIC CONSIDERATIONS

See Anesthetic Considerations following Laparoscopic Hysterectomy, p. 633.

References

1. Chantigian RC, Chantigian PDM: Anesthesia for laparoscopy. In *Complications of Laparoscopy and Hysteroscopy.* Corfman RS, Diamond MP, DeCherney A, eds. Blackwell Scientific Publications, Cambridge: 1993, 11.
2. Luciano AA: Ectopic pregnancy. In *Current Therapy in Obstetrics and Gynecology.* Quilligan EJ, Zuspan PP, eds. WB Saunders, Philadelphia: 1990, 226.
3. Nezhat C, Nezhat F, Luciano AA, et al: *Operative Gynecologic Laparoscopy.* McGraw Hill, New York: 1995, 110.
4. Querleu D, Chapron C: Complications of gynecologic laparoscopic surgery. *Curr Opin Obstet Gynecol* 1995; 7:257-61.

LAPAROSCOPIC MYOMECTOMY

SURGICAL CONSIDERATIONS

Description: Uterine myomata or fibroids are the most common uterine neoplasm, affecting approximately 20-25% of women of reproductive age.[1,6] Their growth is influenced by many factors, such as estrogen acting alone or synergistically with growth hormone and human placental lactogen in pregnancy. The severity of symptoms depends on the number, size and location of the tumors. Symptoms may include constipation, pelvic or abdominal pressure, urinary frequency and, most commonly, menorrhagia. While leiomyomata are seldom the cause of infertility, there is a link between fibroids, fetal wastage and premature delivery.[1] Patients present with profound anemia from menorrhagia or menometrorrhagia, the usual indications for surgery. Other indications include rapidly changing size, ureteral compression, hydroureter or hydronephrosis and size > 12 wk. Size, number and location are the primary factors that will determine surgical approach to myomata.

The simplest approach is a combination of laparoscopy and minilaparotomy for removal of myomas. This approach limits operative time. Three major objectives of laparoscopic myomectomy are: minimizing blood loss, which can be severe; minimizing postop adhesion formation; and maintaining uterine-wall integrity. Preop treatment with GnRH analogues to shrink fibroids has been shown to decrease the size of the myoma and reduce the need for transfusion.[2,5]

Although myomectomy is performed to preserve fertility, postop adhesion formation often jeopardizes this goal. This can be minimized by using a single, vertical, anterior midline uterine incision.[3]

The abdomen is entered in the usual fashion for laparoscopy (e.g., through Veress needle or direct trocar insertion, followed by insufflation and insertion of accessory trocars). To reduce blood loss in pedunculated myomas, diluted vasopressin (3-5 ml) is injected into the base of the stalk where it joins the uterine wall. IV vasopressin can cause ↑BP, myocardial ischemia, dysrhythmias or cardiac arrest and should be avoided. The pedicle is coagulated with the bipolar forceps and cut with CO_2 laser or scissors. For subserosal or intramural myomas, diluted vasopressin is injected between the myometrium and the myoma pseudocapsule. An incision is made on the serosa overlying the myoma using the CO_2 laser or monopolar needle. As the incision is made, the myometrium is retracted away from graspers to expose the tumor. Vessels are coagulated prior to cutting. After the myoma is removed, the myoma bed is irrigated with LR and bleeding points are coagulated again. After closure, the serosa is irrigated with LR. An adhesion barrier may be placed over the incision site to prevent future adhesion formation. Uteroperitoneal fistulae may follow laparoscopic myomectomy because meticulous laparoscopic approximation of all layers of the myometrium is impossible. The use of electrocoagulation for hemostasis inside the uterine defect may also increase this risk.

Removal of the specimen frequently is the most challenging aspect of the operation. The myoma can be removed either by morcellation of the specimen or by extending the suprapubic incision. Alternatively, posterior culdotomy may be performed and the myoma removed via the vagina. A retractor is placed in the vagina and the laser is used to cut along the tented vaginal mucosa. After the myoma is removed, the incision can be closed using laparoscopic suturing. Minilaparotomy or culdotomy facilitate removal but increase postop wound complication risks such as infection or hernia formation. After myoma removal, the abdomen and pelvis are irrigated, the patient is taken out of the Trendelenburg position and any fluid which might have tracked into the upper abdomen is suctioned. The ports are closed in the usual fashion.

Usual preop diagnosis: Uterine myoma, fibroids

SUMMARY OF PROCEDURE

Position	Dorsal lithotomy; steep Trendelenburg to move bowel out of operating field
Incisions	Infraumbilical, 5 mm lateral and 5-12 mm midline suprapubic; minilaparotomy via extension of suprapubic incision or posterior culdotomy for removal of large myomata
Special instrumentation	CO_2 laser; laparoscopic instrumentation
Unique considerations	For large myomata: pretreatment with GnRH analogues (3-6 mo). Intraop injection of dilute vasopressin (1 IU in 100 ml LR) into myometrium to ↓ bleeding.
Antibiotics	Cefotetan 1 g iv
Surgical time	1-3 h
Closing considerations	Close fascia of all 10-12 mm ports; 5 mm ports are closed in a subcuticular fashion. Fascial closure essential in minilaparotomy. Posterior culdotomy requires laparoscopic suturing or vaginal closure.
EBL	100-600 ml
Postop care	1-2 d hospital stay; early ambulation; clear liquids POD 0; gradually advance diet after discharge home.
Mortality	0.08-0.2/1000.[4]
Morbidity	Rates: 1.3-5.9/100[6]
	Peroneal nerve damage from positioning
	Severe bleeding with possible need for transfusion
	Uteroperitoneal fistulae
	Infertility
	Hyponatremia from peritoneal absorption of irrigant
	Air embolism
	Puncture of a major vessel
	Insufflation in the wrong place
	Need for emergent laparotomy
	Uterine rupture in pregnancy: 2%
	Adhesion formation
Pain score	4-6

PATIENT POPULATION CHARACTERISTICS

Age range	Reproductive-age women; myomas shrink in postmenopausal women and are less symptomatic.
Incidence	20-25% of all women
Etiology	Benign transformation and proliferation of a single smooth-muscle cell
Associated conditions	Menorrhagia; anemia; ureteral obstruction; pelvic pain or pressure

ANESTHETIC CONSIDERATIONS

See Anesthetic Considerations following Laparoscopic Hysterectomy, p. 633.

References

1. Buttram VC, Reiter RC: Uterine leiomyomata: etiology, symptomatology and management. *Fertil Steril* 1981; 36:433.
2. Friedman AJ, Rein NS, Harrison-Atlas D, et al: A randomized, placebo-controlled, double blind study evaluating leuprolide acetate depot treatment before myomectomy. *Fertil Steril* 1989; 52:728.
3. Operative Laparoscopy Study Group: Postoperative adhesion development after operative laparoscopy: evaluation at early second-look procedures. *Fertil Steril* 1991; 55:700-4.
4. Querleu D, Chapron C: Complications of gynecologic laparoscopic surgery. *Curr Opin Obstet Gynecol* 1995; 7:257-61.
5. Shaw RW: Mechanism of LHRH analogue action in uterine fibroids. *Horm Res* 1989; 32:150.
6. Vollenhoven BJ, Lawrence AS, Healy DL: Uterine fibroids: a clinical review. *Br J Obstet Gynecol* 1990; 97:285.

LAPAROSCOPIC HYSTERECTOMY

SURGICAL CONSIDERATIONS

Description: Hysterectomy is the second most common gynecologic operation, after cesarean section. The indications for hysterectomy with or without salpingo-oophorectomy include: leiomyomata (38%); malignancy (15%); ovarian tumors (10%); abnormal bleeding (13%); adenomyosis (9%); pelvic pain or adhesions (5%); endometriosis (3%); and uterine prolapse (1%).[3] Other less common indications include parametrial disease, pelvic infection and complications of pregnancy and delivery. Selection of surgical approach to hysterectomy requires consideration of the patient's age, medical history, history of prior pelvic surgery, the presence or possibility of adhesions or endometriosis, uterine size, adnexal pathology and the presence or amount of uterine prolapse.

Laparoscopic hysterectomy offers the advantages of excellent visibility and exposure. There is shorter recovery time, rapid return of bowel function, less pain and a lower wound complication rate. The disadvantages are higher cost and the level of surgical expertise required.[2] The most commonly performed procedure is the **laparoscopically assisted vaginal hysterectomy** (LAVH), in which hysterectomy is begun by laparoscopy, but four or more steps are performed vaginally.[2] Variants include: **total laparoscopic hysterectomy** (TLH), in which all steps are performed laparoscopically; **subtotal laparoscopic hysterectomy** (SLH), a supracervical hysterectomy; and **vaginally assisted laparoscopic hysterectomy** (VALH), in which four steps are completed laparoscopically, and the procedure is completed vaginally. Combinations are usually performed, depending on findings at surgery. A mechanical and antibiotic bowel preparation is advised. Consultation with a urologist, bowel surgeon and oncologist are sought as necessary.

Access to the abdomen is obtained in the usual fashion (e.g., through a Veress needle or direct-trocar insertion, followed by insufflation and insertion of accessory trocars). Diagnostic laparoscopy is performed, adhesions lysed and any endometriosis treated. The course of the ureters is noted through the peritoneum until they are no longer visible at the level of the cardinal ligaments. When ureters cannot be identified clearly because of severe scarring or endometriosis, they are dissected retroperitoneally, and the dissection proceeds as for a radical hysterectomy. At the cardinal ligaments, the peritoneum is opened above or below the ureter and hydrodissection is performed to lift the peritoneum off the ureter without damaging it. Routine hysterectomy using hydrodissection to identify tissue planes and limit blood loss can be performed following identification of the ureters.

If the ovaries are to be spared, the uteroovarian ligament, proximal tube and mesosalpinx are cauterized and cut progressively, and the posterior leaf of the broad ligament is opened with hydrodissection. The bladder is dissected free from the cervix and uterus; and, if bladder trauma is suspected, 5 ml of indigo carmine injected iv (possible ↑BP) may help identify the site of perforation. Next, the uterine vessels are identified, noted to be free of ureter, desiccated and cut. At the level of the cardinal ligaments, the ureters and descending branches of the uterine artery are close to one another and the cervix; therefore, cardinal ligament dissection and cautery must be precise to prevent bleeding and ureteral injury. A small uterus can be removed easily through the vagina. In benign disease, a large uterus can be morcellated and then removed segmentally through the vagina. Pneumoperitoneum will be lost during this procedure, and care must be taken to keep instruments free of bowel or other abdominal structures as this occurs.

If the procedure is to be completed entirely laparoscopically, pneumoperitoneum can be maintained by placing a glove containing two 4" × 4" sponges in the vagina. The vaginal wall is cut circumferentially, and the uterus is pulled to mid vagina, but not removed, to preserve the pneumoperitoneum. Alternatively, the uterus may be morcellated and removed through a 10 mm suprapubic port, or placed in a laparoscopic specimen bag. The suprapubic incision also may be extended into a minilaparotomy incision for specimen removal. The vaginal cuff is closed transversely using laparoscopic sutures, and any coexisting cystocele or enterocele is repaired. Once the uterus is removed and the vaginal cuff closed, the pelvic and abdominal cavities are reevaluated, irrigated and cleared of blood and debris. The skin and fascia are closed in the usual fashion.

Variant procedure: In patients with severe rectovaginal and vesical endometriosis, the retroperitoneal space is entered using hydrodissection, and the external iliac vessels, hypogastric artery and ureter are identified. In cases where extensive dissection and resultant blood loss is anticipated, coagulation or ligation of the hypogastric artery with laparoscopic clips may be performed. Endometriosis of the rectum, rectovaginal septum and uterosacral ligaments is treated by vaporization, excision or a combination of these. Sigmoidoscopy with concurrent laparoscopic visualization of the pelvis may be necessary to rule out the presence of incidental enterotomy. Cystoscopy with ureteral stenting also may be indicated to identify anatomy. (Treatment of bladder and bowel endometriosis have been described in Laparoscopic Surgery for Endometriosis, p. 625.) Once the ureter is identified along its course and entry into the bladder, the uterine vessels are retracted medially and separated from the ureter using a CO_2 laser. The uterus is retracted medially and the ureter laterally as the cardinal and uterosacral ligaments are cauterized and cut with the ureter under direct visualization. After these vascular pedicles have been ligated and all endometriosis treated, the hysterectomy and specimen removal proceed as described above.

Usual preop diagnosis: leiomyomata; malignancy; ovarian tumors; abnormal bleeding; adenomyosis; pelvic pain or adhesions; endometriosis; uterine prolapse; parametrial disease; pelvic infection; complications of pregnancy and delivery

SUMMARY OF PROCEDURE

Position	Dorsal lithotomy; legs in Allen universal stirrups; steep Trendelenburg
Incisions	Intraumbilical; bilateral suprapubic; midline suprapubic (5 or 10 mm)
Special instrumentation	CO_2 laser; laparoscopic instruments
Unique considerations	Extensive ureterolysis and treatment of endometriosis may require addition of cystoscopy, ureteral stent placement and/or sigmoidoscopy.
Antibiotics	Cefotetan 1 g iv
Surgical time	2-6 h. Operative time is increased in cases of extensive adhesiolysis or endometriosis.
Closing considerations	Close fascia of all 10 to 12 mm ports; 5-mm trocar sites closed in a subcuticular fashion. Minilaparotomy closure if needed.
EBL	100-800 ml, depending on anatomy and difficulty of dissection
Postop care	Clear liquid diet; ambulate first POD.
Mortality	0.08-0.2/1000[4]
Morbidity	Overall complication rate: 2.5%[1] Conversion to laparotomy: 4.2/1000[4] Air embolism: Rare Peroneal nerve damage from positioning: Rare Unintended puncture of a viscous: Rare Puncture of a major vessel: Rare Insufflation of incorrect site: Rare Urinary and ureteral trauma, including fistulae: 1.6%
Pain score	6-9

PATIENT POPULATION CHARACTERISTICS

Age range	30s–70s
Incidence	20% of women < 40 yr; 37% of women < age 65[6]
Etiology	See below.
Associated conditions	Myomata; abnormal uterine bleeding; adenomyosis; malignancy; pelvic pain; endometriosis

References

1. Chantigian RC, Chantigian PDM: Anesthesia for laparoscopy. In *Complications of Laparoscopy and Hysteroscopy.* Corfman RS, Diamond MP, DeCherney A, eds. Blackwell Scientific Publications, Cambridge: 1993, 11.
2. Nezhat C, Nezhat F, Luciano AA, et al: *Operative Gynecologic Laparoscopy.* McGraw Hill, New York: 1995, 217-18.
3. Nezhat C, Nezhat F, Nezhat C: Operative laparoscopy (minimally invasive surgery) state of the art. *J Gynecol Surg* 1992; 8:111-41.
4. Querleu D, Chapron C: Complications of gynecologic laparoscopic surgery. *Curr Opin Obstet Gynecol* 1995; 7:257-61.
5. Saidi MH, Sadler RK, Vancaillie TG, Akright BD, Farhart SA, White AJ: Diagnosis and management of serious urinary complications after major operative laparoscopy. *Obstet Gynecol* 1996; 87:272-76.
6. Thompson JD, Warshaw J: Hysterectomy. In *TeLinde's Operative Gynecology.* Rock JA, Thompson JD, eds. Lippincott-Raven Publishers, Philadelphia: 1997, 775.

ANESTHETIC CONSIDERATIONS

(Procedures covered: laparoscopic surgery for endometriosis, ectopic pregnancy, myomectomy, hysterectomy)

PREOPERATIVE

With the exception of tubal pregnancies, most of these cases are done electively in an otherwise healthy patient population.

Respiratory There can be intraop respiratory compromise from ↑intraabdominal pressure 2° CO_2 insufflation; however, patients without significant respiratory disease tolerate the insufflation quite well.
Tests: As indicated from H&P.

Cardiovascular Insufflation of the abdomen (typically with pressures of 14-22 mmHg) → ↑SVR and ↓venous return. ↑$PaCO_2$ → ↑dysrhythmias. These are usually well tolerated in the otherwise healthy patient.
Tests: As indicated from H&P.

Gastrointestinal Patients often have a bowel prep the night before. Check for Sx of dehydration (↓skin turgor, orthostatic ↓BP, ↑HR, etc.) and hypokalemia (e.g., weakness, flattened T waves, dysrhythmias, etc.). The combination of ↑intraabdominal pressure + Trendelenburg position → ↑aspiration risk.
Test: Electrolytes

Hematologic These patients often are having surgery for abnormal uterine bleeding → anemia.
Test: Hct

Laboratory Other tests as indicated from H&P.

Premedication Many of these patients suffer chronic pelvic pain. They can be quite anxious and on chronic anxiolytic medication. Large doses of preop sedatives are often needed 2° extreme anxiety and drug tolerance. For the anxious patient, diazepam 10 mg po 1-2 h prior to surgery is often useful. In addition, midazolam can be titrated to effect (up to 10 mg iv is sometimes needed) in the immediate preop period. Patients with risk factors for regurgitation (e.g., obesity, DM, hiatus hernia) may benefit from Na citrate 15-30 ml po and other full-stomach precautions preinduction (see p. B-5).

INTRAOPERATIVE

Anesthetic technique: GETA—a balanced technique with inhalational agents and narcotics. Neuromuscular blockade allows maximal insufflation of the abdomen with lower intraabdominal pressures.

Induction In order to give the surgeons optimal operating conditions, care must be taken not to inflate the stomach and bowel with gas. Therefore, avoid positive pressure mask ventilation. Preoxygenate 3 min and induce with propofol (1.5-2.5 mg/kg iv) and divided doses of mivacurium (total dose 0.2 mg/kg). If possible, avoid ventilation until after intubation. Following intubation, pass an OG tube to empty the stomach. Rapid-sequence induction (see B-5) usually is indicated for patients with an ectopic pregnancy.

Maintenance	Narcotics and inhalational agents: If the estimated time for the case is > 1 h, do not use N_2O, to avoid bowel distention. Continue neuromuscular blockade. Mivacurium is the preferred neuromuscular blocker (1-15 μg/kg/min) since relaxation is needed until the end of the case and mivacurium will wear off quickly.	
Emergence	Extubation at conclusion of surgery. Reverse neuromuscular blockade if needed; but try to avoid reversal since anticholinesterases may induce nausea. Give prophylactic antiemetic (e.g., metoclopramide 10 mg iv or ondansetron 4 mg iv).	
Blood and fluid requirements	Usually minimal blood loss IV: 18 ga × 1 NS/LR @ 2-4 ml/kg/h	For induction, these patients may need extra fluid 2° dehydration caused by the bowel prep. During surgery large volumes of fluid are sometimes given intraabdominally for irrigation and hydrodissection → fluid overload; therefore, maintenance iv fluid should be kept to a minimum.
Monitoring	Standard monitors (see p. B-1). Foley catheter	
Positioning	✓ and pad pressure points. ✓ eyes.	See Neuropathies, below.
Complications	Hypothermia	2° the large volume of fluid and CO_2 infused into the abdomen. All fluids should be warmed + use a heated forced-air device to warm the patient.
	Extraabdominal insufflation	Occasionally, large volumes of the insufflating gas can enter a vein, hollow viscera, subcutaneous tissue, thorax, mediastinum or pericardium. Fortunately, since the gas is usually CO_2, small volumes are absorbed quickly and usually do not cause major physiologic compromise; however, large volumes may result in cardiopulmonary collapse (e.g., 2° pneumothorax, VAE). Subcutaneous air can compromise the airway in some cases. ✓ airway prior to extubation.
	Neuropathies	These can be long cases, with the patient in lithotomy position. Make sure that the pressure points are padded well and, if the arms are out, relieve stress on the brachial plexus.
	Fluid overload	✓ fluid volume entering and exiting the abdomen. Fluid absorption → fluid overload → CHF, edema.

POSTOPERATIVE

Complications	N/V	↑↑N/V associated with laparoscopic cases. Use prophylactic antiemetics and aggressively treat N/V.
Pain management	Pain control is usually not a major problem.	

References

1. Ding Y, Fredman B, White PF: Use of mivacurium during laparoscopic surgery: effect of reversal drugs on postoperative recovery [see comments]. *Anesth Analg* 1994; 78(3):450-54.
2. Healzer JM, Nezhat C, Brodsky JB, Brock-Utne JG, Seidman DS: Pulmonary edema after absorbing crystalloid irrigating fluid during laparoscopy [letter]. *Anesth Anal* 1994; 78(6):1207.
3. Moore SS, Green CR, Wang FL, Pandit SK, Hurd WW: The role of irrigation in the development of hypothermia during laparoscopic surgery. *Am J Obstet Gyn* 1997; 176(3):598-602.
4. Polati E, Verlato G, Finco G, Mosaner W, Grosso S, Gottin L, Pinaroli AM, Ischia S: Ondansetron versus metoclopramide in the treatment of postoperative nausea and vomiting. *Anesth Analg* 1997; 85(2):395-99.
5. Schwartz RO: Complications of laparoscopic hysterectomy. *Obstet Gyn* 1993; 81(6):1022-24.

Surgeons

Harcharan S. Gill, MD
Fuad S. Freiha, MD, FACS

9.0 UROLOGY

Anesthesiologists

Steven A. Deem, MD
Ronald G. Pearl, MD, PhD

DIAGNOSTIC TRANSURETHRAL (ENDOSCOPIC) PROCEDURES

SURGICAL CONSIDERATIONS

Description: Many urologic diseases are diagnosed and evaluated endoscopically through the urethra with the use of specialized instruments, such as cystoscopes and resectoscopes. With the patient in a lithotomy position, the cystoscope is introduced into the urethra and advanced under direct vision all the way into the bladder (Figs 9-1A,B), allowing inspection of the urethra (**urethroscopy**) and bladder (**cystoscopy**). If pathology is noted, a biopsy can be obtained easily through the cystoscope. It is also possible to introduce small catheters into the ureteral orifices and advance them up to the kidneys for radiologic evaluation (**retrograde pyelography**), to collect urine specimen, or to bypass areas of obstruction. If the upper urinary tract needs to be visualized, a ureteroscope is introduced through the urethra into the bladder and through the ureteral orifice into the ureter and advanced up to the kidney, allowing inspection of the ureter (**ureteroscopy**) and intrarenal collecting system (**nephroscopy**). Often, these procedures precede a major surgical operation.

Usual preop diagnosis: Hematuria; hydronephrosis; benign prostatic hypertrophy; cancer of the urethra, prostate, bladder, ureter and renal pelvis; urinary tract stones; strictures; ureteropelvic junction obstruction; hemorrhagic or interstitial cystitis

SUMMARY OF PROCEDURE

	Urethroscopy/ Cystoscopy	Ureteroscopy/ Nephroscopy
Position	Lithotomy	⇐
Incision	None	⇐
Special instrumentation	Cystoscope	Ureteroscope
Unique considerations	Use of x-ray and fluoroscopy	⇐
Antibiotics	Gentamicin 80 mg iv, slowly	⇐
Surgical time	15 min	45 min
EBL	None	⇐
Postop care	PACU → home	⇐
Mortality	Minimal	⇐
Morbidity	Infection: 5%	⇐ Ureteral perforation: < 5%
Pain score	1	1

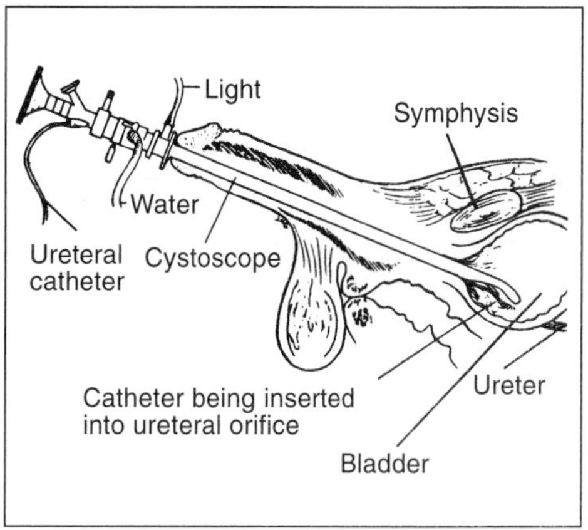

Figure 9-1A. Cystoscope introduced into bladder via urethra, male anatomy. (Reproduced with permission from Hardy JD: *Textbook of Surgery*. JB Lippincott: 1988.)

PATIENT POPULATION CHARACTERISTICS

Age range	All ages	⇐
Male:Female	1:1	⇐
Incidence	30% of all urologic procedures	⇐
Etiology	Hematuria	⇐
	Urethral and bladder tumors	⇐
	Stones	⇐
	Urethral strictures	⇐
		Ureteropelvic junction obstruction
Associated conditions	Prostatic hypertrophy	Hydronephrosis
	Cystitis	⇐

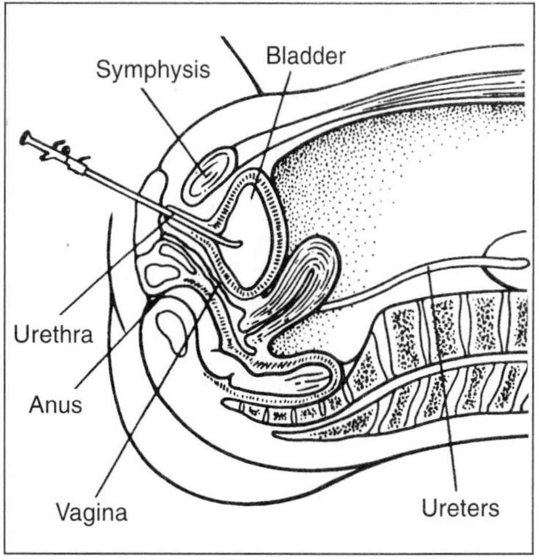

Figure 9-1B. Cystoscope introduced into bladder, female anatomy. (Reproduced with permission from Govan DE: *Roche Manual of Urologic Procedures*. Hoffmann-LaRoche: 1976.)

ANESTHETIC CONSIDERATIONS

See Anesthetic Considerations following Therapeutic Transurethral Procedures (Except TURP), p. 639.

References

1. Carter HB: The urologic examination and diagnostic techniques. In *Campbell's Urology*, 7th edition. Walsh PC, et al, eds. WB Saunders Co, Philadelphia: 1998, Vol 1, Ch 8, 331-41.
2. Huffman JL: Ureteroscopy. In *Campbell's Urology*, 6th edition. WB Saunders Co, Philadelphia: 1992, Vol 3, Ch 61, 2195-2230.

THERAPEUTIC TRANSURETHRAL PROCEDURES (EXCEPT TURP)

SURGICAL CONSIDERATIONS

Description: Therapeutic transurethral procedures, the most common urologic operations, require the use of specialized instruments, such as cystoscopes and resectoscopes. Because of continuously improving instrumentation and fiber optics, the range and complexity of these operations are widening, and more operations are being done transurethrally now than ever before. These operations are: **transurethral resection (TUR)** of any urethral, prostatic or bladder pathology; **fulguration** of bleeding vessels; **instillation of chemicals,** such as oxychlorosene (chloropactin) and formalin into the bladder; **extraction** of stones; and **incision and dilation** of strictures.

With the patient in the lithotomy position, the cystoscope or resectoscope is introduced into the urethra and advanced under direct vision into the bladder, allowing inspection of the urethra and bladder (Figs 9-1A,B). The pathology is identified. If it is a tumor, it is resected piecemeal with the electrode of the resectoscope, using the cutting current and cauterizing the base of the tumor with the coagulating current. If the pathology is a stone, it is extracted with special forceps or a stone basket. Large stones have to be fragmented, prior to extraction, with a mechanical lithotrite, electrohydraulic probe, ultrasound lithotrite or laser (Holmium or pulsed-dye). Chemicals can be instilled through the cystoscope to control interstitial and hemorrhagic cystitis. Bleeding vessels can be coagulated with the electrode. Strictures of the urethra can be dilated or incised with an endoscopic knife. Strictures of the ureter can also be treated endoscopically by dilatation with a balloon catheter or by incision with electrocautery. Balloon catheters with attached cutting electrowires (Accucise) are often used. A temporary ureteral stent is placed at the end of most endoscopic ureteral surgeries.

Variant procedure or approaches: Occasionally, access to the intrarenal collecting system (renal pelvis and calyces) and upper ureter is easier and more appropriately done by a **percutaneous nephrostomy** than a transurethral procedure. The patient is placed in a prone or flank position, a percutaneous stab wound is made at the costovertebral angle and a tube is introduced into the kidney under fluoroscopic control.

Usual preop diagnosis: Tumors of the urinary tract; stones; interstitial or hemorrhagic cystitis; strictures

SUMMARY OF PROCEDURE

	Transurethral	Percutaneous
Position	Lithotomy	Flank or prone
Incision	None	Stab wound
Special instrumentation	Cystoscope; resectoscope; catheters; stents	Percutaneous nephrostomy kit; nephroscope; urethroscope; catheters; stents
Unique considerations	Use of x-rays, fluoroscopy and electrocautery	⇐
Antibiotics	Gentamicin 80 mg iv, slowly	⇐
Surgical time	1 h	2-3 h
EBL	100 ml	500 ml
Postop care	Irrigation of tubes and catheters to clear clots and prevent obstruction	⇐
Mortality	< 1%	⇐

	Transurethral	Percutaneous
Morbidity	Bleeding: 10%	⇐
	Infection: 5%	⇐
	Perforation: 2%	⇐
	Retained stones: 2%	⇐
Pain score	1	3

PATIENT POPULATION CHARACTERISTICS

Age range	All ages	⇐
Male:Female	1:1	⇐
Incidence	10% of urologic diseases involve these procedures	⇐
Etiology	Urethral and bladder tumors; bladder and ureteral stones; interstitial cystitis; hemorrhagic cystitis; urethral stricture	Kidney stones; upper ureteral stones; ureteropelvic junction obstruction

---

ANESTHETIC CONSIDERATIONS FOR TRANSURETHRAL PROCEDURES (EXCEPT TURP)

PREOPERATIVE

Patients of all ages may present for ureteral stone extraction. Paraplegics and quadriplegics have a predilection for nephrolithiasis and may present for repeated cystoscopies. Bladder tumors usually are seen in the older population, who may present for cystoscopy or transurethral resection. These patients may have preexisting medical problems, including CAD, CHF, PVD, cerebrovascular diseases, COPD and renal impairment. Preop evaluation should be directed toward the detection and treatment of these conditions prior to anesthesia.

Neurological Paraplegics and quadriplegics may present for repeated cystoscopies and stone extractions. Note Hx of autonomic hyperreflexia (AH); Sx may include flushing, headache and nasal stuffiness, associated with voiding or noxious stimuli below the level of spinal cord injury (see below).

Musculoskeletal Contractures, pressure sores may make positioning difficult in paraplegics or quadriplegics.

Laboratory Tests as indicated from H&P.

Premedication Sedation prn anxiety (e.g., lorazepam 1-2 mg po 1-2 h before surgery; midazolam 1-2 mg iv in preop area).

INTRAOPERATIVE

Anesthetic technique: Spinal, continuous lumbar epidural and GA are acceptable, with the choice dependent on type and length of procedure, age and coexisting disease and patient preference. Simpler transurethral procedures (e.g., cystoscopy) are amenable to topical anesthesia, while longer and more complex procedures (e.g., ureteral stone extraction) will require regional or GA (see discussion below regarding AH). Note that many of these procedures are done on an outpatient basis; and the anesthetic should be planned appropriately. For regional anesthesia, a sacral block is required for urethral procedures, T9-T10 level for procedures involving the bladder, and as high as T8 for procedures involving the ureters.

Regional anesthesia:

Topical 2% lidocaine jelly

Spinal 0.75% bupivacaine 10-12 mg, 5% lidocaine 50-75 mg (controversial)

Lumbar epidural 1.5-2.0% lidocaine with epinephrine 5 μg/ml, 15-25 ml; supplement with 5-10 ml boluses as needed. Supplemental iv sedation.

General anesthesia:

Induction Standard induction (see p. B-2). ET intubation may not be necessary for shorter procedures; consider LMA. Succinylcholine should be avoided in paralyzed (e.g., paraplegic, quadriplegic) patients 2° ↑K^{++} → VF or asystole.

Maintenance	Pure inhalation anesthetic (e.g., N_2O, sevoflurane/desflurane) for short cases. IV technique (e.g., propofol 100-200 μg/kg/min; supplement with N_2O ± volatile anesthetic ± narcotic). Muscle relaxation not essential. Narcotics unnecessary since postop pain is usually minimal.	
Emergence	No specific considerations	
Blood and fluid requirements	Usually minimal blood loss IV: 18 ga × 1 NS/LR @ 2-4 ml/kg/h	
Monitoring	Standard monitors (see p. B-1).	
Positioning	✓ and pad pressure points. ✓ eyes.	★ **NB**: In lithotomy position, peroneal nerve compression at lateral fibular head → foot drop.
Complications	Anticipate hypotension upon returning from lithotomy position.	Rx: volume (200-500 ml NS/LR) or ephedrine (5 mg iv) may be necessary.
	Autonomic hyperreflexia (**AH**): • Severe HTN • Bradycardia • Dysrhythmias • Cardiac arrest	Patients with spinal cord injury level above T10 are at risk for **AH** associated with stimulation below the level of transection. T6-T10 transection levels may be associated with less severe manifestations. AH can be prevented by GA, spinal or epidural anesthesia. If AH occurs intraop it should be treated by deepening the level of anesthesia, and iv antihypertensive agents (e.g., SNP 0.5-5.0 μg/kg/min, labetalol 5-10 mg iv, phentolamine, 2-5 mg iv), if necessary.

POSTOPERATIVE

Complications	Peroneal nerve injury 2° lithotomy position	Peroneal nerve injury manifested as foot drop with loss of sensation over dorsum of foot. Seek neurology consultation.
	Fever/bacteremia	
	Bladder perforation	Bladder perforation may present as shoulder pain in the awake patient, but may go unnoticed in a patient under GA. Sx include unexplained HTN, tachycardia, hypotension (rare).
Pain management	Pain usually mild.	Rx: morphine 2-4 mg iv q 10-15 min prn, fentanyl 25-50 μg iv, ketorolac 30 mg im or iv.

References

1. Amzallog M: Autonomic hyperreflexia. *Int Clin Anesth* 1993; 31:87-102.
2. Mebust WK: Transurethral Surgery. In *Campbell's Urology*, Vol 2, 7th edition. Walsh PC, Retite AB, Stamey TA, Vaughn ED Jr, eds. WB Saunders Co, Philadelphia: 1998, Ch 49, 1511-28.

TRANSURETHRAL RESECTION OF THE PROSTATE (TURP)

SURGICAL CONSIDERATIONS

Description: **TURP** is one of the most common urologic operations, performed to relieve bladder outlet obstruction by an enlarging prostate gland. It is often preceded by **cystoscopy**, which is used to evaluate the size of the prostate gland and to rule out any other pathology, such as bladder tumor or stone. The operation is performed with the resectoscope, a specialized instrument having an electrode capable of transmitting both cutting and coagulating currents.

The resectoscope is introduced into the bladder (Fig 9-2) and the tissue protruding into the prostatic urethra is resected in small pieces called "chips." Bleeding vessels are coagulated with the coagulating current. The resection is performed with continuous irrigation using an isotonic solution, such as sorbitol 2.7% with mannitol 0.54%. Once the obstructing prostatic tissues are completely resected and bleeding vessels coagulated, the chips are irrigated from the bladder and the resectoscope removed. An indwelling Foley catheter is introduced into the bladder. The time of transurethral resection should not exceed 2 hours because excessive absorption of the irrigating fluid may lead to dilutional hyponatremia, seizures and heart failure. The size of the enlarged prostate or adenoma, therefore, needs to be carefully assessed preop to determine if it is possible to complete the resection within a time limit of 2 hours. If not, an open prostatectomy is performed. This variant approach is discussed under Open Prostate Operations, p. 644.

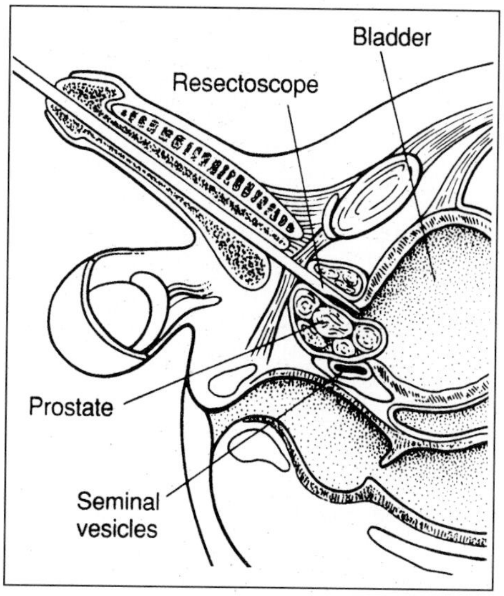

Figure 9-2. Transurethral resection of prostate using a resectoscope. (Reproduced with permission from Govan DE: *Roche Manual of Urologic Procedures*. Hoffmann-LaRoche: 1976.)

Variant procedure or approaches: A number of new techniques have been developed to avoid the morbidity of TURP. These are either vaporization (electrocautery or laser) or thermocoagulation of the prostate (laser, microwave, radio frequency). The following techniques are available and approved:

TUVP: Transurethral vaporization of the prostate with a standard resectoscope using a roller ball electrode at 275-300 watts setting.

VLAP: Visual laser ablation of the prostate is done with Nd:YAG or Ho:YAG laser through a standard cystoscope. All personnel in the OR, including the patient, must wear protective glasses to protect the eyes from inadvertent exposure from a break in the laser fiber.

TUNA: Transurethral needle ablation of the prostate is done with a special disposable device connected to a radio frequency generator.

TUMT: Transurethral microwave thermotherapy is done with a catheter that has a microwave antenna attached to it. A microwave generator is needed for this procedure.

All of the above procedures have several advantages over TURP, including: shorter surgical time, no blood loss, reduced risk of fluid absorption, and all can be done as outpatient procedures.

Usual preop diagnosis: Benign prostatic hypertrophy; prostate cancer

SUMMARY OF PROCEDURE

	TURP	Thermotherapy
Position	Lithotomy	⇐
Incision	None	⇐
Special instrumentation	Cystoscope; resectoscope; catheters; electrocautery	Cystoscope; resectoscope; catheters; electrocautery (standby); laser equipment
Unique considerations	During resection, the patient should be absolutely still because any movement may lead to perforation or injury to the external sphincter, leading to postop incontinence.	During resection, the patient and all personnel should wear protective eyeglasses.
Antibiotics	Gentamicin 80 mg iv, slowly	⇐

	TURP	Thermotherapy
Surgical time	1-2 h (not to exceed 2 h)	1 h
EBL	500 ml	None
Postop care	Irrigation of the Foley catheter to clear it of clots and keep it from being blocked. Determination of serum Na^+	⇐
Mortality	< 1%	⇐
Morbidity	Significant intraop bleeding: 10% Intraop perforation which may require laparotomy: 1% Postop bleeding which may necessitate a return to OR for fulguration of bleeding vessels: 5% Absorption of irrigating fluid which may → dilutional hyponatremia, mental confusion and heart failure: 2%	Postop bleeding: 1% Prolonged catheterization: 10%
Pain score	1	1

PATIENT POPULATION CHARACTERISTICS

Age range	49-90 yr; typically 70s and 80s
Incidence	Very common; 90% of men will develop benign hypertrophy; 20% may need surgical intervention.
Etiology	Aging; benign prostatic hypertrophy; prostate cancer
Associated conditions	COPD (10%); heart disease (10%); HTN (10%); diabetes mellitus (5%); DIC (1-2% of patients with prostate cancer may also have a low-grade, subclinical DIC, which becomes clinically manifest postop).

ANESTHETIC CONSIDERATIONS

PREOPERATIVE

Patients presenting for prostate surgery are generally elderly and may have preexisting medical problems, including CAD, CHF, PVD, cerebrovascular disease, COPD and renal impairment. Preop evaluation should be directed toward the detection and treatment of these conditions prior to anesthesia.

Respiratory	COPD common in this age group. Patients with > 50 pack/year smoking Hx or with any respiratory Sx may need PFTs. For dyspnea with moderate exercise, ✓ VC, FEV_1, MMEF. If VC < 80%, FEV_1 < 60%, or MMEF < 40% predicted, ✓ ABG. If ABG and PFT markedly abnormal, consider postponing surgery until patient's respiratory condition has been optimized. **Tests**: PFT; CXR; ABG, as indicated from H&P.
Cardiovascular	HTN, CAD common in this age group. Assess exercise tolerance by H&P (e.g., should be able to climb a flight of stairs without difficulty or SOB). **Tests**: ECG; others as indicated from H&P.
Neurological	Cerebrovascular disease, Alzheimer's, and other neurologic problems may be present in this age group. Assess mental status to guide evaluation of any intraop or postop changes.
Renal	Anticipate renal impairment 2° chronic obstruction. **Tests**: BUN; creatinine; electrolytes. If ↑BUN and ↑creatinine, ✓ creatinine clearance (normal = 95-140 ml/min).
Musculoskeletal	Various arthritides in this age group may cause problems with positioning for regional anesthesia and surgery.
Endocrine	Increased incidence of diabetes mellitus.

Hematologic Moderate blood loss expected with larger glands. If gland < 30 g, no cross-match necessary; gland 30-80 g, cross-match 2 U of blood; gland > 80 g, cross-match 4 U blood.
Tests: Hct

Laboratory Other tests as indicated from H&P.

Premedication Continue commonly used drugs (e.g., digitalis, β-blockers, NTG) to prevent cardiovascular problems. Sedation prn anxiety (e.g., lorazepam 1-2 mg po 1-2 h before surgery).

INTRAOPERATIVE

Anesthetic technique: Regional or GA. Choice of technique depends on coexisting disease and patient preference. Regional anesthesia may hold some advantage over GA for TURP in that it allows evaluation of mental status and, thus, earlier detection of TURP syndrome. The incidence of postdural puncture headache is very low in this age group (< 1%). A T9 level is optimal. Continuous lumbar epidural anesthesia has no advantage over spinal anesthesia for TURP, since sacral block may be less reliable, the procedure is relatively short, and supplemental doses are usually not necessary.

Regional anesthesia:

Spinal 0.75% bupivacaine, 12 mg in 7.5% dextrose solution (1.6 ml)

General anesthesia:

Induction Standard induction (see p. B-2).

Maintenance Standard maintenance (see p. B-3). Muscle relaxation is not mandatory, although patient movement during the procedure must be avoided.

Emergence Postop pain is usually not significant. Anticipate hypotension when legs are repositioned from lithotomy. Avoid stress on lumbar spine by slowly and simultaneously bringing legs together and returning to supine position.

Blood and fluid requirements	Minimal blood loss (thermotherapy) Moderate blood loss (TURP) IV: 16-18 ga × 1 NS/LR @ 2-4 ml/kg/h	Blood loss can be large (TURP) if venous sinuses are entered; it can also be difficult to quantify because of irrigant. To flush away blood and tissue and to promote visibility during TURP (or thermotherapy), continuous irrigation is used. Irrigating fluid must be nonelectrolytic to prevent dispersion of current, but near isoosmotic to prevent hemolysis of blood. For these reasons, sorbitol (2.7%) with mannitol (0.54%) or glycine (1.5%) are added to distilled water to produce solutions which are slightly hypo-osmolar to blood.
Monitoring	Standard monitors (see p. B-1).	Regional anesthesia allows monitoring of mental status. Invasive monitoring if indicated from H&P.
TURP syndrome	Intravascular volume overload Hyponatremia Hypotonicity 2° absorption of irrigant Symptoms include: • N/V • Visual disturbances • Mental status changes • Coma • Seizures • HTN • Angina • Cardiovascular collapse	Factors which influence the absorption of irrigant include: surgical technique (TURP or thermotherapy), hydrostatic pressure of irrigant (height of bag), number of venous sinuses opened, peripheral venous pressure, duration of surgery, and experience of the surgeon. Resections should optimally be limited to 1 h or less. Some CNS manifestations are 2° glycine and its metabolites. Rx may include observation, diuresis (e.g., furosemide 5-20 mg iv), and administration of hypertonic saline (e.g., 100 ml 3% saline over 1-2 h). Serum sodium < 120 is associated with more severe symptoms, and the goal of therapy is to restore sodium to > 120. In milder cases, observation and water restriction may be sufficient.
Positioning	✓ and pad pressure points. ✓ eyes.	★ **NB**: In lithotomy position, peroneal nerve compression at lateral fibular head → foot drop.
Complications	Bladder perforation TURP syndrome	Bladder perforation may produce shoulder pain in the awake patient. Bladder perforation (and TURP syndrome) may go unnoticed under GA; Sx: ↑BP, ↑HR (occasionally ↓BP).

POSTOPERATIVE

Complications	TURP syndrome Bladder perforation Fever/bacteremia/sepsis Hypothermia	See discussion of TURP syndrome, above.
Pain management	Minimal postop pain	Rx: Morphine 1-4 mg iv prn until comfortable.
Tests	Hct; electrolytes Blood cultures if febrile	Consider serum osmolarity, CXR, ECG in TURP syndrome.

References

1. Abrams PH, Shah PJ, Bryning K, et al: Blood loss during transurethral resection of the prostate. *Anaesthesia* 1982; 37(1):71-73.
2. Jensen V: The TURP syndrome. *Can J Anaesth* 1991; 38(1):90-96.
3. Kabalin JN, Bite J, Doll S: Neodymium:YAG laser coagulation prostatectomy: 3 years of experience with 227 patients. *J Urol* 1996;155:181-185.
4. Mebust WK: Transurethral surgery. In *Campbell's Urology*, 7th edition. Walsh PC, Retite AB, Stamey TA, Vaughn ED Jr, eds. WB Saunders Co, Philadelphia: 1998, Vol 2, Ch 49, 1511-29.

OPEN PROSTATE OPERATIONS

SURGICAL CONSIDERATIONS

Description: Open (in contrast to transurethral or endoscopic) operations on the prostate gland are common. They include: simple prostatectomy; radical prostatectomy; and retropubic exposure of the prostate for brachytherapy through either a midline extraperitoneal incision, which extends from the umbilicus to the symphysis pubis, or through a Pfannenstiel's incision (Fig 9-3, inset).

Simple prostatectomy: When the benign prostatic hypertrophy or adenoma is too large to be resected transurethrally, it is removed by a simple prostatectomy. The prostate gland is exposed through a retropubic approach (Fig 9-3A) and the anterior capsule is incised, exposing the adenoma—the central part of the prostate which is excised, "shelled" out by finger dissection (Fig 9-3B), leaving behind the peripheral prostate and all the associated structures. A Foley catheter is left indwelling in the urethra, and the incision in the prostate capsule is closed. In a **suprapubic prostatectomy**, the incision is made in the bladder and the adenoma shelled from within the bladder.

Radical prostatectomy: The term "radical prostatectomy" may be misleading. It is used to differentiate this cancer operation from a simple prostatectomy (used for benign prostatic hypertrophy). Radical prostatectomy can be achieved through either a **retropubic** or **perineal approach**, the choice being a matter of training, expertise and surgeon's preference. In radical prostatectomy, all of the prostate gland is removed, together with the bladder neck, the seminal vesicles and the ampullae of the vas deferens. A **limited pelvic lymphadenectomy** also is performed. After the prostate gland and its associated structures are removed, the bladder neck is reduced to 1 cm diameter and anastomosed to the membranous urethra over an indwelling Foley catheter. Most of the blood loss occurs during control of the dorsal vein complex. In the past 10 years, attempts have been made to preserve potency by preserving the nerves to the corpora cavernosa.

Usual preop diagnosis: Benign prostatic hypertrophy; prostate cancer

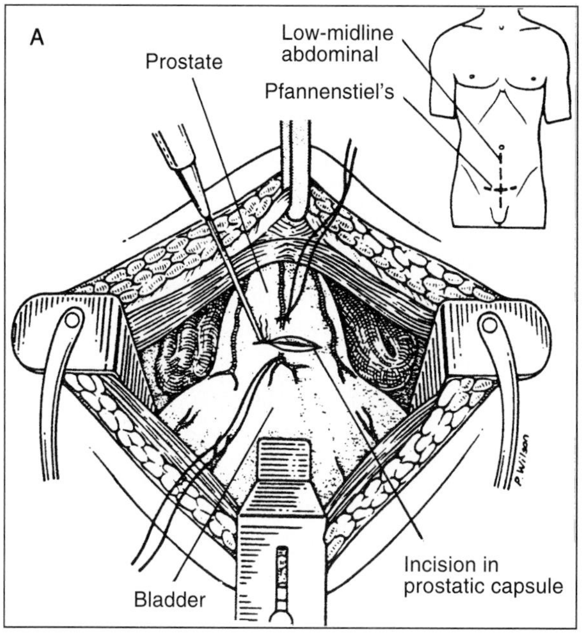

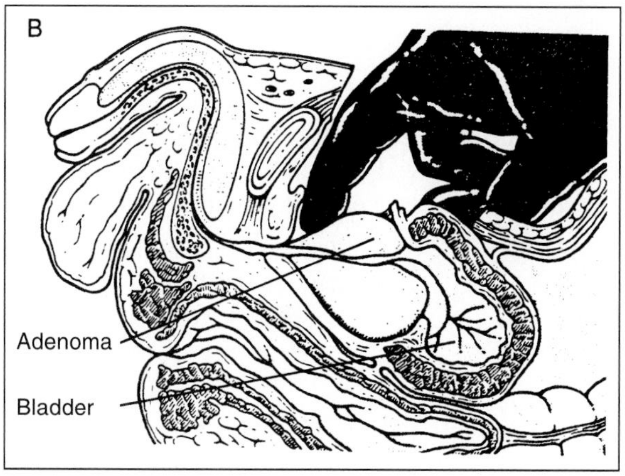

Figure 9-3. Simple retropubic prostatectomy: (A) incision made in the anterior prostatic capsule; (B) adenoma is "shelled out" by finger dissection. (Reproduced with permission from: *Atlas of General Surgery*. Butterworths: 1986.) Inset shows midline abdominal and Pfannenstiel's incisions.

SUMMARY OF PROCEDURE

	Simple Prostatectomy	Radical–Retropubic	Radical–Perineal
Position	Supine	⇐	Lithotomy
Incision	Extraperitoneal, low midline or Pfannenstiel's (Fig 9-3A, inset)	⇐	Perineal (Fig 9-4)
Unique considerations	None	⇐	Extreme hip flexion
Antibiotics	Gentamicin 80 mg iv, slowly	⇐	⇐
Surgical time	1 h	3 h	⇐
EBL	500 ml	1500 ml	500 ml
Postop care	Irrigate catheter to clear blood clots and prevent obstruction, frequently if urine is bloody.	⇐	⇐
Mortality	< 1%	⇐	⇐
Morbidity	Bleeding: 2%	⇐	⇐
	DVT: 2%	⇐	⇐
	Infection: 2%	⇐	⇐
	PE: 1%	⇐	⇐
		Impotence: • Non nerve-sparing: 100% • Nerve-sparing: 50%	
		Lymphocele: 4%	
Pain score	8	8	6

PATIENT POPULATION CHARACTERISTICS

Age range	40-80 yr
Incidence	20% of men will develop symptomatic benign prostatic hypertrophy; 9% will develop clinically evident prostate cancer.
Etiology	Aging
Associated conditions	COPD (10%); CAD (10%); HTN (10%); diabetes mellitus (5%); renal failure (1%)

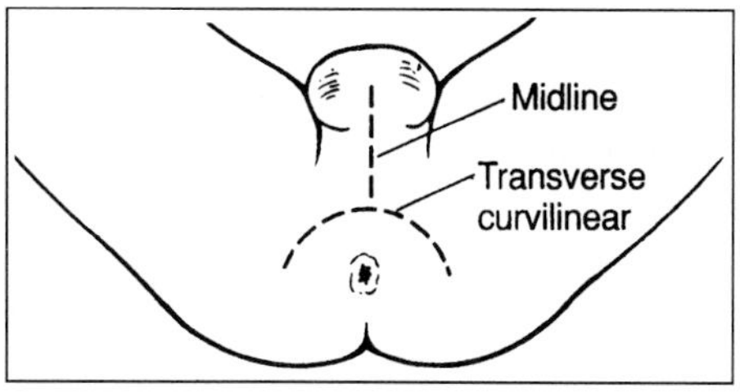

Figure 9-4. Perineal incisions.

ANESTHETIC CONSIDERATIONS

PREOPERATIVE

Patients presenting for prostate surgery are generally elderly and may have preexisting medical problems, including CAD, CHF, PVD, cerebrovascular disease, COPD and renal impairment. Preop evaluation should be directed toward the detection and treatment of these conditions prior to anesthesia.

Respiratory COPD common in this age group. Patients with Hx of >50 pack-year smoking or with respiratory Sx may require PFTs. For dyspnea with moderate exercise, check VC, FEV_1, MMEF. If VC < 80%, FEV_1 < 60%, or MMEF < 40% predicted, check ABG. If ABG and PFT are markedly abnormal, consider postponing surgery until patient's respiratory condition has been optimized.
Tests: PFT; CXR; ABG, as indicated from H&P.

Cardiovascular HTN, CAD common in this age group. Assess exercise tolerance by H&P (e.g., should be able to climb a flight of stairs without difficulty or SOB).
Tests: ECG; others as indicated from H&P.

Neurological Cerebrovascular disease, Alzheimer's and other neurologic problems may be present in this age group. Assess mental status to guide evaluation of any intraop or postop changes.

Renal Anticipate renal impairment 2° chronic obstruction.
Test: Creatinine

Musculoskeletal Various arthritides may cause problems with positioning for regional anesthesia and surgery.

Endocrine Increased incidence of diabetes mellitus.

Hematologic Moderate blood loss expected with larger glands. For glands < 30 g, no cross-match necessary; for glands 30-80 g, cross-match 2 U of blood; for glands > 80 g, cross-match 4 U blood.
Tests: Hct

Laboratory Other tests as indicated from H&P.

Premedication Continue commonly used drugs (e.g., digitalis, β-blockers, diuretics, NTG) to prevent cardiovascular complications. Sedation prn anxiety (e.g., lorazepam 1-2 mg po on call to OR).

INTRAOPERATIVE

Anesthetic technique: Regional (spinal, continuous spinal, continuous lumbar epidural) or GA are acceptable techniques. If regional anesthesia used, optimal block level is T8-T10 (depending on incision site). Advantages of regional anesthesia include potential for lower intraop blood loss, and possible lower incidence of DVT postop. Disadvantages include positioning considerations (see below).

Regional anesthesia:

Spinal Bupivacaine (0.75%) 12 mg in 7.5% dextrose solution (1.6 ml) or hyperbaric tetracaine 10-15 mg with epinephrine 200 μg (0.2 ml of 1:1000 solution).

Epidural 1.5-2% lidocaine with epinephrine 5 μg/ml, 15-25 ml, supplemental iv sedation as necessary. Additional epidural lidocaine (5-10 ml boluses) may be needed, depending on length of procedure.

General anesthesia:

Induction Standard induction (see p. B-2).

Maintenance Standard maintenance (see p. B-3).

Emergence No special considerations

Blood and fluid requirements Moderate-to-large blood loss
IV: 14-16 ga × 1-2
NS/LR @ 4-6 ml/kg/h

Additional requirements dependent on type of anesthesia. Regional techniques are associated with higher fluid requirement because of sympathectomy and systemic vasodilation; it also may be associated with lower blood loss than GA.[2]

Monitoring Standard monitors (see p. B-1).
Depending on underlying disease:

Some patients require CVP to aid in assessment of volume status. Arterial line is often useful for continuous

Monitoring, cont.	± CVP ± Arterial line	BP monitoring and frequent blood draws. Patients at particularly high risk (e.g., Hx of preexisting cardiopulmonary disease) should probably have both.
Positioning	Anticipate hypotension on return from lithotomy position. ✓ and pad pressure points. ✓ eyes.	Rx: volume (200-500 ml NS/LR) or ephedrine (5 mg iv) may be necessary. Elderly patients with arthritis or respiratory impairment may not tolerate the extreme positioning associated with perineal prostatectomy for extended periods of time, thus precluding the use of regional anesthesia (a combined technique with GA may be considered). ★ **NB**: In lithotomy position, peroneal nerve compression at lateral fibular head → foot drop.
Complications	Indigo carmine reaction Hemorrhage Hypothermia VAE	Indigo carmine → false ↓O_2 saturation ± ↑BP; rare allergic reaction → rash + bronchoconstriction + ↓BP.

POSTOPERATIVE

Complications	Peroneal nerve injury 2° lithotomy position DVT	Manifested by foot drop with loss of sensation on dorsum of foot. Seek neurology consultation. Incidence of DVT less with regional than GA. Sx: variable, with pain and tenderness over involved area.
Pain management	Significant postop pain. Rx: morphine 0.1-0.3 mg/kg iv in incremental doses (e.g., 2-4 mg q 10-15 min prn).	Consider epidural narcotic or PCA (see p. C-3).
Tests	Hct	

References

1. Donald JR: The effect of anaesthesia, hypotension, and epidural analgesia on blood loss in surgery for pelvic floor repair. *Br J Anaesth* 1969; 41(2):155-66.
2. Eastham JA, Scardino PT: Radical prostatectomy. In *Campbell's Urology*, 7th edition. WB Saunders Co, Philadelphia: 1998, Vol 3, Ch 85, 2547-64.
3. Gibbons RP: Radical perineal prostatectomy. In *Campbell's Urology*, 7th edition. WB Saunders Co, Philadelphia: 1998, Vol 3, Ch 87, 2589-2604.
4. Hendolin H, Mattila MA, Poikolainen E: The effect of lumbar epidural analgesia on the development of deep vein thrombosis of the legs after open prostatectomy. *Acta Chir Scand* 1981; 147(6):425-29.
5. Oesterling JE: Retropubic and suprapubic prostatectomy. In *Campbell's Urology*, 7th edition. Walsh PC, et al, eds. WB Saunders Co, Philadelphia: 1998, Vol 2, Ch 50, 1529-42.

NEPHRECTOMY

SURGICAL CONSIDERATIONS

Description: Nephrectomies fall into three basic groups: simple, partial and radical. (Surgical anatomy is shown in Fig 9-5.)

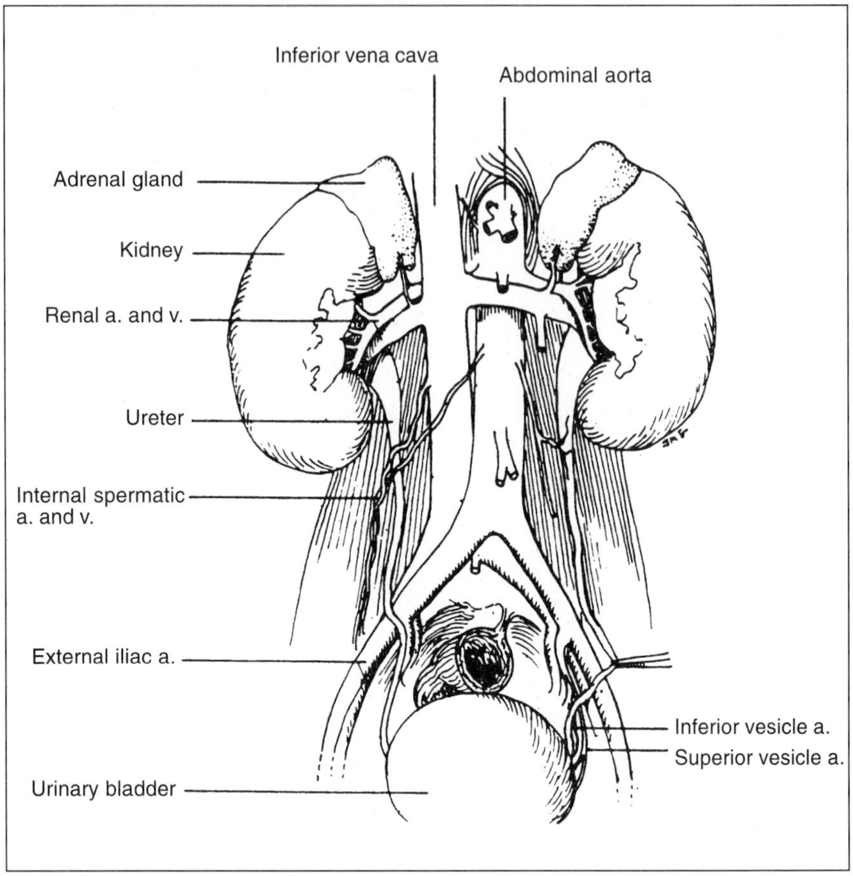

Figure 9-5. Surgical anatomy of the urinary tract. (Reproduced with permission from Hardy JD: *Textbook of Surgery*. Lippincott: 1988.)

Simple nephrectomy, performed for benign conditions, is the surgical excision of the kidney and only a small segment of proximal ureter. The dorsal approach is well suited for this operation and begins with an incision extending from the 12th rib to the iliac crest along the lateral edge of the sacrospinalis muscle and quadratus lumborum muscle. The dorsolumbar fascia is opened, exposing Gerota's fascia and the perinephric fat. The kidney is mobilized until the hilum is exposed. The artery and vein are tied, suture-ligated and transected. The ureter is followed distally as far as possible, tied and transected; and the kidney is delivered out of the incision, which is then closed by approximating the dorsolumbar fascia and the fascia of the sacrospinalis muscle.

Usual preop diagnosis: Chronic hydronephrosis; hypoplastic kidney; renovascular HTN; double collecting system

Partial nephrectomy is the surgical excision of the segment of the kidney harboring the pathology. It is performed for small renal-cell carcinomas and benign tumors of the kidney, such as angiomyolipomas, and for duplicated collecting systems with a diseased moiety. If the partial nephrectomy is being done for renal-cell carcinoma, it may be accompanied with a **regional lymphadenectomy**. The flank approach is well suited for this operation and begins with an incision over the 12th or 11th rib, or in between, and extends anteriorly over the external and internal oblique muscles, which are transected. The transversalis muscle and fascia are opened, exposing Gerota's fascia. The renal capsule is exposed at the planned site of resection. Control of the renal vessels is advised for control of bleeding, if excessive. Incision in the renal parenchyma is made by sharp and blunt dissection, suture-ligating all bleeders. If the collecting system is opened, it should be closed with absorbable sutures. After complete hemostasis, Gelfoam or perinephric fat is used to cover the raw surface of the kidney.

Usual preop diagnosis: Renal-cell carcinoma; double collecting system

Radical nephrectomy is the surgical excision of the kidney, with its surrounding perinephric fat and Gerota's fascia, and the proximal 2/3rds of the ureter, accompanied by paracaval or paraaortic **lymphadenectomy**. It is performed for renal-cell carcinoma. Early control of renal vessels is advised before excessive manipulation of the tumor, to minimize blood loss and hematogenous spread. Transabdominal or flank approaches are best suited for this operation.

Nephroureterectomy is a radical nephrectomy with ureter resection, including the ureteral orifice and a cuff of bladder wall around it. It is accompanied by a regional lymphadenectomy, since it is performed for a cancerous condition. The approach is either transabdominal or extraperitoneal through an extended flank incision, starting at the tip of the 11th rib

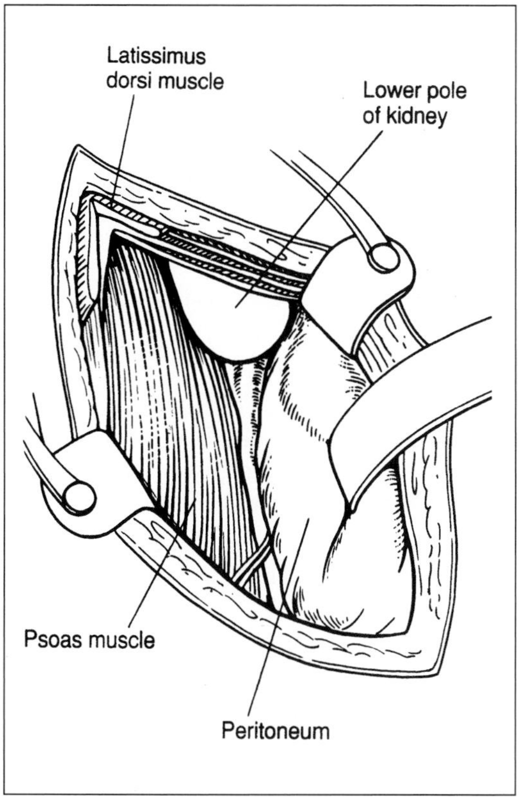

Figure 9-8. Surgical exposure of the lower pole of kidney, renal pelvis and proximal ureter. (Reproduced with permission from *Atlas of General Surgery*. Butterworths: 1986.)

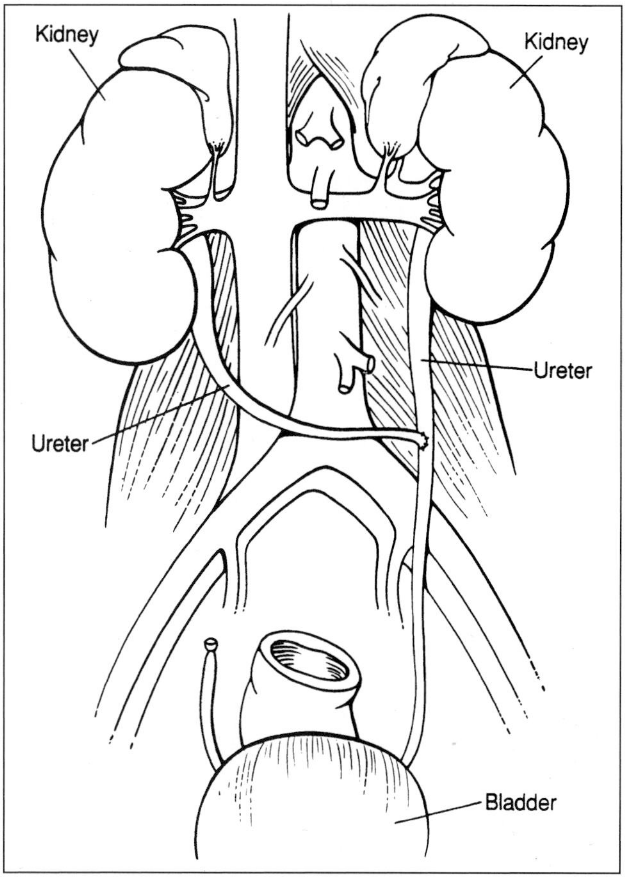

Figure 9-9. Transureteroureterostomy.

PATIENT POPULATION CHARACTERISTICS

	Pyeloplasty	Pyelolithotomy/ Ureterolithotomy	Transureteroureterostomy
Age range	All ages	⇐	⇐
Male:Female	1:1	⇐	⇐
Incidence	Rare	Extremely rare	⇐
Etiology	Ureteropelvic junction obstruction: 80% (of causes of dilated collecting system in the newborn)	Renal pelvic and upper ureteral stone	Traumatic loss of lower ureter; lower ureteral tumor
Associated conditions	Renal failure: 1%		

ANESTHETIC CONSIDERATIONS

(Procedures covered: nephrectomy and operations on the renal pelvis and upper ureter)

PREOPERATIVE

Respiratory Increased postop pulmonary complications because of location of incision. If Hx of pulmonary disease (e.g., asthma, COPD), consider postop respiratory therapy.
Tests: As indicated from H&P.

Cardiovascular Consider possibility of renal HTN.

Hematologic Polycythemia may be seen in association with polycystic kidney disease, renal-cell carcinoma. Consider preop blood donation for autologous transfusion.
Tests: Hct

Laboratory	Electrolytes; BUN; creatinine; other tests as indicated from H&P.	
Premedication	Standard premedication (see p. B-2).	

INTRAOPERATIVE

Anesthetic technique: GA is recommended for these procedures; technique depends on underlying disease. Regional techniques (spinal or epidural) are alternatives, but are less than optimal because of awkward positioning which may lead to patient discomfort and pain resulting from diaphragmatic stimulation.

Induction	Standard induction (see p. B-2).	
Maintenance	Standard maintenance (see p. B-3). If intraperitoneal approach is used, consider limiting N_2O to avoid distention of bowel and interference with operative field.	
Emergence	No specific considerations	
Blood and fluid requirements	Mild-to-moderate blood loss IV: 14-16 ga × 1 NS/LR @ 6-8 ml/kg/h Warm all fluids.	Intraperitoneal approach associated with higher fluid requirements (8-10 ml/kg/h). When renal vessels are to be cross-clamped, mannitol (0.5 g/kg) is often given prior to occlusion (20 min maximum).
Monitoring	Standard monitors (see p. B-1). Urinary catheter Arterial line (partial nephrectomy)	Invasive monitoring if indicated from H&P. CVP line useful for partial nephrectomy in patients with solitary kidneys (↑↑blood loss).
Positioning	Use axillary roll if lateral. Avoid stretching brachial plexus – limit abduction to 90°. If prone, repeatedly ✓ eyes and pressure points. Assure free excursion of abdomen.	The lateral position with kidney rest and table flexion may lead to hypotension, possibly 2° vena cava obstruction. Moderate iv volume administration, as well as gradual assumption of the position, are recommended to avoid this complication.
Complications	Pneumothorax Hypotension with positioning (see above). Indigo carmine → ↑BP, ↑SVR Methylene blue → ↓BP	Sx of pneumothorax include: ↑RR, ↑PIP, hypoxemia, hypercarbia. If in doubt, ✓ CXR.

POSTOPERATIVE

Complications	Postnephrectomy syndrome Eye injury (if prone) Brachial plexus injury (if lateral) Pneumothorax Atelectasis Pneumonia	Postnephrectomy syndrome 2° retractor injury. L1 nerve root damage with resulting pain, dysesthesia and sensory loss in L1 dermatome distribution.
Pain management	Morphine 0.1-0.3 mg/kg iv in incremental doses Consider epidural narcotic, PCA (see pp. C-1 – C-3).	Postop analgesia critical to minimize pulmonary complications.
Tests	Hct; CXR	Others dependent on operative course, coexisting disease.

Reference

1. Franke JJ, Smith JA: Surgery of the ureter. In *Campbell's Urology*, 7th edition. Walsh PC, et al, eds. WB Saunders Co, Philadelphia: 19982, Vol 3, Ch 98, 3062-84.

CYSTECTOMY

SURGICAL CONSIDERATIONS

Description: Open (in contrast to transurethral or endoscopic) bladder operations (cystectomies) account for 15-20% of all urological procedures. They are grouped as simple, partial and radical procedures.

Simple cystectomy is performed for benign conditions of the bladder, such as severe hemorrhagic cystitis, radiation cystitis and contracted bladder. It involves the removal of the bladder only. The operation is performed through a lower abdominal incision. The peritoneal reflections are incised down to the pouch of Douglas; the vasa deferentia are identified, cross-clamped, transected and tied. The superior vesical arteries are identified, cross-clamped near their origin, transected and tied. The ureters are identified, separated from the surrounding tissues, cross-clamped near the bladder, transected and tied. The bladder is bluntly separated from the anterior rectal wall all the way to the apex of the prostate. The lateral pedicles of the bladder are cross-clamped, cut and tied. The endopelvic fascia is incised, separating the prostate from the lateral pelvic wall. The puboprostatic ligaments are transected and the dorsal vein of the penis is suture-ligated. The tied dorsal vein and urethra are incised just distal to the apex of the prostate. The specimen is delivered out of the incision and hemostasis secured with electrocautery. An ileal conduit is then performed (see below).

Partial cystectomy is the excision of only the part of the bladder containing the pathology. This is not a commonly performed operation and is reserved for tumors located in the dome of the bladder of older patients who are poor surgical risks for major operations, such as radical cystectomy. The operation is preceded by a cystoscopy to identify the site of pathology. Beginning with a lower abdominal incision, the dome and lateral walls of the bladder are separated from the surrounding tissues, which are covered by wet packs in order to minimize contamination. An incision is made in the dome of the bladder at least 2 cm away from the pathology. The inside of the bladder is inspected and the pathology identified. The incision in the bladder is continued around, and at least 2 cm away from, the pathology, until the latter is completely excised. Bleeders in the wall of the bladder are electrocoagulated. The bladder wall is then closed in two layers—a through-and-through layer and an inverting layer—using absorbable material. Wet packs are removed, a drain is left in the region and the abdominal incision is closed.

Radical cystectomy (or **radical cystoprostatectomy**) is performed for treatment of invasive bladder cancer. It encompasses the removal of the bladder and the lower ureters, the prostate gland and seminal vesicles in men (Fig 9-10A), and the uterus,

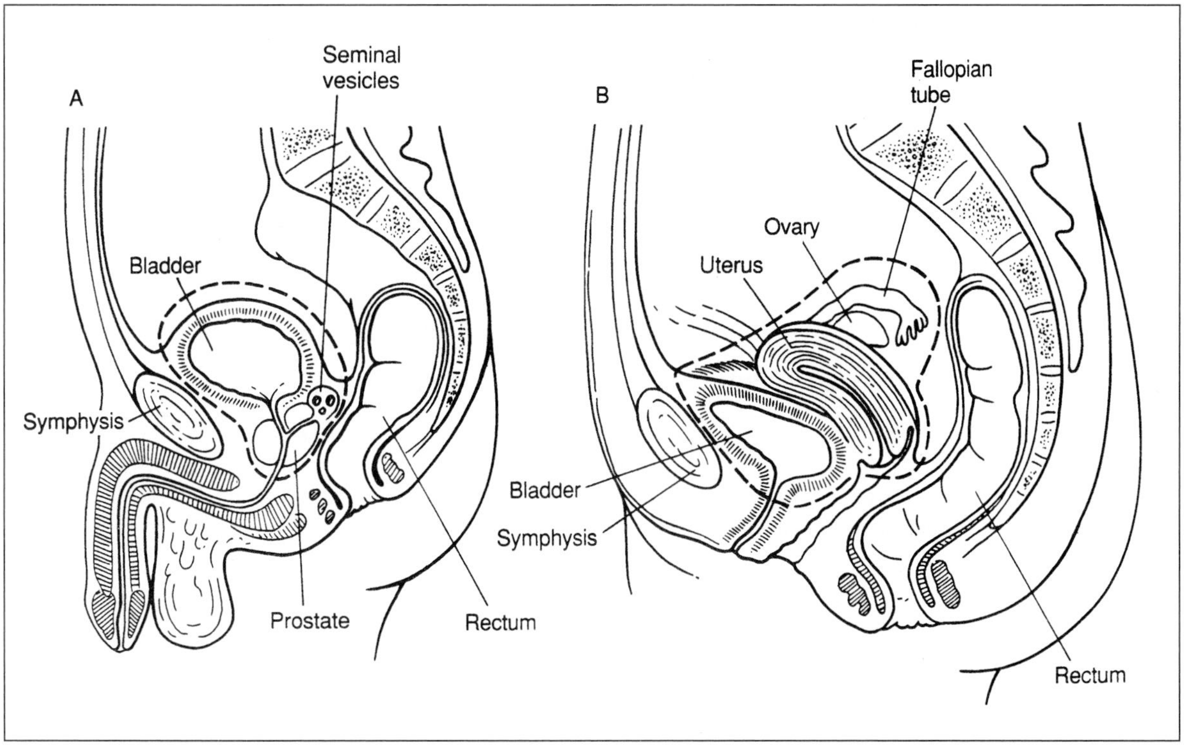

Figure 9-10. Anatomy of the pelvis with tissue to be excised outlined by dashed line: (A) male; (b) female. (Reproduced with permission from *Atlas of General Surgery*. Butterworths: 1986.)

ovaries and anterior vaginal wall in women (Fig 9-10B). Accompanied by a **pelvic lymphadenectomy**, it is performed in the supine position, except when a concomitant **urethrectomy** is required, wherein a lithotomy position is used.

Following cystectomy, whether radical or simple, some form of **urinary diversion** is required. This can be accomplished with either a standard ileal conduit or a bladder substitution. The **ileal conduit** is constructed from 6-8 inches of terminal ileum isolated from the small intestine with its blood supply. The continuity of the small intestine is accomplished by a simple anastomosis. The ureters are implanted into the proximal end of the conduit and the distal end is brought through the abdominal wall as a stoma (Fig 9-11). **Bladder substitution** is a more complex operation wherein a longer segment of bowel is isolated, with its blood supply, and fashioned into a pouch. The ureters are implanted in the pouch and the most dependent part of the pouch is connected to the membranous urethra, avoiding a stoma (Fig 9-12). Not all patients undergoing cystectomies are candidates for bladder substitution. For example, patients who require a urethrectomy are not candidates because of the need to remove the urethra.

Usual preop diagnosis: Bladder cancer; contracted bladder; hemorrhagic cystitis; radiation cystitis; bladder diverticulum

SUMMARY OF PROCEDURE

	Simple Cystectomy	Partial Cystectomy	Radical Cystectomy
Position	Supine	⇐	Supine or lithotomy
Incision	Transperitoneal, midline	⇐	⇐
Antibiotics	Cefotetan or ceftriaxone 1 g	⇐	⇐
Surgical time	4 h	2 h	6 h
EBL	1000 ml	Minimal	1500 ml
Postop care	Care of the stoma	Catheter care	Care of the stoma
Mortality	1%	< 1%	2%
Morbidity	Prolonged ileus: 5%	–	5%
	Infection: 2%	–	2%
		Hematuria: 5%	
Pain score	10	10	10

PATIENT POPULATION CHARACTERISTICS

Age range	40-80 yr	⇐	⇐
Male:Female	3:1	⇐	⇐
Incidence	40,000 new cases of bladder cancer diagnosed/yr; 20% treated with cystectomy.	⇐	⇐
Etiology	Contracted bladder; hemorrhagic and radiation cystitis	Bladder cancer; bladder diverticulum	⇐
Associated conditions	Heart disease (10%); HTN (10%); COPD (5%); diabetes mellitus (5%)	Heart disease (10%)	⇐

ANESTHETIC CONSIDERATIONS

PREOPERATIVE

Respiratory Note Hx of pulmonary disease in older patients.
Tests: As indicated from H&P.

Cardiovascular Note Hx of cardiac disease, HTN in older patients.
Tests: Consider ECG; others as indicated from H&P.

Gastrointestinal Bowel prep likely and may cause dehydration and electrolyte disturbances.
Tests: Electrolytes, if indicated.

Hematologic T&C for 2-4 U PRBC.
Tests: Hct

Laboratory Other tests as indicated from H&P.

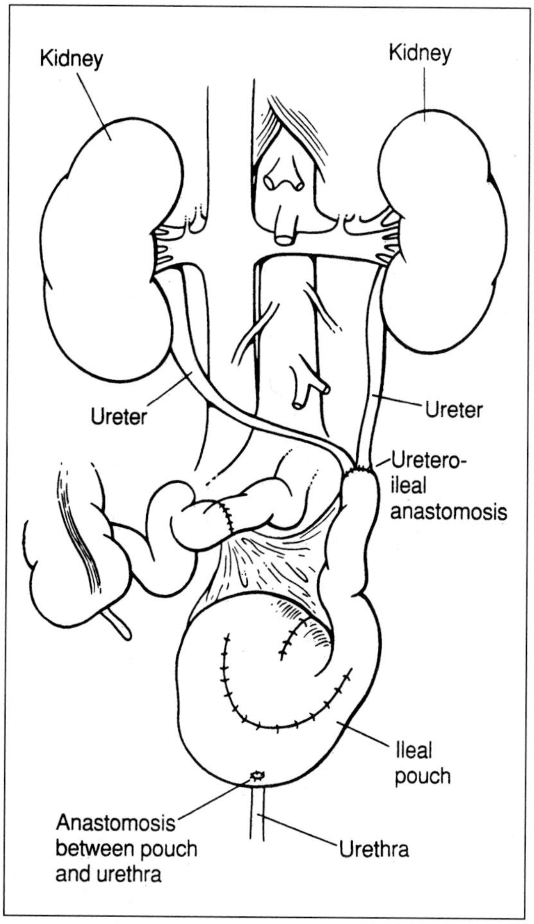

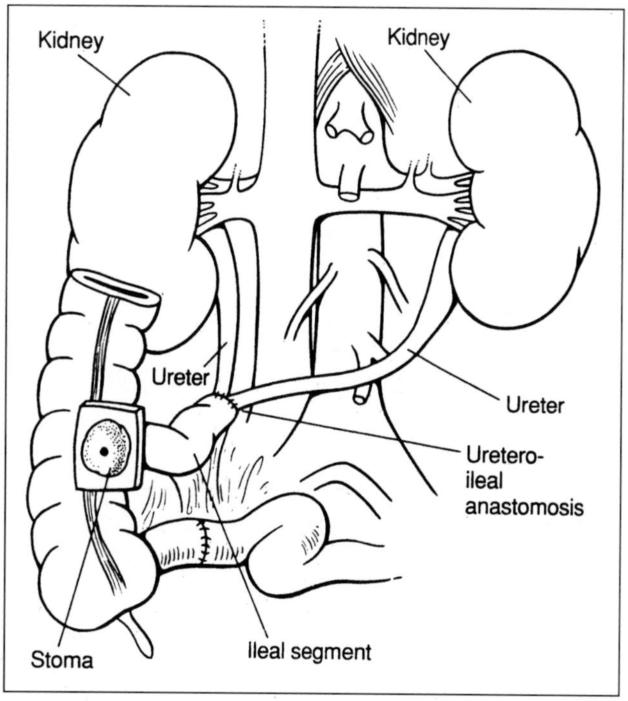

↑ **Figure 9-11.** Ileal conduit. A segment of ileum is isolated from terminal ileum and continuity of the bowel is reestablished with an end-to-end anastomosis. Ureters are joined to the proximal end of the ileal segment and the distal end is brought out to the skin as a stoma.

← **Figure 9-12.** Bladder substitution. A segment of ileum is fashioned into a pouch and anastomosed to the urethra. The ureters are joined to the proximal, nondetubularized segment.

Premedication Sedation prn anxiety in adults (e.g., lorazepam 1-2 mg po 1-2 h preop; midazolam 1-2 mg iv in preop area).

INTRAOPERATIVE

Anesthetic technique: Spinal, continuous lumbar epidural or GA are acceptable, with choice dependent on length of procedure, coexisting disease and patient preference. A combined technique using GA and regional anesthesia may be preferable. A T4 sensory level is recommended since peritoneal stimulation is likely during this procedure.

Regional anesthesia:

Spinal 0.75% bupivacaine 12-15 mg in 7.5% dextrose; hyperbaric tetracaine 10-15 mg with 200 μg epinephrine for procedures longer than 3 h.

Epidural 1.5-2% lidocaine with epinephrine 5 μg/ml, 15-25 ml; supplement with 5-10 ml as needed. Supplemental iv sedation (e.g., midazolam 1 mg iv prn; fentanyl 50 μg iv prn)

General anesthesia:

Induction Standard induction (see p. B-2). These patients may be significantly dehydrated and require volume replacement before induction.

Maintenance Standard maintenance (see p. B-3).

Emergence No specific considerations

Blood and fluid requirements
Significant blood loss possible
IV: 16 ga × 1
NS/LR @ 6-10 ml/kg/h
Warm fluids.
Humidify gases.

Blood loss may be less with regional than GA.

Monitoring	Standard monitors (see p. B-1). Arterial line CVP line	Consider PA catheter in patients with cardiopulmonary disease. UO as measure of volume status may be lost during procedure.
Complications	Major blood loss 3rd-space losses Hypothermia	

POSTOPERATIVE

Complications	Hypothermia	
Pain management	Morphine 0.1-0.3 mg/kg iv in incremental doses Consider epidural narcotics or PCA.	See pp. C1 – C-3.
Tests	Hct	Others as indicated by intraop course.

Reference

1. Marshall FF: Surgery of the bladder. In *Campbell's Urology*, 7th edition. Walsh PC, et al, eds. WB Saunders Co, Philadelphia: 1998, Vol 3, Ch 105, 3274-98.

OPEN BLADDER OPERATIONS (OTHER THAN CYSTECTOMY)

SURGICAL CONSIDERATIONS

Description: Open bladder operations include:

Augmentation cystoplasty (or **enterocystoplasty**): Small, contracted bladders can be enlarged and their size and capacity augmented with a segment of intestine. The bladder is opened widely, anteroposteriorly or from side-to-side, or with a cruciate incision. A segment of intestine—either small bowel, cecum or colon—is isolated from the intestinal tract, detubularized and added on to the bladder.

Variant procedure: The antrum of the stomach can also be used (**gastrocystoplasty**).

Usual preop diagnosis: Contracted bladder from chronic cystitis

Repair of vesicovaginal or enterovesical fistulas: The communication between the vagina and bladder or bladder and bowel is identified and excised, and the edges freshened until normal, noninflamed tissues are exposed. The openings in the bladder and in the vagina or bowel are closed, and omentum is interposed in between to promote healing and prevent recurrences. With enterovesical fistulas, often the diseased segment of the intestine is excised and an end-to-end anastomosis of the intestine is performed.

Variant procedure: Transvaginal repair of vesicovaginal fistula (see Vaginal Operations, p. 668).

Usual preop diagnosis: Vesicovaginal or enterovesical fistula

Ureteral reimplantation, performed to correct vesicoureteral reflux, is more commonly used in the pediatric group than in adults. In adults, it is performed mainly for lower ureteral injuries, iatrogenic or traumatic. The lower ureter is identified and dissected proximally until adequate length is obtained. The bladder is opened and a 2-3 cm submucosal tunnel is created in or near the trigone, and the ureter is brought into the tunnel and fixed with sutures. If there is a large gap between the ureter and the bladder, a psoas hitch procedure is necessary. The bladder is mobilized and stitched to the psoas muscle in order to reach the ureter. In children, if the ureter is dilated, its diameter is reduced by imbrication before reimplantation. In adults, a nonrefluxing implantation is usually not necessary if the operation is being performed for ureteral injury.

Usual preop diagnosis: Vesicoureteral reflux; lower ureteral injuries

SUMMARY OF PROCEDURE

	Augmentation Cystoplasty	Repair of Fistulas	Ureteral Reimplantation
Position	Supine	Supine or lithotomy	Supine
Incision	Low abdominal	⇐	⇐
Antibiotics	Gentamicin 80 mg iv, slowly	⇐	⇐
Surgical time	4 h	3 h	⇐
EBL	Minimal	⇐	⇐
Postop care	Care of catheters and stents	⇐	⇐
Mortality	< 1%	⇐	⇐
Morbidity	Infections: 5%	⇐	⇐
	Urinary leakage: 1%	⇐	⇐
Pain score	10	10	10

PATIENT POPULATION CHARACTERISTICS

Age range	All ages	⇐	⇐
Male:Female	1:4	⇐	⇐
Incidence	Rare	⇐	⇐
Etiology	Contracted bladders from chronic cystitis	Traumatic fistulas; vesicovaginal; regional enteritis; diverticulitis; colon cancer	Vesicoureteral reflux; injury to lower ureters

ANESTHETIC CONSIDERATIONS

PREOPERATIVE

Respiratory Note Hx of pulmonary disease in elderly patients.
Tests: As indicated from H&P.

Cardiovascular Note Hx of cardiac disease in elderly patients.
Tests: Consider ECG; others, if indicated from H&P.

Neurological Paraplegics and quadriplegics may present for operations on the bladder and urinary tract. Obtain Hx of autonomic hyperreflexia (AH). Sx are: flushing, headache, nasal stuffiness, HTN associated with voiding and noxious stimuli below level of transection.

Laboratory Other tests as indicated from H&P.

Premedication Sedation prn anxiety (e.g., lorazepam 1-2 mg po 1-2 h prior to surgery; midazolam 1-2 mg iv in preop area).

INTRAOPERATIVE

Anesthetic technique: Spinal, continuous lumbar epidural or GA are acceptable, with choice dependent on length of procedure, coexisting disease and patient preference. A combined technique using light GA with regional anesthesia is also acceptable. A T10 sensory level is sufficient to provide anesthesia for procedures on the bladder, but a T4 level is recommended if the peritoneum is opened. (See Anesthetic Considerations for Transurethral Procedures [except TURP] p. 640, for patients with AH.)

Regional anesthesia:

Spinal 0.75% bupivacaine 10-15 mg in 7.5% dextrose; 5% lidocaine 75-100 mg (controversial)

Epidural 1.5-2.0% lidocaine with epinephrine 5 μg/ml, 15-25 ml; supplement with 5-10 ml as needed. Supplemental iv sedation.

General anesthesia:

Induction Standard induction (see p. B-2).

Maintenance Standard maintenance (see p. B-3). Consider limiting N_2O for long intraperitoneal procedures to minimize bowel distention.

Emergence	No specific considerations	
Blood and fluid requirements	Minimal-to-moderate blood loss IV: 16-18 ga × 1 NS/LR @ 2-4 ml/kg/h Warm fluids. Humidify gases for lengthy procedures.	Intraperitoneal procedures have considerably higher requirements (e.g., NS/LR @ 6-10 ml/kg/h).
Monitoring	Standard monitors (see p. B-1) for simpler procedures. ± Arterial/CVP lines	UO as a measure of volume status may be lost during the procedure. Consider arterial line, CVP for longer, more complex procedures.
Positioning	✓ and pad pressure points. ✓ eyes.	★ **NB**: In lithotomy position, peroneal nerve compression at lateral fibular head → foot drop.
Complications	AH in spinal cord injured patients	See discussion in Anesthetic Considerations for Transurethral Procedures, p. 640.

POSTOPERATIVE

Complications	Hypothermia Fever, bacteremia	
Pain management	Morphine 0.1-0.3 mg/kg in incremental doses. Consider epidural narcotics or PCA.	See pp. C-1, C-3.
Tests	Hct Blood cultures if febrile	Others as indicated by intraop course.

Reference

1. Marshall FF: Surgery of the bladder. In *Campbell's Urology*, 7th edition. Walsh PC, et al, eds. WB Saunders Co, Philadelphia: 1998, Vol 3, Ch 105, 3274-98.

INGUINAL OPERATIONS

SURGICAL CONSIDERATIONS

Description: Inguinal operations are very common, and are usually performed on an outpatient basis. Groin dissection, however, may necessitate inpatient care.

Inguinal herniorrhaphy: A 3" inguinal incision is made, starting 1" medial to the anterior-superior iliac spine, and ending at the pubic tubercle. The external oblique aponeurosis is excised, opening the external inguinal ring. The spermatic cord and the hernial sac are freed off the inguinal canal (Fig 9-13); then the hernial sac is dissected off the spermatic cord and followed proximally into the internal inguinal ring, where it is suture-ligated and excised. The floor of the inguinal canal is strengthened by approximating the conjoined tendon to the reflected part of the inguinal ligament.

Usual preop diagnosis: Inguinal hernia

Orchiopexy is performed through the same incision as used in herniorrhaphy. Once the inguinal canal is exposed, a search for the undescended testis begins. The testis and cord are dissected free from all surrounding tissue until adequate length is obtained to bring the testis down to the scrotum. Next, a pouch is created in the wall of the scrotum by incising the scrotal skin and dissecting it off dartos fascia. The testis is brought down into the pouch and fixed to the dartos fascia with sutures, and the incisions are closed. Often a **herniorrhaphy** is performed at the same time.

Usual preop diagnosis: Undescended testis

Radical orchiectomy is performed through a herniorrhaphy incision (described above). The spermatic cord is freed and cross-clamped at the internal inguinal ring, transected and suture-ligated. The testis, with its tunica vaginalis, is then delivered through the incision by blunt and sharp dissection and the inguinal incision is closed. Sometimes, a testicular prosthesis is inserted and fixed in the scrotum before the inguinal incision is closed.

Usual preop diagnosis: Testicular cancer

Ligation of spermatic vein is performed through a small, transverse incision 1-2" above the internal inguinal ring. Muscles are split and peritoneum reflected medially to expose the spermatic vessels; the vein is identified and ligated.

Usual preop diagnosis: Varicocele causing infertility

Groin dissection, or **inguinofemoral lymphadenectomy** (lymph node dissection), is the most critical of the inguinal operations. It is performed through either an inguinal incision (Fig 9-13) curved distally over the femoral vessels or through 2 incisions, inguinal and upper-thigh (Fig 9-13), over the femoral triangle. A complete inguinal and femoral lymphadenectomy is performed.

Usual preop diagnosis: Penile cancer

SUMMARY OF PROCEDURE

	Herniorrhaphy, Orchiopexy, Orchiectomy	Ligation of Spermatic Vein	Groin Dissection
Position	Supine	⇐	⇐
Incision	Inguinal (Fig 9-13, inset)	Transverse groin (Fig 9-13, inset)	Inguinal and upper thigh (Fig 9-13, inset)
Antibiotics	None	⇐	⇐
Surgical time	1 h	⇐	3 h
EBL	Minimal	⇐	200 ml
Postop care	PACU → home	⇐	PACU → ward; leg elevation
Mortality	< 1%	⇐	⇐
Morbidity	Wound infection: 2%	⇐	⇐
Pain score	7	5	7

PATIENT POPULATION CHARACTERISTICS

Age range	All ages	Young adults	Middle age
Incidence	Hernia: 5% of population Undescended testis: 0.8% of male children Testis cancer: 6/100,000	1% of young men	Extremely rare, < 1% of all males
Etiology	Unknown; congenital	Varicocele	Penile cancer (very rare)

ANESTHETIC CONSIDERATIONS

PREOPERATIVE

Typically, patients presenting for inguinal operation are healthy, with most returning home on the day of surgery. The most common inguinal operation is herniorrhaphy. In these patients, consider causes of increased intraabdominal pressure during H&P. (Pediatric inguinal operations are discussed in Pediatric General Surgery, pp. 958, 984.) A hernia may strangulate → acute abdomen.

Respiratory Chronic cough is a common precipitating factor.

Gastrointestinal Constipation may be a precipitating factor.

Laboratory Tests as indicated from H&P.

Premedication Sedation for adults prn anxiety (e.g., lorazepam 1-2 mg po 1-2 h before surgery; midazolam 1-2 mg iv in preop area).

INTRAOPERATIVE

Anesthetic technique: Local anesthesia (with sedation), spinal, epidural or GA are acceptable techniques, with choice dependent on patient age and coexisting disease, type and length of procedure and patient preference. Local anesthesia is acceptable for simple herniorrhaphy, although discomfort may be elicited if the peritoneum is manipulated. If a spinal or epidural anesthesia is chosen, a T6 level should be sought. Most inguinal procedures are done on an outpatient basis, and the anesthetic should be planned appropriately.

Regional anesthesia:

Spinal 0.75% bupivacaine, 12-15 mg; 5% lidocaine, 75 mg (controverisal)

Epidural 1.5-2.0% lidocaine with epinephrine 5 μg/ml, 15-25 ml; supplement with 5-10 ml as needed. Supplemental iv sedation with local or regional technique in adults; e.g., midazolam (1-2 mg iv), fentanyl (25-50 μg iv prn anxiety or discomfort); or propofol infusion (25-50 μg/kg/min).

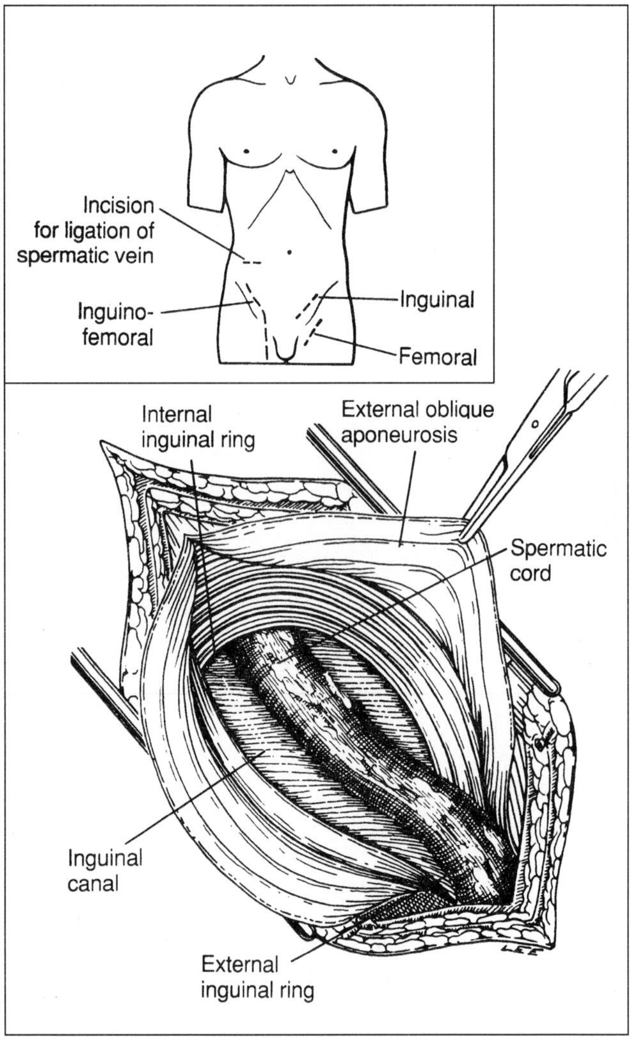

Figure 9-13. Surgical anatomy of the inguinal canal. (Reproduced with permission from *Atlas of General Surgery*. Butterworths: 1986.) Inset shows groin incisions.

General anesthesia:

Induction Standard induction (see p. B-2). ET intubation and/or controlled ventilation may not be needed for shorter cases; consider LMA.

Maintenance Standard maintenance (see p. B-3); consider propofol infusion (100-200 μg/kg/min). Muscle relaxation usually not required.

Emergence No specific considerations

Blood and fluid requirements Usually minimal blood loss
IV: 18 ga × 1
NS/LR @ 1-2 ml/kg/h

Minimize NS/LR to avoid postop urinary retention after herniorrhaphy.

Monitoring Standard monitors (see p. B-1).

POSTOPERATIVE

Complications N/V — May delay discharge from PACU → home.
Failure to void

Pain management Local anesthesia
Ketorolac 30 mg im or iv in adults
± Morphine 2-4 mg iv or fentanyl 25-50 μg iv

Instillation or infiltration of wound with 0.25% bupivacaine or ilioinguinal nerve block provides prolonged postop analgesia and decreases need for narcotics in outpatients. This can be used in both adult and pediatric patients.

References

1. Casey WF, Rice LJ, Hannallah RS, et al: A comparison between bupivacaine instillation versus ilioinguinal/iliohypogastric nerve block for postoperative analgesia following inguinal herniorrhaphy in children. *Anesthesiology* 1990; 72(4):637-39.
2. Goldstein M: Surgical management of male infertility and other scrotal disorders. In *Campbell's Urology*, 7th edition. WB Saunders Co, Philadelphia: 1998, Vol 2, Ch 44, 1331-78.
3. Herr HW: Surgery of penile and urethral carcinoma. In *Campbell's Urology*, 7th edition. WB Saunders Co, Philadelphia: 1998, Vol 3, Ch 108, 3395-409.
4. Rozanski T, Bloom DA, Colodny A: Surgery of the scrotum and testis in childhood. In *Campbell's Urology*, 7th edition. WB Saunders Co, Philadelphia: 1998, Vol 2, Ch 73, 2193-209.

PENILE OPERATIONS

SURGICAL CONSIDERATIONS

Penectomy is the total or partial resection of the penis for squamous-cell carcinoma of the penile skin. If the tumor can be resected with a safe margin of at least 2 cm, partial penectomy is usually enough. A tourniquet is placed at the base of the penis, which is amputated at least 2 cm proximal to the tumor. The corpora cavernosa are sutured and the tourniquet released, followed by inspection for bleeding. The edges of the urethra are sutured to the ventral skin and the lateral and dorsal skin edges are approximated over the ends of the corpora cavernosa. Often, an inguinal lymph node biopsy follows the penectomy.

Usual preop diagnosis: Squamous-cell carcinoma of the penile skin

Insertion of penile prosthesis is performed for impotence. The prosthesis is inserted into the corpora cavernosa (Fig 9-14) through a penile or suprapubic incision. Penile prostheses are either malleable or inflatable. The latter have a reservoir in the retropubic space and a pump in the scrotum.

Usual preop diagnosis: Impotence

Hypospadias repair is performed primarily on children before the age of 5 years. There are many different procedures described, and each has its own application. The aim of any repair is to advance the urethral meatus from its aberrant position to the tip of the glans penis and, at the same time, correct any curvature. These operations require meticulous and careful dissection; magnifying loupes are commonly used.

Usual preop diagnosis: Hypospadias

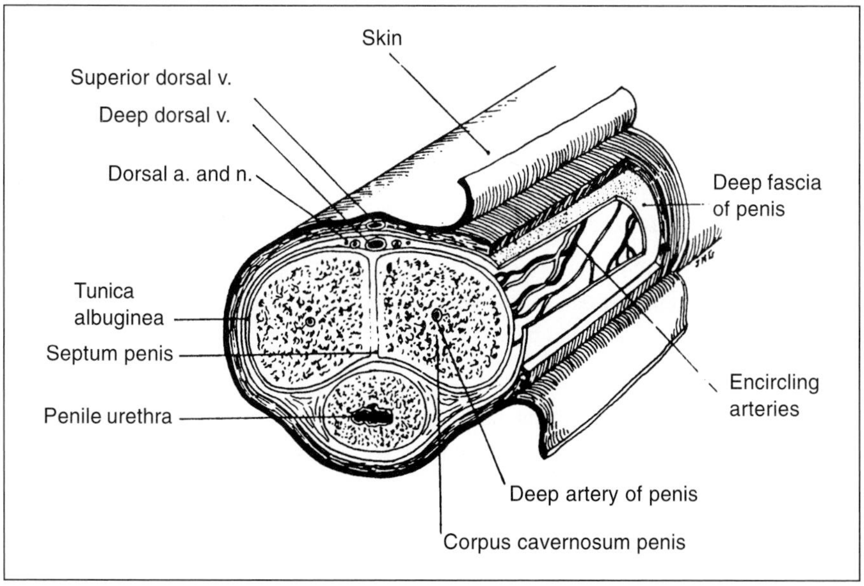

Figure 9-14. Anatomy of the penis. (Reproduced with permission from Hardy JD: *Textbook of Surgery*. JB Lippincott, 1988.)

SUMMARY OF PROCEDURE

	Penectomy	Insertion of Penile Prosthesis	Hypospadias Repair
Position	Supine	⇐	⇐
Incision	Circumferential penile	Bilateral incisions at base of penis	Ventral aspect of penis
Special instrumentation	None	⇐	Magnifying loupes
Unique considerations	None	⇐	Children < 5 yr
Antibiotics	None	Gentamicin 80 mg iv, slowly; ampicillin 2 g iv	None
Surgical time	2 h	⇐	4 h +
Closing considerations	None	⇐	Elaborate pressure dressings
EBL	200 ml	⇐	50 ml
Postop care	PACU → home	⇐	PACU → ward; good sedation
Mortality	< 1%	⇐	⇐
Morbidity	Penile hematoma: 5%	Malfunction: 10%	Urethrocutaneous fistula: 5%
		Edema: 5%	2%
		Infection: 2%	⇐
		Extrusion of the prosthesis: 1%	Hematoma: 2%
Pain score	5	5	5

PATIENT POPULATION CHARACTERISTICS

Age range	Adults	⇐	Children
Incidence	< 1% of all males	1-2% of all males	1:200
Etiology	Poor hygiene	Organic impotence	Congenital

ANESTHETIC CONSIDERATIONS

PREOPERATIVE

Neurological Patients presenting for insertion of a penile prosthesis often have Hx of diabetes or spinal cord injury. Note presence of neuropathy or Hx of autonomic hyperreflexia (AH) (see Anesthetic Considerations for Transurethral Procedures [except TURP], p. 642). Sx suggestive of AH include headache, flushing, nasal stuffiness, HTN associated with voiding or noxious stimuli below the level of transection. It is important to document neurological deficits prior to regional anesthesia.

Hematologic Coagulation defects may be present in patients with priapism. There is a high incidence of priapism in patients with sickle-cell anemia.
Tests: Hct if indicated from H&P.

Laboratory Other tests as indicated from H&P.

Premedication Sedation prn anxiety in adults (e.g., lorazepam 1-2 mg po 1-2 h prior to surgery; midazolam 1-2 mg iv in preop area).

INTRAOPERATIVE

Anesthetic technique: Spinal, caudal, or lumbar epidural and GA are acceptable, with choice dependent on length of procedure, patient age, coexisting disease and patient preference. Sacral anesthesia (saddle block) is sufficient; lumbar epidural anesthesia may be less reliable than spinal or caudal at blocking sacral fibers.

Regional anesthesia:

Spinal 5% lidocaine 50 mg (controversial); 0.75% bupivacaine 10 mg in 7.5% dextrose; hyperbaric tetracaine 10 mg with epinephrine for longer procedures

Caudal 0.5% bupivacaine with epinephrine 5 μg/ml 15-20 ml

Epidural 1.5% lidocaine with epinephrine 5 μg/ml 15-25 ml; supplement with 5-10 ml as needed. Supplemental iv sedation.

General anesthesia:

Induction	Standard induction (see p. B-2). ET intubation may not be necessary for shorter procedures, consider LMA.
Maintenance	Standard maintenance (see p. B-3). Deeper levels of anesthesia are usually required to obtund autonomic reflexes (e.g., HTN, laryngospasm) resulting from intense surgical stimulation that may occur during these procedures.
Emergence	No specific considerations
Blood and fluid requirements	Minimal blood loss IV: 18 ga × 1 NS/LR at 2 ml/kg/h
Monitoring	Standard monitors (see p. B-1).
Complications	AH — See Anesthetic Considerations for Transurethral Procedures, p. 640.

POSTOPERATIVE

Complications	Urinary retention
Pain management	Morphine 0.05-0.1 mg/kg iv or fentanyl 25-50 μg iv prn; ketorolac 30 mg im or iv

References

1. Duckett JW: Hypospadias. In *Campbell's Urology*, 7th edition. WB Saunders Co, Philadelphia: 1998, Vol 2, Ch 68, 2003-2110.
2. Lewis R: Surgery for erectile dysfunction. In *Campbell's Urology*, 7th edition. WB Saunders Co, Philadelphia: 1998, Vol 2, Ch 40, 1215-36.
3. Herr HW: Surgery of penile and urethral carcinoma. In *Campbell's Urology*, 7th edition. WB Saunders Co, Philadelphia: 1998, Vol 3, Ch 108, 3395-3409.

SCROTAL OPERATIONS

SURGICAL CONSIDERATIONS

Description: Scrotal operations are minor, common urologic procedures, performed on an outpatient basis.

Simple orchiectomy is performed as an alternative to medical castration using either estrogens or LH-RH agonists on men with metastatic prostate cancer for androgen ablation. It is always bilateral. A small scrotal incision is made and the testis delivered. The spermatic cord is cross-clamped, transected and suture-ligated.

Usual preop diagnosis: Metastatic prostate cancer

Vasovasostomy is the reestablishment of the continuity of the vas deferens and fertility following a previously performed vasectomy. Through a small scrotal incision, the testis and spermatic cord are delivered. The site of previous vasectomy is identified and excised and the two ends of the vas deferens anastomosed. It is bilateral and requires the use of either the operating microscope or magnifying loupes.

Usual preop diagnosis: Infertility 2° vasectomy

Hydrocelectomy: The testis, with the surrounding hydrocele (Fig 9-15), is delivered through a scrotal incision. The wall of the hydrocele is excised and the edges sutured around the epididymis to prevent recurrence.

Variant procedure or approach: Aspiration used as a temporizing approach since recurrence is almost 100%.

Usual preop diagnosis: Hydrocele

Spermatocelectomy: A spermatocele is a cyst of the epididymis, which is usually excised with that part of the epididymis from which it arises.

Variant procedure: Aspiration as a temporizing maneuver until the operation can be performed.

Usual preop diagnosis: Spermatocele or epididymal cyst

Insertion of testicular prosthesis: A small incision is made in the scrotal skin and a pouch is created by blunt dissection in dartos fascia. The prosthesis is placed in the pouch and fixed to the dartos fascia to prevent prosthesis migration.

Usual preop diagnosis: Absent testis, either congenitally or following orchiectomy

Reduction of testicular torsion is an emergency operation which must be performed within 6 hours of occurrence in order to prevent irreversible ischemic damage to the testis. Through a small scrotal incision, the testis is reduced and fixed to the dartos fascia to prevent retorsion.

Usual preop diagnosis: Acute testicular torsion

SUMMARY OF PROCEDURE

Position	Supine
Incision	Scrotal (Fig 9-15, inset)
Special instrumentation	Operating microscope; magnifying loupe for vasovasostomy
Antibiotics	None
Surgical time	1 h
EBL	Negligible
Postop care	PACU → home
Mortality	< 1%
Morbidity	Scrotal hematoma: 2% Wound infection: 2%
Pain score	4

PATIENT POPULATION CHARACTERISTICS

Age range	All ages
Incidence	Common
Etiology	See preop diagnosis for each procedure, above.

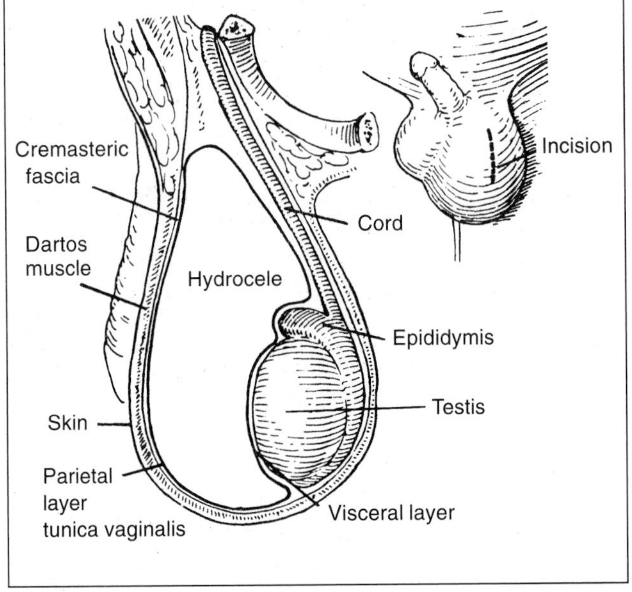

Figure 9-15. Scrotal hydrocele; scrotal incision. (Reproduced with permission from Zollinger RM, Zollinger RM Jr: *Atlas of Surgical Operations*. MacMillan Pub Co: 1983.)

ANESTHETIC CONSIDERATIONS

PREOPERATIVE

Patients presenting for scrotal operations typically fall into two groups: young, otherwise healthy patients and an older population who may present with metastatic prostate cancer accompanied by other medical conditions. The latter group is the focus of the preop evaluation.

Respiratory	Note Hx of pulmonary disease in elderly patients presenting for orchiectomy. **Tests:** As indicated from H&P.
Cardiovascular	Note Hx of cardiac disease in elderly patients presenting for orchiectomy. **Tests:** Consider ECG; others, if indicated from H&P.
Neurological	Document neurological exam prior to regional anesthetic in patients with metastatic prostate carcinoma (spinal-cord or nerve-root compression may be present preop).
Musculoskeletal	Note presence of spinal metastases if orchiectomy is done for palliation of prostate carcinoma. Extensive lumbar metastases may preclude the use of spinal or epidural anesthesia (relative contraindication). **Tests**: L-spine films if Hx suggestive of spinal metastases.

Laboratory	Other tests as indicated from H&P.
Premedication	Sedation prn anxiety (e.g., lorazepam 1-2 mg po 1-2 h prior to surgery; midazolam 1-2 mg iv in preop area).

INTRAOPERATIVE

Anesthetic technique: Local anesthesia (with sedation) is acceptable for simpler operations (vasectomy, orchiectomy). Procedures which are longer or more complex may require spinal, epidural or GA. A sensory level of T10 is required to block pain 2° testicular manipulation. For children undergoing orchiopexy, GA, with or without supplemental caudal blockade, is preferred. Many of these procedures are done on an outpatient basis, and the anesthetic should be appropriately planned.

Regional anesthesia:

Spinal	0.75% bupivacaine 10-12 mg in 7.5% dextrose (1.6 ml); 5% lidocaine 75-100 mg (in dextrose) (controversial) for shorter procedures.
Epidural	1.5-2.0% lidocaine with epinephrine 5 μg/ml, 15-20 ml; supplement with 5-10 ml as needed. Supplemental iv sedation with local or regional techniques (e.g., midazolam 1-2 mg, fentanyl 25-50 μg iv prn anxiety or discomfort).

General anesthesia:

Induction	Standard induction (see p. B-2). Consider use of LMA.	
Maintenance	Standard maintenance (see p. B-3). Muscle relaxation usually not imperative. Deeper levels of anesthesia are usually required to obtund autonomic reflexes (e.g., HTN, laryngospasm) resulting from intense surgical stimulation that may occur during these procedures.	
Emergence	No specific considerations	
Blood and fluid requirements	Minimal blood loss IV: 18 ga × 1 NS/LR @ 2 ml/kg/h	
Monitoring	Standard monitors (see p. B-1).	
Positioning	✓ and pad pressure points. ✓ eyes.	★ **NB**: peroneal nerve compression at lateral fibular head → foot drop.

POSTOPERATIVE

Complications	Peroneal nerve injury 2° lithotomy position	Peroneal nerve injury manifested by foot drop and loss of sensation on dorsum of foot. Seek neurology consultation.
Pain management	Ketorolac 30 mg im or iv in adults ± Morphine 2-4 mg iv or fentanyl 25-50 μg iv prn.	Following orchiopexy, high incidence of postop pain, N/V, which may be reduced by ilioinguinal/iliohypogastric nerve blocks.

References

1. Hannallah RS, Broadman LM, Belman AB, et al: Comparison of caudal and ilioinguinal/iliohypogastric nerve blocks for control of post-orchiopexy pain in pediatric ambulatory surgery. *Anesthesiology* 1987; 66(6):832-34.
2. Rozanski T, Bloom DA, Colodny A: Surgery of the scrotum and testis in childhood. In *Campbell's Urology*, 7th edition. WB Saunders Co, Philadelphia: 1998, Vol 2, Ch 73, 2193-209.

PERINEAL OPERATIONS

SURGICAL CONSIDERATIONS

Urethroplasty: Urethral strictures that do not respond to transurethral dilation and incision are corrected with urethroplasty. A transverse, or longitudinal perineal incision is made and carried down to the urethra, which is dissected free from surrounding tissues. The strictured area is excised and end-to-end anastomosis is performed over a catheter. Repair of a long urethral stricture may require placement of a patch from the scrotum, foreskin or buccal mucosa.

Variant procedure: Transurethral incision and dilation, which is associated with a 30-50% recurrence rate.

Usual preop diagnosis: Urethral stricture, usually posttraumatic

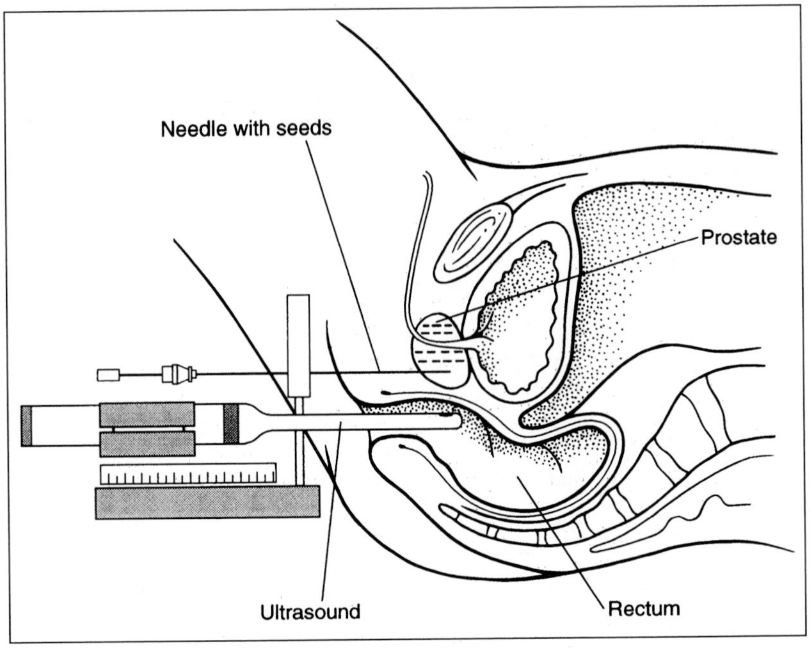

Figure 9-16. Transperineal brachytherapy of prostate gland.

Urethrectomy: Partial or total urethrectomy is done through a longitudinal perineal incision. The urethra is dissected free of surrounding tissues and followed proximally and distally from the membranous urethra to the external urethral meatus. In total urethrectomy, a tubularized skin graft is interposed between membranous urethra and perineal skin.

Usual preop diagnosis: Urethral carcinoma

Insertion of artificial urinary sphincter is performed for incontinence. The operation consists of a perineal incision, through which a cuff is inserted around the bulbar urethra. A suprapubic incision is made to place the reservoir and pump, which inflates and deflates the cuff.

Usual preop diagnosis: Urinary incontinence

Transperineal prostate seed implantation (brachytherapy): High doses of radiation can be delivered to the prostate by implanting radioactive seeds directly into the prostate gland. Using a transrectal ultrasound probe, radioactive seeds (iodine 125 or palladium 103) are implanted into the prostate (Fig 9-16). The patient is placed in lithotomy position, and a rectal ultrasound probe, with a perineal grid attached, is introduced to image the prostate. Radioactive seeds are then placed transperineally using preloaded needles. Preop dosing calculations determine the number and location of the seeds. This procedure is done by a combined team of radiation oncologists and urologists. No special radiation precautions are necessary for the OR team.

Usual preop diagnosis: Prostate cancer

SUMMARY OF PROCEDURE

	Urethroplasty	Urethrectomy	Insertion of Sphincter	Brachytherapy
Position	Lithotomy	⇐	⇐	⇐
Incision	Perineal (Fig 9-4)	⇐	⇐ and scrotal (Fig. 9-15, inset)	None
Antibiotics	Gentamicin 80 mg im/iv	⇐	⇐	⇐
Surgical time	3 h	2 h	3 h	2 h
EBL	100 ml	300 ml	Minimal	⇐
Postop care	PACU → room	⇐	⇐	PACU, outpatient
Mortality	< 1%	⇐	⇐	⇐

	Urethroplasty	Urethrectomy	Insertion of Sphincter	Brachytherapy
Morbidity	Wound infection: 2%	⇐	⇐ Erosion of the urethra: 10% Extrusion of sphincter: 2%	Urinary retention
Pain score	3	3	4	3

PATIENT POPULATION CHARACTERISTICS

Age range	All ages	Adults	Older Adults	50-80 yr
Incidence	< 1% of urologic procedures	⇐	2% of radical prostatectomy	10% of prostate cancer
Etiology	Traumatic strictures	Unknown	Radical prostatectomy (2%); incontinence	Aging

---

ANESTHETIC CONSIDERATIONS

PREOPERATIVE

This is a generally healthy patient population; preop considerations should be based on H&P.

Laboratory Tests as indicated from H&P.

Premedication Sedation prn anxiety in adults (e.g., lorazepam 1-2 mg po 1-2 h prior to surgery; midazolam 1-2 mg iv in preop area).

INTRAOPERATIVE

Anesthetic technique: Spinal or GA are acceptable, with choice dependent on length of procedure, position, patient age, coexisting disease and patient preference. A sacral sensory level (saddle block) is usually sufficient. Lumbar epidural anesthesia may be less reliable at providing sacral anesthesia, and offers no advantages over the above techniques for shorter procedures, although caudal anesthesia may be an acceptable alternative.

Regional anesthesia:

Spinal 0.75% bupivacaine 10 mg in 7.5% dextrose; hyperbaric tetracaine 10 mg (with epinephrine [200 μg] for longer procedures)

Caudal 0.5% bupivacaine with epinephrine 5 μg/ml 15-20 ml. Supplemental iv sedation.

General anesthesia:

Induction Standard induction (see p. B-2). Consider use of LMA.

Maintenance Standard maintenance (see p. B-3); muscle relaxation usually not required. Deeper levels of anesthesia are usually required to obtund autonomic reflexes (e.g., HTN, laryngospasm) resulting from intense surgical stimulation that may occur during these procedures.

Emergence No specific considerations

Blood and fluid requirements Minimal blood loss
IV: 18 ga × 1
NS/LR at 2 ml/kg/h

Monitoring Standard monitors (see p. B-1).

Positioning ✓ and pad pressure points.
✓ eyes.

★ Patients with arthritis or other musculoskeletal disorders may not tolerate the exaggerated lithotomy position, thus precluding the use of a regional technique. **NB**: In lithotomy position, peroneal nerve compression at lateral fibular head → foot drop.

Complications Anticipate hypotension on return from lithotomy position.

Rx: volume (200-500 ml NS/LR) or ephedrine (5 mg iv) may be necessary.

POSTOPERATIVE

Complications	Peroneal nerve injury 2° lithotomy position	Peroneal nerve injury manifested as foot drop with loss of sensation over dorsum of foot. Seek neurology consultation.
Pain management	Mild-to-moderate pain	Rx: morphine 0.05-0.1 mg/kg iv prn

References

1. Duckett JW: Hypospadias. In *Campbell's Urology*, 7th edition. WB Saunders Co, Philadelphia: 1998, Vol 2, Ch 68, 2093-2119.
2. Lewis R: Penile prosthesis. In *Campbell's Urology*, 7th edition. WB Saunders Co, Philadelphia: 1998, Vol 2, Ch 4068, 1216-26.
3. Lynch DF, Schellhammer PF: Tumors of the penis. In *Campbell's Urology*, 7th edition. WB Saunders Co, Philadelphia: 1998, Vol 3, Ch 79, 2453-86.

VAGINAL OPERATIONS

SURGICAL CONSIDERATIONS

Description: Vaginal operations are performed by both urologists and gynecologists. They include the following:

Repair of vesicovaginal fistulas: The vaginal approach is usually recommended for small and distally located vesicovaginal fistulas; otherwise, a transabdominal repair is performed (see Open Bladder Operations, p. 656). An incision is made in the anterior vaginal wall around the fistula, which is excised. Bladder and vaginal walls are separated and closed with interposition of tissues or flaps to separate the incisions and prevent recurrence. A Foley catheter is left indwelling. **Variant approach:** Transabdominal repair of vesicovaginal fistula (see Open Bladder Operations, p. 656).

Usual preop diagnosis: Vesicovaginal fistula

Operations to correct stress urinary incontinence: Many procedures have been designed to correct female urinary incontinence. They fall into two basic groups: (1) operations to correct hypermobility of the urethra, and (2) operations to correct nonfunctioning urethra. The operation most commonly used by urologists to correct hypermobility is the **Stamey procedure** (Fig 9-17), or endoscopic **vesical neck suspension.** The operation is performed through two small suprapubic incisions, one on each side of the midline, and an anterior vaginal incision. A nylon suture is placed in a loop from either side of the bladder neck and not around it. Cystoscopy is done to ensure proper placement and to prevent the suture from transversing the bladder. When the sutures are pulled up and tied over the anterior rectus sheath, they pull the bladder neck up to its original position behind the symphysis pubis and restore the acute posterior ureterovesical angle. A variant of this procedure is the **Raz bladder neck suspension,** where bolsters are not used.

Operations to correct a nonfunctioning urethra include submucosal collagen injection at the bladder neck or construction of a **sling.** Rectus fascia, fascia lata of the thigh or the vaginal wall can be used to construct a sling around the urethra. All these techniques involve a combined suprapubic and vaginal approach.

Variant approach: The **Marshall-Marchetti-Krantz operation**, which is performed retropubically, sutures the anterior portion of the urethra, bladder neck and bladder to the pubic bone.

Usual preop diagnosis: Urinary stress incontinence

Excision of urethral diverticulum: Urethral diverticula are extremely rare and need excision only if they are the cause of recurrent urinary tract infections. An incision is made in the anterior vaginal wall over the urethral diverticulum, which is dissected all around until it is attached only by its neck. It is excised and the neck closed. A Foley catheter is left indwelling, and the vaginal incision is closed.

Usual preop diagnosis: Recurrent urinary tract infections 2° infected urethral diverticulum

Repair of cystocele and rectocele: Some patients with urinary incontinence also present with prolapse of the bladder or rectum into the vagina. These can be repaired at the same time as incontinence surgery. A vaginal incision (anterior for cystocele, posterior for rectocele) is made and dissected laterally to free the bladder or rectum from the vagina. The defect is repaired and the redundant vaginal wall excised.

Usual preop diagnosis: Incontinence with pelvic prolapse, cystocele or rectocele

SUMMARY OF PROCEDURE

	Repair of Vesicovaginal Fistula	Correction of Stress Incontinence	Excision of Urethral Diverticulum
Position	Lithotomy	⇐	⇐
Incision	Anterior vaginal	Anterior vaginal; suprapubic	Anterior vaginal
Special instrumentation	None	Cystoscope	None
Antibiotics	Gentamicin 80 mg iv, slowly	⇐	⇐
Surgical time	2 h	1 h	⇐
EBL	200 ml	500 ml	200 ml
Postop care	PACU → room	⇐	⇐
Mortality	< 1%	⇐	⇐
Morbidity	Infection: 2%	⇐	⇐
	Recurrence: 2%	10%	⇐
Pain score	3	5	3

PATIENT POPULATION CHARACTERISTICS

Age range	20-80 yr	⇐	⇐
Incidence	< 1% of urologic procedures	5% of urologic procedures	< 1% of urologic procedures
Etiology	Traumatic delivery; iatrogenic following hysterectomy (< 1%)	Childbirth	Congenital (extremely rare)

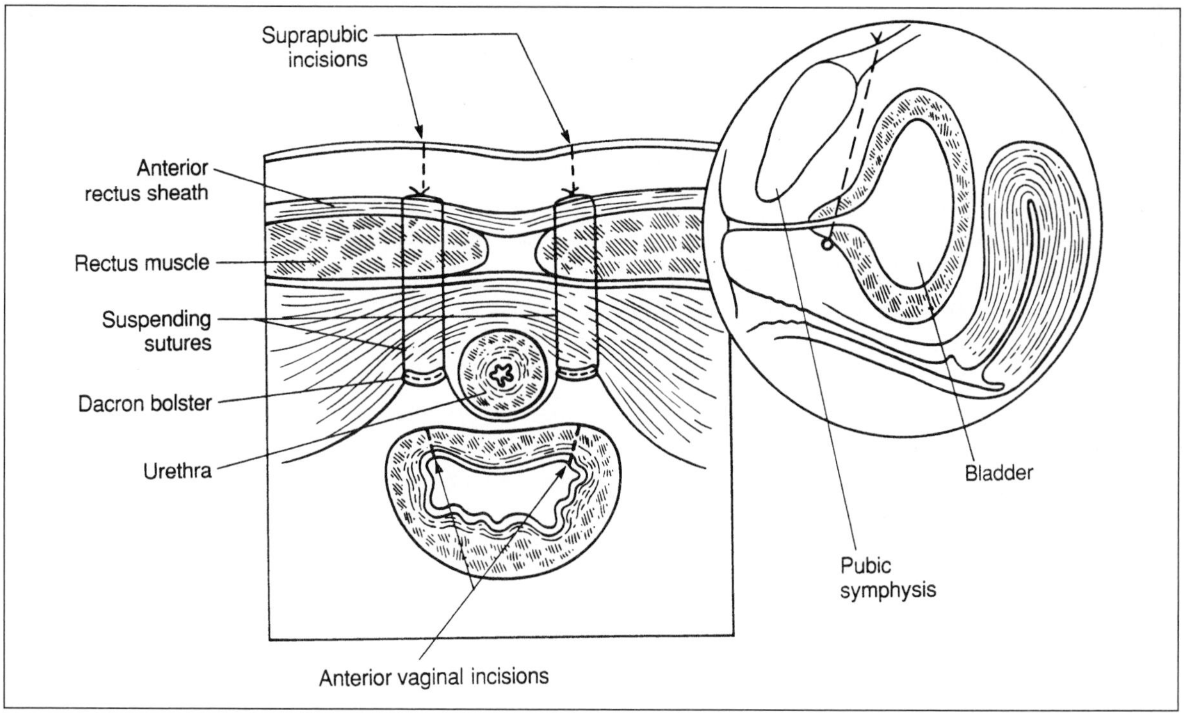

Figure 9-17. Stamey procedure, sectional view; inset shows lateral view.

ANESTHETIC CONSIDERATIONS

PREOPERATIVE

This is a generally healthy patient population. Preop considerations should be based on H&P.

Laboratory	Tests as indicated from H&P.
Premedication	Standard premedication (see p. B-2).

INTRAOPERATIVE

Anesthetic technique: Spinal, continuous lumbar epidural, or GA are acceptable, with choice dependent on age, coexisting disease and patient preference. A block level of T9-T10 is recommended for operations involving the bladder, whereas somewhat higher levels of anesthesia may be necessary if a suprapubic incision is made. Epidural anesthesia may be less reliable than spinal at providing sacral anesthesia.

Regional anesthesia:

Spinal	0.75% bupivacaine 10-12 mg (1.6 ml)	
Epidural	2% lidocaine with epinephrine 5 μg/ml, 15-20 ml. Supplemental iv sedation.	

General anesthesia:

Induction	Standard induction (see p. B-2).	
Maintenance	Standard maintenance (see p. B-3). Muscle relaxation not imperative.	
Emergence	No specific considerations	
Blood and fluid requirements	Minimal blood loss IV: 18 ga × 1 NS/LR @ 2-4 ml/kg/h	
Monitoring	Standard monitors (see p. B-1).	
Positioning	✓ and pad pressure points. ✓ eyes.	★ **NB**: In lithotomy position, peroneal nerve compression at lateral fibular head → foot drop.
Complications	Anticipate hypotension when returning from lithotomy. Bladder perforation	Rx: volume (200-500 ml NS/LR) or ephedrine (5 mg iv) may be necessary. Bladder perforation may present as shoulder pain in the awake patient, but may go unnoticed in the patient under GA. Sx include unexplained HTN, tachycardia, hypotension (rare).

POSTOPERATIVE

Complications	Peroneal nerve injury 2° lithotomy position Bladder perforation (see above).	Peroneal nerve injury is manifested as foot drop with loss of sensation on dorsum of foot. Seek neurology consultation.
Pain management	Consider ketorolac 30 mg iv/im in adults; supplement with morphine 0.05-0.1 mg/kg iv prn.	

References

1. Leach GE, Trockman BA: Surgery for vesicovaginal and urethrovaginal fistula and urethral diverticulum. In *Campbell's Urology*, 7th edition. WB Saunders Co, Philadelphia: 1998, Vol 1 Ch 37, 1135-54.
2. Raz S, Stothers L, Chopra A: Vaginal reconstructive surgery for incontinence and prolapse. In *Campbell's Urology*, 7th edition. WB Saunders Co, Philadelphia: 1998, Vol 1 Ch 32, 1059-94.

10.0 ORTHOPEDIC SURGERY

Surgeons

Gordon A. Brody, MD
Amy L. Ladd, MD (*Epidermolysis bullosa*)

10.1 HAND SURGERY

Anesthesiologists

Talmage D. Egan, MD
Jeffrey D. Swenson, MD
Yuan-Chi Lin, MD, MPH (*Epidermolysis bullosa*)

DARRACH PROCEDURE

SURGICAL CONSIDERATIONS

Description: The Darrach procedure is a resection of the distal ulna. The distal 2 cm of the ulna is resected subperiosteally, and local soft tissues are used to stabilize and cover the remaining ulna. It is commonly performed in patients who have had a disruption of the distal radioulnar joint with subluxation of the ulna. It is also indicated for patients who have had a malunion of a distal radius fracture such that the radius has shortened relative to the ulna or is abnormally angulated, resulting in dorsal subluxation of the ulna and impingement of the ulnar head upon the carpus. This causes painful motion of the wrist and forearm and posttraumatic degenerative arthritis of the ulnar head, carpus and sigmoid notch of the distal radius. Disorders of the distal radioulnar joint and degeneration of the ulnar head, which may lead to attrition rupture of the overlying extensor tendons, are common in rheumatoid arthritis. This dorsal prominence of the ulnar head is treated by **Darrach resection**, combined with a soft-tissue procedure to stabilize the remaining ulna. Osteoarthritic degeneration of the distal radioulnar joint, either 2° trauma (see above) or due to idiopathic osteoarthritis, responds well to this procedure.

Variant procedure or approaches: Modifications of the Darrach procedure, such as the **hemiresection interposition technique of Bowers**, are performed for the same indications as above.

Usual preop diagnosis: Arthritis or derangement of the distal radioulnar joint; rheumatoid arthritis; ulnar impingement syndrome; malunion of Colles' fracture or other fracture of the distal radius

SUMMARY OF PROCEDURE

Position	Supine, with arm extended on hand-surgery table
Incision	Dorsal-ulnar, over distal ulna
Special instrumentation	Pneumatic tourniquet
Antibiotics	Cefazolin 1 g iv
Surgical time	1-2.5 h, depending on associated procedures
Tourniquet	150 mmHg above systolic; max time = 120 min
Closing considerations	Routine skin closure; postop splint placed at conclusion of procedure.
EBL	Minimal; performed under tourniquet control.
Postop care	Elevation to minimize swelling. PACU → home, or overnight stay in observation bed.
Mortality	Minimal
Morbidity	Ulnar nerve injury
	Postop swelling
Pain score	5-7

PATIENT POPULATION CHARACTERISTICS

Age range	Late teens–elderly
Male:Female	Slight predominance of females, due to incidence of malunion of Colles' fractures in women with senile osteoporosis.
Incidence	Not uncommon
Etiology	See Usual Preop Diagnosis, above.
Associated conditions	Rheumatoid arthritis

ANESTHETIC CONSIDERATIONS

See Anesthetic Considerations for Wrist Procedures, p. 683.

Reference

1. Dingman PVC: Resection of the distal end of the ulna. *J Bone Joint Surg* [Am] 1952; 34:893-900.

SURGERY FOR EPIDERMOLYSIS BULLOSA

SURGICAL CONSIDERATIONS

Description: Epidermolysis bullosa (EB) is a disabling inherited condition affecting the skin and submucosa. Recessive dystrophic EB is the most common type requiring surgical treatment. Children develop lesions associated with minimal trauma, which most commonly result in contractures of the hands and feet, mouth and esophagus. Special care is required in handling patients with epidermolysis bullosa, since minor trauma from iv or ECG lead placement can cause severe blistering. Hand surgery typically involves opening up the contracted fingers by removing the cocoon of epidermis. The defects are grafted with full-thickness skin grafts, typically taken from the abdomen. Following sedation or anesthesia, the affected extremity is gently sponged with dilute chlorhexidine solution. A tourniquet is not applied since it is typically not required. A wrist block is administered by the surgeon. The cocoon of scar tissue is removed, the fingers manipulated to expose the defects, and a full-thickness skin graft is harvested. Generous Bactroban ointment and nonadhesive dressings are placed on the hand and a well padded cast is applied at the end of the procedure.

Usual preop diagnosis: EB

SUMMARY OF PROCEDURE

Position	Supine
Incision	As necessary to relieve skin contractures on the hands
Antibiotics	Cefazolin 20-40 mg/kg iv
Surgical time	1-2 h. Positioning, iv placement and sedation/anesthesia are time-consuming, often longer than the procedure itself.
EBL	< 100 ml
Postop care	PACU → home. Return in 2 wk for intraop removal of cast, dressing change and first splint application. Splinting and special gloves are the mainstay of postop treatment.
Mortality	Not associated with procedure
Morbidity	Trauma from positioning and monitoring → new blisters
Pain score	7-9 (similar to 2nd-degree burns)

PATIENT POPULATION CHARACTERISTICS

Age range	1-20 yr; older patients with precancerous or cancerous hand lesions
Male:Female	2-3:1
Incidence	Extremely rare
Etiology	Inherited
Associated conditions	Malnutrition; esophageal strictures; generalized skin contractures

ANESTHETIC CONSIDERATIONS

PREOPERATIVE

EB is a heterogenous group of rare hereditary disorders characterized by blister formation in the skin in response to minor trauma, friction or pressure. The most minor form of EB is EB simplex, in which the blisters heal without scarring. The junctional form is often diagnosed at birth, with blisters caused by the physical trauma of delivery. These patients develop severe scarring and have a short life expectancy. Patients with the recessive dystrophic form may have strictures of the oropharynx, larynx and esophagus. Patients with EB present considerable problems for anesthesiologists.

Airway — A careful airway evaluation is essential, since these patients may have a difficult airway 2° mucous membrane and skin involvement in the area of the oropharynx, face and neck. Patients with EB also may have limited mouth opening and neck movement as the result of scarring and contractures.

Skin — Because of the fragility of skin and mucous membranes in patients with EB, the anesthetic plan should be designed to prevent even the slightest trauma to skin and mucous membranes.

Gastrointestinal — The most common sites of involvement are the oropharynx, esophagus and anus. Dysphagia, esophageal stricture and constipation are common, and are the major causes of morbidity, nutritional deficiencies and growth retardation. Esophageal dilatation, insertion of NG feeding tubes,

Gastrointestinal, cont. gastrostomy and colonic interposition have been performed in patients with EB.[3,14] Esophageal stricture increases the risk of regurgitation and aspiration and precautions to avoid aspiration should be taken (e.g., Na citrate, ranitidine, metoclopramide).

Musculoskeletal Skin lesions can be painful, and some patients will be on chronic opiate medication for pain management.

Hematologic Chronic blood loss from denuded skin can result in anemia and hypoalbuminemia.
Tests: CBC; electrolytes; albumin; coags

Laboratory Other tests as indicated from H&P.

Premedication Adequate premedication is essential to minimize movement during induction. An orally administered combination of midazolam (0.5 mg/kg) and ketamine (3 mg/kg) facilitates the atraumatic placement of iv lines in the OR.

INTRAOPERATIVE

Patients are placed on sheepskin to cushion pressure points. The following should be available: Albolene liquefying cleanser, Surg-O-Flex (flexible tubular bandage), Vaseline gauze, Zeroform, Kerlix, Webril, cotton umbilical tape and Coban wrap. No adhesive tape is used. Adhesive portions of ECG leads and electrocautery dispersion plates are removed; the leads and plates are secured to patients, using Webril or Surg-O-Flex. BP cuffs are applied over multiple layers of cotton padding. Carefully trim the adhesive off the pulse oximetry probe, wrap around the palm or finger, and wrap Coban around the probe. Alternatively, use adult clip-on probe. Anesthesia masks, ETTs, temperature probes and all attached monitoring equipment are lubricated with Albolene. Venipuncture can be difficult, and the iv lines are secured with Vaseline gauze and Coban.

Anesthetic technique: GETA is the preferred method of anesthesia when upper airway manipulation is required or airway protection is compromised. James, et al, reported 309 anesthetics performed on 73 patients with recessive dystrophic EB without the occurrence of laryngeal bullae, postop stridor or "airway embarrassment."[8] The safety of GETA, however, is not well documented in junctional EB patients where columnar epithelium can be involved.[7]

IV anesthesia: Ketamine has been utilized for patients with EB undergoing surgical procedures.[6,13] For iv anesthesia, use a loading dose of midazolam 0.1-0.2 mg/kg with ketamine 0.25-0.5 mg/kg, followed by a continuous infusion of ketamine (1 mg/kg/h) and midazolam (0.1 mg/kg/h). Glycopyrrolate can be used as an antisialagogue in these patients. Alternatively, propofol (50-100 μg/kg/h) with remifentanil (0.05-0.1 μg/kg/h) infusions may be used. Titrate both medications according to patient's response to the surgical stimulation.

Local anesthesia: At our institution, local anesthetic infiltration has not been associated with any serious sequelae; however, Kubota, et al, have recommended against the use of local anesthetic infiltration.[11]

Regional Anesthesia: In some patients with EB, regional anesthesia techniques allow maintenance of airway patency, involve minimal epidermal/dermal damage, and can offer prolonged postop pain relief. Brachial plexus anesthesia,[9,10] epidural anesthesia,[1,15,16] and spinal anesthesia[1,4,15] have been used successfully in patients with EB.

Emergence Adequate postop analgesia and parental presence in the PACU may help prevent excessive struggling and skin trauma during emergence and recovery. Acetaminophen, ketorolac and opiates can be used for postop analgesia. Pruritus, a common side effect of opiates, should be treated promptly.[5,17]

References

1. Broster T, Placek R, Eggers G: Epidermolysis bullosa: anesthetic management for cesarean section. *Anesth Analg* 1987; 66:341-3.
2. Campiglio GL, Pajardi G, Rafanelli G: A new protocol for the treatment of hand deformities and recessive dystrophic epidermolysis bullosa (13 cases). *Ann Chir Main Memb Super* 1997; 16(2): 91-100, discussion 101.
3. Ergun G, Lin A, Dannenberg A, Carter D: Gastrointestinal manifestations of epidermolysis bullosa: a study of 101 patients. *Medicine* 1992; 71(3):121-7.
4. Farber N, Troshynski T, Turco G: Spinal anesthesia in an infant with epidermolysis bullosa. *Anesthesiology* 1995; 83:1364-67.
5. Griffin R, Mayou B: The anesthetic management of patients with dystrophic epidermolysis bullosa. *Anaesthesia* 1993; 48:810-15.
6. Hamann R, Cohen P: Anesthetic management of a patient with epidermolysis bullosa dystrophica. *Anesthesiology* 1971; 34(4): 389-91.
7. Holzman R, Worthen H, Johnson K: Anaesthesia for children with junctional epidermolysis bullosa (letalis). *Can J Anaesth* 1987 34(4):395-99.
8. James I, Wark H: Airway management during anesthesia in patients with epidermolysis bullosa dystrophica. *Anesthesiology* 1982; 56(4):323-6.

9. Kaplan R, Straugh B: Regional anesthesia in a child with epidermolysis bullosa. *Anesthesiology* 1987; 67(2):262-4.
10. Kelly R, Koff H, Rothaus K, Karter D, Artosio J: Brachial plexus anesthesia in eight patients with recessive dystrophic epidermolysis bullosa. *Anesth Analg* 1987; 66:1318-20.
11. Kubota Y, Norton M, Goldenberg S, Robertazzi R: Anesthetic management of patients with epidermolysis bullosa undergoing surgery. *Anesth Analg* 1961; 40(2):244-50.
12. Ladd AL, Kibele A, Gibbons S: Surgical treatment and postoperative splinting of recessive dystrophic epidermolysis bullosa. *J Hand Surg(Am)* 1996; 21(5):888-97.
13. Lee C, Nagel E: Anesthetic management of a patient with recessive epidermolysis dystrophica. *Anesthesiology* 1975; 43(1):122-4.
14. Miline B, Rosales J: Anaesthesia for correction of oesophageal stricture in a patient with recessive epidermolysis bullosa dystrophica: case report. *Can Anaesth Soc J* 1980; 27(2):169-71.
15. Spielman F, Mann E: Subarachnoid and epidural anaesthesia for patients with epidermolysis bullosa. *Can Anaesth Soc J* 1984; 31(5)549-51.
16. Yee C, Gunter J, Manley C: Caudal epidural anesthesia in an infant with epidermolysis bullosa. Anesthesiology 1989; 70:149-51.
17. Yonker-Sell A, Connolly L: Twelve-hour anaesthesia in a patient with epidermolysis bullosa. *Can J Anaesth* 1995; 42(8):735-9.

DORSAL STABILIZATION AND EXTENSOR SYNOVECTOMY OF THE RHEUMATOID WRIST

SURGICAL CONSIDERATIONS

Description: This procedure is indicated for patients with rheumatoid arthritis and extensor tenosynovitis refractory to medical treatment, as well as extensor tendon ruptures and/or intercarpal synovitis. The procedure is performed under tourniquet control through a straight dorsal incision over the wrist. A **radical tenosynovectomy** of the extensor tendons in all six extensor compartments is carried out. Tendon ruptures or impending ruptures are repaired with tendon grafts or side-to-side anastomoses. Bone spurs are removed and a synovectomy of the distal radioulnar joint is carried out. A **modified Darrach procedure**, with resection or osteoplasty of the distal ulna, is usually performed. If there is evidence of synovitis within the wrist joint, a synovectomy is performed through a dorsal arthrotomy. A flap of the extensor retinaculum is transposed beneath the extensor tendons to reinforce the dorsal wrist ligaments and, thus, stabilize the wrist to prevent volar subluxation of the carpus. A posterior interosseous neurectomy is carried out at the same time. The remaining extensor retinaculum is divided into two transverse strips and one is used to stabilize the distal ulna. The second strip is placed dorsal to the extensor tendons so they will not bowstring during wrist extension.

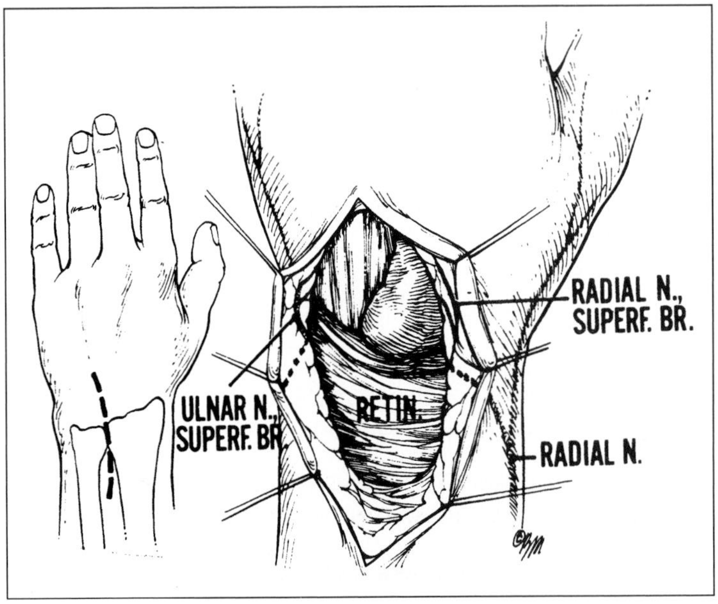

Figure 10.1-1. Incision and exposure for dorsal tenosynovectomy. Note superficial branches of radial and ulnar nerves protected in skin flaps. (Illustration by Elizabeth Roselius, © 1988. Reproduced with permission from Green DP: *Operative Hand Surgery*, 2nd edition. Churchill Livingstone: 1988.)

Usual preop diagnosis: Rheumatoid arthritis with extensor tendon tenosynovitis; extensor tendon rupture; distal radioulnar joint synovitis and/or subluxation

SUMMARY OF PROCEDURE

Position	Supine, with arm extended on hand-surgery table
Incision	Dorsal wrist (Fig 10.1-1)
Special instrumentation	Pneumatic tourniquet
Antibiotics	Cefazolin 1 g iv
Surgical time	2 h
Tourniquet	150 mmHg above systolic; max time = 120 min
Closing considerations	Postop splint
EBL	Minimal; tourniquet used until dressing in place.
Postop care	Admitted overnight for pain control and limb elevation.
Mortality	Minimal
Morbidity	Extremity swelling Delayed healing 2° immunosuppression and steroid use Wound infection
Pain score	3-5

PATIENT POPULATION CHARACTERISTICS

Age range	Procedure uncommon before 4th decade
Male:Female	As in all patients with rheumatoid arthritis, females more common.
Incidence	Not uncommon
Etiology	Connective tissue disorder; rheumatoid arthritis or variant
Associated conditions	All conditions associated with connective tissue disorders, including active rheumatoid arthritis, steroid dependency, immunosuppressive therapy and/or skin fragility

ANESTHETIC CONSIDERATIONS

See Anesthetic Considerations for Wrist Procedures, p. 683.

Reference

1. Millender LH, Nalebuff FA: Preventive surgery—tenosynovectomy and synovectomy. *Orthop Clin North Am* 1975; 6(3):765-92.

METACARPOPHALANGEAL AND INTERPHALANGEAL JOINT ARTHROPLASTY

SURGICAL CONSIDERATIONS

Description: Joint replacement in the hand is most commonly indicated in patients with rheumatoid arthritis with severe joint destruction leading to pain and dysfunction. It is rarely indicated in patients with osteoarthritis. The most common prostheses, made of silicone rubber and popularized by Swanson, differ from total joint replacement in the hip or knee in that they do not function as true joints, but rather as spacers in a **resection arthroplasty**. Most of the stability and motion of these joints depend on meticulous soft-tissue reconstructions involving tendon and ligament transfers, as well as intensive postop physical therapy. To obtain good results, patients must be well motivated and understand their disease process and what will be asked of them during the recovery period. The results for **metacarpophalangeal (MP) arthroplasty** are far better than those obtained in the proximal interphalangeal joints. **Proximal interphalangeal joint arthroplasty** is now indicated only for the central middle and ring digits in patients with good ligamentous and tendinous structures. **Distal interphalangeal (DIP) arthroplasty** is rarely performed, since these patients do well with fusions.

The procedure for the MP joints is performed through a dorsal transverse incision under tourniquet control. The metacarpal heads are removed with an oscillating saw and the intramedullary canals reamed to accept the stems of the prostheses. Once they have been placed with a no-touch technique, the capsule is closed and the supporting ligaments are reconstructed with centralization of extensor tendons. A splint with support for each finger is placed at the conclusion of surgery. Reconstructive procedures of the wrist and fingers can be combined with arthroplasty.

Variant procedure or approaches: Some surgeons favor longitudinal incisions rather than a transverse incision for the approach to the MP joints.

Usual preop diagnosis: Rheumatoid arthritis or other connective-tissue disorder

SUMMARY OF PROCEDURE

Position	Supine, with arm extended on hand-surgery table
Incision	Dorsal hand, transverse or longitudinal
Special instrumentation	MP or PIP joint prostheses and associated instruments for preparing the medullary canal; pneumatic tourniquet
Antibiotics	Cefazolin 1 g iv
Surgical time	2.5 h
Tourniquet	150 mm above systolic; max time = 120 min
Closing considerations	Critical postop splinting
EBL	Minimal; tourniquet used throughout procedure.
Postop care	Admitted to hospital for pain control and limb elevation.
Mortality	Minimal
Morbidity	Swelling Wound infection Prosthesis infection (rare)
Pain score	7

PATIENT POPULATION CHARACTERISTICS

Age range	> 50 yr
Male:Female	As in rheumatoid arthritis, females predominate.
Incidence	Uncommon
Etiology	Rheumatoid arthritis or other connective-tissue disorder
Associated conditions	As in rheumatoid arthritis (e.g., skin fragility, steroid dependency, immunosuppression)

ANESTHETIC CONSIDERATIONS

See Anesthetic Considerations for Wrist Procedures, p. 683.

ARTHRODESIS OF THE WRIST

SURGICAL CONSIDERATIONS

Description: A variety of arthrodeses can be performed about the wrist. These include **radiopancarpal arthrodesis** (total wrist fusion), radiolunate, radioscapholunate and intercarpal arthrodeses (partial wrist fusions). Radiopancarpal is generally performed as a salvage procedure for wrist pathology that cannot be treated with a procedure that preserves wrist motion. These indications include posttraumatic degenerative arthritis following fractures and dislocations, idiopathic osteoarthritis and/or rheumatoid arthritis. In the nonrheumatoid patient, an effective procedure is an arthrodesis using an iliac crest bone graft fixed with plate and screws. More recent techniques with improved plate designs rarely require iliac crest bone graft. Local bone from the distal radius is commonly utilized. Alternative techniques with other forms of fixation are also used. It has been shown that a position of fusion in 10-15° of dorsiflexion provides the greatest grip strength. In the rheumatoid patient, a technique using intramedullary fixation with a large-diameter Steinmann pin is preferred. Rheumatoid bone is osteoporotic, 2° disuse and chronic steroid administration. Screw fixation is not ideal in this soft bone. Bone graft is obtained locally in these patients, usually from the resected ulnar head. **Radiolunate fusion** is also indicated in rheumatoid patients who have progressive ulnar translation of the carpus. The lunate acts to block this translation of the carpus. **Radioscapholunate fusion** is indicated in patients with radiocarpal arthritis. This procedure preserves about 50% of wrist motion which occurs at the midcarpal joint. Bone graft is necessary and is easily obtained from the distal radius through the same incision. There are a variety of **intercarpal arthrodeses**, including **triscaphe** (scaphotrapezialtrapezoid), **scaphocapitate**, **lunotriquetrel** and **four-corner** (capitate-hamate-triquetral-lunate). These procedures are indicated for the treatment of intercarpal arthritis, carpal instabilities due to intercarpal ligament tears and Kienbock's disease. Each procedure requires bone graft, which may be obtained from the distal radius or the iliac crest. The **Cloward cervical spine fusion instrumentation** is useful for obtaining a bicortical plug of bone from the iliac crest with minimal dissection.

Usual preop diagnosis: Posttraumatic arthritis; osteoarthritis or rheumatoid arthritis; Kienbock's disease; carpal instability

SUMMARY OF PROCEDURE

Position	Supine, with arm extended on hand-surgery table. The iliac crest may be prepped and elevated with a sandbag beneath the ipsilateral buttock.
Incision	Dorsal wrist, transverse (for intercarpal fusion) or longitudinal
Special instrumentation	Pneumatic tourniquet
Unique considerations	Bone-graft donor site
Antibiotics	Cefazolin 1 g iv
Surgical time	2 h
Tourniquet	150 mmHg above systolic; max time = 120 min
Closing considerations	Immobilization with splints
EBL	Minimal; procedure is performed under tourniquet control. If iliac crest bone graft is used, there may be up to 500 ml of blood loss.
Postop care	PACU → room for pain and edema control
Mortality	Minimal
Morbidity	Nonunion of fusion ≤ 20%
Pain score	7-9

PATIENT POPULATION CHARACTERISTICS

Age range	> 40 yr
Male:Female	Females predominate in rheumatoid arthritis; males in posttraumatic arthritis.
Incidence	Common
Etiology	Trauma (common); rheumatoid arthritis (common)
Associated conditions	Typical for rheumatoid arthritis (e.g., skin fragility, steroid dependency, immunosuppression)

ANESTHETIC CONSIDERATIONS

See Anesthetic Considerations for Wrist Procedures, p. 683.

Reference

1. Green DP: *Operative Hand Surgery*, 3rd edition. Churchill Livingstone, New York: 1993.

TOTAL WRIST REPLACEMENT

SURGICAL CONSIDERATIONS

Description: The major indication for this procedure is rheumatoid arthritis of the wrist. **Total wrist replacement (TWR)** is often recommended in patients with bilateral wrist disease. An arthrodesis will be carried out on the nondominant helping hand and a TWR on the dominant hand to preserve dexterity. Many surgeons prefer to avoid **bilateral wrist arthrodesis**, although some patients with bilateral fusions have been able to function relatively well. Currently available protheses are suitable only for low-demand patients, and are not indicated for high-demand patients with posttraumatic arthritis. These patients will do better with wrist arthrodesis. Silastic wrist prostheses are associated with a high failure rate and silicone synovitis and their use has been abandoned by many surgeons. The most commonly used prostheses today are metal on ultra-high-molecular-weight polyethylene articulations that are fixed with methylmethacrylate cement or bone ingrowth into porous stems. All of these prostheses depend on intact, normally functioning wrist extensor tendons, especially the extensor carpi radialis brevis, for balance and function. Absence of this tendon is felt by many to be an absolute contraindication to this procedure. Because these tendons are so commonly affected by rheumatoid arthritis, the patient population for this procedure is limited. In addition to functioning tendons, meticulously accurate placement of the components in relation to the centers of rotation of the wrist is critical for success. If the centers of rotation of the prosthesis do not duplicate those of the normal wrist, early component loosening and failure is likely. Intraop radiographs are useful in verifying component position. These patients frequently have other upper extremity deformities which will require reconstruction. Because of the complexity of TWR, other reconstructive procedures are not carried out at the same time.

Usual preop diagnosis: Rheumatoid arthritis

SUMMARY OF PROCEDURE

Position	Supine, with arm extended on hand-surgery table
Incision	Dorsal wrist
Special instrumentation	TWR instrumentation; pneumatic tourniquet
Antibiotics	Cefazolin 1 g iv
Surgical time	2 h
Tourniquet	150 mmHg above systolic; max time = 120 min
Closing considerations	Postop splint
EBL	Minimal; procedure performed under tourniquet control.
Postop care	PACU → room
Mortality	Minimal
Morbidity	Infection
	Poor wound healing
Pain score	4-8

PATIENT POPULATION CHARACTERISTICS

Age range	Rare before 4th decade; most in 6th and 7th decades
Male:Female	Females outnumber males, as in rheumatoid arthritis.
Incidence	Rare
Etiology	Rheumatoid arthritis
Associated conditions	Rheumatoid arthritis

ANESTHETIC CONSIDERATIONS

See Anesthetic Considerations for Wrist Procedures, p. 683.

Reference

1. Green DP: *Operative Hand Surgery*, 3rd edition. Churchill Livingstone, New York: 1993.

THUMB CARPOMETACARPAL JOINT FUSION/ ARTHROPLASTY/STABILIZATION

SURGICAL CONSIDERATIONS

Description: Patients with degenerative arthritis of the carpometacarpal (CMC) joint of the thumb present with subluxation, pain and synovitis of the joint. A **synovectomy and ligament reconstruction** to restore stability will treat pain and prevent further degeneration. This procedure is performed through a curvilinear incision over the joint. A distally attached graft of the radial 1/2 of the flexor carpi radialis tendon is passed through a drill hole in the base of the metacarpal and woven into the joint capsule. In the later stages of degeneration, patients must be treated either with an arthroplasty or an arthrodesis. A variety of **arthroplasty techniques** are available to the surgeon. The most successful methods involve resection of all or part of the trapezium and replacement with a biological spacer—usually a rolled up tendon graft commonly referred to as an "anchovy." These procedures also stabilize the first metacarpal with a tendon transfer through a drill hole in the bone. **Arthrodesis** (fusion) is another alternative. Fixation may be obtained with Kirschner wires and intraosseous compression wires. The time to fusion with this technique is 6 weeks. These patients have very few limitations and perform almost all normal activities of daily living. This procedure requires very little postop hand therapy, compared with arthroplasty techniques. It is also well suited to active patients. In some patients with extensive bone loss and cyst formation, bone graft is necessary and can be obtained from the distal radius.

Usual preop diagnosis: Osteoarthritis of CMC joint; basal joint arthritis; synovitis of CMC joint; CMC joint dislocation; trauma

SUMMARY OF PROCEDURE

Position	Supine, with arm extended on hand-surgery table
Incision	Curvilinear over joint at base of thumb. Tendon graft for interposition can be obtained through multiple small transverse incisions.
Special instrumentation	Pneumatic tourniquet
Antibiotics	Cefazolin 1 g iv
Surgical time	1.5-2 h
Tourniquet	150 mmHg above systolic; max time = 120 min
EBL	Minimal; procedures performed under tourniquet control.
Postop care	Postop splintage; overnight hospital stay for pain control
Mortality	Minimal
Morbidity	Nonunion of arthrodesis occurs as frequently as 20% in some series. Newer techniques, such as the tension-band intraosseous wire and sliding cortical graft, have much lower failure rates. Silicone rubber prostheses are associated with particulate synovitis.
Pain score	8-9

PATIENT POPULATION CHARACTERISTICS

Age range	Joint stabilization in 3rd-5th decades; arthroplasty and arthrodesis in 5th-8th decades
Male:Female	Basal joint instability and arthritis much more prevalent in women
Incidence	Common
Etiology	Trauma may play a role in producing instability. Patients who have had an intraarticular fracture of the base of the first metacarpal with a nonanatomic reduction will have incongruence of the joint and develop posttraumatic arthritis. Rheumatoid arthritis leads to instability and degeneration of the joint. Many patients with congenital ligamentous laxity will have unstable basal joints and will develop arthritis.
Associated conditions	Rheumatoid arthritis; osteoarthritis; carpal tunnel syndrome (CTS)

ANESTHETIC CONSIDERATIONS FOR WRIST PROCEDURES

(Procedures covered: Darrach procedure; dorsal stabilization and extensor synovectomy of the rheumatoid wrist; metacarpophalangeal and interphalangeal joint arthroplasty; arthrodesis of the wrist; total wrist replacement; thumb carpometacarpal joint fusion arthroscopy/stabilization)

PREOPERATIVE

Airway Rheumatoid involvement of the cervical spine, TMJ and cricoarytenoid joint (CAJ) are common in this patient population. Erosion of cervical vertebrae → unstable cervical spine (e.g., atlantoaxial subluxation) necessitates extreme care in head and neck manipulation. Cervical spine fusion (↓neck ROM), TMJ arthritis (↓mouth opening) and CAJ arthritis (laryngeal narrowing, hoarseness, DOE, stridor) portend difficult intubation and may necessitate awake fiber optic intubation. In the case of CAJ arthritis, use of a smaller ETT may be required.

Respiratory Rheumatoid patients may exhibit Sx of pleural effusion (✓ CXR) or pulmonary fibrosis (dyspnea, diffuse rales, ↓diffusing capacity, honeycomb appearance in CXR.
Tests: Consider CXR, PFTs, ABGs in affected patients.

Cardiovascular Rheumatoid patients may suffer from pericarditis, myocarditis, valvular disease and cardiac conduction defects. Because of the physical limitations imposed by the disease process, it may prove difficult to evaluate these patients' cardiovascular status; hence, cardiology consultation, ECG and ECHO may be useful in preparing for surgery.
Tests: Consider ECG and ECHO, especially in patients with severe rheumatoid arthritis.

Neurological Rheumatoid patients may have cervical or lumbar radiculopathies that should be documented carefully preop. In addition, peripheral neuropathy with consequent sensory/motor defects may be present.
Tests: Consider C-spine radiographs to rule out occult subluxations in rheumatoid patients with neck pain or upper extremity radiculopathy.

Musculoskeletal Bony deformities or muscle contractures may necessitate special attention to positioning.

Hematologic Anemia, eosinophilia and thrombocytosis may be present. Venous access may be difficult 2° vasculitis and ↑skin fragility (steroid-induced). Virtually all of these patients will be on some type of anti-inflammatory medication that may result in anemia or Plt inhibition. Ideally, patients should discontinue NSAIDs at least 5 d preop; aspirin, 7 d preop.

Endocrine Rheumatoid patients are likely to be on oral corticosteroids and require supplemental perioperative steroids (e.g., 100 mg hydrocortisone q 8 h iv) to treat adrenal suppression.

Laboratory Hb/Hct serves as a minimum in otherwise healthy rheumatoid patients. Severe rheumatoid patients may require more extensive testing to screen for drug effects, etc. (e.g., serum electrolytes; glucose; kidney function tests; LFTs).

Premedication Standard premedication (p. B-2)

INTRAOPERATIVE

Anesthetic technique: Regional anesthesia, GA, or a combination of the two are commonly used. A brachial plexus block via the axillary approach is excellent for this procedure; it is a means of avoiding tracheal intubation for GA if airway difficulty is anticipated. Intravenous regional anesthesia (Bier block) is most useful for short procedures (< 1 h). If regional anesthesia is contraindicated, rheumatoid patients may require awake fiber optic intubation (see p. B-6).

Regional anesthesia: 1.5% mepivacaine 40-50 ml for routine cases; 0.5% bupivacaine or 1% etidocaine 40 ml for procedures > 2.5 h or if extended analgesia is desired. Epinephrine (2.5-5μg/ml) should be added whenever possible to decrease peak plasma concentrations of local anesthetics.

Axillary block The medial aspect of the upper arm is innervated by the intercostobrachial nerve (T2) and requires a separate subcutaneous field block in the axilla, especially when a tourniquet is used. The lateral cutaneous nerve of the forearm, a sensory branch of the musculocutaneous nerve supplying sensation to the lateral forearm, is frequently missed by the axillary approach to the brachial plexus. Thus, a block of this nerve at the elbow or within the proximal coracobrachialis muscle is sometimes necessary. If sedation is necessary, propofol (50-150 μg/kg/min) by continuous infusion or intermittent bolus injection of opioid/benzodiazepine are good choices.

General anesthesia:

Induction Standard induction (p. B-2) in patients with normal airways

Maintenance Standard maintenance (p. B-3)

Emergence	Skin closure is frequently followed by application of a splint, and the patient should remain anesthetized during the splinting procedure. Cases with difficult airways require awake extubation.	
Blood and fluid requirements	Minimal blood loss IV: 18 ga × 1 NS/LR @ 1.5-3 ml/kg/h	IV placed in the nonoperated upper extremity.
Monitoring	Standard monitors (p. B-1)	
Positioning	Special handling required. ✓ and pad pressure points. ✓ eyes. ✓ C-spine instability.	As with nearly all orthopedic cases, positioning is a subtle, yet crucial aspect of anesthetic management. Rheumatoid patients may have contractures that require special attention. Steroid-dependent patients require special handling because of fragile skin.
Axillary block complications	Inadequate block Intravascular injection Peripheral nerve damage Axillary hematoma Axillary artery thrombosis Pneumothorax	Very minimal doses of local anesthetic can cause CNS toxicity if reverse flow occurs during an intraarterial injection. Axillary thrombosis and pneumothorax are extremely rare.

POSTOPERATIVE

Pain management	PCA (p. C-3), in combination with regional block	Combined regional-general anesthetic techniques are excellent for wrist procedures, especially with respect to postop pain management.
Tests	None routinely indicated.	

References

1. Brockway MS, Wildsmith JA: Axillary brachial plexus block: method of choice? *Br J Anaesth* 1990; 64(2):224-31.
2. Cockings E, Moore PL, Lewis RC: Transarterial brachial plexus blockade using high doses of 1.5% mepivacaine. *Reg Anesth* 1987; 12(4):159-64.
3. Goldberg ME, et al: A comparison of three methods of axillary approach to brachial plexus blockade for upper extremity surgery. *Anesthesiology* 1987; 66(6):814-16.
4. Green DP: *Operative Hand Surgery*, 3rd edition. Churchill Livingstone, New York: 1993.
5. Keenan MA, Stiles CM, Kaufman RL: Acquired laryngeal deviation associated with cervical spine disease in erosive polyarticular arthritis. *Anesthesiology* 1983; 58(5):441-49.
6. Ramamurthy S, Hickey R: Anesthesia. In *Operative Hand Surgery*, 3rd edition. Green DP, ed. Churchill Livingstone, New York: 1993, 25-52.
7. Tuominen MK, Pitkanen MT, Numminen MK, Rosenberg PH: Quality of axillary brachial plexus block. Comparison of success rate using perivascular and nerve stimulator techniques. *Anesthesia* 1987; 42(1):20-2.
8. Vandam LD: Anesthesia for Hand Surgery. In *Flynn's Hand Surgery*, 4th edition. Jupiter JB, ed. Williams and Wilkins, Baltimore: 1991, 46-54.
9. White RH: Preoperative evaluation of patients with rheumatoid arthritis. *Semin Arthritis Rheum* 1985; 14(4):287-99.

EXCISION OF GANGLION OF THE WRIST

SURGICAL CONSIDERATIONS

Description: Ganglion cysts about the wrist most commonly occur dorsally, originating from the scapholunate joint. The second most common site is volar to the scaphotrapezial joint. To prevent recurrence, these synovial fluid-filled outpouchings of the joint capsule must be excised completely. This requires isolating the stalk of the cyst to its origin, and excising a small cuff of normal joint capsule with the cyst. The joint, therefore, must be entered for a complete excision. Older studies found that the recurrence rate was decreased by the use of GA, as opposed to local or regional anesthetics. This was due to the fact that a more complete excision was performed when the patient was under GA. Hand specialists today feel that regional anesthetics are quite acceptable for this procedure, as long as the surgeon performs a meticulous excision. Volar wrist ganglions commonly involve the radial artery, which is at risk during excision. A preop Allen test should be performed to ensure that, if the radial artery is interrupted, there will not be ischemia in the hand.

Usual preop diagnosis: Ganglion cyst, primary or recurrent

SUMMARY OF PROCEDURE

Position	Supine, with arm extended on hand-surgery table
Incision	Longitudinal or transverse directly over cyst
Special instrumentation	Pneumatic tourniquet
Antibiotics	Cefazolin 1 g iv
Surgical time	0.5-1.5 h
Tourniquet	150 mmHg above systolic; max time = 120 min
Closing considerations	Routine skin closure. Large recurrent cysts may require a repair of the wrist capsule. Splint applied in OR.
EBL	Minimal; performed under tourniquet control.
Postop care	Elevation to prevent swelling
Mortality	Minimal
Morbidity	Injury to radial artery: Rare
Pain score	2-4

PATIENT POPULATION CHARACTERISTICS

Age range	Infants–elderly
Male:Female	1:1
Incidence	Very common
Etiology	Unknown. Trauma has been associated with about 50% of ganglion cysts. Underlying carpal instabilities, such as scapholunate instability, have been implicated.
Associated conditions	Carpal instability; trauma (wrist sprains and strains)

ANESTHETIC CONSIDERATIONS

See Anesthetic Considerations following Repair of Flexor Tendon Laceration, p. 689.

PALMAR AND DIGITAL FASCIECTOMY

SURGICAL CONSIDERATIONS

Description: This procedure is indicated for the treatment of Dupuytren's contractures of the digits, which produces a neoplastic thickening of the palmar and digital fascia. These pathologic cords (whose active cell is the myofibroblast) contract and, through their connections with the skin, tendon sheath and phalangeal bone, cause flexion contractures of the metacarpophalangeal, proximal interphalangeal and distal interphalangeal joints. The disease is progressive; and the only treatment is surgical excision of the fascia. In addition to the pathologic changes in the fascia of the hands, many patients also have thickening of the plantar fascia of the foot (Ledderhose's disease) and the dorsal fascia of the penis (Peyronie's disease). Patients with severe contractures that have been neglected may require amputation. Because the pathologic fascia is so intimately connected to the skin, it is sometimes necessary to excise the skin and replace it with full-thickness skin grafts. The groin is an excellent donor site for these grafts.

There are many different surgical approaches, most requiring the creation of Z-plasties for a tension-free closure. The **McCash technique** has been quite successful for the excision of palmar disease. This method consists of excising the palmar fascia through transverse incisions that are not sutured closed, but rather are left open to granulate and contract over a three-week postop period. These patients have a very low complication rate.

Usual preop diagnosis: Dupuytren's contracture

SUMMARY OF PROCEDURE

Position	Supine, with arm extended on hand-surgery table
Incision	Transverse or longitudinal palmar. Groin may be used as a full-thickness skin graft donor site.
Antibiotics	None
Surgical time	1-3 h
Tourniquet	150 mmHg above systolic; max time = 120 min. Because of the need to deflate tourniquet so that hemostasis can be obtained, Bier block is not suitable.
Closing considerations	Must obtain meticulous hemostasis. Z-plasties and skin grafts used frequently.
EBL	Minimal; dissection done under tourniquet control. A small amount of blood loss occurs when tourniquet is released and hemostasis is obtained.
Postop care	Pain control is essential. Patient may be admitted for initial postop period. Limb elevation to minimize swelling. Regional techniques that provide postop pain relief are very useful.
Mortality	Minimal
Morbidity	Hematoma Skin necrosis Infection Digital nerve and artery injury Reflex-sympathetic dystrophy
Pain score	7-8

PATIENT POPULATION CHARACTERISTICS

Age range	Typically, 40-60 yr; can occur in teens.
Male:Female	More common in males
Incidence	Common
Etiology	Definite heritance—associated with strong family Hx. Ethnic diathesis for northern Europeans with fair hair and skin, blue eyes. Almost never seen in Blacks. Experimental studies suggest that microhematomas 2° repetitive trauma may be important in the disease process.
Associated conditions	Cigarette smoking; alcoholism; antiseizure medications

ANESTHETIC CONSIDERATIONS

See Anesthetic Considerations following Repair of Flexor Tendon Laceration, p. 689.

REPAIR OF FLEXOR TENDON LACERATION

SURGICAL CONSIDERATIONS

Description: The prognosis and difficulty of a flexor tendon repair depends on the anatomic site of the laceration. There are five zones of injury in the upper extremity (Fig 10.1-2). Zone I is distal to the flexor digitorum superficialis (FDS) tendon insertion and involves only the flexor digitorum profundus (FDP) tendon. Zone II extends from the entrance to the fibroosseous sheath at the metacarpal head to the FDS insertion. Lacerations usually involve both the FDS and

FDP. These are the most difficult to repair and have the worst prognosis as the tendons are apt to become scarred to each other and limit gliding. Zone III is the palm; Zone IV is within the carpal canal; and Zone 5 is in the forearm. Lacerations in these areas are easier to repair and have good prognoses for restoration of tendon gliding and, thus, digit motion. Associated injuries to the neural structures are common. Digital nerve lacerations are seen in Zone II; median nerve injuries, in Zone IV. Occasionally, nerve injuries occur in Zone V.

In general, nerve injuries are repaired at the time of the tendon repair. Tendons lacerated in the finger are often pulled back into the palm by muscular contraction. A palmar incision is required to retrieve the tendon, which must then be threaded carefully through the pulleys in the digit. Suture techniques for tendon repair create a juncture that is far weaker than an intact tendon. For this reason, the juncture must be protected from mechanical stress for a period of 8 weeks or more. This is done by splinting the hand with the wrist and digits flexed so that the pull on the tendon by its muscle is limited by the tenodesis effect. It is important that the patient emerges gently from anesthesia to limit the stress upon the tendon. The best results are obtained when repair is carried out within 7 days of the injury, although primary repair can be performed up to 3 weeks. After 7 days, the muscle begins to undergo irreversible contracture. If the flexor tendon is advanced after this has occurred, a flexion contracture results. If a flexor tendon laceration is neglected, a palm-to-fingertip tendon graft, using a different flexor tendon, should be performed. If the tendon bed is suitable for gliding, the graft can be accomplished in one stage. If not, a Silastic tendon spacer (rubber rod) must be placed at the first stage. Six to eight weeks later, a palm-to-fingertip graft is placed in the bed prepared with the Silastic rod. Tendon graft donor sites include the palmaris longus tendon and toe extensors.

A variant of the sharp flexor tendon laceration is the FDP avulsion from its insertion in Zone 1. This is the so-called "jersey finger." This injury occurs during forceful grasp, and most commonly affects the ring finger. A common mechanism is the football or rugby player who is grasping the jersey of a ball carrier. The FDP tendon retracts and should be repaired within 7 days. If neglected, these patients should be treated with a **distal interphalangeal (DIP) arthrodesis**. A flexor tendon graft through an intact FDS tendon usually is not indicated, as tendon adhesions will commonly interfere with the function of the FDS, leading to decreased overall active motion of the digit. The most common complication is the development of tendon adhesions, which limit tendon gliding and digit motion. If these patients fail to improve within a 3- to 6-month course of physical therapy, they require an operative tenolysis to lyse the adhesions.

Usual preop diagnosis: Flexor tendon laceration; FDP avulsion ("jersey finger"); digital nerve laceration; median nerve laceration

SUMMARY OF PROCEDURE

Position	Supine, with arm extended on hand-surgery table. The foot may be prepped for a tendon graft.
Incision	Zig-zag hand or wrist
Special instrumentation	Pneumatic tourniquet
Antibiotics	Cefazolin 1 g iv
Surgical time	1-2 h; may be extended for nerve repair and treatment of associated injuries.
Closing considerations	Tendon and nerve repairs must be protected with splints prior to emergence from GA. Smooth extubation (see Emergence).
EBL	Minimal; procedure performed under tourniquet control.
Postop care	PACU → home
Mortality	Minimal
Morbidity	Tendon adhesions: 25% Rupture of tendon repair: < 5% Infection: Rare
Pain score	2-4

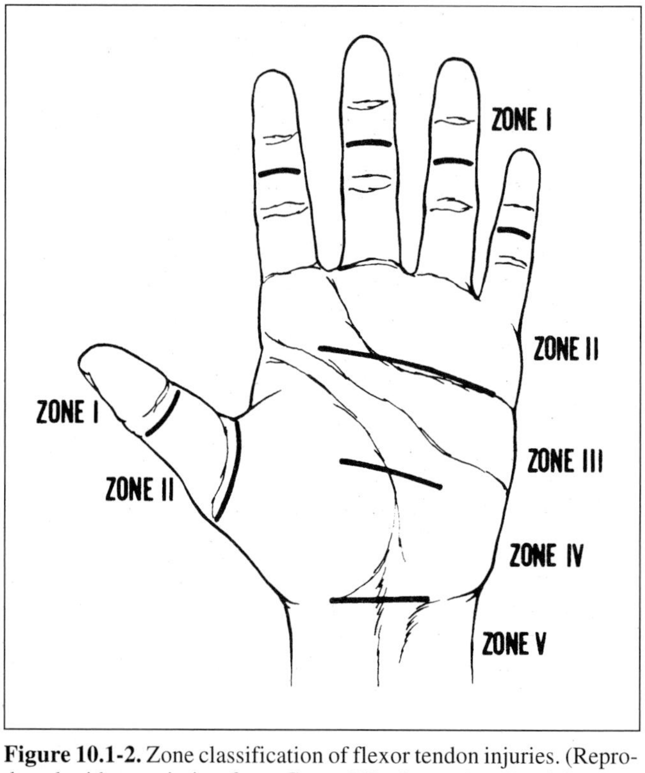

Figure 10.1-2. Zone classification of flexor tendon injuries. (Reproduced with permission from Green DP: *Operative Hand Surgery*, 3rd edition. Churchill Livingstone: 1993.)

PATIENT POPULATION CHARACTERISTICS

Age range	Infant–elderly
Male:Female	Slight male predominance, due to occupational injuries
Incidence	Not uncommon
Etiology	Trauma

ANESTHETIC CONSIDERATIONS

(Procedures covered: excision of ganglion of the wrist; palmar and digital fasciectomy; repair of flexor tendon laceration)

PREOPERATIVE

The majority of patients presenting for these procedures are usually otherwise healthy. Many of them present for elective surgery as a result of progressive functional impairment and pain, and preop workup is routine.

Neurological If regional anesthesia is contemplated, preexisting sensory or motor defects should be carefully documented.

Laboratory Hb/Hct (healthy patients); otherwise, as indicated from H&P.

Premedication Moderate to heavy premedication (e.g., midazolam 0.5-1.0 mg iv q 5 min titrated to effect) is often desirable if regional block is done.

INTRAOPERATIVE

Anesthetic technique: Regional anesthesia (most common), GA or a combination of the two may be used. Intravenous regional anesthesia (Bier block) is most useful for short procedures which last for < 1 h (see Wrist Arthroscopy, p. 693). A brachial plexus block via the axillary approach is excellent for this procedure. Because most of these procedures are done on an outpatient basis, brachial plexus block without GA is usually preferred in order to promote early "street-readiness."

Regional anesthesia: 1.5% mepivacaine 40-50 ml for routine cases; 0.5% bupivacaine or 1% etidocaine 40 ml for procedures > 2.5 h or if extended analgesia is desired. Epinephrine (2.5-5 μg/ml) should be added whenever possible to decrease peak plasma concentrations of local anesthetics.

Axillary block The medial aspect of the upper arm is innervated by the intercostobrachial nerve (T2) and requires a separate subcutaneous field block in the axilla, especially when a tourniquet is used. The lateral cutaneous nerve of the forearm, a sensory branch of the musculocutaneous nerve supplying sensation to the lateral forearm, is frequently missed by the axillary approach to the brachial plexus. Thus, a block of this nerve at the elbow or within the proximal coracobrachialis muscle is sometimes necessary. If sedation is necessary, propofol (50-150 μg/kg/min) by continuous infusion or intermittent bolus injection of opioid/benzodiazepine are good choices.

General anesthesia:

Induction Standard induction (p. B-2)

Maintenance Standard maintenance (p. B-3)

Emergence Standard emergence (p. B-4). Skin closure is frequently followed by application of a splint; patient should remain anesthetized during splinting procedure.

Blood and fluid requirements	Minimal blood loss IV: 18 ga × 1 NS/LR @ 1.5-3 ml/kg/h	An 18 ga iv catheter placed in the nonoperated upper extremity should be adequate.
Monitoring	Standard monitors (p. B-1)	
Positioning	✓ and pad pressure points. ✓ eyes.	
Axillary block complications	Intravascular injection Inadequate block	Minimal doses of local anesthetic can cause CNS toxicity during an accidental intravascular injection. Seizures

Axillary block complications, cont.	Peripheral nerve damage Axillary hematoma CNS toxicity/seizures Axillary artery thrombosis Pneumothorax	should be treated with STP or midazolam titrated to effect, accompanied by airway control. If there is any question of a full stomach, intubation should be accomplished rapidly. Axillary thrombosis and pneumothorax are very rare.

POSTOPERATIVE

Pain management	Oral analgesics are usually sufficient.	The lingering analgesia of the brachial plexus block is often sufficient for pain relief in the recovery room; oral analgesic therapy can be instituted prior to discharging patient to home.
Tests	None routinely indicated.	

References

1. Brockway MS, Wildsmith JA: Axillary brachial plexus block: method of choice? *Br J Anaesth* 1990; 64(2):224-31.
2. Cockings E, Moore PL, Lewis RC: Transarterial brachial plexus blockade using high doses of 1.5% mepivacaine. *Reg Anesth* 1987; 12(4):159-64.
3. Davis WJ, Lennon RL, Wedel DJ: Brachial plexus anesthesia for outpatient surgical procedures on an upper extremity. *Mayo Clin Proc* 1991; 66(5):470-73.
4. Goldberg ME, et al: A comparison of three methods of axillary approach to brachial plexus blockade for upper extremity surgery. *Anesthesiology* 1987; 66(6):814-16.
5. Green DP: *Operative Hand Surgery*, 3rd edition. Churchill Livingstone, New York: 1993.
6. Ramamurthy S, Hickey R: Anesthesia. In *Operative Hand Surgery*, 3rd edition. Green DP, ed. Churchill Livingstone, New York: 1993, 25-52.
7. Tuominen MK, Pitkanen MT, Numminen MK, Rosenberg PH: Quality of axillary brachial plexus block. Comparison of success rate using perivascular and nerve stimulator techniques. *Anesthesia* 1987; 42(1):20-2.
8. Vandam LD: Anesthesia for Hand Surgery. In *Flynn's Hand Surgery*, 4th edition. Jupiter JB, ed. Williams and Wilkins, Baltimore: 1991, 46-54.

WRIST ARTHROSCOPY

SURGICAL CONSIDERATIONS

Description: Wrist arthroscopy may be performed for either diagnostic or therapeutic indications. A smaller diameter version of the standard arthroscope is used for visualizing the wrist joint. All of the entry portals are on the dorsum of the wrist and course between the extensor compartments. Irrigation is used during the procedure and a cannula is routinely placed ulnar to the extensor carpi ulnaris tendon. Unlike the knee joint, where visualization is obtained by distention of the joint, in-the-wrist visualization is obtained by distraction. The digits are placed in finger traps and up to 10 pounds of traction can be placed on the wrist. Specialized instrumentation is available to resect and debride intraarticular structures and to place sutures to repair torn ligaments. The use of the holmium laser and radiofrequency energy generator for debridement, synovectomy and excision of tears of the triangular fibrocartilage has led to shorter operative times. Arthroscopic techniques also can be used to irrigate and debride the infected wrist joint. At Stanford University Medical Center, we have performed over 50 wrist arthroscopies, both diagnostic and therapeutic, under Bier block. All patients tolerated the surgery well and were able to view the procedure on the monitor, and to discuss the findings with the surgeon intraop. Anesthesia time of up to 80 min was well tolerated. If an open procedure, such as repair of an intercarpal ligament, is contemplated following diagnostic arthroscopy, either GA or regional block is preferred.

Variant procedure or approaches: The standard approach is to suspend the forearm vertically in traction. The forearm can also be placed horizontally on the hand table in traction.

Usual preop diagnosis: Internal derangement of the wrist of unknown etiology; tears of the triangular fibrocartilage complex; intercarpal instability due to intercarpal ligament tears; rotatory subluxation of the scaphoid; scapholunate dissociation; luno-triquetral dissociation; fracture of distal radius; ulnar impingement syndrome; rheumatoid synovitis; intraarticular infection

SUMMARY OF PROCEDURE

Position	Supine, with arm extended on hand-surgery table
Incision	Small incisions are made on the dorsum of the wrist for instrument insertion.
Special instrumentation	2.7 mm diameter arthroscope, 0 or 30-degree field of view; light source and video camera; television monitor; surgical power shaver; joint irrigation system; traction device for forearm; pneumatic tourniquet
Unique considerations	Patient is often awake and observes surgery on monitor.
Antibiotics	Cefazolin 1 g iv
Surgical time	30 min-2 h
Tourniquet	150 mmHg above systolic; max time = 120 min
Closing considerations	Arthroscopic portals are each closed with a single skin suture.
EBL	Minimal; procedure performed with tourniquet control.
Postop care	PACU → home
Mortality	Minimal
Morbidity	Infection: < 1%
	Swelling (2° to irrigation fluid): Common
	Nerve and artery damage: Uncommon
Pain score	1-3

PATIENT POPULATION CHARACTERISTICS

Age range	Adolescent–elderly. This procedure is not indicated in children.
Male:Female	1:1
Incidence	Least common form of arthroscopy
Etiology	See Usual Preop Diagnosis, above.
Associated conditions	Degenerative arthritis (posttraumatic and osteo-); rheumatoid arthritis

ANESTHETIC CONSIDERATIONS

See Anesthetic Considerations following Carpal Tunnel Release, p. 692.

Reference

1. Green DP: *Operative Hand Surgery*, 3rd edition. Churchill Livingstone, New York: 1993.

CARPAL TUNNEL RELEASE

SURGICAL CONSIDERATIONS

Description: This is the most commonly performed procedure in hand surgery. It consists of the transection of the transverse carpal ligament through either an open-palmar or an endoscopic approach. The procedure may include synovectomy of the flexor tendons, tendon transfers to restore thumb opposition and the excision of masses from within the carpal canal. In patients with severe synovitis, as in rheumatoid arthritis, a synovectomy should be performed at the same time. If there is advanced thenar atrophy and weakness of thumb opposition, a tendon transfer also should be done at that time. The most common transfer is the **Camitz opponensplasty**, in which the palmaris longis tendon is prolonged with palmar fascia and transferred to the thumb. Transfers of the extensor indicis proprius and superficial flexor tendons also can be performed. Because of the great danger of lacerating a nerve during endoscopic carpal tunnel release, it is recommended that the procedure be performed under a local anesthetic with infiltration only into the skin. Thus, the nerves remain sensate and can be probed and identified by the awake patient. Short-acting sedation can be used during the insertion of the trocar and sheath into the carpal canal.

Usual preop diagnosis: Carpal tunnel syndrome (CTS); median nerve compression at the wrist

SUMMARY OF PROCEDURE

	Open Carpal Tunnel Release	Endoscopic Carpal Tunnel Release
Position	Supine	⇐
Incision	Longitudinal incision in palm; may extend to forearm	2 cm transverse at proximal flexion crease of wrist; 1 cm, mid-palm
Special instrumentation	Pneumatic tourniquet	Endoscopic carpal tunnel release system: endoscope, sheath and trocar, special cutting tools
Unique considerations	None	Danger of intraop injury to digital nerves, median nerve, tendons, superficial vascular arch
Antibiotics	Cefazolin 1 g iv	⇐
Surgical time	0.5-1.5 h	30 min
Tourniquet	150 mmHg above systolic; max time = 120 min	⇐
Closing considerations	Simple skin closure	⇐
EBL	Minimal; performed under tourniquet control.	Minimal
Postop care	Splint, elevation	No splint, early motion, elevation
Mortality	Minimal	⇐
Morbidity	Overall complication rate: 4%	⇐
	Reflex sympathetic dystrophy (RSD): < 5%	Rare
	Hematoma: Rare	Complications of ulnar nerve palsy
	Infection: Uncommon	Tendon and nerve laceration: Rare (< 1%)
		Vascular injury: Less common than nerve injury
Pain score	1-2	1-2

PATIENT POPULATION CHARACTERISTICS

Age range	20-80 yr; 50% are 40-60 yr
Male:Female	1:2
Incidence	Common
Etiology	Compression of the median nerve within the carpal tunnel by synovitis; mass effect 2° tumor or fracture fragments, peripheral neuropathy, gout, anomalous structures, thrombosis of a persistent median artery and idiopathic; repetitive trauma (e.g., computer use)
Associated conditions	Rheumatoid arthritis; thyroid imbalance; diabetes; amyloidosis; multiple myeloma; alcoholism; hemophilia; pregnancy; menopause; gout; fractures of the distal radius; Kienbock's disease

ANESTHETIC CONSIDERATIONS

(Procedures covered: wrist arthroscopy; carpal tunnel release)

PREOPERATIVE

In general, there are two patient populations involved: (1) healthy patients with a history of wrist trauma, and (2) rheumatoid patients. (See Anesthetic Considerations for Wrist Procedures, p. 684, for discussion of preop concerns in the rheumatoid patient.)

Laboratory	Hb/Hct (healthy patients); otherwise, as indicated from H&P.	
Premedication	Moderate to heavy premedication (e.g., midazolam 0.5-1.0 mg iv q 5 min titrated to effect) is often desirable if regional block is done.	

INTRAOPERATIVE

Anesthetic technique: Intravenous regional anesthesia is an excellent technique for procedures that are < 1 hr. For longer procedures, an axillary brachial plexus block is a good alternative. Both of these techniques are especially appropriate for outpatients.

Intravenous regional block	40-50 ml of 0.5% lidocaine is injected intravenously into the exsanguinated limb. This will usually provide up to 1 h of anesthesia before tourniquet pain becomes severe. The use of a double-cuffed tourniquet may help minimize tourniquet pain. For procedures < 40 min, the tourniquet should be deflated briefly (~10 sec), then reinflated while observing the patient for signs of toxicity (60-90 sec) before final deflation. If sedation is needed, propofol (50-150 μg/kg/min) by continuous infusion, or intermittent bolus injection of opioid/benzodiazepine, are good choices.	
Blood and fluid requirements	Minimal blood loss IV: 18 ga × 1 NS/LR @ 1.5-2 ml/kg/h	An 18 ga iv catheter placed in the nonoperated upper extremity should be adequate.
Monitoring	Standard monitors (p. B-1)	
Positioning	✓ and pad pressure points. ✓ eyes.	
Intravenous regional block complications	Systemic toxicity: Tinnitus Dizziness Blurred vision Seizure ↓HR, ↓BP Inadequate block Thrombophlebitis	Systemic toxic reaction to the local anesthetic may occur as a result of tourniquet leak or inadvertent premature (< 20 min) tourniquet release. Treatment is supportive. Seizures are controlled with STP or midazolam with appropriate airway protection. Even with a functioning tourniquet, it is possible to overcome tourniquet pressure by injecting too vigorously. Care must be taken when switching from proximal to distal tourniquet; never deflate proximal tourniquet until verifying that distal tourniquet is working. Finally, never deflate tourniquet(s) until at least 20 min have elapsed.

POSTOPERATIVE

Pain management	Oral analgesics usually sufficient	Residual analgesia with intravenous regional anesthesia is minimal; some iv opioid is usually necessary until the patient is tolerating fluids in the recovery room.
Tests	None routinely indicated.	

References

1. Brown EM, McGriff JT, Malinowski RW: Intravenous regional anaesthesia (Bier block): a review of 20 years' experience. *Can J Anaesth* 1989; 36(3 Pt 1):307-10.
2. Davies JA, Wilkey AD, Hall ID: Bupivacaine leak past inflated tourniquets during intravenous regional analgesia. *Anaesthesia* 1984; 39(10):996-99.
3. Duggan J, Mckeown DW, Scott DB: Venous pressures generated during IV regional anaesthesia. *Br J Anaesth* 1983; 55:1158P-59P.
4. Grice SC, Morell RC, Balestrieri FJ, et al: Intravenous regional anesthesia: evaluation and prevention of leakage under the tourniquet. *Anesthesiology* 1986; 65(3):316-20.
5. Ramamurthy S, Hickey R: Anesthesia. In *Operative Hand Surgery*, 3rd edition. Green DP, ed. Churchill Livingstone, New York: 1993, 25-52.
6. Rosenberg PH, Kalso EA, Tuominen MK, Linden HB: Acute bupivacaine toxicity as a result of venous leakage under the tourniquet cuff during a Bier block. *Anesthesiology* 1983; 58(1):95-8.
7. Sukhani R, Garcia CJ, Munhall RJ, et al: Lidocaine disposition following intravenous regional anesthesia with different tourniquet deflation technics. *Anesth Analg* 1989; 68(5):633-37.
8. Vandam LD: Anesthesia for Hand Surgery. In *Flynn's Hand Surgery*, 4th edition. Jupiter JB, ed. Williams and Wilkins, Baltimore: 1991, 46-54.

REPAIR OF FRACTURES AND DISLOCATIONS OF THE DISTAL RADIUS, CARPUS AND METACARPALS

SURGICAL CONSIDERATIONS

Description: Patients with fractures of the distal radius, carpus and/or metacarpals, which cannot be treated adequately with closed methods, require **open reduction and internal fixation** (ORIF). The criteria for adequate treatment include anatomic reduction of the fracture fragments and stable maintenance of this reduction. Closed, unstable, distal radius fractures often are treated by traction and application of an external fixator in the OR to maintain the reduction by ligamentotaxis. Patients with wrist dislocation and distal radius fractures frequently have signs of neurologic compromise, such as carpal tunnel syndrome (CTS). Vascular compromise of the hand associated with these injuries is rare, usually occurring in patients with severe crush or high-energy injuries. The devascularized hand is a surgical emergency, and revascularization must be carried out as soon as possible. Fractures of these structures are associated with blast and crush injuries, as well as low-velocity gunshot wounds. These injuries have significant soft-tissue components which must be treated. The possibility of a coexisting compartment syndrome should be considered; and a fasciotomy may be needed at the time of surgery. Treatment of these fractures often involves a bone graft from the iliac crest to augment the reduction. A variety of fixation devices, including screws and plates, as well as Kirschner wires, are used. Open fractures are, by definition, contaminated and should be irrigated and debrided within 8 h of the injury. Surgical approaches are direct through longitudinal or transverse incisions. Some fractures of the articular surface of the distal radius are amenable to arthroscopically guided percutaneous pin fixation. Screw fixation of the scaphoid also can be accomplished by arthroscopy. Fluoroscopy is often utilized, as are standard portable radiographs to monitor and assess the quality of the reduction of the fracture.

Soft-tissue coverage of these injuries may be problematic and **local flaps** or **free microvascular tissue transfers** may be indicated. Free transfers can come from the same limb (radial forearm flap, based on the radial artery; lateral upper arm flap, based on the posterior radial collateral artery) or a remote site (latissimus dorsi muscle, based on the thoracodorsal artery; or scapular skin flap, based on the circumflex scapular artery). Remote flaps require special patient positioning and draping. Microsurgical tissue transfers also may need special pharmacological considerations, such as the administration of heparin or dextran to prevent thrombosis of the anastomosis.

Usual preop diagnosis: Fractures of the distal radius (Colles', Barton's, Smith's are common eponyms); wrist dislocations (perilunate, lunate); fractures of the metacarpals; gunshot wounds; crush injuries; blast injuries

SUMMARY OF PROCEDURE

Position	Supine, with arm extended on hand-surgery table. Iliac crest bone graft may be indicated and should be prepped with a sandbag beneath the ipsilateral buttock.
Incision	Longitudinal or transverse
Special instrumentation	Fluoroscopy; wrist arthroscopy instrumentation; internal and external fixation devices and power tools; operating microscope; pneumatic tourniquet
Unique considerations	Associated injuries and soft-tissue problems in high-energy fractures
Antibiotics	Indicated during the treatment of infected fractures. Treatment of both open and closed fractures requires broad spectrum cephalosporin prophylaxis. Special cases of contamination, such as soil and human bite injuries, require specific extended coverage.
Surgical time	30 min-3 h. Microsurgical tissue transfers can have surgical times of 8 h or more.
Tourniquet	150 mmHg above systolic; max time = 120 min
Closing considerations	Some injuries require local flaps or free microsurgical tissue transfers for closure. Fasciotomy wounds are usually left open. Splint applied at surgery.
EBL	Minimal for fracture treatment, as tourniquet control is used. Iliac crest or free-tissue donor sites can result in blood loss of 500-2000 ml.
Postop care	Monitor free-tissue transfers with temperature monitoring and visual inspection.
Mortality	Usually due to associated injuries
Morbidity	Loss of reduction, requiring repair
	Nonunion
	Infection
Pain score	3-9

PATIENT POPULATION CHARACTERISTICS

Age range	All ages. More conservative approaches are used with elderly patients.
Male:Female	1:1
Incidence	Very common
Etiology	Trauma
Associated conditions	Traumatic injuries

ANESTHETIC CONSIDERATIONS

PREOPERATIVE

The majority of patients presenting for these procedures are relatively young and healthy. Most of these patients present for elective repair of a traumatic injury, and preop workup is routine. Replantation and some wrist procedures, such as repair of a compound fracture, require immediate attention and necessitate emergency surgery and full-stomach considerations (see p. B-5).

Neurologic If regional anesthesia is contemplated, preexisting sensory or motor defects should be documented carefully preop.

Laboratory Hb/Hct (healthy patients); otherwise, as indicated from H&P.

Premedication Moderate to heavy premedication (e.g., midazolam 0.5-1.0 mg iv q 5 min titrated to effect) is often desirable if regional block is done.

INTRAOPERATIVE

Anesthetic technique: GETA or regional anesthesia are commonly used. A brachial plexus block via the axillary approach is excellent for short (1-2 h) procedures on the wrist and hand. Regional anesthesia alone is a means of avoiding the risk of aspiration pneumonitis associated with GA in the patient with a full stomach whose operation must be done emergently (see Rapid-Sequence Induction of Anesthesia, p. B-5). Unfortunately, because these cases often require the use of bone grafts harvested from the iliac crest, regional anesthesia alone usually is not feasible. For similar reasons, regional anesthesia also is not appropriate for cases that require a free-tissue transfer.

General anesthesia:

Induction Standard induction (p. B-2)

Maintenance Standard maintenance (p. B-3)

Emergence Skin closure is frequently followed by application of a splint; patient should remain anesthetized during splinting procedure.

Regional anesthesia: 1.5% mepivacaine 40-50 ml for routine cases; 0.5% bupivacaine or 1% etidocaine 40 ml for procedures > 2.5 h or if extended analgesia is desired. Epinephrine (2.5-5 μg/ml) should be added whenever possible to decrease peak plasma concentrations of local anesthetics.

Axillary block The medial aspect of the upper arm is innervated by the intercostobrachial nerve (T2) and requires a separate subcutaneous field block in the axilla, especially when a tourniquet is used. The lateral cutaneous nerve of the forearm, a sensory branch of the musculocutaneous nerve supplying sensation to the lateral forearm, is frequently missed by the axillary approach to the brachial plexus. Thus, a block of this nerve at the elbow or within the proximal body of the coracobrachialis muscle is sometimes necessary. If sedation is needed, propofol (50-150 μg/kg/min) by continuous infusion or intermittent bolus injection of opioid/benzodiazepine (e.g., midazolam 0.5-1.0 mg iv q 5 min and alfentanil 5-10 μg/kg iv q min titrated to effect) can be used.

Blood and fluid requirements Minimal to moderate blood loss
IV: 18 ga × 1
NS/LR @ 1.5-3 ml/kg/h

Minimal to moderate blood loss unless an iliac crest bone graft becomes necessary; these graft donor sites can lose 250-500 ml of blood. An 18 ga iv catheter placed in the nonoperated upper extremity should be adequate.

Monitoring Standard monitors (p. B-1)

Positioning ✓ and pad pressure points.
✓ eyes.

Axillary block complications	Inadequate block Intravascular injection Peripheral nerve damage Axillary hematoma Axillary artery thrombosis Pneumothorax CNS toxicity/seizures	Minimal doses of local anesthetic can cause CNS toxicity during an accidental intravascular injection. Seizures should be treated with STP or midazolam titrated to effect, accompanied by airway control. If there is any question of a full stomach, then intubation should be accomplished rapidly. Axillary thrombosis and pneumothorax are extremely rare.

POSTOPERATIVE

Pain management	PCA (p. C-3), in combination with regional block	Combined regional-general anesthetic techniques are excellent for wrist procedures, especially with respect to postop pain management.
Tests	None routinely indicated.	

References

1. Brockway MS, Wildsmith JA: Axillary brachial plexus block: method of choice? *Br J Anaesth* 1990; 64(2):224-31.
2. Cockings E, Moore PL, Lewis RC: Transarterial brachial plexus blockade using high doses of 1.5% mepivacaine. *Reg Anesth* 1987; 12(4):159-64.
3. Davis WJ, Lennon RL, Wedel DJ: Brachial plexus anesthesia for outpatient surgical procedures on an upper extremity. *Mayo Clin Proc* 1991; 66(5):470-73.
4. Goldberg ME, et al: A comparison of three methods of axillary approach to brachial plexus blockade for upper extremity surgery. *Anesthesiology* 1987; 66(6):814-16.
5. Green DP: *Operative Hand Surgery*, 3rd edition. Churchill Livingstone, New York: 1993.
6. Ramamurthy S, Hickey R: Anesthesia. In *Operative Hand Surgery*, 3rd edition. Green DP, ed. Churchill Livingstone, New York: 1993, 25-52.
7. Tuominen MK, Pitkanen MT, Numminen MK, Rosenberg PH: Quality of axillary brachial plexus block. Comparison of success rate using perivascular and nerve stimulator techniques. *Anesthesia* 1987; 42(1):20-2.
8. Vandam LD: Anesthesia for Hand Surgery. In *Flynn's Hand Surgery*, 4th edition. Jupiter JB, ed. Williams and Wilkins, Baltimore: 1991, 46-54.

DIGIT AND HAND REPLANTATION

SURGICAL CONSIDERATIONS

Description: Patients with traumatic amputations of digits and the hand are candidates for emergency microsurgical replantation of these parts. In children, replantation is attempted for essentially all amputations. In the adult, replantation is carried out for amputations of the thumb, multiple digits, and amputations through the palm. In general, amputations of a single digit are not candidates for replantation because of the minimal loss of function in relation to the long rehabilitation period and expected outcome. Certainly, a single digit amputated proximal to the insertion of the flexor digitorum superficialis (FDS) tendon (Zone II) (Fig 10.1-2) should not be replanted. The condition of the amputated part plays an important role in the decision to proceed with replantation. A severely crushed, contaminated, or burned part cannot be expected to survive and function. The patients may also have associated traumatic injuries which will take preference over replantation (i.e., intraabdominal bleeding with a positive peritoneal lavage, chest injuries). The patient's overall health status must be assessed. A patient with unstable angina should probably not be subjected to a lengthy microsurgical procedure.

There are a variety of reasons that people suffer amputations. Many of these patients are substance abusers or intoxicated at the time of injury. Studies of these patients also have shown a high incidence of psychopathology, along with substance abuse. Because these procedures are emergent, patients often arrive at the hospital with full stomachs. While regional anesthesia techniques provide peripheral vasodilation through their sympatholytic effect, many surgeons prefer general anesthesia because of the unpredictable length of the procedures. While the patient is being readied for induction, the surgeon prepares the amputated part in the OR. At this time, the structures to be repaired are tagged, which saves a great deal of anesthetic time. When the patient is prepped and draped, the hand is irrigated and debrided, and the corresponding structures are tagged in similar manner. The amputated part is brought to the field and the actual replantation is performed. Once arterial blood flow is reestablished, the patient must be kept warm to prevent vasospasm. As with other microsurgical procedures, pharmacologic intervention is indicated to prevent thrombosis; intravenous heparin and dextran are normally administered. Skin grafts for soft-tissue coverage and vein grafts to replace segmental vascular defects are commonly used. Vein grafts can be obtained from the ipsilateral upper extremity or from the lower extremity, especially the dorsum of the foot. The lateral thigh or abdomen are excellent donor sites for split-thickness skin grafts. Rarely is an immediate microsurgical free-tissue transfer indicated for soft-tissue coverage.

Usual preop diagnosis: Traumatic amputation of the digits or hand

SUMMARY OF PROCEDURE

Position	Supine, with arm extended on hand-surgery table
Incision	Extensile exposures of neurovascular structures. Lower extremity prepped and draped as donor site for vein grafts from dorsum of foot, split-thickness skin graft from the thigh.
Special instrumentation	Operating microscope; microsurgical instrumentation
Unique considerations	Emergency procedure
Antibiotics	Cefazolin 1 g iv
Surgical time	3-12 h
Tourniquet	150 mmHg above systolic; max time = 120 min
Closing considerations	Routine volar hand splint
EBL	< 500 ml
Postop care	ICU → requires monitoring in intensive nursing environment. Should be kept pain-free for extended period postop to minimize vessel spasm. Patients will benefit from postop sedation.
Mortality	Minimal
Morbidity	Loss of replanted part (vessel thrombosis): 10% Infection: Rare
Pain score	3-5

PATIENT POPULATION CHARACTERISTICS

Age range	All ages, infant–8th decade
Male:Female	1:1
Incidence	Uncommon
Etiology	Trauma
Associated conditions	Substance abuse; alcoholism

ANESTHETIC CONSIDERATIONS

PREOPERATIVE

In general, there are two patient populations for hand replantation: (1) isolated hand injury patients (common), and (2) multiple trauma victims (rare).

Respiratory	As suggested by coexisting disease or acute trauma injuries. Evidence of occult chest injury, including pneumothorax and pulmonary contusion, should be sought. **Tests:** Consider CXR, ABGs in victims of significant trauma.
Cardiovascular	As suggested by coexisting disease or acute trauma injuries. Look for evidence of occult cardiac or mediastinal injuries, such as myocardial contusion or great vessel rupture. **Tests:** Consider CXR (with NG tube in place to assess mediastinal widening), and ECG in victims of significant trauma.
Neurological	As suggested by coexisting disease or acute trauma injuries. The possibility of closed head injury should be addressed in multiple-trauma victims. Verify integrity of C-spine.

Neurological, cont.	**Tests:** Consider head CT prior to beginning a long procedure under GA in a patient with evidence of head trauma; C-spine x-ray.
Gastrointestinal	All patients should be considered to have full stomachs and, therefore, at increased risk for aspiration pneumonitis. In general, they should receive preop medication to reduce stomach volume and acidity (e.g., metoclopramide 10 mg iv and ranitidine 50 mg iv).
Hematologic	Multiple-trauma victims are likely to suffer from acute blood loss. Although blood loss from these procedures is generally modest, a preop T&C for several U PRBCs is wise for trauma patients. **Tests:** CBC
Metabolic	Approximately 1/2 of trauma victims are intoxicated. Anesthesia-related implications of ethanol intoxication include: decreased anesthetic requirements, diuresis, vasodilation and hypothermia.
Laboratory	As suggested by coexisting disease or acute trauma injuries. In general, most victims of significant trauma are best served by obtaining a wide variety of baseline lab studies to screen for unrecognized injury. These studies normally include: ABGs; UA; renal function tests; LFTs; serum amylase; tox screen.
Premedication	Full-stomach precautions: Na citrate 0.3 M 30 ml, metoclopramide 10 mg iv; H_2-blocker

INTRAOPERATIVE

Anesthetic technique: GETA, after rapid-sequence induction. Because of the unpredictable length of these procedures and the possible need for bone and/or vessel grafts, regional anesthesia is not feasible as the primary technique. A concurrent, continuing brachial plexus block, however, will provide sympathetic blockade, as well as postop analgesia, and catheter placement should be considered prior to inducing GA. The hand injury repair may be done concurrently with other procedures in multiple-trauma victims.

Induction	Rapid-sequence induction is mandatory in emergency cases, unless awake intubation is performed. C-spine fracture patients or those with facial injuries may require awake fiber optic intubation. Hemodynamically unstable, acute-trauma patients may be more safely induced with etomidate or ketamine.
Maintenance	Standard maintenance (p. B-3) for stable patients. Hemodynamically unstable, acute-trauma victims undergoing emergency surgery may be better served by using a combination of medications designed to have minimal hemodynamic consequences (e.g., fentanyl for analgesia, vecuronium for muscle relaxation and scopolamine or midazolam for amnesia). N_2O is best avoided in the unstable patient because of its myocardial depressant effects.
Emergence	Difficult airway or full-stomach cases require awake extubation. Trauma victims who have undergone a prolonged procedure or who have significant associated cardiopulmonary injuries are usually left intubated for postop mechanical ventilation.

Blood and fluid requirements	Significant blood loss IV: 16 ga × 1 NS/LR @ 1.5-3 ml/kg/h + replacement of blood loss Fluid/blood warmers, heating blanket, warmed circuit humidifier	A 16 ga iv catheter in nonoperated upper extremity should be adequate in hemodynamically stable patients. Acute-trauma victims who are unstable require a minimum of 2 large-bore iv catheters.
Monitoring	Standard monitors (p. B-1)	Invasive hemodynamic monitoring should be considered in acute, multiple-trauma victims.
Positioning	✓ and pad pressure points. ✓ eyes.	
Complications	Hemodynamic instability	Previously unrecognized injuries (e.g., pneumothorax, cardiac tamponade, intracranial bleeding) should be considered as a cause of unexplained intraop hemodynamic instability in all acute-trauma victims.

POSTOPERATIVE

Complications	Sepsis ARDS	Many trauma victims survive the initial insult only to die later of sepsis or ARDS.

Pain management PCA (p. C-3)

Tests None routinely indicated.

References

1. Carr DB, Kwon J: Anesthesia techniques and their indications for upper limb surgery. In *Surgery of the Hand and Upper Extremity.* McGraw-Hill, New York: 1996, 199-39.
2. Cullings HM, Hendee WR: Radiation risks in the orthopaedic operating room. *Contemp Orthop* 1984; 8:48-52.
3. Green DP: *Operative Hand Surgery*, 3rd edition. Churchill Livingstone, New York: 1993.
4. Nicholls BJ, Cullen BF: Anesthesia for trauma. *J Clin Anesth* 1988; 1(2):115-29.
5. Ramamurthy S, Hickey R: Anesthesia. In *Operative Hand Surgery*, 3rd edition. Green DP, ed. Churchill Livingstone, New York: 1993, 25-52.
6. Soderstrom CA, Cowley RA: A national alcohol and trauma center survey. Missed opportunities, failures of responsibility. *Arch Surg* 1987; 122(9):1067-71.

POLLICIZATION OF A FINGER

SURGICAL CONSIDERATIONS

Description: This procedure is indicated in the infant with congenital absence or hypoplasia of the thumb. A normal finger with its tendon, nerve and vascular supply is shortened and rotated into the position of the thumb (Fig 10.1-3). Tendon transfers are performed to substitute for the absent or hypoplastic thenar muscles. These patients may have many other associated congenital anomalies, which should be ruled out prior to surgery.

Variant procedure or approaches: There are several different surgical techniques. They all share the basic transposition and rotation of the finger to the thumb position.

Usual preop diagnosis: Aplastic thumb; hypoplastic thumb; radial club hand

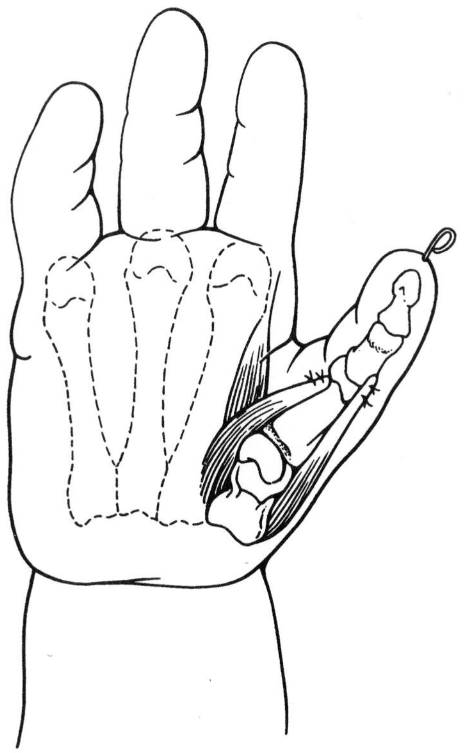

Figure 10.1-3. Pollicization of a finger. (Reproduced with permission from Green DP: *Operative Hand Surgery*, 3rd edition. Churchill Livingstone: 1993.)

SUMMARY OF PROCEDURE

Position	Supine, with arm extended on hand-surgery table
Incision	Multiple incisions on the hand
Special instrumentation	Pneumatic tourniquet
Antibiotics	Cefazolin 1 g iv
Surgical time	2-3 h
Tourniquet	150 mmHg above systolic; max time = 120 min
Closing considerations	Complex skin flaps are necessary. A plaster shell dressing (cast) is placed while the patient is still anesthetized.
EBL	Minimal; performed under tourniquet control.
Postop care	PACU → overnight admission for observation
Mortality	Minimal
Morbidity	Ischemia (loss of digit): Rare Skin flap necrosis: Moderately common
Pain score	1-2

PATIENT POPULATION CHARACTERISTICS

Age range	1-4 yr is ideal time for surgery. Procedure should be done before patient begins school.
Male:Female	1:1
Incidence	Overall, about 1/20,000 live births require a variant of this procedure.
Etiology	Unknown; also associated with thalidomide ingestion.
Associated conditions	Associated congenital anomalies of the upper extremity, spine and lower extremities Absence of radius (radial club hand), common Various forms of syndactylies, common Abnormalities of the hematopoietic system (Fanconi's syndrome), cardiovascular system (ASDs in Holt-Oram syndrome), spine, and GI system, along with hypothyroidism, are frequently associated.

ANESTHETIC CONSIDERATIONS

See Anesthetic Considerations following Pediatric Orthopedic Surgery for Pelvis and Extremities, p. 1020.

SYNDACTYLY REPAIR

SURGICAL CONSIDERATIONS

Description: Syndactyly refers to congenital failure of separation of two or more fingers. It is complete if it extends to the ends of the fingers; incomplete syndactyly extends short of the finger ends. A **simple syndactyly repair** joins fingers by only skin and fibrous tissues. A **complex syndactyly repair** signifies fusion of adjacent phalanges or interposition of accessory phalanges, with frequent abnormalities of the neurovascular structures.[2,4] Surgical separation is performed in the first few years of life for functional, as well as aesthetic reasons. The technique involves creation of a dorsal, proximally based skin flap to recreate the web.[1] A zigzag dorsal and palmar incision is then created, separating from the distal end in a proximal direction. The digital nerve and arteries are dissected proximally as far as possible. Primary closure is almost never possible, and supplemental full-thickness skin graft harvested from the groin is used to complete the closure. Usually only one site is done at a time per hand; and, never should both sides of a digit be released, because of risk to the vascular supply. It is not always possible to save all the bony elements.[2]

Usual preop diagnosis: Syndactyly of fingers; bifid finger, thumb/finger

SUMMARY OF PROCEDURE

Position	Supine
Incision	Zigzag between digits; skin graft donor site from groin
Special instrumentation	Magnification loupes always necessary. Tourniquet is mandatory.
Unique considerations	Groin skin also must be taken for graft closure.
Antibiotics	Usually none
Surgical time	2-4 h
Closing considerations	Above-the-elbow cast to keep incision away from mouth and other hand of the infant or child
EBL	< 20 ml
Postop care	PACU → home, if simple syndactyly
Mortality	Rare
Morbidity	Partial slough of flaps or skin graft Scarring and some stiffness of fingers Angulatory deformities late, occasionally depending on bony elements
Pain score	1-3

PATIENT POPULATION CHARACTERISTICS

Age range	6 mo-5 yr
Male:Female	2:1
Incidence	1/2000 births (the most common significant congenital hand anomaly)
Etiology	Family Hx (10-40%); failure of differentiation in the 6th-8th wk of intrauterine life
Associated conditions	Polydactyly, accessory phalanges; Apert's syndrome; Poland's syndrome

ANESTHETIC CONSIDERATIONS

See Anesthetic Considerations for Pediatric Orthopedic Surgery for Pelvis and Extremities, p. 1020.

References

1. Bauer TB, Tondra JM, Trusler HM: Technical modification in repair of syndactylism. *Plast Reconstr Surg* 1956; 17:385-92.
2. Chapman MW: *Operative Orthopaedics*, 2nd edition. JB Lippincott, Philadelphia: 1993, 1555-58.
3. Flatt AE: *The Care of Congenital Hand Anomalies*. CV Mosby, St. Louis: 1977, 170-212.
4. Morrissy RT: *Atlas of Pediatric Orthopaedic Surgery*. JB Lippincott, Philadelphia: 1992, 703-6.

Surgeon

Amy L. Ladd, MD

10.2 SHOULDER SURGERY

Anesthesiologists

Talmage D. Egan, MD
Jeffrey D. Swenson, MD

SHOULDER ARTHROSCOPY

SURGICAL CONSIDERATIONS

Description: Advances in shoulder arthroscopy permit many procedures to be performed primarily or adjunctively through the arthroscope, replacing a number of procedures that previously were performed through open techniques. The advantages include minimal incisions, decreased postop morbidity and potentially faster rehabilitation. Arthroscopy is frequently employed for diagnostic purposes prior to an open procedure. Diagnostically, the most common uses include verifying a tear of the rotator cuff, capsule or labrum. Examination of the glenohumeral joint and the subacromial bursa also can be performed. Therapeutically, arthroscopy can be used for irrigation in sepsis, synovectomy for rheumatoid arthritis or synovial chondromatosis. It can assist an open procedure, such as limited rotator cuff repair, after the deep and superficial aspects of the tear are identified.[1,2,3,5] Definitive procedures may include anterior stabilization procedures and subacromial decompression in conjunction with a distal clavicle resection. Most surgeons use the lateral decubitus position with the arm abducted approximately 45°, elevated approximately 20° with 5-15 lb of traction applied. The semisitting position, also known as the "beach-chair" or "barber-chair" position,[1] minimizes problems of traction on the brachial plexus seen in the decubitus position. In the beach-chair position, the patient is seated upright, approximately 70° to the horizontal, somewhat more upright than for open shoulder procedures.[2] The surgeon may request a MAP $\leq$ 80 to minimize subacromial bleeding.

Initially, an 18 ga spinal needle is inserted into the glenohumeral joint, passing through the posterior deltoid and infraspinatus muscle and the posterior capsule of the joint (see shoulder anatomy, Fig 10.2-1). Placement is verified by injecting saline to inflate the joint capsule. A stab incision is made using a No. 11 blade in the direction previously

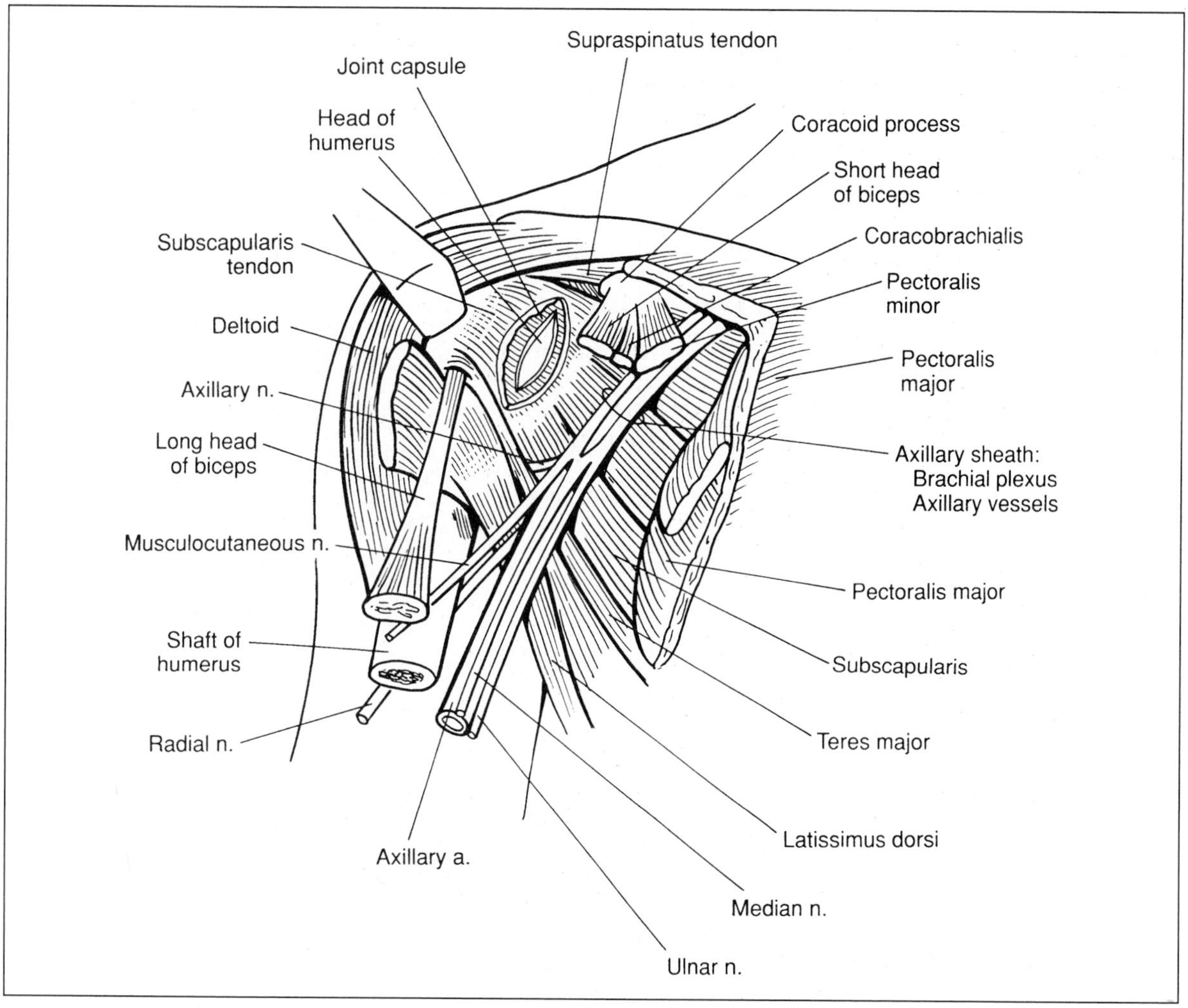

Figure 10.2-1. Anatomy of the shoulder joint, anterior. (Reproduced with permission from Hoppenfeld S, deBoer P, eds: *Surgical Exposures in Orthopaedics: The Anatomic Approach*. JB Lippincott: 1984.)

defined by the finder needle. Sharp, then blunt trocars are used to gain access to the joint and permit insertion of the arthroscopic device. Improper insertion of the instruments can injure the axillary or suprascapular nerves and the cartilage of the glenohumeral joint. An additional anterior portal is used for instrumentation; an anterolateral portal is employed for access to the subacromial space. The joint is continuously irrigated with a LR solution, usually containing epinephrine (1 mg/3 L). At the end of the procedure, the portals are infiltrated with local anesthetic and a drain may be placed within the depth of the wound. The arm is typically placed in a sling or a sling-and-swathe-type immobilization and neurovascular integrity is assessed.

Usual preop diagnosis: Rotator cuff tear; subacromial impingement; glenohumeral instability

SUMMARY OF PROCEDURE

Position	Lateral decubitus or semisitting (beach-chair or barber-chair)[2]
Incision	Posterior arthroscopic portal, anterior instrumentation portal, lateral instrumentation portal for visualizing subacromial bursa; superior portal for semisitting position
Special instrumentation	Arthroscope; power burrs; cutting devices; holmium laser
Unique considerations	Rigid eye patch over ipsilateral eye to prevent corneal abrasion suggested. Positioning of the head with appropriate support, removing upper section of operating table, if possible, for better access with semisitting position. ETT taped to opposite side of face. MAP ≤ 80. VAE possible.
Antibiotics	Cefazolin 1 g iv preop, particularly if bone work performed.
Surgical time	Positioning the patient is time-intensive; can add as much as 45 min. Diagnostic: < 1-1.5 h Reconstructive: 1-4 h
EBL	Minimal – 200 ml (less with use of epinephrine, electrocautery and laser)
Postop care	Frequently outpatient; may be overnight if interscalene or supraclavicular block is given or reconstructive procedure performed.
Mortality	Rare
Morbidity	Extravasation of fluid (NS or LR): > 50% Brachial plexus injury (lateral decubitus position): 5-25% Breakage of instruments: < 1% Infection: 0.04-3.49%
Pain score	5 (diagnostic); 7-8 (reconstruction)

PATIENT POPULATION CHARACTERISTICS

Age range	15-40 yr (instability); 35-75 yr (rotator cuff and acromial pathology)
Male:Female	2:1-4:1
Incidence	Very common – > 50,000/yr
Etiology	Young patients: usually sports-related Older patients: cuff and acromial pathology; age-wear phenomenon Rotator cuff pathology and acromial impingement (frequently coexist)
Associated conditions	Cervical arthritis and radiculopathy with rotator cuff pathology

ANESTHETIC CONSIDERATIONS

See Anesthetic Considerations following Surgery for Shoulder Dislocations or Instability, p. 709.

References

1. Altchek DW, Carson EW: Arthroscopic acromioplasty. Current status. *Orthop Clin Am* 1997; 20(2)157-68.
2. Altchek DW, Warren RF, Skyhar MJ: Shoulder arthroscopy. In *The Shoulder*. Rockwood CA Jr, Matsen FA III, eds. WB Saunders Co, Philadelphia: 1990, 258-77.
3. Bigliani LU, Flatow EL, Deliz ED: Complications of shoulder arthroscopy. *Orthop Rev* 1991; 20(9):743-51.
4. Matthews LS, Fadale PD: *Technique and Instrumentation for Shoulder Arthroscopy: Instructional Course Lectures*. American Academy of Orthopedic Surgeons, Park Ridge, IL: 1989, Vol 38.
5. Segmuller HE, Hays MG, Saies MD: Arthroscopic repair of glenolabral injuries with an absorbable fixation device. *J Shoulder Elbow Surg* 1997; 6(4):383-92.

SURGERY FOR ACROMIAL IMPINGEMENT, ROTATOR CUFF TEARS AND ACROMIOCLAVICULAR DISEASE

SURGICAL CONSIDERATIONS

Description: The terms "acromial impingement," "rotator cuff disease" and "acromioclavicular disease" frequently are used interchangeably, representing a continuum of disease and coexisting conditions, manifest in the fifth decade or later. "Bursitis," "rotator cuff tendinitis" or "bicipital tendinitis" are frequently the first presenting symptoms before a frank rotator cuff tear occurs.

Acromial impingement: Subacromial spurs are associated with subacromial or subdeltoid bursitis and possibly related to outer-thickness rotator cuff tears.

Rotator cuff tears: The rotator cuff is a confluence of four tendons supporting the glenohumeral joint: the subscapularis anteriorly and the supraspinatus, including infraspinatus and teres minor posteriorly. The most common site for rotator cuff tear is the supraspinatus tendon. Rotator cuff repair requires a deltoid-splitting incision. Care is taken not to extend the split more than 5 cm distal to the acromion because of possible injury to the axillary nerve, which innervates the deltoid 5 cm or more from the lateral aspect of the acromion.

Acromioclavicular disease: Acromioclavicular arthritis is frequently associated with this disease, particularly in the older population. "Acromioclavicular arthritis" also can occur in athletes as a result of trauma. An oblique, lateral or saber-type incision is used (see Fig 10.2-1 for shoulder anatomy). Traction of the arm is typically required to identify the extent of acromial impingement or acromioclavicular disease. Similarly, rotation of the arm is required to visualize the extent of the rotator cuff tear. The shoulder girdle is well vascularized; blood loss from these procedures is greater than that from arthroscopy, but usually less than 500 ml. On completion of the procedure, a drain is placed, and a sling-and-swathe-type immobilization splint is applied. Care must be taken in moving the patient. Adequate neuromuscular relaxation permits safe application of dressing and splints (particularly important for rotator cuff repairs).

Usual preop diagnosis: Rotator cuff tears (partial or complete); acromioclavicular disease; impingement; bursitis; bicipital tendinitis

SUMMARY OF PROCEDURE

Position	Semisitting, approximately 40-70°; or lateral decubitus
Incision	Oblique, saber-type incision anteriorly over distal acromion; lateral or deltopectoral incision for wider exposure. Deltoid-splitting incision for rotator cuff tears.
Special instrumentation	Power equipment for bone work; self-retaining retractors for cuff repairs
Unique considerations	Rigid eye protection for ipsilateral eye and careful head positioning
Antibiotics	Cefazolin 1 g iv preop
Surgical time	1-3 hrs
Closing considerations	Muscle relaxation when mobilizing cuff and during closure. Arm in sling and swathe, or abduction pillow for large tears. Immobilizer should be positioned prior to awakening patient to minimize potential for rupture of repair.
EBL	200-400 ml
Postop care	Maintenance of position in sling and swathe; no active motion of shoulder girdle for 2 d - 6 wk, depending on procedure.
Mortality	Rare
Morbidity	Infection: 1-5%
	Breakage of instruments: < 1%
Neurologic morbidity	Axillary nerve damage: < 2%
	Musculocutaneous nerve damage: < 2%
	Brachial plexus damage (position-dependent)
Pain score	5-8

PATIENT POPULATION CHARACTERISTICS

Age range	Rotator cuff tears > 40 yr (younger for athletes)
Male:Female	3:1
Incidence[3,4]	5-30% of general population affected by rotator cuff and acromial conditions, depending on age, thickness of tear, associated conditions
Etiology	Age-related; trauma (70% involved in light work)
Associated conditions	Bursitis; tendinitis; impingement; rotator cuff disease (especially in first-time glenohumeral dislocations > 40 yr); diabetes and renal failure; hypermobility

ANESTHETIC CONSIDERATIONS

See Anesthetic Considerations following Surgery for Shoulder Dislocations or Instability, p. 709.

References

1. Ellman H, Hanker G, Bayer M: Repair of the rotator cuff. End-result study of factors influencing reconstruction. *J Bone Joint Surg* 1986; 68(8): 1136-44.
2. Flatow EL, Altchek DW, Gartsman GM, Ionnotti JP, et al: The rotator cuff. Commentary. *Orthop Clin North Am* 1997; 28(2): 177-94.
3. Ionnotti JP, ed.: *Rotator cuff disorders: evaluation and treatment.* American Academy of Orthopaedic Surgeons, Park Ridge, 1991.
4. Neer CS II: Impingement lesions. *Clin Orthop* 1983; 173:70-7.
5. Tubiana R, McCullough CJ, Masquelet AC: *An Atlas of Surgical Exposures of the Upper Extremity.* JB Lippincott, Philadelphia: 1990.

SURGERY FOR SHOULDER DISLOCATIONS OR INSTABILITY

SURGICAL CONSIDERATIONS

Description: Younger patients, particularly athletes and patients with hypermobility problems, are the most prone to this condition. Recurrent anterior dislocations are the most common, followed by anterior-inferior (A-I) and posterior dislocations, frequently a manifestation of multidirectional instability. First-time dislocators > 40 yr of age have a high incidence of associated rotator cuff tears, while second-time dislocators have a significantly increased chance of recurrent dislocations. Posterior dislocation is most commonly associated with grand mal seizures, significant trauma and multidirectional instability. Frequently, examination under anesthesia will precede the open procedure to better assess the plane of instability.

Typically, the patient is in the semisitting position to allow access to the anterior, lateral and posterior aspects of the glenohumeral joint. Most commonly, the joint is accessed through a deltopectoral (anterior) incision, between the level of the coracoid proximally and the deltopectoral interval distally. Access to the posterior aspect of the glenohumeral joint is through a longitudinal posterolateral incision. In the case of the anterior approach (Fig 10.2-1), the coracobrachialis tendon is retracted medially, and the deltoid is retracted laterally. The joint is entered through a capsular incision and stabilization is performed. Stabilization may require repair of the torn capsule and labrum (**Bankart repair**). A soft-tissue anchor or screw may be inserted to reattach the torn capsule. Or, less frequently, a bone block of the tip of the coracoid with its tendon may be moved to the front of the joint, serving as a sling to prevent dislocations (**Bristow repair**). A drain is placed, and the arm is immobilized. Before awakening the patient, the surgeon will identify special considerations, including the placement of a special brace or splint, and careful positioning to prevent a dislocation.

Usual preop diagnosis: Fractures; Hill-Sachs lesion; glenohumeral instability; A-I dislocation; posterior dislocation

SUMMARY OF PROCEDURE

	Glenohumeral Instability	Anterior-Inferior, Posterior Dislocations
Position	"Beach-chair" or semisitting	Lateral decubitus for posterior stabilization
Incision[5,9]	Deltopectoral	A-I, posterior – splitting of the infraspinatus and teres minor; transverse or longitudinal; posterior – inferior axillary incision
Special instrumentation	Power equipment; special bone-anchoring sutures; glenoid and humeral instrumentation	–
Antibiotics	Cefazolin 1 g iv preop if bone work performed.	⇐
Surgical time	2-4 h	⇐

	Glenohumeral Instability	Anterior-Inferior, Posterior Dislocations
Closing considerations	Repair of cuff, sling and swathe or abduction pillow, as dictated by surgical findings.	⇐
EBL	200-400 ml	⇐
Postop care	No active motion for 6 wk	⇐
Mortality	Minimal	⇐
Morbidity	Axillary nerve palsy: 15% (may be preexisting)	Suprascapular nerve injury
Pain score	8	8

PATIENT POPULATION CHARACTERISTICS

Age range	15-35 yr
Male:Female	1:1
Incidence	Common
Etiology	Trauma; hypermobility; seizures
Associated conditions	Rotator cuff tears; hypermobility syndrome; seizure disorder

ANESTHETIC CONSIDERATIONS

(Procedures covered: shoulder arthroscopy; surgery for acromial impingement, rotator cuff tears and acromioclavicular disease; surgery for shoulder dislocations or instability)

PREOPERATIVE

Typically, three patient populations present for repair of rotator cuff tears or arthroscopy: (1) healthy posttrauma, (2) nonrheumatoid arthritic and (3) rheumatoid arthritic. Individuals presenting for repair of shoulder dislocations also may include those with a joint hypermobility syndrome (e.g., Marfan or Ehlers-Danlos) or seizure disorder patients.

Respiratory Arthritic patients may exhibit Sx of pleural effusion or pulmonary fibrosis. Hoarseness may indicate cricoarytenoid joint (CAJ) involvement → difficult intubation. (See Anesthetic Considerations for Wrist Procedures, p. 683) Seizure disorder patients who suffer from recurrent shoulder dislocation as a result of frequent grand mal seizures also may suffer from occult aspiration pneumonia or pneumonitis.

Tests: Consider CXR; PFTs; ABGs in debilitated rheumatoid patients

Cardiovascular Arthritic patients may suffer from chronic pericardial effusions, valvular disease and cardiac conduction defects. Patients presenting for shoulder stabilization because of joint hypermobility syndromes are likely to have valvular dysfunction and are vulnerable to aortic dissection 2° HTN. These patients may require antibiotic prophylaxis for bacterial endocarditis.

Tests: Consider ECG, ECHO in patients with severe rheumatoid arthritis. Recent ECHO to assess valve function and aortic root size indicated in most patients with Marfan syndrome.

Neurological Arthritic patients may have cervical or lumbar radiculopathies that should be documented carefully preop. For example, head flexion may cause cervical cord compression. Patients with severe seizure disorders can suffer from recurrent shoulder dislocations 2° frequent violent grand mal seizures. Such patients should be maximally treated for seizure disorder prior to elective surgery. Be aware that as many as 15% of shoulder dislocations can be accompanied by axillary nerve palsy, which should be documented carefully preop.

Tests: Consider C-spine radiographs to rule out occult subluxations in arthritic patients with neck complaints or upper extremity radiculopathy. Verify therapeutic levels of antiepileptic medication in seizure disorder patients.

Musculoskeletal Arthritic patients may have limited neck and jaw ROM and may require fiber optic intubation techniques. Bony deformities or muscle contractures may necessitate special attention to positioning. Patients with joint hypermobility syndromes presenting for shoulder surgery may also suffer other joint dislocations 2° positioning problems.

Hematologic Virtually all patients will be on some type of anti-inflammatory medication that may result in anemia or Plt inhibition. Ideally, patients should discontinue NSAIDs at least 5 d preop; aspirin,

Hematologic, cont.	7 d. In addition, selected patients with Ehlers-Danlos are known to have severe coagulation defects that may preclude the use of regional anesthesia. **Tests:** A coagulation profile is mandatory in Ehlers-Danlos patients.	
Endocrine	Rheumatoid patients are likely to be on oral corticosteroids and, thus, require supplemental perioperative steroids (e.g., 100 mg hydrocortisone q 8 h iv) to treat adrenal suppression.	
Laboratory	Hb/Hct (in healthy patients); other tests as indicated from H&P. Patients with Ehlers-Danlos syndrome should always have banked blood available for surgery, except for the most trivial of procedures.	
Premedication	Moderate-to-heavy premedication (e.g., in adults, midazolam 1 mg iv q 5 min titrated to effect) is often desirable prior to placement of regional block.	

INTRAOPERATIVE

Anesthetic technique: GETA or regional anesthesia, or a combination of the two techniques, can be used. The interscalene approach to the brachial plexus is excellent for surgical procedures on the shoulder, either alone or in combination with GA. When logistically feasible, the combined technique is ideal. Unless contraindicated, a long-acting local anesthetic such as bupivacaine should be used in regional anesthesia for shoulder surgery to ameliorate postop pain.

General anesthesia:

Induction	Standard induction (see p. B-2). Arthritic patients may require awake fiber optic intubation.
Maintenance	Standard maintenance (see P. B-3).
Emergence	Management of emergence and extubation should be routine, except in difficult airway cases which require awake extubation.

Regional anesthesia:

Interscalene block	Anesthetics and doses (epinephrine [2.5-5 μg/ml] should be added to local anesthetic whenever possible to decrease peak plasma concentrations): • 3% 2-chloroprocaine 30-40 ml for procedures lasting < 1 h. • 1.5% lidocaine or mepivacaine 30-40 ml for procedures lasting up to 2.5 h. • 1% etidocaine or 0.5% bupivacaine 30-40 ml for procedures lasting > 2.5 h. The skin on the top of the shoulder (C3-C4) and the medial aspect of the upper arm (T2) often require separate subcutaneous field blocks. Phrenic nerve block → hemidiaphragmatic paralysis is an inevitable consequence of the interscalene block, which may not be tolerated by patients with significant preexisting respiratory compromise. Major complications, such as total spinal or pneumothorax resulting from interscalene block, are extremely rare; therefore, this technique is suitable for use in outpatients. Interscalene block is contraindicated in patients with contralateral recurrent laryngeal nerve or phrenic nerve palsy (e.g., post CABG). If sedation is needed, midazolam (0.5-1.0 mg boluses), alfentanil (0.125-0.25 μg/kg/min by infusion) or propofol (50-100 μg/kg/min by infusion), given initially in subanesthetic doses and thereafter titrated to effect, are good choices.

Blood and fluid requirements	Minimal-to-moderate blood loss IV: 18 ga × 1 NS/LR @ 1.5-3 ml/kg/h	IV catheter placed in contralateral upper extremity.
Monitoring	Standard monitors (see p. B-1). ± Precordial Doppler ± Arterial line	To help detect VAE, consider precordial Doppler monitoring when semisitting position used. Consider intraarterial BP monitoring for patients with hypermobility disorders because of risk for aortic dissection 2° HTN.
Positioning	✓ and pad pressure points. ✓ eyes. ↑VAE risk in semisitting position	Postural hypotension is the most common complication of the semisitting position. Changing to this position gradually can help prevent hypotension, as can the use of antiembolism stockings, plus fluid-loading the patient. Marfan and Ehlers-Danlos patients require very gentle positioning to prevent joint dislocations.
Interscalene block complications	Total spinal Accidental epidural injection	Resuscitative equipment, including airway management tools, should be immediately available.

Interscalene block complications, cont.	IV injection (seizures/dysrhythmias) Stellate ganglion block (Horner's syndrome) Laryngeal nerve block Phrenic nerve block Pneumothorax	
Other complications	Hypotension during surgical prep and positioning	Hypotension during long surgical preps normally can be avoided by using light inhalation anesthesia (e.g., isoflurane 0.3-0.5%) to ensure amnesia, with moderate muscle relaxation to prevent bucking on the ETT, and maintaining adequate hydration. Antiembolism stockings will help prevent venous pooling in lower limbs.
	Cardiac dysrhythmia VAE	Dysrhythmias may be 2° to irrigation fluids containing epinephrine.

POSTOPERATIVE

Pain management	PCA (see p. C-3) or regional block techniques.	Combined regional-general anesthetic techniques are excellent for shoulder procedures, especially with respect to postop pain management.
Tests	None indicated routinely.	

References

1. Balas GI: Regional anesthesia for surgery on the shoulder. *Anesth Analg* 1971; 50(6):1036-41.
2. Carron H: Regional anesthesia for upper extremity surgery symposium. *Reg Anesth* 1980; 5:2-9.
3. Dolan P, Sisko F, Riley E: Anesthetic considerations for Ehlers-Danlos syndrome. *Anesthesiology* 1980; 52(3):266-69.
4. Gill TJ, Micheli LJ, Gebhard F, Binder C: Bankart repair for anterior instability of the shoulder. Longterm outcome. *J Bone Joint Surg Am* 1997; 79(6):850-57.
5. Hoppenfeld S: Surgical Exposures in Orthopaedics: *The Anatomic Approach*, 2nd edition. Hoppenfeld S, deBoer P, eds. JB Lippincott, Philadelphia: 1994.
6. Keenan MA, Stiles CM, Kaufman RL: Acquired laryngeal deviation associated with cervical spine disease in erosive polyarticular arthritis. *Anesthesiology* 1983; 58(5):441-49.
7. Reginster JY, Damas P, Franchimont P: Anaesthetic risks in osteoarticular disorders. *Clin Rheum* 1985; 4:30-8.
8. Salathe M, Johr M: Unsuspected cervical fractures: a common problem in ankylosing spondylitis. *Anesthesiology* 1989; 70(5):869-70.
9. Tubiana R, McCullough CJ, Masquelet AC: *An Atlas of Surgical Exposures of the Upper Extremity.* JB Lippincott, Philadelphia: 1990.
10. Urmey WF, Talts KH, Sharrock NE: One hundred percent incidence of hemidiaphragmatic paresis associated with interscalene brachial plexus anesthesia as diagnosed by ultrasonography. *Anesth Analg* 1991; 72(4):498-503.
11. Verghese C: Anaesthesia in Marfan's syndrome. *Anaesthesia* 1984; 39(9):917-22.
12. Wells DG, Podolakin W: Anaesthesia and Marfan's syndrome: case report. *Can J Anaesth* 1987; 34(3+Pt 1):311-14.
13. White RH: Preoperative evaluation of patients with rheumatoid arthritis. *Semin Arthritis Rheum* 1985; 14(4):287-99.
14. Winnie AP: Interscalene brachial plexus block. *Anesth Analg* 1970; 49(3):455-66.

SHOULDER (GLENOHUMERAL) ARTHROPLASTY

SURGICAL CONSIDERATIONS

Description: Shoulder joint replacement is most commonly performed for end-stage arthritis or following trauma. Osteoarthritis is far less common in the glenohumeral joint than in the hip and knee joints. Inflammatory conditions, such as rheumatoid arthritis and psoriatic arthritis, may require shoulder replacement for correction and pain relief, and are frequently associated with massive rotator cuff tears.

Hemiarthroplasty, or replacement of the humeral side only, is commonly done for osteoarthritis. Comminuted fractures about the shoulder joint may require **arthroplasty**, particularly in the older patient. As with total hip and total knee replacements, bone cement (polymethylmethacrylate), as well as special implants for improved bone fixation, may be used.

The most common type of arthroplasty is the **unconstrained** (separate glenoid and humeral components), while **constrained** or **hinged devices** rarely are used. During arthroplasty, the humeral component is placed within the shaft of the humerus after the humeral head is removed. The glenoid component requires resurfacing of the glenoid, the most difficult aspect of this procedure. Similar to other total joint replacements, revision surgery may be required, adding to the operative time and blood loss.

Through a deltopectoral incision (Fig 10.2-1), the interval between the coracoid and the deltoid insertion are developed. This is followed by making an oblique incision of approximately 10 cm between the deltoid muscle and the pectoralis muscle. The coracobrachialis tendon is retracted, the capsule of the glenohumeral joint is divided and the joint is identified. Removal of the humeral head is performed, and the humeral component is replaced. If the glenoid is replaced, the surface is fashioned to accept a glenoid component. Similar to total hip surgery, this requires sizing of the canal of the humerus, as well as determining the size and position of the humeral head and the size of the glenoid cavity. A provisional reduction is performed, with the humeral component or the humeral and glenoid components in place, at which time the fit is preliminarily assessed. Cement (polymethylmethacrylate) may be used for fixing the components in place. Following final positioning, the joint is reduced and the wound is closed over suction drainage. The shoulder girdle is well vascularized and blood loss may exceed a unit. A sling-and-swathe-type immobilization is applied; revision surgery may require a special splint. A specific program of protected rehabilitation typically lasts 6-12 wk.

Usual preop diagnosis: Osteoarthritis; inflammatory arthritis; trauma

SUMMARY OF PROCEDURE

Position	Semisitting
Incision	Deltopectoral incision or extended incision
Special instrumentation	Glenoid and humeral instrumentation, in addition to usual shoulder instruments; mixing and introduction of cement
Unique considerations	Systemic illnesses of the patient; systemic complications of use of cement in the patient; precautions in pregnant staff working with methylmethacrylate; usage of laminar flow or UV lighting for total joint precautions, depending on the surgeon's preference and capabilities of the OR.
Antibiotics	Cefazolin 1 g iv preop, if bone work performed.
Surgical time	2-5 h
Closing considerations	Drain; sling and swathe
EBL	200-1000 ml
Postop care	No postop active motion for approximately 4-6 wk
Mortality	< 1%
Morbidity	Blood loss Nerve injury Hypotension Infection
Pain score	8

PATIENT POPULATION CHARACTERISTICS

Age range[3]	45-80 yr
Male:Female	1:1
Incidence	Uncommon
Etiology	Osteoarthritis; inflammatory arthritis; trauma; avascular necrosis; systemic disease
Associated conditions	Inflammatory disease; systemic disease; alcoholism; rotator cuff pathology; arthritis and radiculopathy; cervical arthritis

ANESTHETIC CONSIDERATIONS

PREOPERATIVE

Typically, three patient populations present for shoulder arthroplasty: (1) healthy posttrauma, (2) nonrheumatoid arthritic and (3) rheumatoid arthritic.

Respiratory Rheumatoid arthritic patients may exhibit Sx of pleural effusion or pulmonary fibrosis. Hoarseness may indicate cricoarytenoid joint (CAJ) involvement → difficult intubation. (See Anesthetic Considerations for Wrist Procedures, p. 683.)
Tests: Consider CXR; PFTs; ABGs in debilitated rheumatoid patients

Cardiovascular Rheumatoid arthritic patients may suffer from chronic pericardial effusions, valvular disease and cardiac conduction defects.
Tests: Consider ECG and ECHO in patients with severe rheumatoid arthritis.

Neurological Arthritic patients may have cervical or lumbar radiculopathies that should be documented carefully preop. For example, head flexion may cause cervical cord compression.
Tests: C-spine radiographs to rule out occult subluxations in rheumatoid patients with neck complaints or upper extremity radiculopathy

Musculoskeletal Arthritic patients may have limited neck and jaw ROM that may require special intubation techniques. Bony deformities or muscle contracture may necessitate special attention to positioning.

Hematologic Virtually all nontrauma patients will be on some type of anti-inflammatory medication that may result in anemia or Plt inhibition. Ideally, patients should discontinue NSAIDs at least 5 d preop.

Endocrine Rheumatoid patients are likely to be on oral corticosteroids and, thus, require supplemental perioperative steroids (e.g., 100 mg hydrocortisone q 8 h iv) to treat adrenal suppression.

Laboratory Hb/Hct (healthy patients); other tests as indicated from H&P.

Premedication Moderate-to-heavy premedication (e.g., midazolam 0.5-1 mg iv q 5 min titrated to effect) is desirable if regional block is done.

INTRAOPERATIVE

Anesthetic technique: GETA or regional anesthesia, or a combination of the two, can be used. The interscalene approach to the brachial plexus is excellent for surgical procedures on the shoulder, either alone or in combination with GA. Unless contraindicated, a long-acting local anesthetic such as bupivacaine should be used in regional anesthesia for shoulder surgery to ameliorate postop pain.

General anesthesia:

Induction Standard induction (see p. B-2). Rheumatoid patients may require awake fiber optic intubation.

Maintenance Standard maintenance (see p. B-3). Because of the typically long duration of these cases, the opioid selected as part of the balanced anesthetic technique is best given, perhaps, by continuous infusion (e.g., iv sufentanil [0.25-1.0 μg/kg/h]). Some surgeons prefer muscle relaxation beyond that provided by volatile anesthetic.

Emergence Management of emergence and extubation should be routine except in difficult airway cases which require awake extubation. Emergence from anesthesia should be delayed until patient's shoulder is securely immobilized in the sling and swathe to prevent undesired movement of the newly placed prosthesis.

Regional anesthesia:

Interscalene block Typical anesthetics and doses. Note that epinephrine [2.5-5 μg/ml] should be added to the local anesthetic whenever possible to decrease peak plasma concentrations:
- 1.5% lidocaine or mepivacaine 30-40 ml for procedures lasting up to 2.5 h.
- 1% etidocaine or 0.5% bupivacaine 30-40 ml for procedures lasting > 2.5 h.

The skin on the top of the shoulder (C3-C4) and the medial aspect of the upper arm (T2) often require separate subcutaneous field blocks. Phrenic nerve block → hemidiaphragmatic paralysis is

Interscalene block, cont.	an inevitable consequence of the interscalene block, which may not be tolerated by patients with significant preexisting respiratory compromise. Major complications, such as total spinal or pneumothorax resulting from interscalene block, are extremely rare. Interscalene block is contraindicated in patients with contralateral recurrent laryngeal nerve or phrenic nerve palsy. If sedation is needed, midazolam (0.5-1.0 mg boluses), alfentanil (0.125-0.25 μg/kg/min by infusion) or propofol (50-100 μg/kg/min by infusion), given initially in subanesthetic doses, and thereafter titrated to effect, are good choices.	
Blood and fluid requirements	Moderate-to-significant blood loss IV: 16 ga × 1 NS/LR @ 1.5-3.0 ml/kg/h	RBC recovery and reinfusion techniques (e.g., Cell Saver) are advisable because blood loss can be considerable. IV in nonoperated upper extremity.
Monitoring	Standard monitors (see p. B-1). Precordial Doppler	Consider invasive, hemodynamic monitoring in the debilitated or elderly patient. Since VAE is a possible complication of the semisitting position, consider using precordial Doppler for cases done in this position.
Positioning	✓ and pad pressure points. ✓ eyes. ↑VAE risk	Postural hypotension is the most common complication of the semisitting position. Changing patient to this position gradually can help prevent hypotension, as can the use of antiembolism stockings and fluid-loading the patient.
Interscalene block complications	Total spinal Epidural anesthesia IV injection (seizures/dysrhythmias) Stellate ganglion block (Horner's syndrome) Laryngeal nerve block Phrenic nerve block Pneumothorax	Resuscitative equipment, including airway management tools, should be immediately available.
Other complications	Potential for embolic event Hypotension during prep and positioning	Because of the increased risk of VAE during shoulder arthroplasty, N_2O may be D/C'd during placement of humeral component. Use of methylmethacrylate cement has been associated with the sudden onset of hypotension and even cardiac arrest, presumably due to profound vasodilation ± associated VAE. ↓BP during long surgical prep usually can be avoided by using light inhalation anesthesia (isoflurane 0.3-0.5%) to ensure amnesia, with moderate muscle relaxation to prevent bucking on ETT, and maintaining adequate hydration.

POSTOPERATIVE

Pain management	PCA (see p. C-3) or regional block techniques.	Combined regional-general anesthetic techniques are excellent for shoulder procedures, especially with respect to postop pain management.
Tests	None indicated routinely.	

References

1. Andersen KH: Air aspirated from the venous system during total hip replacement. *Anaesthesia* 1983; 38(12):1175-78.
2. Balas GI: Regional anesthesia for surgery on the shoulder. *Anesth Analg* 1971; 50(6):1036-41.
3. Cofield RH: Degenerative and arthritic problems of the glenohumeral joint. In *The Shoulder*. Rockwood CA Jr, Matsen FA III, eds. WB Saunders Co, Philadelphia: 1990, 678-749.
4. Keenan MA, Stiles CM, Kaufman RL: Acquired laryngeal deviation associated with cervical spine disease in erosive polyarticular arthritis. *Anesthesiology* 1983; 58(5):441-49.
5. Neer CS II, Watson KC, Stanton FJ: Recent experience in total shoulder replacement. *J Bone Joint Surg* [Am] 1992; 64:319-37.

6. Newens AF, Volz RG: Severe hypotension during prosthetic hip surgery with acrylic bone cement. *Anesthesiology* 1972; 36(3):298-300.
7. Reginster JY, Damas P, Franchimont P: Anaesthetic risks in osteoarticular disorders. *Clin Rheum* 1985; 4:30-8.
8. Salathe M, Johr M: Unsuspected cervical fractures: a common problem in ankylosing spondylitis. *Anesthesiology* 1989; 70(5):869-70.
9. White RH: Preoperative evaluation of patients with rheumatoid arthritis. *Semin Arthritis Rheum* 1985; 14(4):287-99.

SHOULDER GIRDLE PROCEDURES

SURGICAL CONSIDERATIONS

Description: Trauma about the shoulder girdle in young patients ranges from athletic injuries to life-threatening trauma. Some of these injuries include common athletic injuries such as **acromioclavicular joint separations** which rarely require surgery unless there is associated **acromial** or **clavicular fractures. Posterior sternoclavicular dislocations** may warrant surgical stabilization if the trachea is compressed. **Clavicle fractures**, frequently associated with **scapular fractures**, occasionally require open reduction.

Scapular fractures involving the glenoid also may require surgical stabilization. Extreme fractures involving the shoulder girdle (**scapulothoracic dissociations**) include scapular fracture, clavicle fracture, subclavian or axillary artery disruption and brachial plexus injury. These may coexist with **proximal humerus fractures**, rib fractures and pneumothorax. In the older, debilitated patient, the most common injury is proximal humeral fracture, which may be amenable to surgical stabilization, or may be so comminuted as to warrant hemi- or total arthroplasty.

For each of these fractures, the incision is made over the appropriate site, the fracture or dislocation is identified and reduced under manual or manipulative traction, and appropriate fixation proceeds. For instance, a displaced proximal humerus fracture in a young person may require fixation with a plate and screws through a deltopectoral approach (see Surgery for Shoulder Dislocations or Instability, p. 708, and Shoulder Arthroplasty, p. 711). A scapular fracture in a scapulothoracic dissociation would be stabilized with a plate and screws via a posterior approach (see Surgery for Shoulder Dislocations or Instability, p. 708) after vascular repair of the subclavian artery and fixation of the clavicle, if necessary. Typically, a sling or sling-and-swathe-type immobilization is required. As with other shoulder procedures, relaxation is necessary upon awakening the patient.

Usual preop diagnosis: Trauma about the shoulder girdle

SUMMARY OF PROCEDURE

	Anterior	Posterior
Position	Semisitting or prone	Lateral decubitus (scapula)
Incision	Anterior, superior or oblique for acromioclavicular; supraclavicular for clavicle; deltopectoral for proximal humerus and glenoid	Posterior lateral border or medial border of scapula, spinous scapula, depending on location
Special instrumentation	Plates and screws; tension band wiring for comminuted fractures	⇐
Unique considerations	Multiple trauma warrants early stabilization; may require vascular repair and brachial plexus exploration.	⇐
Antibiotics	Cefazolin 1 g iv	⇐
Surgical time	2-10 h	⇐
Closing considerations	Fracture-dependent; most commonly requires application of sling-and-swathe.	⇐
EBL	200-1200 ml or greater, depending on trauma	⇐

	Anterior	Posterior
Postop care	May require ICU for multiple-trauma patients.	⇐
Mortality	Mortality dependent on associated conditions: Infection Neurologic injury Respiratory failure Massive blood loss Unrecognized pneumothorax Cardiac tamponade	⇐
Morbidity	Nerve injury (axillary, brachial plexus)	Axillary and suprascapular
	Stiffness	⇐
	Poor healing	⇐
Pain score	6-10	6 (clavicle and AC joint); 8 (scapula and proximal humerus)

PATIENT POPULATION CHARACTERISTICS

Age range	15-80 yr, depending on nature of trauma
Male:Female	5:1
Incidence	Common
Etiology	Trauma
Associated conditions	Axillary nerve palsy; musculocutaneous nerve palsy; brachial plexus injury; arterial disruption in high-energy trauma; brachial and great vessel injuries and posterior sternoclavicular dislocation pneumothorax

ANESTHETIC CONSIDERATIONS

See Anesthetic Considerations following Brachial Plexus Surgery, p. 717.

References

1. Collins DN, Harryman DT II: Arthroplasty for arthritis and rotator cuff deficiency. *Orthop Clin North Am* 1997; 20(2):225-39.
2. Imatani RJ: Fractures of the scapula: a review of 53 fractures. *J Trauma* 1975; 15(6):473-78.
3. Neer CS II: Fractures about the shoulder. In *Fractures in Adults*. Rockwood CA Jr, Green DP, eds. JB Lippincott, Philadelphia: 1984, 713-21.
4. Neer CS II and Rockwood CA Jr: Fractures and dislocations of the shoulder. In *Fractures in Adults*. Rockwood CA Jr, Green DP, eds. JB Lippincott, Philadelphia: 1984, 675-985.
5. Neviaser RJ: Injuries to the clavicle and acromioclavicular joint. *Orthop Clin North Am* 1987; 18(3):433-38.
6. Richards RR, Sherman RM, Hudson AR, Waddell JP: Shoulder arthrodesis using a pelvic-reconstruction plate. A report of eleven cases. *J Bone Joint Surg* [Am] 1988; 70(3):416-21.
7. Rockwood CA Jr: Injuries to the sternoclavicular joint. In *Fractures in Adults*. Rockwood CA Jr, Green DP, eds. JB Lippincott, Philadelphia: 1992, 910-48.
8. Rockwood CA Jr, Matsen FA III, eds: *The Shoulder*. WB Saunders Co, Philadelphia, 1990.

BRACHIAL PLEXUS SURGERY

SURGICAL CONSIDERATIONS

Description: Brachial plexus injuries occur most commonly in two groups: traumatic birth injuries and high-energy trauma. Surgery ranges from exploration with neurolysis to repairs to cable nerve grafting. Typically, the latter requires grafting with the sural nerve, and nerve pedicle transfer, such as transfer of the spinal accessory nerve to denervated paralyzed muscle, combined with muscle transfers. C5-C6 is most commonly injured in obstetrical (Erb's) palsy. Injuries in adults are more commonly closed-traction. Similar to obstetrical palsy, they occur with an outstretched, abducted arm with the neck rotated in the opposite direction. The most severe form includes complete avulsion at the preganglionic level, presenting with a Horner's syndrome, winging of the scapula and a flail arm. These are typically "supraclavicular" injuries, and have a poorer prognosis. Surgical exposure may proceed above the clavicle similar to an anterior neck dissection, or may require an extension below the clavicle. Occasionally, an osteotomy of the clavicle for extensive dissection is required. For axillary nerve dissection, a posterior approach is also used. Open injuries, such as gunshot or knife wounds, are typically "infraclavicular" and have a better prognosis. (See diagram of brachial plexus, Fig 10.2-2.)

Usual preop diagnosis: Obstetrical palsy; adult trauma – most commonly motorcycle accident

SUMMARY OF PROCEDURE

Position	Lateral decubitus or semisitting
Incision	Supra- or infraclavicular, extensile to include deltopectoral incision. Clavicle osteotomy incision will provide for improved exposure. Supraclavicular incision used for supraclavicular brachial plexus.
Special instrumentation	Nerve stimulator
Unique considerations	Associated trauma
Antibiotics	Cefazolin 1 g iv preop
Surgical time	4-10 h
Closing considerations	Other incisions if nerve grafts obtained.
EBL	400-2000 ml
Mortality	Minimal
Morbidity	Bleeding Hematoma Pneumothorax Clavicular nonunion
Pain score	8

PATIENT POPULATION CHARACTERISTICS

Age range	Infants and children: 3 mo-8 yr; adults: 20-40 yr
Male:Female	Adult: 5:1
Incidence	Infants: 0.3-8/1000 births; adults: Commonly associated with motorcycle accidents
Etiology	Obstetrical palsy; trauma
Associated conditions	None known

ANESTHETIC CONSIDERATIONS

(Procedures covered: shoulder girdle procedures; brachial plexus surgery)

PREOPERATIVE

With the exception of traumatic birth injuries, most of these patients are healthy males who have suffered major blunt or penetrating trauma. For the acute and subacute trauma victim, the major anesthesia-related concerns center around associated traumatic injuries. Many adult trauma victims with brachial plexus injuries will be operated on in the first few days after their injury. For infants (usually operated on at 6-12 mo), the major anesthesia-related concerns are those routinely associated with pediatric anesthesia. Approximately half of all trauma victims are intoxicated. The anesthesia-related implications of ethanol intoxication include: decreased anesthetic requirements, diuresis, vasodilation and hypothermia.

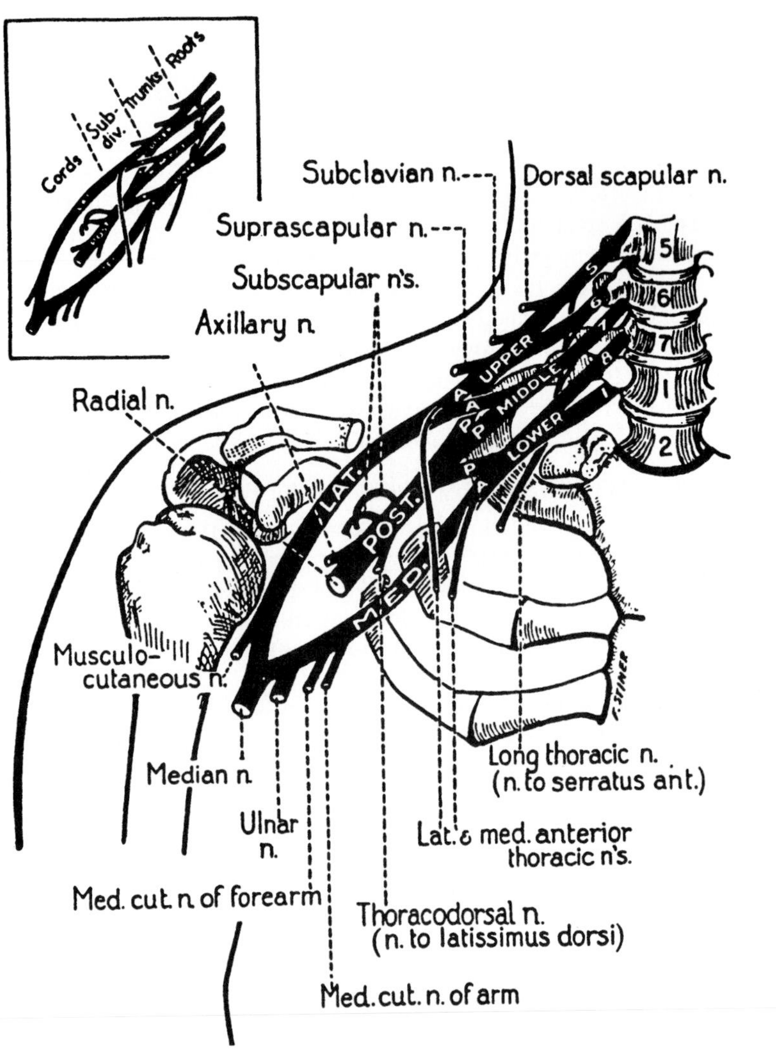

Figure 10.2-2. Diagram of the brachial plexus. (Reproduced with permission from Haymaker W, Woodhall B: *Peripheral Nerve Injuries*. WB Saunders: 1956.)

Respiratory As suggested by coexisting disease or acute trauma injuries. Look for evidence of occult chest injury, including pneumothorax (tachypnea, wheezing, ↓BP, ↓PaO_2, CXR changes) and pulmonary contusion (multiple rib fracture, ↓PaO_2).

Tests: Consider CXR and ABGs in victims of significant trauma; other tests as indicated from H&P.

Cardiovascular As suggested by coexisting disease or acute trauma injuries. Look for evidence of occult cardiac or mediastinal injuries, such as myocardial contusion (e.g., ECG abnormalities typically consistent with ischemia) or great vessel rupture (e.g., widened mediastinum).

Tests: Consider CXR (with NG tube in place to access mediastinal widening) and ECG in victims of significant trauma; others as indicated from H&P.

Neurological Victims of shoulder trauma are vulnerable to brachial plexus damage. Look for evidence of upper extremity nerve dysfunction and document any injuries preop. The possibility of closed-head injury also should be considered.

Tests: Head CT prior to beginning a procedure under GA in a patient with evidence of head trauma.

Musculoskeletal As suggested by coexisting disease or acute trauma injuries. The amount of force necessary to produce a brachial plexus injury mandates a C-spine series to rule out C-spine fracture in all victims of brachial plexus trauma.

Laboratory In general, most victims of significant trauma are best served by obtaining a wide variety of baseline lab studies to screen for unrecognized injury. These studies generally should include: Hct; CBC; ABGs; UA; renal function tests; LFTs; serum amylase.

Premedication None

INTRAOPERATIVE

Anesthetic technique: GETA is preferred over regional techniques because of the unpredictable and prolonged length of these procedures and the need to evaluate brachial plexus function postop.

Induction Rapid-sequence induction is mandatory in unscheduled cases, unless awake FOL intubation is performed (see Anesthetic Considerations for Thoracolumbar Neurosurgical Procedures in Neurosurgery, p. 64). C-spine fracture patients or those with facial injuries may require awake fiber optic intubation or other special airway techniques as indicated from H&P. Hemodynamically unstable, acute-trauma patients can be induced more safely with etomidate (0.3-0.4 mg/kg iv) or ketamine (1-3 mg/kg iv).

Maintenance Balanced anesthesia with low-dose isoflurane (0.4-0.6%), iv sufentanil (0.25-1.0 μg/kg/h) and N_2O in O_2 is suitable for stable patients. Hemodynamically unstable, acute-trauma victims undergoing emergency surgery are not likely to tolerate this regimen and are better served by using a combination of medications designed to have minimal hemodynamic consequences (e.g., fentanyl for analgesia, vecuronium for muscle relaxation and scopolamine or midazolam for amnesia). N_2O, with its myocardial depressant effects, is best avoided in the unstable patient. For brachial plexus surgery, some surgeons prefer minimal muscle relaxation after tracheal intubation so that a nerve stimulator can be used to help identify surgical anatomy.

Emergence Management of emergence and extubation should be routine except in difficult airway or full-stomach cases, which require that extubation be delayed until the patient's airway reflexes have returned and the patient is fully awake.

Blood and fluid requirements	Significant blood loss IV: 14-16 ga × 1-2 NS/LR @ 1.5-3 ml/kg/h + replacement of blood loss @ 3 × volume Fluid warmer Airway humidifier	IV catheter placed in the nonoperated upper extremity is usually adequate in hemodynamically stable patients. Unstable, acute-trauma victims require a minimum of 2 large-bore iv catheters.
Monitoring	Standard monitors (see p. B-1). ± SSEP	Invasive hemodynamic monitoring should be considered in acute, multiple-trauma victims. Some surgeons request SSEP to make continuous assessment of preop intact brachial plexus possible. When using SSEP monitoring, high doses of volatile anesthetic agents should generally be avoided because they adversely affect SSEP readings.
Positioning	✓ and pad pressure points. ✓ eyes. VAE risk	Postural hypotension is the most common complication of the semisitting position, particularly during the surgical prep period. SCD or antiembolism stockings may be beneficial. VAE is a potential complication of this position.
Complications	Hemodynamic instability	Previously unrecognized injuries (e.g., pneumothorax, cardiac tamponade, intracranial bleeding) should be considered as a cause of unexplained intraop hemodynamic instability in all acute-trauma victims.
	Possible VAE	VAE risk is increased with patient in semisitting position.

POSTOPERATIVE

Complications	Sepsis ARDS	Many trauma victims survive the initial insult only to die later of sepsis or ARDS.
Pain management	PCA (see p. C-3).	
Tests	None routinely indicated.	

References

1. Balas GI. Regional anesthesia for surgery on the shoulder. *Anesth Analg* 1971; 50(6):1036-41.

2. Grundy BL: Intraoperative monitoring of sensory-evoked potentials. *Anesthesiology* 1983; 58(1):72-87.
3. Leifert RD: Neurological problems. In *The Shoulder.* Rockwood CA Jr, Matsen FA III, eds. WB Saunders Co, Philadelphia: 1990, 750-58.
4. Mahla ME, Long DM, McKennett J, Green C, McPherson RW: Detection of brachial plexus dysfunction by somatosensory evoked potential monitoring–a report of two cases. *Anesthesiology* 1984; 60(3):248-52.
5. Nanakas AO: Injuries to the brachial plexus. In *The Pediatric Upper Extremity: Diagnosis and Treatment.* Bora FW Jr, ed. WB Saunders Co, Philadelphia: 1986, 247-58.
6. Nicholls BJ, Cullen BF: Anesthesia for trauma. *J Clin Anesth* 1988; 1(2):115-29.
7. Soderstrom CA, Cowley RA: A national alcohol and trauma center survey. Missed opportunities, failures of responsibility. *Arch Surg* 1987; 122(9):1067-71.
8. Thompson RW, Petrinec D, Toursarkissian B: I. Surgical treatment of thoracic outlet compression syndromes. II. Supraclavicular exploration and vascular reconstruction. *Ann Vasc Surg* 1997; 11(4):442-51.

ARM SURGERY

SURGICAL CONSIDERATIONS

Description: Surgical procedures on the arm are primarily for trauma or tumor surgery. Other procedures include extended approaches from the shoulder for significant trauma or tendon transfer. Exploration of peripheral nerves, most commonly of the radial nerve, are also included in this category, as are distal extensile approaches from the elbow for trauma or for lateral epicondylitis ("tennis elbow"). Depending on the lesion or fracture, the incision is developed through an internervous or intramuscular compartment. Procedures include **excisional biopsy** for soft tissue or bone tumors of the arm; **tumor excision**, which may be marginal, wide or radical, depending on the tumor encountered; **tendon transfers**, such as pectoralis transfer to replace biceps function, used primarily for brachial plexus injuries; **fractures and nonunion fractures of the humerus** and other bony procedures. Depending on the location of pathology, appropriate incisions as outlined are used.

Usual preop diagnosis: Trauma; tumor

SUMMARY OF PROCEDURE

Position	Supine; semisitting position for extended deltopectoral; lateral decubitus
Incision	Anterolateral approach; posterior approach in the lateral decubitus position
Special instrumentation	Plate and screws; external fixators; IM rods; occasionally, PMMA (methylmethacrylate cement) for tumor surgery
Unique considerations	CT-guided sclerotherapy preop for vascular tumors. Longitudinal incisions for biopsy and tumor excisions (not violating fascial planes).
Antibiotics	Cefazolin 1 g iv preop
Surgical time	45 min-4 h
Closing considerations	Drain frequently required.
EBL	Minimal-500+ ml, depending on pathology
Mortality	Varies with pathology
Morbidity	Bleeding Shoulder stiffness Nerve injury
Pain score	4-7

PATIENT POPULATION CHARACTERISTICS

Age range	Varies with procedure
Male:Female	Varies with procedure
Incidence	Procedure-dependent
Etiology	Fractures; nerve entrapment (radial) following trauma; tumors
Associated conditions	Radial nerve injury with humeral fractures

ANESTHETIC CONSIDERATIONS

PREOPERATIVE

With the exception of tumor patients, the majority of patients presenting for arm procedures are relatively young and healthy. Most of these patients present for elective repair of a traumatic injury; thus, the preop workup is routine. Some arm procedures, such as repair of a compound fracture, require immediate attention and necessitate emergency surgery and full-stomach considerations.

Laboratory Hb/Hct (healthy patients); other tests as indicated from H&P.

Premedication Moderate-to-heavy premedication (e.g., midazolam 0.5-1.0 mg iv q 5 min titrated to effect) is often desirable if regional block is used.

INTRAOPERATIVE

Anesthetic technique: GETA or regional anesthesia, or a combination of the two, can be used for surgical procedures on the arm. A brachial plexus block via the supraclavicular approach is excellent for procedures on the distal arm. The interscalene approach to the brachial plexus is perhaps best for more proximal procedures near the shoulder. Regional anesthesia alone is a means of avoiding the risk of aspiration pneumonitis associated with GA in the patient with a full stomach.

General anesthesia:

Induction Standard induction (see p. B-2) except in acute-trauma patients, where rapid-sequence induction is appropriate (see p. B-5).

Maintenance Standard maintenance (see p. B-3).

Emergence Management of emergence and extubation should be routine, except in difficult airway cases, which require awake extubation. Skin closure is frequently followed by application of a splint; patient should remain anesthetized during splinting procedure.

Regional anesthesia:

Interscalene block Typical anesthetics and doses. Note that the addition of epinephrine [2.5-5 μg/ml] will reduce peak plasma anesthetic concentrations:

- 3% 2-chloroprocaine 30-40 ml for procedures lasting < 1 h.
- 1.5% lidocaine or mepivacaine 30-40 ml for procedures lasting up to 2.5 h.
- 1% etidocaine or 0.5% bupivacaine 30-40 ml for procedures lasting > 2.5 h.

Skin on the top of the shoulder (C3-C4) and the medial aspect of the upper arm (T2) often require separate subcutaneous field blocks. Phrenic nerve block → hemidiaphragmatic paralysis is an inevitable consequence of the interscalene block, which may not be tolerated by patients with significant preexisting respiratory compromise. Major complications (e.g., total spinal or pneumothorax) resulting from interscalene block, are very rare; therefore, this technique is suitable for outpatients. Interscalene block is contraindicated in patients with contralateral recurrent laryngeal nerve or phrenic nerve palsy. If sedation is needed, midazolam (0.5-1.0 mg boluses), alfentanil (0.125-0.25 μg/kg/min by infusion) or propofol (50-100 μg/kg/min by infusion) given initially in subanesthetic doses, and thereafter titrated to effect, are good choices.

Supraclavicular block 1.5% mepivacaine or lidocaine 40 ml for routine cases. 1% etidocaine 40 ml for procedures estimated to last > 2.5 h. The upper arm medial aspect is innervated by the intercostobrachial nerve (T2) and requires a separate subcutaneous field block in the axilla, especially with tourniquet use.

Supplemental sedation Supplemental sedation may be accomplished with use of propofol by continuous infusion (50-150 μg/kg/min) or intermittent bolus injection of opioid/benzodiazepine (e.g., midazolam 0.5-1.0 mg iv q 5 min and alfentanil 5-10 μg iv q 5 min) titrated to effect.

Blood and fluid requirements Minimal blood loss
IV: 18 ga × 1
NS/LR @ 1.5-3 ml/kg/hr

IV catheter should be placed in the contralateral upper extremity.

Monitoring Standard monitors (see p. B-1).

Positioning ✓ and pad pressure points.
✓ eyes.

Complications: Interscalene block	Total spinal Epidural anesthesia IV injection (seizures/dysrhythmias) Stellate ganglion block (Horner's syndrome) Laryngeal nerve block Phrenic nerve block Pneumothorax	Resuscitative equipment, including airway management tools, should be immediately available.
Supraclavicular block	Inadequate block Intravascular injection Peripheral nerve damage Hematoma Horner's syndrome Phrenic nerve paralysis Recurrent laryngeal nerve paralysis Pneumothorax	If accidental intraarterial injection occurs, minimal doses of local anesthetic can cause CNS toxicity. Pneumothorax is an important concern when the supraclavicular approach is used. A large pneumothorax may become symptomatic quickly; most take many hours to develop and may be without Sx. The possibility of pneumothorax associated with the supraclavicular block makes this approach less suitable for use with outpatient procedures.

POSTOPERATIVE

Pain management	PCA (see p. C-3). ± Regional block	Combined regional-general anesthesia is excellent for arm procedures, especially with respect to postop pain management.
Tests	None routinely indicated.	

References

1. Henry AK: *Extensile Exposure*, 2nd edition, Churchill Livingstone, Edinburgh: 1973.
2. Hoppenfeld S, deBoer, eds: *Surgical Exposures in Orthopaedics: The Anatomic Approach.* JB Lippincott, Philadelphia: 1984.
3. Moorthy SS, Schmidt SI, Dierdorf SF, Rosenfeld SH, Anagnostou JM: A supraclavicular lateral paravascular approach for brachial plexus regional anesthesia [see comments]. *Anesth Analg* 1991; 72(2):241-44.
4. Moran MC: Modified lateral approach to the distal humerus for internal fixation. *Clin Orthop* 1997; (340):190-97.

Surgeons

John J. Csongradi, MD
(Knee, Lower Leg, Ankle/Foot Procedures)
Stuart B. Goodman, MD, MSC, FRCS(C), FACS
(Hip, Pelvis, Upper Leg, Knee Procedures)

10.3 SURGERY OF THE LOWER EXTREMITIES

Anesthesiologist

Frederick G. Mihm, MD

OPEN REDUCTION AND INTERNAL FIXATION (ORIF) OF PELVIS OR ACETABULUM

SURGICAL CONSIDERATIONS

Description: ORIF procedures of the acetabulum and pelvis are some of the most challenging operations in orthopedic surgery. They are long and tedious procedures, requiring special training, several surgical assistants, and a whole armamentarium of plates, screws, reduction clamps and different devices. The patient usually arrives in OR in balanced traction, with either a tibial or femoral traction pin. Stabilization of anterior pelvic ring (pubic symphysis) may be performed acutely by the orthopedic surgeon, using plates and screws applied to the pubic rami during **exploratory laparotomy** by a general/trauma surgeon. The procedures involve obtaining a reduction by open means through one or more long incisions.

Anterior approaches to the pelvis include the suprapubic Pfannenstiel's incision for plating the symphysis, and the ilioinguinal and iliofemoral incisions for reaching the anterior and medial portion of the acetabulum. Lateral approaches to the acetabulum may be combined with a **trochanteric osteotomy**, for wider exposure. Posterior incisions over the buttock expose the posterior column and also can be combined with a trochanteric osteotomy for wider exposure of the acetabular dome. **Extensile exposures** utilize larger dissections in order to visualize both anterior and posterior columns of the acetabulum and pelvis. The aim is to secure a congruous, anatomically sound reduction that is maintained by the application of plates and screws. Bone grafting is used to bridge defects. The patient is usually on protected, weight-bearing crutches for several months in the postop period. (Also see Closed Reduction and External Fixation of Pelvis, p. 729.)

Usual preop diagnosis: Fractures of pelvis/acetabulum; nonunion/malunion of the pelvis/acetabulum

SUMMARY OF PROCEDURE

Position	Supine (anterior); lateral decubitus (transtrochanteric); lateral decubitus or prone (posterior)
Incision	Ilioinguinal, iliofemoral over hip joint (anterior); straight lateral, posterior with anterior extension (with transtrochanteric); posterolateral (posterior)
Special instrumentation	Fracture table; plates, screws, reduction clamps, etc. Cell Saver recommended.
Antibiotics	Cefazolin or cefamandole 1 g iv q 6-8 h × 48 h
Surgical time	3-6 h (anterior); 4-6 h (with transtrochanteric); 3-6 h (posterior)
Closing considerations	May require reapplication of balanced traction.
EBL	1000 ml or more
Postop care	Multiple-trauma victim → ICU; others → PACU
Mortality	10%+, dependent on extent of multiple trauma
Morbidity	Ileus: Virtually 100%
	Sacroiliac pain (pelvic fractures): 25-50%
	Lumbosacral plexus or sciatic nerve injury (usually peroneal branch): 15-25%
	Heterotrophic ossification: 10-25% (↓with NSAIDs)
	Avascular necrosis: 5-20%
	Genitourinary problems, including bladder and urethral rupture: 5-15%
	Gynecological and colorectal injuries: 3-7%
	Leg-length discrepancy: 3-5%
	Nonunion: 3-5%
	Vascular complications: 1%
	Respiratory distress: Common
	Delayed union: Not uncommon
	Osteomyelitis
	↓BP 2° to retroperitoneal hematoma: Not uncommon
	Malunion: Not uncommon
	Residual instability: Not uncommon
	Rupture of diaphragm: Rare
Pain score	9

PATIENT POPULATION CHARACTERISTICS

Age range	Any age, but predominance of males < 30 yrs
Male:Female	5:1
Incidence	1-2%
Etiology	Motorcycle and motor vehicle accidents (60-80%); falls (10-15%); crush injury (5%); others (5%)
Associated conditions	Frequently associated with trauma to other organ systems, including head and neck, chest, abdomen and extremities. These often will be addressed concurrently with pelvic or acetabular fracture.

ANESTHETIC CONSIDERATIONS

See Anesthetic Considerations for Procedures About the Pelvis and Hip, p. 731.

References

1. Bucholz RW, Brumback RJ: Fractures of the shaft of the femur. In *Fractures in Adults*, 4th edition. Rockwood CA Jr, Green DP, Bucholz RW, Heckman JD, eds. JB Lippincott, Philadelphia: 1996, 1827-1918.
2. Burgess AR, Tile M: Fractures of the pelvis. In *Fractures in Adults*, 3rd edition. Rockwood CA Jr, Green DP, Bucholz RW, eds. JB Lippincott, Philadelphia 1991, 1399-1479.
3. Guyton JL: Fractures of hip, acetabulum, and pelvis. In *Campbell's Operative Orthopaedics*, 9th edition. Canale ST, ed. Mosby-Year Book, St. Louis: 1998, Vol 3, 2181-2280.
4. Jones A, Reinert C, Bucholz R: Complications of fractures of the pelvic ring and acetabulum. In *Complications in Orthopaedic Surgery*, 3rd edition. Epps CH Jr, ed. JB Lippincott, Philadelphia: 1994, 749-62.
5. LaVelle DG: Delayed union and nonunion of fractures. In *Campbell's Operative Orthopaedics*, 9th edition. Canale ST, ed. Mosby-Year Book, St. Louis: 1998, Vol 3, 2537-78.
6. Mears DC, Rubash HE: *Pelvic and Acetabular Injuries*. Slack Inc., Thorofare NJ: 1986.
7. Tile M: *Fractures of the Pelvis and Acetabulum*, 2nd edition. Williams and Wilkins, Baltimore: 1995, 549-54.

OSTEOTOMY AND BONE GRAFT AUGMENTATION OF THE PELVIS

SURGICAL CONSIDERATIONS

Description: Patients undergoing this procedure have acetabular insufficiency (acetabular dysplasia), i.e., poor coverage of the femoral head by the acetabulum without advanced arthrosis of the hip. The aim of the operation is to expand the bony roof of the acetabulum to enable a broader contact surface for the hip joint. In children, bone grafting alone may be sufficient; in adults, however, cutting of the pelvis (osteotomy) to reorient or broaden the weight-bearing surface is necessary. A supplemental bone graft to expand the weight-bearing surface may be added. The osteotomy usually is fixed internally with screws or pins to allow early mobilization without displacement. Weight-bearing is permitted after healing of the osteotomy—about 8 wk postop.

Usual preop diagnosis: Acetabular dysplasia or deficiency; subluxation of the hip

SUMMARY OF PROCEDURE

Position	Supine
Incision	Anterior: ilioinguinal or iliofemoral
Special instrumentation	Pelvic retractors; power or Gigli saw; screws and other instrumentation
Unique considerations	Intraop radiographs
Antibiotics	Cefazolin or cefamandole 1 g iv q 6-8 h × 48 h
Surgical time	3 h
EBL	500+ ml
Postop care	PACU → room; usually on protected, weight-bearing walker or crutches × 8 wk
Mortality	Minimal
Morbidity	Ileus: 100% Leg-length discrepancy: Uniformly present after pelvic osteotomy Neurological deficit: Injury to lateral cutaneous nerve: Common (50%) Sciatic nerve: Uncommon (1%) Thromboembolism: 5-10% Wound infection: Septic arthritis, osteomyelitis: 1-7% Delayed union, nonunion, malunion: 1-2% Genitourinary problems—urinary retention requiring catheterization: Common Hematoma: Common Hypotension 2° to retroperitoneal hematoma: Rare Vascular complications: Rare
Pain score	8

PATIENT POPULATION CHARACTERISTICS

Age range	0-50 yrs
Male:Female	3-4 × higher incidence in females for congenital hip dysplasia; equal incidence for other causes
Etiology	Congenital hip dysplasia; neuromuscular disorders—cerebral palsy, meningomyelocele; pediatric trauma to acetabular growth plate
Associated conditions	Depends on etiology (e.g., neuromuscular disorder)

ANESTHETIC CONSIDERATIONS

See Anesthetic Considerations for Procedures About the Pelvis and Hip, p. 731.

References

1. Chiari K: Iliac osteotomy in young adults. In *The Hip: Proceedings of the 7th Open Meeting of the Hip Society*. CV Mosby, St. Louis: 1979, 260-77.
2. Salter RB, Thompson GH: The role of innominate osteotomy in young adults. *In The Hip: Proceedings of the 7th Open Meeting of the Hip Society*. CV Mosby, St. Louis: 1979, 278-312.
3. Sutherland DH, Greenfield R: Double innominate osteotomy. *J Bone Joint Surg* [Am] 1977; 59(8):1082-91.

ARTHRODESIS OF THE SACROILIAC JOINT

SURGICAL CONSIDERATIONS

Description: In this procedure, a painful and/or unstable sacroiliac (SI) joint is fused, usually by excising the joint through a **posterior approach** and employing an iliac crest bone graft. Supplemental screw fixation of the joint often is used. The SI joint may be exposed through a dorsal vertical incision directly over the posterior pelvis. The posterior muscles are reflected from the medial aspect of the pelvis, and the SI joint is easily identified. The joint is debrided of cartilage and packed with strips of cancellous bone. Alternatively, the procedure may be performed through an **anterior approach**, sweeping the abdominal contents medially and approaching the SI joint anteriorly. The incision follows just inferior to the iliac crest; and the abdominal muscle insertions are detached from the iliac crest. The pelvis is exposed subperiosteally, posterior to the SI joint. Then the joint cartilage is excised and packed with cancellous bone strips.

Variant procedure or approaches: Anterior or posterior approach

Usual preop diagnosis: Arthritis or arthrosis of the SI joint; pelvic instability

SUMMARY OF PROCEDURE

Position	Usually prone; rarely supine (when concomitantly fixing an acetabular fracture through an anterior approach)
Incision	Posterior, usually; anterior, rarely
Special instrumentation	Special pelvic retractors, screws and plates; intraop x-ray
Unique considerations	Intraop radiographs or use of image intensifier
Antibiotics	Cefazolin or cefamandole 1 g iv q 6-8 h × 48 h)
Surgical time	2-3 h
EBL	250-500 ml
Postop care	Usually on protected, weight-bearing walker or crutches × 6-8 wk
Mortality	Extremely low
Morbidity	Ileus: Virtually always Osteomyelitis: < 1% Wound infection: < 1% Genitourinary problems; urinary retention requiring catheterization: Common Delayed union, nonunion, malunion, leg-length discrepancy: Not uncommon Neurological deficit; injury to lumbosacral plexus: Rare, unless present preop; L5 nerve root susceptible in anterior approaches Hypotension 2° to retroperitoneal hematoma: Rare Injury to bowel: Rare Vascular complications; injury to iliac arteries: Rare Thromboembolism
Pain score	7

PATIENT POPULATION CHARACTERISTICS

Age range	20-50 yr
Male:Female	Increased incidence in males (trauma)
Incidence	Rare
Etiology	Trauma—postpelvic fracture dislocation; painful septic arthritis

ANESTHETIC CONSIDERATIONS

See Anesthetic Considerations for Procedures About the Pelvis and Hip, p. 731.

References

1. Christian CA, Donley BG: Arthrodesis of the ankle, knee and hip. In *Campbell's Operative Orthopaedics*, 9th edition. Crenshaw AH, ed. Mosby-Year Book, St. Louis: 1998, Vol 1, 145-88.
2. Guyton JL: Fractures of hip, acetabulum, and pelvis. In *Campbell's Operative Orthopaedics*, 9th edition. Crenshaw AH, ed. Mosby-Year Book, St. Louis: 1998, Vol 3, 2042-80.
3. Jones A, Reinert C, Bucholtz R: Complications of fractures of the pelvic ring and acetabulum. In *Complications in Orthopaedic Surgery*, 3rd edition. Epps CH Jr, ed. JB Lippincott, Philadelphia: 1994, 749-62.

CLOSED REDUCTION AND EXTERNAL FIXATION OF THE PELVIS

SURGICAL CONSIDERATIONS

Description: This procedure entails manipulating the pelvis to obtain an acceptable reduction by closed means under GA, and then applying an anterior external fixation device to maintain the reduction. The pins for the external fixator are inserted into the iliac crest either percutaneously or through small incisions. During this procedure, either radiographs or the image intensifier is used to confirm that an acceptable reduction has been obtained. In some centers, this procedure is done in the emergency department as a life-saving procedure.

Usual preop diagnosis: Displaced fracture of the pelvis; unstable fracture of the pelvis

SUMMARY OF PROCEDURE

Position	Supine
Incision	Done percutaneously or through small incisions along the iliac crest.
Special instrumentation	External fixation device of surgeon's choice; often performed on a radiolucent table using the image intensifier.
Antibiotics	Cefazolin or cefamandole 1 g iv q 6-8 h × 48 h. Combination antibiotics, if multiple severe, open fractures or other significant injuries are present.
Surgical time	1-1.5 h
EBL	Negligible from surgical procedure; however, anticipate large blood losses (4+ U) from the pelvic fracture alone.
Postop care	Multiple-trauma victim → ICU; others → PACU
Mortality	10% or more, depending on extent of multiple trauma; 50% in open fractures
Morbidity	Ileus: Virtually 100% SI pain: 15-30%+ Genitourinary problems, including bladder or urethral rupture: 13% Neurological deficit to lumbosacral plexus: 1-10% Malunion/severe deformity: 5% Leg-length discrepancy: 3-5% Impotence: 1-5% Residual instability: 1-3% Vascular complications: 1% Hypotension 2° to retroperitoneal hematoma: Common Respiratory distress: Common Gynecological and colorectal injuries: More common with open fractures/dislocations Delayed union, nonunion: Not uncommon Osteomyelitis: Rare Rupture of diaphragm: Rare
Pain score	7-10

PATIENT POPULATION CHARACTERISTICS

Age range	Any age, but predominance of males < 30 yr
Male:Female	5:1
Incidence	Common
Etiology	Motorcycle and motor vehicle accidents (60-80%); falls (10-15%); crush injury (5%); other (5%)
Associated conditions	Frequently associated with trauma to other organ systems, including head and neck, chest, abdomen and extremities. Patient sustaining a pelvic fracture also has a probability of having other injuries, including: musculoskeletal (85%); respiratory (60%); CNS (40%); GI (30%); urologic (12%); CVS (6%). These will often be addressed concurrently with the pelvic fracture.

ANESTHETIC CONSIDERATIONS

See Anesthetic Considerations for Procedures About the Pelvis and Hip, p. 731.

References

1. Bucholz RW, Brumback RJ: Fractures of the shaft of the femur. In *Fractures in Adults*, 4th edition. Rockwood CA Jr, Green DP, Bucholz RW, Heckman JD, eds. JB Lippincott, Philadelphia: 1996, 1827-1918.
2. Guyton JL: Fractures of hip, acetabulum, and pelvis. In *Campbell's Operative Orthopaedics*, 9th edition. Crenshaw AH, ed. Mosby-Year Book, St. Louis: 1998, Vol 3, 2042-80.
3. Jones A, Reinert C, Bucholtz R: Complications of fractures of the pelvic ring and acetabulum. In *Complications in Orthopaedic Surgery*, 3rd edition. Epps CH Jr, ed. JB Lippincott, Philadelphia: 1994, 749-62.
4. Mears DC, Rubash HE: *Pelvic and Acetabular Injuries*. Slack Inc, Thorofare NJ: 1986.
5. Tile M: *Fractures of the Pelvis and Acetabulum*, 2nd edition. Williams and Wilkins, Baltimore: 1995, 549-54.

AMPUTATIONS ABOUT THE HIP AND PELVIS: DISARTICULATION OF THE HIP AND HINDQUARTER AMPUTATION

SURGICAL CONSIDERATIONS

Description: These surgical procedures accomplish an excision of the entire lower extremity. In a **hip disarticulation**, the amputation is performed through the hip joint. An anterior, racquet-shaped incision is made and all muscles crossing the hip joint are incised or detached. The femoral artery, vein and nerve, obturator vessels, sciatic nerve and deep vessels are isolated and ligated. The gluteal flap is brought anteriorly and sewn to the anterior portion of the incision. In a **hindquarter amputation**, excision of the lower extremity, hip joint and a portion of the pelvis is performed. Anterior and posterior incisions are used; and the iliac wing is divided posteriorly and the symphysis pubis is disarticulated anteriorly. Either the common iliac or external iliac vessels are ligated, as are all nerves to the lower extremity. Usually the gluteal flap is drawn anteriorly for closure. These procedures are performed very rarely—for severe trauma, tumor or infection—and are often life-saving surgeries. They often are performed in conjunction with a general surgeon, and standard bowel prep is done. The operations are long and tedious, with extensive blood loss, in patients who are usually systemically ill.

Usual preop diagnosis: Malignant tumor of femur, hip or pelvis; traumatic amputation to femur, hip or pelvis; uncontrollable infection to leg, hip or pelvis (e.g., clostridia)

SUMMARY OF PROCEDURE

	Hip Disarticulation	Hindquarter Amputation
Position	Supine	Lateral decubitus; stabilized by bean bag and/or kidney rests.
Incision	Anterior racquet type (rare)	Anterior and posterior
Unique considerations	Urinary catheter should be placed.	Urinary catheter, NG tube; scrotum strapped to opposite thigh; anus stitched closed/sealed.
Antibiotics	Cefazolin or cefamandole 1 g iv q 6-8 h	⇐
Surgical time	3-4 h	4-5 h
EBL	1000-2000 ml (intraop blood salvage system recommended, except for tumors.)	2000-3000 ml
Postop care	ICU	⇐
Mortality	Rare in patients undergoing elective amputation for trauma or localized tumor; higher for patients with debilitated trauma, chronic infection or extensive invasive malignant tumor; highest in clostridial infections: ~50%+.	⇐
Morbidity	Anemia: Common	⇐
	Electrolyte abnormalities: Common	⇐
	Hematoma: Common	⇐

	Hip Disarticulation	Hindquarter Amputation
Morbidity, cont.	Neurological injury to lumbosacral plexus or peripheral nerves: Common	⇐
	Paralytic ileus: Common	⇐
	Psychosocial problems: Common	⇐
	UTI: Common	⇐
	Flap necrosis: Not uncommon	⇐
	Incomplete excision with recurrence of tumor or infection: Not uncommon	⇐
	Injury to peritoneal or retroperitoneal contents, including bowel and bladder: Not uncommon	⇐
	Vascular injury—iliac, other vessels: Not uncommon	⇐
Pain Score	10	10

PATIENT POPULATION CHARACTERISTICS

Age range	Any age
Male:Female	Similar, except higher incidence in males for traumatic etiologies
Incidence	Uncommon
Etiology	Malignant tumor; trauma; infection—clostridial myonecrosis, chronic osteomyelitis, etc.

ANESTHETIC CONSIDERATIONS FOR PROCEDURES ABOUT THE PELVIS AND HIP

(Procedures covered: ORIF of pelvis or acetabulum; osteotomy and bone graft augmentation of pelvis; arthrodesis of SI joint; closed reduction and external fixation of pelvis; amputations about hip and pelvis: disarticulation of hip and hindquarter amputation)

PREOPERATIVE

Patients presenting for pelvic surgery generally fall into two categories: 1) Major trauma—pelvic fracture requires substantial force and seldom occurs alone. These patients require aggressive fluid therapy with large-bore ivs and invasive monitors (arterial line and CVP). If the patient can be made hemodynamically stable with volume resuscitation, a thorough evaluation for coexisting neurological, thoracic or abdominal trauma should be undertaken prior to anesthesia. 2) Tumor resection and amputation of thigh, hip and pelvis. Because of large intraop blood loss and 3rd-spacing of fluids, invasive hemodynamic monitoring is necessary. Although epidural anesthesia is seldom adequate for surgery, postop epidural analgesia is an effective means of controlling the tremendous pain caused by this type of surgery. Other patient populations covered in this section include otherwise healthy patients with congenital or acquired hip dysplasia presenting for augmentation procedures.

Respiratory Trauma patients are at risk for hemothorax, pneumothorax, pulmonary contusion, fat embolism and aspiration. A chest tube will be needed prior to surgery if either a hemothorax or pneumothorax is present. Pulmonary fat embolus occurs in 10-15% of patients with long bone fractures, and can occur after isolated pelvic fractures. Sx include hypoxemia, tachycardia, tachypnea, respiratory alkalosis, mental status changes, conjunctival petechiae, fat bodies in the urine and diffuse pulmonary infiltrates. Sx of pulmonary aspiration are similar to those of fat embolism. Preop therapy for either should include supplemental O_2 to correct hypoxemia (may necessitate mechanical ventilation) and meticulous fluid management to prevent worsening of pulmonary capillary leak.
Tests: CXR, or others as indicated from H&P.

Cardiovascular Blunt chest trauma can produce both cardiac contusion and aortic tear. Preop ECG and CPK isoenzymes will help evaluate the presence of myocardial injury. A wide mediastinal silhouette suggests aortic tear, which requires evaluation with TEE or angiography.
Tests: Consider ECG; CPK isoenzymes; others as indicated from H&P.

Neurological The possibility of coexistent neurologic trauma necessitates a thorough preop mental status review

Neurological, cont.	and peripheral sensory exam. A CT scan of the head is indicated for any patient with loss of consciousness prior to anesthesia.
Musculoskeletal	For trauma patients, cervical spine films will evaluate the stability of the cervical spine prior to neck manipulation during ET intubation. Thoracic and lumbar x-rays also should be evaluated for the presence of traumatic spinal deformity or instability that would require special stabilization in the anesthetized patient. **Tests:** C-spine x-rays or others as indicated from H&P.
Hematologic	Restore Hct to 25% prior to inducing anesthesia. Have available 1 blood volume (70 ml/kg) or 1 total erythrocyte mass (20 ml/kg) for intraop transfusion. Transfusions of more than 1 blood volume will require monitoring and possible replacement of platelets and coagulation factors. The incidence of DVT is very high in these patients, and prophylaxis with SCDs or low-dose subcutaneous heparin is indicated whenever feasible.
Renal	Renal injury commonly results from trauma to the collecting system, myoglobinuria from rhabdomyolysis and ischemic, acute, tubular necrosis from hypovolemia or aortic dissection. Foley catheters should be placed only after urologic consultation for possible urethral tear. Suprapubic catheters are often necessary. Monitoring of UO is mandatory to detect intraop compromise of the collecting system, and to monitor adequacy of renal perfusion. **Tests:** Consider UA; BUN; creatinine; others as indicated from H&P.
Laboratory	Hct; electrolytes; other tests as indicated from H&P.
Premedication	Pain can be treated with morphine (1-2 mg iv q 10 min titrated to pain relief) prior to anesthesia.

INTRAOPERATIVE

Anesthetic technique: GETA is indicated due to the duration and extent of the surgery, as well as the varied positions that are necessary to accomplish pelvic fixation. Regional anesthesia is generally inadequate for major pelvic surgery; however, in elective surgeries, serious consideration should be given to postop epidural analgesia.

Induction	A rapid-sequence induction (see p. B-5) is necessary for trauma patients to minimize aspiration risk. Elective cases can undergo a standard induction (see p. B-2).
Maintenance	Standard maintenance (see p. B-3).
Emergence	Extubate trauma patients when fully awake and protective airway reflexes have returned. Do not extubate patients with evolving pulmonary injuries (fat embolism, aspiration or contusion). Monitoring in an ICU usually is indicated for trauma and cancer patients. Prolonged stays can be anticipated for patients with severe coexistent trauma.

Blood and fluid requirements	Large blood loss IV: 14-16 ga × 2 NS/LR @ 8-12 ml/kg/h 2-4 U PRBC in OR Warm fluids. Humidify gases.	Expect large blood losses (from 0.5-2 or more blood volumes) with all but augmentation procedures. Cell scavenging techniques are useful to reduce the requirement for blood. Care should be taken to ensure that cells have been adequately washed to minimize ↓BP on reinfusion.
Control of blood loss	Deliberate hypotension Hemodilution	Patients with severe cardiovascular disease or carotid artery stenosis are not candidates for hypotension. Full replacement of any volume deficit is mandatory prior to inducing hypotension. Commonly used agents are isoflurane (1-3%) or esmolol (50-200 μg/kg/min) ± SNP (0.25-3 μg/kg/min). These agents are titrated to produce a 30% ↓ in preop MAP (but not < 60 mmHg).
Monitoring	Standard monitors (see p. B-1). Arterial line CVP line ± PA catheter UO	Patients with myocardial dysfunction should have fluid and inotropic/pressor therapy, guided by a PA catheter. Patients for shelf procedures may require only standard monitoring.
Positioning	✓ and pad pressure points. ✓ eyes.	Meticulous padding of the chest, pelvis and extremities is imperative to prevent nerve injury and ischemia of the extremities. ↓BP → risk of neurovascular injury.

Complications	Hypothermia Damage to urinary collecting system Major blood loss Coagulopathy	Warming of hypothermic patient may unmask severe volume depletion that will increase fluid requirement to well above apparent losses.

POSTOPERATIVE

Complications	Nerve root damage Peripheral nerve damage	Preop or intraop damage to L4-S5 nerve roots and cauda equina, resulting in hemiplegia and bladder and bowel dysfunction. Neuropathy of the femoral, genitofemoral and lateral femoral cutaneous nerves can result from pressure on the ilioinguinal ligament during surgery.
Pain management	IV morphine Spinal opiates	Morphine 1-2 mg iv q 10 min prn
Tests	Hct, CXR, coagulation profile, as indicated.	Epidural hydromorphone 50 μg/ml infused at 100-250 μg/hr, ± bupivacaine 0.125-0.25% at 4-8 ml/h, provides excellent analgesia.

References

1. McCollough NC III: Complications of amputation surgery. In *Complications in Orthopaedic Surgery,* 3rd edition. Epps CH Jr, ed. JB Lippincott, Philadelphia: 1994.
2. Tooms RE: Amputations of lower extremity. In *Campbell's Operative Orthopaedics*, 9th edition. Crenshaw AH, ed. CV Mosby, St. Louis: 1998, Vol 1, 532-47.

ARTHROPLASTY OF THE HIP

SURGICAL CONSIDERATIONS

Description: **Total hip arthroplasty** is one of the most successful procedures in orthopedic surgery. In this procedure, the hip joint (Fig 10.3-1) is approached through one of several standard incisions. The femoral head is dislocated from the acetabulum, and the arthritic femoral head and a portion of the neck are excised. The acetabulum is reamed to accept a cemented or cementless cup made of metal and plastic. The femoral stem and head are usually modular, allowing for numerous shapes, sizes, lengths, etc. The metallic femoral component may be cemented or cementless. A hybrid total hip combines a cemented femoral stem and a cementless acetabular cup. After relocation of the new prosthetic hip joint and closure of the tissues, the patient usually is placed in traction or positioning devices to prevent dislocation. Mobilization takes place over the ensuing days.

Variant procedure or approaches: **Unipolar** (only the femoral side is replaced); **bipolar** (both the femoral side and the acetabular side are replaced; the acetabular cup is not fixed to the pelvis). **Revision procedures** are more arduous and time-consuming, as the "failed" or loose component(s) must be removed and the bone prepared to accept new cemented or cementless components. These procedures require more specialized equipment for extracting prostheses and cement, and rebuilding the femoral or acetabular bone stock (allografts, autografts, etc.). Often, special components are needed for implantation of a new prosthesis. In the **Girdlestone procedure** (**resection arthroplasty**), the components are removed, but not replaced. This procedure is usually performed for infection.

Usual preop diagnosis: Fracture of femoral neck; arthritis of hip; arthrosis of hip; loose (or malpositioned) hip prosthesis; chronic dislocation of hip arthroplasty; infected hip arthroplasty

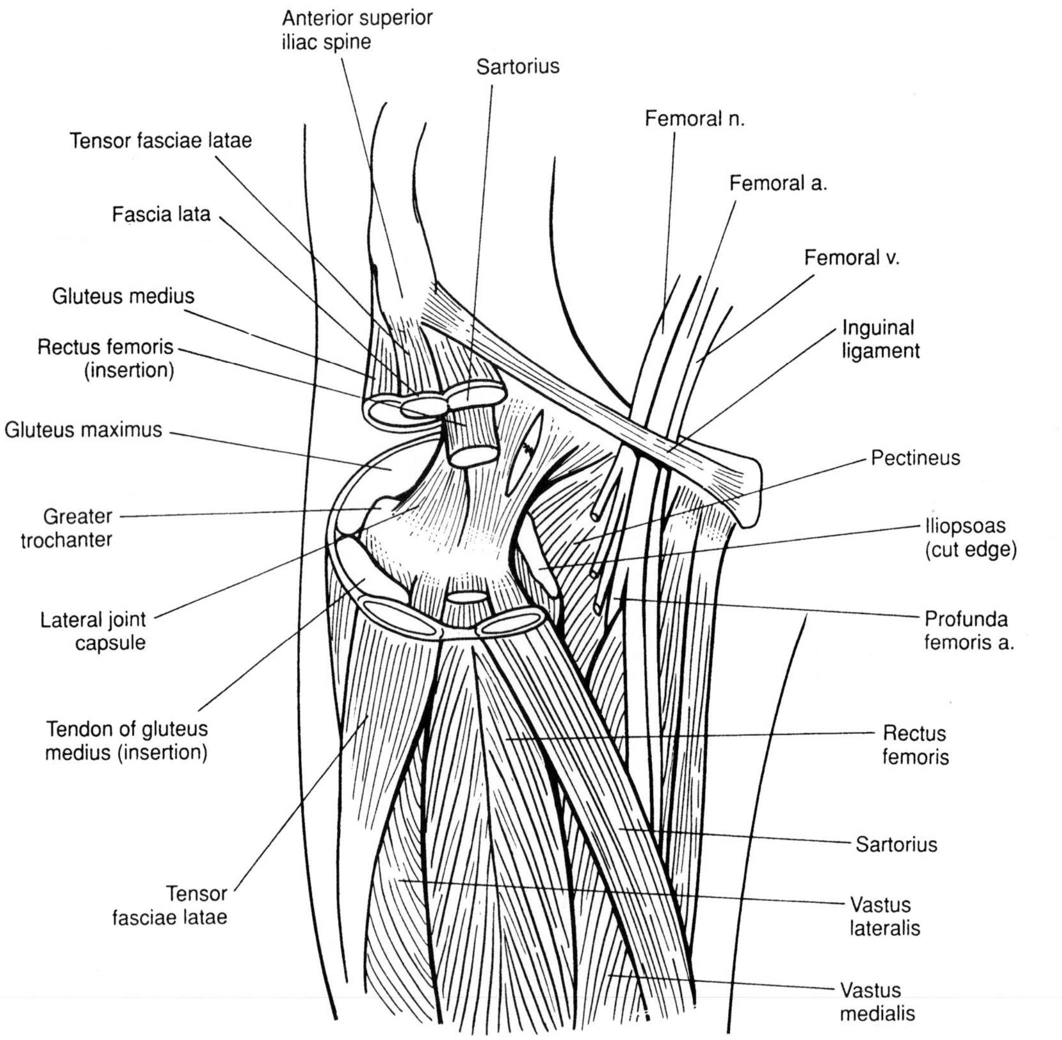

Figure 10.3-1. Surgical exposure of the hip joint: The hip joint may be exposed through a number of approaches. The relevant anatomical landmarks are shown here. (Reproduced with permission from Hoppenfeld S, deBoer P: *Surgical Exposures in Orthopaedics*. JB Lippincott: 1984.)

SUMMARY OF PROCEDURE

	Unipolar, Bipolar, Total Hip Replacement	Revision, Total Hip Replacement	Girdlestone Resection Arthroplasty
Position	Supine (for anterior or anterolateral approaches); lateral decubitus position (for lateral or posterior approaches)	⇐	⇐
Incision	Anterolateral, lateral or posterolateral over hip joint	⇐	⇐
Special instrumentation	Appropriate prostheses and instrumentation	Special instruments for excising cement	⇐
Unique considerations	In lateral decubitus position, patient is usually stabilized by bean bag and/or kidney rests. SCDs used.	A trochanteric osteotomy is frequently performed.	⇐
Antibiotics	Cefazolin or cefamandole 1 g iv q 6 h × 48 h	⇐	⇐ after intraop cultures

	Unipolar, Bipolar, Total Hip Replacement	Revision, Total Hip Replacement	Girdlestone Resection Arthroplasty
Surgical time	2-3 h	3-6 h or more	3 h or more
EBL	500-750 ml (intraop blood retrieval system may be useful).	≥ 1000 ml; intraop blood retrieval recommended.	⇐
Postop care	Patient's legs immobilized between abduction wedge; or operated leg suspended in a splint or placed in traction.	⇐	⇐
Mortality	1-2% (increasing with age)	⇐	⇐
Morbidity	DVT:	⇐	⇐
	Without prophylaxis: ≥ 50%	⇐	⇐
	With low-molecular-weight heparin, coumadin, SCDs or antiembolism stockings: 10-20%	⇐	⇐
	Heterotopic ossification: 3-50% (average, 13%; significant, 4-5%)	> 3-50%	⇐
	Intraop cementless fracture: 5-20%	⇐	⇐
	UTI: 7-14%	⇐	⇐
	Late aseptic loosening requiring revision: 5-10% (after 10 yr)	> 5-10%	⇐
	Wound infection: 1%	3-10%	⇐
	Primary psoriatic and diabetic patients: 5-10%		
	Primary OA: 1%		
	Hematoma (major): < 5%	⇐	5-10%
	Femoral/sciatic nerve injury: 0.7-3.5%	⇐	⇐
	PE: 1.8-3.4% (if no prophylaxis)	⇐	⇐
	Intraop cemented fracture: 1-3%	2-3%	1-3%
	Postop subluxation/dislocation: 0.5-3%	⇐	–
	Vascular injury to iliac vessels: < 0.5%	> 0.5%	⇐
	Urinary retention requiring catheterization: Common	⇐	⇐
	GI bleed, MI, cholecystitis: Rare	⇐	–
			Neurological injury: 3-10%
Pain score	7	8	8

PATIENT POPULATION CHARACTERISTICS

Age range Hip fracture and cases of arthrosis of the hip joint, generally > 60 yr; arthritis of the hip (e.g., rheumatoid arthritis or juvenile rheumatoid arthritis, traumatic arthritis), all ages

Male:Female Dependent on disease etiology

Incidence Common: approximately 200,000/yr in U.S.

Etiology Osteoarthritis; seropositive or seronegative arthritis; avascular necrosis; traumatic arthritis; congenital dislocation of the hip

Associated conditions Dependent on primary conditions (e.g., rheumatoid arthritis patients may have numerous deformities, cardiorespiratory disease, etc.)

ANESTHETIC CONSIDERATIONS

See Anesthetic Considerations for Hip Procedures, p. 738.

References

1. Bierbaum BE, Pomeroy DL, Berklacich FM: Late complications of total hip replacement. In *The Hip and its Disorders*. Steinberg ME, ed. WB Saunders Co, Philadelphia: 1991, 1061-96.
2. Harkey JW: Arthroplasty of hip. In *Campbell's Operative Orthopaedics*, 9th edition. Crenshaw AH, ed. Mosby-Year Book, St. Louis: 1998, Vol 1, 473-520.
3. Ranawat CS, Figgie MP: Early complications of total hip replacement. In *The Hip and its Disorders*. Steinberg ME, ed. WB Saunders Co, Philadelphia: 1991, 1042-60.
4. Shaw JA Greer RB III: Complications of total hip replacement. In *Complications in Orthopaedic Surgery*, 3rd edition. Epps CH Jr, ed. JB Lippincott, Philadelphia: 1994, 1013-1106.

ARTHRODESIS OF THE HIP

SURGICAL CONSIDERATIONS

Description: In adults, this procedure is accomplished by fusing the femur to the acetabulum. Some form of internal fixation is usually employed; a spica cast is sometimes placed immediately postop or a few days later. The patient is usually not a good candidate for total hip arthroplasty (e.g., a young, healthy male with unilateral traumatic arthritis). The hip is usually fused in 30° of flexion, 10-30° of external rotation, and neutral-to-slight adduction. The surgical procedure may be performed through anterior, lateral or posterior incisions, with the lateral being most common. A **trochanteric osteotomy** facilitates exposure. After excising the cartilage surfaces, internal fixation, using screws ± a plate, is performed (Fig 10.3-2).

Usual preop diagnosis: Arthritis or arthrosis of the hip; previous septic arthritis of the hip; recurrent subluxation or dislocation of the hip

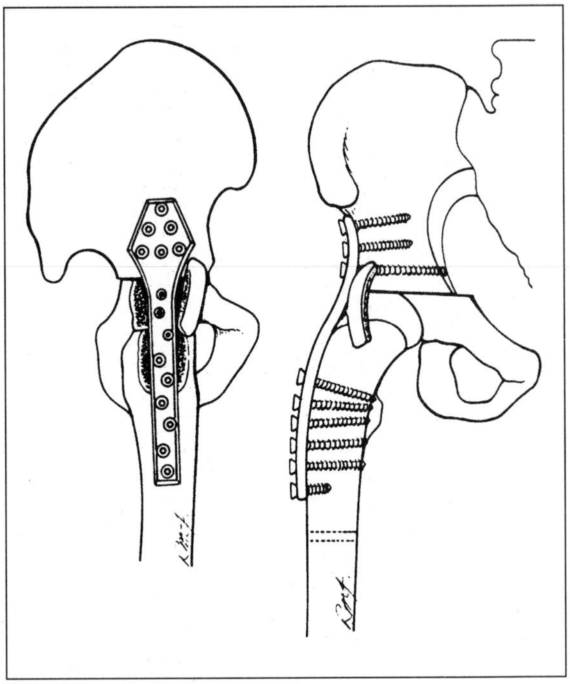

Figure 10.3-2. Arthrodesis of the hip using an AO Cobra plate. (Reproduced with permission from Crenshaw AH: *Campbell's Operative Orthopaedics*, Vol I. Mosby-Year Book: 1992. Redrawn from Muller ME, et al: *Manual of internal fixation*. Techniques recommended by AO group, 2nd edition. Springer-Verlag: 1979.)

SUMMARY OF PROCEDURE

Position	Usually supine; occasionally lateral decubitus
Incision	Anterior or lateral thigh
Special instrumentation	Plates and screws or other internal fixation; reamers from surface replacement arthroplasty set may also be useful; intraop x-ray; fracture table
Unique considerations	Intraop radiographs or image intensifier used with patient on fracture table
Antibiotics	Cefazolin or cefamandole 1 g iv q 6-8 h × 48 h
Surgical time	3-4 h
EBL	500-1000 ml; Cell Saver recommended.

Postop care	Spica cast
Mortality	Extremely low
Morbidity	Limb shortening: Some shortening is always present Thromboembolism: 10-50% Delayed union, nonunion, malunion: 10-15% Femoral shaft fracture: 5-10% Wound infection: < 1% Genitourinary problems: urinary retention requiring catheterization: Common Ileus: Common Late degenerative arthritis of other lower extremity joints or back: Common, many yr later Injury to iliac or femoral vessels: Rare Neurological deficit; injury to lateral cutaneous nerve, sciatic or femoral nerves: Not uncommon Osteomyelitis: Rare Vascular complications: Rare Superior mesenteric artery syndrome causing duodenal obstruction: Extremely rare
Pain score	9

PATIENT POPULATION CHARACTERISTICS

Age range	18-50 yr
Male:Female	Usually males > females
Incidence	Rare
Etiology	Trauma, general; neuromuscular disorders—cerebral palsy, meningomyelocele; trauma to acetabular growth plate; congenital hip dysplasia
Associated conditions	Depends on etiology

ANESTHETIC CONSIDERATIONS

See Anesthetic Considerations for Hip Procedures, p. 738.

References

1. Carnesale PG, Stewart MJ: Complications of arthrodesis surgery. In *Complications in Orthopaedic Surgery*. Epps CH Jr, ed. JB Lippincott, Philadelphia: 1986, 1289-1306.
2. Russell TA: Arthrodesis of the lower extremity and hip. In *Campbell's Operative Orthopaedics*. Crenshaw AH, ed. CV Mosby, St. Louis: 1987, Vol 2, 1091-1130.

SYNOVECTOMY OF THE HIP

SURGICAL CONSIDERATIONS

Description: An **arthrotomy** of the hip joint is performed through one of several standard approaches (anterior, anterolateral, lateral, posterior). A **capsulotomy** is performed, and is closed with reabsorbable sutures later in the case. Generally, the hip is not dislocated, but the cartilage surfaces are inspected and documented. The synovium, as well as any loose bodies, cartilage flaps and osteophytes, are excised. Although weight-bearing is usually protected, ROM and strengthening exercises are begun early.

Usual preop diagnosis: Chronic synovitis of hip; loose bodies in hip; juvenile and adult rheumatoid arthritis; pigmented villonodular synovitis

SUMMARY OF PROCEDURE

Position	Supine for anterior or anterolateral surgical approaches; lateral decubitus for posterior approaches
Incision	Overlying hip joint, depending on specific surgical approach
Unique considerations	Patient may have systemic disease (e.g., rheumatoid arthritis); careful positioning of limbs is necessary to avoid fracture or skin slough.
Antibiotics	Cefazolin or cefamandole 1 g iv q 6-8 h
Surgical time	2 h
EBL	< 500 ml
Mortality	Rare
Morbidity	Thromboembolism: 10-50% Neurovascular injury—femoral or sciatic nerve, or iliac vessels: < 3% Wound infection or dehiscence: < 3% Septic arthritis and osteomyelitis: < 1% (unless synovectomy is performed for infection). Avascular necrosis of femoral head: Rare (if hip is not dislocated). Hematoma: Rare (if drainage tubes employed). Inability to void, requiring urinary catheterization: Common
Pain score	7-8

PATIENT POPULATION CHARACTERISTICS

Age range	< 60 yr
Male:Female	Dependent on disease etiology (e.g., preponderance of females in rheumatoid arthritis)
Incidence	Rare
Etiology	Septic arthritis (very common); rheumatoid arthritis, juvenile/adult (rare); pigmented villonodular synovitis (rare); trauma (rare)
Associated conditions	See Etiology, above.

ANESTHETIC CONSIDERATIONS FOR HIP PROCEDURES

(Procedures covered: arthroplasty; arthrodesis; synovectomy)

PREOPERATIVE

Osteoarthritis is the most common indication for hip arthroplasty. These patients are usually elderly and their anesthetic management is tailored to any concurrent disease. Rheumatoid and other inflammatory arthritides form another group of candidates for these procedures, and the special anesthetic considerations for these patients are outlined below. Avascular necrosis of the hip is seen in patients with sickle-cell disease and in heart transplant patients.

Respiratory Patients with rheumatoid arthritis frequently have associated pulmonary complications. SOB on performing activities of daily living or exercise such as climbing a flight of stairs warrants further evaluation with PFTs. Pulmonary effusions are common. Pulmonary fibrosis (rare) often manifests as cough and dyspnea. Rheumatoid arthritis involvement of the cricoarytenoid joints may produce glottic narrowing (requiring small ETT) and manifest as hoarseness. Arthritic involvement of the TMJ limits mouth opening and may necessitate special techniques (e.g., fiber optic or light wand) for ET intubation.
Tests: As indicated from H&P.

Cardiovascular The severity of the arthritis often limits exercise; thus, a dobutamine stress ECHO and/or dipyridamole/thallium imaging may be necessary for adequate cardiac evaluation in patients with poor exercise tolerance. HTN and cardiovascular disease are common in elderly patients (dysrhythmias/TIAs → fall → hip fracture). Rheumatoid arthritis is associated with pericardial effusion, cardiac valve fibrosis, cardiac conduction abnormalities and aortic regurgitation (AR). An ECG is indicated in all rheumatoid arthritis patients, and ECHO is indicated for patients with physical Sx suggestive of tamponade or cardiovascular disease.
Tests: As indicated from H&P.

Neurological In patients with rheumatoid arthritis, a thorough neurological exam preop often yields evidence of cervical nerve-root compression. Patients with arthritis involving the cervical spine should have

Neurological cont. lateral neck films preop to determine the stability of the atlantooccipital joint. After the stability of the spine has been established, full ROM of the neck should be evaluated for evidence of further nerve-root compression or cerebral ischemia (suggesting vertebral artery compression). Evidence of cerebral ischemia mandates a neurovascular evaluation to plan intraop BP management.
Tests: As indicated from H&P.

Musculoskeletal Pain and decreased joint mobility make positioning and regional anesthesia difficult in patients with arthritis.

Hematologic Rheumatoid arthritis patients often have anemia. Also, anemia may be 2° NSAID gastritis. Patients with Hb > 12 g/dL are candidates for preop autologous blood donation. Hip fracture → potential large volume blood loss at fracture site. DVT is common after hip surgery, and prophylaxis for its occurrence reduces mortality. Effective preventive measures include SCDs and subcutaneous heparin. NSAID-induced coagulopathy may preclude the use of regional anesthesia.
Tests: As indicated from H&P.

Renal In order to predict the clearance of anesthetics and adjuvants in this elderly population, a preop estimation of renal function may be useful.
Tests: As indicated from H&P.

Laboratory Other tests as indicated from H&P.

Premedication In the absence of limited pulmonary reserve or severe cardiac disease, a standard premedication (see p. B-2) is appropriate. Full-stomach precautions may be necessary for patients in acute pain.

INTRAOPERATIVE

Anesthetic technique: GETA or regional anesthesia (may be difficult 2° pain on positioning).

General anesthesia:

Induction The lateral position may mandate ET intubation for patients undergoing GA. A careful preop airway evaluation will determine the need for special airway techniques (e.g., fiber optic intubation or light wand). Aggravation of cricoarytenoid arthritis that is common in rheumatoid arthritis patients can be minimized if a small ETT (6-7 mm cuffed) is used. For otherwise healthy patients, standard induction (see p. B-2) is appropriate.

Maintenance Standard maintenance (see p. B-3). Neuromuscular blockade facilitates the placement and testing of the prosthesis. In otherwise healthy patients, induced hypotension (e.g., ↓20%) → ↓blood loss.

Emergence No special considerations

Regional anesthesia: Induction of regional anesthesia, with its attendant positioning requirements, can be uncomfortable in patients with limited joint mobility. Rheumatoid arthritis patients, however, rarely have involvement of the lumbar spine, and regional anesthesia offers the advantages of decreased perioperative DVT, decreased intraop blood loss and no need for airway manipulation. Anesthesia to T10 is adequate. Full motor blockade is essential for placement of the prosthesis and assessment of the passive ROM. Lumbar epidural block (15-20 ml 2% lidocaine with epinephrine 1:200,000, administered over 15 min) has the advantage of slow onset, allowing time to treat the induced cardiovascular changes. Postop epidural opiates can provide excellent analgesia. Spinal anesthesia, with 15 mg of bupivacaine 0.5% and morphine 0.2 mg placed at L3-L4, has a more rapid onset than epidural anesthesia and yields analgesia for up to 24 h postop.

Blood and fluid requirements	Major blood loss IV: 14-16 ga × 2 NS/LR @ 4-8 ml/kg/h	Cell scavenging helps reduce total transfusion requirement. Care should be taken to ensure that cells have been adequately washed to minimize ↓BP on reinfusion.
Control of blood loss	Regional anesthesia Controlled hypotension	These techniques may be appropriate in selected patient populations.
Monitoring	Standard monitors (see p. B-1). ± CVP line ± Arterial line	Invasive monitoring is indicated in the presence of exercise-limiting cardiac or pulmonary disease.
Positioning	Axillary roll, bean bag ✓ and pad pressure points. ✓ eyes.	Meticulous padding of extremities and maintaining a neutral neck position are mandatory. A bean bag and axillary roll also are necessary to stabilize patient in the lateral position and to protect dependent arm from neurovascular compression injuries.

Complications	Methylmethacrylate: ↓BP 2° vasodilation ↓PaO_2 2° embolization Cardiovascular collapse VAE Major blood loss DVT (femoral vein: 80%) Nerve damage Femur fracture	Embolization of air, fat, bone fragments and cement may occur during insertion of the femoral prosthesis. Systemic hypotension and pulmonary HTN may occur. Care should be taken to ensure that patient is adequately hydrated prior to procedure, and pressors may be necessary to maintain BP (ephedrine 5-20 mg iv or epinephrine 10-100 μg iv and increasing the dose as necessary).

POSTOPERATIVE

Complications	Nerve damage DVT Continued blood loss	Sciatic nerve injury is evidenced by foot drop and an inability to flex the knee.
Pain management	Spinal opiates Epidural analgesia	Epidural hydromorphone 50 μg/ml infused at 100-250 μg/hr provides excellent analgesia.
Tests	Hct CXR, if CVP was placed. Monitor UO	

Reference

1. Dutkowsky JP: Miscellaneous nontraumatic disorders. In *Campbell's Operative Orthopaedics*, 9th edition. Crenshaw AH, ed. Mosby-Year Book, St. Louis: 1998, Vol 1, 787-856.

OPEN REDUCTION AND INTERNAL FIXATION (ORIF) OF PROXIMAL FEMORAL FRACTURES

(FEMORAL NECK, INTERTROCHANTERIC, SUBTROCHANTERIC FRACTURES)

SURGICAL CONSIDERATIONS

Description: Fractures of the proximal femur are seen in two distinct populations: most commonly in elderly patients as the result of falls, and in younger patients following trauma. In elderly patients, the fracture occurs through osteoporotic bone in the femoral neck, intertrochanteric or subtrochanteric area (Fig 10.3-3). Displaced femoral neck fractures are usually treated by **prosthetic replacement**. Nondisplaced or minimally displaced femoral neck fractures are usually treated by **closed reduction and percutaneous pinning** of the fracture. Intertrochanteric and subtrochanteric fractures, whether displaced or nondisplaced, are usually treated by ORIF with a nail/plate or nail/rod device. Prosthetic replacement is performed only rarely. Elderly patients frequently have numerous medical problems, which means that the fractures require prompt internal fixation/prosthetic replacement to facilitate early mobilization. In younger patients (16-40 yr), proximal femoral fractures are almost always treated by ORIF with screws, plates and screws, or intramedullary devices. These are normally much higher energy fractures, often associated with multiple trauma.

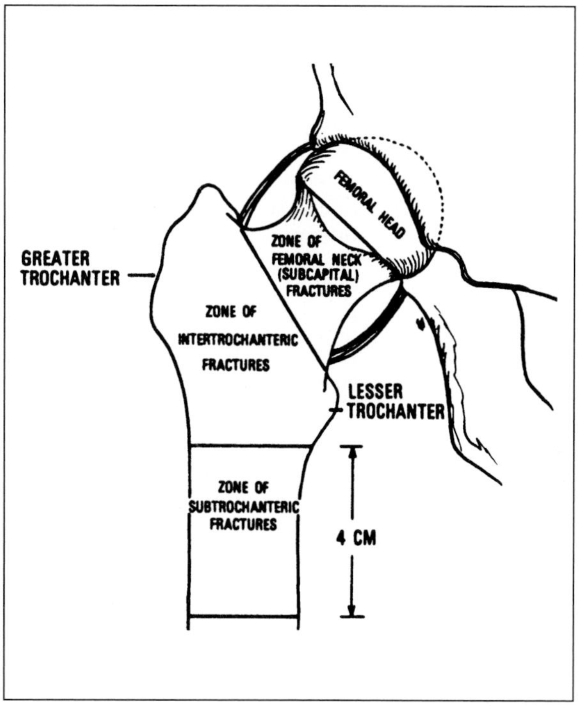

Figure 10.3-3. Anatomical classification of fractures of the proximal femur. (Reproduced with permission from Hardy JD: *Hardy's Textbook of Surgery* 2nd edition. JB Lippincott: 1988.)

Variant procedure or approaches: **Percutaneous pinning** of nondisplaced femoral neck fracture; **ORIF of displaced femoral neck fracture** (also see Arthroplasty for the Hip, p. 733); **ORIF of intertrochanteric or subtrochanteric fracture** are variants.

Usual preop diagnosis: Nondisplaced femoral neck fracture; displaced femoral neck fracture (those not requiring prosthetic replacement); intertrochanteric ± subtrochanteric fracture

SUMMARY OF PROCEDURE

	Nondisplaced Femoral Neck Fracture	Displaced Femoral Neck Fracture	Intertrochanteric ± Subtrochanteric Fracture
Position	Supine, on fracture table	⇐	⇐
Incision	Proximal lateral thigh	⇐	⇐
Special instrumentation	Usually multiple percutaneous pins	Multiple screws or other devices	Screw plate device or intramedullary device
Unique considerations	Fracture table and image intensifier used.	⇐	⇐
Antibiotics	Broad-spectrum cephalosporin (e.g., cefazolin or cefamandole 1 g iv q 6-8 h × 48 h)	⇐	⇐
Surgical time	1 h. Percutaneous pinning may be accomplished with local anesthesia only.	1.5-2 h, including placing patient on fracture table and obtaining adequate reduction of fracture	1.5-3 h
EBL	< 100 ml	250-500 ml	500+ ml
Postop care	Generally PACU → room; if medically unstable, → ICU	⇐	⇐

	Nondisplaced Femoral Neck Fracture	Displaced Femoral Neck Fracture	Intertrochanteric ± Subtrochanteric Fracture
Mortality	10-30% in first 12 mo postop in elderly; in younger patients, depends on multiple trauma.	⇐	⇐
Morbidity	Dysrhythmias: ~50%	⇐	⇐
	MI: ~50%	⇐	⇐
	Respiratory failure: ~50%	⇐	⇐
	Urinary retention requiring catheterization: ~50%	⇐	⇐
	UTI: ~50%	⇐	⇐
	Thromboembolism: 40%+	⇐	⇐
	Avascular necrosis and late segmental collapse: 10-20%	≥15-35%	1%
	Infection, deep: 2-17%	⇐	⇐
	Infection, superficial: 2-17%	⇐	⇐
	Septic arthritis: 2-17%	⇐	⇐
	Nonunion: 5-5%	20-30%	2%
	Malunion: < 10%	> 10%	10-20%
	Loss of reduction: < %5	> 10%	10%
	Hematoma	–	–
	Intraop comminution of the fracture	–	–
	Neurological injury: Rare	⇐	⇐
	Vascular injury: Rare	⇐	⇐
Pain score	5-6	7	8

PATIENT POPULATION CHARACTERISTICS

Age range Usually > 60 yr (patients with an intertrochanteric fracture average 65-70 yr); occasionally, younger patients, 16-35 yr (as part of multiple-trauma situation)

Male:Female Elderly 1:4-5

Incidence Extremely common—about 5-100 per 100,000; femoral neck fractures are about twice as common as intertrochanteric fractures.

Etiology Accidents and falls (may be 2° TIA, stroke, MI, dysrhythmia); pathological fracture; multiple trauma (younger patients); stress fracture

Associated conditions Numerous serious medical conditions often present in elderly; senile dementia; multiple trauma often

ANESTHETIC CONSIDERATIONS

See Anesthetic Considerations for Lower-Extremity Procedures, p. 785.

References

1. Guyton JL: Fractures of the hip, acetabulum, and pelvis. In *Campbell's Operative Orthopaedics*, 9th edition. Crenshaw AH, ed. CV Mosby, St. Louis: 1998, Vol 3, 2181-2280.
2. Kyle RF, Schmidt AH, Campbell SJ: Complications of the treatment of fractures and dislocations of the hip. In *Complications in Orthopaedic Surgery*, 3rd edition. Epps CH Jr, ed. JB Lippincott, Philadelphia: 1994, 443-86.
3. LaVelle DG: Delayed union and nonunion of fractures. In *Campbell's Operative Orthopaedics*, 9th edition. Crenshaw AH, ed. CV Mosby, St. Louis: 1998, Vol 3, 2579-2630.

OPEN REDUCTION AND INTERNAL FIXATION (ORIF) OF DISTAL FEMUR FRACTURES

SURGICAL CONSIDERATIONS

Description: ORIF of the distal femur fracture involves a longitudinal incision along the femoral shaft, obtaining reduction by direct visualization of the fracture fragments, and applying plates and screws along the femur for rigid internal fixation. An iliac crest bone graft may be necessary. Some intramedullary devices are also available for fixation of these fractures.

Usual preop diagnosis: Fracture of the distal femur; nonunion/malunion of the distal femur; degenerative arthritis of knee, with deformity

SUMMARY OF PROCEDURE

Position	Supine. Patient usually arrives at OR in balanced traction if fracture is acute.
Incision	Anterior knee, lateral or medial thigh along the femoral shaft
Special instrumentation	Special plates, screws, rods, reduction clamps; radiolucent table; intraop blood salvage
Unique considerations	Usually requires intraop radiographs; tourniquet.
Antibiotics	Broad-spectrum cephalosporin (e.g., cefazolin or cefamandole 1 g iv q 6-8 h × 48 h)
Surgical time	3 h (or more, depending on difficulty)
EBL	750 ml or more
Postop care	Multiple-trauma victim → ICU; others → PACU
Mortality	~3-4%, depending on the extent of multiple trauma
Morbidity	Nonunion: 4-33% Malunion: 4-31% Infection, osteomyelitis, septic arthritis; closed/open: Grade I: 1-5% Grade II: 5-20% Grade III: > 20% Delayed union: 0-17% Vascular complications: 2-3% Neurological deficit to peripheral nerves, peroneal nerve: ~3% Compartment syndrome: Rare Hypotension: Rare Leg-length discrepancy: Rare Respiratory distress and fat embolism: Rare
Pain score	8

PATIENT POPULATION CHARACTERISTICS

Age range	Any age; predominance of males < 40 yr (trauma); degenerative arthritis of knee < 60 yr. Special rare case is elderly patient with a supracondylar fracture above a total knee replacement.
Male:Female	5:1
Incidence	Common in trauma center patients; rare in cases of degenerative arthritis of knee (osteotomy) or elderly patient with a supracondylar fracture above a total knee replacement.
Etiology	Motorcycle and motor vehicle accidents; falls; industrial injury; degenerative arthritis of knee
Associated conditions	Frequently associated with trauma to other organ systems.

ANESTHETIC CONSIDERATIONS

See Anesthetic Considerations for Lower-Extremity Procedures, p. 785.

References

1. LaVelle DG: Delayed union and nonunion of fractures. In *Campbell's Operative Orthopaedics*, 9th edition. Crenshaw AH, ed. CV Mosby, St. Louis: 1998, Vol 3, 2579-2630.
2. Mize R, Johnson EE, Hohl M: Complications of fractures and dislocations of the knee. In *Complications in Orthopaedic* Surgery, 3rd edition. Epps CH Jr, ed. JB Lippincott, Philadelphia: 1994, 525-56.

3. Whittle AP: Fractures of lower extremity. In *Campbell's Operative Orthopaedics*, 9th edition. Crenshaw AH, ed. CV Mosby, St. Louis: 1998, Vol 3, 2042-2180.
4. Whittle AP: Malunited fractures. In *Campbell's Operative Orthopaedics*, 9th edition. Crenshaw AH, ed. Mosby, St. Louis: 1998, 2579-2630.
5. Wiss DA, Watson JT, Johnson EE: Fractures of the knee. In *Rockwood and Green's Fractures in Adults*, 4th edition. Rockwood CA Jr, Green DP, Bucholz RW, Hickman JD, eds. JB Lippincott, Philadelphia: 1996, 1919-2000.

OPEN REDUCTION AND INTERNAL FIXATION (ORIF) OF THE FEMORAL SHAFT WITH PLATE

SURGICAL CONSIDERATIONS

Description: ORIF of the femoral shaft involves obtaining a reduction by open means, usually through a longitudinal lateral incision along the length of the femur, and applying plates and screws along the femur to maintain the reduction. An iliac crest bone graft may be necessary.

Usual preop diagnosis: Fracture of femur

SUMMARY OF PROCEDURE

Position	Supine or lateral decubitus
Incision	Lateral thigh along length of femur, ± iliac crest incision
Special instrumentation	Special plates, screws; reduction clamps; blood salvage device
Unique considerations	Fracture or radiolucent table; image intensifier. Patient usually arrives at OR in balanced traction.
Antibiotics	Broad-spectrum cephalosporin (e.g., cefazolin or cefamandole 1 g iv q 6-8 h)
Surgical time	3 h or more, depending on difficulty
EBL	750 ml; Cell Saver recommended.
Postop care	Multiple-trauma victims: ICU; others: PACU
Mortality	Dependent on extent of multiple trauma
Morbidity	Knee stiffness: 20-30% Delayed union, nonunion, malunion: 5-21% Leg-length discrepancy: 0-11% Failure of fixation: 5-10% Infection, osteomyelitis: < 5% Hypotension: Not uncommon Respiratory distress and fat embolism: Not uncommon, often subclinical Compartment syndrome: Rare Neurological deficit to peripheral nerves: Rare Vascular complications: Rare
Pain score	9

PATIENT POPULATION CHARACTERISTICS

Age range	Any age, but predominance of males < 30 yr
Male:Female	5:1
Incidence	Unknown
Etiology	Motorcycle and motor vehicle accidents; falls; industrial injuries
Associated conditions	Frequently associated with trauma to other organ systems

ANESTHETIC CONSIDERATIONS

See Anesthetic Considerations for Lower-Extremity Procedures, p. 785.

References

1. Azer R, Rankin EA: Complications of femoral shaft fractures. In *Complications in Orthopaedic Surgery*, 3rd edition. Epps CH Jr, ed. JB Lippincott, Philadelphia: 1986, 487-524.
2. Bucholz RW, Brumback RJ: Fractures of the shaft of the femur. In *Rockwood and Green's Fractures in Adults*, 4th edition. Rockwood CA Jr, Green DP, Bucholz RW, Heckman JD, eds. JB Lippincott, Philadelphia: 1996, 1827-1918.
3. LaVelle DG: Delayed union and nonunion of fractures. In *Campbell's Operative Orthopaedics*, 9th edition. Crenshaw AH, ed. CV Mosby, St. Louis: 1998, Vol 3, 2579-2630.
4. Whittle AP: Malunited fractures. In *Campbell's Operative Orthopaedics*, 9th edition. Crenshaw AH, ed. Mosby, St. Louis: 1998, 2579-2630.

INTRAMEDULLARY NAILING OF FEMORAL SHAFT

SURGICAL CONSIDERATIONS

Description: This procedure, performed acutely for fracture or later for a nonunion or malunion of the femoral shaft, involves obtaining a reduction by closed or open means, and inserting an intramedullary nail from proximal to distal in the femur, typically through a small incision in the lateral thigh (closed technique). An iliac crest bone graft may be necessary for nonunions. The procedure is usually performed using a fracture table and image intensifier. Through a small incision just proximal to the greater trochanter, the piriformis fossa (just lateral to the femoral neck) is exposed. Reaming of the medullary canal is performed, and a long nail (rod) is inserted proximal to distal (Fig 10.3-4). Screws are usually inserted through the rod if the fracture is comminuted and unstable. Some surgeons recommend delayed nailing if a femoral fracture is associated with chest trauma.

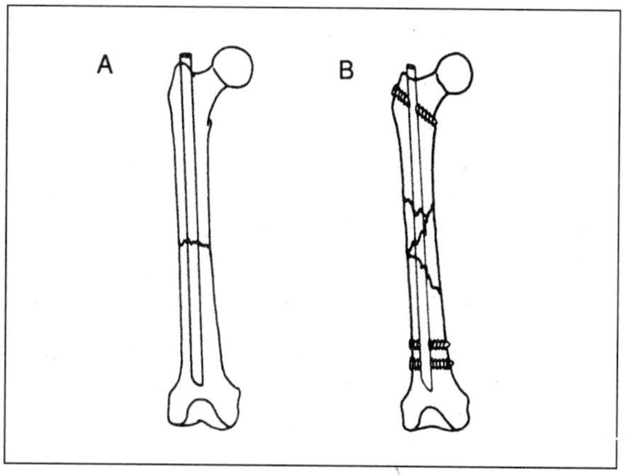

Figure 10.3-4. (A) Simple and (B) locked intramedullary fixation of femoral shaft. (Reproduced with permission from Hardy JD: *Hardy's Textbook of Surgery*, 2nd edition. JB Lippincott: 1988.)

Usual preop diagnosis: Femoral shaft fracture; nonunion/malunion of the femur; leg-length discrepancy

SUMMARY OF PROCEDURE

Position	Supine or lateral decubitus
Incision	Proximal lateral thigh
Special instrumentation	Intramedullary nails and interlocking screws; intramedullary saw for closed femoral shortening of femur
Unique considerations	If fracture is acute, patient may be a multiple-trauma case with other injuries. Most surgeons use fracture table with image intensifier. Patient may arrive at OR in balanced traction.
Antibiotics	Broad-spectrum cephalosporin (e.g., cefazolin or cefamandole 1 g iv q 6-8 × 48 h)
Surgical time	2-3 h; 3+ h for nonunion/malunion of femur or closed femoral shortening of femur
EBL	250-500 ml; 750 cc or more for nonunion/malunion of femur or closed femoral shortening of femur (Cell Saver recommended).

Postop care	If surgery performed acutely, patient is usually a multiple-trauma victim with numerous injuries and extensive blood loss; usually goes to ICU.
Mortality	Dependent on extent of trauma
Morbidity	Respiratory distress and fat embolism: 10% Malunion: 5-10% Infection, osteomyelitis: Closed technique: 0-1% Open technique: 1-10% Neurological deficit to peripheral nerves: 2% Vascular complication: ~2% (up to 15% have occult vascular-flow abnormalities) Delayed union: 1% Nonunion: 1% Hypotension: Common in multiple-trauma situations Knee stiffness: Common Leg-length discrepancies: Not uncommon Compartment syndrome: Rare Failure of fixation: Rare
Pain score	6

PATIENT POPULATION CHARACTERISTICS

Age range	Any age, but predominance of males < 30 yr
Male:Female	5:1
Incidence	Very common
Etiology	Motorcycle and motor vehicle accidents (60-80%); falls (5-10%); industrial injuries (5-10%); previous trauma (rare)
Associated conditions	Frequently associated with trauma to other organ systems.

ANESTHETIC CONSIDERATIONS

See Anesthetic Considerations for Lower-Extremity Procedures , p.785.

References

1. Bucholz RW, Brumback RJ: Fractures of the shaft of the femur. In *Rockwood and Green's Fractures in Adults*, 4th edition. Rockwood CA Jr, Green DP, Bucholz RW, Heckman JD, eds. JB Lippincott, Philadelphia: 1996, 1827-1918.
2. LaVelle DG: Delayed union and nonunion of fractures. In *Campbell's Operative Orthopaedics*, 9th edition. Crenshaw AH, ed. CV Mosby, St. Louis: 1998, Vol 3, 2579-2630.
3. Azer R, Rankin EA: Complications of femoral shaft fractures. In *Complications in Orthopaedic Surgery*, 3rd edition. Epps CH Jr, ed. JB Lippincott, Philadelphia: 1986, 487-524.
4. Whittle AP: Malunited fractures. In *Campbell's Operative Orthopaedics*, 9th edition. Crenshaw AH, ed. Mosby, St. Louis: 1998, 2579-2630.

REPAIR OF NONUNION/MALUNION OF PROXIMAL THIRD OF FEMUR, PROXIMAL FEMORAL OSTEOTOMY FOR OSTEOARTHRITIS

SURGICAL CONSIDERATIONS

Description: Operations for nonunion/malunion of the proximal femur entail realigning the bones with a femoral osteotomy (as necessary); stabilizing the reduction with internal fixation (using a nail/plate-nail/rod device); and supplementing this with a bone graft. In young patients (< 50 years) in whom early osteoarthritis (OA) of the hip spares some of the cartilage, the hip may be realigned with **proximal femoral osteotomy**. This entails cutting the bone at the level of the lesser trochanter, realigning the hip and stabilizing the osteotomy with internal fixation.

Variant procedure or approaches: Osteotomy of proximal 1/3 of femur for degenerative arthritis of hip

Usual preop diagnosis: Nonunion/malunion of proximal 1/3 of femur; early degenerative arthritis of hip

SUMMARY OF PROCEDURE

	Repair Nonunion/Malunion	Proximal Femoral Osteotomy
Position	Supine or lateral decubitus	⇐
Incision	Proximal lateral thigh	⇐
Special instrumentation	Plates, screws; reduction clamps; occasionally, an intramedullary device. Cell Saver recommended. Some surgeons use fracture or radiolucent table with image intensifier.	⇐
Antibiotics	Broad-spectrum cephalosporin (e.g., cefazolin or cefamandole 1 g iv q 6-8 h)	⇐
Surgical time	2 h for bone grafting alone; 3 h or more if difficult malunion	3 h
EBL	500-750 ml or more	500 ml +
Mortality	Rare: < 1%	⇐
Morbidity	Leg-length discrepancy: Common	–
	Technical complications/fixation failure: 1-5%	⇐
	Superficial, deep infection/osteomyelitis: 1%	⇐
	Malunion: Not uncommon	–
	Compartment syndrome: Rare	⇐
	Neurological deficit to peripheral nerves: Rare	⇐
	Vascular complications: Rare	⇐
		Progressive pain/arthritis (by 5-10 yr): 40-50%
		Delayed union: 5-10%
		Nonunion: 1-5%
Pain score	8	8

PATIENT POPULATION CHARACTERISTICS

Age range	Any age	⇐
Male:Female	1:1	⇐
Incidence	Rare	⇐
Etiology	Previous surgery (rare); previous trauma (rare)	Early degenerative arthritis of the hip: Not uncommon
Associated conditions	May accompany multiple traumas	⇐

ANESTHETIC CONSIDERATIONS

See Anesthetic Considerations for Lower-Extremity Procedures, p. 785.

References

1. LaVelle DG: Delayed union and nonunion of fractures. In *Campbell's Operative Orthopaedics*, 9th edition. Crenshaw AH, ed. CV Mosby, St. Louis: 1998, Vol 3, 2579-2630.
2. Whittle AP: Malunited fractures. In *Campbell's Operative Orthopaedics*, 9th edition. Crenshaw AH, ed. CV Mosby, St. Louis: 1994, Vol 3, 2537-78.
3. Kyle RF, Schmidt AH, Campbell SJ: Complications of the treatment of fractures and dislocations of the hip. In *Complications in Orthopaedic Surgery*, 3rd edition. Epps CH Jr, ed. JB Lippincott, Philadelphia: 1994, 443-86.

CLOSED REDUCTION AND EXTERNAL FIXATION OF FEMUR

SURGICAL CONSIDERATIONS

Description: This procedure entails manipulating the femur to obtain an acceptable reduction by closed or limited-open means, then applying an external fixation device to maintain the reduction. The pins for the external fixator are inserted percutaneously or through small incisions. This method of treatment may be used for severe open fractures (e.g., Grade III) with extensive bone and soft-tissue injury.

Usual preop diagnosis: Displaced, open fracture of the femur

SUMMARY OF PROCEDURE

Position	Supine or lateral
Incision	Done percutaneously or through small incisions
Special instrumentation	External fixation device of surgeon's choice; radiolucent table with image intensifier
Unique considerations	Fracture is usually an open, extremely comminuted fracture in a multiple-trauma patient.
Antibiotics	Broad-spectrum cephalosporin (e. g., cefazolin or cefamandole 1 g iv q 6-8 h) + gentamicin (80 mg iv q 8 h until wound closed); adjust for renal status for Grade III open fractures.
Surgical time	1 h
EBL	Operative blood loss usually 100-200 ml; however, blood loss may be extensive prior to surgery.
Postop care	Multiple-trauma victims → ICU; others → PACU
Mortality	Dependent on extent of trauma
Morbidity	Refracture: 2-12% Hypotension 2° blood loss and other injuries: Common Stiffness of knee: Common Delayed union, nonunion, malunion: More common in comminuted, open fractures Leg-length discrepancy: More common in severely comminuted fractures Osteomyelitis: More common in open fractures Respiratory distress: More common in multiple-trauma situations Amputation: Rare Compartment syndrome: Rare Neurological deficit to peripheral nerves: Rare Vascular complications: Rare
Pain score	9-10 (due to extensive open fracture)

PATIENT POPULATION CHARACTERISTICS

Age range	Any age, but predominance of males < 30 yr
Male:Female	5:1
Incidence	Common
Etiology	Motorcycle and motor vehicle accidents; falls; industrial injury
Associated conditions	Frequently associated with trauma to other organ systems, including head and neck, chest, abdomen, and extremities; these will often be treated simultaneously with the femur fracture.

ANESTHETIC CONSIDERATIONS

See Anesthetic Considerations for Lower-Extremity Procedures, p. 785.

References

1. Azer SN, Rankin EA: Complications of femoral shaft fractures. In *Complications in Orthopaedic Surgery*, 3rd edition. Epps CH Jr, ed. JB Lippincott, Philadelphia: 1986, 487-524.
2. Bucholz RW, Brumback RJ: Fractures of the shaft of the femur. In *Rockwood and Green's Fractures in Adults*, 4th edition. Rockwood CA Jr, Green DP, Bucholz RW, Heckman JD, eds. JB Lippincott, Philadelphia: 1996, 1827-1918.
3. LaVelle DG: Delayed union and nonunion of fractures. In *Campbell's Operative Orthopaedics*, 9th edition. Crenshaw AH, ed. CV Mosby, St. Louis: 1998, Vol 3, 2579-2630.
4. Whittle AP: Malunited fractures. In *Campbell's Operative Orthopaedics*, 9th edition. Crenshaw AH, ed. CV Mosby, St. Louis: 1994, Vol 3, 2537-78.

ARTHROPLASTY OF THE KNEE

SURGICAL CONSIDERATIONS

Description: In this procedure, an arthrotomy of the knee joint is performed, and metallic and plastic components are used for replacement of the knee joint surfaces (**total knee replacement**). The femur, patella and tibia are exposed; cartilage and minimal bone are excised with a saw. The new components may be cemented or uncemented. Alternatively, arthroplasty may be performed on only one compartment of the knee (i.e., medial/lateral **unicompartmental knee replacement**). In **revision procedures**, one or more components of the old joint are removed and new components are placed. In a **resection or excision arthroplasty** of the knee, normally done for infection of the prosthesis, the components are removed but not replaced.

Usual preop diagnosis: Arthritis of knee; arthrosis of knee; loose (or malpositioned) knee prosthesis; infected knee

SUMMARY OF PROCEDURE

	Knee Replacement	Revision	Resection/Excision
Position	Supine	⇐	⇐
Incision	Anterior or anteromedial over patella	⇐	⇐
Special instrumentation	Appropriate prostheses and instrumentation	Special instruments for excising cement	⇐
Unique considerations	± Tourniquet; ± SCD	⇐	⇐
Antibiotics	Broad-spectrum cephalosporin (e.g., cefazolin or cefamandole 1 g iv q 6-8 h × 48 h)	Broad spectrum cephalosporin after cultures taken	⇐
Surgical time	2 h	3-4 h or more	3 h
Closing considerations	In infected or complex revision cases (rare), a local or free flap is required.	⇐	⇐
EBL	300-500 ml	500-1000 ml	⇐
Postop care	Bulky dressing or splint; or continuous passive motion is begun, using a machine.	⇐	Splint/cast
Mortality	Rare	⇐	⇐
Morbidity	DVT, without prophylaxis: 50-75%	⇐	⇐
	DVT, with prophylaxis (e.g., low molecular weight heparin, coumadin, SCD, antiembolism stockings): 10-20%	⇐	⇐
	Postop subluxation/dislocation of patella: ≤ 35%	> 35%	–
	Superficial wound necrosis: 10-15%	> 10-15%	≥ 10-15%
	Wound infection: Primary rheumatoid or psoriatic arthritis, diabetes: 5-10% Primary osteoarthritis (OA): 1%	> 5-10%	Rare
	PE: 1-7%	⇐	⇐
	Postop subluxation/dislocation of knee joint: 1-6%	≥ 1-6%	–
	Late aseptic loosening requiring revision after ~10 yr: 5%	–	–
	Peroneal nerve injury: 1-5%	> 1-5% (more common in difficult revisions)	1-5%

	Knee Replacement	Revision	Resection/Excision
Morbidity, cont.	Urinary retention requiring catheterization: Common	–	–
	Hematoma: Rare (1%)	–	–
	Hypotension	–	–
	Knee stiffness	–	–
	Intraop fracture: Rare	⇐	⇐
	Wound dehiscence: Rare	–	–
	Fat embolism: Extremely rare	–	–
	Vascular injury to popliteal vessels: Extremely rare	–	–
Pain score	7	8	9

PATIENT POPULATION CHARACTERISTICS

Age range	Generally, > 60 yr. Arthritis of the knee (e.g., rheumatoid arthritis or juvenile rheumatoid arthritis), hemophilia, ≥18 yr
Male:Female	1:1
Incidence	Common—approximately 150,000/yr in U.S.
Etiology	Arthrosis of the knee (degenerative joint disease [DJD] or OA); seropositive or seronegative arthritis; traumatic arthritis; hemophiliac arthropathy of the knee
Associated conditions	Dependent on primary condition

ANESTHETIC CONSIDERATIONS

See Anesthetic Considerations For Knee Procedures, p. 759.

References

1. Blaster RB, Matthews LS: Complications of prosthetic knee arthroplasty. In *Complications in Orthopaedic Surgery*, 3rd edition. Epps CH Jr, ed. JB Lippincott, Philadelphia: 1994, 1057-86.
2. Guyton JL: Arthroplasty of the ankle and knee. In *Campbell's Operative Orthopaedics*, 9th edition. Crenshaw AH, ed. Mosby-Year Book, St. Louis: 1998, Vol 1, 232-94.
3. Insall JN: Total knee replacement. In *Surgery of the Knee*. Insall JN, ed. Churchill Livingstone, New York: 1984, 587-695.

ARTHRODESIS OF THE KNEE

SURGICAL CONSIDERATIONS

Description: In this procedure, the femur is fused to the tibia, obliterating the knee joint. Through a midline incision and anterior arthrotomy, the cartilage surface and a small amount of bone are excised. The cut ends are opposed and aligned in 0-20° of flexion and 5-10% of valgus. The bones are stabilized with plates, screws, an intramedullary rod or an external fixator.

Usual preop diagnosis: Arthritis or other arthrosis of the knee; previous septic arthritis of the knee, failed or infected knee arthroplasty

SUMMARY OF PROCEDURE

Position	Usually supine
Incision	Anterior midline over knee
Special instrumentation	External fixator; internal fixation with plates and screws or intramedullary nail
Unique considerations	Intraop radiographs or image intensifier; tourniquet
Antibiotics	Cefazolin or cefamandole 1 g iv q 6-8 h × 48 h
Surgical time	3 h (+ 1 h, if necessary, to excise total knee arthroplasty)
Closing considerations	Cast or splint while anesthetized
EBL	< 100 ml, if tourniquet and local fixation used. 500-1000 ml, if no tourniquet used, or if intramedullary procedures are used.
Mortality	Rare, but depends primarily on age and medical condition of patient.
Morbidity	Thromboembolism – ≥ incidence following total knee replacement: DVT (without prophylaxis): 50-75% DVT (if prophylaxis used): 10-20% PE (if no prophylaxis; reduced if anticoagulation or SCDs used): 1-7% Failure of fusion (nonunion), malunion: 10%; higher after failed knee replacement: 19-44%; with Charcot joint, as high as 50%) Pin tract infection: ≥ 1 - 10% Wound infection: 5% Deep infection and osteomyelitis Urinary retention requiring catheterization, UTI: Common Breakage or failure of internal or external fixation: Rare Fat embolism: Rare GI bleed, MI: Rare Hematoma: Rare Hypotension: Rare Intraop femoral or tibial fracture: Rare Neurological injury, usually popliteal nerve or peroneal nerve: Rare Superficial wound necrosis and wound dehiscence: Rare Vascular injury to popliteal vessels: Rare Amputation: Extremely rare (usually due to acute arterial occlusion or uncontrollable local sepsis)
Pain score	9

PATIENT POPULATION CHARACTERISTICS

Age range	Any age
Male:Female	1:1
Incidence	Rare
Etiology	Failed or infected total knee replacement (probably most common etiology); trauma to knee—unreconstructable, intraarticular fractures; total unstable knee or failed ligament repairs with severe DJD in a young patient

ANESTHETIC CONSIDERATIONS

See Anesthetic Considerations For Knee Procedures, p.759.

References

1. Blaster RB, Matthews LS: Complications of prosthetic knee arthroplasty. In *Complications in Orthopaedic* Surgery, 3rd edition. Epps CH Jr, ed. JB Lippincott, Philadelphia: 1994, 1057-86.
2. Carnesale PG, Stewart MJ: Complications of arthrodesis surgery. In *Complications in Orthopaedic Surgery*, 3rd edition. Epps CH Jr, ed. JB Lippincott, Philadelphia: 1994, 1279-1308.
3. Christian CA, Donley BG: Arthrodesis of the ankle, knee, hip. In *Campbell's Operative Orthopaedics*, 9th edition. Canale ST, ed. Mosby-Year Book, St. Louis: 1998, Vol 1, 145-88.
4. Mize R, Johnson EE, Hohl M: Complications of fractures and dislocations of the knee. In *Complications in Orthopaedic Surgery*, 3rd edition. Epps CH Jr, ed. JB Lippincott, Philadelphia: 1994, 525-56.

OPEN REDUCTION AND INTERNAL FIXATION (ORIF) OF PATELLAR FRACTURES

SURGICAL CONSIDERATIONS

Description: In ORIF of patellar fractures, a short incision over the patella is used to perform a reduction by direct visualization of the fracture fragments of the patella. Since this is generally an intraarticular fracture, the fragments should be reduced precisely. The torn quadriceps retinaculum is also repaired. Part or all of the patella may be excised; pins, wires and/or screws are normally used to fix the patellar fragments together internally. Thereafter, the knee is casted, or early motion of the knee is started.

Usual preop diagnosis: Fracture of patella; severe degenerative arthritis of patellofemoral joint

SUMMARY OF PROCEDURE

Position	Supine
Incision	Anterior over patella
Special instrumentation	Wire, pins, screws as necessary
Unique considerations	Intraop radiographs may be obtained; tourniquet
Antibiotics	Cefazolin or cefamandole 1 g iv q 6 h × 48 h
Surgical time	1.5-2 h
Closing considerations	Splint or cast usually applied.
EBL	< 100 ml
Mortality	< 1%
Morbidity	Late degenerative arthritis of patellofemoral joint: ~50-60% DVT: ~5% Wound infection, septic arthritis, osteomyelitis: ~5% Delayed union, nonunion, malunion: ~2-5% Knee stiffness: Common Weakness: Common Avascular necrosis: Rare Sympathetic dystrophy: Rare Following patellectomy—quadriceps strength: ~75% of normal
Pain score	7

PATIENT POPULATION CHARACTERISTICS

Age range	Any age; frequently seen in young, active, healthy adults.
Male:Female	1:1
Incidence	~1% of all skeletal injuries
Etiology	Trauma: falls (60%); motorcycle and motor vehicle accidents (25-35%); industrial injury (6%); degenerative arthritis of patellofemoral joint (rare)

ANESTHETIC CONSIDERATIONS

See Anesthetic Considerations for Knee Procedures, p.759.

References

1. Hohl M, Johnson EE, Wiss DA. Fractures of the knee. In *Rockwood and Green's Fractures in Adults*, 3rd edition. Rockwood CA Jr, Green DP, Bucholz RW, eds. JB Lippincott, Philadelphia: 1991, 1725-97.
2. Mize R, Johnson EE, Hohl M: Complications of fractures and dislocations of the knee. In *Complications in Orthopaedic Surgery*, 3rd edition. Epps CH Jr, ed. JB Lippincott, Philadelphia: 1994, 525-56.
3. Whittle AP: Fractures of lower extremity. In *Campbell's Operative Orthopaedics*, 9th edition. Canale ST, ed. Mosby-Year Book, St. Louis: 1998, Vol 3, 2042-2180.
4. Whittle AP: Malunited fractures. In *Campbell's Operative Orthopaedics*, 9th edition. Canale ST, ed. Mosby-Year Book, St. Louis: 1998, Vol 3, 2537-78.

REPAIR OR RECONSTRUCTION OF KNEE LIGAMENTS

SURGICAL CONSIDERATIONS

Description: Collateral ligaments are usually repaired by direct suture or by stapling the torn ligaments to bone. Cruciate tears are generally repaired only if bone is avulsed at one end of the ligament, again with direct suture, staples or screws. For collateral ligament repair, a longitudinal incision is made directly over the ligament medially or laterally. The ligament is exposed by deep dissection and elevation of skin flaps. The torn ligament is repaired by direct suture or by fixing it to bone with a screw or staple. Following closure, the knee is immobilized with a long leg splint or cast. Cruciate ligaments are repaired in similar fashion except for the approaches: medial parapatellar (with anterior arthrotomy) for the anterior cruciate ligament (ACL) and posteromedial (with posterior arthrotomy) for the posterior cruciate ligament (PCL). Cruciate ligament reconstruction is performed for instability 2° intrasubstance tears of these ligaments. Homografts, such as a portion of the patellar tendon or semitendinosus tendon, normally are used, but allografts or synthetics also are available. (The ligaments of the knee are illustrated in Figs 10.3-5, 10.3-6.)

Usual preop diagnosis: Trauma

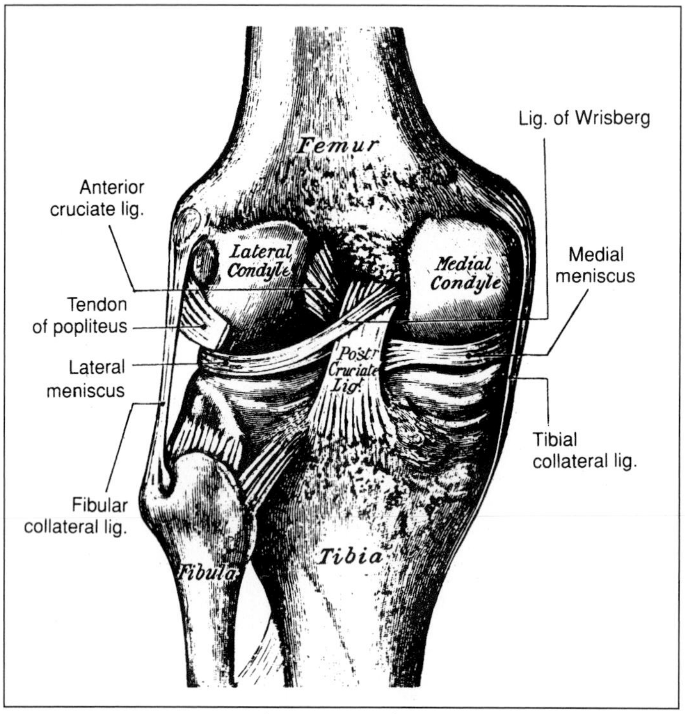

Figure 10.3-5. Left knee joint (from behind), showing interior ligaments. (Reproduced from Goss CM, ed: *Gray's Anatomy of the Human Body*, 27th edition. Lea & Febiger: 1959.)

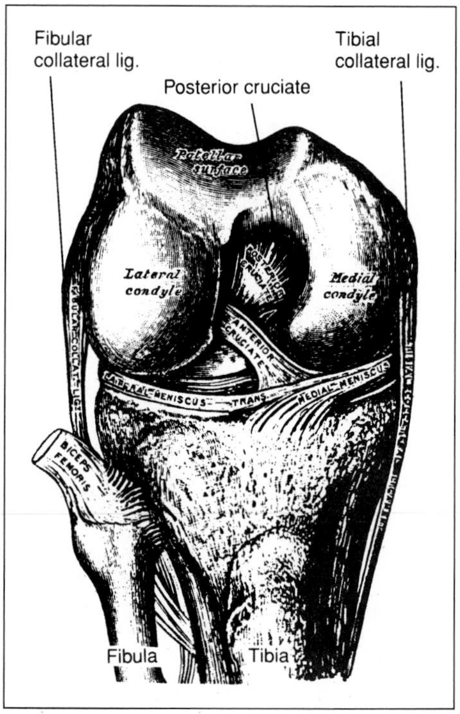

Figure 10.3-6. Right knee joint, dissected from the front. (Reproduced from Goss CM, ed: *Gray's Anatomy of the Human Body*, 27th edition. Lea & Febiger: 1959.)

SUMMARY OF PROCEDURE

	Repair or Collateral Reconstruction	Repair or Cruciate Reconstruction
Position	Supine	⇐
Incision	Over collateral ligament	Anterior and lateral ACL or medial PCL
Special instrumentation	Staples	Drill guides, staples, screws
Unique considerations	Often arthroscopically assisted; tourniquet	⇐
Antibiotics	Cefazolin 1 g iv preop	⇐
Surgical time	2 h	⇐
Closing considerations	Splint or cast while anesthetized	⇐
EBL	100 ml	⇐
Postop care	PACU → room or home	⇐

	Repair or Collateral Reconstruction	Repair or Cruciate Reconstruction
Mortality	Minimal	⇐
Morbidity	Infection: < 1%	⇐
	Thrombophlebitis: < 5%	⇐
Pain score	4	7

PATIENT POPULATION CHARACTERISTICS

Age range	Young adult
Male:Female	2:1
Incidence	Common
Etiology	Trauma: 100%

ANESTHETIC CONSIDERATIONS

See Anesthetic Considerations for Knee Procedures, p .759.

Reference

1. Canale ST, ed: *Campbell's Operative Orthopaedics*, 9th edition. Mosby-Year Book, St. Louis: 1998.

PATELLAR REALIGNMENT

SURGICAL CONSIDERATIONS

Description: The goal of this procedure is prevention of chronic subluxation or dislocation of the patella. Soft tissue components of the surgery include incision (release) of the lateral patellar retinaculum and reefing or tightening of the medial retinaculum (Fig 10.3-7). In cases of severe malalignment of the extensor mechanism, the insertion of the patellar tendon may be moved to a new, more medial location (**tibial tubercle transfer**). In this procedure, the tibial tubercle generally is detached with a saw or osteotomes, leaving a bone pedicle attached distally. The tubercle is then rotated medially on the pedicle and fixed in its new position with a screw. Many surgeons routinely perform an anterior compartment fasciotomy to prevent postop compartment syndrome.

Usual preop diagnosis: Chronic patellar subluxation or dislocation

SUMMARY OF PROCEDURE

	Patellar Realignment	Tibial Tubercle Transfer
Position	Supine	⇐
Incision	Anteromedial or anterolateral to knee	⇐
Special instrumentation	None	Screws or staples
Unique considerations	Tourniquet	⇐
Antibiotics	None	Cefazolin 1 g iv preop
Surgical time	1 h	1.5 h
Closing considerations	None	Splint or cast while anesthetized
EBL	50 ml	100 ml
Postop care	PACU → room or home	⇐
Mortality	Minimal	⇐

Figure 10.3-7. Anatomy of the patellar retinaculum. (Reproduced with permission from Hoppenfeld S, deBoer P: *Surgical Exposures in Orthopaedics: The Anatomic Approach.* JB Lippincott: 1984.)

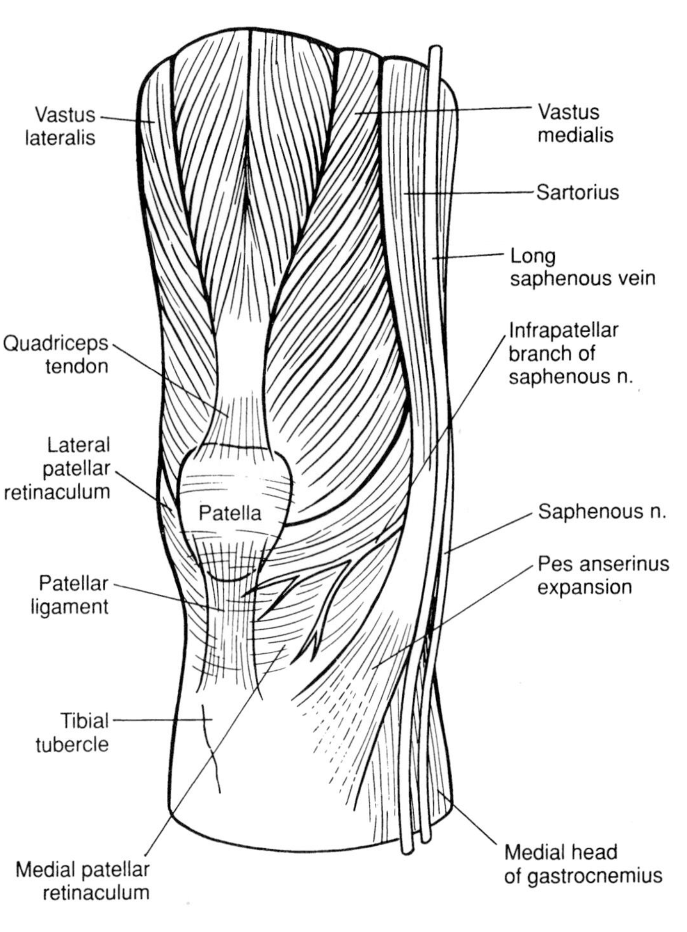

	Patellar Realignment	Tibial Tubercle Transfer
Morbidity	Hemarthrosis: 100%	5%
	Redislocation: 20%	25%
	Thrombophlebitis: 10-20%	⇐
	Compartment syndrome: < 1%	⇐
	Infection: < 1%	⇐
Pain score	6	7

PATIENT POPULATION CHARACTERISTICS

Age range	Usually young adult
Male:Female	1:2
Etiology	Trauma (70%); congenital (30%)
Associated conditions	Patellofemoral dysphasia (60-70%)

ANESTHETIC CONSIDERATIONS

See Anesthetic Considerations for Knee Procedures, p. 759.

Reference

1. Epps CH Jr, ed: *Complications in Orthopaedic Surgery*, 3rd edition. JB Lippincott, Philadelphia: 1994.

ARTHROSCOPY OF THE KNEE

SURGICAL CONSIDERATIONS

Description: **Knee arthroscopy** is used to diagnose and treat intraarticular problems, most commonly torn meniscus, but the procedure is also used for ligament injuries (Fig 10.3-5, 10.3-6), osteochondral fractures, loose bodies, arthritis and infections. In knee arthroscopy, multiple portals or entry points for the arthroscope and instruments generally are used. The most common portals are anteromedial and anterolateral adjacent to the patellar ligament. Other portals may be suprapatellar, parapatellar and posterior. Portals are made by making a stab wound with a knife and then entering the joint with a combination of sharp and blunt trochars. A diagnostic inspection from one of the anterior portals is normally performed at the outset. A second portal is used with a nerve hook to manipulate intraarticular tissues. If resection or repair is performed, the appropriate instruments are inserted through one of the portals. Meniscus repair and cruciate reconstruction may require separate longitudinal incisions, which are usually posteromedial or posterolateral, for placement of sutures and/or drill holes.

Meniscectomy and/or **debridement** are often performed in conjunction with arthroscopy. **Cruciate ligament reconstruction** usually is performed with arthroscopic assistance. At the end of the procedure, the knee joint is copiously irrigated with NS or LR solution through one of the portals. Portals are closed with Steri-Strips or a single suture; compression bandages are applied; and often a knee immobilizer is used.

Usual preop diagnosis: Torn meniscus; cruciate ligament tear; arthritis

SUMMARY OF PROCEDURE

	Arthroscopy	Meniscectomy/Debridement	Cruciate Reconstruction
Position	Supine	⇐	⇐
Incision	3-4.5 cm portals	⇐	⇐ + Anterior midline and lateral
Special instrumentation	Arthroscopic video system; small biters and graspers	⇐ + Shaver	⇐ + Drill guides and drills; fixation screws
Unique considerations	Thigh holder; foot of table 90°; ± tourniquet	⇐	⇐
Antibiotics	None	⇐	Cefazolin 1 g iv preop
Surgical time	0.5 h	1-2 h	2-3 h
Closing considerations	No splint; local anesthetic injected	⇐	⇐
EBL	Minimal	⇐	50 ml
Postop care	PACU → home	⇐	⇐ Or overnight
Mortality	< 0.1%	⇐	⇐
Morbidity	Hemarthrosis: 5-20%	5%	⇐
	Thrombophlebitis: < 2%	⇐	⇐
	Infection: 0.1%	⇐	⇐
	Stiffness: < 0.1%	< 4%	⇐
Pain score	3	4	6

PATIENT POPULATION CHARACTERISTICS

Age range	10-70 yr (usually 20-40 yr)
Male:Female	2:1
Incidence	The most common arthroscopic procedure (85% of total)
Etiology	Trauma (~85%); arthritis (~10%); infection (~5%)
Associated conditions	Usually healthy; systemic arthritis (< 5%)

ANESTHETIC CONSIDERATIONS

See Anesthetic Considerations for Knee Procedures, p. 759.

Reference

1. McGinty JB, ed: *Operative Arthroscopy*. 2nd edition. Raven Press, New York: 1995.

KNEE ARTHROTOMY

SURGICAL CONSIDERATIONS

Description: **Arthrotomy** of the knee is the opening of the joint for drainage, excision of intraarticular tissue (synovium, meniscus, loose bodies), ligament repair/reconstruction or fracture fixation. The knee is generally opened with a parapatellar incision, either medial or lateral, and the joint capsule is incised just adjacent to the patella. After the intraarticular pathology is addressed, a tight capsular closure is performed, followed by subcutaneous tissue and skin closure.

Variant procedure or approaches: **Arthrotomy with debridement** may be used for infection or arthropathy which produces debris. In both cases, **synovectomy** may be necessary.

Usual preop diagnosis: Infection; trauma (fracture, sprain, torn meniscus); arthritis

SUMMARY OF PROCEDURE

	Arthrotomy	Arthrotomy with Debridement	Arthrotomy with Synovectomy
Position	Supine	⇐	⇐
Incision	Medial or lateral parapatellar	⇐	⇐
Special instrumentation	Tourniquet	⇐	⇐
Antibiotics	Cefazolin 1 g iv preop	⇐	⇐
Surgical time	1 h	2 h	2-3 h
Closing considerations	Compressive dressing; may be splinted; suction drain	⇐	⇐
EBL	100 ml	⇐	⇐
Postop care	PACU → room	⇐	⇐
Mortality	Minimal	⇐	⇐
Morbidity	Hemarthrosis: 100%	⇐	⇐
	Degenerative arthritis: 5-20%	⇐	⇐
	Stiffness: 5%	⇐	⇐
	Thrombophlebitis: 5%	⇐	⇐
	Infection: 1%	10%	20%
Pain score	7	7	8

PATIENT POPULATION CHARACTERISTICS

Age range	Infant–elderly (usually young adult)
Male:Female	1:1
Incidence	Common
Etiology	Infection; trauma; arthritis
Associated conditions	Inflammatory arthritis (20%)

ANESTHETIC CONSIDERATIONS

See Anesthetic Considerations for Knee Procedures, p. 759.

Reference

1. Epps CH Jr, ed: *Complications in Orthopaedic Surgery*, 3rd edition. JB Lippincott, Philadelphia: 1994.

REPAIR OF TENDONS—KNEE AND LEG

SURGICAL CONSIDERATIONS

Description: Acute ruptures of tendons in the lower limb are repaired by **direct suture** and sometimes reinforced with part of another tendon. At the knee, patellar tendon ruptures are most common; at the ankle, Achilles tendon ruptures are most common. A longitudinal incision generally is made directly over the tendon. The tendon sheath is opened and tendon ends reapproximated with a nonabsorbable tendon stitch. If necessary, the repair may be augmented by synthetic tape or fascia or protected with a wire which takes tension off the repair. The tendon sheath is closed separately from the skin incision; and a cast or splint is applied. **Achilles tendon repair** and **posterior tibial tendon repair** require different positioning. For an Achilles tendon repair, the patient is placed prone, and a longitudinal incision is made just medial to the tendon, spanning the rupture. The tendon sheath is incised and carefully protected. Torn ends of the tendon are approximated with multiple tendon stitches and may be protected with a fascial flap developed from the gastrocnemius fascia. The tendon sheath is carefully closed, followed by skin wound closure. A splint or cast is applied with the foot in equinus.

Usual preop diagnosis: Tendon rupture

SUMMARY OF PROCEDURE

	Posterior Tendon Repair	Achilles Tendon Repair
Position	Supine	Prone
Incision	Over tendon	⇐
Special instrumentation	Wire or synthetic tape for augmentation	⇐
Unique considerations	Tourniquet	⇐
Antibiotics	If young, none; in elderly or infirm, cefazolin 1 g iv preop	⇐
Surgical time	1 h	⇐
Closing considerations	Splint or cast while anesthetized	⇐
EBL	Minimal	⇐
Postop care	PACU → room or home	⇐
Mortality	Minimal	⇐
Morbidity	Weakness: ~10%	⇐
	Wound slough: 5%	⇐
	Adhesions: < 1%	⇐
	Infection: < 1%	⇐
		Rerupture: 5-10%
Pain score	3	3

PATIENT POPULATION CHARACTERISTICS

Age range	Any age
Male:Female	1:1
Incidence	Uncommon
Etiology	Trauma (90%); chronic tendinitis (10%)
Associated conditions	Obesity; diabetes mellitus (DM); inflammatory arthritis

ANESTHETIC CONSIDERATIONS FOR KNEE PROCEDURES

(Procedures covered: arthroplasty; arthrodesis; ORIF of patellar fractures; repair/reconstruction of ligaments; patellar realignment; arthroscopy; arthrotomy; tendon repair—knee and leg)

PREOPERATIVE

Trauma and osteoarthritis (OA) are the most common indications for these procedures. Trauma patients (e.g., those with sports injuries) are often young and healthy, whereas arthritic patients are often elderly and anesthetic management must be tailored to any concurrent disease. Patients with rheumatoid and other inflammatory arthritides form another group of candidates for these procedures; the special anesthetic considerations for these patients are described in Anesthetic Considerations for Hip Procedures, p. 738. A final group of patients undergoing these procedures are hemophiliacs, who develop arthritis from recurrent bleeding into their joints. The hematologic management of these patients is discussed below.

Respiratory These patients often have rheumatoid arthritis and associated pulmonary conditions. For example, pulmonary effusions are common. Limited respiratory reserve warrants further evaluation. Pulmonary fibrosis (rare) often manifests as a cough and dyspnea. Rheumatoid arthritis involving the cricoarytenoid joints may manifest as hoarseness, glottic narrowing and difficult intubation. Arthritic involvement of the TMJ and cervical spine may further complicate airway management.
Tests: As indicated from H&P.

Cardiovascular The severity of the arthritis often limits exercise and makes assessment of cardiovascular status difficult. Dobutamine stress, ECHO and dipyridamole thallium imaging may be necessary for an adequate cardiac evaluation. Rheumatoid arthritis is associated with pericardial effusion, cardiac valve fibrosis, cardiac conduction abnormalities and aortic regurgitation (AR).
Tests: ECG and others as indicated from H&P.

Neurological In arthritic patients, a thorough preop neurological exam often yields evidence of cervical nerve root compression. After the stability of the neck has been established, the full range of neck motion should be evaluated for evidence of nerve compression and cerebral ischemia (suggesting vertebral artery compression). Consider preop lateral neck films to determine stability of atlantooccipital joint.
Tests: As indicated from H&P.

Musculoskeletal Pain and decreased joint mobility may make positioning and regional anesthesia difficult in this patient population.

Hematologic Hemophiliacs require restoration of clotting factors preop. Administer 1 U of factor concentrate/kg body weight for each 2% increase necessary to achieve clotting factor activity of 40% normal. FFP contains 1 U/ml and cryoprecipitate 20 U/ml. Hemophilia B, but not hemophilia A, can be treated with prothrombin complex concentrate; however, these products can activate clotting factors and → DIC. Approximately 10% of hemophiliacs develop antibodies to exogenous clotting factors, and the care of these patients should be guided by a consulting hematologist.
Tests: Hct; other tests as indicated from H&P.

Laboratory Other tests as indicated from H&P.

Premedication Diazepam 5-10 mg po 1 h preop. Preop patellar pain is effectively treated with a femoral nerve block at the inguinal ligament using 10 ml of lidocaine 1.5% epinephrine 1:200,000.

INTRAOPERATIVE

Anesthetic technique: For many of these patients, regional anesthesia may be the preferred technique, offering the advantages of ↓blood loss, ↓DVT, minimal respiratory impairment and effective postop analgesia. Patients with rheumatoid arthritis rarely have involvement of the lumbar spine. Since rheumatoid arthritis frequently affects the cervical spine, however, these patients may have limited range of neck motion, an unstable atlantooccipital joint, and cricoarytenoid and TMJ arthritis. Careful airway evaluation, therefore, is important to determine the appropriateness of special intubation techniques (e.g., fiber optic, light wand).

Regional anesthesia: Either subarachnoid or epidural blocks are useful techniques, depending on the patient population (e.g., younger patients may be at ↑risk of spinal headache following SAB). Anesthesia extending from S2 to T12 (T8 if tourniquet is used) is adequate for knee surgery. Full motor blockade is essential for fixation of the patella, or placement of the joint prosthesis and assessment of the passive ROM of the prosthesis. Typical drugs and doses include: subarachnoid—15 mg of 0.75% bupivacaine with morphine 0.2 mg; epidural—15-20 ml 2% lidocaine with epinephrine 1:200,000 in divided doses.

General anesthesia:

Induction Standard induction (see p. B-2) is appropriate for patients with normal airways.

Maintenance Standard maintenance (see p. B-3). Neuromuscular relaxation facilitates the placement of the prosthesis. Hemophiliacs will require infusion of clotting factors. For hemophilia A and von Willebrand's disease, 1.5 U/kg/h; for hemophilia B, 0.75 U/kg/h.

Emergence The tourniquet is deflated around the time of emergence. In patients with moderate-to-severe lung disease, controlled ventilation should be continued until after the lactic acid that has accumulated in the leg has been metabolized (3-5 min), since these patients may be unable to increase ventilation to buffer this acid load.

Blood and fluid requirements	IV: 14-16 ga × 1 NS/LR @ maintenance during the case, and 5-10 ml/kg bolus prior to tourniquet deflation	A tourniquet blocks intraop blood loss. When it is deflated, prepare for a 1-2 U blood loss over the ensuing h; more, if the posterior tibial artery has been damaged in the dissection.
Control of blood loss	Tourniquet	Inflation pressure is typically 100 mmHg > systolic pressure. Maximum "safe" tourniquet time is 1.5-2 hr, followed by a 5-to-(preferably) 15-min reperfusion interval, if further tourniquet time is necessary.
Monitoring	Standard monitors (see p. B-1). ± CVP line	A CVP line is indicated in the presence of significant cardiac or pulmonary disease.
Positioning	✓ and pad pressure points. ✓ eyes.	In rheumatoid arthritic patients, meticulous padding of the extremities is mandatory.
Complications	Posterior tibial artery trauma Peroneal nerve palsy	A 20% fall in mean BP is common on tourniquet deflation. Additional crystalloid (5-10 ml/kg) may be necessary to replace edema fluid and blood loss to the leg.

POSTOPERATIVE

Complications	Hemorrhage from the posterior tibial artery Peroneal nerve palsy → foot drop Tourniquet-related nerve injury Post-tourniquet syndrome (PTS)	✓ surgical drain output. Examine patient for evidence of neurologic dysfunction and notify surgeons as necessary. PTS is a self-limiting condition in which the affected limb is edematous, pale and weak.
Pain management	Spinal opiates: • Epidural anesthesia • Spinal anesthesia	Epidural hydromorphone 50 μg/ml infused at 100-250 μg/h provides excellent analgesia. Intrathecal morphine 0.2-0.3 mg provides analgesia for up to 24 h after administration.
Tests	Hct; other studies as indicated.	

Reference

1. Epps CH Jr, ed: *Complications in Orthopaedic Surgery*, 3rd edition. JB Lippincott, Philadelphia: 1994.

OPEN REDUCTION AND INTERNAL FIXATION (ORIF) OF THE TIBIAL PLATEAU FRACTURE

SURGICAL CONSIDERATIONS

Description: **ORIF of the tibial plateau** or proximal tibia fracture involves making a longitudinal incision along the proximal leg lateral to the knee, obtaining a reduction by direct visualization of the fracture fragments, and applying plates and screws along the tibia for rigid internal fixation. An iliac crest bone graft may be necessary. A **proximal tibial osteotomy** involves correcting malalignment (valgus and varus) of the lower extremity by excising a wedge of bone from the tibia and correcting the mechanical axis.

Usual preop diagnosis: Tibial plateau or proximal tibial fracture; nonunion/malunion of the tibial plateau or proximal tibia; degenerative arthritis of the knee, with varus or valgus deformity

SUMMARY OF PROCEDURE

	ORIF Tibial Plateau Fracture	Proximal Tibial Osteotomy
Position	Supine	⇐
Incision	Lateral to knee, usually; medial, rarely	Transverse or lateral incision
Special instrumentation	Special plates, screws; reduction clamps; radiolucent table	⇐
Unique considerations	Intraop radiographs or image intensifier; tourniquet	⇐
Antibiotics	Cefazolin or cefamandole 1 g iv q 6-8 h × 48 h	⇐
Surgical time	Approximately 2.5-3 h; more, depending on difficulty	⇐
Closing considerations	Splint, cast while anesthetized	⇐
EBL	< 200 ml	⇐
Postop care	Multiple-trauma victim → ICU; others → PACU; ± continuous passive motion	PACU → ward
Mortality	Rare, except in severe multiple trauma	None
Morbidity	Compartment syndrome: 10-20%	< 25%
	Wound infection: 7-15%	~2%
	DVT (symptomatic): 3-5%	2%
	Delayed union, nonunion, malunion: < 5%	⇐
	Peripheral nerve damage: 3%	0.2%
	Intraarticular fracture: 2%	
	Hypotension (multiple trauma)	
	Leg-length discrepancy	
	Osteomyelitis, septic arthritis	
	Respiratory distress and fat embolism	
	Vascular complications	
Pain score	7	7

PATIENT POPULATION CHARACTERISTICS

Age range	Any age; fracture most common in younger trauma patients and elderly Degenerative arthritis of knee, < 60 yr
Male:Female	1:1
Incidence	Common
Etiology	Trauma: falls, motorcycle and motor vehicle accidents, industrial injuries Degenerative: arthritis of knee

ANESTHETIC CONSIDERATIONS

See Anesthetic Considerations for Lower-Extremity Procedures, p. 785.

References

1. Aglietti P, Chambat P: Fractures of the knee. In *Surgery of the Knee*. Insall JN, ed. Churchill Livingstone, New York: 1984, 395-490.

2. Hohl M, Johnson EE, Wiss DA: Fractures of the knee. In *Rockwood and Green's Fractures in Adults*, 3rd edition. Rockwood CA Jr, Green DP, Bucholz, eds. JB Lippincott, Philadelphia: 1991.
3. LaVelle DG: Delayed union and nonunion of fractures. In *Campbell's Operative Orthopaedics*. Canale ST, ed. CV Mosby, St. Louis: 1998, Vol 3, 2579-2630.
4. Mize R, Johnson EE, Hohl M: Complications of fractures and dislocations of the knee. In *Complications in Orthopaedic Surgery*, 3rd edition Epps CH Jr, ed. JB Lippincott, Philadelphia: 1994, 525-56.
5. Whittle AP: Malunited fractures. In *Campbell's Operative Orthopaedics*. Canale ST, ed. Mosby, St. Louis: 1998, 2537-78.

INTRAMEDULLARY NAILING, TIBIA

SURGICAL CONSIDERATIONS

Description: In intramedullary nailing of the tibia, a metal nail is placed into the medullary canal of the tibia to stabilize (or prevent) a fracture. The affected leg generally is placed in traction, on a fracture table, via stirrup or calcaneal pin. Following the incision, an awl is used to make an entry hole in the proximal metaphysis of the tibia, through which a guide wire is introduced. The guide wire is placed across the aligned fracture, and the nail is introduced and driven over the guide wire. Prior to nail insertion, the medullary canal is often reamed to allow use of a larger nail. Most nails are interlocked both proximally and distally with screws which pass from the bone through holes in the nail.

Usual preop diagnosis: Fracture, nonunion or malunion of the tibia

SUMMARY OF PROCEDURE

Position	Supine, on fracture table. Consider inducing anesthesia before moving patient.
Incision	Proximal longitudinal incision over the patellar tendon; stab wound for screws
Special instrumentation	Nails, screws and insertion instruments; intramedullary reamers; image intensifier
Antibiotics	Cefazolin 1 g iv preop
Surgical time	2 h
Closing considerations	No splint or cast
EBL	200 ml
Postop care	PACU → room
Mortality	Minimal
Morbidity	Compartment syndrome: < 5%
	Infection: < 2%
	Neuropraxia: < 1%
Pain score	5

PATIENT POPULATION CHARACTERISTICS

Age range	> 16 yr
Male:Female	5:1
Etiology	Trauma (95%); tumor (5%)
Associated conditions	Multiple trauma (50%); compartment syndrome (5%)

ANESTHETIC CONSIDERATIONS

See Anesthetic Considerations for Lower-Extremity Procedure, p. 785.

Reference

1. Rockwood CA Jr, Green DP, Bucholz RW, Heckman JD, eds: *Rockwood and Green's Fractures in Adults*, 4th edition. JB Lippincott, Philadelphia: 1996.

EXTERNAL FIXATION, TIBIA

SURGICAL CONSIDERATIONS

Description: Fractures of the tibia are fixed with percutaneous pins which are clamped to an external frame. Stainless steel pins are drilled into the proximal and distal fragments of the fracture through stab wounds in the skin and subcutaneous tissues. Usually 2-3 pins are placed on either side of the fracture. Pin clamps and an external frame are attached and the fracture aligned with the assistance of the image intensifier or under direct vision. Following fracture alignment, the pin clamps and frames are tightened to hold fracture alignment. External fixation is often used with open fractures. **Small-pin fixators** (e.g., Ilizarov) are used for fracture fixation, leg lengthening and treatment of bony defects. Wound irrigation and debridement often accompany application of the fixation frame.

Usual preop diagnosis: Tibia fracture; tibial nonunion or malunion; tibial shortening

SUMMARY OF PROCEDURE

Position	Supine
Incision	Stab wounds. Small-pin fixator may require metaphyseal incision for osteotomy.
Special instrumentation	Pins; fixation frame; image intensifier
Antibiotics	Cefazolin 1 g iv preop
Surgical time	0.5-1 h Small-pin fixator: 3-5 h
Closing considerations	May be open fracture (usually left open)
EBL	50 ml; small-pin fixator, 100 ml
Postop care	PACU → room
Mortality	Minimal
Morbidity	Infection: 15% Compartment syndrome: < 2% Neuropraxia: < 1%
Pain score	2-3

PATIENT POPULATION CHARACTERISTICS

Age range	All ages
Male:Female	5:1
Incidence	Common
Etiology	Trauma (95%); shortened limb (< 2%); ununited or malunited fracture (< 2%)
Associated conditions	Open fracture (95%); compartment syndrome (< 2%); congenital anomaly (< 1%)

ANESTHETIC CONSIDERATIONS

See Anesthetic Considerations for Lower-Extremity Procedures, p. 785.

Reference

1. Rockwood CA Jr, Green DP, Bucholz RW, Heckman JD, eds: *Rockwood and Green's Fractures in Adults*, 4th edition. JB Lippincott, Philadelphia: 1996.

OPEN REDUCTION AND INTERNAL FIXATION (ORIF) OF DISTAL TIBIA, ANKLE, AND FOOT FRACTURES

SURGICAL CONSIDERATIONS

Description: ORIF is nearly always required for displaced fractures involving the ankle or joints in the foot. A longitudinal incision is made over the fractured medial and/or lateral malleoli. Dissection is carried directly down to the bone and the fracture is identified and reduced under direct vision. Open fractures may require irrigation and debridement. The fractures are realigned under direct vision and fixed and stabilized with pins, plates and/or screws. An intraop radiograph is obtained to confirm reduction and placement of hardware. The incisions are closed and a splint or cast is applied.

Usual preop diagnosis: Fracture of the distal tibia, ankle or foot

SUMMARY OF PROCEDURE

	ORIF Ankle	With Irrigation and Debridement
Position	Supine	⇐
Incision	Longitudinal over fracture site	⇐ + Extension of existing wound
Special instrumentation	Pins, plates and screws; tourniquet; x-ray or image intensifier	⇐
Antibiotics	Cefazolin 1 g iv preop	⇐
Surgical time	2 h	2-3 h
Closing considerations	Splint or cast while anesthetized	Splint or cast; may leave wound open.
EBL	50 ml	100 ml
Postop care	PACU → room	⇐
Mortality	Minimal	⇐
Morbidity	Wound dehiscence: 10%	⇐
	Loss of reduction: 7%	⇐
	Infection: 3%	15%
Pain score	4	4

PATIENT POPULATION CHARACTERISTICS

Age range	Infant–elderly (usually > 60 yr)
Male:Female	1:1
Incidence	~ 250,000 cases/yr in U.S.
Etiology	Trauma: 100%
Associated conditions	Alcohol abuse; obesity; diabetes mellitus (DM)

ANESTHETIC CONSIDERATIONS

See Anesthetic Considerations for Lower-Extremity Procedures, p. 785.

References

1. Carragee EJ, Csongradi JJ, Bleck EE: Early complications in the operative treatment of ankle fractures. Influence of delay before operation. *J Bone Joint Surg* [Br] 1991; 73(1):79-82.
2. Epps CH Jr, ed: *Complications in Orthopaedic Surgery*, 3rd edition. JB Lippincott, Philadelphia: 1994.
3. Rockwood CA Jr, Green DP, Bucholz RW, Heckman JD, eds: *Rockwood and Green's Fractures in Adults*, 4th edition. JB Lippincott, Philadelphia: 1996.

REPAIR NONUNION/MALUNION, TIBIA

SURGICAL CONSIDERATIONS

Description: This procedure is used to treat a fracture that has not healed or was misaligned upon healing. The fracture is mobilized, usually grafted with autogenous or allograft bone, and realigned. With an anterior approach, a longitudinal incision is made anteromedial or anterolateral to the shaft of the tibia. Dissection is carried directly down to the bone and the nonunion identified. If the tibia is approached with a posterolateral incision, the patient is turned prone and a longitudinal incision is made just posterior to the fibula. Dissection is carried down posteriorly to the interosseous membrane, to the tibia, and the procedure becomes identical to the anterior approach. Tissue interposed between the bone ends may or may not be debrided. The cortex of the bone adjacent to the nonunion is roughened with an osteotome. Autogenous or allograft bone is placed adjacent to or in the nonunion site. In the case of a malunion, the bone may be osteotomized with a saw or osteotomes to allow realignment. If skeletal fixation is used, a plate may be attached to the bone through the same incision. Alternatively, an intramedullary nail may be placed through an incision anterior to the tibial tubercle. If an intramedullary device is used, the canal may be reamed with intramedullary reamers prior to placement of the nail. A third type of **skeletal fixation** is the external fixator that stabilizes the nonunion via percutaneous pins placed into the proximal and distal tibia, which are then spanned by a device with pin clamps at both ends. An intraop x-ray is often used to confirm fixation and placement of devices; alternatively, an image intensifier may be used.

Variant procedure or approaches: Autogenous **bone grafting from the iliac crest** is commonly used to stimulate healing. An incision is made directly over the iliac crest and muscles are stripped from the crest and table of the ilium. Osteotomes and gouges are used to remove either the inner or outer table of the ilium and cancellous bone between the two tables. The wound is closed over a suction drain.

Usual preop diagnosis: Ununited or malunited fracture

SUMMARY OF PROCEDURE

	Basic Repair	With Iliac Graft	With Skeletal Fixation
Position	Supine (prone with posterior lateral graft)	⇐	⇐
Incision	Anteromedial or posterolateral to shaft of tibia	Anteromedial, parallel to iliac crest	⇐
Special instrumentation	Tourniquet; x-ray or image intensifier	⇐	Pins, plates, screws, rods, external fixator; tourniquet; x-ray or image intensifier
Antibiotics	Cefazolin 1 g iv preop. (If infected nonunion anticipated, antibiotics are withheld until cultures are obtained.)	⇐	⇐
Surgical time	2 h	2.5 h	3 h
Closing considerations	Splint or cast applied while anesthetized.	⇐	No splint or cast
EBL	100 ml	200-300 ml	⇐
Postop care	PACU → room	⇐	⇐
Mortality	Minimal	⇐	⇐
Morbidity	Thrombophlebitis: 5%	⇐	⇐
	Compartment syndrome: 1%	⇐	⇐
	Infection: 1%	⇐	⇐
	Hematoma: < 1%	5%	1-3%
Pain score	5	8	5-8

PATIENT POPULATION CHARACTERISTICS

Age range	10-80 yr (usually 20-40 yr)
Male:Female	5:1
Incidence	5-10% of tibia fractures; 50-75% of open fractures
Etiology	Trauma: 100%
Associated conditions	Poor nutrition (50%); infection (10%); metabolic disease (10%)

ANESTHETIC CONSIDERATIONS

See Anesthetic Considerations for Lower-Extremity Procedures, p. 785.

References

1. Csongradi JJ, Maloney WJ: Ununited lower limb fractures. *West J Med* 1989; 150(6):675-80.
2. Epps CH Jr, ed: *Complications in Orthopaedic Surgery*, 3rd edition. JB Lippincott, Philadelphia: 1994.

ARTHROSCOPY OF THE ANKLE

SURGICAL CONSIDERATIONS

Description: **Ankle arthroscopy** is usually a diagnostic procedure, although it may be used for debridement or removal of loose bodies. The ankle joint is generally inspected through anterolateral and anteromedial portals (entry wounds). Posterolateral and posteromedial portals also may be used. Each portal is made via a 5 mm stab wound in the skin (Fig 10.3-8); then instrumentation is placed, using trochars. If the ankle joint is tight, a mechanical distractor (external fixator distraction apparatus spanning the ankle joint) may be used. The distractor is attached to the bones via percutaneous pins, as in the case of the application of an external fixator. The portals are closed with sterile tape or a single suture. **Debridement** may be used to reduce local or generalized articular damage.

Usual preop diagnosis: Trauma; infection; arthritis

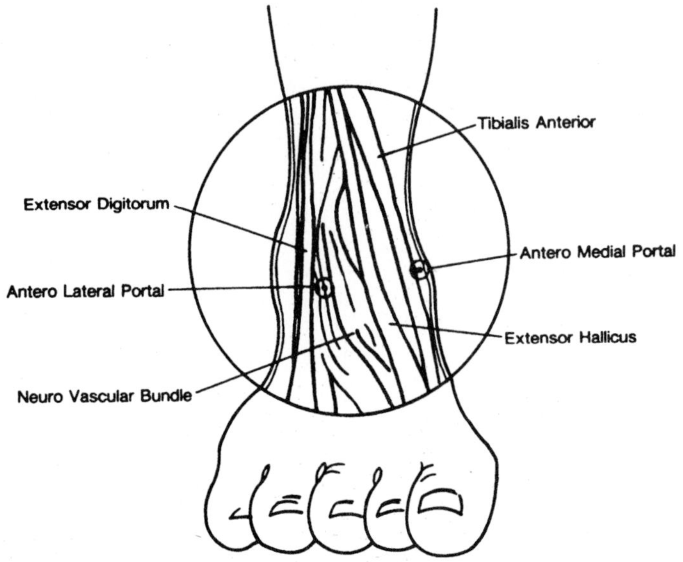

Figure 10.3-8. Portals for ankle arthroscopy. (Reproduced with permission from Chapman MW, ed: *Operative Orthopaedics*. JB Lippincott: 1988.)

SUMMARY OF PROCEDURE

	Arthroscopy	Arthroscopy + Debridement
Position	Supine	⇐
Incision	0.5 cm portals (incisions)	⇐
Special instrumentation	Arthroscopic video system; small biters and graspers	⇐ + Shaver
Unique considerations	± Tourniquet. May use distractor with pins through tibia and calcaneus.	⇐
Antibiotics	Cefazolin 1 g iv preop (optional)	⇐
Surgical time	1 h	1-2 h
Closing considerations	No splint; incisions injected with local anesthetic.	⇐
EBL	Minimal	50 ml
Postop care	PACU → home	⇐
Mortality	< 0.01%	⇐
Morbidity	Hemarthrosis: 5%	⇐
	Thrombophlebitis < 2%	⇐
	Infection: < 1%	⇐
Pain score	2-3	3

PATIENT POPULATION CHARACTERISTICS

Age range	12-70 yr (usually 20-40 yr)
Male:Female	1:1
Incidence	Uncommon
Etiology	Trauma (70%); arthritis (20%); infection (5%)
Associated conditions	Usually healthy; may have systemic arthritis.

ANESTHETIC CONSIDERATIONS

See Anesthetic Considerations for Lower-Extremity Procedures, p. 785.

Reference

1. McGinty JB, ed: *Operative Arthroscopy*, 2nd edition. Raven Press, New York: 1995.

ANKLE ARTHROTOMY

SURGICAL CONSIDERATIONS

Description: Arthrotomy of the ankle is the opening of the joint for drainage, debridement or fracture treatment. The joint is usually opened with an anterolateral, midline or an anteromedial longitudinal incision. Tendons and neurovascular structures are carefully retracted to expose the joint capsule, which is then opened in line with the skin incision. After intraarticular pathology is addressed, careful closure of the capsule is performed, taking care to obtain good hemostasis.

Usual preop diagnosis: Infection; trauma; arthritis

SUMMARY OF PROCEDURE

Position	Supine
Incision	Anterior midline or anteromedial longitudinal
Special instrumentation	Tourniquet
Antibiotics	Cefazolin 1 g iv preop
Surgical time	1 - 2 h
Closing considerations	± Splint while anesthetized; may have suction drain.
EBL	Minimal
Postop care	PACU → room
Mortality	Minimal
Morbidity	Hemarthrosis: 20%
	Thrombophlebitis: 5%
	Infection: 1%
Pain score	5

PATIENT POPULATION CHARACTERISTICS

Age range	Infant – elderly
Male:Female	1:1
Incidence	Rare
Etiology	Trauma (70%); arthritis (20%); infection (10%)
Associated conditions	Inflammatory arthritis; multiple trauma; immunosuppression

ANESTHETIC CONSIDERATIONS

See Anesthetic Considerations for Lower-Extremity Procedures, p. 785.

Reference

1. Crenshaw AH, ed: *Campbell's Operative Orthopaedics*, 8th edition. Mosby-Year Book, St. Louis: 1992.

ANKLE ARTHRODESIS

SURGICAL CONSIDERATIONS

Description: An **ankle fusion** may need to be performed for severe pain 2° arthritis of the ankle. In most cases, an anterior approach is made to the ankle joint. An alternative approach is through the medial malleolus. The ankle joint is exposed and the surfaces of the joint are debrided either with osteotomes or a burr. Cancellous bone is exposed on the distal tibia and talus and the joint is clamped together either with a simple external fixation device with pins going through the distal tibia and talus or with bone screws that go from the distal tibia into the talus. The wound is closed over a drain, and a splint may be applied.

Usual preop diagnosis: Arthritis of the ankle

SUMMARY OF PROCEDURE

Position	Supine
Incision	Anterior midline over distal tibia
Special instrumentation	Tourniquet; external fixator or bone screws
Unique considerations	Intraop radiographs
Antibiotics	Cefazolin 1 g iv preop
Surgical time	2 h
Closing considerations	May be splinted; suction drain.
EBL	100 ml
Postop care	PACU → room
Mortality	Minimal
Morbidity	Nonunion (late): 15% Thrombophlebitis: 10% Hematoma: 5% Wound dehiscence: 5% Infection: 1%
Pain score	8

PATIENT POPULATION CHARACTERISTICS

Age range	All adult
Male:Female	1:1
Etiology	Degenerative arthritis; trauma; avascular necrosis of talus; septic arthritis
Associated conditions	Inflammatory arthritis; any disease requiring steroids

ANESTHETIC CONSIDERATIONS

See Anesthetic Considerations for Lower-Extremity Procedure, p. 785.

References

1. Chapman MW, ed: *Operative Orthopaedics*. 2nd edition. JB Lippincott, Philadelphia: 1993.
2. Crenshaw AH, ed: *Campbell's Operative Orthopaedics*, 8th edition. Mosby-Year Book, St. Louis: 1992.

REPAIR/RECONSTRUCTION OF ANKLE LIGAMENTS

SURGICAL CONSIDERATIONS

Description: Lateral ankle ligaments may be repaired acutely, but generally are reconstructed at a later date, if necessary, with the peroneus brevis used in most reconstructions. An incision is made posterior to the distal fibula, curving around the lateral malleolus and ending in the anterolateral foot. The peroneus brevis tendon is identified and detached from its musculotendinous junction in the leg, and the peroneus brevis muscle is sutured to the peroneus longus tendon. A hole is drilled from anterior to posterior in the distal lateral malleolus; then the detached end of the peroneus brevis tendon is threaded through the hole. It is then attached to either the calcaneus or the talus, anterior to the lateral malleolus, with a staple or by suturing into a hole in the bone. The skin and subcutaneous tissues are closed and a splint or cast is applied.

Usual preop diagnosis: Lateral instability of the ankle

SUMMARY OF PROCEDURE

Position	Supine or lateral decubitus
Incision	Posterolateral aspect of ankle
Special instrumentation	Bone staples; tourniquet
Antibiotics	Cefazolin, 1 g iv preop
Surgical time	2 h
Closing considerations	Splint or cast while still anesthetized.
EBL	Minimal
Postop care	PACU → room or home
Mortality	Minimal
Morbidity	Infection: < 1% Rerupture: < 1% Wound dehiscence: < 0.1%
Pain score	5

PATIENT POPULATION CHARACTERISTICS

Age range	Young adults
Male:Female	2:1
Etiology	Ankle sprain
Associated conditions	Alcohol abuse; obesity; diabetes mellitus (DM)

ANESTHETIC CONSIDERATIONS

See Anesthetic Considerations for Lower-Extremity Procedures, p. 785.

Reference

1. Epps CH Jr, ed: *Complications in Orthopaedic Surgery*, 3rd edition. JB Lippincott, Philadelphia: 1994.

AMPUTATION THROUGH ANKLE (SYME)

SURGICAL CONSIDERATIONS

Description: **Syme amputation** (Fig 10.3-9) is ankle disarticulation with closure, using a posterior flap, including the heel pad. It is more functional than below-knee amputation because patients can bear weight on the end of the stump; however, success is poor in patients with vascular disease or peripheral neuropathy. The posterior flap is dissected directly from the calcaneus, carefully preserving the tough heel pad and its blood supply. The heel pad is sutured directly to the distal tibia to prevent migration and to cover the bone end. The posterior flap is then sutured to the anterior flap with interrupted sutures and a compression dressing applied.

Usual preop diagnosis: Trauma; infection

SUMMARY OF PROCEDURE

Position	Supine
Incision	Anterior and posterior flaps
Special instrumentation	Tourniquet
Antibiotics	Cefazolin 1 g iv preop
Surgical time	1.5-2 h
Closing considerations	Bulky dressing; if infection present, wound may be left open.
EBL	100 ml
Postop care	PACU → room
Mortality	Minimal
Morbidity	Phantom pain: 90% Infection: 10-15% Wound breakdown: 10-15% Pneumonia: 12% MI: 7% PE: 6% Hematoma: 5% Stroke: 5%
Pain score	5

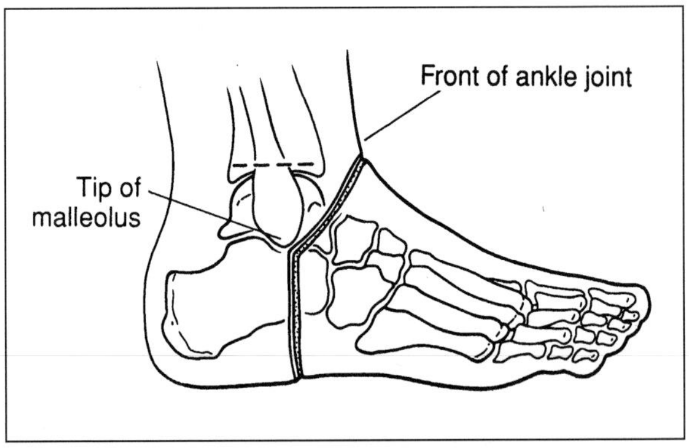

Figure 10.3-9. Incision for Syme amputation. (Reproduced with permission from Chapman MW, ed: *Operative Orthopaedics*. JB Lippincott: 1988. Redrawn from Wagner WF Jr: The Syme amputation. In *American Academy of Orthopaedic Surgeons: Atlas of limb prosthetics*. Mosby-Year Book: 1981.)

PATIENT POPULATION CHARACTERISTICS

Age range	Typically, > 60 yr
Male:Female	3:1
Incidence	20,000-30,000/yr
Etiology	Trauma (50%); infection (30%); congenital anomaly (5%)
Associated conditions	Peripheral vascular disease (30-40%); diabetes mellitus (DM) (< 20%)

ANESTHETIC CONSIDERATIONS

See Anesthetic Considerations for Lower-Extremity Procedures, p. 785.

Reference

1. Epps CH Jr, ed: *Complications in Orthopaedic Surgery*, 3rd edition. JB Lippincott, Philadelphia: 1994.

AMPUTATION, TRANSMETATARSAL

SURGICAL CONSIDERATIONS

Description: This amputation, usually for infection or ischemic necrosis of the toes, is performed at the midmetatarsal level, leaving the patient able to walk without a prosthesis. A transverse dorsal incision is made at the transmetatarsal level, and a plantar incision is made beginning at the corners of the dorsal incision and extending distally to the metatarsal heads to create a long plantar flap. The plantar flap is reflected proximally to the midmetatarsal level and tapered distally. The metatarsals are sectioned with a saw, and nerves and tendons are sectioned proximal to the osteotomies. The plantar flap is then brought over the ends of the bones and sutured with interrupted sutures to the dorsal flap. A compression dressing is applied.

Variant procedure or approaches: Other partial-foot amputations, such as **midtarsal** and **ray amputation**, are much less common. They are managed in a fashion similar to that of the transmetatarsal amputation.

Usual preop diagnosis: Gangrene of the toes; infection

SUMMARY OF PROCEDURE

Position	Supine
Incision	Dorsal and plantar flaps
Special instrumentation	Tourniquet
Antibiotics	Cefazolin 1 g iv preop
Surgical time	1-2 h
Closing considerations	Bulky dressing
EBL	50 ml
Postop care	PACU → room
Mortality	Minimal
Morbidity	Phantom pain: 90% Infection: 10-15% Wound breakdown: 10-15% Hematoma: 5%
Pain score	5

PATIENT POPULATION CHARACTERISTICS

Age range	> 60 yr
Male:Female	3:1
Incidence	20,000-30,000 total amputations/yr
Etiology	Vascular disease (70%); infection (25%) trauma (< 5%); congenital anomalies (< 1%)
Associated conditions	Vascular disease (70%); diabetes mellitus (30%); pulmonary disease (30%)

ANESTHETIC CONSIDERATIONS

See Anesthetic Considerations for Lower-Extremity Procedures, p. 785.

References

1. Crenshaw AH, ed: *Campbell's Operative Orthopaedics*, 8th edition. Mosby-Year Book, St. Louis: 1992.
2. Epps CH Jr, ed: *Complications in Orthopaedic Surgery*, 3rd edition. JB Lippincott, Philadelphia: 1994.

LENGTHENING OR TRANSFER OF TENDONS, ANKLE AND FOOT

SURGICAL CONSIDERATIONS

Description: In cases of motor imbalance from neuromuscular disease or trauma, tendons are lengthened or transferred to a new insertion to partially restore balance or normalize joint motion. For **tendon lengthening**, a longitudinal incision generally is made directly over the tendon. Subcutaneous tissues and tendon sheath are incised to expose the tendon, which is transected with a Z-type incision. The tendon is placed in its lengthened position and the ends of the Z are closed with absorbable suture. If present, the tendon sheath is closed separately from the skin closure. In a **tendon transfer**, the tendon is usually cut close to its insertion and transferred to a new bony insertion, which often requires a separate incision. The tendon is attached to the bone either with a metal staple or by suturing it into a drill hole in the bone.

Variant procedure or approaches: **Achilles tendon lengthening** is used to bring the ankle out of equinus. A **posterior tibial tendon lengthening** and/or **posterior ankle capsulotomy** may accompany the procedure.

Usual preop diagnosis: Contracture of muscle

SUMMARY OF PROCEDURE

	Tendon Lengthening	Achilles Tendon Lengthening
Position	Supine	Prone
Incision	Over tendon; sometimes multiple incisions	Over tendon
Special instrumentation	Tourniquet	⇐
Antibiotics	If young, none; in elderly or infirm, cefazolin 1 g iv preop	⇐
Surgical time	2 h	1 h
Closing considerations	Splint or cast while anesthetized	⇐
EBL	10 ml	⇐
Postop care	PACU → room	PACU → room or home
Mortality	Minimal	⇐
Morbidity	Infection: < 1%	⇐
Pain score	4	3

PATIENT POPULATION CHARACTERISTICS

Age range	Any age
Male:Female	1:1
Incidence	Rare
Etiology	Neuromuscular disease (80%); trauma (20%)
Associated conditions	Static encephalopathy/cerebral palsy (75%); other neuromuscular disease (25%)

ANESTHETIC CONSIDERATIONS

See Anesthetic Considerations for Lower-Extremity Procedures, p. 785.

Reference

1. Crenshaw AH, ed: *Campbell's Operative Orthopaedics*, 8th edition. Mosby-Year Book, St. Louis: 1992.

AMPUTATION ABOVE THE KNEE

SURGICAL CONSIDERATIONS

Description: In above-the-knee amputations, the distal part of the lower extremity is excised, starting just above the knee at the level of the distal third of the femur (Fig 10.3-10). A stump is fashioned, and will require prosthetic fitting at a later time. The most commonly performed stumps incorporate anterior and posterior flaps of equal length. The underlying muscles (hamstrings and quadriceps) are either sewn to each other (**myoplasty**) or to bone (**myodesis**). In a **guillotine**, or **open amputation**, the stump is not fashioned (tissues are not closed) until later. This is a multistage procedure used for dirty, traumatic amputations, infection, or above-knee amputations with questionable survival, and is usually done as a life-saving measure. Internal fixation of part of the remaining femur may be indicated in traumatic amputations. The patient returns to the OR every 1-3 d for redebridement until closure of the clean stump can be performed.

Usual preop diagnosis: Peripheral vascular disease or gangrene of lower extremity; trauma to lower extremity; open-femur fracture with traumatic amputation; tumor of lower extremity

SUMMARY OF PROCEDURE

Position	Supine
Incision	Anterior and posterior on thigh
Special instrumentation	Amputation saw and rasp; drill for myodesis
Unique considerations	Patient often very ill from sepsis, chronic disease or trauma
Antibiotics	Cefazolin or cefamandole 1 g iv q 6-8 h), ± gentamicin (80 mg iv q 8 h); adjust dosage for renal status, ± penicillin (1-2 million U iv q 4 h).
Surgical time	1- 2 h
Closing considerations	Compressive dressing ± special stump sock
EBL	250 ml or more; higher for traumatic amputations
Postop care	Generally PACU → room (if medically unstable → ICU)
Mortality	Approximately 10-20%; higher in PVD (10-39%)
Morbidity	Phantom limb: 85-95%
	Phantom pain: 2-15%
	Wound infection ± deep infection: < 15% in PVD
	Respiratory failure or pneumonia: 10-15%
	MI: 7-10%
	Thromboembolism: 6-10%
	Cerebrovascular accident: 5-10%
	Failure to heal ± wound dehiscence: Uncommon
	Contractures – flexion and abduction contracture: Common
	Urinary retention requiring catheterization: Common
	Hematoma: Rare
	Reamputation: Rare
	Neuromas: Rare
	UTI: Rare
	Contralateral amputation, especially in diabetics and those with PVD
	Postop depression
Pain score	7-10

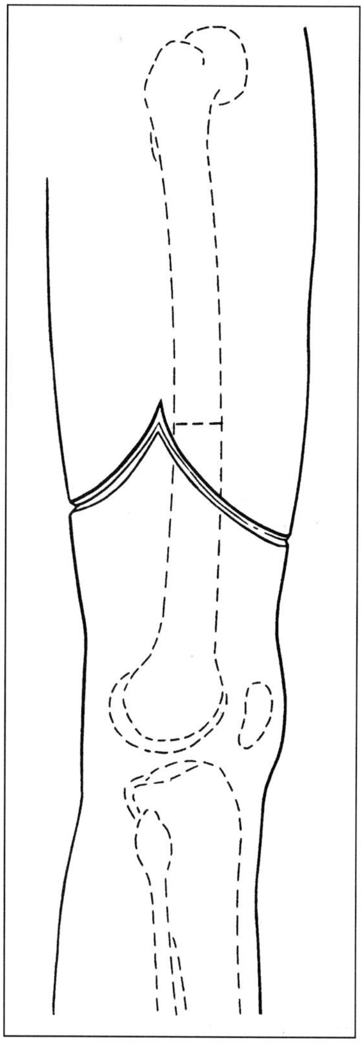

Figure 10.3-10. Amputation through middle third of thigh. (Reproduced with permission from Crenshaw AH: *Campbell's Operative Orthopaedics*, 7th edition. CV Mosby: 1987.)

PATIENT POPULATION CHARACTERISTICS

Age range	70-90% > 60 yr: PVD, diabetic gangrene 18-35 yr: multiple trauma with traumatic amputation; tumor of lower extremity
Male:Female	Overall 3-9:1 Elderly, predominance of males Multiple trauma, 4-5:1 Tumor 1:1
Incidence	Common for PVD patients; rare for trauma or tumor
Etiology	PVD and diabetic gangrene (70-90%); multiple trauma (younger patients) (rare—usually with severe Grade IIIC injuries with neurovascular severance); tumor (rare); uncontrollable infection (e.g., gas gangrene) (rare)
Associated conditions	Diabetes (70-80% of patients presenting for this procedure); numerous other serious medical conditions; multiple trauma in younger patients

ANESTHETIC CONSIDERATIONS

See Anesthetic Considerations for Above- and Below-Knee Amputation, p. 778.

References

1. McCollough NC III, Epps CH Jr, Banks WJ Jr: Complications of amputation surgery. In *Complications in Orthopaedic Surgery*, 3rd edition. Epps CH Jr, ed. JB Lippincott, Philadelphia: 1994, 1279-1308.
2. Tooms RE: Amputations of lower extremity. In *Campbell's Operative Orthopaedics*, 9th edition. Canale ST, ed. Mosby-Year Book, St. Louis: 1998, Vol 1, 532-41.

AMPUTATION BELOW THE KNEE

SURGICAL CONSIDERATIONS

Description: **Below-the-knee amputation** is ablation of the lower limb, usually at the level of the midleg. A long, posterior flap normally is used to cover the stump. The condition of the soft tissues may dictate the level and/or type of flaps used. The procedure begins with an anterior transverse incision made over the midtibia. A long posterior flap, which is 2-3 times the diameter of the leg in length, is then made. The bone is exposed anteriorly and the anterolateral neurovascular structures and muscles are transected and ligated as appropriate (Fig 10.3-11). The bone is then transected with a bone saw, and the posterior structures are transected and ligated as appropriate. The amputated leg and foot are then removed from the table and the posterior flap is tapered and shaped for closure. Deep sutures are placed to secure the posterior muscles to the anterior tibia. The skin opening and subcutaneous tissues are closed with interrupted sutures (Fig 10.3-12). Finally, a drain is placed (sometimes), and either a compression dressing or an immediate postop cast is applied.

Variant procedure or approaches: **Guillotine amputation** may be used as the first of a two-stage procedure in infected or contaminated cases. With a guillotine amputation, the bone and soft tissues are transected very quickly in guillotine fashion at the midtibial level. Neurovascular structures are ligated as appropriate. These wounds are usually left open and a compression dressing applied.

Usual preop diagnosis: Dysvascular limb; infection; trauma

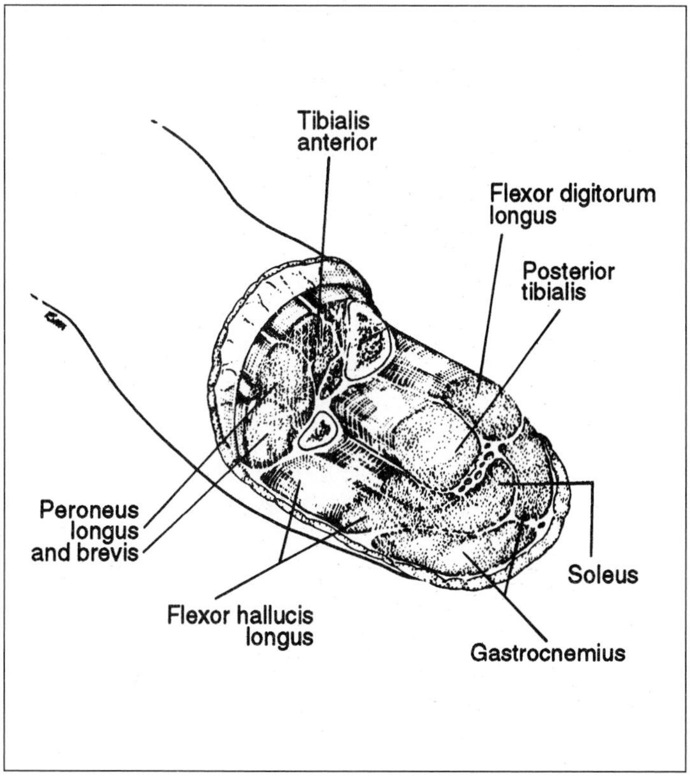

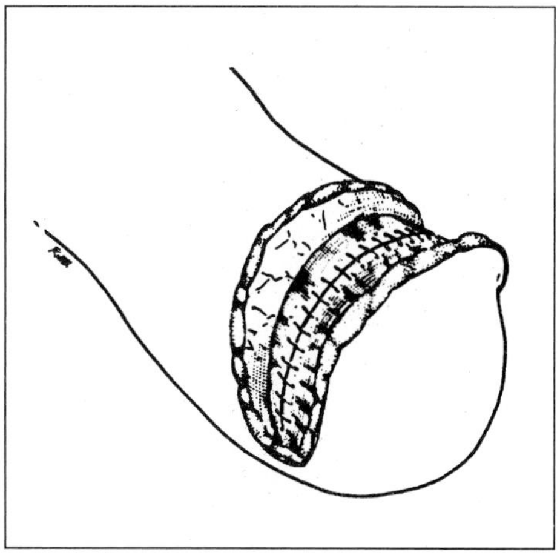

↑ **Figure 10.3-12.** Suture of flap to deep fascia and periosteum anteriorly.

← **Figure 10.3-11.** Below-knee amputation prior to closure.

(Both figures reproduced with permission from Crenshaw AH: *Campbell's Operative Orthopaedics*, 8th edition. CV Mosby: 1992. Redrawn from Burgess EM and Zettl JH: *Artif Limbs* 1969; 13:1.)

SUMMARY OF PROCEDURE

Position	Supine
Incision	Anterior and posterior flaps; for guillotine amputation, circumferential incision
Special instrumentation	Bone saw; tourniquet, if traumatic (tourniquet contraindicated if infected or avascular)
Antibiotics	Cefazolin 1 g iv preop
Surgical time	1.5 h; for guillotine amputation, 0.5 h
Closing considerations	May use cast; drain. Bulky dressing needed for guillotine amputation.
EBL	200 ml
Postop care	PACU → room
Mortality	10%
Morbidity	Phantom pain: 90%
	Infection: 10-15%
	Wound breakdown: 10-15%
	Pneumonia: 12%
	MI: 7%
	PE: 6%
	Hematoma: 5%
	Stroke: 5%
Pain score	5

PATIENT POPULATION CHARACTERISTICS

Age range	Usually, > 60
Male:Female	3:1
Incidence	20,000-30,000 total amputations/yr
Etiology	Dysvascular limb (70%); trauma (20%); infection (5%); tumor (5%); congenital anomaly (< 1%)
Associated conditions	Vascular disease (70-80%); malnutrition (50%); diabetes mellitus (30%); pulmonary disease (30%)

ANESTHETIC CONSIDERATIONS FOR ABOVE- AND BELOW-KNEE AMPUTATION

PREOPERATIVE

Vascular disease and tumors are the two most common indications for these surgeries. Patients presenting for amputations often have severe systemic vascular disease. Their inability to perform exercise limits the usefulness of preop history in evaluating cardiopulmonary reserve, and often necessitates invasive studies for full evaluation.

Respiratory — Smoking is a risk factor common to both vascular and pulmonary diseases. Chronic bronchitis or COPD patients should have maximum medical therapy (e.g., inhaled bronchodilators, theophylline and steroids, when appropriate) prior to anesthesia. Regional anesthesia is an excellent choice for patients with severe pulmonary disease.
Tests: As indicated from H&P.

Cardiovascular — Significant cardiovascular disease is present in 30% of patients presenting for vascular surgery. Particularly in diabetics, CAD is often silent. Dipyridamole thallium imaging of the heart can reveal the preop myocardium at risk of ischemia; however, therapy of stenotic coronary arteries usually can be undertaken only after the amputation. Medical management, to include ß-blockers when tolerated, will reduce perioperative MIs.
Tests: ECG; others as indicated from H&P.

Neurological — Peripheral and autonomic neuropathies may be present in the diabetic patient. Hence, these patients may be more susceptible to injury from malpositioning and are less able to tolerate the hemodynamic changes associated with regional anesthesia. Preexisting neurological deficits should be carefully documented.

Musculoskeletal — Rhabdomyolysis can occur in the presence of partial ischemia. (See Renal, below.)

Hematologic — Often a trial of heparin, warfarin or thrombolytic therapy will have been undertaken prior to amputation. Coagulation studies, including PT, PTT and bleeding time are, therefore, often necessary to determine the appropriateness of epidural or intrathecal anesthesia. Warfarin-induced elevation of the PT can be reversed preop with FFP 5-10 ml/kg body weight. This therapy may induce fluid overload in patients with poor cardiac reserve. For these patients, diuretics should be administered to maintain normovolemia.
Tests: As indicated from H&P.

Renal — Limb ischemia can result in myoglobinemia from rhabdomyolysis. Evidence of progressive renal failure or rising CPK-MM fractions should be treated with hydration, forced alkaline diuresis and prompt amputation.
Tests: Consider creatinine; BUN; CPK enzymes, if creatinine is elevated.

Laboratory — Diabetic patients require preop control of blood glucose and perioperative glucose monitoring.

Premedication — Standard premedication (see p. B-2).

INTRAOPERATIVE

Anesthetic technique: Either regional or GA may be appropriate.

Regional anesthesia: Both SAB and epidural blocks are useful techniques. Subarachnoid anesthesia has the advantage of limited spread of the block above the level of surgery, while obtaining adequate blockade of the sacral roots that are resistant to low-dose epidural techniques. Epidural anesthesia allows for extending the duration of anesthesia and for the administration of postop epidural analgesia. Anesthesia from T12 (T8 with tourniquet) is adequate. Full motor blockade is not necessary. Typical drugs and doses include: subarachnoid—75 mg of 5% lidocaine in 5% dextrose (controversial) with morphine 0.2 mg; epidural—12-15 ml 2% lidocaine with epinephrine 1:200,000 in divided doses.

General anesthesia:

Induction — Standard induction (see p. B-2) is appropriate for patients with normal airways. Intubation is indicated for diabetic patients with gastroparesis.

Maintenance — Standard maintenance (see p. B-3).

Emergence — No special considerations

Blood and fluid requirements	Moderate blood loss IV: 16 ga × 1 NS/LR @ 4-6 ml/kg/h	Expect 100-200 ml blood loss, mostly during cleaning of wound made while developing a flap.
Control of blood loss	Tourniquet may be used.	Inflation pressure is typically 100 mmHg > systolic pressure. Maximum "safe" tourniquet time is 1.5-2 h, followed by a 5- to- (preferably) 15-min reperfusion interval, if further tourniquet is necessary.
Special considerations	Tourniquet deflation and limb reperfusion	Mild hypotension is common. In patients with moderate-to-severe lung disease, continue controlled ventilation until after the lactic acid accumulated in the ischemic leg is metabolized (3-5 min), since these patients may be unable to increase ventilation adequately to buffer this acid load.
Monitoring	Standard monitors (see p. B-1). ± CVP line ± Arterial line	Invasive monitoring is indicated in the presence of severe cardiac or pulmonary disease. Serial blood glucose determination should be made in the diabetic patient.
Positioning	✓ and pad pressure points. ✓ eyes.	Meticulous padding of the extremities is necessary to prevent ischemic skin ulceration in patients with vascular insufficiency.

POSTOPERATIVE

Complications	Hematoma Bleeding	✓ drains.
Pain management	Spinal opiates Epidural analgesia	Epidural hydromorphone 50 μg/ml infused at 50-200 μg/h provides excellent analgesia.
Tests	CXR if CVP was placed	Other studies as indicated.

Reference

1. McCollough NC III, Epps CH Jr, Banks WJ Jr: Complications of amputation surgery. In *Complications in Orthopaedic Surgery*, 3rd edition. Epps CH Jr, ed. JB Lippincott, Philadelphia: 1994, 1279-1308.

FASCIOTOMY OF THE THIGH

SURGICAL CONSIDERATIONS

Description: Increased intracompartmental pressure in the thigh requires surgical release of tight skin and fascial structures (Fig 10.3-13). This usually occurs after severe trauma to the thigh (e.g., crush injury, comminuted fracture, etc.) or, after prolonged vascular surgery, with ischemia to the thigh. Compartment syndrome is a true emergency and must be treated within minutes of recognition. Failure to do so may result in loss of limb or death. Conventional devices may be used to measure intracompartmental pressure, which usually is abnormal if > 30-35 mmHg (normal = < 30 mmHg). **Fasciotomy of the thigh** involves incising the skin and fascia over the thigh and debriding any necrotic tissue. The wound is left open for later redebridement, delayed primary closure or skin grafting. Thus, the fasciotomy begins a multistage procedure of incision and debridement, with subsequent reconstruction.

Usual preop diagnosis: Compartment syndrome of thigh; crush injury to thigh

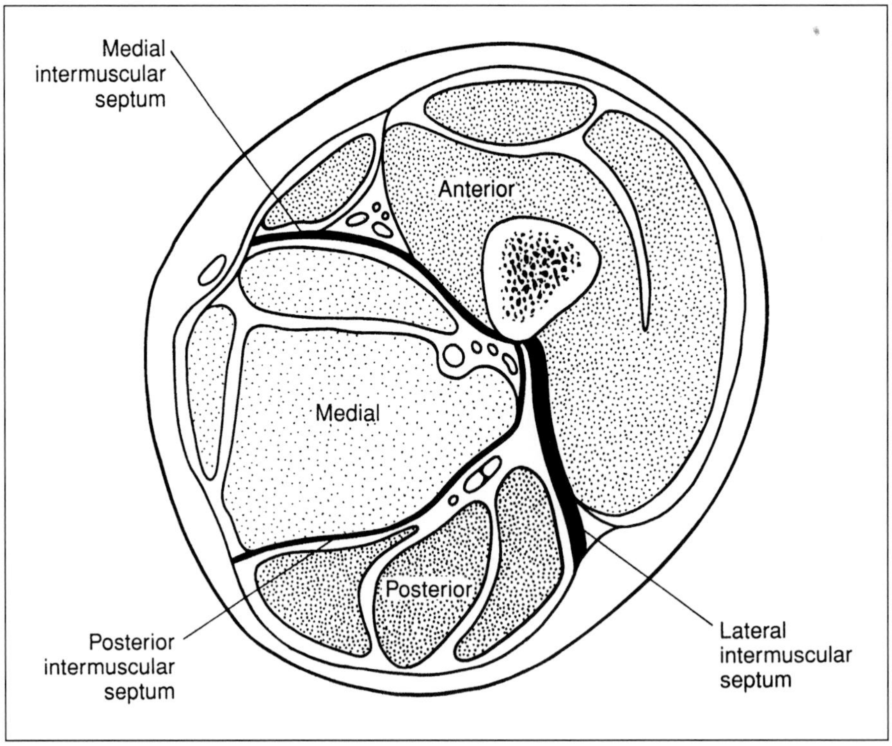

Figure 10.3-13. Cross-section of the thigh showing the 3 major compartments. (Reproduced with permission from Tarlow SD, Achterman C, Hayhurst J, Ovadin D: Acute compartment syndrome of the thigh. *J Bone Joint Surg* [Am] 1986; 68:1441.)

SUMMARY OF PROCEDURE

Position	Supine or lateral decubitus
Incision	Lateral thigh
Unique considerations	Patient may be very ill. If an ipsilateral femoral fracture is present with a compartment syndrome, the surgeon may want to perform ORIF, intramedullary nailing, or external fixation of the fracture.
Antibiotics	Cefazolin or cefamandole 1 g iv q 6 h
Surgical time	1.5-2 h for fasciotomy alone
Closing considerations	Wound left open and covered by sterile dressings.
EBL	250-500 ml
Postop care	If surgery is performed acutely, patient frequently will be a multiple-trauma victim with numerous injuries and extensive blood loss, and usually goes to ICU.
Mortality	Dependent on extent of multiple trauma
Morbidity	Hypotension and fluid loss: Common Neurological deficit to peripheral nerves: Common, if decompression delayed Respiratory distress and fat embolism: Not uncommon, if concomitant femur fracture Vascular complications: Not uncommon Amputation: Rare if decompression prompt Systemic sepsis: Rare Wound infection: Rare New compartment syndrome; insufficient fasciotomy: Rare
Pain score	7-8

PATIENT POPULATION CHARACTERISTICS

Age range	Any age, but predominance of males < 30 yr
Male:Female	5:1
Incidence	Extremely rare
Etiology	Trauma – motorcycle and motor vehicle accidents, falls, industrial injury, crush injuries; postsurgery – local hematoma and swelling; thrombosis or disruption of blood supply to thigh (e.g., failed proximal vascular bypass surgery, aortic dissection, etc.); massive infection of thigh compartment (e.g., gas gangrene)
Associated conditions	Burns; drug and alcohol overdose; frequently associated with trauma to other organ systems

ANESTHETIC CONSIDERATIONS

See Anesthetic Considerations following Fasciotomy of the Leg, p. 782.

References

1. Mubarak SJ: Compartment syndromes. In *Operative Orthopaedics*, 2nd edition. Chapman MW, et al, eds. JB Lippincott, Philadelphia: 1993, 379-96.
2. Dutkowsky JP: Miscellaneous nontraumatic disorders. In *Campbell's Operative Orthopaedics*, 9th edition. Canale ST, ed. Mosby-Year Book, St. Louis: 1998, Vol 1, 787-856.

FASCIOTOMY OF THE LEG

SURGICAL CONSIDERATIONS

Description: This procedure is the surgical decompression of fascial compartments for treatment or prevention of compartment syndrome. Patients are often very ill and unstable with other injuries or disease. Compartment syndrome is a true emergency and must be treated within minutes of recognition. Failure to do so may result in loss of limb or death. There are four compartments in the leg: anterior, lateral, deep posterior and superficial posterior (Fig 10.3-14). Generally, all four compartments are released during the procedure. A four-compartment fascial decompression can be performed through two incisions—medial and lateral. A medial longitudinal incision is made just posterior to the tibia; through this incision, the superficial and deep posterior compartments are identified and the fascia incised in longitudinal fashion. A straight, lateral, longitudinal incision is made and the deep fascia overlying the anterior and lateral compartments is identified. The fascia of each compartment is then incised longitudinally. Skin incisions are rarely closed because of the swelling. A compression dressing is applied and splints may be used.

Usual preop diagnosis: Compartment syndrome; vascular trauma

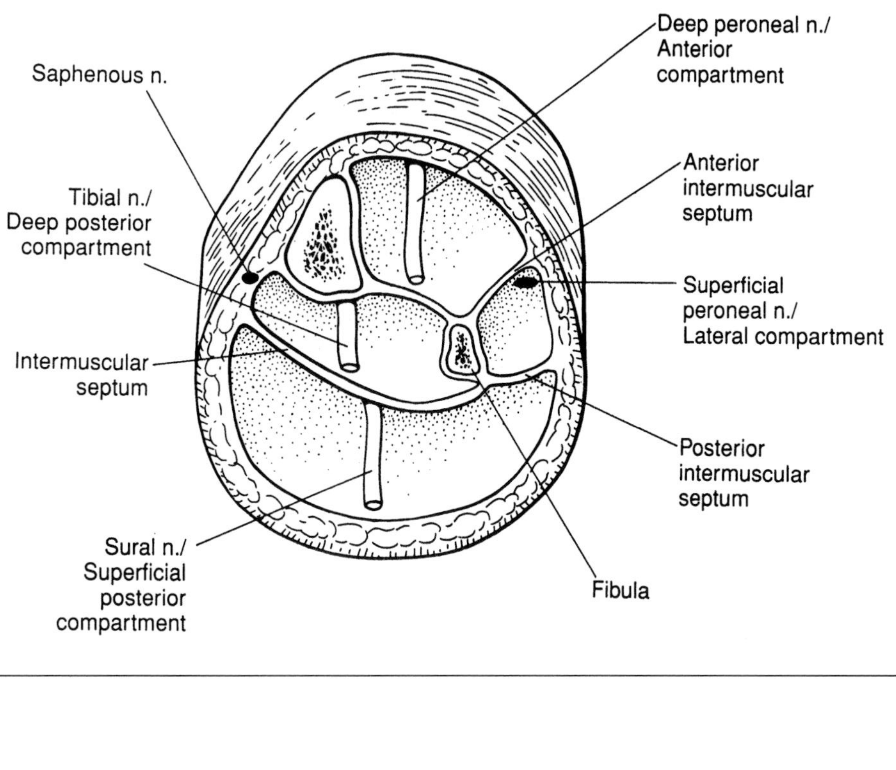

Figure 10.3-14. Cross-section of the left leg, middle lower third, showing the 4 compartments with associated peripheral nerves. (Reproduced with permission from Mubarak SJ, Owen CA: Double-incision fasciotomy of the leg for decompression in compartment syndromes. *J Bone Joint Surg* [Am] 1977; 59:184-87.)

SUMMARY OF PROCEDURE

Position	Supine
Incision	Medial and lateral parallel to tibia
Unique considerations	Often associated with fracture; may require fixation.
Antibiotics	Cefazolin 1 g iv preop
Surgical time	0.5+ h
Closing considerations	Wounds left open; splint may be required.
EBL	100 ml
Postop care	PACU → room; vascular monitoring is carried out clinically via a pulse oximeter on toes
Mortality	Minimal
Morbidity	Myonecrosis: 50% Thrombophlebitis: 10-20% Infection: 10-15%
Pain score	3

PATIENT POPULATION CHARACTERISTICS

Age range	All ages
Male:Female	1:1
Incidence	~5% of tibia fractures
Etiology	Trauma – blunt fracture, vascular (90%); drug overdose (10%); burns (< 5%); revascularization (< 5%)
Associated conditions	Multiple trauma (60%); vascular disease (15%)

ANESTHETIC CONSIDERATIONS FOR FASCIOTOMY OF THIGH AND LEG

PREOPERATIVE

Compartment syndromes and necrotizing fasciitis are the indications for these procedures. Patients with compartment syndrome often have no systemic disease, while patients with necrotizing fasciitis have a rapidly life-threatening infection that requires prompt surgical debridement and often is complicated by rhabdomyolysis and DIC.

Respiratory	Usually no special considerations, unless massive sepsis.
Cardiovascular	Sepsis is uniformly present in patients with necrotizing fasciitis. Management includes antibiotics and hemodynamic support with dopamine (5-15 μg/kg/min) or epinephrine (0.02-0.25 μg/kg/min) with therapy guided by invasive hemodynamic monitoring, which may include PA catheter.
Neurological	If fasciotomy is for compartment syndrome, there may be compromise of distal nerves and blood flow. Perform a thorough neurologic exam of the involved extremity to document preop deficits.
Hematologic	If infection is the indication for the fasciotomy, DIC is likely. Evaluate for pathologic bleeding. Administer factors necessary to correct coagulopathy during the procedure. **Tests:** CBC; PT; PTT; fibrinogen; fibrin split products; Plt count
Renal	Both necrotizing fasciitis and compartment syndrome often cause myoglobinuria and rhabdomyolysis. Myoglobinuria can be inferred from urine that is dipstick-positive for occult blood but microscopically free of RBCs in the absence of hemolysis.
Laboratory	Hct; serial K^+ levels if there is an active diuresis; other studies as indicated from H&P.
Premedication	Diazepam 5-10 mg po 1 hr preop

INTRAOPERATIVE

Anesthetic technique: Regional techniques are appropriate for compartment syndrome decompression, unless there is evidence of DIC. These surgeries are usually of short duration (< 1 h). Sepsis and hemodynamic instability usually mandate GETA for fasciotomy in patients with necrotizing fasciitis.

Regional anesthesia: Either subarachnoid or epidural blocks are useful in the absence of infection or severe coagulopathy. Subarachnoid anesthesia has the advantage of adequate blockade of the sacral roots that are resistant to low-dose epidural techniques. Anesthesia from T10-S2 is adequate. Typical drugs and dosages include: subarachnoid—15 mg of 0.5% bupivacaine; epidural—12-15 ml 2% lidocaine with epinephrine 1:200,000 in divided doses.

General anesthesia:

Induction	Standard induction (see p. B-2).	
Maintenance	Standard maintenance (see p. B-3).	
Emergence	Consider postop ventilation for patients with impaired oxygenation or ongoing hemodynamic instability; otherwise, no special considerations.	
Blood and fluid requirements	IV: 16 ga × 1 (compartment syndrome) 14-16 ga × 2 (necrotizing fasciitis) NS/LR @ 4-6 ml/kg/h	To prevent renal damage, insure adequate circulatory volume; induce osmotic diuresis with mannitol 0.25 g/kg iv. Furosemide 10-100 mg also may be necessary to maintain diuresis. Replace UO with 0.5 NS + 50 mEq bicarbonate/L, or as guided by invasive monitoring.
Monitoring	Standard monitors (see p. B-1). UO ± Arterial line ± CVP or PA catheter	Patients with necrotizing fasciitis require an arterial line and either a CVP or PA catheter to guide fluid and inotropic/pressor therapy.
Positioning	✓ and pad pressure points. ✓ eyes.	

POSTOPERATIVE

Complications	DIC Renal failure 2° rhabdomyolysis Hypo/hyperkalemia Sepsis syndrome including ARDS	
Pain management	PCA or epidural analgesia	See pp. C-3, C-1.
Tests	Hct Electrolytes UA (dipstick and microscopic)	For patients with sepsis: coagulation profile, including PT/PTT, fibrin split products and Plt count

References

1. Epps CH Jr, ed: *Complications in Orthopaedic Surgery*, 3rd edition. JB Lippincott, Philadelphia: 1994.
2. Rockwood CA Jr, Green DP, Bucholz RW, Heckman JD, eds: *Rockwood and Green's Fractures in Adults*, 4th edition. JB Lippincott, Philadelphia: 1996.

BIOPSY, LEG AND FOOT

SURGICAL CONSIDERATIONS

Description: Biopsy is performed to excise tissues for pathologic evaluation, usually through a small, longitudinal wound. For **incisional biopsy**, a longitudinal incision is made over the mass. Overlying soft tissues are incised with minimal undermining. The area in question is incised and the biopsy removed, with care being taken to prevent spillage into the adjacent tissues. The pathologist often is asked to perform a frozen section to determine whether diagnostic tissue is present. The wound is closed with interrupted sutures and a compression dressing applied. A splint or cast may be used if a significant amount of bone has been removed. If the lesion is small, x-ray control or image intensification may be necessary for localization. **Needle biopsy** may be used for distinct osseous lesions to obtain small amounts of tissue for culture or histology. **Excisional biopsy** may be used for benign lesions like exostoses or lipomas.

Usual preop diagnosis: Tumor; infection

SUMMARY OF PROCEDURE

	Incisional Biopsy	Needle Biopsy	Excisional Biopsy
Position	Supine	⇐	⇐
Incision	Short longitudinal	Stab wound	Stab wound
Special instrumentation	Bone-cutting instruments; x-ray or image intensifier	Trephine (e.g., Craig needle); x-ray or image intensifier	X-ray or image intensifier
Unique considerations	Tourniquet	⇐	⇐ (Bone graft may be necessary.)
Antibiotics	None (May be given postop.)	⇐	⇐
Surgical time	1 h	0.5 h	0.5-2 h
Closing considerations	May be splinted.	Usually no splint	May be splinted.
EBL	50 ml	Minimal	100-200 ml
Postop care	PACU → room or home	⇐	PACU → room
Mortality	Minimal	⇐	⇐
Morbidity	Hematoma: 5%	⇐	⇐
	Tumor spread: < 5%	⇐	⇐
	Infection: < 1%	⇐	⇐
Pain score	3	2	3

PATIENT POPULATION CHARACTERISTICS

Age range	All ages
Male:Female	1:1
Incidence	Rare
Etiology	Tumor (75%); infection (25%)
Associated conditions	Metastatic disease; immune compromise

ANESTHETIC CONSIDERATIONS

See Anesthetic Considerations for Lower-Extremity Procedures, p. 785.

Reference

1. Enneking WF: *Musculoskeletal Tumor Surgery*. Churchill Livingstone, New York: 1983.

BIOPSY OR DRAINAGE OF ABSCESS/EXCISION OF TUMOR

SURGICAL CONSIDERATIONS

Description: This procedure involves obtaining a piece of tissue for histologic and/or bacteriologic diagnosis by closed, percutaneous means or by open biopsy. Subsequently, the area may be drained (abscess or infection) or an open excision of a tumor may follow (with or without internal fixation). For excision of tumors of the pelvis, acetabulum or femur, please consult the appropriate section describing fractures of the area. Each case must be individualized.

Variant procedure or approaches: Excision of infection or tumor of proximal or distal femur, femoral shaft, pelvis or acetabulum.

Usual preop diagnosis: Femur: biopsy of mass; infection; osteomyelitis. Pelvis or acetabulum: biopsy of pelvis or acetabulum; drainage of abscess or infection of pelvis or acetabulum; osteomyelitis of pelvis or acetabulum; septic arthritis of acetabulum

SUMMARY OF PROCEDURE

Position	Supine or lateral decubitus
Incision	Percutaneous, short or long; location depends on surgical approach.
Special instrumentation	Biopsy needles and instruments to take core biopsy; bone cement may be used to plug biopsy site. Some surgeons use fracture table or radiolucent table with image intensifier.
Unique considerations	May require intraop frozen section and gram stain.
Antibiotics	After tissue has been obtained, cefazolin or cefamandole 1 g iv q 6 h × 48 h. A gram stain will help decide immediate antibiotic coverage, but cultures and sensitivities are ultimately necessary.
Surgical time	1 h for simple procedures; much longer (up to 12 h) for more extensive excisional procedures ± further reconstruction.
EBL	100-1000 ml or more
Postop care	If procedure is extensive with much blood loss, or the patient is unstable or ill from chronic sepsis or invasive tumor, it is prudent to send patient to ICU.
Mortality	Dependent on extent of procedure. Biopsy or drainage of a small, localized abscess in soft tissue or bone is rarely life-threatening. Wide/radical excision of a malignant tumor in the pelvis or extremities is frequently life/limb-threatening.
Morbidity	The following are dependent on site and procedure: Intraop fracture Nonunion Chronic osteomyelitis Compartment syndrome Residual instability of pelvis or hip joint Fracture of pelvis or acetabulum, nonunion Chronic osteomyelitis or septic arthritis Hypotension 2° to blood loss Respiratory distress Neurological injury to lumbosacral plexus, sciatic nerve or other peripheral nerves Vascular injury to iliac or other vessels Injury to GI, genitourinary or gynecological organs
Pain score	2-10

PATIENT POPULATION CHARACTERISTICS

Age range	Any age; predominance of elderly patients with tumors
Male:Female	1:1
Incidence	Rare
Etiology	Benign and malignant tumors (common); infection (rare); previous surgery (rare); previous trauma (rare)
Associated conditions	Metastatic disease or other foci of infection

ANESTHETIC CONSIDERATIONS FOR LOWER-EXTREMITY PROCEDURES

(Procedures covered: ORIF of femur, tibia, ankle and foot; intramedullary nailing of femur and tibia; closed reduction and external fixation of femur and tibia; distal tibial and ankle procedures; repair nonunion/malunion of femur and tibia; ankle arthroscopy, arthrotomy, arthrodesis; amputation of ankle and foot; tendon lengthening; biopsy of leg and foot; biopsy or drainage of abscess/excision of tumor)

PREOPERATIVE

Trauma victims comprise the largest group of patients for these procedures. Minimizing the time between fracture and surgery for open wounds significantly reduces the incidence of wound infection. Evaluations for other injury, adequacy of fluid resuscitation and preexisting conditions need to be undertaken promptly and used as a guide for anesthetic management. Patients with bone cancer form another subset of patients and often have concurrent medical conditions and have undergone chemotherapy or radiation therapy preop.

Respiratory Pulmonary fat embolus occurs in 10-15% of patients following bone fracture. Sx include hypoxemia, ↑HR, tachypnea, respiratory alkalosis, mental status changes and conjunctival petechiae. Lab analysis may reveal fat in the urine. Preop therapy for this condition should include supplemental O_2 with mechanical ventilation, to correct hypoxemia, and meticulous fluid management to prevent worsening pulmonary capillary leak.
Tests: Consider CXR; others as indicated from H&P.

Cardiovascular Cardiac contusion or tamponade are possible if blunt chest trauma has occurred during the injury. A large volume of blood can be hidden around a long bone fracture site. ↑HR, orthostasis or ↓BP indicate hypovolemia, and this should be corrected with crystalloid (10-40 ml/kg) or blood if Hct < 24%. In patients with a tibial or distal femur fracture, and who are presenting with hemodynamic instability and ongoing blood loss, consider applying a tourniquet to the thigh prior to induction.
Tests: Consider ECG; CPK enzyme levels and ECHO will help evaluate the presence of cardiac injury.

Neurological Perform a thorough neurological evaluation, including mental status and peripheral sensory exams. A CT scan of the head is indicated for any patient with prolonged loss of consciousness prior to anesthesia. Drug abuse is common in trauma patients and they should be asked specifically about any drug use.
Tests: Patients with inappropriate behavior or a positive drug abuse Hx should undergo a urine and plasma drug screen.

Musculoskeletal Consider cervical instability and obtain spine films if mechanism of injury included rapid deceleration or trauma to the head or neck. Myoglobinemia and ↑K^+ may result from crush injury.

Hematologic Patients with cancer who have undergone chemotherapy and multiple transfusions often develop sensitivities to blood products and may require specialized blood products such as leukocyte-poor PRBC or red cells negative for a particular antigen. The availability of these blood products should be confirmed prior to surgery.
Tests: Hct and others as indicated from H&P.

Renal **Tests:** UA

Laboratory Other tests as indicated from H&P.

Premedication Due to the risk of gastric aspiration, minimal or no premedication is given to trauma victims. For other patients, diazepam 5-10 mg po 1 h preop. Narcotic premedication (morphine 1-2 mg iv q 10 min titrated to effect) is appropriate for patients experiencing pain with movement.

INTRAOPERATIVE

Anesthetic technique: For trauma patients, regional anesthesia permits evaluation of mental status, provides intact airway reflexes and ↓blood loss. Combative patients, those requiring multiple concurrent surgical procedures or prolonged (> 2 h) procedures are often managed with GETA.

Regional anesthesia: Either subarachnoid or epidural blocks are useful techniques. Subarachnoid anesthesia has the advantage of adequate blockade of the sacral roots that are resistant to low-dose epidural techniques. Epidural anesthesia allows for the administration of postop epidural analgesia. Anesthesia from T12 (T8 with tourniquet) to S2 is adequate. Full motor blockade is desirable. Typical drugs and doses include: subarachnoid—15 mg of 0.5% bupivacaine with morphine 0.2 mg (omit if outpatient); epidural—12-15 ml 2% lidocaine with epinephrine 1:200,000 in divided doses (Na bicarbonate 0.1 mg/ml will speed onset of block).

General anesthesia:

Induction Standard induction (see p. B-2) is appropriate for patients with normal airways. Trauma patients require a rapid-sequence induction (see p. B-5) and intubation with cricoid pressure to prevent gastric aspiration.

Maintenance Standard maintenance (see p. B-3). Trauma patients are often cold and require active warming if < 35°C (convection blanket and active humidifier). Warming the patient may unmask severe hypovolemia that should be corrected.

Emergence	Trauma patients should have full return of protective airway reflexes and, given the possibility of fat embolus, evidence of adequate oxygenation on 50% O_2 prior to extubation.	
Blood and fluid requirements	IV: 14-16 ga × 2 NS/LR @ 4-8 ml/kg/h Warm fluids. Humidify gases.	Some fractures can involve large (30 ml/kg) blood losses that are hidden in the leg or thigh. Clinical signs of hypovolemia and serial Hct determination should guide fluid therapy.
Control of blood loss	Tourniquet	Inflation pressure is typically 100 mmHg greater than systolic pressure. Maximum "safe" tourniquet time is 1.5-2 h, followed by a 5- to- (preferably) 15-min reperfusion interval, if further tourniquet time is necessary.
Monitoring	Standard monitors (see p. B-1). ± Arterial line ± CVP line	Arterial/CVP lines indicated for patients with ↓BP not readily correctable with crystalloid infusion, massive blood loss (> 1 blood volume) or the need for postop ventilation.
Positioning	✓ and pad pressure points. ✓ eyes.	
Special considerations	Release of tourniquet	A 20% fall in mean BP is common on tourniquet deflation. Additional crystalloid (5-10 ml/kg) may be necessary to replace edema fluid and blood loss to the leg.
Complications	Fat embolism Myoglobinemia	

POSTOPERATIVE

Complications	Hypoxemia	May be 2° fat embolism.
Pain management	Spinal opiates: Epidural anesthesia Spinal anesthesia	Epidural hydromorphone 50 μg/ml infused at 100-250 μg/h provides excellent analgesia. Intrathecal morphine 0.2-0.3 mg provides analgesia for up to 24 h after administration. (Monitor for delayed respiratory depression.)
Tests	Hct CXR, if CVP placed or oxygenation is impaired.	Other studies as indicated.

References

1. Carnesale PG: General principles of tumors. In *Campbell's Operative Orthopaedics*, 9th edition. Canale ST, ed. Mosby-Year Book, St. Louis: 1998, Vol 1, 643-82.
2. Warner WC Jr: General principles of infections. In *Campbell's Operative Orthopaedics*, 9th edition. Canale ST, ed. Mosby-Year Book, St. Louis: 1998, Vol 1, 563-77.
3. Kyle RF, Schmidt AH, Campbell SJ: Complications of the treatment of fractures and dislocations of the hip. In *Complications in Orthopaedic Surgery*, 3rd edition. Epps CH Jr, ed. JB Lippincott, Philadelphia: 1994, 443-86.

Surgeon

Eugene J. Carragee, MD

10.4 SPINE SURGERY

Anesthesiologists

Stanley I. Samuels, MB, BCh, FFARCS
Richard A. Jaffe, MD, PhD

MINIMALLY INVASIVE POSTERIOR LUMBAR DISCECTOMY (MICRODISCECTOMY)

SURGICAL CONSIDERATIONS

Description: Since the mid-1990s, a number of techniques have been developed to allow the decompression of lumbar roots (removal of disc material) with as little trauma to the nerves and surrounding tissues as possible. In most instances, little or no bone is removed and, therefore, this is not technically a laminectomy or laminotomy. These minimally invasive procedures typically are carried out in healthy young or middle-aged persons with sciatica and are not done for more involved pathology such as deformity, tumor or infection. Transpedicular fixation and short-segment fusions may be attempted using modifications of these techniques.

Microdiscectomy approach: This can be done under GA, regional (epidural or spinal) or local anesthesia. The patient is placed in a prone or kneeling position and the posterior landmarks are palpated to identify the approximate level (e.g., L4/5); then the overlying skin is infiltrated with local anesthetic. A spinal needle is placed to the level of the lamina and an x-ray or fluoroscopic image is taken to confirm the level. A 1" incision is made over the proposed interspace and, using either traditional or specialized retractors, the soft tissue is displaced to expose the ligamentum flavum. With the use of an operating microscope, the ligamentum flavum is removed, the nerve retracted and the extruded disc excised. For a single level this should take between 30-90 min, depending on the size of the patient and whether there is any scarring or adhesions from previous surgery.

Variant approach: Percutaneous discectomy through a posterolateral approach is usually reserved for "contained discs"—protrusions into, but not through, the outer anulus of the disc. These are usually done under a MAC with local anesthetic. The percutaneous instruments may be positioned using fluoroscopic guidance with or without a fiber optic light source and camera/monitor setup. The disc space is entered posterolaterally. The surgeon usually avoids anesthetizing the area around the nerve root so that the patient can alert the team if the root is struck by an instrument (quite painful). Once the disc space is entered, fluoroscopic or camera images are used to guide the surgeon in the removal of herniated disc. The disc material can be removed with specialized grabbers or automatic power-driven shavers.

Usual preop diagnosis: Chronic back pain 2° herniated lumbar disc; lumbar retinopathy

SUMMARY OF PROCEDURE

	Microdiscectomy	Percutaneous
Position	Prone or kneeling with bolster or frame support. The abdomen must hang free to decompress the epidural veins.	Prone or lateral decubitus
Incision	Posterior midline or slightly off midline at the appropriate vertebral level	About 8-12 cm lateral to the midline at the appropriate vertebral level
Special instrumentation	Microscope; light source; specialized retraction and dissection instruments for working in a small, deep incision	Percutaneous instruments, including trocars, sounds and arthroscopic-type grabbers and shavers; fluoroscopy and, sometimes, camera/monitor and fiber optic light setup
Unique considerations	Often outpatient procedure	Patient must be alert enough to respond to pain if nerve roots are encountered.
Antibiotics	Cefazolin 1 g iv	⇐
Surgical time	0.5-1.5 h	1-2 h
Closing considerations	Minimal suturing	Usually no closure (Bandaids)
EBL	25-100 ml	Minimal
Postop care	PACU. Mobilization as soon as tolerated. Usually discharged within 24 h.	PACU → home. Mobilization as tolerated.
Mortality	Very rare	⇐
Morbidity	Nerve injury	Failure to decompress the nerve adequately
	Dural laceration	–
	Infection	⇐
Pain score	4	2

PATIENT POPULATION CHARACTERISTICS

Age range	16-60 yr
Male:Female	3:2
Incidence	Common
Etiology	Degenerative; trauma (rare)

ANESTHETIC CONSIDERATIONS

PREOPERATIVE

Typically, this is an otherwise healthy patient population.

Musculoskeletal Since these patients may have chronic back pain with radiculopathy, they may not be suitable candidates for regional anesthetic techniques. Postop exacerbation of symptoms may be incorrectly ascribed to the anesthetic technique. A careful motor and sensory evaluation of the lower extremities should be documented.

Hematologic If regional anesthetic is planned and the patient is taking aspirin or NSAID, check Plt count and Hx for easy bleeding or bruising (relative contraindications to regional anesthesia).
Tests: Hct; Plt

Laboratory Other tests as indicated from H&P.

Premedication Standard premedication (see p. B-2).

INTRAOPERATIVE

Anesthetic technique: Microdiscectomies are commonly done under GA; however, local or regional anesthetic techniques are suitable in selected patients. Percutaneous discectomies typically require only MAC with sedation. These patients must be awake in order to alert the surgeon to inadvertent nerve root contact. In some centers, regional anesthesia (spinal or epidural) is the anesthetic of choice.

General Anesthesia:

Induction Standard induction (see p. B-2).

Maintenance Standard maintenance (see p. B-3).

Emergence No special considerations

MAC See p. B-4.

Regional anesthesia:

Spinal Patient in sitting, lateral decubitus or prone position for placement of subarachnoid block. Doses of local anesthetics should be adequate to provide a high lumbar level of sensory anesthesia (e.g., lidocaine 5%, 50-75 mg (controversial), tetracaine 10-14 mg, or bupivacaine 8-12 mg).

Epidural Patient in sitting or lateral decubitus position for placement of epidural catheter. A test dose (e.g., 3 ml of 1.5% lidocaine with 1:200,000 epinephrine [5 μg/ml]) is administered and the patient is observed for development of subarachnoid block or Sx of an intravascular injection. Titrate 2% lidocaine with epinephrine (3-5 ml at a time) until desired surgical level is obtained.

Blood and fluid requirements	IV: 18 ga × 1 NS/LR @ 5-8 ml/kg/h	Blood not likely to be required.
Monitoring	Standard monitors (see p. B-1).	
Positioning	✓ and pad pressure points. ✓ eyes.	Chest support or bolsters to optimize ventilation in the prone or kneeling position. Take care in positioning patient's extremities and genitals. Avoid pressure on eyes and ears after turning patient.

POSTOPERATIVE

Complications	Urinary retention Atelectasis Cauda equina syndrome	Rx: Catheterize until return of urinary function. Cauda equina syndrome is characterized by varying degrees of urinary/fecal incontinence, sensory loss in the perineal area and lower extremity motor weakness.
Pain management	PCA (p. C-3) Epidural analgesia (p. C-1)	PO analgesics may be suitable: acetaminophen and codeine (Tylenol #3 1-2 tab q 4-6 h) or oxycodone and acetaminophen (Percocet 1 tab q 6 h)
Tests	As indicated by patient status.	

References

1. Bookwalter J III, Busch M, Nicely D: Ambulatory surgery is safe and effective in radicular disc disease. *Spine* 1994; 19:526-30.
2. Carragee E, Helms E, O'Sullivan G: Are post-operative activity restrictions necessary after posterior lumbar discectomy? A prospective study of outcomes in 50 consecutive cases. *Spine* 1996; 21:1893-97.
3. Kambin P, Zhou L: Arthroscopic discectomy of the lumbar spine. *Clin Orthop* 1997; 337:49-57.
4. Kambin P, Zhou L: History and current status of percutaneous arthroscopic disc surgery. *Spine* 1996; 21:62S-68S.
5. McCulloch JA: Microdiscectomy. In *The Adult Spine.* Frymoyer J, ed. Raven Press, New York: 1991, 1765-84.
6. Zahrawi F: Microlumbar discectomy: Is it safe as an outpatient procedure? *Spine* 1994;1070-73.

ANTERIOR SPINAL RECONSTRUCTION AND FUSION—THORACIC AND THORACOLUMBAR SPINE

SURGICAL CONSIDERATIONS

Description: Most spinal procedures have traditionally been approached posteriorly. The advent of surgical treatment for vertebral TB and postpolio spinal deformities during the 1960s saw the development of surgical approaches to the anterior spine.[2] Initially, these procedures were reserved for patients with significant deformities, especially kyphosis. More recently, the treatment of traumatic, neoplastic and degenerative conditions have been included in the anterior approach. Regardless of the condition under treatment, the approach is similar for a given level. There are several more or less distinct types of surgical exposures, depending on the level.

Cervicothoracic approach: Most cephalad and difficult is the approach to the upper thoracic spine (T1-T3). This generally includes a modified anterior cervical exposure with a caudal extension, including a resection of the clavicle, part of the manubrium and sometimes the rib at the thoracic outlet. Dangers in this exposure are to the great vessels at the thoracic outlet, trachea (rare) and esophagus (more common), lung parenchyma, sympathetic ganglia, lymphatic duct (on the left) and brachial plexus. Once the spine is exposed and the discs and/or vertebrae are removed, the spinal cord is at risk. This procedure occasionally involves entering the thoracic cavity, in which case it is usually done intrapleurally, that is, through the parietal pleura. The lung needs to be collapsed at least partially. Spinal cord monitoring is usually performed; wake-up tests are not.

Transthoracic approach: Further down the spine, the levels from T5-T10 are more easily reached via a transthoracic approach. This involves a typical thoracotomy with the resection of a rib. The level of the rib resection is usually 1-2 levels above the highest vertebral level being approached. The great vessels and lung parenchyma are at risk, as is the thoracic duct (on the left) (Fig 10.4-1). The patient is in the lateral decubitus position and the mediastinum and heart usually fall to the opposite side, out of harm's way. Risk to the spinal cord depends on the difficulty and extent of the vertebral disease and the reconstruction. Spinal cord monitoring usually is performed intraop. The need for the lung to be deflated varies with the extent of the exposure. In centers where this procedure is frequently performed and the surgeons are accustomed to the respiratory motion during operation, DLTs are not routinely used. Since there is no (intended) violation of the lung parenchyma, air leaks and parenchymal repairs are not common.

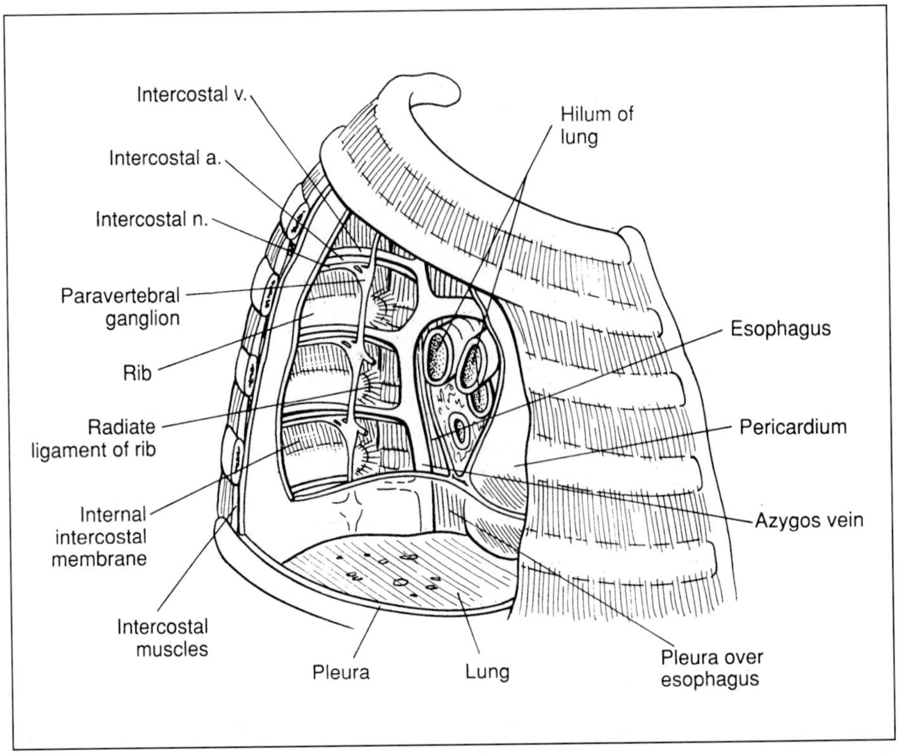

Figure 10.4-1. Surgical anatomy of the transthoracic approach. (Reproduced with permission from Hoppenfeld S, deBoer P: *Surgical Exposures in Orthopaedics*. JB Lippincott: 1984.)

Transdiaphragmatic approach: When the exposure must transverse the diaphragm, a combined retroperitoneal and transthoracic approach is used. This requires the diaphragm to be sectioned circumferentially from the chest wall and spine. If only the very low segments of the thoracic spine (T10-T12) are exposed, the required deflation of the involved lung is minimal. The risks are the same as those encountered with the transthoracic or retroperitoneal approaches alone. Regardless of the level of exposure, the operating table is normally used during the procedure to manipulate the spine for better exposure and to "lock in" implants, bone grafts, etc. Usually, the area of the spine to be exposed is centered above the "breaking" joint and kidney rests of the table (Fig 10.4-2). After the initial exposure, the table is angled in the center with the head and legs pointing down and kidney rests elevated to "open up" the section of spine facing the surgeon. After removal of the disk, abscess or tumor, a reconstruction—using bone graft, metal implants, bone cement, or a combination of these—is performed. The operating table is straightened and, with the spine in neutral alignment, the stability of the reconstruction is tested. This maneuver may need to be repeated several times.

The **morbidity** of these procedures depends primarily on the nature of the underlying disease. Obviously, bleeding and visceral injury are more likely when debriding a grapefruit-sized Potts abscess with several destroyed vertebrae than in removing a degenerated lumbar disk for fusion.

In some instances, the anterior procedure may be followed with a posterior fusion, either immediately or after 5-7 d of convalescence. If done immediately after, the patient needs to be repositioned prone, and the second procedure done through a midline exposure. Sometimes anterior and posterior surgery are performed simultaneously by two surgical

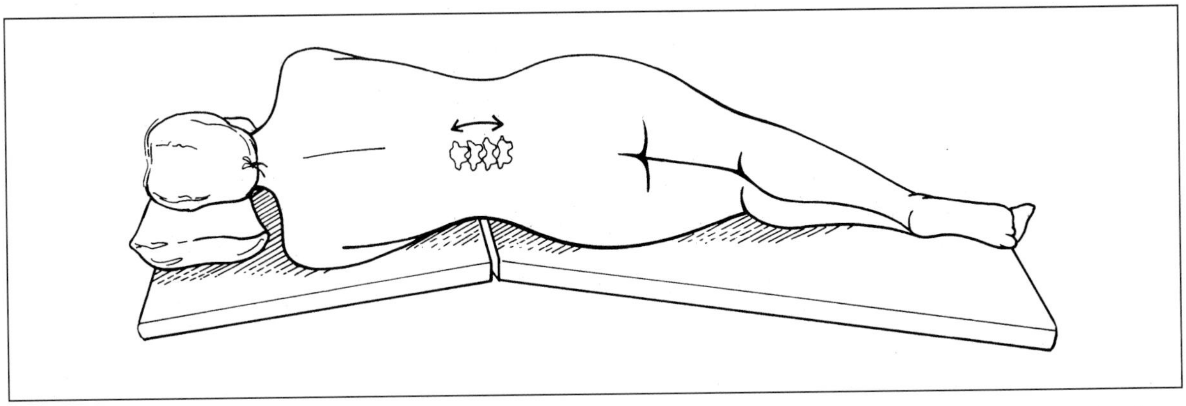

Figure 10.4-2. Patient position for transdiaphragmatic or retroperitoneal approach. (Reproduced with permission from Hoppenfeld S, deBoer P: *Surgical Exposures in Orthopaedics*. JB Lippincott, Philadelphia: 1984.)

teams. The most common reason for a staged anterior/posterior procedure (in the U.S.) is scoliosis; however, fractures at the thoracolumbar junction, after anterior decompression and reconstruction, are often instrumented and fused posteriorly.

Usual preop diagnosis: Fractures (usually at thoracic lumbar junction); idiopathic scoliosis; primary neoplasm or metastatic disease to the spine; pyogenic or TB osteomyelitis of the spine; Scheuermann's kyphosis

SUMMARY OF PROCEDURE

	Cervicothoracic Approach	Transthoracic Approach	Transdiaphragmatic Approach
Position	Supine; towel roll placed between shoulder blades, head slightly extended and turned away from operated side	Lateral decubitus; intended segments over the table break and kidney rests; axillary roll (Fig 10.4-2)	⇐
Incision	Inverted "L" longitudinally along manubrium to sternal notch, then transversely above clavicle	Along a rib 2 levels above the highest segment to be exposed	⇐
Special instrumentation	Instrumentation rarely used. Strut grafts, using rib, fibula, clavicle or cement, may be used to replace excised vertebrae.	For thoracolumbar scoliosis, a Zielke-type rod and screws may be used; more rigid instrumentation sometimes used in fractures.	⇐ (More common to use instrumentation at the affected level than above.)
Unique considerations	Difficulty and dangers of exposure to vessels and viscera (described above); postop respiratory distress well described.	In performing spinal reconstruction, manipulation of operating table is essential to "lock in" graft or implant (see above).	⇐
Antibiotics	Cefazolin 1 g iv (+ gentamicin 80 mg iv, if indwelling bladder catheter)	⇐	⇐
Surgical time	2-6 h	⇐	⇐
Closing considerations	Patient usually transferred to bed prior to being aroused; sudden jerking motions may dislodge graft or implant.	⇐	⇐
EBL	200-5000 ml. Blood loss is extremely variable; when bleeding occurs, it may be torrential from the aorta, vena cava or iliac vessels and branches. In nontumor or infection cases, 200-400 ml is usual.	⇐	⇐
Postop care	Chest drain, NG suction usually needed; short period of ICU observation is usual.	⇐	⇐
Mortality	< 0.1%, except in cases of malignancy or sepsis	⇐	⇐
Morbidity	For elective degenerative cases: 5-10% overall	⇐	⇐
	DVT: 6%	⇐	⇐
	Neurological: 3%	⇐	⇐
	Infection: 1%	⇐	⇐
	Sexual dysfunction	⇐	⇐
	For sepsis or tumor: 50-80% (overall)	⇐	⇐
	Cardiorespiratory failure	⇐	⇐
	Sepsis	⇐	⇐
Pain score	7-8 (if patient sensate at level of surgery)	7-8 (if patient sensate at level of surgery)	7-8 (if patient sensate at level of surgery)

PATIENT POPULATION CHARACTERISTICS

Age range	12-30 yr (scoliosis surgery); > 40 (tumor and infection surgery); 15-35 yr (fractures)
Male:Female	1:1, except more scoliosis surgery in females (1:4) and more fractures in males
Incidence	20,000/yr
Etiology	Scoliosis, idiopathic (50%); trauma (20%); scoliosis, neuromuscular (15%); infections, tumors (10%); scoliosis, congenital (5%)
Associated conditions	Pulmonary HTN and impaired pulmonary function; neuromuscular scoliosis (poliomyelitis, CP, muscular dystrophy, Friedreich's ataxia); aspiration; cardiomyopathy

ANESTHETIC CONSIDERATIONS

See Anesthetic Considerations for Spinal Reconstruction and Fusion, p. 799.

References

1. Emery SE, Chan DP, Woodward HR: Treatment of hematogenous pyogenic vertebral osteomyelitis with anterior debridement and primary bone grafting. *Spine* 1989; 14(3):284-91.
2. Hodgson AR, Stock FE, Fang HSY et al: Anterior spinal fusion: the operative approach and pathological finding in 412 patients with Potts disease of the spine. *Br J Surg* 1980; 48:172-86.
3. Hoppenfeld S, deBoer P: *Surgical Exposures in Orthopaedics: An Anatomic Approach,* 2nd edition. JB Lippincott, Philadelphia: 1994, 215-302.
4. Kostuik JP, Carl A, Ferron S: Anterior Zielke instrumentation for spinal deformity in adults. *J Bone Joint Surg* [Am] 1989; 71(6):898-906.
5. Kurz LT, Pursel SE, Herkowitz HN: Modified anterior approach to the cervicothoracic junction. *Spine* 1991; 16(10 Suppl):S542-47.
6. Sundaresan N, Shah J, Feghali JG: A transsternal approach to the upper thoracic vertebrae. *Am J Surg* 1984; 148(4):473-77.

ANTERIOR SPINAL RECONSTRUCTION AND FUSION—LUMBOSACRAL SPINE

SURGICAL CONSIDERATIONS

Description: The same general considerations apply here as in thoracolumbar reconstruction segments. The thoracic cavity is not entered, nor is the diaphragm sectioned. Careful preop assessment is needed, as these patients vary greatly in morbidity. The same operative procedure is performed for removal of a degenerative disk in a healthy patient as is carried out to decompress the caudae equinae in a debilitated patient with metastatic breast carcinoma.

Retroperitoneal approach: Below the diaphragm, exposure of the lumbar spine L2-S1 can be performed through a retroperitoneal approach (Fig 10.4-3). This involves a flank incision, often with resection of the 11th or 12th rib. The patient lies in a decubitus or partial decubitus position. At risk here are the great vessels above and below the bifurcation of the aorta (L4-L5). The ureter crosses the operative field and must be identified and protected. The sympathetic chain may be damaged along the vertebra, but the consequences of this are minimal. The presacral plexus further down may be injured and result in persistent retrograde ejaculation.

Regardless of the level of exposure, the operating table normally is used during the procedure to manipulate the spine for better exposure and to "lock in" implants, bone grafts, etc. Usually the area of the spine to be exposed is centered above the "breaking" joint and kidney rests of the table (Fig 10.4-2). After initial exposure, the table is angled in the center with the head and legs pointing down and the kidney rests elevated to open up the section of spine facing the surgeon. After the removal of the disc, abscess or tumor, a reconstruction—using bone graft, metal implants, bone cement, or a

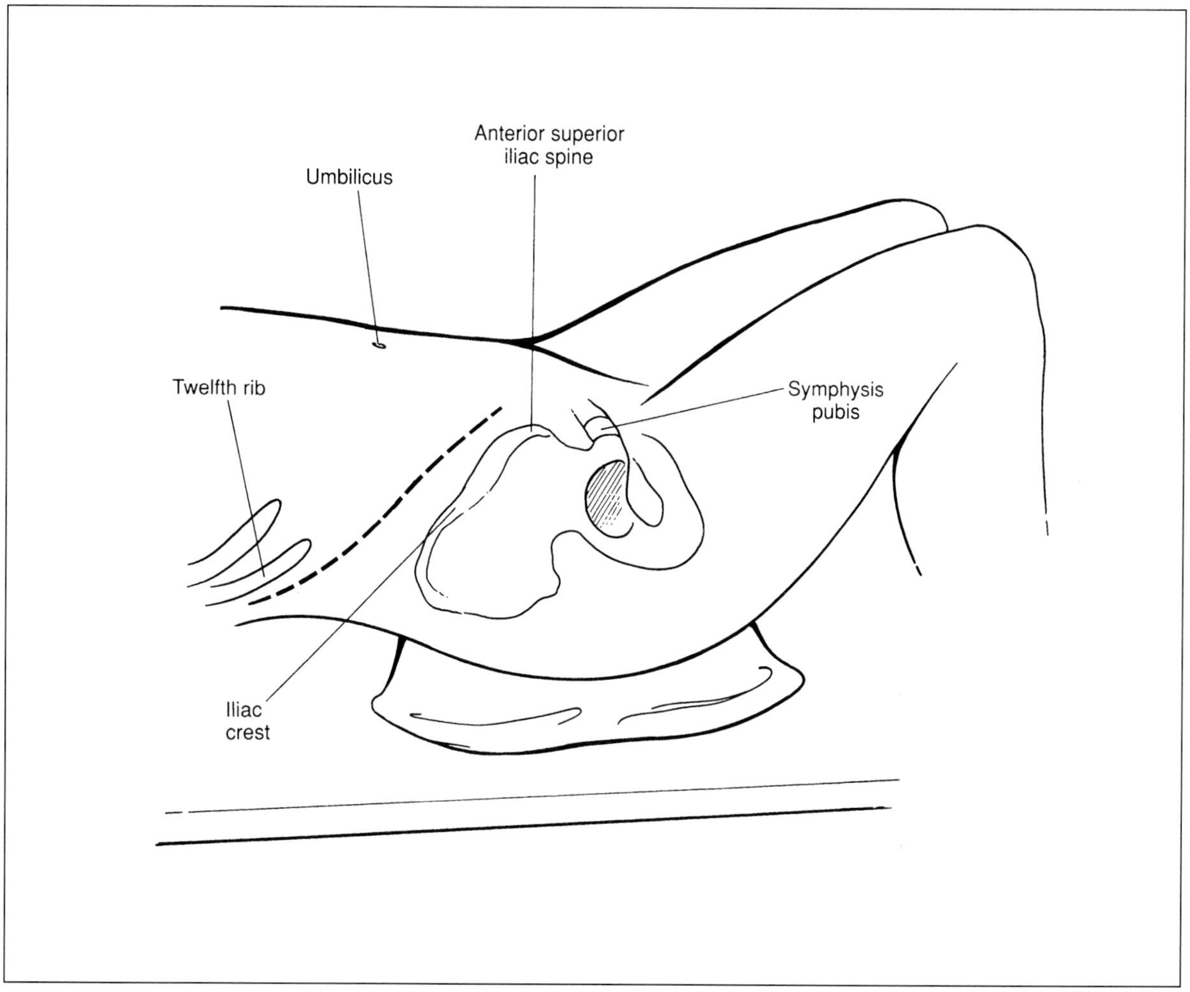

Figure 10.4-3. Retroperitoneal approach to lumbar spine. (Reproduced with permission from Hoppenfeld S, deBoer P: *Surgical Exposures in Orthopaedics*. JB Lippincott: 1984.)

combination of these—is performed. The table is then straightened; and with the spine in neutral alignment, the stability of the reconstruction is tested by this maneuver, which may need to be repeated several times.

In some instances, the anterior reconstruction and fusion is followed with a **posterior fusion**, either immediately or after 5-7 d of convalescence. If done immediately after, the patient needs to be positioned prone on the operating table, and the second procedure done through a midline exposure. Sometimes anterior and posterior surgeries can be performed simultaneously by two surgical teams. The most common reason for a staged anterior/posterior procedure (in the U.S.) is scoliosis. Recent trends in degenerative lumbar disk surgery indicate that anterior and posterior fusions are becoming more common, with some evidence suggesting better results in fusion and pain relief.

Variant procedure or approaches: When the L5 vertebra and sacrum need to be widely exposed, a **transperitoneal approach** may be needed. This involves a laparotomy or Pfannenstiel's incision, displacement of the bowels out of the pelvis and exposure of the lumbosacral junction (Fig 10.4-4). The patient is supine for this procedure and the surgical risks are similar, as with other intraabdominal approaches.[11]

In a recent modification to the retroperitoneal approach, the patient is placed in the supine position. In this **supine retroperitoneal approach,** an incision is made in either a longitudinal or transverse fashion between the umbilicus and the pubis. The rectus abdominus fascia is incised and the rectus abdominus is retracted medially or laterally, allowing access to the retroperitoneal space without violating the peritoneal cavity. The advantage of this approach over the transperitoneal approach includes decreased need for bowel manipulation, → ↓3rd-space loss of fluid and ↓heat loss.

Usual preop diagnosis: Degenerative disc disease; segmental instability,[14,15] vertebral fractures requiring decompression; vertebral osteomyelitis or tuberculosis;[4,10] neoplastic disease of the lumbar spine[11]

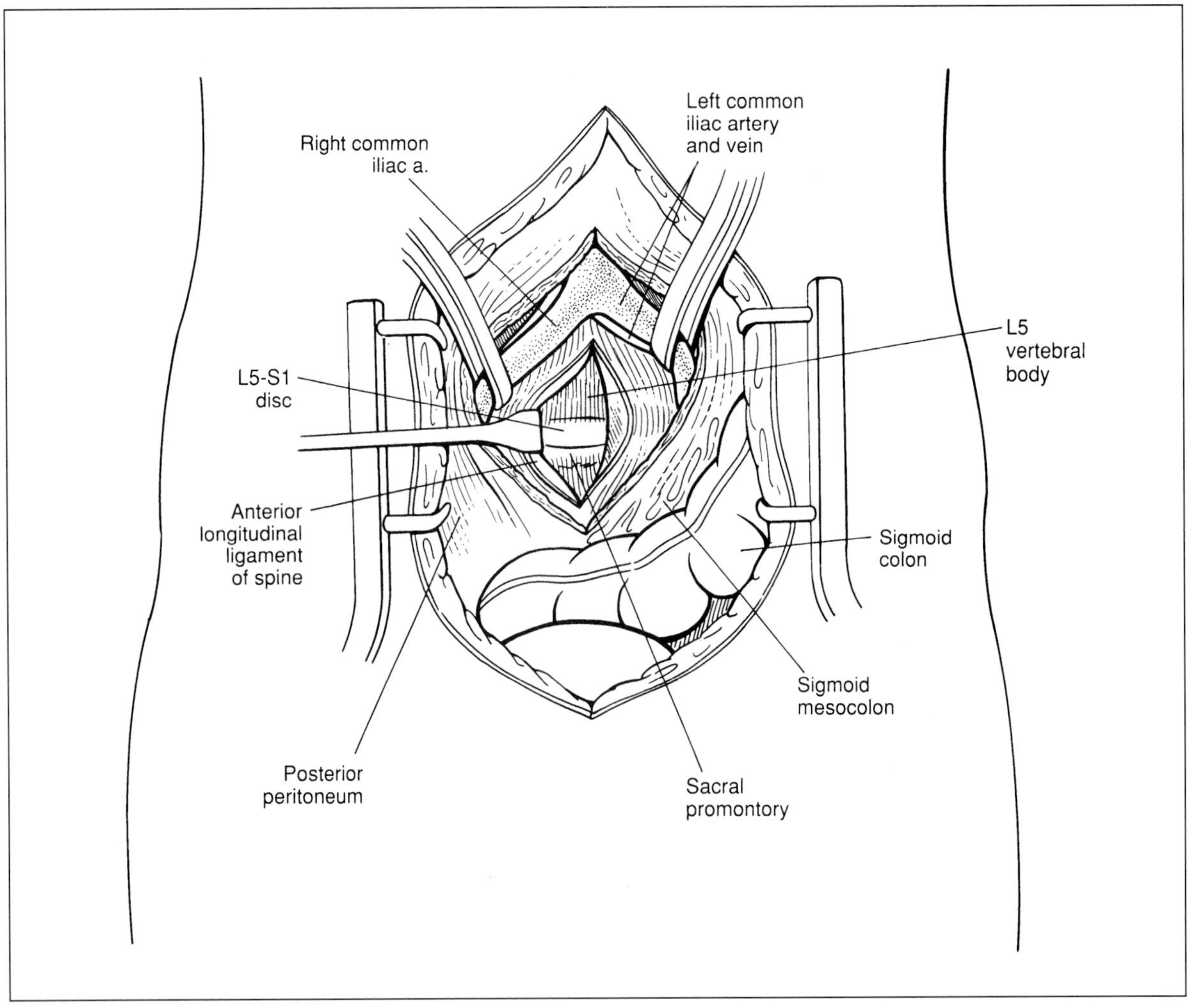

Figure 10.4-4. Transperitoneal approach to lumbosacral junction. (Reproduced with permission from Hoppenfeld S, deBoer P: *Surgical Exposures in Orthopaedics*. JB Lippincott: 1984.)

SUMMARY OF PROCEDURE

	Retroperitoneal Approach (Lateral)	Transperitoneal Approach
Position	Lateral decubitus, affected side up. The up hip and knee are flexed to relax psoas muscle and allow its reflection to expose the lumbar vertebral bodies.	Supine
Incision	Flank incision curving anteriorly to the lateral margin of the rectus abdominus (Fig 10.4-3)	Pfannenstiel's above the pubis
Special instrumentation	Occasional use of anterior instrumentation to stabilize fractures or to reconstruct the spine when entire vertebrae are removed	⇐
Unique considerations	In performing spinal reconstruction, manipulation of operating table is essential to "lock in" graft or implant (see above).	⇐ + A general bowel prep usually is performed preop.
Antibiotics	Cefazolin 1 g iv (+ gentamicin 80 mg iv, if indwelling bladder catheter already in place); exception is when infection is suspected and specific cultures are obtained intraop.	⇐
Surgical time	3-6 h	⇐
Closing considerations	The spine may be more or less stable after reconstruction, and patient usually trans-	⇐

	Retroperitoneal Approach (Lateral)	Transperitoneal Approach
Closing considerations, cont.	ferred to bed prior to being awakened. Sudden jerking motions, etc., may dislodge graft or implant.	
EBL	200-5000 ml. Blood loss extremely variable. When bleeding occurs, it may be torrential from the aorta, vena cava or iliac vessels and branches. In nontumor/infection cases, 200-400 ml is usual.	⇐
Postop care	Patients with degenerative conditions and elective surgeries normally recover in PACU and return to ward. Patients with infections, fractures and tumors are usually observed in ICU for 24 h postop. Ileus for 24-72 h is usual; NG suction usually continues until bowel sounds and passing flatus are present. Generally, mobilization depends on final stability.	⇐
Mortality	Malignancy or sepsis: 1-2%	⇐
	Elective: < 0.1%	⇐
Morbidity	In patients with malignancy, sepsis or fractures with caudae equinae compression, overall serious complications: 25-50%	⇐
	Cardiopulmonary failure	⇐
	Neurologic deficit	–
	Pneumothorax	–
	Sepsis	⇐
Pain score	6	6

PATIENT POPULATION CHARACTERISTICS

Age range	Variable (infant–adult)
Male:Female	1:1, except more scoliosis surgery in females (1:4)
Incidence	Uncommon
Etiology	Infection (osteomyelitis, TB); trauma; congenital; neoplasia; idiopathic

ANESTHETIC CONSIDERATIONS FOR SPINAL RECONSTRUCTION AND FUSION

(Procedures covered: anterior and posterior spinal reconstruction and fusion: thoracic, thorocolumbar and lumbar [Harrington, Luque or rod-screw instrumentation, Dwyer, Zielke])

PREOPERATIVE

Patients presenting for spinal reconstruction most commonly will have either idiopathic or acquired scoliosis, a complex deformity involving both lateral curvature and rotation of the spine, as well as an associated deformity of the rib cage. Types of scoliosis include: idiopathic, congenital, neuromuscular, myopathic, traumatic, tumor-related and mesenchymal disorders. The majority of cases are idiopathic, with a male:female ratio of 1:4. Normally, the cervical spine and lumbar spine are lordotic, while the thoracic spine is kyphotic. Surgery is indicated when the curvature is severe (angulation beyond 40° in the thoracic or lumbar spine[7]) or progressing rapidly. Nonscoliotic patients presenting for this surgery may have spinal instability as a result of trauma, metastatic carcinoma or infection (e.g., TB). These patients are usually healthy apart from their underlying pathology. The patients with disseminated lung or breast cancer may need a careful workup with regard to respiratory, nutritional and chemotherapeutic status. (See Anesthetic Considerations for Lobectomy, Pneumonectomy, p. 175, or Mastectomy, p. 469.)

Respiratory Respiratory impairment proportional to angle of lateral curvature (Cobb angle) (Fig 10.4-5)[21]

Cobb Angle	30°-60°	60°- 90°	>90°
VC	↓25%	↓50%	↓70%
TLC	↓27%	↓37%	↓50%

Respiratory, cont. Restrictive pattern: $\downarrow$TLC + $\downarrow\downarrow$VC
• If VC > 70% predicted, respiratory reserve is adequate.
• If VC < 40% predicted, postop ventilation usually is required.
Expect further significant (~40%) $\downarrow$VC immediately postop requiring 7-10 d to resolve.
$\uparrow$RR + $\downarrow$TV $\rightarrow$ $\uparrow$dead space + $\downarrow$alveolar ventilation $\rightarrow$ V/Q mismatch $\rightarrow$ hypoxemia.[12]
Patients with scoliosis of neuromuscular origin are more susceptible to aspiration and respiratory failure.
Tests: CXR; ABG; PFT; assess exercise tolerance by Hx.

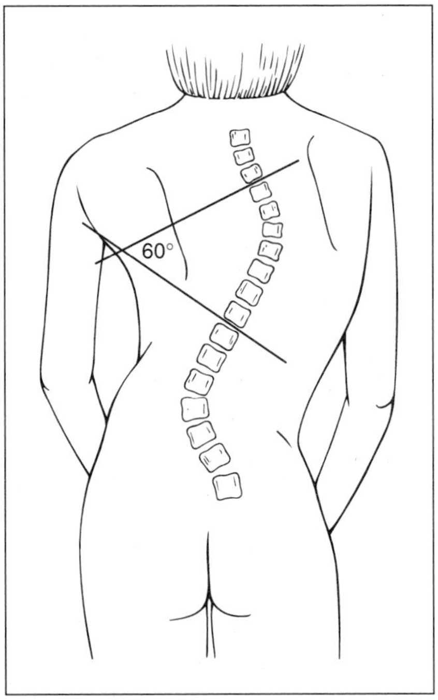

Figure 10.4-5. Cobb angle.

Cardiovascular ★ $\uparrow$PVR (**NB**: independent of severity of scoliosis). High incidence of CHD and mitral valve prolapse.
Tests: ECG; ECHO—consult cardiologist if apical systolic murmur or other evidence of cardiovascular impairment is present.[12]

Neurological Some surgeons may request that the patient be awakened intraop to test anterior (motor) cord function. Practice wakeup testing preop to reveal any baseline deficits and reassure the patient that no pain will be felt during intraop testing. Tuberculous spondylitis (Pott's disease) frequently presents with focal neurological lesions ranging from loss of bowel and bladder control to paraplegia. Careful preop documentation of the neurological status is essential as surgery may worsen these symptoms.

Musculoskeletal When the Cobb angle > 25°, the degree of respiratory impairment will be significant and the need for postop ventilatory support becomes more likely. Patients with muscular dystrophy may be more sensitive to myocardial depression from anesthetic agents and also may require postop ventilation 2° muscle weakness. Succinylcholine may cause severe rhabdomyolysis with hyperkalemia. These patients also may be at risk for MH.

Hematologic Avoid use of Plt inhibitors for 2-3 wk before surgery. Encourage autologous blood donation. (If Hb > 11 g/dL, may repeat donation q 3-7 d up to 14 d before surgery). Consider use of intraop hemodilution, controlled hypotension and Cell Saver. Be aware that patients with previously placed spinal support (e.g., Milwaukee brace) for correction of scoliosis may have more blood loss than would otherwise occur.

Laboratory Hb/Hct; clotting profile: investigate all abnormalities before surgery. Other tests as indicated from H&P.

Premedication Standard premedication (see p. B-2), if appropriate.

INTRAOPERATIVE

Anesthetic technique: GETA. For pediatric cases, preheat room to 78° F. For anterior reconstruction, consider placement of thoracic/lumbar epidural catheter to supplement GA and for postop pain management.

Induction Standard induction (p. B-2). A DLT may facilitate surgical access in the patient undergoing an anterior correction. The smallest available DLT is size 28 Fr (OD = 8.9 mm), typically suitable for a child aged 12-14 yr.

Maintenance Standard maintenance (p. B-3). It is important to use low concentrations and minimize changes of potent inhalational agents during measurement of SSEPs. Continue muscle relaxation. Droperidol is avoided as its α-blocking effect reduces the effectiveness of the epinephrine injected at the beginning of surgery to reduce incisional bleeding.

Emergence Surgeons may place epidural catheter before wound closure for postop pain management to compliment the previously placed spinal opiates. Patients are usually extubated; however, some

Emergence, cont.	may require continued intubation and admission to ICU (e.g., preop medical condition or massive intraop blood loss). Especially careful handling of the patient is necessary during transfer from OR table to bed.	
Blood and fluid requirements	Anticipate large blood loss. IV: 14-16 ga × 2 NS/LR @ 8-10 ml/kg/h Warm all fluids. Humidify gases. T&C 2-4 U PRBC.	Blood loss is a major consideration during scoliosis surgery. Profuse bleeding may occur when the erector spinal muscles are stripped and when large areas of cancellous bone are exposed. It may vary from 25%- >100% of the patient's blood volume, although blood loss is usually less with the anterior approach (Dwyer's).
Control of blood loss	Position to prevent venous engorgement. ↓MAP to 60-70 mmHg. ↓Hct to 25-28%.	Controlled hypotension (to MAP = 60-70 mmHg) in the fit patient has been shown to dramatically reduce blood loss, although there may be some ↑risk of spinal-cord ischemia. In addition, deliberate hemodilution to Hct = 25%-28% may prove useful. Maintain UO at 0.5-1.0 ml/kg/h during controlled hypotension.[20]
Monitoring	Standard monitors (p. B-1) Arterial line CVP line Urinary catheter ± SSEP	Trends in CVP may be more reliable than measurement of UO to assess changes in volume status in patients in the prone or lateral positions.
Positioning	✓ and pad pressure points. ✓ eyes, neck.	Pressure points must be carefully padded and checked frequently, especially during controlled hypotension.
Wakeup test	40-60 min advance warning from surgeons is needed. • Decrease inhalational agents. • Reverse muscle relaxants (and narcotics, if necessary). • Monitor train of four. • Request hand squeeze; if present, elicit bilateral foot movement. • Reinduce anesthesia with STP or propofol (1 mg/kg). **Dangers:** Air embolus Dislodgement of spinal instrumentation Accidental extubation[23]	The wakeup test assesses integrity of motor pathways in the ventral cord. Uncontrolled patient movement during wakeup test can result in accidental extubation or dislodgement of the spinal instrumentation. Unrestrained inspiratory efforts may provoke venous air embolism. The anesthesiologist must be prepared to rapidly reanesthetize the patient.
SSEP and MEPs	SSEP: Dorsal cord function only MEPs: Ventral cord function Use N_2O/narcotic anesthetic.	SSEPs are required to test sensory pathways in the dorsal cord. In some centers, SSEPs are followed throughout surgery. The SSEP technician should be informed of changes in the level of anesthesia. SSEPs very sensitive to changes in volatile anesthetic in a dose-dependent manner. Sevoflurane and desflurane complicate EP monitoring 2° rapidity with which brain levels may change.
Complications	Spinal cord ischemia Massive blood loss Fat embolism	SSEP indications of spinal cord ischemia should be treated by restoring normal BP and by ↓ cord traction. Prompt transfusion may be necessary and blood should be available in the room (2-4 U PRBC).

POSTOPERATIVE

Complications	Pulmonary insufficiency Hypothermia Pneumothorax Dislodgement of internal fixation	Postop ventilation may be required in patients with severe respiratory impairment (see Preoperative Considerations, above). In addition, thoracotomy, surgical trauma to the diaphragm and fat embolism may further ↑ the risk

Complications, cont.		of postop pulmonary insufficiency. Careful handling of patient in transfer is mandatory.
	Neurologic sequelae	Neurologic sequelae probably remain the most feared complication, and it is important to document postop neurologic exam.
Pain management	Intrathecal morphine 0.1-0.25 mg by surgeon intraop, dependent on age of patient. PCA (p. C-3) Thoracic/lumbar epidural opiates	Pain is a significant problem for postop scoliosis patients. Most need analgesia × 3-4 d. Preop consultation with patient (and parents) about different pain management techniques is important. See p. C-1.
Tests	CXR; ABG; Hct	✓ for pneumothorax and line placement.

References

1. Brown JC, Swank S, Specht L: Combined anterior and posterior spine fusion in cerebral palsy. *Spine* 1982; 7(6):570-3.
2. Chapman MW: *Operative Orthopaedics*, 2nd edition. JB Lippincott, Philadelphia: 1993, 2899-2913.
3. Dwyer AF, Schafer MF: Anterior approach to scoliosis. Results of treatment in fifty-one cases. *J Bone Joint Surg* [Br] 1974; 56(2):218-24.
4. Emery SE, Chan DK, Woodward HR: Vertebral osteomyelitis. *Spine* 1989; 14:284-91.
5. Ferguson RL, Allen BL Jr: Staged correction of neuromuscular scoliosis. *J Pediatr Orthop* 1983; 3:555-62.
6. Floman Y, Penny JN, Micheli LJ, Riseborough EJ, Hall JE: Combined anterior and posterior fusion in seventy-three spinally deformed patients: indications, results and complications. *Clin Orthop* 1982; 164:110-22.
7. Goldstein LA, Waugh TR: Classification and terminology of scoliosis. *Clin Orthop* 1973; 93:10-22.
8. Goodarzi M, Shier N, Ogden J: Epidural versus patient-controlled analgesia with morphine for postoperative pain after orthopedic procedures in children. *J Pediatr Orthop* 1993; 13:663-67.
9. Hagberg CA, Welch WC, Bowman-Howard ML: Anesthesia and surgery for spine and spinal cord procedures. In *Textbook of Neuroanesthesia with Neurosurgical and Neuroscience Perspectives.* Albin MS, ed. McGraw-Hill: New York: 1997, 1039-82.
10. Hodgson AR, Stock FE, Fang HSY et al: Anterior spinal fusion: the operative approach and pathological finding in 412 patients with Potts disease of the spine. *Br J Surg* 1980; 48:172-86.
11. Hoppenfeld S, deBoer P: *Surgical Exposures in Orthopaedics: the anatomic approach,* 2nd edition. JB Lippincott, Philadelphia: 1994, 215-302.
12. Kafer ER: Respiratory and cardiovascular functions in scoliosis and the principles of anesthetic management. *Anesthesiology* 1980; 52(4):339-51.
13. Kostuik JP, Carl A, Ferron S: Anterior Zielke instrumentation for spinal deformity in adults. *J Bone Joint Surg* [Am] 1989; 71(6):898-906.
14. Kozak JA and O'Brien JP: Simultaneous combined anterior and posterior fusion. An independent analysis of a treatment for the disabled low-back pain patient. *Spine* 1990; 15(4):322-28.
15. Leong JCY: Anterior interbody fusion. In *Lumbar Interbody Fusion*. Lin PM and Gill K, eds. Aspen Pub, Rockville: 1989, 133-47.
16. McMaster MJ: Anterior and posterior instrumentation and fusion of thoracolumbar scoliosis due to myelomeningocele. *J Bone Joint Surg* [Br] 1987; 69(1):20-5.
17. Morrissy RT: *Atlas of Pediatric Orthopaedic Surgery*. JB Lippincott, Philadelphia: 1992, 75-97.
18. O'Brien JP, Yau AC, Gertzbein S, Hodgson AR: Combined staged anterior and posterior correction and fusion of the spine in scoliosis following poliomyelitis. *Clin Orthop* 1975; 110:81-9.
19. O'Brien T, Akmakjian J, Ogin G, Eilert R: Comparison of one-stage versus two-stage anterior/posterior spinal fusion for neuromuscular scoliosis. *J Pediatr Orthop* 1992; 12(5):610-15.
20. Phillips WA, Hensinger RN: Control of blood loss during scoliosis surgery. *Clin Orthop* 1988; 229:88-93.
21. Smyth RJ, Chapman KR, Wright TA, Crawford JS, Rebuck AS: Pulmonary function in adolescents with mild idiopathic scoliosis. *Thorax* 1984; 39(12):901-4.
22. Smyth RJ, Chapman KR, Wright TA, Crawford JS, Rebuck AS: Ventilatory patterns during hypoxia, hypercapnia, and exercise in adolescents with mild scoliosis. *Pediatrics* 1986; 77(5):692-97.
23. Sudhir KG, Smith RM, Hall J, Hall JE, Hansen DD: Intraoperative awakening for early recognition of possible neurologic sequelae during Harrington-rod spinal fusion. *Anesth Analg* 1976; 55(4):526-28.

11.0 RECONSTRUCTIVE SURGERY

Surgeons

Andrew E. Turk, MD
Annette C. Cholon, MD
Lars M. Vistnes, MD, FRCS(C) (*Abdominoplasty, mammoplasty*)

11.1 AESTHETIC SURGERY

Anesthesiologists

Rona G. Giffard, MD, PhD (*Abdominoplasty, mammoplasty*)
Terri D. Homer, MD (*Liposuction*)
Bruce D. Halperin, MD (*Liposuction*)
George W. Commons, MD (*Liposuction*)

ABDOMINOPLASTY

SURGICAL CONSIDERATIONS

Description: Abdominoplasty is most commonly performed for true abdominal skin and wall laxity. Such laxity is often found in conjunction with a diastasis of the recti muscles and a partial herniation of abdominal contents into the abdominal wall through this diastasis. The procedure is often performed in combination with abdominal **liposuction** (see p. 812) to get rid of excess fat in the panniculus adiposis found in both men and women. Abdominoplasty is less commonly performed than it was prior to the advent of liposuction.

It is performed through an incision made just above the pubic hairline, and extended bilaterally to the area of both anterior and superior iliac spines. The operation involves total undermining of the flap that is raised at the level of the abdominal wall musculature, extending as far up as the costal margin on both sides. Then the excess skin is pulled down and resected, which usually requires the placement of the umbilicus at a new site in the abdominal wall. In the case of morbidly obese persons undergoing abdominoplasty, the procedure is essentially as described above, but consists more of a **wedge resection** of skin and fat with minimal to no amount of undermining. The individual who has had liposuction is usually up and about with a girdle and quite comfortable within 24-48 h, whereas the abdominoplasty patient who has suction drains and a very tight closure usually ambulates with some difficulty for the first 7-10 d after surgery.

Usual preop diagnosis: Abdominal laxity; rectus diastasis

SUMMARY OF PROCEDURE

Position	Supine
Incision	Extended Pfannenstiel's; periumbilical
Antibiotics	Cefazolin 1 g iv
Surgical time	2.5 h
Closing considerations	Flex table to facilitate closure.
EBL	200-600 ml; greater in morbidly obese
Postop care	Pillows under knees; head of bed raised to maintain flexed position.
Mortality	0-1%
Morbidity	Ileus: 10% Infection: 2-3% Dehiscence: 1% Fat embolism: 1%
Pain score	4-6

PATIENT POPULATION CHARACTERISTICS

Age range	30-55 yr
Male:Female	1:5
Incidence	10,000+/yr (This procedure is one of the most commonly performed of all plastic surgical operations.)
Etiology	Overeating
Associated conditions	Morbid obesity

ANESTHETIC CONSIDERATIONS

PREOPERATIVE

Typically, there are two patient populations for abdominoplasty: the generally healthy, and the morbidly obese. Some patients have Hx of amphetamine, cocaine or thyroid hormone abuse,[2] and increased incidence of hiatal hernia. The following considerations focus on the morbidly obese patient (body weight [kg] $\geq 2 \times$ ideal weight. Ideal body weight [kg] is estimated by subtracting 100 [male] or 105 [female] from height in cm).

Respiratory In the morbidly obese patient, findings include[1]: ↑O_2 consumption, ↑CO_2 production, restrictive lung disease, ↓FRC, ↓ERV, ↓VC, ↓IC, and ↓PaO_2. These changes are exacerbated by the supine position. Younger patients may show alveolar hyperventilation in response to hypoxemia; older

Respiratory, cont.	patients may not, and may retain CO_2. Patients may have obesity hypoventilation syndrome (Pickwickian syndrome) and sleep apnea: intermittent airway obstruction, hypoxemia and hypercarbia during sleep, which may → pulmonary HTN. Obese patients are at increased risk of pulmonary aspiration due to increased incidence of hiatal hernia, gastroesophageal reflux and increased gastric volumes (typically > 25 ml with pH < 2.5). See Premedication, below, for aspiration prophylaxis. **Tests:** Consider CXR, room-air ABG and PFT (helpful, but generally do not predict postop complications, e.g., atelectasis, pneumonia).
Cardiovascular	↑CO and ↑blood volume → LVH. Chronic hypoxia and pulmonary compromise may produce right heart failure, ↓↓exercise tolerance, ↑risk of CAD and pulmonary systemic HTN. Patients with LVH may have ↑dysrhythmias. Some patients may have previously taken fenfluramine alone or in combination with phentermine for weight loss. Those patients should be evaluated for pulmonary HTN (e.g., dyspnea, central cyanosis, right axis deviation and CXR changes) and valvular heart disease. **Tests:** ECG (↑HR, conduction abnormalities, LVH); CXR (cardiomegaly)
Metabolic	Increased incidence of diabetes, hypercholesterolemia, hypertriglyceridemia, liver abnormalities; ↓plasma folate, B_{12}; ↑incidence of cholelithiasis, nephrolithiasis. Determine whether electrolyte abnormalities are present in patient S/P ileojejunal bypass. **Tests:** As indicated from H&P.
Hematologic	Polycythemia suggests chronic hypoxemia (see Respiratory, above). **Tests:** Hb/Hct
Laboratory	Other tests as indicated from H&P.
Premedication	Sedative premedication is avoided in the morbidly obese due to their pulmonary compromise. Aspiration prophylaxis is essential: ranitidine 100 mg po or iv the evening before, and 60-90 min before surgery, plus nonparticulate antacid (Na citrate 0.3 M, 30 ml po) preinduction. Additionally, metoclopramide 10 mg iv may be given, although it has not been shown to be more effective in combination with an H_2-blocker than the H_2-blocker alone. For the healthy outpatient, midazolam 1-2 mg iv immediately preop may lessen anxiety.

INTRAOPERATIVE

Anesthetic technique: GETA. Morbidly obese patients may not tolerate the supine position for an extended period of time.

Induction	Standard induction (p. B-2) for healthy patients. Special considerations for the morbidly obese include prophylaxis for aspiration (see above), followed by rapid-sequence induction in an appropriately positioned patient (see Fig 7.2-6). If mandibular and cervical mobility are decreased by excessive soft tissue, plan awake fiber optic intubation with the patient sitting. Anticipate rapid O_2 desaturation during periods of hypoventilation, even with adequate preoxygenation.
Maintenance	Standard maintenance (p. B-3). Calculate drug dosage on basis of lean body mass. In the obese, increased plasma fluoride concentrations are found after anesthesia with halothane and enflurane; controlled ventilation with large TV and high inspired O_2 concentration is recommended. Since epinephrine infiltration generally is used to decrease blood loss, isoflurane is recommended as the ★ least dysrhythmogenic of the inhalation agents in the presence of epinephrine. **NB:** Midazolam has a prolonged half-life in obese patients, but awakening times from inhalational or narcotic-based anesthetics are comparable to those of nonobese patients.
Emergence	Smooth emergence with minimal bucking, coughing or retching to minimize tension on the suture line; give antiemetics (metoclopramide 10 mg or droperidol 1 mg iv) 1 h before conclusion of surgery. Maintenance of flexed position will minimize tension on suture line. Small additional doses of narcotic (e.g., meperidine 10 mg) may be titrated to RR if patient is allowed to resume spontaneous respiration before the end of the case.
Blood and fluid requirements	Moderate blood loss IV: 16-18 ga × 1 NS/LR @ 6-10 ml/kg/h

Monitoring	Standard monitors (see p. B-1). ± Arterial line ± CVP line	Additional monitoring for the morbidly obese patient may include arterial and CVP lines.
Positioning	Flexed position Pillows under knees ✓ and pad pressure points. ✓ eyes.	Flexed position minimizes tension on suture line. Morbidly obese may require 2 OR tables side-by-side. Supine position may be poorly tolerated; monitor ventilation closely.
Complications	Fat emboli	Fat emboli are more common during liposuction.

POSTOPERATIVE

Complications	Patients may have postop ileus of 1-2 d duration.	The morbidly obese should not be outpatients; they have an increased incidence of wound infection, DVT, PE and postop pulmonary complications. Provide supplemental O_2 for the first 2 d postop. Keep patient in semisitting or flexed position to avoid undue stress on wound.
Pain management	Epidural narcotics or PCA may be used (pp. C-1, C-3).	Monitor patient for postop respiration depression.
Tests	Pulse oximetry	Maximum reduction of arterial saturation may occur on postop day 2-3.[3]

References

1. Cooper JR, Brodsky JB: Anesthetic management of the morbidly obese patient. *Semin Anesth* 1987; Vol VI: 260-70.
2. Klein JA: Anesthesia for liposuction in dermatologic surgery. *J Dermatol Surg Oncol* 1988; 14(10):1124-32.
3. Shenkman ZZ, Shir Y, Brodsky JB: Perioperative management of the obese patient. *Br J Anaesth* 1993; 70(3):349-59.
4. Vaughan RW, Wise L: Postoperative arterial blood gas measurements in obese patients: effects of position on gas exchange. *Ann Surg* 1975; 182(6):705-9.
5. Vistnes, LM: *Procedures in Plastic and Reconstructive Surgery: How They Do It.* Little, Brown, Boston: 1991.

MAMMOPLASTY AND RELATED SURGERY

SURGICAL CONSIDERATIONS

Description: There are at least four patient population categories for mammoplasty: those presenting for breast augmentation, breast lift or reduction mammoplasty, and those presenting for reconstruction of breast, usually following cancer surgery.

Augmentation mammoplasty, by definition, is an operation in which the skin and mammary tissues are augmented by the placement of a prosthesis. The most commonly used prosthesis at the present time is a saline-filled silicone prosthesis. Placement of the prosthesis may be above or below the pectoralis muscle, depending on surgeon's choice and amount of tissue available. The operation can be done under local anesthesia or GA.

Breast lift: There is usually enough ptosis of the breast that it is necessary to replace the ptotic breast tissue at a higher level. This requires resection of the skin and placement of a nipple areolar complex at a higher level on the chest wall. It may be combined with a modest augmentation—e.g., placement of a prosthesis above or below the pectoralis major muscle—at the same time. This is a more extensive operation than augmentation mammoplasty and requires more time.

Breast reduction: Depending on the size of the breast to be reduced, the amount of tissue removed from each breast may be anywhere from 200-1000 g. The nipple is usually transplanted to a higher site, based on an inferior pedicle of dermis and breast tissue. If the reduction is in the 1000 g range, however, the nipple is usually transplanted as a free graft.

Breast reconstruction: Done in three basic ways: (1) Reconstruction using tissue expansion, with the eventual placement of a breast implant. (2) Use of a breast implant and augmentation by local flaps, such as a latissimus dorsi musculocutaneous flap, in order to make up for tissue lost at the time of the surgery. (3) Use of total autogenous tissue, usually with a transverse rectus abdominis muscle (TRAM) flap. In this procedure, a wedge of abdominal wall skin and subcutaneous tissue is moved on its blood supply of one or both of the recti muscles to the new site on the chest wall, fashioned in such a way as to construct a new breast. This is the longest and most complicated procedure. In some situations it can be done as a free (microsurgical) flap. All three procedures are discussed in more detail in Breast/Chest Wall Reconstruction, Functional Restoration, p. 832.

Usual preop diagnosis: Hypomastia; hypermastia; breast ptosis; S/P mastectomy

Breast implant removal: Patients with capsular contractures or thick scar tissue around the breast implant will require capsulotomy (incision) or capsulectomy (excision) to remove the implant. Compared to breast augmentation, these patients may experience increased blood loss; otherwise, these procedures are similar.

Usual preop diagnosis: Capsular contracture of breast; ruptured breast implant; malposition of breast implant; silicone implant replacement

SUMMARY OF PROCEDURE

	Breast Augmentation	Breast Lift	Reduction Mammoplasty	Reconstruction Of Breast
Position	Supine	⇐	⇐	⇐
Incision	Inframammary, subareolar, or axillary incisions	⇐	⇐	⇐
Unique considerations	May place patient in sitting position during procedure.	⇐	⇐	May need to turn patient on side if reconstruction involves use of latissimus dorsi flap.
Antibiotics	Cefazolin 1 g iv intraop	⇐	⇐	⇐
Surgical time	1 h	1.5 h	2-3 h	2-8 h (implant vs TRAM)
Closing considerations	May need patient sitting up for application of dressing.	⇐	⇐	⇐
EBL	Minimal	Usually requires transfusion of 1 U autologous blood.	⇐	1-2 U, particularly if combined with breast resection.
Postop care	None	Suction drains	⇐	⇐
Mortality	Minimal	0-0.1%	0-0.5%	⇐
Morbidity	Prosthesis failure: 5%	⇐	N/A	5%
	Infection: 1%	⇐	⇐	⇐
	Dehiscence: < 1%	⇐	1%	⇐
			Graft failure: 2%	Flap failure: 2%
Pain score	2-3	2-4	2-4	3-5

PATIENT POPULATION CHARACTERISTICS

Age range	17-45 yr
Incidence	5000+/yr in U.S.
Etiology	Absence of development; atrophy 2° childbearing
Associated conditions	None common

Reference

1. Vistnes LM: *Procedures in Plastic Surgery: How They Do It.* Little, Brown, Boston: 1991.

ANESTHETIC CONSIDERATIONS

PREOPERATIVE

Typically, three patient populations present for mammoplasty: 1) healthy individuals, for reduction/augmentation mammoplasty or removal of an implant; 2) morbidly obese, for reduction mammoplasty; 3) breast cancer patients, for reconstruction after mastectomy. (For preop considerations in the morbidly obese patient, see Anesthetic Considerations for Abdominoplasty, p. 807.) Breast cancer patients undergoing mastectomy with immediate reconstruction will not have had either chemotherapy or radiation. The following considerations are for breast cancer patients undergoing delayed reconstruction postchemotherapy.

Respiratory — Pulmonary fibrosis may complicate chemotherapy. Alkylating agents (e.g., cyclophosphamide and melphalan), used to treat breast cancer, have some pulmonary toxicity. Consider pulmonary fibrosis in a patient reporting dyspnea, nonproductive cough and fever.
Tests: Consider CXR; ABG, PFTs as indicated from H&P.

Cardiovascular — Cardiomyopathy and CHF may result from chemotherapy, especially doxorubicin (Adriamycin) > 550 mg/m^2.
Tests: Consider ECG; ECHO, if indicated from H&P.

Neurological — Note any previous damage to long thoracic nerves, as evidenced by winged scapula deformity.

Musculoskeletal — Avoid iv and BP cuff on mastectomy side.

Hematologic — Leukopenia, thrombocytopenia and anemia from chemotherapy may be present.
Tests: CBC; Plt count

Renal/Hepatic — Methotrexate can produce some renal and hepatic dysfunction.
Tests: Creatinine; LFTs

Laboratory — Other tests as indicated from H&P, prior chemotherapy, obesity.

Premedication — Midazolam 1-2 mg iv immediately preop or Valium 5-10 mg po 1 h preop

INTRAOPERATIVE

Anesthetic technique: GETA

Induction — Standard induction (p. B-2). ✓ with surgeons regarding use of a nerve stimulator during dissection (and the need to avoid muscle relaxants).

Maintenance — Standard maintenance (p. B-3). Surgeons may want patient sitting for part of the procedure. Pneumothorax should be considered with any change in lung inflation pressure, O_2 saturation, or BP.

Emergence — During some of the procedure and for application of dressing, patient may be moved to sitting position, with consequent coughing, bucking, etc. (Rx: deeper anesthesia, e.g., propofol 0.5 mg/kg or lidocaine 1 mg/kg.) Watch BP carefully and treat orthostatic hypotension if it occurs, usually with a fluid bolus if the patient is not fluid sensitive (Hx of CHF or renal failure).

Blood and fluid requirements	IV 16-18 ga × 1 NS/LR @ 4-8 ml/kg/h	Minimal blood loss for simple reconstruction, augmentation or reduction; larger blood losses anticipated for combined procedures (mastectomy with immediate reconstruction or flap reconstruction).
Monitoring	Standard monitors (p. B-1)	Arterial line in the morbidly obese
Positioning	Patient may need to be sitting for application of dressing.	Avoid HTN, bucking and straining; these may cause or exacerbate bleeding at reconstruction site.

POSTOPERATIVE

Complications — Pneumothorax

Pain management — PCA (p. C-3)

References

1. Desidero DP, Kross RA, Bedford RF: Evaluation of the patient with oncologic disease. In *Principles and Practice of Anesthesiology*, 2nd edition. Longnecker DE, Tinker JH, Morgan GE Jr, eds. Mosby-Year Book, St. Louis: 1998, 379-96.
2. Shenkman Z, Shir Y, Brodsky JB: Perioperative management of the obese patient. *Br J Anaesth* 1993; 70(3):349-59.

LIPOSUCTION

SURGICAL CONSIDERATIONS

Description: Liposuction—suction-assisted lipectomy—is currently the most commonly performed aesthetic surgical procedure in the U.S. Initially a procedure used to contour small areas, it has become an efficient and popular tool not only for contouring, but also for the removal of large volumes of excess fat. With the introduction of superwet and tumescent techniques in the mid 1980s, early operative concerns of excessive blood loss are no longer an issue. These concerns are, however, replaced by the serious considerations of fluid balance and serum lidocaine and epinephrine levels. For this reason, close cooperation between the surgeon and anesthesiologist is vital for assuring patient safety and comfort. Traditional liposuction technique involves the use of metal suction cannulas of varying diameters and lengths introduced through strategically placed stab incisions to aspirate fat following the infusion of tumescent fluid. Suctioning is accomplished with a mechanical aspirator or by utilizing a syringe technique.

The surgical procedure itself may be performed under local, MAC or GETA, depending on the amount of expected aspirate and corresponding length of the surgical procedure. Preop antibiotics are given. Patient positioning varies according to the body region in question, and often intraop repositioning is necessary to reach both dorsal and ventral aspects of the patient. Surgeon preference dictates positioning, and various combinations of supine, prone and bilateral decubitus are often used, thus necessitating a secure airway.

The **tumescent technique** involves the infusion of crystalloid, lidocaine and epinephrine into subcutaneous tissues to provide hemostasis and facilitate the ease of fat evacuation. Varying amounts of fluid may be used, and this has been categorized into **dry** (no tumescent injection), **wet** (< 1 ml injectate infiltrated/ml expected aspirate) and **superwet** (> 1 ml injectate/ml of expected aspirate) techniques. Though exact formulas of tumescent infusate remain individualized, it is generally agreed that maximum lidocaine levels should remain below 35 mg/kg, to assure that patient serum concentrations remain in nontoxic levels. Total infusion volumes may vary from 1-15 L of tumescent infusion, depending on the number of body regions undergoing suctioning, as well as on the size of the patient. Studies have shown that this fluid is absorbed and eliminated over a 48 h period postop. For this reason, iv fluid hydration should be kept to an absolute minimum; and communication between the surgeon and anesthesiologist should be frequent in assessing patient fluid status.

Tumescent infusate is introduced into the subcutaneous tissues region-by-region throughout the course of the procedure. Each infusion is followed by a 10 min waiting period for hemostasis to take maximal effect. Fat evacuation is then accomplished through either traditional or ultrasonic techniques. The procedure is completed with the closure of the small incisions and the placement of 1-5 layers of compressive garments onto the treated areas. For larger tumescent infusions, a Foley catheter is left in place in the postop period.

The newer technique of **ultrasonic liposuction** incorporates the use of ultrasonic energy through a slightly larger cannula to lyse adipose cells. The resultant liquefied fat emulsion is suctioned during the ultrasonic process, as well as in a postultrasonic evacuation period. Ultrasonic liposuction is easier to perform surgically and allows better skin retraction postop, which leads to improved body contouring. The use of ultrasonic energy has been shown to increase tissue temperatures; thus, room temperature infusate is recommended. For more extensive surgery, the infusion of large quantities of low-temperature fluid may affect the patient's core body temperature. A warm room, as well as a table warmer and Bair Hugger, may be necessary to maintain patient temperature.

Following completion of the liposuction procedure (whether traditional or ultrasonic), surgical compression garments are applied in multiple layers to minimize hematoma and seroma formation. Subcutaneous space created by the liposuction surgery is virtually eliminated by use of these garments. Drains may be used to remove serous or blood collection in the surgical areas. Drain use is more common following the use of the ultrasonic liposuction technique than in traditional liposuction.

Usual preop diagnosis: Obesity

SUMMARY OF PROCEDURE

Position	According to body region (repositioning often required)
Incision	Multiple stab incisions
Special instrumentation	Suction cannulae; ultrasonic aspirator
Unique considerations	Potential for lidocaine/epinephrine toxicity and volume overload
Antibiotics	Cefazolin 1 g
Surgical time	5-9 h, depending on extent of procedure
Closing considerations	Compressive dressings/garments
EBL	≤ 1000 ml (although transfusion rarely required)
Postop care	PACU → home

Mortality	Rare (frequently related to lidocaine toxicity)
Morbidity	Fluid overload → CHF/pulmonary edema Lidocaine toxicity Abdominal perforation ± visceral injury Blood loss Hematoma formation Pneumothorax Respiratory compromise 2° pain or restriction garments Fat embolism
Pain score	4-5

PATIENT POPULATION CHARACTERISTICS

Age range	Teens–60 yr
Male:Female	F > M
Etiology	Quest for eternal youth

ANESTHETIC CONSIDERATIONS

PREOPERATIVE

Patients considering liposuction surgery should be healthy and in ASA category I or II. Liposuction is relatively contraindicated in morbidly obese patients; however, larger volumes of resection—in excess of 10,000 ml—may be appropriate for some patients. Preop consultation with the surgical team is necessary for finalizing the anesthetic plan. Patient positioning will be determined by the areas being liposuctioned. Most tumescent fluid recipes include lidocaine 500-1000 mg/L with epinephrine 1:1,000,000. Tumescent injection may range from 0.75-2 ml of solution/1 ml of anticipated fat aspiration. IV fluid administration will depend on the volume of tumescent fluid used and the hydration status of the patient during surgery. Large-volume tumescent injections will require limiting iv fluids during surgery.

Respiratory	Postop discomfort following chest and back liposuction may interfere with respiration. Restrictive compression garments applied to the chest or upper abdomen also may restrict breathing. Patients with respiratory impairment (e.g., smokers) may not be candidates for this procedure.
Cardiovascular	Patients with Hx of CHF or those with MVP may not be candidates for high-volume liposuction. Fluid management is based on volume status and the quantity of tumescent fluid injected during surgery. Tumescent solution injected into the subcutaneous tissue is absorbed over 48 h. Postop pulmonary edema has been reported 2° fluid overload in patients receiving larger volumes of tumescent injection. Some patients may have previously taken fenfluramine alone or in combination with phentermine for weight loss. Those patients should be evaluated for pulmonary HTN (e.g., dyspnea, central cyanosis, right axis deviation and CXR changes) and valvular heart disease.
Neurologic	Preop neurologic exam should be normal. Local anesthetic administration during tumescent injection may cause areas of numbness postop.
Hematologic	Transfusion therapy, which was common during the early days of liposuction, is now rarely needed. Tumescent injection with low-concentration epinephrine solutions causes vasoconstriction in the surgical areas and minimizes blood loss. **Tests:** Hct
Laboratory	Other tests as indicated from H&P.
Premedication	Midazolam 1-2 mg or oral benzodiazepine (e.g., lorazepam 1 mg po 1-2 h preop)

INTRAOPERATIVE

Anesthetic technique: Local or regional anesthesia have been used for small-volume resections, but there are questions regarding vasodilation → ↑blood loss and ↑risk of fat embolization. GETA is commonly used for larger-volume resections.

Induction	Standard induction (see p. B-2).
Maintenance	Standard maintenance (see p. B-3) with volatile anesthetics ± propofol infusion. Neuromuscular blockade as appropriate. Anesthesia should be maintained during application of compression garments. Typically, dexamethasone 8 mg is given at the start of the case.

Emergence	Antiemetic prophylaxis with metoclopramide (10 mg) and ondansetron (4 mg) is appropriate. Careful monitoring of respiratory function is necessary when surgery has been performed on the chest, back or upper abdomen, since compression garments may limit respiration.	
Blood and fluid requirements	IV: 18 ga × 1 NS/LR ≤ 1 L/case Measure I/O.	IV rate based on tumescent technique and blood loss. Transfusion rarely needed. Autologous blood transfused only after 6000 ml aspirate. Consider furosemide 5-10 mg if patient > 2000 ml positive fluid balance.
Monitoring	Standard monitors (see p. B-1). ± Foley catheter	$ETCO_2$ useful for detecting air/fat emboli. UO during large-volume resections will help evaluate intravascular volume status.
Positioning	✓ and pad pressure points. ✓ eyes. Repeat ✓s frequently.	Frequent intraop position checks are needed as patient position will change during surgery → potential for peripheral nerve injury.
Complications	Local anesthetic toxicity Excess blood loss Volume overload Abdominal cavity perforation Pneumothorax Peripheral nerve injury	Lidocaine 35-55 mg/kg has been shown to produce safe serum levels when used with epinephrine for tumescent injection during liposuction.[6,10] Peak plasma lidocaine level occurs 4-12 h after infusion.
	Hypothermia	Vigorous efforts needed to maintain body temperature (e.g., fluid warmer, Bear Hugger).

POSTOPERATIVE

Complications	Hypoxemia	Consider fat embolism, pneumothorax of pulmonary edema in differential diagnosis (DDx).
	HTN	Consider epinephrine effect in DDx.
	Respiratory compromise	May be 2° compression garments and pain.
Pain management	PO analgesics IV opiates	Patients often will be comfortable 2° residual local anesthesia, which may persist for 8-24 h. Oral analgesics are usually satisfactory for postop pain control.
Tests	Hct	✓ Hct following large-volume procedures.

References

1. Burk RW III, Guzman-Stein G, Vasconez LO: Lidocaine and epinephrine levels in tumescent technique liposuction. *Plast Reconstr Surg* 1996; 97:1379.
2. Courtiss EH, Choucair RJ, Donelan MB: Large-volume suction lipectomy: an analysis of 108 patients. *Plast Reconstr Surg* 1992; 89:1068.
3. Hunstad JP: Body contouring in the obese patient. *Clin Plast Surg* 1996; 23(4):647-70.
4. Kaplan B, Moy RL: Comparison of room temperature and warmed local anesthetic solution for tumescent liposuction. *Dermatol Surg* 1996; 22(8):707-9.
5. Klein JA: Tumescent technique for local anesthesia improves safety in large volume liposuction. *Plast Reconstr Surg* 1993; 92:1085-100.
6. Klein JA: Tumescent technique for regional anesthesia permits lidocaine doses of 35 mg/kg for liposuction. *J Dermatol Surg Oncol* 1990; 16:248-63.
7. Maxwell GP: Ultrasound assisted lipoplasty update. *Aesth Surg Quart* 1995; Fall:20-21.
8. Meister F: Possible association between tumescent technique and life-threatening pulmonary complications. *Clin Plast Surg* 1996; 23:642.
9. Ostad A, Kageymis N, Moy RL: Tumescent anesthesia with a lidocaine dose of 55 mg/kg is safe for liposuction. *Dermatol Surg* 1996; 22:921-27.
10. Pitman GH, Aker JS, Tripp ZD: Tumescent liposuction: a surgeon's perspective. *Clin Plast Surg* 1996; 23(4):633-41.
11. Samdal F, Amland PF, Bugge JF: Blood loss during liposuction using the tumescent technique. *Aesthetic Plast Surg* 1994; 18(2):157-60.
12. Samdal F, Amland PF, Bugge JF: Plasma lidocaine levels during suction-assisted lipectomy using large doses of dilute lidocaine with epinephrine. *Plast Reconstr Surg* 1994; 93(6):1217-22.
13. Zocchi M: Ultrasonic assisted lipoplasty. Technical refinements and clinical evaluations. *Clin Plast Surg* 1996; 23(4):575-98.

Surgeons

Barry H. J. Press, MD, FACS
Lynn D. Solem, MD

11.2 BURN SURGERY

Anesthesiologist

Rona G. Giffard, MD, PhD

FREE SKIN GRAFT FOR BURN WOUND

(WITH TANGENTIAL EXCISION, EXCISION TO FASCIA, OR DEBRIDEMENT)

SURGICAL CONSIDERATIONS

Description: Until the mid 1970s, management of burn wounds involved daily debridement, hydrotherapy and spontaneous eschar separation, with subsequent skin grafts applied to the granulated tissue. Recently, operative management has become much more aggressive with the description of **tangential excision** (TE) by **Janzekovic**[5]. This surgical approach to the burn wound involves operative excision of eschar (burned necrotic tissue). Thin slices of burned tissue are removed with either manual or power dermatomes until a healthy wound bed is developed. Assessment of the wound bed is done with visualization of bleeding and/or the clinical appearance of the excised bed.

It has become apparent that early eschar excision is advantageous even if wounds are so extensive they cannot be closed with autografts. In this situation, TE or **excision to fascia** is performed, but the wounds are closed with the application of cadaver allograft, Integra (preferred); porcine xenograft, Dermagraft; or synthetic/biologic dressings. The wound is maintained in this way, with further debridement and changing of the biologic dressings as necessary, until autograft becomes available. The recently developed ability to apply cultured keratinocytes to these wounds has added another option for definitive coverage of excised burns.

In patients with serious burns (>40% total body surface area [TBSA]), excision usually commences on postop d 2-5, after completion of fluid resuscitation. In serious burns, repeated excisions and coverage as described above are performed every 2-3 d, as the patient's condition permits. If eschar excision can be completed before secondary sepsis supervenes, management of the patient is easier and the complications and morbidity are lessened considerably. For deep burns in high-risk patients, **excision to fascia** can be performed. This generally is done with a cutting electrocautery or cold knife, and involves removal of all burned and unburned tissue down to the investing muscle fascia. Generally, the fascia is viable and will support a skin graft. Fascial excision can be performed more rapidly and with less blood loss than TE. Its disadvantages, however, are the marked cosmetic deformities that occur because of the loss of all soft tissue overlying the musculature and, often, functional limitations for the same reason. TE is the more frequently performed procedure.

Usual preop diagnosis: Thermal burn; electrical or chemical burn

SUMMARY OF PROCEDURE

Position	Supine, prone or lateral. Prone generally is preferred for early excisions so that large areas, such as the back, buttocks and posterior legs, can be excised initially for maximum reduction of eschar load. Patients tolerate the prone position better before secondary sepsis or pulmonary complications have supervened. Position changes may be necessary intraop if, for example, donor skin is to be harvested from the back for application to the anterior surface of the body.
Incision	Anywhere eschar is to be excised.
Special instrumentation	Dermatomes, as determined by the surgeon. Manual dermatomes include Weck, Humby and Eschmann knives. Powered dermatomes (generally used in the U.S. for harvesting skin grafts) include Padgett, Zimmer and Brown. Because blood loss is generally diffuse and can be massive, several techniques are used to minimize it. TEs of extremities can be performed by experienced surgeons under pneumatic tourniquet control.
Temperature considerations	Due to loss of skin integrity and large exposed surfaces, these patients lose heat rapidly. Fluids, gases and the OR should be warm, although there is no demonstrable benefit to warming the OR past the point of isothermic neutrality (~82°F [28°C]).[4] Many surgeons, however, will maintain the room at ~100°F (38°C). All areas not in the operative field should be covered, and a warming blanket (Bair Hugger) frequently is used.
Unique considerations	In excising burn eschar or harvesting skin grafts, depending on location of recipient and donor sites, many surgeons use subcutaneous infiltration of NS to smooth out irregularities (e.g., underlying ribs) to physically improve the ease of taking skin grafts. Substantial amounts of NS can be infiltrated subcutaneously (e.g., up to 2-3 L). In a small child, this may be a significant fluid bolus and should be figured into the total fluids administered to patient by anesthesiologist.
Antibiotics	Cefazolin (adult = 1g; child = 15 mg/kg) iv on induction of anesthesia
Surgical time	★ **NB**: The endpoints for surgical excision are: (1) a **time of 2-3 h**; (2) **core temperature of 35°C**; or (3) **blood loss of 10 U PRBC**. The violation of any of these parameters invites coagulopathy and increasing problems with hemostasis and vital sign stability. Adverse affects occurring after 3-4 h of operative time are more closely associated with massive transfusion or hypothermia than with time itself.

Closing considerations After excision of wounds and attainment of hemostasis, wounds are closed, using either autograft, allograft, xenograft or synthetic biologic dressings (described above). Uncontrolled patient movement poses a problem for graft security; however, most of the time grafts are secured with circumferential dressings (to protect against this eventuality). Application of these dressings and splints may be very time-consuming, and any uncontrolled patient movement is detrimental to graft positioning.

EBL Varies with magnitude of procedure, but the goal is to **keep it under 10 U PRBC**. Blood ordered varies with surgeon and procedure, and whether pneumatic tourniquet control is used. Bleeding is also controlled with the application of dilute solutions of epinephrine (e.g., 1:200,000). Substantial absorption occurs and very high plasma epinephrine levels have been measured in these patients. Complications from this, however, are minimal in patients with severe burns because of high

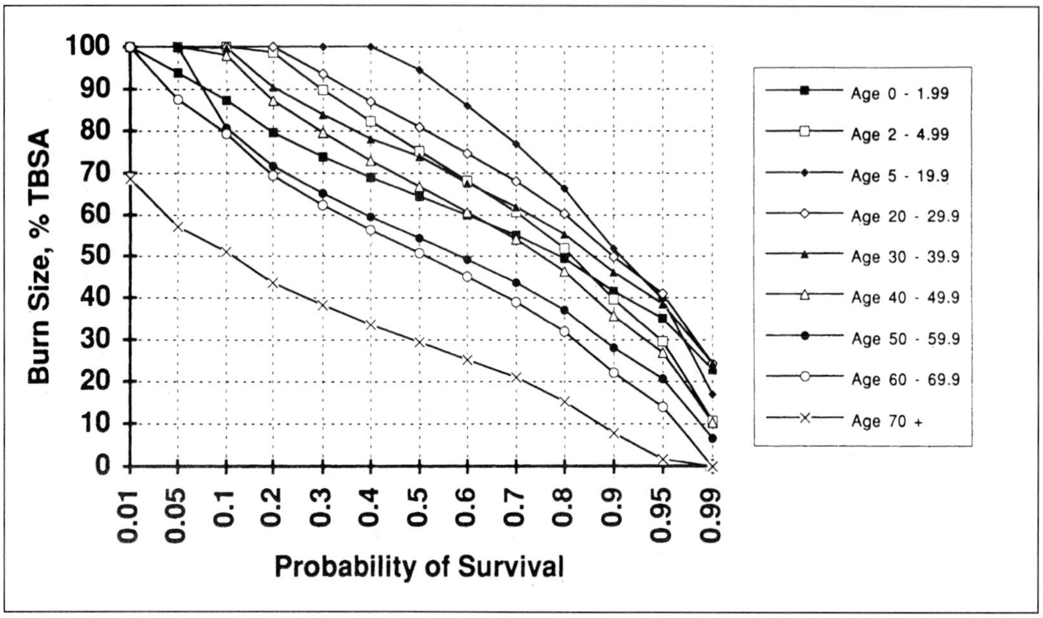

Figure 11.2-1. Probit Survival Curves for 6,417 patients by age groups. (Both Probit Survival figures reproduced with permission from Saffle JR, Davis B, Williams P, et al: Recent outcomes in the treatment of burn injury in the United States: A report from the American Burn Association Patient Registry. *J Burn Care Rehab* 1995; 16:219-32.)

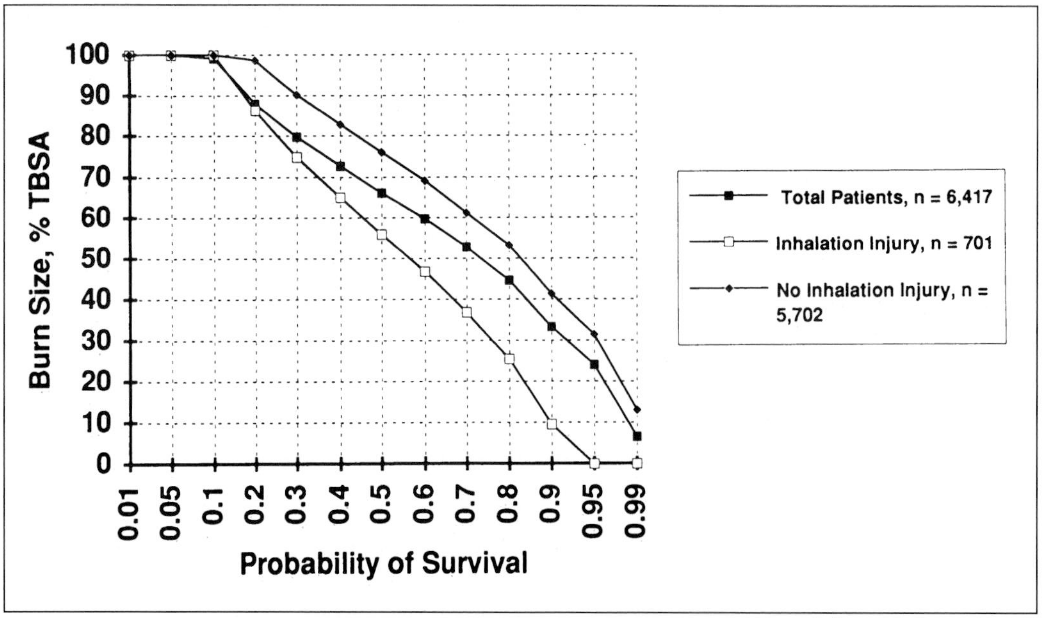

Figure 11.2-2. Probit Survival for patients with and without inhalation injury.

EBL, cont.	endogenous catecholamine secretion. Other topical agents used for hemostasis include thrombin and microcrystalline collagen. These modalities are often combined with compressive wraps and elevation of excised extremities to promote hemostasis. Because blood loss may be massive and difficult to control, close communication between anesthesiologist and surgeon is essential. In large excisions, blood replacement often is begun prior to excision so that the anesthesiologist does not get behind in blood replacement. As a rule, replacement with blood and crystalloid is preferable to artificial plasma expanders such as hetastarch or dextran.
Postop care	Generally, patients can be extubated at the end of these procedures, recovered in the PACU and returned to the burn center. If patient remains intubated, generally he/she is transported directly back to the burn center, where body temperature can be maintained more easily.
Mortality	18-40% (Mortality is a function of the burn size, plus other associated conditions, especially inhalation injury: see Figs 11.2-1 and 11.2-2.)
Morbidity	Massive blood loss Sepsis Infection 2° to catheters and lines
Pain score	2-5 (Most patients are maintained on methadone, sustained-release or iv morphine, for perioperative pain control.)

PATIENT POPULATION CHARACTERISTICS

Age range	All
Male:Female	More commonly male
Incidence	500,000/yr
Etiology	Scald; flame burns; chemicals; electric burns
Associated conditions	Generally few, except in elderly patients

ANESTHETIC CONSIDERATIONS

PREOPERATIVE

The extent of physiologic derangement depends on the percent of TBSA burned, time since burn was sustained and treatment received in the interval. Patients are usually young and healthy; older patients generally have a poorer prognosis. Generally, after major burns, the patient is fluid-resuscitated and stabilized, then brought to the OR on about the 3rd d to begin TE and coverage of the burned area with skin grafts. Blood loss and hypothermia are the predominant considerations during surgery on burn patients. Blood loss can be rapid and massive, as much as 8 U in 15 min, and can be difficult to estimate as it generally is not collected into the suction.

Respiratory	**Upper airway**: A patient with burns around the airway should be intubated early as subsequent intubation may become more difficult, or even impossible. Careful assessment of airway, face, head and neck is essential to anticipate problems with subsequent airway management. **Lower airway**: Patients may suffer from ARDS, and ventilator settings should be noted preop. High PIP and minute-volume requirements may necessitate the use of an ICU-type ventilator in OR. Patients with extensive burns can be severely hypermetabolic (a patient with 40% TBSA burns may have twice the normal metabolic rate) with ↑CO_2 production. These patients may require high minute-ventilation (as much as 30 L/min), and high levels of PEEP to maintain normocarbia. Other possible effects of severe burns include: ↓lung and chest-wall compliance, ↓FRC, ↑A-a gradient, ↑carboxyhemoglobinemia and ↑methemoglobinemia. **Tests:** ABG, depending on pulmonary status; CXR
Cardiovascular	The hypermetabolism associated with burns increases cardiac demand, and burn patients have greatly elevated circulating levels of catecholamines → ↑HR. **Tests:** As indicated from H&P.
Neurological	Evaluate for burn encephalopathy. Characterize baseline mental status before anesthesia to allow evaluation of recovery postop.
Musculoskeletal	Damaged muscle → ↑acetylcholine receptor density, resulting in ↓sensitivity to nondepolarizing muscle relaxants and potentially fatal elevations of K in response to succinylcholine. In burns

Musculoskeletal, cont. >5% TBSA, avoid succinylcholine after the 4th d postburn. Recovery of normal response to muscle relaxants does not occur until burns have healed completely.

Hematologic Coagulopathies may result directly from the burn injury, as well as from rapid replacement of blood loss during operative procedures.
Tests: Hb/Hct; electrolytes; coagulation profile

IV access May be difficult; assess preop. Consider central line placement with a large-bore catheter such as a Cordis.

Laboratory Other tests as indicated from H&P.

Premedication Adequate analgesia should be given (titrate dose to effect) to allow transport and movement to OR table.

Transport For patients with severe ARDS, transportation from burn unit to OR may pose formidable challenges with regard to ventilation. Cardiopulmonary monitoring must be continued during transport; the ventilation system used in transport must be capable of delivering high minute-volumes, PEEP and inspiratory pressures. These requirements may not be satisfied by standard bag-valve systems and may require a high-quality transport ventilator.

INTRAOPERATIVE

Anesthetic technique: GETA

Induction Thiopental (3-5 mg/kg) or propofol (1.5-2.5 mg/kg iv), if patient is already volume-resuscitated; otherwise, use etomidate 0.3 mg/kg or ketamine 1-3 mg/kg. Pancuronium (0.15 mg/kg) or vecuronium (0.3 mg/kg) for intubation. In patients with extensive burns, 1.5 times the usual intubation dose may be required. If the face is burned, mask induction or awake FOL may be necessary. The ETT should be sutured in place or wired to the teeth by the surgeon to avoid dislodging it, especially during procedures in the prone position. Alternatively, the tube may be secured with umbilical tape or a Tube Tamer.

Maintenance Standard maintenance (see p. B-3). These patients may require minute-volumes > 30 L/min, high inspiratory pressures and PEEP for adequate ventilation. For these cases a Siemens or ICU-type ventilator is recommended. Surgeons may give epinephrine topically to decrease blood loss. Epinephrine is well absorbed from the disrupted skin surface → ↑↑plasma catecholamine levels; thus, isoflurane is preferred over halothane to decrease the risk of dysrhythmias.

Emergence Estimation of an adequate dose of narcotic to provide good postop analgesia may be difficult as these patients are often on high doses of narcotics preop.

Blood and fluid requirements

Extensive blood loss
IV: 14-16 ga × 2 or a Cordis
NS/LR @ 8-10 ml/kg/h
Keep UO @ 0.5-1 ml/kg/h.
Blood: ~200 ml/1% BSA excised and grafted.[5]
Fluid warmer
T&C 2-4 U PRBC (to keep ahead).

Blood must be in OR prior to induction. The major blood loss generally is associated with eschar excision, usually the first part of the procedure. For patients without contraindications to hemodilution, it is often better to delay PRBC transfusion until major blood loss is complete. IV hyperalimentation should be continued during surgery; or, replace the same volume with 10% dextrose infusion to avoid hypoglycemia. If sudden ↓BP occurs during very rapid infusion of blood (>150 ml/min), consider using calcium to counteract the chelating effect of citrate. Avoid fluid overload, especially if patient has ARDS, is a small child, or is elderly. As the surgical site is superficial, there is not much 3rd-space loss. It may be necessary to have an additional person available to help administer blood.

Thermal considerations

Room = 80-82°F
Warm all fluids.
Humidify gases.
Warming blanket
Reflective head cover

Temperature must be monitored throughout the case. The surgeon should be notified if patient's core temperature is dropping.

Monitoring

Standard monitors (see p. B-1).
± CVP line, PA catheter

ECG may require needle electrodes or alligator clip electrodes to skin graft if there is no skin availability to apply

Monitoring, cont.		adhesive electrodes. Patients who are hemodynamically unstable should be monitored with PA catheters.
Positioning	✓ and pad pressure points. ✓ eyes.	The burn patient may be uniquely susceptible to laryngeal or upper airway edema in the prone position, so examination of the upper airway before extubation is recommended to avoid emergent reintubation.
Complications	Massive blood loss	

POSTOPERATIVE

Complications	Hypothermia Coagulopathy	May occur as the result of massive blood loss and replacement.
Transport	Continue cardiopulmonary monitoring. High minute-ventilation requirements ↑PIP ↑PEEP	Verify adequacy of transport ventilation system before departing OR.
Pain management	Oral methadone or sustained-release Morphine sulfate IV fentanyl or morphine sulfate	Titrate analgesia to effect.
Tests	Hct, ABG, electrolytes, PT, PTT, Plt, if massive transfusion given.	

References

1. Burke JF, Quinby WC Jr, Bondoc CC: Primary excision and prompt grafting as routine therapy for the treatment of thermal burns in children. *Surg Clin North Am* 1976; 56(2):477-94.
2. Caan LM, Miller SM: Trauma and burns. In *Clinical Anesthesia.* Barash PG, Cullen BF, Stoelting RK, eds. Lippincott-Raven Publishers, Philadelphia: 1997, 1173-1204.
3. Heimbach DM: Early burn excision and grafting. *Surg Clin North Am* 1987; 67(1):93-107.
4. Jankovich GH, Austin EN: Environmental Injuries. In *Surgery: Scientific Principles and Practice.* Greenfield LJ, et al, eds. JB Lippincott, Philadelphia: 1993, 359.
5. Janzekovic Z: A new concept in the early excision and immediate grafting of burns. *J Trauma* 1970; 10(2):1103-8.
6. Moran KT, O'Reilly TJ, Furman W, Munster AM: A new algorithm for calculation of blood loss in excisional burn surgery. *Am Surg* 1988; 54(4):207-8.
7. Pavlin EG: *Surgical Management of the Burn Wound.* Heimbach DM, Engrav LH, eds. Raven Press. New York: 1985, Ch 9, 139-53.

Surgeon

Stephen A. Schendel, MD, DDS

11.3 FUNCTIONAL RESTORATION

Anesthesiologists

Stanley I. Samuels, MB, BCh, FFARCS
Richard A. Jaffe, MD, PhD

REPAIR OF FACIAL FRACTURES

SURGICAL CONSIDERATIONS

Description: Facial fractures are characterized by location. Fractures of the maxilla are classified either as **LeFort I**, **II** or **III**, depending on the level of the fracture (Fig 11.3-1). **LeFort III** is essentially a disassociation of the cranium and face. **LeFort II** is a triangular fracture with a fracture line across the nose, through the infraorbital rims, and extending to the entire lower maxillary structures. **LeFort I** is a horizontal fracture, separating the teeth and maxillary components from the upper facial structures. In these cases, the maxilla is usually mobile, or impacted posteriorly, occasionally closing off the posterior airway. Associated fractures in the maxillary region include fractures of the zygoma. Orbital fractures (most common is the orbital floor fracture), isolated nasal fractures, and nasal orbital ethmoid fractures (usually with severe comminution of the upper face and telecanthus, and possible intracranial fractures) have the potential for CSF rhinorrhea.

Fractures of the mandible are classified by the type of fracture and location (Fig 11.3-2), the most common being the subcondylar fracture. Fractures involving the mandibular body, such as the parasymphyseal fracture, may end up with a mobile mandible. In cases of bilateral mandibular body fractures associated with symphyseal fractures, the mandible can be flail and fall posteriorly in the supine position, blocking off the airway. All the fractures involving change in occlusion (LeFort maxillary and all mandibular fractures), require reestablishment of a normal occlusion by intermaxillary wiring and the application of arch bars. This may be combined with rigid fixation, most commonly internal plates. Many approaches are possible, requiring, for example, external excisions under the eyelid, along the inferior border of the mandible, or, in extreme cases, a bicoronal incision, depending on the extent of the fracture and associated facial lacerations. Oral incisions may be associated with external incisions.

Usual preop diagnosis: Facial trauma

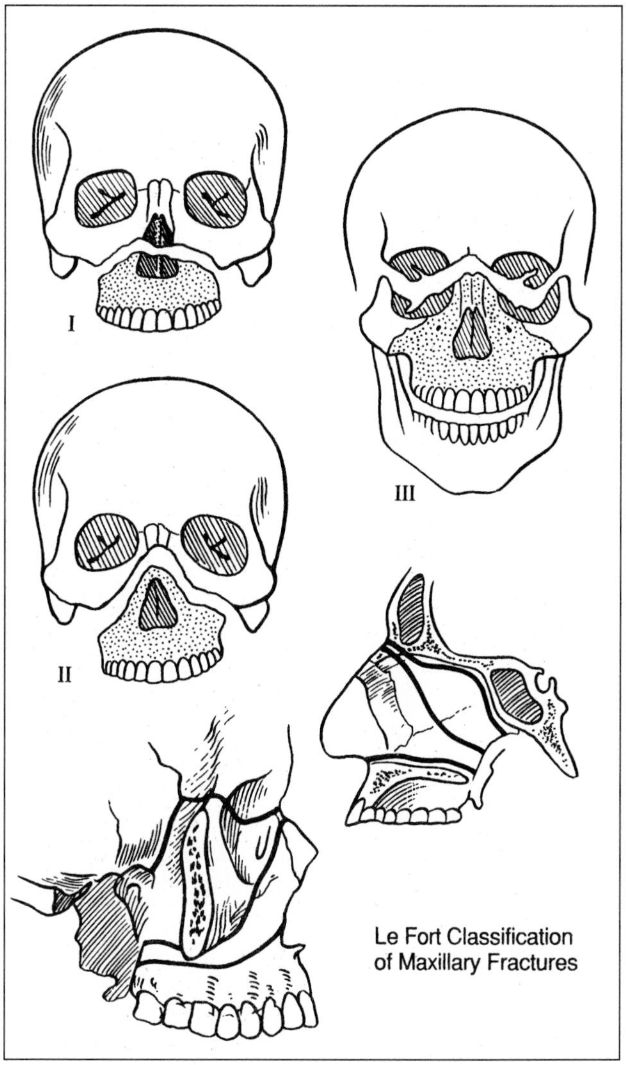

Figure 11.3-1. LeFort I is a horizontal fracture involving mobilization of the dentition and maxilla. LeFort II is a pyramid-shaped fracture including the dentition and nasal structures. LeFort III fracture involves separation of the cranium from facial bone structure. (Reproduced with permission from Schultz RC: *Facial Injuries.* Yearbook Medical Pub: 1988.)

SUMMARY OF PROCEDURE

	Mandibular	Maxillary Orbital/Zygomatic	Nasal
Position	Supine	⇐	⇐
Incision	Intraoral; lateral submandibular	Intraoral, ± subciliary incisions); possibly coronal	Closed reduction; possibly intranasal
Special instrumentation	Air power tools; plate fixation; headlight	⇐	⇐

	Mandibular	Maxillary Orbital/Zygomatic	Nasal
Unique considerations	Nasal RAE; throat pack; ETT	Fractures not involving change in occlusion (e.g., orbital zygomatic, nasal fractures) can be handled by oral intubation. All fractures with a change in occlusion should undergo nasal intubation, with either RAE or 60° curved connector.	⇐
Antibiotics	Cefazolin 1 g iv q 4-6 h × 5-7 d	⇐	⇐
Surgical time	1-3 h	1-6 h	1 h
EBL	Minimal	50-600 ml	Minimal
Postop care	PACU (uncomplicated fractures); ICU (large fractures ± intracranial trauma)	⇐ + Patient may wake up with jaws wired together.	⇐
Mortality	Minimal	⇐	⇐
Morbidity	Pain	⇐	⇐
	Swelling	⇐	⇐
	Infection	⇐	⇐
	Bone loss	⇐	⇐
	Poor occlusal or cosmetic result	–	–
	Visual problems	⇐	–
Pain score	5	4	4

PATIENT POPULATION CHARACTERISTICS

Age range > 4 yr

Male:Female 1:1

Incidence The most common bones to be fractured are nasal bones, followed by the zygoma and arch, mandible and orbital floor; 2/3 of patients involved in motor vehicle accidents (MVAs).[1]

Etiology MVAs (54%); home accidents (17%); athletic injuries (11%)

Associated conditions Dental fractures; intracranial injury; cervical spine fractures (10%); shock; globe injuries

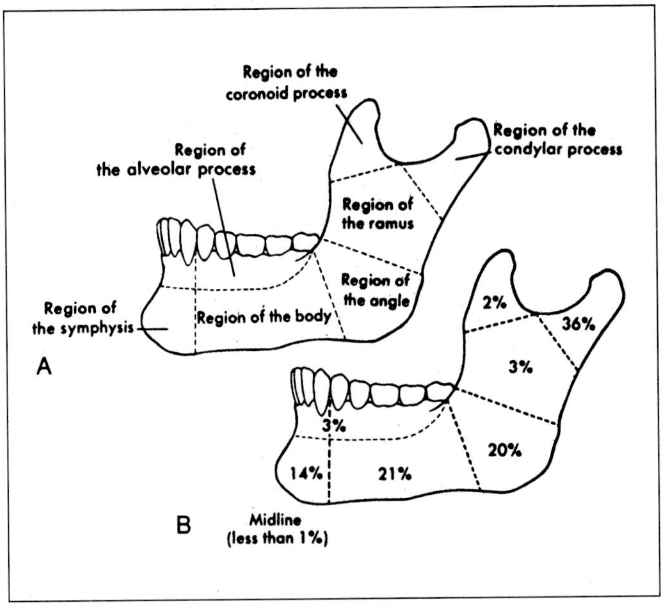

Figure 11.3-2. (A) Mandibular regions. (B) Percentage of fractures occurring in each region. (Reproduced with permission from Kruger GO: *Textbook of Oral and Maxillofacial Surgery*, 6th edition. CV Mosby Co: 1984.)

ANESTHETIC CONSIDERATIONS

PREOPERATIVE

The forces required to produce facial fractures are considerable and frequently result in other associated trauma (e.g., cervical spine injury, subdural hematoma, pneumothorax, intraabdominal bleeding). Soft-tissue injury to the tongue or larynx can make airway management difficult. When in doubt, a tracheostomy under local anesthesia or awake intubation should be considered. In mandible or maxillary fractures, nasal intubation is usually best, because the patient will be placed in intermaxillary fixation (IMF) (teeth brought together via wires or rubber bands) at the conclusion of the procedure. In malar or nasal bone fractures, the fixation may be precarious, making it undesirable to use masked ventilation at the termination of the procedure and necessitating awake extubation. Facial nerve monitoring or observation may be required, contraindicating the use of muscle relaxants.

Frequently, the anesthesiologist's first encounter with these patients is in the ER where prompt airway management decisions are essential, often before diagnostic imaging studies are complete. These patients should be treated with full-stomach precautions (see p. B-5) and may have already aspirated. Patients may be unable to open their mouths 2° pain or mechanical factors. The cause of limited mouth opening should be determined before induction of anesthesia. Several options exist. Often, the airway can be managed simply by inserting an oropharyngeal airway; failing this, an emergency intubation will be necessary. Blind nasal intubation should be avoided in patients with CSF rhinorrhea or other evidence of nasopharyngeal trauma, where the potential for creating false passages and additional trauma is significant. An awake oral intubation with topical anesthesia is often the safest approach. Emergency oral intubation may be complicated by an unstable C-spine and limited jaw opening, together with blood and debris in the oropharynx, making visualization difficult, if not impossible. Often the only recourse is tracheostomy under local anesthesia. As with any trauma victim, attention is first directed toward maintaining the airway and restoration of fluid volume. The repair of the facial fracture may be carried out incidentally to the primary trauma surgery or, more often, is deferred until the patient's condition is stabilized. This preop assessment will focus on the patient coming to the OR for semielective repair of a facial fracture.

Airway

Semielective: Usually facial swelling and intraoral bleeding will have resolved, although mouth opening may be limited 2° pain or mechanical factors. Airway management requires knowledge of the fracture site(s). Patients with a maxillary fracture may benefit from an oral intubation to allow inspection of the nasopharynx before nasal intubation and definitive repair. The possibility of an awake fiber optic intubation (see p. B-6) should be discussed with the patient. Patients with an isolated orbital, zygomatic or nasal fracture do not usually present airway management problems. The surgeon should be consulted regarding the preferred intubation route.

Trauma: Airway and nasal obstruction following trauma can be extreme, as a result of soft-tissue swelling and accumulated blood and secretions. The extent of facial fractures, particularly in the midface, should be identified as they may preclude nasal intubation. Mandibular fractures may make access to the oropharynx difficult. In the case of massive trauma to the face, urgent tracheostomy should be considered.

Tests: As indicated from H&P.

Respiratory

Evaluate for associated trauma and respiratory insufficiency 2° aspiration. ✓ that chest tubes are functioning properly.

Tests: CXR; others as indicated from H&P.

Cardiovascular

Blunt chest trauma may be associated with myocardial contusion and pericardial effusion/tamponade. **Semielective:** Typically, several days will have elapsed since the initial trauma and the patient should be hemodynamically stable.

Tests: ECG; others as indicated from H&P.

Neurological

Semielective: Document any neurological deficit and altered mental status. Meningitis may occur in patients with persistent rhinorrhea or pneumocephalus.

Trauma: Intracranial injury may be associated with facial fractures. Patients with head trauma may have ↑ICP; therefore, appropriate methods (e.g., CO_2 ↓, fluid ↓, smooth induction/intubation) are used to prevent further ↑ICP. Basilar skull fractures preclude passage of nasotracheal and NG tubes. In the presence of otorrhea or rhinorrhea, positive-pressure mask ventilation is inadvisable, due to the potential for causing pneumocephalus.

Tests: Review skull and C-spine x-rays.

Musculoskeletal

Semielective: May be associated with other fractures and soft-tissue trauma which may affect patient positioning.

Trauma: Cervical spine injuries are commonly associated with facial injuries. The C-spine should be cleared by x-ray exam prior to transport to OR. If C-spine cannot be cleared, intubation should be done with the head in a neutral position (splinted or with axial traction), using direct FOL (see p. B-6).

Hematologic

Trauma: Maxillary surgery may be associated with major blood loss and, for elective cases, autologous donation should be encouraged.

Tests: Hct; others as indicated from H&P.

Laboratory Other tests as indicated from H&P.

Premedication Standard premedication (see p. B-2) is appropriate for nontrauma, neurologically intact patients with normal airways.

Trauma: Trauma patients should be considered to have full stomachs, and sedative premedications are best avoided. Aspiration prophylaxis with 0.3 M Na citrate (30 ml po), ± metoclopramide 10 mg iv ± ranitidine 50 mg iv, should be considered.

INTRAOPERATIVE

Anesthetic technique: The majority of patients presenting for elective procedures are healthy and have normal airways. In the case of facial trauma, however, intubation of the trachea may be impossible. Hence, a tracheostomy under local anesthesia may be life-saving.

Induction If there is any doubt regarding the ease of intubation, an awake FOL should be performed (see p. B-6). Nasal intubation is preferred for patients with mandibular and maxillary (LeFort) fractures involving a change in occlusion. Patients with orbital, zygomatic or nasal fractures are usually intubated orally. In patients with normal airways, a standard induction (see p. B-2) is appropriate. Nasal or oral ETTs (RAE), or anode ETTs are commonly used to minimize intrusion into the surgical field.

Maintenance Standard maintenance (see p. B-3); muscle relaxation is usually required. Administration of an antiemetic (e.g., metoclopramide 10 mg iv or ondansetron 4 mg iv) is beneficial in patients who have their jaws wired or banded together.

Emergence Patients with difficult airways or with jaws wired together should be extubated when fully awake. Extubation over a tube-changer may be appropriate. A wire cutter (or scissors for elastic bands) should be at the bedside at all times. Ensure that all throat packing has been removed before extubation. Some patients with multiple trauma or extensive soft-tissue swelling may require continued postop intubation and mechanical ventilation.

Blood and fluid requirements	Moderate blood loss IV: 16-18 ga × 1 **Trauma:** NS/LR @ 6-8 ml/h **Other:** NS/LR @ 2-4 ml/h	Blood loss from facial fractures or orthognathic procedures can be extensive. T&C patient so blood is immediately available in OR.
Monitoring	Standard monitors (see p. B-1). ± Arterial line	Invasive monitoring may be required in patients with intracranial or other trauma, or for controlled hypotension.
Control of blood loss	Surgical hemostasis Topical vasoconstrictors Posterior oropharyngeal packing Controlled hypotension	Surgical hemostasis should control most bleeding in these procedures. Topical vasoconstrictors such as phenylephrine or cocaine can be applied on the surgical field. Posterior oropharyngeal packing can keep blood from passing undetected into the upper GI tract. Controlled ↓BP can be achieved simply by increasing volatile anesthetic levels.
Positioning	✓ and pad pressure points. ✓ eyes.	Some surgeons prefer that the OR table be rotated 90° or 180°. Be prepared with long hoses and appropriate connectors. Protect eyes with an ophthalmic ointment.
Complications	ETT damage	Nasal ETT may be wired inadvertently to the maxilla, making extubation difficult. In case of ETT damage, be prepared to reestablish the airway rapidly by reintubation, usually over an intubating stylet or gum elastic bougie.

POSTOPERATIVE

Complications	Airway obstruction	Wire cutters (or scissors) should be available at bedside to facilitate emergent reintubation or other form of airway management. Consider retained throat pack.
	N/V	Vigorous treatment of nausea is important.
Pain management	Parenteral narcotics (see p. C-1) or PCA with antiemetics (see p. C-3).	Local anesthetic infiltrated at end of procedure.

References

1. Manson PN: Facial Injuries. In *Plastic Surgery*, Vol 2. McCarthy JG, ed. WB Saunders Co, Philadelphia: 1990, 867-1141.
2. Stanley RB. Jr: Maxillofacial trauma. In *Otolaryngology—Head and Neck Surgery,* Vol I, 2nd edition. Cummings CW, Krause CJ, eds. Mosby-Year Book, St. Louis: 1993, 374–402.

LEFORT OSTEOTOMIES

SURGICAL CONSIDERATIONS

Description: LeFort osteotomies are used to correct maxillary deformities. The most common is the **LeFort I**, a transverse osteotomy, above the apices of the teeth, used to correct maxillary retrusion or maxillary vertical excess. An intraoral vestibular incision is used for this approach, followed by an osteotomy of the maxilla, with either a burr or a saw, and completed with osteotomes. The osteotomy goes through both sinuses and frequently into the nasal cavity. **LeFort II** or, occasionally, **LeFort III maxillary osteotomies** (Fig 11.3-1) may be used to correct severe midfacial retrusion with an orbital component. In these cases, infraorbital incisions are used with either brow or coronal incisions. With maxillary advancements, iliac or cranial bone grafts are often necessary. Most of these patients have orthodontic appliances and will require maxillary fixation with either wire or elastics at the end of the procedure. The maxilla is usually rigidly fixed in the new position with small miniplates.

Usual preop diagnosis: Facial deformities

SUMMARY OF PROCEDURE

	LeFort I	LeFort II	LeFort III
Position	Supine; table may be rotated 90° or 180°	⇐	⇐
Incision	Intraoral	Intraoral and facial or coronal	⇐
Special instrumentation	Miniplates and screws for maxilla	⇐	⇐
Unique considerations	Jaw frequently closed, either by wires or elastics, at end of procedure; RAE or armored tube used.	⇐	⇐
Antibiotics	Cefazolin 1 g iv × 5 d	⇐	⇐
Surgical time	3-6 h	⇐	⇐
EBL	400-800 ml	⇐	⇐
Postop care	PACU → room	ICU × 1 d	⇐
Mortality	Rare	⇐	⇐
Morbidity	Relapse	⇐	⇐
	Infection	⇐	⇐
	Bone/tooth loss: Uncommon	⇐	⇐
	Intraop bleeding: Uncommon	⇐	⇐
Pain score	4	5	5

PATIENT POPULATION CHARACTERISTICS

Age range	15 yr–adulthood, usually < 30 yr
Male:Female	1:1
Incidence	Up to 5% of population
Etiology	Usually developmental in nature
Associated conditions	None, unless part of a recognized condition (e.g., Apert's syndrome, Crouzon's disease). May be associated with congenital anomalies, such as cleft lip and palate.

ANESTHETIC CONSIDERATIONS

See Anesthetic Considerations following Mandibular Osteotomies/Genioplasty, p. 831.

References

1. Lanigan DT, Hey JH, West RA: Major vascular complications of orthognathic surgery: hemorrhage associated with LeFort I osteotomies. *J Oral Maxillofac Surg* 1990; 48(6):561-73.
2. Hilley MD, Ghali GE, Giesecke AU: Anesthesia for orthognathic surgery in modern practice. In *Orthognathic Reconstructive Surgery*, 2nd edition. Bell WH, ed. WB Saunders Co, Philadelphia: 1992, 128-53.
3. Scully JR, Matheson JD: Emergency airway management in the traumatized patient. In *Oral and Maxillofacial Trauma,* 2nd edition. Fonseca RJ, Walker RV, eds. WB Saunders, Philadelphia: 1997, 105-37.

MANDIBULAR OSTEOTOMIES/GENIOPLASTY

SURGICAL CONSIDERATIONS

Description: Mandibular deformities include either a retruded mandible or a prognathic mandible involving a malocclusion (Class II or III) and may be combined with a small chin (microgenia). Surgical correction of the basic mandibular deformity involves either advancing or retruding the mandible. The most common procedure for this is the **sagittal ramus split osteotomy** (**Obwegesser**). This may be combined with a **genioplasty** to correct the chin deformity. Genioplasty also may be performed as an isolated procedure, the most common type being one in which a horizontal osteotomy of the inferior mandible is performed and the chin segment repositioned. A variety of approaches for mandibular osteotomies often involve the ramus area of the mandible and are performed via an intraoral approach.

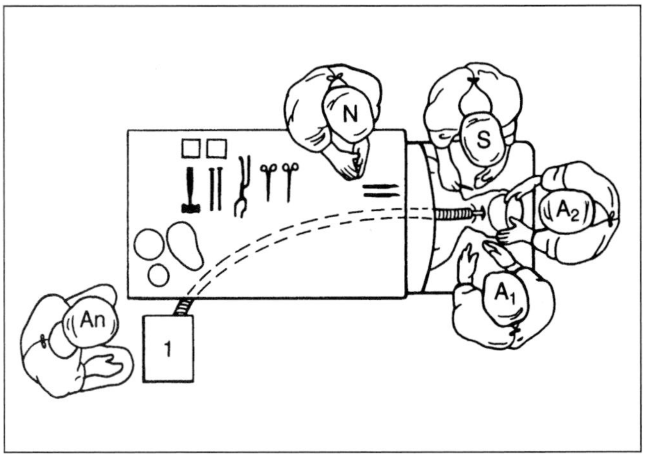

Figure 11.3-3. Standard anesthesia and surgical setup for a maxillofacial surgical procedure and certain craniofacial surgical procedures. The table may be rotated 90°-180° with anesthesia equipment and personnel at the foot or off to one side. (Reproduced with permission from Bell WH, ed: *Modern Practice of Orthognathic Surgery*, Vol I. WB Saunders: 1990.)

In some very large deformities, an external incision (**Risdon** type) and bone graft placement may be necessary to complete the mandibular ramus reconstruction. Occasionally, deformities may be corrected by mandibular body osteotomies. **Rigid fixation** of mandibular osteotomies is often accomplished by the use of small miniplates or screws. Fixation also can be accomplished with elastic traction (rarely, wire fixation) between mandible and maxilla, placed either at the time of surgery, or several days following, and held in position for 1-2 wk. **Distraction osteogenesis** is being used more frequently in treating certain congenital jaw deformities. This involves a partial mandibular osteotomy and application of a distraction device, usually extraoral. Microgenia may be corrected by placement of an implant without performing an osteotomy. This procedure can be done either via the oral route or the extraoral route through a small submental incision. Most frequently this isolated procedure is performed with local anesthesia and sedation.

Usual preop diagnosis: Mandibular deformity

SUMMARY OF PROCEDURE

Position	Supine; table may be rotated 90° or 180°.
Incision	Usually oral, but may be in the submental or posterior mandibular area externally.
Special instrumentation	Miniplates and screws; distractor for distraction osteogenesis
Unique considerations	Postop, patient may have bimaxillary fixation with inability to open the mouth.
Antibiotics	Cefazolin 1 g iv
Surgical time	Genioplasty: 0.5-1 h Mandibular osteotomy: 2-4 h
EBL	Genioplasty: 50 ml Mandibular osteotomy: 100-200 ml
Postop care	PACU → room
Mortality	Rare
Morbidity	Mandibular relapse: ≤ 30% Mental nerve paresthesia: 5-20%
Pain score	4

PATIENT POPULATION CHARACTERISTICS

Age range	4 yr–adult
Male:Female	Unknown
Incidence	Unknown
Etiology	Developmental (90%); acquired (10%)

ANESTHETIC CONSIDERATIONS

(Procedures covered: LeFort osteotomies; mandibular osteotomies/genioplasty)

PREOPERATIVE

These surgeries are usually performed on patients with facial disproportion. In general, this patient population is young and healthy; however, many of them will present with challenging airway management problems. In addition, facial disproportion will alter congenital anomalies (e.g., Crouzon's disease, Apert's syndrome). (For discussion of specific syndromes, see Anesthetic Considerations for Pediatric Orthopedic Surgery of the Pelvis and Lower Limbs, p. 1020).

Airway As usual, a careful airway evaluation is essential since many of these patients have abnormal airway anatomy. Visual inspection often reveals the reasons for the surgery and allows the anesthesiologist to determine the safest approach to intubation. When a difficult intubation is anticipated, the need for awake fiber optic intubation should be discussed with the patient.

Respiratory/ cardiovascular Consider the anesthetic implications of associated congenital syndromes in this patient population.
Tests: As indicated from H&P.

Hematologic Encourage autologous blood donation for maxillary procedures.
Tests: Hct

Laboratory Other tests as indicated from H&P.

Premedication Standard premedication (see p. B-2) is usually appropriate.

INTRAOPERATIVE

Anesthetic technique: GETA

Induction If there is any doubt regarding the ease of intubation, an awake FOL should be performed (see p. B-6). Nasal intubation is preferred for patients undergoing mandibular or maxillary osteotomies, as well as genioplasty. In patients with normal airways, a standard induction (see p. B-2) is appropriate. Nasal or oral ETTs (RAE), or anode ETTs, are commonly used to minimize intrusion into the surgical field.

Maintenance Standard maintenance (see p. B-3); muscle relaxation is usually required. Administration of an antiemetic (e.g., metoclopramide 10 mg iv or ondansetron 4 mg iv) is essential in patients who have their jaws wired or banded together.

Emergence	Patients with difficult airways or with their jaws wired (or banded) together should be extubated when fully awake. A wire cutter (or scissors for elastic bands) should be at the bedside at all times. Ensure that all throat packing has been removed before extubation.	
Blood and fluid requirements	Moderate blood loss IV: 16 ga × 1 NS/LR @ 5-8 ml/kg/h	Maxillary osteotomies may be associated with major blood loss (e.g., 1500-2000 ml). Deliberate hypotension (SBP < 90) may be useful during maxillary surgery and blood should be readily available.
Monitoring	Standard monitors (see p. B-1). ± Arterial line ± CVP line or 2nd iv	Direct arterial pressure measurements are useful for deliberate hypotension. Central venous access or a 2nd peripheral iv may be useful for vasodilator infusions.
Positioning	✓ and pad pressure points. ✓ eyes.	Eyes should be protected with an ophthalmic ointment and possible tarsorrhaphy by the surgeons. Some surgeons prefer to have the OR table rotated 90° or 180°. Be prepared with circuit-extension tubing.
Complications	ETT damage Hemorrhage	ETT may be cut during maxillary osteotomy, necessitating rapid reintubation.

POSTOPERATIVE

Complications	Airway obstruction	Wire cutters (or scissors) should be available at bedside to facilitate emergent reinduction or other form of airway management. Consider retained throat pack.
	N/V	Vigorous treatment of nausea is important.
Pain management	Parenteral narcotics (see p. C-1) or PCA with antiemetics (see p. C-3).	

BREAST/CHEST-WALL RECONSTRUCTION

SURGICAL CONSIDERATIONS

Description: Breast defects are usually the result of mastectomy for cancer. Congenital defects (e.g., Poland syndrome) are rare. Chest-wall defects occasionally are seen following cardiovascular surgery, or they can be radiation-induced.

There are three approaches to **breast reconstruction**: **tissue expansion** of the overlying skin by placement of an expander, followed by a permanent prosthesis; **transfer of a flap**, such as a latissimus dorsi myocutaneous flap, to the defect, followed by placement of a breast prosthesis; and complete **soft-tissue reconstruction**, most frequently using a pedicled or free rectus abdominis flap. Breast reconstruction following breast ablation can be accomplished using a latissimus dorsi myocutaneous flap as shown in Fig 11.3-4. The flap and skin pedicle are transferred from the ipsilateral back to the anterior chest where they are inserted into position. It is always necessary to use an implant with a latissimus dorsi reconstruction as the flap itself is not of adequate size to totally reconstruct an absent breast. Alternatively, the breast may be reconstructed by using the TRAM flap, which is a rectus abdominis muscle myocutaneous flap. This flap can be transferred with the superior epigastric vessels as a pedicled flap of either the contralateral or ipsilateral side, although the contralateral is preferred. The TRAM flap also may be transferred as a free flap with microvascular anastomoses, as demonstrated in Fig 11.3-5. **Chest-wall reconstruction** is frequently accomplished by rotation or transfer of the pectoralis muscles, followed by advancement of skin pedicles with split-thickness skin grafts. Occasional defects will need a pedicular or a free-rectus flap for adequate coverage.

Usual preop diagnosis: Carcinoma of the breast; radiation therapy; cardiovascular surgery; Poland syndrome

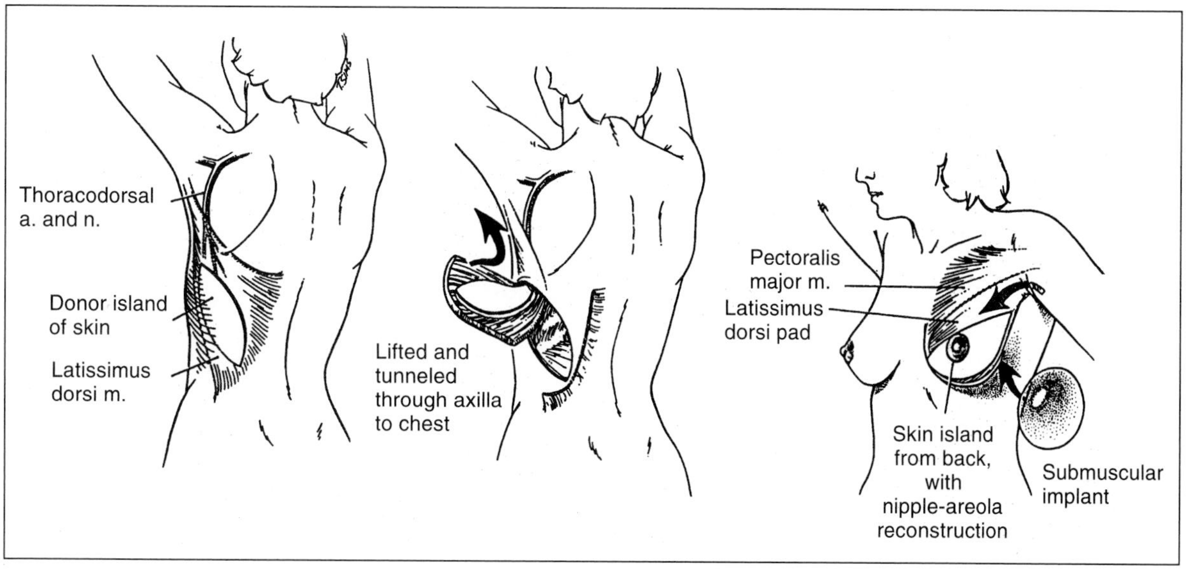

↑**Figure 11.3-4.** Breast reconstruction using latissimus dorsi myocutaneous flap. (Reproduced with permission from Barton FE Jr: Breast cancer, preventive mastectomy, and breast reconstruction. *SRPS* 1991; 6(30):14.)

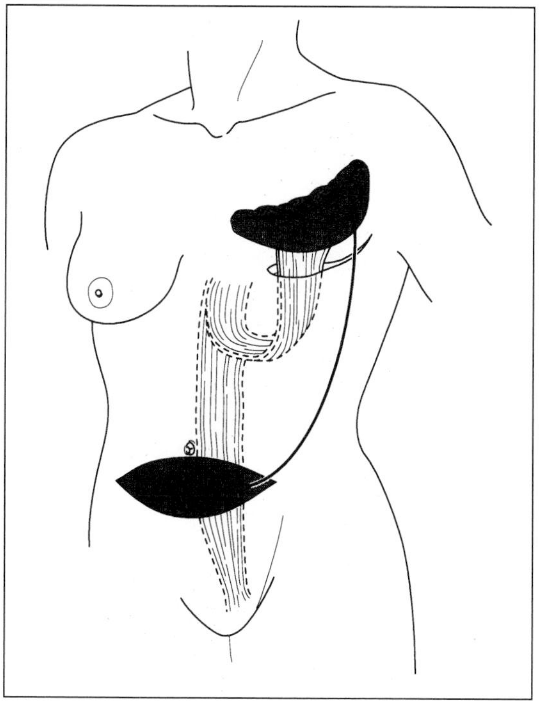

←**Figure 11.3-5.** Breast reconstruction using free TRAM flap. (Reproduced with permission from Greenfield, LJ, et al, eds: *Surgery: Principles and Practice*, 2nd edition. Lippincott-Raven Publishers, Philadelphia: 1997, 2283.)

SUMMARY OF PROCEDURE

	Tissue Expander/Prosthesis	Latissimus Flap	Rectus Flap (TRAM)
Position	Prone	Lateral decubitus; prone	Prone; table flexed
Incision	Breast	⇐	⇐
Antibiotics	Cefazolin 1 g q 4-6 h iv × 5-7 d	⇐	⇐
Surgical time	1 h	3 h	4-6 h
Closing considerations	Extensive dressing required	⇐	⇐
EBL	Minimal-100 ml	200-400 ml	300-500 ml
Postop care	PACU → room	⇐	⇐
Mortality	Rare	⇐	⇐
Morbidity	Capsular contraction: ± 30%	–	–
	Decreased sensation: 15%	⇐	⇐

	Tissue Expander/Prosthesis	Latissimus Flap	Rectus Flap (TRAM)
Morbidity, cont.	Hematoma: 2.2%	⇐	⇐
	Fat/skin necrosis: 1.7-1.9%	⇐	⇐
	Nipple areola necrosis: 1.4%	⇐	⇐
		Flap loss: Rare	⇐
		Abdominal hernia: Infrequent	⇐
Pain score	4-5	4-5	4-5

PATIENT POPULATION CHARACTERISTICS

Age range	30-45 yr
Male:Female	Breast reconstruction: mostly female
Incidence	Breast reconstruction is performed in 9% of female population; incidence of chest wall unknown
Etiology	Cancer; trauma; idiopathic; radiation or postcardiovascular surgery (chest-wall reconstruction)
Associated conditions	Breast cancer; cardiovascular disease; S/P chemotherapy; pulmonary disease

ANESTHETIC CONSIDERATIONS

PREOPERATIVE

Typically, this surgery is carried out on patients presenting for reconstruction following cancer surgery, such as radical neck dissection and mastectomy (see Anesthetic Considerations for the primary procedure). The following considerations are for cancer patients undergoing delayed reconstruction post-chemotherapy.

Respiratory Pulmonary fibrosis may complicate chemotherapy. Bleomycin (> 200 mg/m^2) has the greatest pulmonary toxicity, but alkylating agents, including cyclophosphamide and melphalan, used to treat breast cancer, have some pulmonary toxicity. Avoid high FiO_2 (> 40%) with bleomycin. Consider pulmonary fibrosis in a patient reporting dyspnea, nonproductive cough and fever.
Tests: CXR; ABG and PFTs as indicated from H&P.

Cardiovascular Cardiomyopathy and CHF may result from chemotherapy, especially doxorubicin (Adriamycin) > 550 mg/m^2.
Tests: ECG; ECHO, if indicated from H&P.

Neurological Note any previous damage to long thoracic nerves, as evidenced by winged scapula deformity.

Musculoskeletal It is traditional to avoid iv and BP cuff on mastectomy side.

Hematologic Leukopenia, thrombocytopenia and anemia from chemotherapy can be present.
Tests: CBC; Plt count; coagulation profile; Hb/Hct

Renal/Hepatic Methotrexate can produce renal and hepatic dysfunction.
Tests: Electrolytes; BUN; creatinine; LFTs

Laboratory Other tests as indicated from H&P, prior chemotherapy.

Premedication Midazolam 1-2 mg iv immediately preop, or valium 5-10 mg po 1 h preop

INTRAOPERATIVE

Anesthetic technique: GETA

Induction Standard induction (see p. B-2) and intubation.

Maintenance Standard maintenance (see p. B-3). Muscle relaxation is usually appropriate. These patients should be kept warm and well hydrated to minimize peripheral vasoconstriction, which might impair graft perfusion.

Emergence During some of the procedure and for application of dressing, patient may be moved to sitting position, with consequent coughing, bucking, etc. (Rx: deeper anesthesia, e.g., propofol 0.5 mg/kg or lidocaine 1 mg/kg.) Watch BP carefully and treate orthostatic hypotension if it occurs, usually with a fluid bolus if the patient is not fluid sensitive (e.g., Hx of CHF or renal failure).

Blood and fluid requirements	IV: 16 ga × 1 NS/LR @ 4-6 ml/kg/h Warm fluids. Humidify gases.	Keep patient warm and maintain a positive fluid balance. Hypothermia may impair flap perfusion.
Monitoring	Standard monitors (see p. B-1). UO	
Positioning	✓ and pad pressure points. ✓ eyes.	
Complications	Pneumothorax	Pneumothorax should be considered with any ↑lung inflation pressure, ↓O_2 saturation or ↓BP.
	Decubitus ulcer	Pressure necrosis can occur in as little as 2 h. Carefully pad and repeatedly ✓ pressure points.
	Dextran reaction	Prophylactic use of very low molecular weight dextran (Promit) usually prevents allergic reactions to higher molecular weight dextrans. Adult dose = 20 ml (pediatric dose = 0.3 ml/kg) iv 1-2 min (maximum 15 min) before dextran infusion.

POSTOPERATIVE

Complications	Pneumothorax ↓ Flap perfusion	
Pain management	Parenteral opiates (see p. C-1). PCA (see p. C-3).	Pain should be treated promptly to minimize reflex peripheral vasoconstriction and impaired graft perfusion.

PRESSURE-SORE AND WOUND RECONSTRUCTION

SURGICAL CONSIDERATIONS

Description: Pressure sores are frequently seen in para/quadriplegics or other nonambulatory patients. In the supine patient, pressure sores are commonly located in the sacral and trochanteric areas. Ischial ulcers are most commonly found in the wheelchair-bound patient. Surgical reconstruction of pressure sores in these patients involves debridement of the wound and transposition of adjacent tissue flaps. Other areas in which pressure sores are frequently found are the heel and knee. Closure of these involves rotation of flaps and, occasionally, skin grafting of the donor site or flap.

Variant procedure or approaches: Rotation or transposition myocutaneous flap, fasciocutaneous flap, or muscle flaps covered by split-thickness skin grafts

Usual preop diagnosis: Pressure sores

SUMMARY OF PROCEDURE

	Sacral	Ischial	Trochanteric
Position	Prone, flexed at waist; (occasionally lithotomy)	Prone, flexed at waist	Lateral decubitus
Incision	Back or gluteal	Back, gluteal or thigh	Posterior or lateral thigh
Antibiotics	Cefazolin 1 g iv until drains removed, 7-14 d	⇐	⇐
Surgical time	2-4 h	⇐	⇐

	Sacral	Ischial	Trochanteric
Closing considerations	No sheer forces or pressure to surgical area. Patient may be transferred to a nonpressure bed immediately postop.	⇐	⇐
EBL	100-400 ml	⇐	⇐
Postop care	PACU → room; occasionally, spinal rehabilitation unit	⇐	⇐
Mortality	Rare	⇐	⇐
Morbidity	Infection	⇐	⇐
	Wound breakdown	⇐	⇐
	Late recurrence of ulcer	⇐	⇐
Pain score	2	2	2

PATIENT POPULATION CHARACTERISTICS

Age range	20-40 yr
Male:Female	Predominantly male
Incidence	Typically in paraplegic or quadriplegic patients
Etiology	Prolonged bed rest with pressure in traumatized patients or those with altered sensation
Associated conditions	Infection; paraplegia; debilitation; quadriplegia

ANESTHETIC CONSIDERATIONS

PREOPERATIVE

These surgeries are carried out on nonambulatory or quadriplegic/paraplegic patients who develop decubitus ulcer. Anesthesia for plegic patients may well present several challenges, as discussed below.

Respiratory Plegic patients may have intercostal muscle weakness → atelectasis and ↓clearance of secretions → recurrent URIs and V/Q mismatching → hypoxemia.
Tests: PFT; ABG; others as indicated from H&P.

Cardiovascular Autonomic hyperreflexia (AH) may occur in patients with an injury level of T10 or above. Manifestations include ↑BP, ↓HR, dysrhythmia and vasodilatation in response to stimulation below the lesion. Seizures and cerebral hemorrhage also have been reported. Identify triggering stimuli (e.g., bowel or bladder distension, cutaneous stimulation). T4 or higher lesions → ↓BP on induction of general or regional anesthesia, initiation of IPPV or postural changes.
Tests: ECG; others as indicated from H&P.

Neurological ✓ level of cord injury. AH in patient with spinal cord injury (see Cardiovascular, above) may manifest as headaches, sweating, facial flushing or syncope. Hyperreflexia below injury level.

Musculoskeletal Immobility → skeletal muscle atrophy, osteoporosis and decubitus ulcer formation.

Gastrointestinal Spinal cord injury → ↓GI function → constipation/full stomach.

Renal Chronic spinal cord injury → recurrent UTIs and calculi → renal failure. Foley catheter placement may → autonomic hyperreflexia (AH).
Tests: UA; BUN; creatinine; others as indicated from H&P.

Laboratory Immobility → ↑Ca^{++} → dysrhythmia and nausea.
Tests: Others as indicated from H&P.

Premedication Standard premedication (see p. B-2) is usually appropriate. Patients with limited respiratory reserve should receive minimal sedation. Nifedipine (10 mg sublingually 5 min or po 20 min before induction) may be used to blunt AH.

INTRAOPERATIVE

Anesthetic technique: GETA. If flap donor and recipient sites are confined to the lower half of the body, regional anesthesia may be considered for short procedures. Spinal or epidural anesthesia will minimize AH; however, anesthetic level may be difficult to assess and regional anesthesia may not be tolerated for prolonged surgery. Lighter levels of GA will not prevent AH.

Induction Standard induction (see p. B-2) and intubation. Avoid succinylcholine in patients with muscle paralysis (2° ↑K^+). AH may occur with Foley catheter placement.

Maintenance Standard maintenance (see p. B-3). Muscle relaxation is usually appropriate and may be necessary to reduce muscle spasticity. Plegic patients are prone to hypothermia. These patients should be kept warm and well hydrated to minimize peripheral vasoconstriction, which might impair graft perfusion.

Emergence AH 2° distended bladder or rectum may occur on emergence from anesthesia.

Blood and fluid requirements	IV: 16 ga × 1 NS/LR @ 4-6 ml/kg/h Warm fluids. Humidify gases.	Keep patient warm and maintain a positive fluid balance. Hypothermia may impair flap perfusion.
Monitoring	Standard monitors (see p. B-1). UO ± Arterial line	An arterial line may be useful in patients susceptible to AH and for prolonged procedures where regular ABGs and blood chemistries will be useful.
Positioning	✓ and pad pressure points. ✓ eyes.	Many of these patients may be osteoporotic, so great care should be used in moving and positioning.
Complications	Hypothermia	Patients with spinal cord injury often have impaired thermoregulation. Maintain normal body temperature with warming blankets, fluid and airway warmers.
	AH	AH should be promptly controlled with SNP bolus (5-50 μg) and infusion while anesthesia is deepened.
	Decubitus ulcer	Pressure necrosis can occur in as little as 2 h. Carefully pad and repeatedly ✓ pressure points.
	Dextran reaction	Prophylactic use of very low molecular weight dextran (Promit) usually prevents allergic reactions to higher molecular weight dextrans. Adult dose = 20 ml (pediatric dose = 0.3 ml/kg) iv 1-2 min (maximum 15 min) before dextran infusion.

POSTOPERATIVE

Complications	Respiratory insufficiency	Quadriplegic patients may have ↓VC and ↓ERV and be uniquely susceptible to residual respiratory depressant effects.
	AH	AH may occur 2° distended bladder or rectum. Rx: phentolamine 1 mg iv q 1 min and/or SNP bolus/infusion; removal of stimulus.
Pain management	Parenteral opiates (see C-1). PCA (see C-3).	Pain should be promptly treated to minimize reflex peripheral vasoconstriction and impaired graft perfusion.

Surgeons

William C. Lineaweaver, MD, FACS
Kenneth C. W. Hui, MD, FACS

11.4 FUNCTIONAL RESTORATION—MICROSURGERY

Anesthesiologists

Richard A. Jaffe, MD, PhD
Stanley I. Samuels, MB, BCh, FFARCS

MICROSURGERY—FLAP PROCEDURES

SURGICAL CONSIDERATIONS

Description: Microsurgical flap operations have revolutionized reconstructive surgery. In these operations, the surgeon brings distant flap tissue to a defect. The survival of the flap depends on the successful attachment of critical flap vessels to vessels near the defect, thereby establishing a blood supply to the flap. Skin, muscle, bone, nerve and combinations of these tissues can be utilized for repair of defects which could not be repaired satisfactorily (or at all) by conventional procedures using tissue adjacent to the defect. Microsurgical flap procedures are applied to all body regions (see Table 11.4-1). The most common sites of these operations include the mandible, breast and extremities.

Each of these cases will have a recipient site and a donor site. The recipient site is the location of the defect, and the patient's positioning must be appropriate to the procedure planned for this recipient site, be it debridement of an open tibial fracture, a mastectomy or a mandibulectomy with neck dissection. The donor site is the location (see Fig 11.4-1) from which the flap will be harvested. Whenever possible, the patient should be positioned so that the recipient and donor sites are simultaneously accessible. Occasionally, recipient and donor sites that are positionally incompatible will require one or more intraop procedures.

Complicated immediate reconstructions can require multiple surgical teams operating in sequence. Breast reconstruction for cancer, for example, requires mastectomy by general surgeons, followed by axillary vessel exploration, TRAM flap harvest, flap anastomosis and inset, and donor site repair by microsurgeons. Some of these cases require use of vein grafts and skin grafts. These sites must be accessible.

The anesthesiologists must work closely with the surgical team to coordinate the many elements of these cases. First, patient position should be clearly planned. All operative sites must be identified, and iv lines, arterial lines and monitors placed compatibly with planned surgery. ETT placement and tracheostomy procedures should be anticipated in head and neck cases. The anesthesiologist should also understand the sequence of procedures in a multiple-team operation.

Perioperative use of anticoagulants should be discussed by the anesthesiologist and the microsurgeon. Most patients undergoing microsurgical procedures will receive dextran to promote tissue perfusion by reducing blood viscosity. Some complex cases may be partially or completely heparinized, which may preclude the use of epidural anesthesia. Although some microsurgeons feel that epidural anesthesia may improve blood flow to the site of reconstruction, experimental and clinical evidence for this opinion is lacking, and anticoagulation may lead to complications at the epidural site.

Finally, large surgical fields, wide exposures and long operations can lead to significant hypothermia. While warming fluids and taking other measures, the anesthesiologist should remind the surgeon to cover areas of the surgical field whenever possible.

Usual preop diagnosis: tumor; trauma; chronic infection; facial palsy; congenital defects

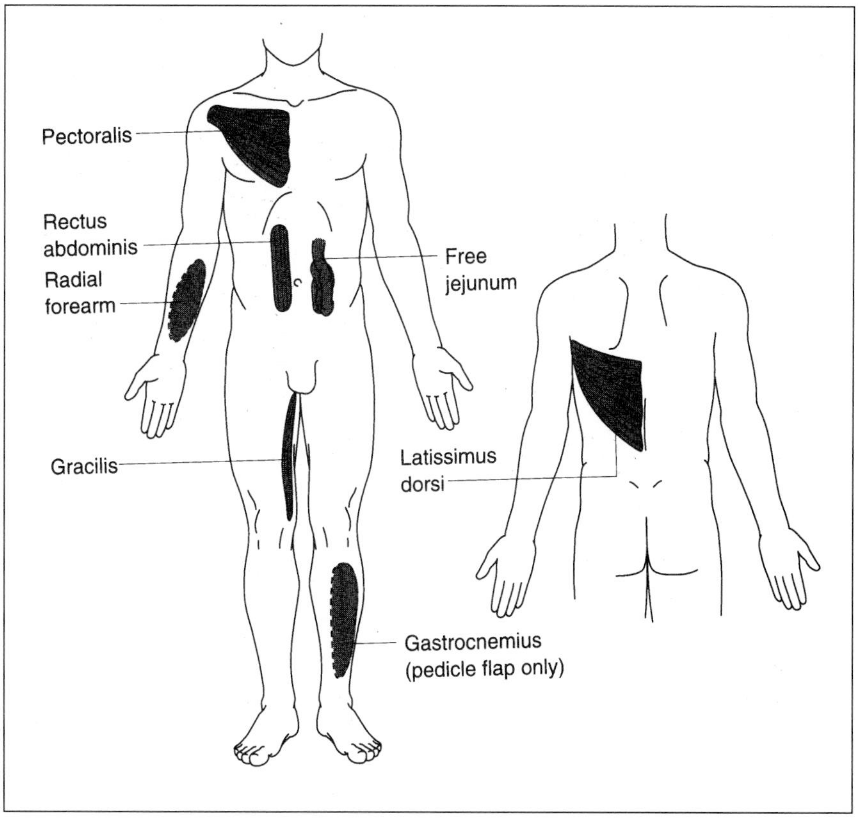

Figure 11.4-1. Locations of commonly used flaps. (Reproduced with permission from Greenfield, LJ, et al, eds: *Surgery: Principles and Practice*, 2nd edition. Lippincott-Raven Publishers, Philadelphia: 1997, 2283.)

SUMMARY OF PROCEDURE

Position	Requirements of the recipient site take precedence; optimal position for the donor site is then considered (see Table 11.4-2).
Incision	Each site will have specific incision.
Special instrumentation	Microscope; tourniquet for extremities
Unique considerations	Multiple surgical teams; hypothermia; ± anticoagulation; if intraop nerve stimulation is planned, muscle relaxants should be avoided.
Antibiotics	Cefazolin (1g iv) in uncomplicated cases; broader coverage in complicated circumstances
Surgical time	Simple flap: 4-6 h Complex cases: 8-12 h
Closing considerations	Splints and dressings should be secured before emergence.
EBL	Skin flap: 200 ml Muscle flap: 200-500 ml Bone flap: 500-1000 ml
Postop care	ICU for flap perfusion monitoring
Mortality	< 2% (usually associated with coexisting disease)
Morbidity	Soft-tissue complications: 20-30% Vascular complication requiring reexploration: 5-10% Flap failure: 5%
Pain score	3-5

PATIENT POPULATION CHARACTERISTICS

Age range	2-90 yr
Male:Female	1:1
Incidence	50-200/yr/major center
Etiology	Malignancy; trauma; chronic infection
Associated conditions	Complications of underlying disease (e.g., anemia)

Table 11.4-1 Common Recipient Sites and Flap Reconstruction

Region	Defect	Flap
Head and neck	Scalp, skull	Latissimus dorsi, scapula
	Skull base	Latissimus dorsi, serratus anterior, rectus abdominus, radial forearm
	Orbit, midface	Serratus anterior, rectus abdominis, lateral arm scapula, radial forearm, fibula, iliac crest
	Palate	Radial forearm, radial forearm osteocutaneous
	Mandible	Fibula, iliac crest, radial forearm, radial forearm osteocutaneous, scapula, scapular osteocutaneous
	Cervical esophagus	Jejunum, radial forearm
	Facial palsy	Gracilis, serratus anterior
Trunk	Breast	Transverse rectus myocutaneous (TRAM)
	Pelvis, perineum, genitalia	Latissimus dorsi, radial forearm
	Avascular necrosis, femoral head	Fibula
Upper extremity	Thumb	Great toe
	Finger	Second, third toes
	Palm	Lateral arm
	Dorsum of hand	Rectus abdominis, serratus anterior
	Forearm, wrist	Rectus abdominis, gracilis
	Elbow	Rectus abdominis
	Bone	Fibula, iliac crest
Lower extremity	Heel, foot	Lateral arm, radial forearm, rectus
	Leg	Rectus, latissimus dorsi
	Knee	Latissimus dorsi

Table 11.4-2 Common Flaps and Harvest Positions

Flap type	Flap	Ideal position for harvest
Skin	Lateral arm	Patient on side, donor arm up.
	Radial forearm (± bone)	Patient supine, donor arm on hand table.
	Scapular (± bone)	Patient on side, donor side up.
Bone	Fibula (± skin)	Patient supine, or on side, with donor leg up.
	Iliac crest (± skin)	Patient supine; both groins, abdomen prepared.
Muscle	Latissimus dorsi	Patient on side, donor side up.
	Serratus anterior	Patient on side, donor side up.
	Rectus abdominis, TRAM	Patient supine; both groins, abdomen prepared.
	Gracilis	Patient supine, donor leg abducted at hip.
Toe	Great toe, other toes	Patient supine; foot and leg prepared.
Jejunum	Jejunum	Patient supine; abdomen prepared.

ANESTHETIC CONSIDERATIONS

PREOPERATIVE

These surgeries are carried out on patients who have sustained major soft-tissue losses and require a flap procedure to cover the defects. There are typically three patient populations presenting for surgery: (1) those presenting for reconstruction following cancer surgery, such as radical neck dissection and mastectomy; (2) patients following trauma, usually with upper or lower-limb defects; and (3) patients with congenital defects. In general, these patients should present few problems for the anesthesiologist. In a patient with a congenital lesion, however, it is prudent to look for evidence of CHD, musculoskeletal deformities and airway problems.

Respiratory Exposure of the thorax to radiation may produce pathologic changes in the lungs and related structures, including pneumonitis (→ dyspnea, hypoxemia) that may progress to fibrosis (→ ↓pulmonary compliance). Tracheal or bronchial fibrosis may → partial airway obstruction. Patients with breast cancer may have been treated with chemotherapeutic agents (e.g., methotrexate, cyclophosphamide, bleomycin) that can be pulmonary toxins producing fibrosis, interstitial infiltrates and pleural effusions.
Tests: Consider PFT and pulmonary consult.

Cardiovascular Exposure of the heart to radiation may produce pathologic changes in the heart and related structures, including accelerated atherosclerotic changes, myocardial fibrosis, pericarditis and valvular dysfunction. Patients with breast cancer may have been treated with doxorubicin (Adriamycin), which may produce cardiomyopathy (usually seen at total doses > 550 mg/m^2) → CHF. XRT increases the incidence of clinically significant cardiomyopathy.

Hematologic Patients may be anemic 2° chemotherapeutic agents.
Tests: CBC, with differential and Plt count

Laboratory Other tests as indicated from H&P.

Premedication Standard premedication (see p. B-2).

INTRAOPERATIVE

Anesthetic technique: GETA. Regional anesthesia alone is usually inappropriate, given the surgical sites and the length of the procedure. Adjunctive regional techniques have been advocated to promote vasodilation and thereby ↑ blood flow through the flap.

Induction Standard induction (see p. B-2) and intubation.

Maintenance Standard maintenance (see p. B-3). Muscle relaxation is usually required. The patient must be kept warm and well hydrated to minimize peripheral vasoconstriction, which might impair graft perfusion.

Emergence	Smooth emergence to avoid disrupting the surgical repair. Patients are usually transported to the ICU for continuous monitoring of flap perfusion.	
Blood and fluid requirements	Moderate blood loss IV: 16 ga × 1 NS/LR @ 4-5 ml/kg/h Warm fluids. Humidify gases.	Keep patient warm, and maintain a positive fluid balance. An Hct of 30-35% will provide adequate O_2 transport while minimizing viscosity. Dextran 40 is usually used to further ↓ viscosity, thereby ↑ flap blood flow.
Monitoring	Standard monitors (see p. B-1). UO ± Arterial line	An arterial line may be useful for prolonged procedures where regular ABGs and blood chemistries will be needed.
Positioning	✓ and pad pressure points. ✓ eyes.	These can be very lengthy surgeries and careful monitoring of pressure points is essential.
Complications	Hypothermia	Maintain normal body temperature with warming blankets, fluid and airway warmers.
	Decubitus ulcer	Pressure necrosis can occur in as little as 2 h. Carefully pad and repeatedly ✓ pressure points.
	Dextran reaction	Prophylactic use of very low molecular weight dextran (Promit) usually prevents allergic reactions to higher molecular weight dextran. Adult dose = 20 ml 1-15 min before dextran infusion.

POSTOPERATIVE

Complications	Arterial thrombosis Hematoma	May require reexploration. May require reexploration.
Pain management	Parenteral opiates (see p. C-1). PCA (see p. C-3).	Pain should be treated promptly to minimize reflex peripheral vasoconstriction and impaired graft perfusion.

References

1. Banic A, Krejei V, Erni D, Petersen-Felix S, Sigurdsson G: Effects of extradural anaesthesia on microcirculatory blood flow in free latissimus dorsi musculocutaneous flaps in pigs. *Plast Reconstr Surg* 1997; 100:945.
2. Buncke HJ, ed. *Microsurgery.* Lea & Febiger, Philadelphia: 1991.
3. Hynynen M, Eklund P, Rosenberg PH: Anaesthesia for patients undergoing prolonged reconstructive and microvascular plastic surgery. *Scand J Plast Surg* 1982; 16:201.
4. Jones NF: Resection and reconstruction of extensive and complex tumors of the head and neck. In *Excision and Reconstruction in Head and Neck Cancer.* Soutar D, Tiwari R, eds. Churchill Livingstone, Edinburgh: 1994, 405.
5. Lineaweaver W: Microsurgery. In *Plastic Surgery.* Ruberg RL, Smith DJ, eds. CV Mosby, St. Louis: 1994, 65.
6. Lineaweaver W, Ching P, Siko P, Yim K, Alpert B, Buncke GM, Buncke H: Transfusion requirements for clinical elective muscle transplantation. In *Trans Third Vienna Muscle Symposium.* Frelinger G, Deutinger M, eds. Blackwell MZV, Vienna: 1992, 378.
7. Scott GR, Rothkopf DM, Walton RL: Efficacy of epidural anaesthesia in free flaps of the lower extremity. *Plast Reconstr Surg* 1993; 91:673.

MICROSURGERY—REPLANTATION

SURGICAL CONSIDERATIONS

Description: Replantation of amputated parts is the most common emergency application of microsurgery. Replantation procedures can range from reattachment of a single amputated finger to repair of an avulsed scalp or a devascularized foot. Cases involving the upper extremities make up the vast majority of replantations.

All replantation cases present the same general challenge to the surgeon: reestablishment of arterial and venous circulation and optimum emergency repairs of skeletal and soft-tissue injuries. These procedures require close communication between the surgeon and the anesthesiologist.

The patient and surgeon must reach an understanding regarding the possibility and desirability of replantation. At the same time, the anesthesiologist must make a rapid assessment of the patient's general medical condition and any specific problems (simultaneous injuries, blood loss) that could complicate a prolonged replantation procedure. Discovery of serious illness or injuries may lead to abandonment of replantation.

Replantation may be done under general or regional anesthesia, although regional anesthesia offers no clear benefit. In the OR, the surgeon and anesthesiologist should plan patient positioning together. Injured extremities are placed on an extremity table, and other sites may be designated for vein and skin grafting. Placement of lines, monitors and warming devices can then be made in coordination with the surgical sites.

Specific variations of replantation procedures have unique features, as follows.

Replantation of fingers and hands: Generally, two surgeons work simultaneously. One surgeon at the back table explores the amputated parts, tagging significant nerves, vessels and tendons. A second surgeon debrides the amputation sites and identifies the stumps of reparable structures. The surgeons then proceed with replantation. Generally, bone fixation and tendon repairs are performed first. Vessel and nerve repairs are performed next, using a microscope. The need for vein grafting and anticoagulation is determined intraop. Blood transfusions are rarely needed except when using anticoagulants. (Also see Digit and Hand Replantation, p. 696.)

Replantation of extremities: Replantation of arms or legs must be handled very efficiently since irreversible muscle damage occurs within 4 h of ischemia. Generally, the sequence of surgery is similar to finger replantation, with the exception being that a temporary arterial circulation (using a dialysis shunt) is established as soon as possible to minimize ischemia time in an amputated part. Ongoing venous blood loss occurs while skeletal repairs are done, and transfusion is frequently required. Definitive vessel repairs (often requiring vein grafts) and nerve repairs are done under the microscope.

Scalp replantation: Scalp avulsions are caused by entanglement of hair in machinery. These amputations are frequently replantable, sparing the patient a grotesque and unstable deformity. Initial evaluation should include careful assessment of the cervical spine since the patient transiently hangs by the neck until the scalp separates. Initial blood loss can be significant and should be replaced preop. Replantation proceeds by identifying matching vessels at the margin of the defect and the avulsed scalp. The superficial temporal vessels are most commonly repaired, and use of vein grafts should be anticipated. Following the first artery repair, brisk bleeding generally occurs at the scalp margin until vein repairs are completed. This blood loss should be anticipated.

Usual preop diagnosis: Trauma

SUMMARY OF PROCEDURE

	Fingers/Hands	Extremities	Scalp
Position	Supine, injured arm extended	Supine	Supine or side (depending on vessel position)
Incision	Conventional hand exposure	Extension of injury; fasciotomies may be done.	Preauricular
Special instrumentation	Microscope; hand table; tourniquet	Microscope; tourniquet	Microscope; neurosurgical headrest
Unique considerations	Anticoagulation	⇐	RAE or anode tube; table, 180°
Antibiotics	Cefazolin 1g iv	⇐	⇐
Surgical time	1st finger: 3-4 h; 2 h/subsequent finger Hand: 4 h	4-8 h	4 h
Closing considerations	Splint applied before emergence.	Cast or splint applied before emergence.	Elevate head as much as possible.
EBL	100-200 ml	2-6 U	2-8 U
Postop care	ICU for monitoring	⇐	⇐
Mortality	None	Rare	None
Morbidity	Replant failure: 5-15%	Failure: 10-20%	Vascular occlusion, reexploration
Pain score	5-6	5-6	3-5

PATIENT POPULATION CHARACTERISTICS

Age range	Childhood-old age	⇐	Young adult
Male:Female	> 10:1	⇐	1:2
Incidence	250/yr/major center	Rare	⇐
Etiology	Trauma	⇐	⇐
Associated conditions	Other injuries	Other injuries, blood loss	Cervical spine injuries, blood loss

ANESTHETIC CONSIDERATIONS FOR REPLANTATION

PREOPERATIVE

In general, there are two patient populations for replantation procedures: (1) isolated limb and scalp injury patients (common), and (2) multiple trauma victims (rare). Most patients are otherwise healthy and the preop workup is routine.

Gastrointestinal All of these patients should be considered to have full stomachs and, therefore, are at increased risk for aspiration pneumonitis. In general, they should receive preop medication to reduce stomach volume and acidity (e.g., metoclopramide 10 mg iv and ranitidine 50 mg iv) 30-60 min before induction, time permitting.

Metabolic Approximately 50% of trauma victims are intoxicated. Anesthesia-related implications of acute ethanol intoxication include: decreased anesthetic requirements, diuresis, vasodilation and hypothermia.

Laboratory As suggested by coexisting disease.

Premedication Standard premedication (see p. B-2). Full-stomach precautions: Na citrate 0.3 M 30 ml immediately before induction of anesthesia.

INTRAOPERATIVE

Anesthetic technique: GETA, after rapid-sequence induction. These procedures are often lengthy and regional anesthesia is usually not appropriate as the primary technique. A concurrent, continuous regional anesthetic, however, will provide sympathetic blockade, as well as postop analgesia. Brachial plexus or lumbar epidural catheter placement should be considered prior to inducing GA.

Induction Rapid-sequence induction (see p. B-5) is mandatory in emergency cases, unless awake intubation is performed. C-spine fracture patients or those with facial injuries may require awake fiber optic intubation (see p. B-6).

Maintenance Standard maintenance (see p. B-2) for stable patients.

Emergence Difficult airway or full-stomach cases require awake extubation.

Blood and fluid requirements	Significant blood loss possible IV: 16 ga × 1-2 (extremity/scalp) IV: 18 ga × 1 (digit) NS/LR @ 1.5-3 ml/kg/h + 3 × blood loss Fluid/blood warmers, heating blanket, warmed circuit humidifier	A 16 ga iv catheter in a nonoperated upper extremity should be adequate in hemodynamically stable patients.
Monitoring	Standard monitors (see p. B-1). ± Arterial line, CVP	Invasive hemodynamic monitoring should be considered in cases where large blood loss is anticipated.
Positioning	✓ and pad pressure points. ✓ eyes.	
Control of blood loss	Tourniquet may be used.	Inflation pressure is typically 100 mmHg greater than systolic pressure. Maximum "safe" tourniquet time is 1.5-2 h, followed by a 5 to (preferably) 15 min reperfusion interval, if further tourniquet time is necessary.

Special considerations	Tourniquet deflation and limb reperfusion	Mild hypotension is common. In patients with moderate-to-severe lung disease, continue controlled ventilation until after the lactic acid that has accumulated in the ischemic limb is metabolized (3-5 min), since these patients may be unable to increase ventilation adequately to buffer this acid load.
Complications	Hemodynamic instability	Previously unrecognized injuries (e.g., pneumothorax, cardiac tamponade, intracranial bleeding) should be considered as a cause of unexplained intraop hemodynamic instability in all acute-trauma victims.

POSTOPERATIVE

Complications	Reperfusion failure	May require immediate reexploration.
Pain management	PCA (p. C-3)	
Tests	None routinely indicated.	Reimplant perfusion must be monitored.

References

1. Alpert BS, Lineaweaver W, Buncke HJ: Surgical treatment of the avulsed scalp. In *Hair Transplantation,* 3rd edition. Unger WP, ed. Marcel Dekker, New York: 1995, 777.
2. Buncke HJ, Whitney TM, Valauri F, Alpert B: Replantation. In *Microsurgery.* Buncke HJ, ed. Lea & Febiger, Philadelphia: 1991, 1:594.
3. Carr DB, Kwon J: Anesthesia techniques and their indication for upper limb surgery. In *Surgery of the Hand and Upper Extremity.* Peimer CA, ed. McGraw-Hill, New York: 1996, 119-39.
4. Furnes H, Lineaweaver W, Buncke HJ: Blood loss associated with anticoagulation of patients with replanted digits. *J Hand Surg* 1992; 17A:226.
5. Gayle L, Lineaweaver W, Buncke GM, Oliva A, Alpert BS, Billys J, Buncke HJ: Lower extremity replantation. *Clin Plastic Surg* 1992; 18:437.
6. Livingston KG: Safety of dextran in relation to other colloids—ten years' experience with hapten inhibition. *Infusionsther, Transfusionsmed* 1993; 20:206.
7. Partington M, Lineaweaver W, O'Hara M, Kitzmiller J, Valauri F, Buncke GM, Alpert BS, Buncke HJ: Unrecognized injuries in patients referred for emergency microsurgery. *J Trauma* 1993; 34:238.
8. Raggi RP: Balanced regional anesthesia for hand surgery. *Orthop Clin North Am* 1986; 17:473.
9. Sanders N, Anderson KR: Anesthesia for microsurgery. In *Microsurgery.* Buncke HJ, ed. Lea & Febiger, Philadelphia: 1991, 729.
10. Strauch B, Greenstein B, Goldstein R, Liebling RW: Problems and complications encountered in replantation surgery. *Hand Clin* 1986; 2:389.
11. Tamai S: Twenty years' experience of limb replantation: A review of 293 upper extremity replants. *J Hand Surg* 1982; 6:549.

12.0 PEDIATRIC SURGERY

Surgeons

Stephen L. Huhn, MD
Lawrence M. Shuer, MD (*Craniofacial surgery*)
Gary K. Steinberg, MD, PhD (*Vein of Galen surgery*)

12.1 PEDIATRIC NEUROSURGERY

Anesthesiologist

C. Philip Larson, Jr, MD

CRANIOFACIAL SURGERY

SURGICAL CONSIDERATIONS

Description: Craniofacial surgery is a broad term which refers to both cranial and/or facial surgery for the correction of cranial dysostosis or craniofacial dysmorphism. Cranial dysostosis is the maldevelopment of the cranial base and/or vault, 2° to premature fusion of cranial sutures. This is commonly referred to as **craniosynostosis** and the surgical procedure involves removal of the affected suture(s). Craniosynostosis may involve one or more suture, and resulting deformities are characteristic and well recognized. For example, scaphocephaly, the most common form of craniosynostosis, is caused by premature fusion of the sagittal suture. This results in an increase in the AP diameter of the head. The most common surgical procedure for correction of this condition is a **linear craniectomy**. Common cranial dysostoses and their corrective procedures include: scaphocephaly—linear craniectomy (sagittal); trigonocephaly—linear craniectomy (metopic); posterior plagiocephaly—linear craniectomy (lambdoid); anterior plagiocephaly—lateral canthal advancement; brachycephaly—bilateral canthal advancement (coronal).

Head growth to adult size occurs by 2-3 yr of age; by this time, normal sutures have developed a fibrous union, which ossifies at 6-8 yr. Craniosynostosis, therefore, is a developmental abnormality which presents within the first yr of life. Early recognition and surgical correction are well correlated with improved cosmetic outcome.[1-2] Most elective procedures are scheduled prior to 6 mo of age; but many centers prefer surgical correction at approximately 3 mo. Patient weight, blood volume and expected blood loss must be considered when surgery is scheduled. Most craniosynostoses (single and multiple) are sporadic, although a predisposition has been reported. In addition, several inheritable conditions exist, the most common being Crouzon's disease and Apert's syndrome, in which craniosynostosis is one of multiple genetic defects. Because of abnormalities in development of the cranial base, facial dysmorphism occurs, resulting in shallow, misplaced orbits and midface hypoplasia. Surgical correction today follows the guidelines established by **Tessier** and colleagues.[5,6,7] Surgical repair is often staged with correction of the cranial vault and base within the first yr of life and advancement of the midface after primary dentition is complete. Multiple procedures are often required.

Positioning of patient, type of headrest and incision all vary, depending on location of the suture abnormality. Most commonly, the child is supine and a padded horseshoe headrest is used. A bicoronal, biparietal or Meisterschnitt incision is used. This provides good access to the anterior skull base, the pterion, the anterior fontanel and the coronal sutures. When the occipital region is involved (i.e., sagittal and/or lambdoidal craniosynostosis), the child may be placed prone and a biparietal or midsagittal incision used. Occasionally, the entire cranial vault needs to be exposed (multiple suture craniosynostosis), and a special headrest applied to the cheeks and suboccipital region is used. Pin fixation cannot be used safely in children < 2 yr old.

Once the skin incision is made, blood loss should be minimized by the use of Raney clips along the skin edge. The craniectomy is performed, preferably with a high-speed craniotome such as the Midas Rex. The extent of bone removal varies by the degree and number of sutures involved. Blood loss from bone edges should be controlled with bone wax. Injury to the superior sagittal or transverse sinus may occur, and the need for massive transfusion, although rare, should be anticipated. The procedure is extradural and any defects in the dura should be repaired to prevent CSF leak. Increased ICP may result if reduction of the cranial vault is excessive and must be corrected prior to closure. Drains are placed in the sagittal subgaleal space prior to skin closure.

Usual preop diagnosis: Craniosynostosis (sagittal, coronal, metopic, lambdoidal); craniofacial dysmorphism; Apert's syndrome; Crouzon's disease

SUMMARY OF PROCEDURE

Position	Supine or prone (less common); or table 180°
Incision	Bicoronal, biparietal, Meisterschnitt, midsagittal
Special instrumentation	Midas Rex craniotome; mini- or microplates/screws
Unique considerations	↑ICP and/or hydrocephalus may coexist. ↑ICP is usually seen with multiple-suture synostosis; it also occurs in single-suture craniosynostosis,[4] but is rare (< 5-10%). Hydrocephalus is typically seen in monogenic conditions (e.g., Apert's syndrome, Crouzon's disease). Most neurosurgeons shunt the hydrocephalus and treat the ↑ICP prior to craniosynostosis surgery.
Antibiotics	Vancomycin (13-15 mg/kg) or cloxacillin (25-50 mg/kg) for cranial surgery. Vancomycin or cloxacillin and cefotaxime (25-30 mg/kg) for craniofacial surgery involving nasal sinuses.
Closing considerations	Watch for increased blood loss from the scalp after hemostatic skin clips are removed. To prevent excessive blood loss, reapproximate only one portion of the scalp at a time.

EBL	Highly variable; must be minimalized. Amount depends on the number of sutures involved, age of the patient and the magnitude of the repair. Operative injury to the superior sagittal sinus may be catastrophic if hemostasis cannot be achieved or volume loss is excessive.
Postop care	ICU. Postop Hct and Hb levels required. Blood transfusion often necessary in infants (< 10 kg).
Mortality	< 1-2%
Morbidity	Meningitis CSF rhinorrhea ↑ICP (2° skull reshaping) Venous thrombosis Neurological injury: Rare
Pain score	1-3

PATIENT POPULATION CHARACTERISTICS

Age range	Newborn–young adult
Male:Female	1.2:1
Incidence	1/2,000/yr
Etiology	Sporadic; heritable (monogenic and chromosomal syndromes); environmentally induced (amniotic bands, iatrogenic)
Associated conditions	Congenital defects (limbs, heart, brain, kidneys); hydrocephalus; encephalocele (sincipital/basal); fibrous dysplasia; craniometaphyseal dysplasia; holoprosencephaly

ANESTHETIC CONSIDERATIONS

PREOPERATIVE

Craniofacial surgery encompasses a wide variety of procedures, with the two most common being linear craniectomy for craniosynostosis (or premature closure of the cranial sutures) and reconstructive (cosmetic surgery) for congenital deformities of the forehead, orbit ridges and nose. Craniosynostosis usually manifests itself in the first yr of life, while surgery for other congenital deformities of the face and skull is usually performed from ages 1-6 yr.

Respiratory As a result of their craniofacial deformities, some children may present difficult intubations. Their airways should be carefully evaluated preop.

Neurological Presenting Sx in infants with craniosynostosis include: progressively increasing irritability, crying, failure to eat and failure to grow in head circumference. These Sx may be due in part to ↑ICP. On physical examination, one or more of the cranial sutures are fused. Infants with other types of craniofacial deformity usually have no Sx related to their abnormalities.

Laboratory Tests as indicated from H&P.

Premedication For children, midazolam 0.5 mg/kg po (see p. D-2) generally provides satisfactory preop sedation after ~30 min. For young children (< 5 yr) refusing po meds, instillation of midazolam 0.3 mg/kg intranasally provides rapid amnesia, sedation and easy separation from the parents.[3]

INTRAOPERATIVE

Anesthetic technique: GETA.

Induction Standard pediatric induction (see p. D-2). Orotracheal tubes are preferred over nasotracheal tubes because the surgery may involve reflection of the scalp down over the eyes and nose, in which case a nasal tube would be in the way. Verify ETT placement (see p. D-3). Tape the tube firmly in place at one side of the mouth using benzoin adherent. Ventilation is controlled to $PetCO_2$ = 35-40 mmHg with a mechanical ventilator, from the start of anesthesia until the surgical wound is closed. When craniofacial surgery is performed, the surgeon usually places plastic corneal shields in the eyes and sutures the lids shut to protect eyes from injury.

Maintenance Standard maintenance (see p. D-3). Muscle relaxation is usually provided. Maintain a near normal BP. Maintain normal temperature by keeping the OR warm (78°F) and using warming lights as needed.

Emergence	No specific considerations. The ETT is removed at the conclusion of the anesthetic. Patient usually goes to ICU.	
Blood and fluid requirements	Large blood loss IV: 18-20 ga × 1-2 NS/LR @ 4 ml/kg/h 5% albumin Fluid warmer	Administer crystalloid via a continuous infusion pump. Blood is usually necessary. It is advisable to begin transfusion at the start of surgery, to avoid getting behind. Generally, it is better to administer warmed blood by syringe, in 10 ml increments. Serial Hct determinations are useful.
Monitoring	Standard monitors (see p. D-1). ± Foley catheter ± Doppler ± Arterial line ± CVP line	If operation is anticipated to last several h, a Foley catheter should be inserted. If patient is semisitting, a Doppler ultrasound probe should be placed on the chest to monitor for air embolism. Invasive monitoring is often appropriate. ↑K^+ and ↓Ca^{++} are most common following transfusions with whole blood or FFP.
Positioning	OR table rotated 180° ✓ and pad pressure points. ✓ eyes.	
Complications	Major blood loss VAE	 VAE may occur if dural sinus entered.

POSTOPERATIVE CONSIDERATIONS

Complications	Bleeding Hypovolemia	Major complications from these operations are uncommon.
Pain management	Parenteral opioids (see p. E-1). Avoid oversedation.	Fentanyl 1-2 μg/kg q 60 min
Tests	Hct	Hct determinations are necessary to determine adequacy of blood replacement.

References

1. Hoffman HJ: Congenital malformations of the spine and skull. In *Practice of Surgery*. Goldsmith HS, ed. Harper & Row, New York; 1980.
2. Hoffman HJ, Hendrick EB: Early neurosurgical repair in craniofacial dysmorphism. *J Neurosurg* 1979; 51(6):796-803.
3. Karl HW, Keifer AT, Rosenberger JL, Larach MG, Ruffle JM: Comparison of the safety and efficacy of intranasal midazolam or sufentanil for preinduction of anesthesia in pediatric patients. *Anesthesiology* 1992: 76(2):209-15.
4. Shillito J Jr, Matson DD: Craniosynostoses: a review of 519 surgical patients. *Pediatrics* 1968; 41(4):829-53.
5. Tessier P: Relationship of craniostenoses to craniofacial dysostoses and to faciostenoses: a study with therapeutic implications. *Plast Reconstr Surg* 1971; 48(3):224-37.
6. Tessier P: Total facial osteotomy. Crouzon's syndrome, Apert's syndrome: oxycephaly, scaphocephaly, turricephaly. *Ann Chir Plast* 1967; 12(4):273-86.
7. Tessier P, Guiot G, Rougerie J, Delbet JP, Pastoriza J: Cranio-naso-orbito-facial osteotomies. Hypertelorism. *Ann Chir Plast* 1967; 12(2):103-18.

REPAIR OF MYELOMENINGOCELE

SURGICAL CONSIDERATIONS

Description: Myelomeningocele is a type of spina bifida consisting of an exposed neural placode requiring early closure. The condition represents failure of primary neurulation, resulting in an open, unfolded spinal cord (placode). The defect may be detected before birth by high resolution ultrasound and/or elevated maternal serum α-fetoprotein. The myelomeningocele consists of the neural placode within an open dural sac and skin defect, whereas a meningocele represents an outpouching of the dural tissue without neural elements. Despite a very thin parchment of epithelium over the neural tissue, most myelomeningoceles typically leak CSF from the time of birth. The defects, which can vary in size, are commonly located in the sacral or lumbar spine: thoracic and cervical lesions are far less common. Associated CNS conditions include the Chiari II malformation and hydrocephalus. Children with myelomeningoceles have a higher incidence of other congenital anomalies, including hydronephrosis, malrotation of the gut, ventricular or atrial septal defects (ASDs) and craniofacial defects.

The fundamental goals of surgery are preservation of neural tissue, reconstitution of normal intrathecal environment and complete skin closure to prevent CSF leak. Delay in closure increases the risk of ventriculitis and motor dysfunction. Most defects are, therefore, closed within the first 24 h of life, pending evaluation of potential associated renal and/or cardiac lesions. During the procedure, the child should be in the prone position. The defect is dissected so that the various anatomic layers can be separated. The neural elements are identified and often the placode can be imbricated. The dura is dissected from the adjacent fascia and closed. An attempt may be made to close the lumbosacral fascia as a separate layer; however, in most cases, the subcutaneous and skin layers comprise the only covering over the dura. If the cutaneous defect is large, local rotated skin or myocutaneous flaps may be required to adequately close the skin.

Approximately 15% of patients with myelomeningoceles will present with hydrocephalus at birth, requiring early treatment. Some surgeons may elect to insert a ventriculoperitoneal shunt at the time of myelomeningocele closure. In addition, some patients may have an associated prominent vertebral angulation, or kyphosis, which could necessitate partial vertebrectomies in order to reestablish normal spinal alignment.

Usual preop diagnosis: Myelomeningocele; meningocele; myelodysplasia; spina bifida

SUMMARY OF PROCEDURE

Position	Prone
Incision	Surrounding the defect, preserving skin which can be utilized in the closure
Special instrumentation	Loupes or operating microscope (optional)
Unique considerations	Concomitant hydrocephalus, lower brain stem dysfunction. Need for blood replacement rare in straightforward cases.
Antibiotics	Cefotaxime (25-30 mg/kg iv), vancomycin (13-15 mg/kg iv, slowly)
Surgical time	1.5-3 h
Closing considerations	Skin closure may be complex and require rotation of flaps or aid of plastic surgeon.
EBL	Negligible–25 ml (in most cases)
Postop care	Neonatal nursery. Postop, child often nursed on stomach or side. Head size is monitored for development of hydrocephalus, which may require shunting at a later date.
Mortality	Approaching zero
Morbidity	Meningitis/ventriculitis Hind brain dysfunction Wound infection CSF leak Massive blood loss
Pain score	3-5

PATIENT POPULATION CHARACTERISTICS

Age range	Newborn (diagnosed at birth)
Male:Female	~1:1
Incidence	1/1000 live births
Etiology	Congenital
Associated conditions	Hydrocephalus; lower extremity weakness; bowel and/or bladder dysfunction (neurogenic bladder); scoliosis; Chiari II malformations; congenital cardiac anomalies

ANESTHETIC CONSIDERATIONS

PREOPERATIVE

Myelomeningoceles are congenital abnormalities of the spinal cord which result in a saccular protrusion near the base of the spine. The sac, containing neural elements and CSF, can vary in size from very small to a volume that occupies the whole lower spinal region. The diagnosis may be suspected by fetal ultrasound, and is confirmed at birth. It is generally believed that immediate removal of the sac and covering of the defect with skin is desirable to preserve neurological function and avoid infections. These newborns, therefore, are usually brought to surgery within 24 h after birth.

Cardiovascular May have associated congenital anomalies.
Tests: ECHO

Neurological Although difficult to assess at this age, newborns may have motor and/or sensory deficits in the lower extremities, neurogenic bladder and lower cranial nerve dysfunction.

Renal May have associated congenital anomalies.
Tests: Renal ultrasound

Laboratory Routine preop studies

Premedication None necessary

INTRAOPERATIVE

Anesthetic technique: GETA

Induction Standard pediatric induction (see p. D-2), followed by establishment of iv access, and then ET intubation (3.0-4.0 ETT) with the use of a muscle relaxant (e.g., vecuronium 0.15 mg/kg or rocuronium 1 mg/kg). Before intubation, administer atropine (0.1-0.2 mg) to decrease secretions and prevent reflex bradycardia during manipulation of the airway. Sevoflurane is preferred because of its low blood-gas-partition coefficient and absence of airway irritability, thus allowing for a smooth, rapid induction. Verify ETT placement (see p. D-3). Tape tube firmly in place at one side of the mouth using benzoin adherent.

Maintenance Sevoflurane 2-3% or halothane 1% or less with N_2O or air/O_2 mixture to maintain arterial O_2 sat at 95-96%. Depending on the duration of operation, additional doses of vecuronium (0.1 mg/kg) or rocuronium (0.3 mg/kg) may be needed. Maintain a near-normal BP. Maintain normal temperature by keeping OR warm (78°F) and using warming lights as needed. Ventilation is controlled to maintain $PetCO_2$ = 35-40 mmHg with a mechanical ventilator, or manually from the start of anesthesia until surgical wound is closed.

Emergence The ETT is removed at the conclusion of the anesthetic. The newborn is nursed in the prone or lateral positions for the first few d postop.

Blood and fluid requirements
IV: 22-24 ga × 1
D10 @ 2-4 ml/kg/h (newborn)
D10 1/4 NS @ 4 ml/kg/h (> 24 h)
Warm fluids.

Administer crystalloid, usually D10 1/4 NS via a continuous infusion pump, etc. Blood is rarely, if ever, necessary.

Monitoring Standard monitors (see p. D-1).

Positioning
✓ and pad pressure points.
✓ eyes.

Prone with shoulders and hips on bolsters to elevate abdomen off operating table. Head turned to the side which results in the tube being furthest from the bed. ✓ tube placement by listening to breath sounds after positioning.

POSTOPERATIVE

Complications
CSF leak
Hydrocephalus

Pain management Parenteral opiates (see p. E-1).

Reference

1. Reigel DH, Rotenstein D: Spinal bifida. In *Pediatric Neurosurgery: Surgery of the Developing Nervous System,* 3rd edition. Cheek WR, Marlin AE, McLone DG, eds. WB Saunders, Philadelphia: 1994, 51-76.

SURGICAL CORRECTION OF SPINAL DYSRAPHISM

SURGICAL CONSIDERATIONS

Description: Various congenital deformities of the spine classified as spinal dysraphism include: lipoma of the filum, lipomyelomeningocele, diastematomyelia, dermal sinus tract and myelocystocele. Each of these conditions involve some sort of tethering of the spinal cord that can cause progressive neurologic dysfunction and/or pain over time. A prophylactic operation is advisable prior to the onset of neurological dysfunction. The procedure usually requires a **laminectomy** (see Lumbar Laminectomy, p. 62), to expose the defect, which has been imaged preop by appropriate radiologic studies. The cord is untethered by careful dissection of the neural elements from the offending structure. In the case of lipoma of the filum or simple tethering of the cord, it may be necessary only to incise the filum. In the case of diastematomyelia, there is a bone or cartilaginous spicule within the spinal canal between the two hemicords. The spicule is resected and the cords are untethered in the process. In the case of the lipomyelomeningocele, the surgeon debulks the mass of fat which usually is contiguous from the subcutaneous tissues through the fascial planes, through a defect in the spinal canal (spina bifida) and dura, and ultimately attached to the spinal cord. The cord is freed through careful dissection of the fat mass. The surgeon must be careful not to sacrifice any of the nerve roots which traverse the most dependent portion of the lipoma toward the exiting root sleeves. The operating microscope and a CO_2 laser are often useful. A dural graft is required to close the defect created by the lipoma.

Usual preop diagnosis: Tethered spinal cord; fat filum terminale; lipomyelomeningocele; lipoma of the filum; diastematomyelia; spinal dysraphism; dermal sinus tract; caudal agenesis

SUMMARY OF PROCEDURE

Position	Prone
Incision	Posterior midline centered over abnormality
Special instrumentation	Operating microscope; laser
Unique considerations	Blood replacement with loss of significant amount of blood in the infant
Antibiotics	Cefotetan (25-30 mg/kg iv) and vancomycin (13-15 mg/kg iv slowly), appropriate for weight
Surgical time	1.5-5 h (longer for diastematomyelia and lipomyelomeningocele)
Closing considerations	Surgeon often wants to test integrity of dural closure with Valsalva maneuver: sustained (10-20 sec) inspiratory pressure at 20-40 cmH_2O.
EBL	5-100 ml
Postop care	Patient often kept flat postop to protect dural closure.
Mortality	Approaching zero
Morbidity	Infection Neurological deficit Aseptic meningitis CSF leak Massive blood loss
Pain score	3-5

PATIENT POPULATION CHARACTERISTICS

Age range	Newborn–adults
Male:Female	~1:1
Incidence	Uncommon
Etiology	Congenital
Associated conditions	Ankle/foot deformity (talipes); neurologic impairment; scoliosis; vertebral abnormalities; VACTERL/VATER association (vertebral, anal, cardiac, tracheoesophageal, renal and limb anomalies); cutaneous anomaly over spine; syringomyelia; caudal agenesis; neurogenic bowel/bladder

ANESTHETIC CONSIDERATIONS

PREOPERATIVE

A variety of spinal abnormalities fall under the category of spinal dysraphism, the most common being a tethered cord or a lipoma of the spinal cord. In the case of the tethered cord, there is usually a Hx of myelomeningocele repair at birth. Most patients range from 3-16 yr of age.

Neurological	Presenting Sx are usually those of pain in the lower back radiating into the legs and/or progressively worsening motor or sensory deficits in the anal region or involving the lower extremities (document carefully).
Musculoskeletal	Lower extremity sensory or motor deficits may be present and should be carefully documented.
Renal	Renal function may be impaired in patients with Hx of recurrent UTIs. **Tests:** UA; BUN; Cr; others as indicated from H&P.
Laboratory	Other tests as indicated from H&P.
Premedication	For children, midazolam 0.5 mg/kg po (see p. D-2) generally provides satisfactory preop sedation after ~30 min. For young children (< 5 yr) refusing po meds, instillation of midazolam 0.3 mg/kg intranasally provides rapid amnesia, sedation and easy separation from the parents.
Latex allergy	Meningomyelocele patients may have developed a latex allergy (see Appendix F).

INTRAOPERATIVE

Anesthetic technique: GETA

Induction	The two most common induction techniques are: (1) Standard induction (see p. D-2). (2) Inhalation induction with sevoflurane or halothane, N_2O, O_2, followed by establishment of iv access, and then ET intubation (3.0-4.0 ETT) with the use of a muscle relaxant (e.g., vecuronium 0.15 mg/kg or rocuronium 1 mg/kg). Sevoflurane is preferred because of its rapid, smooth induction. If the ETT is cuffed, palpate the cuff in the sternal notch. Tape the tube firmly in place at one side of the mouth using benzoin adherent.
Maintenance	Standard maintenance (see p. D-3). Upon completion of placement of the dural graft, and before closure of the wound, the surgeon will want to check the integrity of the graft to eliminate any CSF leaks. The surgeon will ask that positive pressure be applied to the airway to at least 20 cmH_2O for 10-20 sec. If graft leaks are detected, they will be repaired and the test repeated.
Emergence	The ETT is removed at the conclusion of the anesthetic. The patient is nursed flat in the prone or lateral position for the first few days postop to lessen the chance of a CSF leak developing.

Blood and fluid requirements	IV: 18-20 ga × 1 NS/LR @ 4-6 ml/kg/h	In children, administer fluids via a continuous infusion pump. Blood is rarely, if ever, necessary.
Monitoring	Standard monitors (see p. D-1). ± UO ± Foley catheter	If the operation is anticipated to last several h, a Foley catheter should be inserted.
Positioning	✓ and pad pressure points. ✓ eyes.	Prone with the shoulders and hips on bolsters to elevate the abdomen off the operating table. Head turned to the side, resulting in the tube being furthest from bed. ✓ tube placement by listening to breath sounds after positioning.
Complications	Severe bradycardia Latex allergy	Manipulation of the spinal cord may produce ⇊HR reflexly. See Appendix F for latex allergy considerations.

POSTOPERATIVE

Complications	Possible neurological deficits Infection CSF leak	Major complications from this operation are uncommon, but include new neurological deficits from irritation of the spinal cord during surgery, localized infection and CSF leak from the wound site.
Pain management	Parental opiates or PCA (see pp. E-1, E-3).	

References

1. Oakes WJ: Management of spinal cord lipomas and lipomyelomeningoceles. In *Neurosurgery Update II*. Wilkins RH, Rengachary S, eds. McGraw-Hill, New York: 1991, 345-52.
2. Pang D: Tethered cord syndrome: newer concepts. In *Neurosurgery Update II*. Wilkins RH, Rengachary SS, eds. McGraw-Hill, New York: 1991, 336-44.
3. Reigel DH: Sacral agenesis and diastematomyelia. In *Pediatric Neurosurgery: Surgery of the Developing Nervous System*. McLaurin R, Epstein F, eds. Grune & Stratton, New York: 1982, 79-90.

CRANIOTOMY FOR VEIN OF GALEN ANEURYSM

SURGICAL CONSIDERATIONS

Description: A vein of Galen aneurysm is a large, arteriovenous fistula between arteries of the posterior cerebral circulation and a massively enlarged vein of Galen (deep venous drainage of the brain). Patients can present with CHF (infants), hydrocephalus (infants, children, adults) or intracranial hemorrhage (adults).

Treatment is directed at staged occlusion of the arterial feeders to the arteriovenous fistula and thrombosis of the fistula itself from the venous side, using open microsurgical techniques, endovascular methods, or both. With reduction of aneurysmal flow, CO will decrease with ↑SVR and ↓mixed venous PO_2. **Subtemporal**, **midline occipital** or **bilateral occipital craniotomies** can be used to isolate and occlude arterial feeders to the vein of Galen aneurysm. Sometimes a **burr hole** is placed over the torcula (confluence of venous sinuses) for direct retrograde placement of thrombogenic coils into the arteriovenous fistula. Surgery generally is not undertaken until the CHF has been medically controlled.

Usual preop diagnosis: Vein of Galen aneurysm; intracranial hemorrhage; hydrocephalus; progressive neurologic deficits

SUMMARY OF PROCEDURE

Position	Lateral decubitus, Concorde (modified prone), or semisitting; for burr hole, lateral
Incision	Temporal or occipital; for burr hole, occipital
Special instrumentation	Operating microscope, microscopic instruments; intraop angiography; for burr hole, endovascular catheters and equipment
Unique considerations	Careful attention to blood loss in infants
Antibiotics	Vancomycin (1 g iv slowly q 12 h for adults; 10-15 mg/kg iv slowly q 6 h for children); cefotaxime (1 g iv q 6 h for adults; 40 mg/kg iv q 6 h for children)
Surgical time	3-5 h
Closing considerations	Meticulous hemostasis; avoid hypotension or HTN (MAP 80-90 adults, 70-80 children).
EBL	< 250 ml
Postop care	Monitor for ↑ICP (using ventricular or subdural catheters) as a result of venous HTN 2° with rapid occlusion of arteriovenous fistula. ICU × 1-3 d.
Mortality	Approaches 100% if in CHF
Morbidity	Deep venous infarct: 5-10% Hydrocephalus Stroke Subdural hygroma Infection: Rare
Pain score	3-4

PATIENT POPULATION CHARACTERISTICS

Age range	1 mo–3 yr (typically)
Male:Female	1:1
Incidence	Rare
Etiology	Congenital
Associated conditions	Other intracranial vascular malformations; high-output CHF

ANESTHETIC CONSIDERATIONS

PREOPERATIVE

Vein of Galen aneurysms are rare congenital abnormalities representing less than 1% of all aneurysms.[1] They are usually diagnosed in infants because they cause an abnormal increase in head size due to the aneurysmal dilatation and obstruction of the dural sinus. The abnormal vasculature constitutes a high-flow shunt, much like an arteriovenous malformation (AVM). If left untreated, the morbidity and mortality are high; however, treatment with radiologic embolization and/or surgical excision is also associated with high morbidity and mortality rates.

Cardiovascular Because these lesions constitute high-flow shunts through the brain, the infants are prone to develop CHF, which is fatal in more than 40% of patients.

Neurological Infants usually present with an abnormal head size, seizure disorder or bizarre neurological signs such as high-pitched crying, posturing, failure to eat or thrive, etc.

Laboratory CT; MRI; cerebral angiography. The infant may need sedation and anesthetic management to obtain adequate diagnostic studies.

Premedication None

INTRAOPERATIVE

Anesthetic technique: GETA, with the goals being the same as those for intracranial vascular malformations (IVMs).

Induction Whenever possible, an iv induction is preferred. STP 2-3 mg/kg, propofol 1-2 mg/kg, fentanyl 2-3 μg/kg, and vecuronium 0.1 mg/kg or rocuronium 1 mg/kg are satisfactory induction agents.

Maintenance STP $\leq$ 5 mg/kg, fentanyl $\leq$ 5 μg/kg, isoflurane $\leq$ 1% with N_2O or air 60-70% to keep O_2 sat = 95-98%. Additional doses or nondepolarizing neuromuscular blocking drug may be administered as needed to maintain a single-twitch response to nerve stimulation.

Emergence Plan to leave ETT in place for at least 24 h postop; infant should receive controlled ventilation and sedation during that interval. If infant does not show evidence of serious neurological injury postop, the ETT may be removed within 1-2 d.

Blood and fluid requirements	IV: 20-22 ga ×1-2 20 ga CVP, either IJ or subclavian	Replace blood as it is lost. Limit crystalloid fluid therapy to no more than 10 ml/kg above UO.
Control of brain volume	Same as for IVMs (see page 19).	
Monitoring	Same as for IVMs (see p. 19).	
Control of BP	Goal = normal range for age Neonate: 55-70/40 (HR = 180) 1 yr: 70-100/60 (HR = 140)	BP should be kept in the normal range for the infant with close monitoring from an arterial catheter. If HR becomes excessive, esmolol infusion is useful.
Positioning	Same as for IVMs (see p. 19).	
Complications	Coagulopathy	If large volumes of blood are needed, a coagulopathy may ensue. Monitoring of coagulation status during surgery may be necessary.
	Hypothermia	Once the aneurysm is surgically corrected, immediate efforts must be made to return infant to a normal body temperature by the conclusion of the operation.

POSTOPERATIVE

Complications Neurological deficits
Intracranial hemorrhage
Heart failure

Pain management Codeine 1-1.5 mg/kg im

Tests Same as for IVMs (see p. 20).

References

1. Lasjaunias P, Rodesch G, Pruvost P, Laroche FG, Landrieu P: Treatment of vein of Galen aneurysmal malformation. *J Neurosurg* 1989; 70(5):746-50.
2. Moriarity JL, Steinberg GK: Surgical obliteration for vein of Galen malformation: a case report. *Surg Neurol* 1995; 44:365-70.
3. Ojemann RG, Ogilvy CS, Heros RC, Crowell RM: *Surgical Management of Cerebrovascular Disease*. Williams & Wilkins, Baltimore: 1995.
4. Schmidek HH, Sweet WH, eds: *Operative Neurosurgical Techniques, Indications, Methods, Results*. Grune & Stratton, Orlando: 1995.
5. Wilkins RL, Rengachary SS, eds: *Neurosurgery*. McGraw-Hill, New York: 1996.
6. Youmans JR, ed: *Neurological Surgery*, Vol 1-6. WB Saunders Co, Philadelphia: 1990.

VENTRICULOSCOPY AND THIRD VENTRICULOSTOMY

SURGICAL CONSIDERATIONS

Description: Ventriculoscopy is the technique of intraop visualization of the lateral, third and, occasionally, fourth ventricles using fiber optic endoscopes inserted through standard cranial burr holes. The ventriculoscope permits direct inspection and limited navigation within the ventricle for both diagnostic and therapeutic purposes, and is most commonly applied in the setting of hydrocephalus. In addition to CT scans, preop MRI exam of the brain is often obtained to better depict the anatomy of the ventricular system, which is often distorted by congenital lesions. The enlarged ventricles produced by the hydrocephalus contribute to the safety and feasibility of most endoscopic techniques. The dilated ventricles allow selective endoscopic navigation, enabling a variety of procedures.[1,2,7] The endoscope can be used to fenestrate multicompartmental periventricular or arachnoid cysts, position ventricular catheters during shunt insertion, biopsy intraventricular tumors and, in some cases, resect intraventricular tumors. Neuroendoscopy does not help in the initial cannulation of the ventricle (a common misconception).

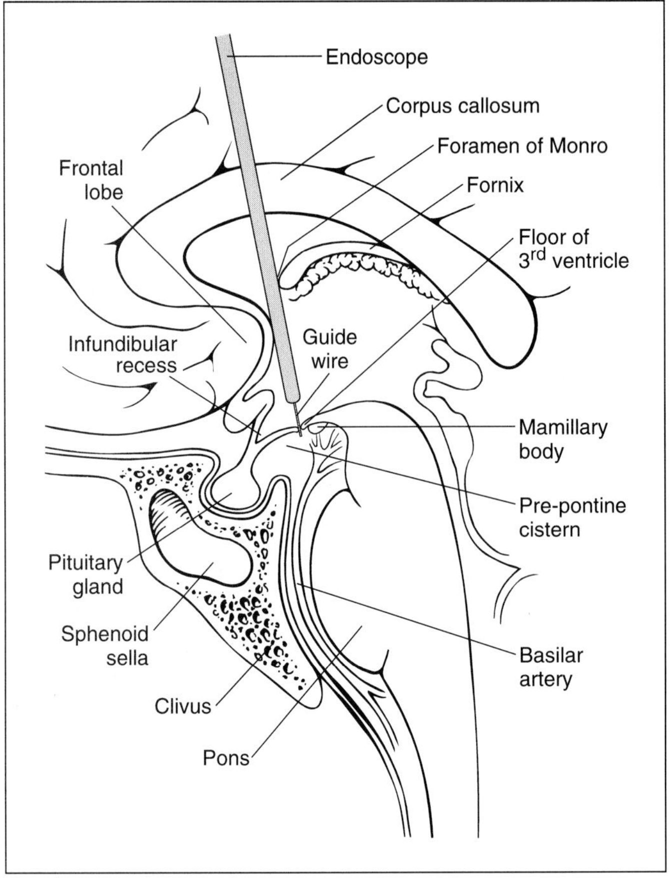

Figure 12.1-1. Endoscopic third ventriculostomy. The figure depicts fenestration of the floor of the third ventricle by a blunt probe inserted through the endoscope.

Endoscopic ventriculoscopy may be performed through either frontal or parietal-occipital approaches, with the patient typically supine with the neck slightly flexed. Standard small incisions similar to shunt insertions are used. A twist drill or burr hole is created and the ventricle cannulated by insertion of the shunt catheter or an introducer with a peel-away sheath (for larger endoscopes). The endoscopes vary in size from 1.1 mm, for use inside a standard shunt catheter, to larger endoscopes, equipped with working channels, for more complex intraventricular procedures.[3] The endoscope is attached to a camera cable and light source and the image is displayed on a conventional video monitor. After the ventricle is "tapped" through conventional methods, the endoscope can be inserted and the ventricular anatomy identified. Once the intraventricular anatomic landmarks—such as the choroid plexus—are recognized, the scope can be navigated to the site of interest. Smaller endoscopes are used to position the catheter in the optimal ventricular location during shunt placement or revision. Larger endoscopes equipped with channels for instrumentation are used for biopsy, tumor resection, cyst aspiration or fenestration procedures. Most scope systems have a separate channel for fluid irrigation if minor bleeding or debris obscure visibility. Patients undergoing third ventriculostomy may also be prepped for shunt insertion in the event the ventriculostomy is aborted because of unfavorable third ventricular anatomy. A temporary extraventricular drain (EVD) may be left in place following some procedures in order to control CSF drainage postop and/or to allow assessment of ICP.

Intraop complications associated with neuroendoscopic procedures include: minor or major intraventricular hemorrhage; air entrapment (pneumocephalus); injury to paraventricular structures (basal ganglia, hypothalamus, brain stem); cardiorespiratory depression; and delayed arousal from anesthesia. Intraventricular hemorrhage is caused by direct or indirect injury to ependymal and extraependymal blood vessels. Fortunately most bleeding encountered is minor, but may be sufficient to interfere with visualization and illumination of the ventricle. Cardiorespiratory depression and cardiac arrhythmia are due, at least in part, to phenomena attributed to ↑ICP from excessive irrigation without equal extracranial egress, rate of fluid installation, and/or nonisothermic irrigant irritating the hypothalamic nuclei adjacent to third ventricle.[4] **Third ventriculostomy** refers to fenestration of the floor of the third ventricle in order to create a communication between the third ventricle and the basilar cistern (Fig 12.1-1). The technique is most commonly applied to patients with obstructive, or noncommunicating, hydrocephalus, although broader indications are being explored.[5,6] This form of hydrocephalus results from impaired CSF flow through the Sylvian aqueduct or fourth ventricle outlets. For patients with noncommunicating hydrocephalus, successful third ventriculostomy allows CSF communication between the third ventricle and the interpeduncular subarachnoid space, thereby alleviating the hydrocephalus and avoiding shunt placement. The fenestration is conducted first by direct visualization of the floor of the third ventricle and then by perforation of the ependymal and arachnoid tissue between the mammillary bodies and the infundibular recess. The perforation can be dilated by inflation of a balloon catheter passed through the fenestration. Because of the proximity to the brain stem—in addition to the complications encountered with ventriculoscopy—third ventriculostomy carries the additional risk of mesencephalic injury, hypothalamic dysregulation, cranial nerve injury and hemorrhage from the basilar artery and adjacent perforating vessels. Minor bleeding can be controlled easily by steady irrigation. In the event of excessive bleeding, conversion to an open craniotomy is unlikely to improve control of the hemorrhage.

Usual preop diagnosis: Obstructive hydrocephalus; shunt malfunction; loculated multicompartmental hydrocephalus; intraventricular mass; arachnoid cyst; retained catheter

SUMMARY OF PROCEDURE

Position	Supine with head turned; table 90° or 180°
Incision	Small frontal or parietal-occipital
Special instrumentation	Endoscope (1.1-6 mm diameter); video system
Unique considerations	Hydrocephalus, ↑ICP; suspicion of latex allergy in patients with spina bifida
Antibiotics	Nafcillin (25 mg/kg q 4-6 h iv) or cefazolin (25 mg/kg q 8 h iv)
Closing considerations	Monitor for delayed intraventricular or subdural hemorrhage, ventricular collapse, acute hydrocephalus, CSF leak.
Postop care	Floor or ICU setting with cardiac and O_2 sat monitoring × 24 h. Measurement of serum sodium. Fluid intake/output recording. CT to r/o hemorrhage and to evaluate ventricular volume may be necessary. EVD used in cases of third ventriculostomy for drainage of CSF and testing of ICP.
Mortality	0-7% (most series report 0%)
Morbidity	Intraventricular hemorrhage Acute hydrocephalus CSF leak/pneumocephalus Meningitis/ventriculitis Subdural effusions or hematoma Cranial nerve palsy Hemiparesis Diabetes insipidus SIADH Temperature dysregulation
Pain score	2-4

PATIENT POPULATION CHARACTERISTICS

Age range	Newborn–adult
Male:Female	1:1
Incidence	3/1000 live births (congenital only)
Etiology	Congenital and acquired
Associated conditions	Hydrocephalus; spinal dysraphism; Chiari malformation; posthemorrhagic hydrocephalus; arachnoid cyst

ANESTHETIC CONSIDERATIONS

Anesthetic management is similar to that for Ventricular Shunt Procedures, p. 45.

References

1. Drake JM: Ventriculostomy for treatment of hydrocephalus. In *Neurosurgery Clinics of North America.* Butler AB, McLone DG, eds. 1993; 4(4):657-66.
2. Grant JA, McLone DG: Third ventriculostomy: A review. *Surg Neurol* 1997; 47:210-12.

3. Grotenhuis JA. *Manual of Endoscopic Procedures in Neurosurgery.* Uitgeverij Machaon, Nijmegen, The Netherlands: 1995.
4. Handler MH, Abbott R, Lee M: A near-fatal complication of endoscopic third ventriculostomy: case report. *Neurosurg* 1994; 35(3): 525-28.
5. Jones RFC, Kwok BCT, Stening WA, Vonau M: The current status of endoscopic third ventriculostomy in the management of non-communicating hydrocephalus. *Minim Invasive Neurosurg* 1994; 37:28-36.
6. Jones RFC, Kwok BCT, Stening WA, Vonau M: Third ventriculostomy for hydrocephalus associated with spinal dysraphism: indications and contraindications. *Eur J Pediatr Surg* 1996; 6(Suppl 1):5-6.
7. Walker ML, Petronio J, Carey CM: Ventriculoscopy. In *Pediatric Neurosurgery: Surgery of the Developing Nervous System.* Cheek WR, Marlin AE, McLone DG, Reigel DH, Walker ML, eds. WB Saunders, Philadelphia: 1994, 572-81.

Surgeon

Anna H. Messner, MD

12.2 PEDIATRIC OTOLARYNGOLOGY

Anesthesiologists

Gregory B. Hammer, MD
Cathy R. Lammers, MD

PEDIATRIC OTOLARYNGOLOGY

INTRODUCTION—SURGEON'S PERSPECTIVE

ANESTHESIOLOGIST/SURGEON COOPERATION

Pediatric otolaryngology/head and neck surgery procedures frequently involve the oral cavity, pharynx, larynx and tracheobronchial tree. This can result in competition for the airway between the anesthesiologist and pediatric otolaryngologist. Preop, a ventilation plan should be discussed and agreed upon to avoid a poor outcome. Neither specialist should assume that the other intuitively knows which combination of anesthesia and ventilation is best for an individual case. Frequently, the table will be turned 90° during the procedure. Close communication must be maintained throughout the procedure.

TUBE POSITIONING

Many head and neck procedures require turning of the head during the procedure. This necessitates that the tube be securely fastened to the face, but not tightly anchored to the bed or chest. Delays can be avoided if the anesthesiologist and surgeon have discussed the positioning of the ETT (nasal or oral, taped to the left corner of mouth, etc.) preop. If a tracheotomy is to be performed, the tape around the tube should be loosened prior to draping so that the anesthesiologist can easily remove the tube without visualizing the tape under the drapes.

SPONTANEOUS VENTILATION AND MUSCLE RELAXATION

If vocal cord function is to be visualized or the trachea examined for tracheomalacia, spontaneous ventilation of the patient is preferred. In some head and neck cases—such as parotidectomy or mastoidectomy—muscle relaxation is contraindicated to avoid interference with facial nerve monitoring, and so that facial movements can be seen. In other cases—such as esophagoscopy—muscle relaxation aids the surgeon in passing the esophagoscope through the cricopharyngeus. It is always best to discuss the use of muscle relaxants preop.

LASER CASES

If any foreign object, such as an ETT, is in the airway, the FiO_2 should not be raised above 0.3, in order to avoid an airway fire. All OR personnel need to be prepared to wear protective glasses during the case.

MYRINGOTOMY AND TYMPANOSTOMY TUBE PLACEMENT

SURGICAL CONSIDERATIONS

Description: Tympanostomy (PE or pressure equalizing) tubes are placed in the patient with chronic serous otitis media (fluid in the middle ear for > 3 mo) or recurrent acute otitis media (6 or more episodes of otitis media over the prior yr). Occasionally, PE tubes are placed in a child with meningitis of otitic origin or with acute otitis media that is unresponsive to antibiotics. The patient is supine and the OR table in the 0-degree position. The microscope is positioned over the bed and the head turned to expose the ear. An ear speculum is inserted into the ear canal, cerumen is removed, and an incision is made in the tympanic membrane. Fluid is sometimes suctioned from the middle ear; then, a tympanostomy tube is inserted into the ear, straddling the tympanic membrane. Antibiotic ear drops frequently are inserted into the external auditory canal. The surgeon changes to the other side of the table, the microscope is repositioned, the head is turned, and the procedure is repeated on the other ear.

Usual preop diagnosis: Chronic serous otitis media; acute otitis media

SUMMARY OF PROCEDURE

Position	Spine; head to anesthesia
Incision	Tympanic membrane
Special instrumentation	Operating microscope
Antibiotics	No parenteral antibiotics (except for SBE prophylaxis); topical antibiotic ear drops
Surgical time	10-30 min. Patients with small ear canals (e.g., Down syndrome) can take longer.
EBL	None
Postop care	PACU → home
Mortality	Rare
Morbidity	Bleeding from ear Purulent drainage from ear (otorrhea)
Pain score	1-3

PATIENT POPULATION CHARACTERISTICS

Age range	3 mo+ (most common, 1-3 yr)
Male:Female	1:1
Incidence	Most common surgical procedure requiring GA
Etiology	Chronic middle ear infections
Associated conditions	Cleft palate

ANESTHETIC CONSIDERATIONS

PREOPERATIVE

The majority of children presenting for PE tubes are < 3 yr and generally in good health. Many of these children, however, have recurrent URI, which contributes to edema of the eustachian tubes, predisposing to episodes of acute otitis media. Intervals between URI may be brief, and scheduling surgery during these interludes is often impractical. Children with mild URI generally can be anesthetized safely for PE tube placement if tracheal intubation is not performed. Surgery should be delayed for patients with acute, febrile illnesses, and in those with Sx referable to the lower airways (e.g., productive cough, wheezing).

Respiratory Surgery in patients with URI Sx referable to the extrathoracic airway alone is generally not delayed. These Sx include nasal congestion and/or discharge and mild conjunctivitis. Fever, productive cough and wheezing are Sx of lower respiratory tract involvement and should prompt rescheduling of the procedure 2-3 wk after these Sx have abated. In borderline cases (e.g., those with rales auscultated on chest exam but no other lower tract Sx), O_2 sat may be measured by pulse oximetry. Procedures in patients with $SpO_2 < 95\%$ should be deferred.

Laboratory None

Premedication Some practitioners advocate withholding premedication, as the duration of action of the premed may outlast the surgery. In general, however, we administer oral midazolam with acetaminophen to those patients > 9-12 mo (see p. D-2) and have not found a significant, related delay in discharge from PACU. Alternatively, acetaminophen with codeine (1 mg/kg) may be given to provide mild sedation and postop analgesia.

INTRAOPERATIVE

Anesthetic technique: GA via face mask

Induction A standard inhalation induction with sevoflurane or halothane, N_2O and O_2 is performed with routine monitoring. An oral airway commonly is inserted, as soft tissue obstruction may occur when the head is turned fully to the side during surgery. CPAP 5-8 cmH_2O also may be useful in maintaining airway patency. Following induction, rectal acetaminophen (10-15 mg/kg) may be given for postop analgesia.

Maintenance If sevoflurane was used for induction, consider switching to halothane or isoflurane. Marked agitation has been noted following emergence from sevoflurane. An iv catheter is not placed routinely.

Emergence	For bilateral procedures, the inhalational anesthetic is D/C before or during the 2nd myringotomy to facilitate prompt emergence. N_2O is continued until the completion of surgery. As the patient is awakening, gentle oropharyngeal suctioning is performed.	
Blood and fluid requirements	None	
Monitoring	Standard monitors (see p. D-1).	
Positioning	✓ and pad pressure points. ✓ eyes.	
Complications	Laryngospasm	Secretions → laryngospasm 2° irritation of the vocal cords, especially in children with URI. Rx: 100% O_2 and CPAP or manual ventilation with PEEP ≤ 20-25 cmH_2O. Rarely, succinylcholine (1-2 mg/kg im) may be needed if a significant decrease in SpO_2 occurs and ventilation is not possible. Atropine (0.1-0.2 mg/kg) should be given in the same syringe to mitigate bradycardia 2° effects of succinylcholine. Oropharyngeal suctioning and manual ventilation usually result in resolution of the laryngospasm. Rarely, tracheal intubation may be indicated for recurrent laryngospasm.

POSTOPERATIVE

Complications	Laryngospasm	Laryngospasm may occur, and should be treated as described above.
Pain management	Acetaminophen 10-15 mg/kg po ± Codeine 1 mg/kg or hydrocodone 0.15 mg/kg	Consider previously administered po and/or pr dosing.

References

1. Tait AR, Knight PR: The effects of general anesthesia on upper respiratory tract infections in children. *Anesthesiology* 1987; 67:930-35.
2. Tobias JD, Lowe S, Hersey S, et al: Analgesia after bilateral myringotomy and placement of pressure equalization tubes in children: acetaminophen vs acetaminophen with codeine. *Anesth Analg* 1995; 81:496-500.

TONSILLECTOMY AND ADENOIDECTOMY

SURGICAL CONSIDERATIONS

Description: The dissection is carried out with the patient supine, shoulders elevated by a shoulder roll (typically, a rolled towel) and head stabilized by a "doughnut." A mouth gag is inserted, and a small suction catheter is passed through the nose and brought out the mouth to elevate the soft palate and expose the nasopharynx. The adenoids are viewed with a mirror and/or palpated. A curette, adenotome or suction Bovie is used to remove the adenoids; then, typically, the nasopharynx is packed. The tonsillectomy is performed by grasping the tonsil with Allis forceps and drawing it medially. A vertical incision is made in the anterior tonsillar pillar with a sickle knife, scissors or electrocautery instruments; then, the tonsil is dissected from the surrounding tissue and removed. A snare may be used to amputate the inferior pole of the tonsil prior to removal. Hemostasis is obtained through use of packs and suction electrocautery. After hemostasis has been obtained in the tonsillar fossae, the pack is removed from the nasopharynx, and hemostasis is achieved in the nasopharynx using suction electrocautery.

Usual preop diagnosis: Obstructive sleep apnea (OSA); chronic tonsillitis and/or adenoiditis; tonsillar and adenoid hypertrophy; asymmetric enlargement of tonsils (to r/o cancer)

SUMMARY OF PROCEDURE

Position	Supine, shoulder roll, head extended; table turned 90°; surgeon at head of table
Incision	Intraoral mucosal
Special instrumentation	Mouth gag (McIvor, Crowe-Davis, Dingman)
Unique considerations	Observe for compression of ETT or accidental extubation when mouth gag is manipulated. Patients with Down syndrome must be evaluated preop for possible atlantoaxial subluxation, as the neck is typically extended. Steroids used routinely by some practitioners (e.g., dexamethasone 0.7-1 mg/kg).
Antibiotics	Not used routinely.
Surgical time	45-90 min
EBL	25-200 ml. Monitor closely.
Postop care	Lateral position; suction in midline only. Most commonly, PACU → home.
Mortality	Rare
Morbidity	Bleeding: 4% Aspiration: Rare Tooth damage: Rare
Pain score	Adenoidectomy, 3-5; tonsillectomy, 6-9

PATIENT POPULATION CHARACTERISTICS

Age range	8 mo+
Male:Female	1:1
Incidence	500,000 cases/yr in U.S.
Etiology	OSA; chronic infection; peritonsillar abscess; snoring. (R/O lymphoma, carcinoma, lymphoproliferative disease.)
Associated conditions	Down syndrome

ANESTHETIC CONSIDERATIONS

PREOPERATIVE

While most children presenting for tonsillectomy and/or adenoidectomy are healthy, a variety of related medical problems may exist. Severe adenoidal hyperplasia may cause nasopharyngeal obstruction, obligate mouth breathing, failure to thrive 2° poor feeding and disturbances of speech and sleep. Chronic nasal obstruction may → narrowing of the upper airway and dental and facial changes (so-called "adenoidal facies"). Tonsillar hyperplasia may cause airway obstruction, sleep apnea, CO_2 retention and cor pulmonale, and failure to thrive. Most of these changes are reversible with removal of the adenoids and tonsils. Children presenting for adenoidectomy/tonsillectomy also frequently have URI (see Myringotomy and Tympanostomy Tube Placement, p. 868).

Respiratory	See discussion under Anesthetic Considerations for Myringotomy and Tympanostomy Tube Placement, p. 868.
Dental	Examination of the airway should include inspection of the teeth, and parents should be advised that loose teeth may be dislodged during placement of the mouth gag or laryngoscopy.
Cardiovascular	In children with severe sleep apnea, CXR and ECG should be done to evaluate the presence of cor pulmonale. If significant RVH and/or cardiomegaly are present, consider ECHO and consultation by pediatric cardiologist.
Hematologic	A careful Hx is taken for Sx of easy bruising or bleeding. If present, a CBC with Plt count, as well as PT, PTT and bleeding time are performed. In patients with a negative Hx, we order no preop lab tests.
Premedication	Children with severe sleep apnea (airway obstruction) generally should not be premedicated. Patients who are very anxious may receive a reduced dose of oral midazolam (see p. D-2) in a well monitored environment (e.g., with an experienced RN or member of the anesthesia team present). SpO_2 should be monitored, if possible, following administration of premedication.

INTRAOPERATIVE

Anesthetic technique: GETA

Induction	A standard inhalational induction (see p. D-2); however, airway obstruction during induction is common in these patients, and is usually alleviated with placement of an oral airway and administration of CPAP 10-20 cmH_2O. An iv catheter should be placed as soon as possible to facilitate administration of muscle relaxant ± glycopyrrolate (4-6 μg/kg) to reduce oral secretions. An oral RAE ETT is used and taped securely in the midline position to facilitate placement of the mouth gag. A cuffed ETT may be desirable because, in combination with a throat pack, it minimizes the risk of entry of blood and oral secretions into the trachea during surgery. Bilateral breath sounds and chest excursion should be confirmed after placement of the mouth gag, which may cause kinking and obstruction of the ETT. Acetaminophen (10-15 mg/kg) may be given pr after induction.	
Maintenance	Standard maintenance (see p. D-3). An intermediate-acting, nondepolarizing muscle relaxant (e.g., vecuronium 0.1 mg/kg) is given to facilitate tracheal intubation. Opioids are given for postop analgesia (e.g., fentanyl 2-3 μg/kg, morphine sulfate 0.1-0.15 mg/kg). The use of propofol instead of anesthetic vapor may reduce the incidence of postop N/V, which is common following adenoidectomy/tonsillectomy. For children with Hx of postop N/V, administration of ondansetron (0.1 mg/kg up to 4 mg) should be considered.	
Emergence	Blood and secretions should be suctioned from the oropharynx and stomach following the completion of surgery. The patient should be fully awake prior to tracheal extubation, which may be performed supine or in the lateral position with the head down. Verify removal of throat packs.	
Blood and fluid requirements	IV: 22 or 20 ga × 1 NS/LR @ 5-10 ml/h	Blood loss is typically ~4 ml/kg and may accumulate in the stomach → N/V.
Monitoring	Standard monitors (see p. D-1).	
Positioning	✓ and pad pressure points. ✓ eyes.	
Complications	Airway obstruction ETT dislodgement/kinking	 Usually caused by insertion/manipulation of mouth gag.

POSTOPERATIVE

Complications	Airway obstruction	Retention of throat pack → airway obstruction. Remove with Magill forceps. Recurrent airway obstruction may require application of positive pressure via face mask (CPAP vs manual ventilation with PEEP) ± placement of an oral airway. Severe postop airway obstruction is more common in patients < 2 yr. In these patients, admission to PICU may be necessary. CPAP via face mask or nasal mask may be helpful. On rare occasion, tracheal intubation and mechanical ventilation are required until swelling of the airway resolves.
	Hemorrhage	Bleeding may occur in the immediate postop period or several days later. Patients present with anemia and hypovolemia, as well as airway compromise and a full stomach 2° swallowed blood. IV fluid, including blood, should be given. Rapid-sequence intubation should be performed with cricoid pressure in preparation for surgical treatment.
Pain management	Morphine 0.025-0.05 mg/kg	May be given incrementally in PACU. Subsequently, acetaminophen with codeine 1 mg/kg or hydrocodone 0.15 mg/kg is given.

References

1. Colclasure JB, Grahamm SS: Complications of outpatient tonsillectomy and adenoidectomy: a review of 3,340 cases. *Ear Nose Throat J* 1990; 69:155-60.
2. Linden BE, Gross CW, Long TE, et al: Morbidity in pediatric tonsillectomy. *Laryngoscope* 1990; 100:120-24.
3. Mather SJ, Peurtrell JM: Postoperative morphine requirements, nausea and vomiting following anaesthesia for tonsillectomy. Comparison of intravenous morphine and non-opioid analgesic techniques. *Paediatr Anaesth* 1995; 5:185-88.

BRONCHOSCOPY/ESOPHAGOSCOPY

SURGICAL CONSIDERATIONS

Description: Flexible bronchoscopy is performed when the dynamics of the larynx and trachea need to be visualized. The child is supine on the OR table, which is turned 90°-180°. With the child sedated or under GA, but breathing spontaneously, the bronchoscope is passed through the nose into the pharynx by way of an adapter attached to a standard anesthesia mask. The larynx is viewed with the patient under "light anesthesia" so that vocal cord movement can be observed; then the anesthesia is deepened and the bronchoscope passed into the trachea. The trachea and bronchi are viewed and, when indicated, bronchoalveolar lavage or bronchial biopsy can be performed.

Rigid bronchoscopy is preferred when direct ventilation of the trachea is required and/or when foreign bodies need to be removed. It also can be used for diagnosis of airway lesions. Direct laryngoscopy is performed; then the rigid bronchoscope is passed through the vocal cords into the trachea. The anesthesia tubing is connected to the bronchoscope and the patient is ventilated through the scope. If a foreign body is present, the telescope within the bronchoscope will be removed and optical forceps inserted through the bronchoscope to remove the foreign body. During the time when the telescope is being changed, a leak will be present in the ventilation system.

Usual preop diagnosis: Airway obstruction; bronchial foreign body; pneumonia (requiring bronchoalveolar lavage); tracheal or bronchial lesion

Flexible or rigid esophagoscopy can be performed for diagnostic or therapeutic (removal of foreign body) purposes. Flexible esophagoscopy can be performed under conscious sedation; however, GETA is preferred for rigid esophagoscopy. The esophagoscope is inserted through the mouth into the esophagus, and the entire length of the esophagus is viewed. If a foreign body is to be removed with the rigid esophagoscope, the telescope and forceps are passed through the lumen of the esophagoscope. If a foreign body (especially food stuff) is to be removed with the flexible esophagoscope, the scope may need to be passed several times.

Esophageal dilation may be performed in one of several ways. Balloon dilation can be performed with the flexible esophagoscope. Alternatively, a guide wire can be passed through the esophagoscope, then Savary/Gilliard dilators in successively larger sizes are passed over the wire. Another option is to remove the esophagoscope after the stenosis has been visualized; then, Maloney or Hurst dilators are passed blindly through the mouth and into the esophagus. Care must be taken to avoid accidental extubation of the patient while the dilators are being inserted and removed.

Usual preop diagnosis: Gastroesophageal reflux; esophageal foreign body; esophageal stricture

SUMMARY OF PROCEDURE

	Bronchoscopy	Esophagoscopy
Position	Patient supine; table turned 90°	⇐
Unique considerations	Ventilate through rigid bronchoscope. Ventilate via mask with adapter for flexible bronchoscope. Dexamethasone (0.7-1 mg/kg) may be indicated, if glottic or subglottic edema is present.	Observe for accidental extubation. ETT taped to left side of mouth.
Antibiotics	None	⇐
Surgical time	10 min-1.5 h	15 min-1 h
EBL	None	< 10 ml
Postop care	Watch for airway compromise; PACU.	PACU
Mortality	Rare	⇐
Morbidity	Laryngospasm Laryngeal edema Dental trauma	Esophageal perforation Bleeding Dental trauma
Pain score	3-4	3-4

PATIENT POPULATION CHARACTERISTICS

Age range	Newborn+
Male:Female	1:1
Incidence	Common

Associated conditions	Bronchoscopy requiring bronchial alveolar lavage (BAL): immunocompromised patient Esophageal stricture: tracheoesophageal fistula (TEF) Esophageal foreign body: esophageal stricture

ANESTHETIC CONSIDERATIONS

See Anesthetic Considerations following Laryngoscopy, Supraglottoplasty, Excision of Laryngeal Lesions, p. 874.

LARYNGOSCOPY, SUPRAGLOTTOPLASTY, EXCISION OF LARYNGEAL LESIONS

SURGICAL CONSIDERATIONS

Description: Flexible laryngoscopy typically is performed in the clinic setting, but may be performed in the OR in the unstable or uncooperative child. The patient should be breathing spontaneously and will be in a sitting (with support) or supine position. Topical anesthesia and vasoconstrictors are applied to the nose; then the scope is passed through the nose into the pharynx, and the larynx is viewed. Vocal cord function is best assessed with the child only mildly sedated.

Diagnostic direct laryngoscopy is performed with the child in a supine position, table turned 90°, with a small shoulder roll in place. The laryngoscope is introduced and, with a lifting motion, a thorough exam of the oropharynx, hypopharynx and larynx is performed. If more than a brief exam is to take place, the vocal cords are anesthetized with topical lidocaine to help prevent laryngospasm. A telescope (often connected via camera to a video monitor) may be passed through the vocal cords to observe the trachea and major bronchi.

Microlaryngoscopy with removal/ablation of laryngeal lesions—most commonly papillomas, nodules or polyps—is accomplished by suspending the laryngoscope from the Mayo stand or OR table, using a suspension apparatus. The patient continues to breath spontaneously or is paralyzed and jet ventilated. When the laser is used, the patient's eyes and face are covered with a damp cloth. OR personnel must wear protective glasses. A microscope with the laser attached is positioned so that the laser beam passes through the laryngoscope onto the vocal folds.

Young infants with severe laryngomalacia may undergo a **supraglottoplasty** for relief of airway obstruction. The laryngoscope is suspended and the laser or microlayrngeal instruments are used to remove redundant aryepiglottic fold tissue.

Usual preop diagnosis: Diagnostic laryngoscopy: hoarseness; airway obstruction, stridor. Operative laryngoscopy: laryngeal papillomas; laryngeal nodules; laryngeal web; laryngeal polyps; subglottic hemangioma or cysts; severe laryngomalacia.

SUMMARY OF PROCEDURE

Position	Supine; table turned 90°
Special instrumentation	± Jet ventilation; laryngoscope suspension apparatus; video equipment
Unique considerations	Potential laser precautions; patient not usually intubated; dexamethasone 0.7-1.0 mg/kg to prevent laryngeal edema; laryngeal topical lidocaine 0.4 mg/kg.
Antibiotics	None
Surgical time	15 min-1.5 h
EBL	< 5 ml
Postop care	Observe for airway obstruction in PACU.
Mortality	Rare
Morbidity	Laryngospasm Laryngeal edema Dental trauma
Pain score	3-5

PATIENT POPULATION CHARACTERISTICS

Age range	Newborn +
Male:Female	1:1
Incidence	Occasional
Etiology	Papillomas: Most commonly, viral infection contracted from mother at time of vaginal delivery) Nodules, polyps: Vocal abuse, gastropharyngeal reflux Subglottic hemangioma: Unknown Subglottic cyst: Prior intubation Laryngeal cysts, webs: Congenital malformation Laryngomalacia: Unknown
Associated conditions	Chronic hoarseness, stridor; GERD; FTT

ANESTHETIC CONSIDERATIONS

(Procedures covered: laryngoscopy; bronchoscopy; supraglottoplasty; excision of laryngeal lesions)

PREOPERATIVE

Direct laryngoscopy (DL) is most commonly performed for patients with stridor. In infants, stridor is most often 2° laryngomalacia, with vocal cord paralysis being less common. Patients with severe laryngomalacia and those with posttransplant lymphoproliferative disease involving the epiglottis may undergo supraglottoplasty utilizing electrocautery and/or laser excision. Older children may present with stridor 2° laryngeal masses or papillomatosis, for which laser therapy also may be performed. A careful H&P is contributory to the diagnosis, after which flexible laryngoscopy in the ENT clinic can be confirmatory.

Laryngoscopy and **rigid bronchoscopy** also are performed for the removal of airway foreign bodies (FB). A Hx of choking and/or coughing while eating is usually elicited. Children may present with agitation, wheezing and cyanosis. This condition constitutes a true surgical emergency and the patient should be taken to the OR as soon as possible.

Airway/ Respiratory Stridor usually is worsened with crying or agitation, and often less severe during sleep.

Dental Loose teeth, if present, may be dislodged.

Laboratory No routine tests are indicated. In stable patients with suspected FB aspiration, CXR may be obtained.

Premedication Because stridor often is decreased during quiet breathing and sleep, premedication with oral midazolam is usually beneficial in patients > 9-12 mo. Children with FB aspiration generally should not be given po medications. They may benefit from small doses of iv midazolam.

INTRAOPERATIVE

Anesthetic technique: GA. Primary and backup plans for airway management during the procedure should be discussed in detail with the ENT surgeon in advance of anesthetic induction.

Induction Mask induction is followed by placement of an iv catheter, if not already in place. In cases where vocal cord function must be evaluated, spontaneous breathing is maintained under halothane or sevoflurane in 100% O_2.

Maintenance Prior to removal of the face mask for DL, a deep level of anesthesia is achieved. During DL, blow-by O_2 is administered.

For patients in whom vocal cord function must be assessed, gradual offset of inhalational anesthesia should → ↑vocal cord excursion. Supraglottoplasty and laser excision of laryngeal lesions may be performed with intermittent mask anesthesia. Propofol with or without remifentanil may be used, although the risk of apnea is increased with these agents as compared with inhalational anesthesia. In general, even a small ETT will interfere with the surgical procedure. Alternatively, muscle relaxant may be given and jet ventilation maintained using a Sanders jet ventilator (see Fig 3-4, p. 126). Intermittent jets of 100% O_2 are delivered with a high-pressure (40-55 psi) gas source through a tube incorporated into the laryngoscope blade. As the jet is pointed toward the glottic opening, air is entrained by the Venturi effect. Manual ventilation is performed while chest excursion is observed to ensure that excessive inflating pressures and volumes are avoided. During jet ventilation, anesthesia is maintained with iv agents. Propofol 150-200 μg/kg/min is infused with remifentanil 0.15-0.40 μg/kg/min. (Remifentanil 0.1 mg is added to each 10 ml of propofol in a single syringe; e.g., for a propofol infusion of 100 μg/kg/min, remifentanil 0.1 μg/kg/min is delivered.)

★ **NB:** fire hazard during laser surgery is minimal in the absence of a combustible material (e.g., plastic) in the field. An FiO_2 of 1.0 may, therefore, be used safely, unless a plastic ETT is in place. For selected laser procedures involving the tissues around the glottis, a metal or metal-wrapped ETT may be used.

During rigid bronchoscopy, ventilation is performed through a side port of the bronchoscope. Assisted, spontaneous ventilation under deep inhalational anesthesia may be maintained. Alternatively, iv anesthesia and muscle relaxation may be preferred, as described above. For FB cases, maintenance of spontaneous ventilation generally is preferred to avoid distal displacement of the FB. Gentle, assisted ventilation may be required, however, to ensure adequate oxygenation and ventilation.

Emergence	A conventional ETT is placed after removal of the laryngoscope or bronchoscope, as laryngospasm following these procedures is common. Tracheal extubation is performed with the patient fully awake and following complete reversal of neuromuscular blockade, if applicable.	
Blood and fluid requirements	IV: 22 ga × 1 NS/LR @ 3-5 ml/kg/h	Blood loss is minimal.
Monitoring	Standard monitors (see p. D-1).	
Positioning	Table rotated 90°	Shoulder roll/neck extension for surgery
	✓ and pad pressure points.	
	✓ eyes.	Eyes covered with wet sponges or goggles when laser in use.
Complications	Hypoventilation	Adjust Sanders jet; mask ventilation prn.
	Hypoxemia	
	Airway injury	2° jet ventilation, DL/bronchoscope
	Pneumothorax	
	Eye trauma	
	Laryngospasm	Rx: 100% O_2, CPAP vs manual ventilation/PEEP
	Eye injury	
	Airway fire	Remove ETT; irrigate with NS; resume ventilation with 100% O_2 when fire extinguished.

POSTOPERATIVE

Complications	Dental trauma Bleeding Eye trauma Pneumothorax	
Pain management	Acetaminophen (10-15 mg/kg) ± Hydrocodone 0.15 mg/kg or codeine 1 mg/kg q 4 h	
Tests	CXR	If respiratory distress, ↓SpO_2 present.

References

1. Weeks DG: Laboratory and clinical description of the use of jet-venturi ventilator during laser microsurgery of the glottis and subglottis. *Anesth Rev* 1985; 12:32-6.
2. Zalzal GH: Stridor and airway compromise. *Pediatr Clin North Am* 1989; 36:1389-1402.

REMOVAL OF BRANCHIAL CLEFT CYST OR THYROGLOSSAL DUCT CYST

SURGICAL CONSIDERATIONS

Description: Branchial cleft cysts and tracts typically present in the lateral neck; thyroglossal duct cysts, in the midline. Removal consists of making an incision in the neck around the opening of the tract (if present), or over the palpable cyst, and following the tract superiorly to its origin. A **Sistrunk procedure** is performed in the case of a thyroglossal duct cyst, and involves the removal of the middle section of the hyoid bone.

Usual preop diagnosis: Branchial cleft cyst; thyroglossal duct cyst

SUMMARY OF PROCEDURE

Position	Supine; head 180° from anesthesia; oral intubation
Incision	Horizontal neck
Antibiotics	Clindamycin 10 mg/kg
Surgical time	45 min-1.5 h
EBL	< 20 ml
Postop care	Routine
Mortality	Rare
Morbidity	Bleeding/neck hematoma Infection Recurrence of cyst Damage to CN XI, XII
Pain score	4-6

PATIENT POPULATION CHARACTERISTICS

Age range	Newborn-adult
Male:Female	1:1
Etiology	Congenital
Associated conditions	Branchio-oto-renal (BOR) syndrome

ANESTHETIC CONSIDERATIONS

See Anesthetic Considerations following Incision/Drainage of Deep Neck Abscess, p. 877.

INCISION/DRAINAGE OF DEEP NECK ABSCESS

SURGICAL CONSIDERATIONS

Description: Children with deep neck abscesses (retropharyngeal, parapharyngeal, peritonsillar) are at risk for acute airway obstruction; therefore, the abscesses are drained on an emergent basis. Retropharyngeal and peritonsillar abscesses typically are drained through an intraoral approach; parapharyngeal abscesses, through an external neck approach. In each case, the child must be intubated orally and placed in the supine position. The anesthesiologist or otolaryngologist who is intubating the child must be prepared for abnormal pharyngeal anatomy 2° the abscess. Care must be taken that the abscess is not ruptured in the intubation process. A tracheotomy tray should be in the OR at the time of intubation. In most cases, the child can be extubated immediately after the abscess is drained; however, in a small number of cases, the child may need to remain intubated until the pharyngeal edema subsides.

Usual preop diagnosis: Retropharyngeal, parapharyngeal or peritonsillar abscess

SUMMARY OF PROCEDURE

Position	Supine; table turned 90°-180°; oral intubation
Incision	Intraoral (retropharyngeal or peritonsillar abscess); lateral neck (parapharyngeal abscess)
Unique considerations	Acute airway obstruction can occur with induction. Care must be taken to avoid rupture of abscess on intubation; ± dexamethasone 1 mg/kg.
Antibiotics	Clindamycin 10 mg/kg
Surgical time	30-90 min
EBL	< 30 ml
Postop care	May remain intubated postop.
Mortality	Rare
Morbidity	Aspiration (if abscess ruptures spontaneously) Airway obstruction 2° aspiration or edema Bleeding
Pain score	5

PATIENT POPULATION CHARACTERISTICS

Age range	Most common, 6 mo-3 yr; can occur at any age.
Male:Female	1:1
Incidence	Uncommon
Etiology	URI

ANESTHETIC CONSIDERATIONS

(Procedures covered: excision of branchial cleft and thyroglossal duct cyst; incision/drainage of neck abscess)

PREOPERATIVE

These patients generally are otherwise healthy children. A cystic hygroma (cystic lymphangioma), as with other neck masses, may cause airway obstruction and difficult intubation.

Respiratory The size and extent of the neck mass should be defined carefully in an effort to detect the potential for airway compromise and to avoid soft-tissue trauma during intubation, with consequent acute airway obstruction. Inspiratory stridor suggests supraglottic obstruction, while expiratory stridor is associated with subglottic/intrathoracic obstruction. The patients should have had prior CT/MRI imaging; anesthesia records for these studies should be reviewed.
Tests: CXR; CT/MRI

Cardiovascular Cervical masses may be adherent to and/or cause compression of the great vessels.
Tests: CT/MRI

Hematologic T&C for cystic hygroma, or if a cervical mass involves great vessels or extends into the mediastinum (~3%).
Tests: Hct

Laboratory Other tests as indicated from H&P.

Premedication If > 9-12 mo and asymptomatic, midazolam (0.5-0.75 mg po) 30 min prior to arrival in OR. Avoid all premedication in patients with significant potential for airway compromise.

INTRAOPERATIVE

Anesthetic technique: GETA

Induction Standard pediatric induction (see p. D-2) in patients without airway compromise. When airway obstruction is present, iv should be secured prior to mask induction, which may be done with halothane or sevoflurane in 100% O_2. As plane of anesthesia deepens, gently assist ventilation.

Induction, cont.	Give atropine (0.01-0.02 mg/kg iv) prior to laryngoscopy. If partial airway obstruction exists, maintain spontaneous ventilation with CPAP and perform laryngoscopy at ~3 MAC of volatile agent. FOB should be available. Have full range of ETT sizes available, since airway narrowing may be present. Once airway is secured, proceed with neuromuscular blockade (e.g., vecuronium 0.1 mg/kg).	
Maintenance	Standard pediatric maintenance (see p. D-3). Surgeon may infiltrate incision with local anesthetic. Limit lidocaine to 5 mg/kg when used without epinephrine, or 7 mg/kg when used with epinephrine, and bupivacaine to 2.5 mg/kg.	
Emergence	Reverse neuromuscular blockade with neostigmine (0.07 mg/kg iv) and atropine (0.02 mg/kg iv). Confirm air leak around ETT and extubate when fully awake.	
Blood and fluid requirements	Minimal blood loss IV: 20-22 ga × 1 Great vessel involvement: IV: 20 ga × 1-2 NS/LR @ 3 ml/kg/h	Minimal 3rd-space losses. Each ml blood loss can be replaced with 3 ml NS/LR. When great vessels involved, place at least 1 iv in lower extremity. Blood loss can be quite sudden; have blood available in OR.
Monitoring	Standard monitors (see p. D-1). ± Arterial line, 22 ga	An arterial line is used when there is risk of large blood loss or perioperative airway compromise.
Positioning	✓ and pad pressure points. ✓ eyes.	
Complications	ETT dislodged/loss of airway Laryngospasm Bronchospasm Hemorrhage	ETT must be secured carefully. Liberal use of benzoin adherent. Avoid tension on ETT by circuit hoses. Hold ETT during surgeon's intraoral examination to prevent accidental extubation.

POSTOPERATIVE

Complications	Subglottic edema Upper airway obstruction from edema related to tumor resection Recurrent laryngeal nerve injury	Dexamethasone (0.5-1 mg/kg iv) and nebulized racemic epinephrine (1.25%) with mist O_2 to treat subglottic edema.
Pain management	Morphine (0.025-0.1 mg/kg iv q 2-4 h Acetaminophen (10-15 mg/kg po/pr q 4 h)	The majority of these procedures are performed on outpatient basis (except cystic hygroma).

References

1. Gregory GA, ed: *Pediatric Anesthesia*, 3rd edition. Churchill Livingstone, New York: 1994.
2. Motoyama EK, Davis PC, eds: *Smith's Anesthesia for Infants and Children*, 5th edition. CV Mosby, St. Louis: 1990.
3. Tapper D: Head and neck-sinuses and masses. In *Pediatric Surgery*. Ashcraft KW, Holder TM, eds. WB Saunders, Philadelphia: 1993, 923-34.

CRICOID SPLIT, LARYNGOTRACHEOPLASTY

SURGICAL CONSIDERATIONS

Description: A **cricoid split** is most commonly performed in the NICU baby who fails extubation due to subglottic stenosis. **Diagnostic bronchoscopy** is performed; then the baby is reintubated or the bronchoscope is left in the airway and the procedure is performed over the bronchoscope. A horizontal neck incision is made over the cricoid cartilage. The strap muscles are separated in the midline; the laryngeal cartilage and trachea are exposed; and a vertical incision is made through the inferior portion of the thyroid cartilage, through the cricoid cartilage and first tracheal ring. Typically, an ETT 1/2 size larger than the previously placed ETT is inserted.

A **laryngotracheoplasty** is performed in the patient with moderate-to-severe subglottic stenosis. In most of these patients, a tracheotomy will already be present. During the procedure, the tracheotomy tube may be switched for an anode tube, which is sutured or taped to the chest. After the airway is exposed as above, a costal cartilage, auricular cartilage or laryngeal cartilage graft will be harvested. The graft(s) are sutured into the anterior and/or posterior airway and, in some children, a stent will be positioned within the larynx and trachea. The tracheotomy tube may or may not be removed, depending on the plan for a single-stage vs multiple-stage procedure (the tracheotomy tube is not removed at the initial procedure if a stent is used).

Usual preop diagnosis: Subglottic stenosis

SUMMARY OF PROCEDURE

Position	Supine
Incision	Horizontal neck
Unique considerations	After the cut is made into the airway, a leak may be present, depending on position of the cuff (if present).
Antibiotics	Clindamycin 10 mg/kg
Surgical time	Cricoid split: 45 min Laryngotracheoplasty: 1.5-4 h
EBL	5-30 ml
Mortality	Rare
Morbidity	Pneumothorax Bleeding Infection Stent dislodgement Residual/recurrent subglottic stenosis
Pain score	4-6

PATIENT POPULATION CHARACTERISTICS

Age range	Newborn-adult
Male:Female	1:1
Incidence	Rare
Etiology	Endotracheal intubation; congenital
Associated conditions	Prematurity with prolonged NICU course

ANESTHETIC CONSIDERATIONS

PREOPERATIVE

These procedures are performed in patients with subglottic stenosis with a lesion that is either congenital or acquired. Congenital subglottic stenosis varies with regard to the length of trachea involved and the degree of stenosis. Segmental stenosis may occur in the region of the cricoid cartilage, midtrachea or just above the carina. Sx are severe retractions, especially with agitation or intercurrent URI, dyspnea and stridor. If the stenotic segment is short and severe, excision with primary anastomosis may be performed. If the involved segment is long, tracheoplasty is usually performed.

Acquired subglottic stenosis occurs as a complication of prolonged tracheal intubation and mechanical ventilation, most commonly in neonates born prematurely with severe lung disease associated with prematurity (infant respiratory distress syndrome [IRDS]). The stenotic lesion usually is limited to the level of the cricoid cartilage, and is treated with the cricoid split procedure. In addition to tracheal stenosis, tracheomalacia may be present.

Respiratory — Patients may be intubated and mechanically ventilated in the PICU. A variable degree of lung disease may be present; some patients may be on minimal ventilatory support, while others may be receiving relatively high FiO_2 and/or inflating pressures. Some patients will have an indwelling tracheostomy tube that bypasses the stenotic lesion, and may be cared for at home.
Tests: As indicated from H&P.

Cardiovascular	Although not common, cor pulmonale with RVH may be present 2° chronic lung disease.
Hematologic	Anemia is common, especially in infants with chronic lung disease. **Tests:** Hct
Premedication	Infants in PICU usually are receiving a regimen of sedative and analgesia drugs. These should be continued until induction of anesthesia, with supplemental doses given preop as needed. Tolerance may be present, and drug doses should be titrated to achieve an adequate level of sedation.

INTRAOPERATIVE

Anesthetic technique: GETA

Induction	In intubated patients with iv access, an iv induction is performed; otherwise, induction is done with inhalation agents. In the absence of an ETT, a mask induction is performed, with care being taken to preserve upper airway patency, as even mild obstruction tends to exacerbate tracheal collapse. Following neuromuscular blockade, tracheal intubation is performed with an ETT smaller than normal for age. In patients with severe stenosis, an ETT as small as 2.5 mm may be required. If a tracheostomy tube is in place, it is removed at the time of ETT placement. If prolonged sedation and mechanical ventilation are planned postop, central venous access should be considered.
Maintenance	Plans for postop mechanical ventilation are discussed with the surgeon. In those patients for whom mechanical ventilation is planned for > 24 h, high-dose opioid anesthesia is appropriate (e.g., fentanyl 20-50 μg/kg), as well as a long-acting muscle relaxant (pancuronium). A mixture of air and O_2 is used to keep $SpO_2 \leq 95\%$ to minimize O_2 toxicity.
Emergence	The majority of patients are transported to the PICU with indwelling ETT with residual sedation, narcosis and neuromuscular blockade. IV sedation may be achieved with midazolam, lorazepam or diazepam prior to completion of surgery.

Blood and fluid requirements	IV: 24 or 22 ga × 1 NS/LR @ maintenance	Blood loss < 30 ml
Monitoring	Standard monitors (see p. D-1).	
Positioning	✓ and pad pressure points. ✓ eyes.	
Complications	Tracheal edema Injury to neck structures: Trachea Vascular structures Recurrent laryngeal nerve injury	Rx: dexamethasone (0.5-1 mg/kg)

POSTOPERATIVE

Complications	Tracheal disruption (leak)	Presents with subcutaneous emphysema of the neck, face and chest wall.
	Recurrent laryngeal nerve injury	May cause vocal cord dysfunction.
Sedation/ analgesia	Heavy sedation	To minimize head and neck movement and tracheal wound disruption while ETT is in place.

References

1. Allen TH, Stevens IM: Prolonged endotracheal intubation in infants and children. *Br J Anaesth* 1985; 37:566-73.
2. Cotton RT: Pediatric laryngotracheal stenosis. *J Pediatr Surg* 1984; 19:699.
3. Vinograd I, Klim B, Efrati Y: Airway obstruction in neonates and children: surgical treatment. *J Cardiovasc Surg* 1994; 35:7-12.

CHOANAL ATRESIA REPAIR

SURGICAL CONSIDERATIONS

Description: Infants born with bilateral choanal atresia typically have severe airway distress shortly following birth because neonates are obligate nose breathers. The distress resolves after the child is intubated or a McGovern nipple (large nipple with cross-cuts in the end) or oral airway is positioned in the oral cavity. These infants undergo primary repair of the atresia within the first few d of life. Children with unilateral choanal atresia usually do not have any respiratory distress and, thus, surgery is often postponed until a later age.

Intranasal repair involves opening up the atretic area with nasal dilators or urethral sounds and placing an intranasal stent. If a transpalatal repair is performed, a Dingman mouth gag is placed in the mouth, a palatal flap is raised and the posterior portion of the hard palate and posterior septum is removed. A stent is positioned in the nose. The infant should be able to breathe spontaneously through the nose at completion of either procedure.

Usual preop diagnosis: Bilateral or unilateral choanal atresia

SUMMARY OF PROCEDURE

Position	Supine; head 90°-180° from anesthesia
Incision	Intranasal or intraoral
Special instrumentation	Nasal dilators; Dingman mouth gag
Antibiotics	Clindamycin 10 mg/kg
Surgical time	30 min-2 h
EBL	< 10 ml
Postop care	Observation in PICU for respiratory distress
Mortality	Rare
Morbidity	Bleeding Infection Airway obstruction if stents become malpositioned
Pain score	3-6

PATIENT POPULATION CHARACTERISTICS

Age range	Newborn-young child
Male:Female	1:1
Incidence	Rare
Etiology	Congenital
Associated conditions	Coloboma, heart disease, atresia choanae, retarded growth, genital anomalies and ear deformities (CHARGE) association (see Anesthetic Considerations, below).

ANESTHETIC CONSIDERATIONS

PREOPERATIVE

Because many neonates are nasal breathers, choanal atresia may present with cyanosis at rest, resolving with crying or placement of an oral airway. Unilateral atresia is usually asymptomatic; bilateral lesions usually → respiratory distress in the newborn period, but occasionally are asymptomatic. Although choanal atresia is most commonly an isolated anomaly, it may present as part of the CHARGE association.

Respiratory	Classic findings include cyanosis at rest, resolving with crying.
Cardiovascular	When part of the CHARGE association, cardiac defects include tetralogy of Fallot, ASD, VSD, PDA, AV canal or right-side aortic arch.
Neurologic	When part of the CHARGE association, a variety of CNS abnormalities may be present. Hypoxia 2° airway obstruction may cause CNS impairment and seizures.
Premedication	Repair of choanal atresia usually is performed in infancy, and premedication is not indicated.

INTRAOPERATIVE

Anesthetic technique: GETA

Induction	Standard pediatric induction (see p. D-2). Airway obstruction may develop during induction of anesthesia. Early placement of an oral airway, facilitated by topical anesthesia of the tongue with viscous lidocaine prior to induction, may prevent or relieve the obstruction. An oral RAE ETT is preferred, especially if a transpalatal repair is planned using a Dingman mouth retractor.	
Maintenance	Inhalational anesthesia is maintained during the procedure. During the first mo of life, opioids should be avoided generally because of the risk of postop respiratory depression. For infants undergoing repair after the first mo of life, small doses of fentanyl (1-2 μg/kg) or morphine sulfate (0.05-0.1 mg/kg) may be given. Muscle relaxation does not need to be maintained following tracheal intubation.	
Emergence	Nasal stents placed following the repair must be secure and free of secretions prior to tracheal extubation. Patients must be fully awake and capable of maintaining patency of their oropharynx in the event of postop swelling and transient obstruction of the nasopharynx.	
Blood and fluid requirements	IV: 24 or 22 ga × 1 NS/LR @ maintenance	Blood loss is < 10 ml; may be greater in older infants.
Monitoring	Standard monitors (see p. D-1).	
Positioning	✓ and pad pressure points. ✓ eyes.	
Complications	Airway obstruction	2° swelling of the nasopharynx or obstruction or displacement of nasal stents
	Bleeding	Especially in older infants

POSTOPERATIVE

Complications	See Intraop Complications, above.	
Pain management	Acetaminophen po/pr	Small doses of opioid may be given iv immediately postop, with special attention to avoid respiratory depression/obstruction.

References

1. Harris J, Robert E, Kfallfen B: Epidemiology of choanal atresia with special reference to the CHARGE association. *Pediatrics* 1997; 99:363-67.
2. Menasse-Palmer L, Bogdanow A, Marion RW: Choanal atresia. *Pediatr Rev* 1995; 16:475-76.
3. Prescott CA: Nasal obstruction in infancy. *Arch Dis Child* 1995; 72:287-89.

PEDIATRIC TRACHEOTOMY

SURGICAL CONSIDERATIONS

Description: A **tracheotomy** is performed in the infant or child with upper airway obstruction (subglottic stenosis, laryngeal web, etc.) or in the child in whom prolonged mechanical ventilation is anticipated. In most cases, the child will already be intubated and the procedure will be performed over the ETT. In selected infants, the tracheotomy can be performed with a rigid bronchoscope in the airway through which the patient is being ventilated. A midline horizontal neck incision is made just inferior to the cricoid cartilage. The dissection is carried out in the midline until the trachea is reached. In children, the tracheal incision is vertical; and the patient typically has a large air leak. As the ETT or bronchoscope is being removed, a tracheotomy tube is inserted in the neck. The ventilation tubing will be exchanged for new sterile tubing and the tracheotomy tube secured with neck sutures and/or ties around the neck. Stay sutures may be placed around the tracheal wall and taped to the right and left sides of the chest. In the case of accidental decannulation postop, these sutures can be used to pull open the tracheal incision to aid in replacement of the tracheotomy tube.

Usual preop diagnosis: Ventilator dependence; subglottic stenosis

SUMMARY OF PROCEDURE

Position	Supine; head to anesthesia
Incision	Horizontal neck
Special instrumentation	Tracheotomy hook
Unique considerations	Have ETT tube tape loosened for easy removal underneath the drapes. When trachea is opened, a large air leak may be present.
Antibiotics	Clindamycin 10 mg/kg
Surgical time	30 min-1 h
EBL	< 10 ml
Postop care	Close observation in PICU. CXR immediately following procedure to r/o pneumothorax.
Mortality	2-5%, usually 2° tracheotomy tube plugging or dislodgement
Morbidity	Pneumothorax Subcutaneous emphysema Bleeding Infection Plugging Skin abrasion around trach edges in patient with short, chubby neck
Pain score	3-5

PATIENT POPULATION CHARACTERISTICS

Age range	Newborn-adult
Male:Female	1:1
Incidence	Uncommon
Etiology	Anatomical airway obstruction; ventilatory dependence; high, spinal-cord or head injury
Associated conditions	Prematurity; trauma

ANESTHETIC CONSIDERATIONS

See Anesthetic Considerations following Tracheostomy, in Chapter 3.0 Otolaryngology, p. 149.

Surgeons

David D. Yuh, MD
Bruce A. Reitz, MD

12.3 PEDIATRIC CARDIOVASCULAR SURGERY

Anesthesiologist

Kristi L. Peterson, MD

SURGERY FOR ATRIAL SEPTAL DEFECT (OSTIUM SECUNDUM)

SURGICAL CONSIDERATIONS

Description: Atrial septal defects (ASDs) are among the most common congenital cardiac defects. ASDs vary widely in size and location and are broadly classified as **ostium secundum, ostium primum, sinus venosus,** and **coronary sinus** types. Ostium secundum defects—the most common (80%)—result from a developmental failure of the septum secundum and are usually located in the midportion of the atrial septum. A L→R shunt results in augmented pulmonary blood flow which, if left uncorrected, may lead to pulmonary vascular occlusive disease (PVOD), pulmonary HTN, RV failure and atrial arrhythmias. In 1953, Gibbon successfully repaired an ASD using a pump-oxygenator and, in doing so, ushered in the era of open cardiac surgery.

Secundum ASDs that fail to spontaneously close should be electively closed in early childhood to avoid long-term complications. Currently, ASD closure is performed through a standard median sternotomy on CPB. A right anterolateral thoracotomy through the 4th intercostal space also provides satisfactory exposure and provides female patients with better cosmesis. Once CPB and cardioplegic arrest have been instituted, a right atriotomy is created and the ASD is visualized.

Repair is effected by direct suture closure or patch closure using autologous pericardium or prosthetic material (i.e., Gore-Tex, Dacron). After the repair is completed and the atriotomy is closed, the aortic cross-clamp is released, standard deairing maneuvers are performed, and CPB is discontinued. The chest is then closed in the standard fashion.

Variant procedure or approaches: Several centers have been gaining experimental experience with a percutaneously introduced and minimally invasive "clamshell" device for ASD closure.

Usual preop diagnosis: ASD; ostium secundum defect

SUMMARY OF PROCEDURE

Position	Supine; right lateral decubitus (thoracotomy)
Incision	Standard median sternotomy; right anterolateral thoracotomy (4th intercostal space)
Unique considerations	R→L shunt → systemic embolization
Antibiotics	Cefazolin 15-30 mg/kg q 8 h
Surgical time	Aortic cross-clamp: 20-30 min Total: 2 h
Closing considerations	Routine closure with chest tube in pericardial space; temporary atrial pacing wire (older patients); possible left atrial line for monitoring
EBL	Minimal
Postop care	Extubation in OR or within several h; 24 h monitoring in ICU; older patients may have high left atrial pressures early after repair.
Mortality	Rare
Morbidity	Hemorrhage Atrial arrhythmias
Pain score	8-10

PATIENT POPULATION CHARACTERISTICS

Age range	Neonate–early adulthood
Male:Female	1:2
Incidence	10-15% of congenital heart defects
Etiology	Developmental failure of the septum secundum to cover the foramen ovale
Associated conditions	ASD may coexist with nearly any of the other recognized congenital cardiac anomalies, but is more commonly associated with pulmonary stenosis (10%), partial anomalous pulmonary venous return (7%), VSD (5%), PDA (3%) and mitral stenosis (2%). ASDs are also part of other malformations, including tricuspid atresia, total anomalous pulmonary venous connection (TAPVC) and mitral atresia.

ANESTHETIC CONSIDERATIONS

PREOPERATIVE

Pathophysiology L→R shunt → ↑pulmonary blood flow (Q_P) → ↑PA pressures → ↑PVR → RV overload → RV failure. The larger the area of the defect, the greater the shunt. When Q_P/Q_S ratio (systemic flow) < 1.5, it is often well tolerated and the patient may be asymptomatic. When Q_P/Q_S ratio > 3, dyspnea, fatigue and poor feeding occur. In early infancy there is little shunting; however, as PVR decreases and RV compliance increases, the L→R shunt will increase. Most infants with ASD are asymptomatic, but 5% have CHF and failure to thrive (FTT). Pulmonary HTN is rare in infants. The incidence of significant pulmonary vascular disease increases with age. It is very rare for a patient to progress to Eisenmenger's syndrome (severe pulmonary HTN → shunt reversal [R→L]). Among adults not corrected, 14% develop CHF and 20% develop dysrhythmias.

Unlike VSDs, ASDs rarely close spontaneously, although closure can occur in the 1st yr of life. Small ASDs generally do not adversely affect life span. Closure is advocated by some because of the small ↑ incidence of bacterial endocarditis and paradoxical embolism.

Cardiovascular and respiratory Most patients are relatively asymptomatic. Young children often have Hx of frequent URI. Older children may c/o dyspnea and fatigue. The systolic murmur of an ASD is heard best in the pulmonic area. Fixed splitting of 2nd heart sound. If a patient is cyanotic, shunt reversal may have occurred and these patients may be inoperable.

Tests: ECG: incomplete RBBB + RVH may be present. CXR: cardiomegaly and ↑pulmonary vascular markings. ECHO: documents size and position of defect and L→R shunt; cardiac catheterization: rarely indicated except in patients with severe pulmonary HTN.

Laboratory Hb/Hct; T&C; other tests as indicated from H&P.

Premedication Generally not necessary for patients < 1 yr of age. Midazolam 0.5-0.7 mg/kg po 30 min prior to induction very effective. The goal is to maintain cardiovascular and respiratory stability in a nonstruggling patient.

INTRAOPERATIVE

Anesthetic technique: GETA ± regional anesthesia. An early extubation may be appropriate in these patients. Patients receiving epidural anesthesia will have the catheter placed 1 h prior to heparinization (see Epidural analgesia, Tetralogy of Fallot [TOF], p. 905).

Induction Infants may generally tolerate an inhalation induction; however, the presence of heart failure or other medical problems may make an iv induction more appropriate (fentanyl 10 μg/kg or ketamine 1-2 mg/kg, followed by muscle relaxant). An iv induction should be used in patients with significant pulmonary HTN and/or RV failure.

Smaller children generally tolerate an inhalation induction with halothane or sevoflurane in 50% N_2O + O_2. After induction, iv access is established and pancuronium 0.1 mg/kg, followed by remifentanil 1 μg/kg, is given. In patients with difficult iv access, im succinylcholine 4 mg/kg with atropine 0.01 mg/kg may be given. The patient is then intubated orally. If the patient is to remain intubated postop, however, nasal intubation is preferred for comfort and ETT stability. Well sedated older children generally tolerate placement of an iv (especially with the use of EMLA cream); and iv induction is accomplished with STP 2-4 mg/kg or propofol 2 mg/kg, followed by a muscle relaxant (e.g., vecuronium 1 mg/kg).

Maintenance In patients in whom immediate postop extubation is planned, anesthesia is maintained using a volatile agent in air + O_2, combined with epidural anesthesia. N_2O is turned off after induction to avoid expansion of any intraop VAE. In patients with pulmonary HTN, RV failure and/or other medical conditions requiring postop mechanical ventilation, a high-dose narcotic technique is appropriate (e.g., fentanyl 100-200 μg/kg ± inhalation agent).

Emergence Patients may be extubated awake or in a deep plane of anesthesia. An effective regional anesthetic is essential for early awake extubation. BP is controlled with an SNP or NTG infusion. Patients extubated while deeply anesthetized rarely require BP control. For patients returning to the ICU intubated and ventilated, portable monitoring equipment, O_2, bag, mask, airway equipment and emergency drugs should be available during transport.

Blood and fluid requirements	IV: appropriate for patient's size × 1-2 LR @ TKO Blood warmer ✓ for air bubbles. T&C 1 U PRBC.	★ **NB:** It is critical to avoid iv air bubbles in these patients. ✓ iv tubing and stopcocks for adherent bubbles. Have blood ready in OR although transfusion not usual for secundum repairs.
Monitoring	Standard monitors (see p. D-1). Arterial line CVP line Urinary catheter ACT monitoring ± TEE	ABG, electrolytes and Hct should be checked as needed during the procedure. Place at least 2 O_2 probes to ensure readings during critical times. Avoid dorsalis pedis and posterior tibial arterial lines (inaccurate 2° spasm post CPB). Femoral arterial line may be used. Double lumen CVP in IJ preferable. Distal port reserved for vasoactive infusions. TEE monitoring may be used to assess repair and anatomy in sinus venous defects and more complicated intraatrial baffles. Humidify gases to minimize heat loss during rewarming.
Positioning	✓ and pad pressure points. ✓ eyes.	
Pre CPB	Heparinization (3 mg/kg) ✓ ACT > 400. ✓ pupils (constricted OK). ✓ NMB. ✓ UO.	
CPB	Hypothermia ✓ adequate flow and pressure during CPB. Ventilation stopped ✓ face for venous congestion. ✓ ABG and ACT. ✓ UO. Infusions stopped Blood should be available.	The patient is not actively cooled for secundum ASD repair. The temperature generally drifts to about 33-34°C. For more complex repairs, active cooling to 24-26°C is done or DHCA (13-17°C) may be required.
Transition off CPB	Rewarming Vasoactive infusions restarted Flush lines. Rezero transducers. Suction ETT. Resume ventilation. Observe inflation of both lungs.	Surgeon will deair heart, and this maneuver can be monitored with TEE. Aerosolized albuterol is usually given after suctioning.
Post CPB	Reversal of heparin with protamine ✓ UO.	1 mg of protamine will reverse 100 U of residual heparin.
	Modified ultrafiltration (MUF)	MUF uses the CPB machine to remove excess water and inflammatory mediators. It has been shown to ↓ postop edema and improve cardiopulmonary function.
	↓Pulmonary HTN ✓ pupils.	For patients with pulmonary HTN, institute maneuvers to ↓PVR (see TOF, p. 906).
Complications	Air embolism (VAE) Supraventricular dysrhythmias	 Potential for paradoxical embolization
	Heart block Ventricular dysfunction Pulmonary HTN/RV failure	Likely 2° atriotomy

POSTOPERATIVE

Complications	Bleeding Epidural or spinal hematoma	 In regional anesthesia patients

Tests	ABG Electrolytes; Hct; coags CXR

References

1. Baue AE, Geha AS, Hammond GL, Laks H, Naunheim KS: *Glenn's Thoracic and Cardiovascular Surgery,* 6th edition. Appleton & Lange, Stamford: 1996.
2. Castaneda AR, Jonas RA, Mayer JE Jr, Hanley FL: Atrial septal defect. In *Cardiac Surgery of the Neonate and Infant.* WB Saunders, Philadelphia: 1994, 143-55.
3. Cooper JR, Goldstein MT: Septal and endocardial cushion defects and double outlet right ventricle perioperative management. In *Pediatric Cardiac Anesthesia,* 3rd edition. Lake CL, ed. Appleton & Lange, Stamford, CT: 1998, 285-301.
4. Kambam J: Endocardial cushion defects. In *Cardiac Anesthesia for Infants and Children.* Kambam J, Fish FA, Merrill WH, eds. CV Mosby, St. Louis: 1994, 203-10.
5. Kirklin JW, Barrett-Boyes BG: Atrial septal defect and partial anomalous pulmonary venous connection. In *Cardiac Surgery,* 2nd edition. Churchill Livingstone, New York: 1993, 609-44.
6. Kopf GS, Laks H: Atrial septal defects and cor triatriatum. In *Glenn's Thoracic and Cardiovascular Surgery,* 6th edition. Baue AE, ed. Appleton & Lange, Stamford: 1996: 1115-25.

SURGERY FOR ATRIOVENTRICULAR CANAL DEFECT

SURGICAL CONSIDERATIONS

Description: Atrioventricular (A-V) canal defects comprise a spectrum of congenital cardiac anomalies stemming from the embryonic maldevelopment of endocardial cushions. This leads to the absence of septal tissue immediately above and below the level of the A-V valves and defects in the A-V valves in continuity with these septal defects. **Partial A-V canal defects** (or **ostium primum atrial septal defects**) involve the atrial septum, while **complete A-V canal defects** involve the atrial and ventricular septa. Pathophysiologically, these defects result in L → R shunting at the atrial and/or ventricular levels, leading to pulmonary HTN and CHF. A-V valvular insufficiency is also frequently observed with these defects, contributing to the early development of CHF.

Palliative repair of A-V canal defects consists of **pulmonary artery banding** to reduce excessive pulmonary blood flow. **Palliation** is rare and is reserved for very small infants with complicating conditions, such as CHF and pneumonia. **Total correction** is now performed routinely, even in neonates. Repair consists of the closure of atrial and ventricular septal defects (VSDs) with or without closure of the defect in the anterior leaflet of the mitral valve, and repair of associated defects, such as a patent ductus arteriosus (PDA) or secundum atrial septal defect (ASD). The septal defects may be repaired with either a **"two-patch technique,"** consisting of a Dacron patch on the ventricular septum and pericardial patch on the atrial septum, or a single Dacron patch covering both atrial and ventricular septal defects. The ASD is frequently closed by placing the coronary sinus return on the left atrial side to avoid suturing in close proximity to the bundle of His.

Partial A-V canal defects: Exposure is obtained through a standard median sternotomy. CPB is instituted with aortic cross-clamping and cardioplegic arrest. Through a right atriotomy, the mitral valve cleft is sutured. A pericardial patch is placed across the top of the ventricular septum, around the coronary sinus orifice, and along the free edge of the superior portion of the ASD. The atriotomy is then closed and the aorta unclamped. Cardiac resuscitation and deairing procedures are initiated and routine closure is commenced.

Complete A-V canal defects: Following median sternotomy, CPB is instituted with aortic cross-clamping and cardioplegic arrest. Through a right atriotomy, the two-patch technique is used to close the ventricular and atrial components of the septal defect and division of the single common A-V valve into left-sided "mitral" and right-sided "tricuspid" valves. These new valves are attached to the top of the ventricular septal patch and the septal commissure in the left-sided valve is closed. Closure of the right atrium, aortic unclamping, rewarming and resuscitation of the heart are commenced and CPB is discontinued. Closure proceeds in the standard fashion.

Usual preop diagnosis: AV canal defect: common, complete and partial A-V canal; ostium primum ASD

SUMMARY OF PROCEDURE

	Partial A-V Canal Defect	Complete A-V Canal Defect
Position	Supine	⇐
Incision	Standard median sternotomy	⇐
Unique considerations	None	Repair performed through a right atriotomy; no ventriculotomies required.
Antibiotics	Cefazolin 15-30 mg/kg q 8 h	⇐
Surgical time	Aortic cross-clamp: 30-40 min Total: 2-3 h	Aortic cross-clamp: 60-80 min Total: 3-4 h
Closing considerations	Chest tube in pericardial space; temporary ventricular pacing wire; possibly right or left atrial line for monitoring	⇐
EBL	Moderate	⇐
Postop care	ICU for 1-2 d, with 12-24 h assisted ventilation; minimal need for inotropes.	1-3 d assisted ventilation; pulmonary HTN protocol, including hyperventilation and sedation; use of pulmonary vasodilators (e.g., isoproterenol, PGE_1, NO); use of inotropes for adequate CO. Avoid excessive volume to prevent distension and mitral valve regurgitation.
Mortality	0-1%	2-4%
Morbidity	Hemorrhage Infection Transient heart block	Pulmonary vasospasm Right heart dysfunction Mitral valve regurgitation Low CO Hemorrhage Heart block Residual VSD
Pain score	8-10	8-10

PATIENT POPULATION CHARACTERISTICS

Age range	1-20 yr (usually 4-5 yr)	2 mo-1 yr
Male:Female	1:1	⇐
Incidence	0.5-1% of congenital heart defects	⇐
Etiology	Frequently associated with Down syndrome: Rare (in patients with partial A-V canal defect)	Frequently associated with Down syndrome: Common (75% in patients with complete A-V canal defect)
Associated conditions	Left A-V valve insufficiency	Pulmonary HTN, left A-V valve insufficiency, minor associated cardiac anomalies (e.g., PDA or ASD)

ANESTHETIC CONSIDERATIONS

PREOPERATIVE

Pathophysiology Partial A-V canal involves a defect in the atrial septum with L→R shunting at the atrial level. There is usually a cleft in the anterior leaflet of the mitral valve causing MR. Patients with large shunts are at risk for developing pulmonary HTN. Patients with small shunts can remain asymptomatic and may present much later. Complete A-V canal involves an interatrial communication, interventricular communication cleft in the mitral valve and abnormally developed tricuspid valve. Large L→R shunts may lead to early onset of pulmonary HTN and subsequent cardiac failure. Pulmonary vascular changes are usually reversible up to 2 yr of age.

Respiratory Look for pulmonary congestion or any infectious process. Pulmonary HTN can be present in partial or complete A-V canal.

Tests: CXR: enlarged heart + increased pulmonary markings

Cardiovascular Partial A-V canal → RV volume overload and MR. Complete A-V canal → CHF and biventricular failure. Both partial and complete A-V canal are associated with Down syndrome.

Cardiovascular, cont. — **Tests:** ECG: RAE, RVE; ECHO diagnostic; cardiac cath may be indicated to assess PVR.

Down syndrome — Commonly associated with complete A-V canal defect. Mental retardation (100%), hearing loss (50%), small trachea (25%), frequent pulmonary infection, airway obstruction (intrathoracic and extrathoracic). Possibly difficult intubation in this patient population. All patients with Down syndrome should be considered at risk from atlantoaxial instability, and one should avoid excessive neck flexion or rotation.

Neurological — Neck pain, torticollis, gait disturbance, hyperreflexia, limb weakness or paresthesia suggest atlantoaxial subluxation (neurology consultation prior to surgery).

Laboratory — As indicated from H&P.

Premedication — Midazolam 0.5-0.75 mg/kg po. Occasionally, older children with Down syndrome will not cooperate for oral premed; consider ketamine (4-6 mg/kg im) + glycopyrrolate 10 μg/kg in same syringe.

INTRAOPERATIVE

Anesthetic technique: GETA ± regional anesthesia

Induction — Typically, mask halothane or sevoflurane in N_2O and O_2. If iv in place, fentanyl 10 μg/kg and pancuronium 0.2 mg/kg. Nasal intubation preferred since ETT less likely to dislodge when placing and removing TEE. Verify ETT position (see p. D-3). In children with Down syndrome, anticipate difficult airways and atlantoaxial instability. Avoid excessive neck flexion. If early or immediate extubation is planned, a regional anesthetic is placed soon after induction. In this population, candidates for early or immediate extubation have only partial A-V canals and small shunts. (See Tetralogy of Fallot Induction, p. 905).

Maintenance — In patients with regional anesthesia in whom immediate or early extubation is planned, a volatile anesthetic in O_2 is given. In patients requiring postop mechanical ventilation, fentanyl 100-200 μg/kg total, pancuronium prn and midazolam (0.1-0.2 mg/kg) ± volatile agent (FiO_2 = 1) is used for anesthesia.

Emergence — For patients with regional anesthetics and a smooth intraop course, immediate extubation can be done in a deep or awake state. Age, child's activity level and npo status must be considered to determine at what level of anesthesia a patient may be extubated. BP is tightly controlled with SNP or NTG prn. Patients extubated in deep state of anesthesia rarely require BP control with dilators. Transport to ICU.

Blood and fluid requirements — See Tetralogy of Fallot (TOF), p. 905.

Monitoring — See TOF, p. 905.

Monitoring	TEE	TEE is used to assess left A-V valve regurgitation, valvular function, residual shunt and ventricular function.
CPB	Management of CPB is discussed in Intraoperative Considerations for TOF, p. 906.	
Complications	Air embolism	Avoid air embolism in A-V canal patients (shunt reversal → paradoxical embolization).
	LVOTO	Reduce LV afterload if left A-V valve regurgitation is present.
	Ventricular dysfunction or failure	
	A-V block, sinus node dysfunction	A-V block may be temporary 2° edema and/or cardioplegic arrest. Permanent injury can occur to the conduction system at the A-V node or bundle of His with repair of the VSD. Temporary atrial and ventricular pacing wires are placed.
	Systemic desaturation	If coronary sinus drainage is directed surgically to LA, then systemic sat = 92-96%.
	Persistent bleeding	
	Hypothermia	
	Pulmonary HTN	To reduce PVR, see Post CPB, TOF, p. 906. NO may be necessary for refractory pulmonary HTN.

POSTOPERATIVE

Complications	Residual lesions → left A-V valve regurgitation, residual VSD/ASD, A-V valve stenosis	
Tests	ABG; electrolytes; Hct; coags CXR TEE	Analysis of post repair function is best done by TEE.

References

1. Baue AE, Geha AS, Hammond GL, Laks H, Naunheim KS: *Glenn's Thoracic and Cardiovascular Surgery,* 6th edition. Appleton & Lange, Stamford: 1996.
2. Castaneda AR, Jonas RA, Mayer JE Jr, Hanley FL: Atrioventricular canal defect. In *Cardiac Surgery of the Neonate and Infant.* WB Saunders, Philadelphia: 1994, 167-86.
3. Kambam J: Endocardial cushion defects. In *Cardiac Anesthesia for Infants and Children.* Kambam J, Fish FA, Merrill WH, eds. CV Mosby, St. Louis: 1994, 203-10.
4. Kirklin JW, Barrett-Boyes BG: Atrioventricular canal defect. In *Cardiac Surgery,* 2nd edition. Churchill-Livingstone, New York: 1993, 693-74.
5. Lowe DA, Stayer SA, Rehman MA: Abnormalities of the atrioventricular valves. In *Pediatric Cardiac Anesthesia,* 3rd edition. Lake CL, ed. Appleton & Lange, Stamford, CT: 1998, 407-30.
6. Stark J, Lofland GK: Atrioventricular septal defects. In *Glenn's Thoracic and Cardiovascular Surgery,* 6th edition. Baue AE, ed. Appleton & Lange, Stamford: 1996, 1163-77.
7. Vick WG, Titus JL: Defects of the atrial septum including the atrioventricular canal. In *The Science and Practice of Pediatric Cardiology.* Garson A, Bricker JT, McNamara DG, eds. Lea & Febiger, Philadelphia: 1990.

SURGERY FOR VENTRICULAR SEPTAL DEFECT

SURGICAL CONSIDERATIONS

Description: Ventricular septal defects (VSDs) are the most common congenital cardiac anomaly. Physiologically, these defects result in L→R shunting in proportion to the defect size. Untreated, this defect can lead to RV volume overload and CHF in infancy and irreversible pulmonary HTN later in life. As PVR rises, shunt reversal to a R→L shunt can occur, producing hypoxemia and cyanosis; this is known as **Eisenmenger's syndrome** and occurs in about 10% of untreated, nonrestrictive VSDs. Moderate-to-large VSDs which remain open beyond 1 yr of age should be closed. Severe, intractable CHF in infants refractory to medical therapy (i.e., diuretics, digoxin), or ↑PVR in infants > 6 mo are indications for earlier VSD repair.

Lillehei, Varco and colleagues first successfully performed VSD repairs using normothermic cross-circulation in 1955. Kirklin subsequently described successful VSD closure using extracorporeal circulation in 1957. VSD repair is performed through a median sternotomy on CPB with bicaval cannulation. In young infants (< 8 kg), profound hypothermia (18° C) and total circulatory arrest with a single venous cannula facilitate the repair. Once CPB and cardioplegic arrest have been instituted, a right atriotomy is created and the VSD is visualized by retracting the tricuspid valve leaflets. The VSD is then closed with a prosthetic patch (e.g., Gore-Tex, Dacron), with care being taken not to place sutures through the nearby conduction fiber bundles. After the repair is completed and the atriotomy is closed, the aortic cross-clamp is released, standard deairing maneuvers are performed, and CPB is discontinued. The chest is then closed in the standard fashion.

Variant procedure or approaches: Supracristal defects may be more easily exposed through a pulmonary arteriotomy, while some inferiorly located muscular VSDs may be better accessed through a right ventriculotomy.

Usual preop diagnosis: VSD

SUMMARY OF PROCEDURE

Position	Supine
Incision	Standard median sternotomy
Antibiotics	Cefazolin 15-30 mg/kg q 8 h
Surgical time	Aortic cross-clamp: 20-30 min Total: 2 h
Closing considerations	Routine closure with chest tube in the pericardial space; temporary ventricular pacing wire; possibly right/left atrial and/or pulmonary arterial lines for monitoring
EBL	Minimal-to-moderate
Postop care	Extubation in OR or within several h; 24 h monitoring in ICU. Older patients may have high left atrial pressures early after repair.
Mortality	5-10%
Morbidity	Hemorrhage Acute cardiac failure Ventricular arrhythmias Complete atrioventricular heart block Residual shunting
Pain score	8-10

PATIENT POPULATION CHARACTERISTICS

Age range	Neonate – adult
Male:Female	1:1
Incidence	20% of congenital heart defects; 2/1000 births
Associated conditions	PDA (6%); coarctation of the aorta (5%); congenital AS (2%); congenital mitral valve disease (2%); also part of other malformations, including TOF, TGA, DORV, tricuspid atresia

ANESTHETIC CONSIDERATIONS

PREOPERATIVE

Pathophysiology VSDs are classified by their location (Types I-IV) and whether shunt flow is restricted or nonrestricted. Large VSDs offer little resistance to flow (nonrestrictive) and, therefore, RV pressures = LV pressures. The Q_P/Q_S ratio or shunt is determined primarily by the ratio of PVR to SVR. In small VSDs, flow is restrictive and the Q_P/Q_S ratio is determined by the size of the defect. The RV pressure is normal-to-mildly-elevated and the Q_P/Q_S ratio is rarely > 1.5. Moderate-size VSDs cause ↑RV systolic pressure, and the Q_P/Q_S ratio is generally in the range of 2.5-3.0.

Infants with VSD will have ↑L→R shunt as their PVR decreases. At this time, symptoms of CHF may develop, and approximately 30% of these infants will require surgery. Spontaneous closure is thought to occur in 30-40% of all VSDs within the 1st yr of life. A large VSD left untreated will cause PVOD or Eisenmenger's syndrome (pulmonary HTN + R→L shunt).

Cardiovascular and respiratory Infants may present with feeding difficulty and failure to thrive (FTT). Children with small VSDs may be asymptomatic, while children with larger VSDs may have ↓exercise tolerance, fatigue, frequent URIs and Sx of CHF. A holosystolic murmur can be heard best at the left lower sternal border. Cyanosis is absent unless there is R→L shunting (suggesting pulmonary HTN).

Tests: ECG: small VSD → no changes; moderate VSD → LAE + LVH; large VSD → LAE + BVH. CXR: findings vary with size of VSD. ↑pulmonary vascular markings with ↑PA size. ECHO: diagnostic, documents size and position of VSD, valvular function, shunt magnitude and direction, and an estimate of PA pressures. Cardiac cath: Useful in selected patients–measurement of PA pressures, calculation of Q_P/Q_S ratio and PVR.

Laboratory Hct; electrolytes (children on diuretic Rx); others as indicated from H&P.

Premedication See ASD, p. 888.

INTRAOPERATIVE

Anesthetic technique: GETA ± epidural anesthesia. The anesthetic management of patients with VSD is similar to that for patients with ASD (see p. 888). Specific differences are presented below.

Blood and fluid requirements	IV: appropriate for patient size × 1-2 LR @ TKO Blood warmer T&C 1 U PRBC.	Minimize administration of iv fluids. The LV is volume-overloaded in small VSDs and both ventricles are volume-overloaded in large VSDs.
Monitoring	Standard monitors (see p. D-1). Arterial line	
	Surgical LA line Urinary catheter ACT monitoring TEE	A LA line may be placed by the surgeon if there is concern about LV dysfunction. Humidify gases to reduce heat loss during rewarming.
Pre CPB	See ASD, p. 889.	
CPB	See ASD, p. 889.	Most VSDs are closed under hypothermic conditions (25-28°). Deep hypothermic cardiac arrest is rarely used except in the smallest infants with A-V canal-type VSDs and multiple muscular septal defects.
Transition off CPB	See ASD, p. 889.	
Post CPB	Careful replacement of blood loss Maintenance of adequate filling pressure (LA = 5-10 mmHg)	
	Temporary pacemaker wires	Placed in patients with conduction disturbances; pacemaker wires also may be placed prophylactically in patients with NSR.
	TEE	✓ for residual shunt and ventricular and valvular function.
	Pulmonary HTN (see TOF, p. 906).	NO may be necessary for refractory pulmonary HTN.

POSTOPERATIVE

Complications	Persistent bleeding	
	Heart block: RBBB; bifascicular block	May appear early or later in postop course.
	Pulmonary HTN	If patient is treated with NO, monitor methemoglobin concentration.
	Ventricular dysfunction/failure	Especially in patients with ventriculotomy
	Residual shunt	Dx: TEE
Tests	ABGs Electrolytes; Hct; coags prn CXR	

References

1. Baue AE, Geha AS, Hammond GL, Laks H, Naunheim KS: *Glenn's Thoracic and Cardiovascular Surgery,* 6th edition. Appleton & Lange, Stamford, CT: 1996.
2. Castaneda AR, Jonas RA, Mayer JE Jr, Hanley FL: Ventricular septal defect. In *Cardiac Surgery of the Neonate and Infant.* WB Saunders, Philadelphia: 1994, 187-201.
3. Cooper JR, Goldstein MT: Septal and endocardial cushion defects and double outlet right ventricle perioperative management. In *Pediatric Cardiac Anesthesia,* 3rd edition. Lake CL, ed. Appleton & Lange, Stamford, CT: 1998, 285-301.
4. Kambam J: Endocardial cushion defects. In *Cardiac Anesthesia for Infants and Children.* Kambam J, Fish FA, Merrill WH, eds. CV Mosby, St. Louis: 1994, 203-10.
5. Kirklin JW, Barrett-Boyes BG: Ventricular septal defect. In *Cardiac Surgery,* 2nd edition. Churchill-Livingstone, New York: 1993, 749-824.
6. Lowe DA, Stayer SA, Rehman MA: Abnormalities of the atrioventricular valves. In *Pediatric Cardiac Anesthesia,* 3rd edition. Lake CL, ed. Appleton & Lange, Stamford, CT: 1998, 407-30.
7. Tchervenkov CI, Shum-Tim D: Ventricular septal defect. In *Glenn's Thoracic and Cardiovascular Surgery,* 6th edition. Baue AE, ed. Appleton & Lange, Stamford: 1996, 1127-36.

SURGERY FOR PATENT DUCTUS ARTERIOSUS

SURGICAL CONSIDERATIONS

Description: Patent ductus arteriosus (PDA) is usually located between the proximal descending thoracic aorta and the main PA. Pathophysiologically, this results in L→R shunting and augmented pulmonary blood flow which, if left untreated, may lead to pulmonary HTN and CHF. A relatively common congenital heart anomaly, comprising 12-15% of CHDs, PDA was first successfully ligated by Gross in 1938. Early administration of indomethacin may promote ductal closure in many premature infants, obviating surgical intervention; however, this mode of therapy is generally contraindicated in the setting of renal insufficiency or intracranial bleeding.

Surgical ductal closure is indicated for significant L→R shunting. The ductus usually can be exposed via a small, left, posterolateral thoracotomy in the 4th intercostal space without CPB. The ductus is identified and dissected, with special care taken to avoid injury to the phrenic and left recurrent laryngeal nerves (Fig 12.3-1). The ductus is interrupted with a surgical clip in neonates; in older children, the ductus is divided between vascular clamps and the ends are oversewn. A small thoracostomy tube is placed, and the thoracotomy is closed. The thoracostomy tube is removed in the OR immediately after the chest is closed or a few h later.

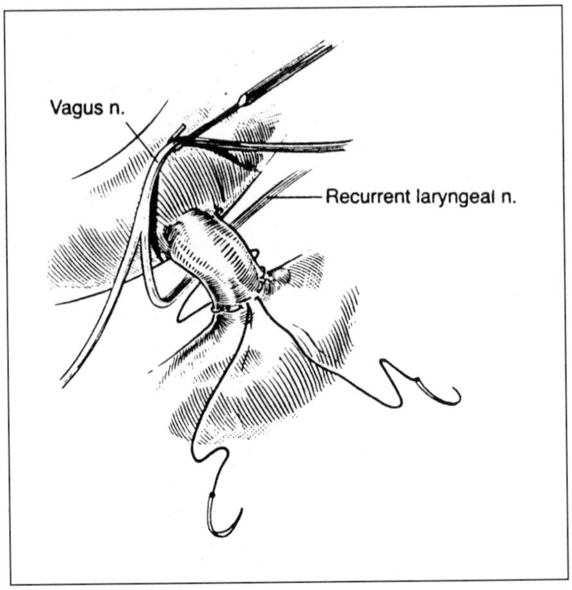

Figure 12.3-1. Ligature of PDA. Note vagus and recurrent laryngeal nerves. (Reproduced with permission from Castaneda AR, et al: Patent ductus arteriosus. In *Cardiac Surgery of the Neonate and Infant.* WB Saunders, Philadelphia: 1994, 209.

Variant procedure or approaches: Percutaneous coil embolization and thoracoscopic clip ligation are alternative approaches for PDA closure.

Usual preop diagnosis: PDA

SUMMARY OF PROCEDURE

Position	Right lateral decubitus
Incision	Left posterolateral thoracotomy, 4th intercostal space
Antibiotics	Cefazolin 15-30 mg q 8 h
Surgical time	30-60 min
Closing considerations	Routine closure with left thoracostomy tube
EBL	Minimal
Postop care	24 h observation in ICU; extubation in the OR or within several h
Mortality	Rare
Morbidity	Hemorrhage, recurrent laryngeal or phrenic nerve injury
Pain score	6-8

PATIENT POPULATION CHARACTERISTICS

Age range	1 mo–adulthood
Male:Female	1:2
Incidence	12-15% of congenital heart defects
Etiology	Failure of complete ductal closure

ANESTHETIC CONSIDERATIONS

PREOPERATIVE

Two different patient populations present for PDA ligation: the term-infant or child for elective closure and the premature infant requiring more immediate surgery. Closure of PDA can be done in the catheterization lab via transcatheter closure or in the OR using video-assisted thoracoscopic (VAT) techniques or an open thoracotomy. The following discussion for anesthetic management covers open thoracotomy only. The premature infant requiring surgical closure of PDA typically presents because indomethacin Rx has failed or is contraindicated. Premature infants often have primary pulmonary disease and multisystem organ problems. Most of these infants are mechanically ventilated, have iv access established and require hemodynamic support. To avoid a hazardous transport to the OR with an unstable infant, the surgical closure of PDA is often done in the NICU. The ductus functionally closes in the majority of term infants within 24 h after birth. If the ductus remains patent in the full-term infant, it is unlikely to close spontaneously. This is in contrast to premature infants in whom spontaneous closure frequently occurs as maturation continues. Permanent anatomic closure usually occurs within the first mo.

PDA results in a shunt between aorta and PA (L→R). As the PVR ↓ postnatally, the shunt will ↑. The hemodynamic manifestations of a small PDA are minimal. If the ductus is large, the shunt flow is determined by the PVR-SVR difference. L→R shunt → severe CHF + ↑PVR (as early as 6 mo) → progression to Eisenmenger's syndrome.

Cardiovascular Clinical presentation depends on the size of the ductus. An infant with a large ductus can present in CHF with tachypnea, tachycardia, diaphoresis, failure to thrive (FTT) and hepatosplenomegaly. A continuous systolic murmur heard best at the left upper sternal border and widened pulse pressure with bounding pulses may be present. The older infant may have minimal shunt 2° ↑PVR. There may be lower body cyanosis 2° ductal flow becoming R→L. A small PDA may be detected by a murmur only.

Tests: CXR: Normal or cardiomegaly with ↑PA size and ↑pulmonary vascular markings. ECG: Normal or LVH/BVH. ECHO diagnostic: documents patency, evaluates left-sided cardiac chamber sizes and aortic arch anatomy and estimates size of shunt. Cardiac cath: Rarely indicated except for defining status of pulmonary vasculature. Contraindicated for premature infants.

Laboratory Hct; others as indicated from H&P.

Premedication Not indicated in premature infants. Midazolam 0.5-0.7 mg orally 30 min prior to induction for children > 9 mo having routine PDA closure.

INTRAOPERATIVE

Anesthetic technique: GETA ± epidural anesthesia. Children presenting for elective operation generally tolerate an inhalation induction with sevoflurane or halothane in 50% N_2O + O_2. Once the patient is anesthetized, iv access is established, followed by oral intubation, either with deep volatile anesthesia or with administration of a muscle relaxant (e.g., vecuronium 1 mg/kg) and then remifentanil (1 μg/kg). Administering the muscle relaxant prior to the narcotic avoids chest-wall rigidity. Most children presenting for elective closure of PDA are candidates for epidural anesthesia unless they have significant pulmonary HTN (see Epidural anesthesia section in TOF, p. 905). In patients > 25 kg, placement of a DLT for selective ventilation of the right lung will improve surgical access. Avoid hyperoxia and hyperventilation → ↑SVR + ↓PVR → ↑ L→R shunt. In neonates, because of their high PVR, it is important to avoid further ↑ PVR (hypoventilation and hypoxemia) because the L→R shunt can reverse to a R→L shunt.

Maintenance In patients for whom immediate postop extubation is planned, anesthesia is maintained with isoflurane in air + O_2. In premature infants or patients with pulmonary HTN, a high-dose narcotic technique (fentanyl 50 μg/kg) is appropriate.

Emergence Patients may be extubated awake or in a deep plane of anesthesia. An effective regional anesthetic is essential for early awake extubation. BP is controlled with SNP or NTG infusion. Patients extubated while deeply anesthetized rarely require BP control. For patients returning to the NICU intubated and ventilated, portable monitoring equipment, O_2, bag/mask airway equipment and emergency drugs should be available during transport.

Blood and fluid requirements	IV: 22-24 × 1-2 Continue iv dextrose. Blood warmer T&C 1 U PRBC.	Blood loss may become significant if the ductus is torn during ligation. Have blood ready for rapid transfusion.
	✓ for air bubbles.	Clear air bubbles from iv tubing and stopcocks (potential bidirectional shunt → paradoxical embolism).
Monitoring	Standard monitors (see p. D-1). ± Arterial line ± CVP line	Place BP cuff on the right arm and pulse oximeter on the foot to monitor flow in the ascending and descending aorta. Inadvertent aortic occlusion → ↓LE pulses/pres-

Monitoring, cont.		sure/perfusion. Inadvertent PA occlusion → ↓SpO_2 + ↓$ETCO_2$. Bradycardia may occur during manipulation of the ductus and should be treated with atropine (0.01-0.03 mg/kg). An esophageal stethoscope allows auscultation of the murmur, which will disappear when the ductus is ligated. The diastolic BP will ↑ postligation.
Positioning	✓ and pad pressure points. ✓ eyes.	
Complications	↓SpO_2/↓HR Occlusion of aorta or PA Torn ductus → hemorrhage Residual PDA Lung trauma ± pneumothorax Cardiac tamponade	Indicates compromised infant. Should hand ventilate; may require stopping surgery and removal of retractors.

POSTOPERATIVE

Complications	Pneumonia Chylothorax Recurrent laryngeal nerve injury Vagus nerve injury	
Tests	Hct CXR	Other tests as indicated.

References

1. Baue AE, Geha AS, Hammond GL, Laks H, Naunheim KS: *Glenn's Thoracic and Cardiovascular Surgery,* 6th edition. Appleton & Lange, Stamford: 1996.
2. Castaneda AR, Jonas RA, Mayer JE Jr, Hanley FL: Patent ductus arteriosus. In *Cardiac Surgery of the Neonate and Infant.* WB Saunders, Philadelphia: 1994, 203-13.
3. Haas G: Patent ductus arteriosus and aortopulmonary window. In *Glenn's Thoracic and Cardiovascular Surgery,* 6th edition. Baue AE, ed. Appleton & Lange, Stamford: 1996, 1137-61.
4. Kambam J: Endocardial cushion defects. In *Cardiac Anesthesia for Infants and Children.* Kambam J, Fish FA, Merrill WH, eds. CV Mosby, St. Louis: 1994, 203-10.
5. Kirklin JW, Barrett-Boyes BG: Patent ductus arteriosus. In *Cardiac Surgery,* 2nd edition. Churchill-Livingstone, New York: 1993, 841-59.
6. Rosen DA, Rosen KR: Anomalies of the aortic arch and valve. In *Cardiac Anesthesia,* 3rd edition. Lake CL, ed. Appleton & Lange, Stamford: 1997.

SURGERY FOR COARCTATION OF THE AORTA

SURGICAL CONSIDERATIONS

Description: Coarctation of the aorta is a congenital narrowing of the upper descending aorta, typically located between the left subclavian artery and the ligamentum/ductus arteriosus (Fig 12.3-2). Coexisting intracardiac defects are not uncommon. Surgical repair of aortic coarctation, first performed by Crafoord in 1944, consisted of resection of the narrowed aortic segment followed by an **end-to-end repair.** The same year, Blalock and Park proposed an alternative technique in which the left subclavian artery was divided distally and sutured into the descending thoracic aorta, creating a bypass. Subsequently, the use of an onlay prosthetic graft to widen the area of coarctation and the use of a **subclavian artery flap** were described by Waldhausen. Prosthetic interposition tube graft repairs have been described in patients with diffuse aortic hypoplasia. Patients with an associated intracardiac L→R shunt (e.g., VSD) may require concomitant pulmonary artery banding following repair of the coarctation.

In infants, a left posterolateral thoracotomy approach is used. The lung is retracted anteriorly and the pleura is incised vertically over the aorta along the left subclavian artery. The aorta and ductus/ligamentum arteriosus are cleared above and below the level of coarctation. The transverse aortic arch is then clamped proximally and distally to the coarctation. The ductus/ligamentum arteriosus is ligated and the coarctation excised. The proximal anastomosis may extend under the aortic arch. If a subclavian flap angioplasty is performed, the distal left subclavian artery is ligated and opened longitudinally down into the aorta, across the coarctation and into the descending aorta. Patch aortoplasty is performed by creating a longitudinal aortotomy above and below the coarctation and suturing a generously sized patch onto the defect. Following repair, the aortic cross-clamps are released, with careful monitoring of distal aortic pressures. The pleura is then sutured over the aorta and standard closure is commenced.

Variant procedure or approaches: In children or adults, a left posterolateral thoracotomy is used, the lung is retracted anteriorly, and the pleura is opened longitudinally. The aorta, including the distal transverse arch and proximal left subclavian artery, is dissected clear. Most repairs then proceed with resection of the coarctation and end-to-end anastomosis. Occasionally, an onlay prosthetic patch or tube graft (for diffuse aortic narrowing) are used for repair.

Usual preop diagnosis: Coarctation of the aorta

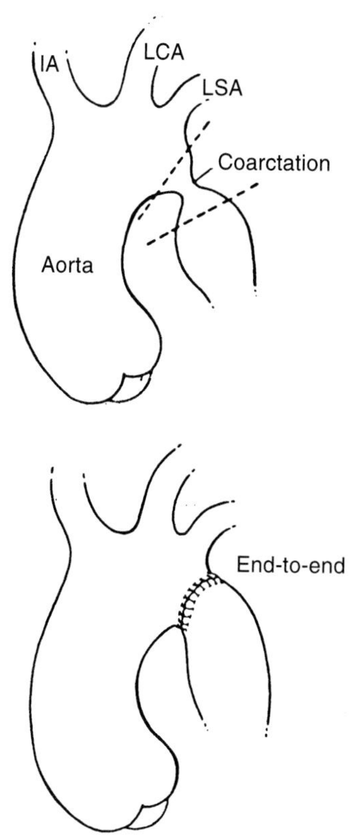

→ **Figure 12.3-2.** Coarctation of the aorta. (Reproduced with permission from Hardy JD: *Hardy's Textbook of Surgery*, 2nd edition. JB Lippincott, Philadelphia: 1988.)

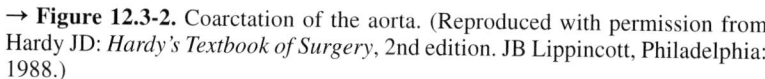

SUMMARY OF PROCEDURE

	Infant	Child or Adult
Position	Right lateral decubitus	⇐
Incision	Posterolateral left thoracotomy, 3rd-4th interspace	⇐
Unique considerations	For subclavian flap angioplasty, avoid iv or arterial lines in left arm. If arterial line is in an upper or lower extremity, the opposite site should have a BP cuff for simultaneous monitoring.	Collateral circulation is adequate if distal aortic MAP > 50 mmHg. In rare cases of inadequate collateral circulation, left atrial-to-descending-aorta or femoral bypass should be considered. Mild hypothermia of 33-34° may be useful.
Antibiotics	Cefazolin 15-30 mg/kg q 8 h	⇐
Surgical time	Aortic cross-clamp: 12-20 min Total: 1-1.5 h	Aortic cross-clamp: 15-30 min Total: 2-2.5 h
Closing considerations	Thoracostomy tube	⇐
EBL	Minimal	1-2 ml/kg
Postop care	Early extubation in ICU; consider intercostal nerve block or epidural analgesia; careful control of MAP may require SNP or esmolol infusion.	⇐
Mortality	2-4%	< 1%
Morbidity	Bleeding	⇐
	Infection	⇐
	Paraplegia: < 0.5%	⇐
Pain score	8-10	8-10

PATIENT POPULATION CHARACTERISTICS

	Infant	Child or Adult
Age range	1 wk–1 yr	1 yr–adult
Male:Female	2:1; 1:1 for coarctations with associated defects	⇐
Incidence	5-8% of congenital heart defects	5% of congenital heart defects
Etiology	Possibly due to localized aortic narrowing with ductal closure	⇐
Associated conditions	PDA (50%); VSD (36%); congenital mitral stenosis (7%); single ventricle (7%); TGA/VSD (7%)	Usually an isolated defect. When repaired at a later age, bicuspid aortic valve.

ANESTHETIC CONSIDERATIONS

PREOPERATIVE

Pathology Coarctation, or narrowing of a portion of the aortic arch and/or isthmus, most commonly occurs at the junction of the ductus arteriosus. Flow reduction also can occur as a result of a more proximal obstruction, such as at the aortic valve or LV outflow tract (LVOT), or as a result of a defect (e.g., VSD) causing L→R shunt. The clinical presentation of the neonate or infant with coarctation depends upon: (1) degree of obstruction, (2) rate at which high-grade stenosis develops, (3) patency of the ductus, (4) PVR, and (5) associated cardiac anomalies. Patients with mild-to-moderate stenosis and no associated abnormalities will be asymptomatic with HTN and diminished lower extremity pulses. The ductus will often be closed. Neonates with critical stenosis will demonstrate ductal-dependent aortic flow. With the ductus open and ↑PVR, the neonate may be asymptomatic. R→L ductal flow, enhanced by ↑PVR, may result in palpable lower extremity pulses, obscuring the diagnosis. As the ductus closes, lower torso hypoperfusion will become significant (acidemia, gut ischemia, cold lower extremities). In the absence of a VSD, rapid ductal closure will result in an acute rise in LV afterload without time for compensatory LVH, causing LV failure. If there is a significant VSD, ductal closure and a concomitant ↓PVR will result in a huge L→R shunt and LV failure from volume overload. In infants with more complex associated anomalies (e.g., cerebral aneurysms, bicuspid aortic valve), the coarctation is just one of several problems that need careful consideration.

Respiratory In the neonate, dyspnea and tachypnea may suggest LV failure.
Tests: CXR (cardiomegaly, characteristic aorta, PE)

Cardiovascular **Neonates:** Patients present with ↑BP, a pressure gradient between upper and lower extremities and a systolic murmur. Most neonates also present with "critical" coarctation and are ductal dependent. If the ductus is closing, PGE_1 may reopen the duct or at least relax juxtaductal tissue and improve perfusion. PGE_1 treatment may allow time for ECHO assessment of associated lesions.
Symptomatic infants: Young infants admitted with Sx of shock are medically managed until they have stabilized. Generally, small or moderate-size VSDs will not be addressed at first operation. If an associated lesion is to be repaired with the coarctation, the approach will be through a median sternotomy, using CPB.
Asymptomatic infants: Collateral flow may reduce the pressure gradient, thereby eliminating the murmur. As a general rule, surgery is indicated when ECHO or MRI scan demonstrates > 50% narrowing at the coarctation site, or > 20 mmHg resting gradient by cuff measurement.
Older children: Often present with HTN, epistaxis or headache, and diminished or absent femoral pulses. Often, they are on β-blockers or Ca^{++} channel blockers. The indication for operation is similar to that of asymptomatic infants. Controversy exists as to the long-term benefit of repair of moderate coarctation in older children, as systemic HTN and LVH frequently do not resolve following repair.
Tests: ECHO; ECG; ABG; CXR—rib notching 2° collateral vessels

Renal Renal failure may occur 2° CHF/renal hypoperfusion.
Tests: BUN, Cr, electrolytes

Laboratory Hct and others as indicated by H&P.

Premedication Generally not necessary for children < 9 mo old. Not appropriate in severely ill infants. Otherwise, midazolam 0.5-0.7 mg/kg po (maximum of 15 mg). For children > 25 kg, diazepam 5-10 mg po or other routine preanesthetic medication.

INTRAOPERATIVE

Anesthetic technique: GETA ± epidural anesthesia

Induction The type of induction must take into consideration patient's age, severity of coarctation, cardiac function and associated problems (e.g., ASD/VSD). In very sick neonates and symptomatic infants, an iv induction with fentanyl 10 μg/kg and vecuronium 0.1 mg/kg is appropriate. Avoid ↓SVR and myocardial depression while maintaining a normal HR. Inhalation induction (sevoflurane or halothane in 50% N_2O and O_2) is well tolerated in asymptomatic patients. IV access is established and followed by muscle relaxation and oral intubation (nasal intubation if postop ventilation is anticipated). Patients may have an epidural anesthetic placed to help control BP during surgery as well as provide postop analgesia (see p. 905). Regional anesthesia in coarctation patients, however, is controversial because coincidental neurologic injury may occur when cord blood flow is decreased from aortic cross-clamping. A standard induction in older children may be appropriate (see p. D-2). In most infants and children, single-lumen ETT is sufficient. In children > 25 kg, selective ventilation of the right lung with a DLT will facilitate surgery.

Maintenance When early postop extubation is planned, maintain anesthesia with a volatile agent (e.g., isoflurane) in N_2O/O_2. A high-dose narcotic technique (50-100 μg/kg fentanyl ± volatile agent) is appropriate for critically ill patients. Consider mild hypothermia (34-35°C) for CNS protection. The operation is usually done through a left thoracotomy. The aortic arch, isthmus and descending aorta are mobilized. 100 U/kg of heparin may be given. The ductus arteriosus is ligated, then the aortic arch and descending aorta are occluded. The anesthesiologist should observe the arterial line trace closely during proximal occlusion and immediately inform the surgeon of any damping. Upper and lower extremity cuff pressures are measured. In our experience, no single objective method exists to assess the adequacy of repair in the OR. The most important factor is the feeling by the surgeon that the best possible technical repair was performed. Concern should be raised if: (1) the surgeon feels that the technical reconstruction was suboptimal, (2) the cuff gradient or proximal/distal arterial line gradient is substantially > 20 mmHg, (3) the surgeon feels a harsh thrill at the level of the suture line, or (4) there is a "diastolic runoff" pattern on TEE.

Emergence Infants and children undergoing elective operation usually can be extubated in the OR. In neonates or infants with compromised cardiac function, extubation should be delayed until their clinical status has improved. SNP, dopamine or milrinone are usually continued postop and the patient gradually weaned. In young infants, systolic pressure consistently > 120 mmHg should be treated. A chest tube is left in place to monitor blood loss, or the appearance of a chylous effusion.

Blood and fluid requirements

IV: appropriate for patient size × 1-2
LR @ TKO (D-5 LR in neonates)
Blood warmer
T&C 1-2 U.

As a rule, infants and children undergoing coarctation repair will not require transfusion. Infrequently, however, sudden and substantial blood loss can occur, necessitating rapid transfusion. Adequate iv access, and immediate availability of blood is essential in this operation.

Monitoring

Standard monitors (see p. D-1).
RUE arterial line
± CVP
BP cuffs × 2 (UE + LE)
± SSEP

BP must be monitored above and below to level of coarctation. A right, radial arterial line allows BP monitoring during occlusion of the aortic arch. If a percutaneous radial arterial line cannot be placed, a surgical cutdown should be performed or a right axillary arterial line should be placed. Both upper and lower extremity cuff pressures should be monitored to avoid HTN above and hypotension below the cross-clamp, and to assess the repair.
✓ ABG, glucose, Hct at intervals.

Control of BP

Anesthetic depth
SNP

In neonates and infants, GA is usually sufficient to control BP during aortic cross-clamp; however, SNP may be necessary to control BP in some patients. In infants with

Control of BP, cont.		a large VSD, extreme ↑afterload will be prevented by the L→R shunt → ↑pulmonary blood flow → ↓systemic blood flow.
Aortic cross-clamping	±Heparin 100 U/kg Ductus arteriosus ligated Aorta cross-clamped × 2 ✓ arterial line for damping. Ischemia time = 10-20 min Maintain distal perfusion. Lactic acidosis → ↓SVR + ↓BP.	Aortic cross-clamping presents an acute afterload to the LV. Ischemia may occur → ↓ contractility and ± VF. Consider low-dose inotropic support. Right RA damping may suggest ↓CBF 2° innominate artery occlusion. Maintain normocarbia. After the clamp is removed, lactic acid washout occurs → ↓SVR + ↓BP (usually transient, no Rx required).
Positioning	✓ and pad pressure points. ✓ eyes.	
Complications	Spinal cord ischemia HTN Bleeding Hypothermia Residual coarction	

POSTOPERATIVE

Complications	Paraplegia	Incidence = 0.14-0.4%. The cause is likely 2° spinal cord ischemia. If a regional anesthetic was placed preop, spinal or epidural hematoma must be r/o.
	HTN Bleeding	
	GI bleed	Occurs infrequently. Attributable to mesenteric arteritis.
	Abdominal pain and ileus Recurrent laryngeal or phrenic nerve injury Chylous effusion Residual or recurrent coarction	
Tests	CXR, Hct, ABGs	
Pain management	Epidural opiates ± local anesthesia	Adequate analgesia is helpful for controlling HTN.

References

1. Backer CL, Mavroudis C: Coarctation of the aorta and interrupted aortic arch. In *Glenn's Thoracic and Cardiovascular Surgery,* 6th edition. Baue AE, ed. Appleton & Lange, Stamford: 1996, 1253-69.
2. Baue AE, Geha AS, Hammond GL, Laks H, Naunheim KS: *Glenn's Thoracic and Cardiovascular Surgery,* 6th edition. Appleton & Lange, Stamford, 1996.
3. Castaneda AR, Jonas RA, Mayer JE Jr., Hanley FL: Aortic coarctation. In *Cardiac Surgery of the Neonate and Infant.* WB Saunders, Philadelphia: 1994, 333-52.
4. Kambam J: Endocardial cushion defects. In *Cardiac Anesthesia for Infants and Children.* Kambam J, Fish FA, Merrill WH, eds. CV Mosby, St. Louis: 1994, 203-10.
5. Kirklin JW, Barrett-Boyes BG: Coarctation of the aorta. In *Cardiac Surgery,* 2nd edition. Churchill-Livingstone, New York: 1993, 1263-1326.
6. Morriss MJH, McNamara DG: Coarctation of the aorta and interrupted aortic arch. In *Science and Practice of Pediatric Cardiology.* Garson A, Bricker JT, McNamara DG, eds. Lea & Febiger, Philadelphia: 1990.
7. Rosen DA, Rosen KR: Anomalies of the aortic arch and valve. In *Pediatric Cardiac Anesthesia,* 3rd edition. Lake CL, ed. Appleton & Lange, Stamford: 1997, 431-70.

SURGERY FOR TETRALOGY OF FALLOT

SURGICAL CONSIDERATIONS

Description: In **tetralogy of Fallot (TOF)**, the RV infundibulum is underdeveloped, resulting in RV outflow tract obstruction (RVOTO), a large malalignment (overriding aorta) VSD, RVH (see Fig 12.3-3) and, occasionally, an ASD (pentalogy of Fallot). TOF is the most common cyanotic congenital cardiac defect, comprising approximately 10% of surgically correctable defects. Pathophysiologically, RVOTO leads to significant R→L shunting across a nonrestrictive VSD, which, in turn, leads to inadequate pulmonary blood flow and varying degrees of cyanosis. The variation in presentation depends primarily on the type of RVOTO.

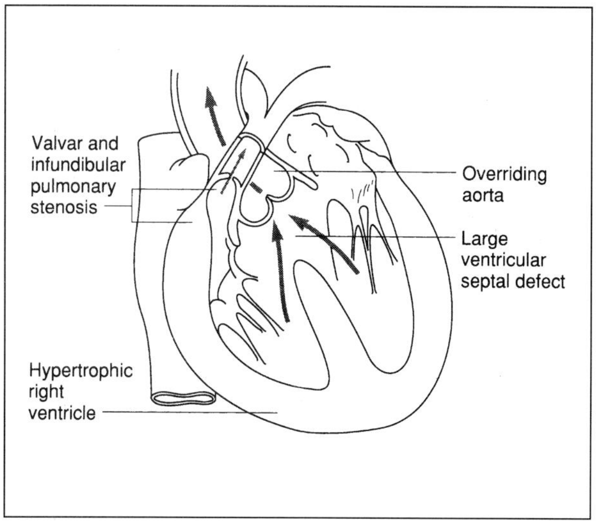

Figure 12.3-3. Anatomic features of tetralogy of Fallot. The primary morphologic abnormality, anterior and superior displacement of the infundibular septum, results in malalignment VSD, overriding the aortic valve and obstructing RV outflow. RV hypertrophy is a secondary occurrence. (Reproduced with permission from Greenfield LJ, et al, eds: *Surgery: Scientific Principles and Practice*, 2nd edition. Lippincott-Raven Publishers, 1997, 1489.)

Patients with TOF were first treated palliatively beginning in 1944, with the introduction of the **Blalock-Taussig** (B-T) systemic-to-pulmonary artery shunt. This procedure augments pulmonary blood flow and, hence, systemic oxygenation. Currently, however, most cases of TOF are treated routinely with early complete correction between 3-12 mo of age. Initial palliation with the Blalock-Taussig procedure is now reserved for patients with severe pulmonary arterial hypoplasia and/or an anomalous left anterior descending coronary artery originating from the right coronary artery.

Surgical correction is performed through a standard median sternotomy on standard CPB with moderate hypothermia. During cooling, the modified Blalock-Taussig shunt, if present, is ligated and divided, followed by aortic cross-clamping, cardioplegic arrest, and topical cooling. The pulmonary valve and RVOT are accessed through a longitudinal pulmonary arteriotomy and the tricuspid valve (via a right atriotomy), respectively. RVOTO is treated as necessary by infundibular muscle resection, pulmonary valvotomy or valvectomy, and patch augmentation of the main PA or its branches. Autologous pericardium, Gore-Tex or other type of biologic membrane material may be used for patch widening the RVOT at any level, from the RV to the PAs. The VSD, accessed through the tricuspid valve, is closed with a Dacron patch in the standard fashion, with care being taken to avoid injury to the bundle of His.

Variant procedure or approaches: In patients with severe hypoplasia or atresia of the RVOT, or in patients with an anomalous origin of the LAD coronary artery from the right coronary artery, a **Rastelli procedure** is performed. This operation consists of patch closure of the VSD and reconstruction of the RVOT in which a conduit, in the form of a cryopreserved homograft or valved prosthesis, is placed between the RV and the PA.

Usual preop diagnosis: TOF; cyanotic CHD; severe cyanotic spells; failure to thrive (FTT)

SUMMARY OF PROCEDURE

	Neonate Repair	Infant and Adult Repair With Standard CPB
Position	Supine	⇐
Incision	Standard median sternotomy	⇐
Unique considerations	R→L shunt → systemic embolization	⇐
Antibiotics	Cefazolin 15-30 mg/kg q 8 h	⇐
Surgical time	Aortic cross-clamp: 60 min	60-90 min
	CPB: 80-100 min	80-120 min
	Total: 3-4 h	3-4 h
Closing considerations	Chest tube in pericardial (and possibly pleural) space, if opened; temporary ventricular pacing wires; possibly right- or left-atrial line for monitoring.	⇐

	Neonate Repair	Infant and Adult Repair With Standard CPB
EBL	Moderate	⇐
Postop care	NICU × 2-3 d. 1-2 d assisted ventilation; inotropes for RV dysfunction.	PICU/SICU for 2-3 d
Mortality	4-5%	2-4%
Morbidity	Hemorrhage	⇐
	Infection	⇐
	Low CO	⇐
	Stroke	⇐
	Heart block	⇐
	Residual VSD	⇐
	Transient, right-side CHF	⇐
Pain score	8-10	8-10

PATIENT POPULATION CHARACTERISTICS

Age range 2 mo-65 yr (usually < 5 yr)

Male:Female 3:2

Incidence 10% of congenital cardiac defects

Etiology No apparent correlation with any specific genetic disorder; higher than expected prevalence of older maternal age at time of conception of affected children.

Associated conditions A-V canal; PDA; previous systemic-to-pulmonary arterial shunt; anomalous left coronary artery from pulmonary artery (ALCAPA); metabolic acidosis (profound hypoxia); right-sided aortic arch

---

ANESTHETIC CONSIDERATIONS

PREOPERATIVE

Pathophysiology VSD + RV outflow obstruction = R→L shunting → systemic desaturation (hypoxemia) → further ↑R→L shunting by:
- ↑systemic venous return (tachypnea)
- ↑RVOTO (↑↑ in PVR, infundibular spasm, volume depletion)
- ↓SVR (acidosis, arteriolar dilation)

"TET" spells **Hypercyanotic ("TET") spells:** etiology uncertain. Probably initiated by ↑O_2 demand (e.g., 2° crying, feeding, exercise) → ↓PaO_2, ↓pH and ↑$PaCO_2$ → ↑RR → ↑venous return + ↑R→L shunt. Volume depletion, infundibular spasm and ventricular dysfunction also may initiate an episode. Preventive measures: sedative premed to ↓ anxiety and ↓ O_2 consumption. Keep patient hydrated. Rx: Rapid and vigorous treatment often essential to break a potentially fatal cycle.
- "Squatting" (knees-to-chest) → ↑SVR and ↓venous return → ↓ R→L shunting.
- Phenylephrine bolus (10 μg/kg) → ↑SVR. Infusion @ 2-5 μg/kg/min may be necessary.
- $NaHCO_3$ 1-2 mEq/kg → correction of acidosis → ↑SVR.
- Propranolol (β-blockade) → ↓HR and ↓inotropy → ↑RVESV and ↓RVOTO → ↓ R→L shunt.
- Morphine sedation (0.1 mg/kg) → ↓infundibular spasm, → ↓R→L shunt.
- Hyperventilation → ↓$PaCO_2$ → ↓PVR. Give supplemental O_2. Manual abdominal compression → ↑SVR.

Respiratory Infectious/asthmatic pulmonary processes will complicate preop and postop cardiopulmonary function. Optimize pulmonary function preop.
Tests: CXR: ↓pulmonary vascular markings and characteristic heart shape.

Cardiovascular CHF is rare in young patients except in infants without a pulmonary valve, but more common in older children/adults 2° RV cardiomyopathy, chronic hypoxia and functionally induced aortic insufficiency. An understanding of the patient's anatomic defects and their pathophysiology (e.g., is RVOTO fixed or dynamic?) is essential for formulating the anesthetic plan.

Cardiovascular, cont.

Tests: ABG; ECG: ✓ for RVH, right axis deviation (RAD) ± complete or incomplete RBBB. CXR: ✓ heart size, "coeur en sabot" (elevation of apex 2° RVH, RAE). Cardiac cath and ECHO: Locate site of pulmonary outflow obstruction, VSD, bronchopulmonary collaterals, PDA, abnormal patency of previous surgical shunts (e.g., B-T shunt). Define aortic arch anatomy, abnormal coronary or subclavian arteries, tricuspid regurgitation/aortic insufficiency (TR/AI), ventricular function.

Hematologic

Polycythemia (typical with chronic O_2 sat < 90%) → ↑blood viscosity → thromboembolic events. Polycythemia → ↓Plt + coagulopathy. Extreme polycythemia (> 70) may require isovolemic hemodilution preop or intraop.
Tests: CBC; Plt; bleeding time; coagulation profile

Laboratory

Electrolytes if on diuretics; otherwise, tests as indicated from H&P.

Premedication

As required to ↓ anxiety, avoid TET spells and facilitate separation from parents. Midazolam 0.5-0.75 mg po 30 min prior to induction.

INTRAOPERATIVE

Anesthetic technique: GETA ± regional anesthesia/analgesia. Children are brought into prewarmed OR (80°F, isothermal for infants). If iv is placed preinduction (implying very fragile hemodynamics), it will be used for iv induction, thereby avoiding potent inhalational agents. Avoid air bubbles in iv tubing/stopcocks. DHCA may be required to facilitate surgical repair in some patients.

Induction

Typically mask induction with halothane or sevoflurane, O_2 ± N_2O. If iv in place, fentanyl (10 μg/kg) and pancuronium (0.2 mg/kg) ± volatile agent. Avoid ↓↓SVR. Intubation via nasal route (ETT less likely to be dislodged when placing and removing TEE). Verify ETT position (see p. D-3). For children in whom early or immediate ("on the table") extubation is planned, a regional anesthetic is placed soon after induction. In older children and adults, the regional block is often placed before induction. In any case, the block should be placed at least 1 h before heparinization. This technique is controversial because of the risk of epidural or spinal hematoma; more than 250 epidural blocks have been done at Stanford without evidence of hematoma or other complications.

Epidural analgesia

Single-shot or catheter techniques are acceptable. In single-dose epidurals, morphine sulfate is generally used because it is longer acting. For spinal anesthesia at L_{2-5}, use 0.5% tetracaine 0.2 mg/kg + 5 μg/kg of preservative-free morphine. Our preferred regional technique is a thoracic epidural at T_{6-12}, using 0.25% bupivacaine (0.5 ml/kg) + hydromorphone (5-10 μg/kg). This approach provides: (1) segmental anesthesia at level of incision; (2) short threading distance for catheter and, therefore, less vein disruption; (3) decreased incidence of paresthesia; (4) no LE motor blockade—can test motion early; (5) better analgesia.

Maintenance

In patients with regional anesthesia and where extubation is planned, anesthetic is maintained with isoflurane or sevoflurane—otherwise fentanyl (100-200 μg/kg total, in divided doses), pancuronium (0.2 mg/kg prn), midazolam (0.1-0.2 mg/kg as hemodynamically tolerated) ± volatile agent. FiO_2 = 1. TET spells can occur 2° surgical manipulation. Rx as in preop spells ± direct aortic compression.

Emergence

For patients with regional anesthesia and a smooth intraop course, immediate extubation can be done in a deep or awake state. Age, child's activity level and npo status must be considered to determine at what level of anesthesia a patient may be extubated. BP is tightly controlled with SNP or NTG. Patients extubated in deep state of anesthesia rarely require BP control with vasodilators. Patients requiring postop ventilation are transported to the ICU intubated and ventilated.

Blood and fluid requirements

IV: 22-24 ga × 2
LR @ TKO
T&C PRBC or whole blood.
Warm fluids.
Humidify and warm gases.

Blood in OR before incision. For redo chests, make blood ready for immediate administration. Avoid air bubbles: R→L shunt → systemic embolization of air.

Monitoring

Standard monitors (see p. D-1).
Urinary catheter
Arterial line (usually radial)
CVP line: 4 Fr double-lumen (usually right IJ)

Double-lumen CVP placed in IJ, femoral or subclavian vein. Distal port reserved for vasoactive infusions and proximal port for blood sampling, pressure measurements, drug and volume administration. Usually a 22 ga catheter is placed percutaneously in the radial artery (avoid

Monitoring, cont.	TEE Additional SpO_2 monitors ± surgical LA line: have spare transducer available.	Blalock-Taussig shunt side—usually right side). On infants, a fiber optic transilluminator may facilitate arterial cannulation. Dorsalis pedis and posterior tibial arteries are avoided, due to problems with spasm and clotting when coming off CPB. Femoral arteries are cannulated as a last resort, using a 2½ or 3 Fr 2-4 cm catheter. If all else fails, a surgical cutdown is performed. Older children (> 20 kg) may receive adult-size central lines, as well as PA catheters, if medically indicated. Multiple SpO_2 sites ensure continuous O_2 monitoring during critical events.
Infusions	EACA load: 150 mg/kg over 30 min	EACA infusion: 20 mg/kg/h × 5 h, starting at induction
Pre CPB	Heparinization (3 mg/kg) ACT > 400 sec MAP ~70 mmHg ✓ muscle relaxation. Drips off ✓ pupils. ✓ UO.	In the pre CPB period, crystalloid and/or 5% albumin is administered as needed to compensate for bleeding and 3rd-space losses. Blood replacement is reserved for major blood loss situations associated with redo's and/or surgical entry into major vessels/heart chambers.
CPB	Ventilation stopped. Hypothermia: 24-26°C ± DHCA (13-17°C nasopharynx) Hct 20-25 typical during CPB ✓ adequate flow/pressure. ✓ anesthetic/NMB levels. ✓ pupils. ✓ face for venous congestion. ✓ ABG, electrolytes, UO, Hct and ACT q 30 min.	Drugs are injected into the pump reservoir as appropriate. Ice packs placed around head for DHCA. Phentolamine (0.2 ml/kg) given into pump prior to cooling and warming. Methylprednisolone 30 mg/kg for DHCA. Lasix (0.5-1 mg/kg) for ↓UO and hemoconcentration. Perfusion pressure, CVP and flow rates are monitored in tandem with the perfusionists. Observation for venous congestion is ongoing during the procedure.
Transition off CPB	Rewarming Vasoactive infusions started at 34°C. Flush lines. TEE Rezero transducers. Suction ETT. Resume ventilation. Observe lung inflation. ✓ bilateral breath sounds. ✓ ABGs, electrolytes, Hct (~30). ✓ ACT (> 400). ✓ ECG: pacing may be necessary. Supplement NMB and deepen anesthesia.	Aerosolized albuterol given with bronchopulmonary toilet. Surgeons deair heart, which can be monitored by TEE. A measurement of the RV and LV pressure ratio helps to judge adequacy of repair of the RVOTO. TEE is also used to evaluate the anatomy, the repair, and pressures. If question of residual VSD, can ✓ PA and mixed venous sats to look for step-up. Full-flow CPB at normothermia is often allowed to rebuild myocardial ATP stores. The cross-clamp is removed and the empty heart (vented) is allowed to beat. The vent is D/C and the heart is gradually allowed to work with progressively less "pump" support.
Post CPB	Inotropic support (dopamine, dobutamine, epinephrine) Rx pulmonary HTN (↓PVR): $FiO_2 = 1$ $PaCO_2$ ~30 NTG ± PGE_1 Minimize mean airway pressure. AV sequential pacemaker (heart block not uncommon). Surgical PA or LA line usually placed to monitor cardiac status. Reverse anticoagulation. Rx coagulopathy: fresh (< 48 h old);	↓RV compliance is expected (↑RVEDP = RV failure). This RV "failure" is 2° to RVH, CPB, hypothermic arrest, infundibulotomy and pulmonary regurgitation, as well as general surgical manipulation of the RV. RV afterload reduction is essential, initially through ventilatory efforts: clear unobstructed ventilation; do not allow wheezing (albuterol prn); use gentle hyperventilation on 100% O_2. If these maneuvers are not sufficient, then NTG/PGE_1 are used. Rarely, NO may be required to control pulmonary HTN. Inotropic support of RV also typically is used—dopamine/dobutamine initially and epinephrine reserved for severe RV dysfunction. Inotropic support, especially dopamine and epinephrine, may ↑ PVR, thus confound-

Post CPB, cont.	whole blood preferred. FFP/Plt/cryo/EACA, as necessary. Modified ultrafiltration (MUF)	ing overall resuscitation. MUF uses the CPB machine to remove excess H_2O and inflammatory medications (↓edema and imporved cardiopulmonary function).
Positioning	✓ and pad pressure points. ✓ eyes.	
Complications	See Postoperative Complications, below.	

POSTOPERATIVE

Complications	Persistent bleeding Persistent RVOTO Hypothermia RV failure Pneumothorax/hemothorax Cardiac tamponade Dysrhythmias	Sometimes a PFO will be left surgically open, especially if RV failure is severe, in order to allow RV decompression via a R→L intraatrial shunt. This often will result in profound systemic O_2-Hb desaturation (preferable to uncompensated RV failure). ECHO will confirm the existence of intraatrial shunting.
Tests	ABGs Electrolytes Coag profile CXR: ✓ line, ETT placement. TEE ECHO	TEE monitoring is an invaluable anatomical and physiological monitor.

References

1. Baue AE: *Glenn's Thoracic and Cardiovascular Surgery,* 6th edition. Appleton & Lange, Stamford: 1996.
2. Castaneda AR, Jonas RA, Mayer JE Jr, Hanley FL: Tetralogy of Fallot. In *Cardiac Surgery of the Neonate and Infant.* WB Saunders, Philadelphia: 1994, 215-34.
3. Karl TR: Tetralogy of Fallot. In *Glenn's Thoracic and Cardiovascular Surgery,* 6th edition. Baue AE, ed. Appleton & Lange, Stamford: 1996, 1211-19.
4. Samuelson PN, Lell WA: Tetrology of Fallot. In *Pediatric Cardiac Anesthesia,* 3rd edition. Lake CL, ed. Appleton & Lange, Stamford: 1998, 303-14.

SURGERY FOR TOTAL ANOMALOUS PULMONARY VENOUS CONNECTION

SURGICAL CONSIDERATIONS

Description: Total anomalous pulmonary venous connection (TAPVC) is a rare congenital cardiac malformation in which the entire pulmonary venous return empties into the right atrium, usually via a common pulmonary venous sinus (Fig 12.3-4). An interatrial R→L shunt, in the form of a PFO or an ASD, is required to maintain systemic output and, hence, survival in the postnatal period. The objective of surgical correction is to redirect the entire pulmonary venous return to the left atrium.

TAPVC was first successfully repaired in 1956 by Lewis and Varco at the University of Minnesota, by joining of the pulmonary venous sinus to the left atrium and closure of the ASD. Although mortality for this lesion was initially quite high, particularly in infants with obstruction of the pulmonary veins, recent improvements in intraop and postop management have permitted successful correction in most neonates and infants. There are four TAPVC drainage patterns, as defined by Darling and associates. These include **supracardiac** (45%), **cardiac** (25%), **infracardiac** (25%), and **mixed** (5%) patterns of venous drainage. The anomalous drainage in supracardiac TAPVC is usually by a left vertical vein into the innominate vein. In cardiac TAPVC, drainage is usually into the coronary sinus and occasionally into the right atrium. In infracardiac TAPVC, drainage is usually into the portal vein. The mixed type consists of combinations of the other three varieties of TAPVC.

When pulmonary venous drainage is obstructed, patients present with cyanosis, severe pulmonary edema, pulmonary HTN, and ↓CO. Symptomatic TAPVC is repaired at any age, frequently with induced hypothermia and circulatory arrest. Critically ill neonates with obstructed pulmonary venous return must undergo urgent correction after stabilization (i.e., intubation/ ventilation, diuretics).

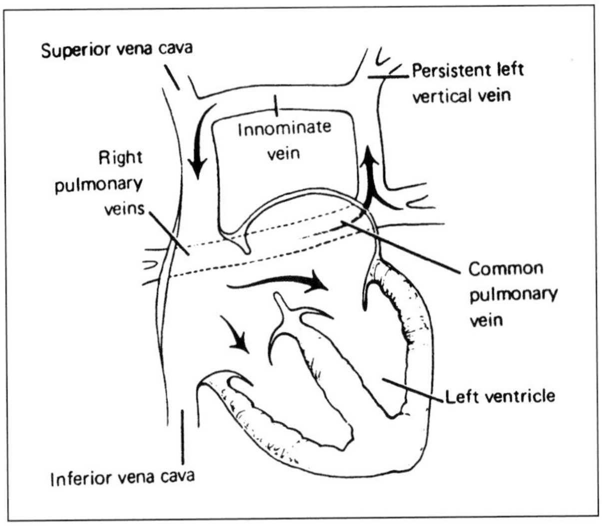

Figure 12.3-4. Total anomalous pulmonary venous (TAPV) connection. Supracardiac TAPV connection with pulmonary venous drainage into left vertical vein, which, in turn, drains into the innominate vein. (Reproduced with permission from Way LW: *Current Surgical Diagnosis and Treatment*, 10th edition. Lange Medical Publications: 1973, 398.)

In most cases, the right and left pulmonary veins drain into a common pulmonary venous sinus, allowing for its anastomosis to the left atrium for a definitive repair. Through a standard median sternotomy, the aortic and venous cannulae are placed and CPB with cooling is initiated. The aorta is cross-clamped, immediately followed by cardioplegic arrest. After CPB is stopped, the venous cannulae are removed, the cardiac apex is reflected anteriorly, and the pulmonary veins are dissected superiorly through the posterior pericardium. The left atrium is then opened transversely with extension out onto the left atrial appendage, followed by the direct anastomosis of the pulmonary venous confluence to the left atrium. Finally, via a right atriotomy, the ASD or PFO is closed and CPB with rewarming is started.

Successful outcomes are often dependent upon adequate control of elevated PVR in the early postop period. Placement of a transthoracic PA catheter is often very helpful in this regard.

Variant procedure or approaches: Alternatively, repair of TAPVC may be accomplished through a right atriotomy and across the atrial septum, constructing the anastomosis between the pulmonary venous confluence and left atrium from within the left atrium.

Usual preop diagnosis: TAPVC; total anomalous venous return; total anomalous pulmonary venous drainage—all of these ± obstruction and either supracardiac, cardiac, or mixed types

SUMMARY OF PROCEDURE

Position	Supine
Incision	Standard median sternotomy
Unique considerations	Patients often require urgent or emergency surgery. Obligatory R→L shunting → risk of systemic embolization. Myocardial preservation using blood or crystalloid cardioplegia, in addition to topical myocardial hypothermia, is used.
Antibiotics	Cefazolin 15-30 mg/kg q 8 h
Surgical time	Aortic cross-clamp: 40 min Circulatory arrest: 30-35 min Total: 2.5-3 h
Closing considerations	A fine polyvinyl catheter inserted through the free wall of the right ventricle and advanced into the pulmonary trunk will permit drug infusions for pulmonary HTN. A chest tube is inserted into the pericardial space; temporary ventricular pacing wires are placed.
EBL	Moderate
Postop care	2-4 d of assisted ventilation, sedation and hyperventilation; pulmonary vasodilators, including isoproterenol, PGE_1, SNP; inotropes as needed for right heart dysfunction.
Mortality	2-20%, depending on presence of preop pulmonary venous obstruction and metabolic acidosis.

Morbidity	Pulmonary vasospasm: 25-40% Low CO: 10% Hemorrhage: 2-3%
Pain score	8-10

PATIENT POPULATION CHARACTERISTICS

Age range	1 d–20 yr (usually < 1 mo)
Male:Female	4:1 in infracardiac type; equal distribution in other types
Incidence	0.5%-2% of congenital heart defects
Etiology	Failure of fusion of the pulmonary vein evagination (from posterior left atrium) with the pulmonary venous plexus surrounding the lung buds.
Associated conditions	PDA present in nearly all infants within the first few wk of life and in about 15% of cases overall. VSD occasionally occurs (may be associated with TOF, DORV, interrupted aortic arch and other lesions).

ANESTHETIC CONSIDERATIONS

PREOPERATIVE

Pathophysiology Some degree of cyanosis is always present. The L→R shunt must be compensated for by a R→L shunt through a PFO or ASD. The anomalous connection of all the pulmonary veins to the right atrium or its tributaries are frequently stenosed and, therefore, obstructed. The result is severe pulmonary venous congestion, which causes pulmonary HTN. If the atrial septal communication and R→L shunt is small → RV overload and dilation → RV failure. Patients with pulmonary venous obstruction and pulmonary HTN present early in infancy with tachypnea, cyanosis, pulmonary edema and acidosis. Some of these patients may require ECMO. Patients with unobstructed total anomalous pulmonary veins have minimal cyanosis and often present later.

Respiratory In patients with obstructed TAPVC, expect severe pulmonary edema and pulmonary HTN.
Tests: ✓ CXR: ↑heart size, ↑pulmonary vascularity, "figure-of-8" or "snowman" cardiac silhouette.

Cardiovascular ECHO findings: large RV and small LA. Interventricular cath for balloon or blade septostomy in patients with restrictive ASD may be necessary to improve R→L shunting.
Tests: ✓ ECG for right axis deviation (RAD), RAE and RVH.

Laboratory ABG and Hct; other tests as indicated from H&P.

Premedication Generally not indicated and not necessary in severely ill infants.

Transport to OR Patients are transported from the ICU in a heated transport unit. ECG, SpO_2 and arterial line monitoring via a portable monitor. If neonate is intubated, ventilation is assisted with a Jackson Rees setup. Resuscitative drugs and airway equipment should accompany the patient.

INTRAOPERATIVE

Anesthetic technique: GETA. DHCA may be required to facilitate surgical repair in some patients.

Induction Infants are often severely ill and come to the OR intubated and ventilated, with invasive lines and inotropic support. Verify ETT placement. Patients are subject to rapid cardiovascular decompensation. Pancuronium (0.1-0.2 mg/kg) or vecuronium (0.1 mg/kg) is given prior to fentanyl (10 μg/kg) to avoid chest rigidity. Volatile agents are rarely tolerated in obstructed TAPVC.

Maintenance Fentanyl (100-200 μg/kg) in divided doses. Pancuronium prn, midazolam 0.1-0.2 mg/kg ± volatile agent as tolerated. FiO_2 = 1.0. Ventilation maneuvers to ↓PVR. (See Post CPB, p. 906.)

Emergence Transport to ICU intubated and ventilated. If NO used in OR, must have delivery system ready for transport to ICU). There may be continued requirement for inotropic support.

Blood and fluid requirements	IV: 22-24 ga × 2 taped securely LR @ TKO Continue iv dextrose in neonates. 5% albumin	Avoid air bubbles with R→L shunt—can cause systemic embolization of air. ✓ blood glucose. Avoid hyperglycemia, especially during deep hypothermia circulatory arrest (DHCA).

Blood and fluid, cont.	Fresh, whole blood, if available, or PRBC Blood warmer Humidify gases.	
Monitoring	Standard monitors (see D-1). See TOF (p. 905).	Severely ill infants usually present with invasive monitoring and ETT. ✓ correct placement of UAC and UVC preop.
Positioning	✓ & pad pressure points. ✓ eyes	
CPB	Management of CPB is discussed in Intraoperative Considerations for TOF, p. 906.	
Complications	Refractory pulmonary HTN	Pulmonary HTN may be difficult to control. Ventilation maneuvers (see TOF, p. 906), vasodilators, and deep anesthesia to ↓PVR. NO is started for refractory pulmonary HTN; if NO is unsuccessful, ECMO may be instituted. Bradycardia must be avoided because the CO is HR dependent. The LV is noncompliant due to under filling in fetal life.
	RV failure Persistent bleeding Hypothermia Bradycardia and dysrhythmias	Inotropic rapport of RV: dopamine/dobutamine, initially; then epinephrine, if necessary.
	Overdose of NO → methemoglobinemia	✓ metHb while on NO therapy.

POSTOPERATIVE

Complications	See above.	
Tests	ABG Hct; electrolytes; coags	
	Methemoglobin	Only if on NO
	CXR	

References

1. Baue AE: *Glenn's Thoracic and Cardiovascular Surgery,* 6th edition. Appleton & Lange, Stamford: 1996.
2. Castaneda AR, Jonas RA, Mayer JE Jr, Hanley FL: Total anomalous pulmonary venous connection. In *Cardiac Surgery of the Neonate and Infant.* WB Saunders, Philadelphia: 1994, 157-66.
3. Drinkwater DC Jr, D'Agostino HJ Jr: Anomalous pulmonary and systemic venous connections. In *Glenn's Thoracic and Cardiovascular Surgery, 6th edition.* Baue AE, ed. Appleton & Lange, Stamford: 1996, 1105-14.
4. Kambam J: Endocardial cushion defects. In *Cardiac Anesthesia for Infants and Children.* Kambam J, Fish FA, Merrill WH, eds. CV Mosby, St. Louis: 1994, 203-10.
5. Kirklin JW, Barrett-Boyes BG: Total anomalous pulmonary venous connection. In *Cardiac Surgery,* 2nd edition. Churchill-Livingstone, New York; 1993, 645-73.
6. Lake CL: Anamolies of the systemic and pulmonary venous returns. In *Pediatric Cardiac Anesthesia,* 3rd edition. Appleton & Lange, Stamford: 1998, 353-71.
7. Mazzucco A, Bartolo HIU, Stellin G, Gallucci V: Anomalies of the systemic venous return: A review. *J Cardiac Surg* 1990; 5:122-33.

SURGERY FOR COMPLETE TRANSPOSITION OF THE GREAT ARTERIES

SURGICAL CONSIDERATIONS

Description: Complete **transposition of the great arteries (TGA)** is a congenital cardiac defect in which the aorta arises from the RV and the PA arises from the LV (Fig 12.3-5). TGA is associated with an intact ventricular septum (TGA/IVS) or a ventricular septal defect (TGA/VSD). Pathophysiologically, this discordant ventriculoarterial configuration results in systemic and pulmonary circulations placed in a parallel (normally in series) configuration. Thus, a L→R shunt in the form of an atrial septal defect (ASD), VSD, or patent ductus arteriosus (PDA) is required to permit oxygenated blood to enter the "right-sided" systemic circulation. The earliest surgical treatment for TGA was described by **Blalock** and **Hanlon** in 1950, with a procedure in which an **atrial septectomy** was performed, improving the mixing of pulmonary and systemic blood at the atrial level. In the 1950s, a variety of partial physiologic corrections were developed in which the pulmonary veins or the vena cava were transposed to the alternate atria. Palliative treatment was advanced by **Rashkind's** description of a **balloon atrial septostomy** in 1966. More complete palliation was obtained by **atrial switch** operations, described by **Senning** in 1959 and **Mustard** in 1963, in which systemic and pulmonary venous return were baffled to the appropriate ventricles. Postop complications with the atrial switch operations, however, led to the development of the more "anatomic" **arterial switch** operations described by **Jatene**, **Yacoub** and others beginning in the 1970s. By 1987, the arterial switch operation in neonates was widely accepted as the standard approach to TGA.

Total correction is now performed routinely in the first 3 wk of life. The heart is exposed through a standard median sternotomy and CPB is instituted. The aortic cross-clamp is applied, followed by cardioplegic arrest and induced hypothermia. The ascending aorta is transected at its midportion and the pulmonary trunk is transected just proximal to its bifurcation. Two buttons from the "neopulmonary artery" (former aortic root) containing the origins of the left and right coronary arteries are transposed and anastomosed to the "neoaorta" (former main pulmonary trunk). The distal aortic segment is swung beneath the pulmonary artery bifurcation. Pericardial patches are used to repair the defects resulting from excision of the coronary artery buttons and any associated ASDs and/or VSDs are repaired. The distal aortic segment is anastomosed to the neoaorta and the distal bifurcated pulmonary artery segment is anastomosed to the neopulmonary artery. If hypothermia has been induced, a brief period of circulatory arrest facilitates repair of the ASD and/or VSD, if present. The aortic cross-clamp is removed and rewarming is begun during the neopulmonary arterial anastomosis. CPB is then discontinued and closure is routine.

Usual preop diagnosis: Complete TGA; transposition of the great vessels; transposition ± VSD; ASD; PDA

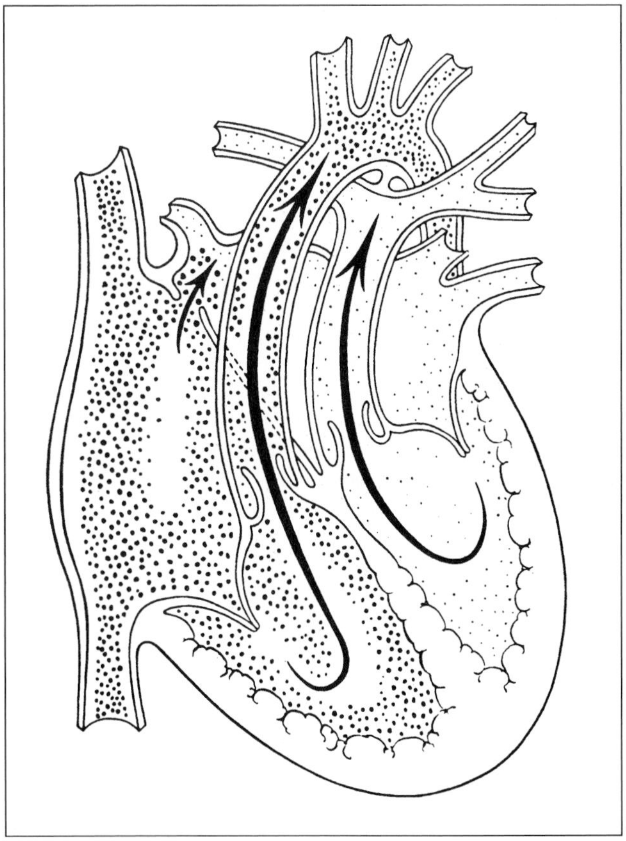

Figure 12.3-5. Transposition of the great arteries. (Reproduced with permission from Waldenhausen JA, Pierce WS: Transposition of the great arteries. In Hardy JD, ed: *Rhoads Textbook of Surgery, 5th ed.* JB Lippincott: 1977.)

SUMMARY OF PROCEDURE

Position	Supine
Incision	Standard median sternotomy
Unique considerations	Operation to be performed before LV pressure falls substantially 2° ↓PVR.
Antibiotics	Cefazolin 15-30 mg/kg q 8 h
Surgical time	Aortic cross-clamp: 45-70 min Circulatory arrest: 10-15 min Total: 3 h
Closing considerations	Routine closure with chest tube in the pericardial space; temporary ventricular pacing wire; possible right or left atrial line for monitoring.

EBL	Minimal
Postop care	24-48 h of assisted ventilation; pulmonary HTN protocol consisting of hyperventilation and sedation and use of pulmonary vasodilators; inotropes for adequate CO
Mortality	5%
Morbidity	Hemorrhage Coronary artery kinking and myocardial ischemia Pulmonary vasospasm
Pain score	8-10

PATIENT POPULATION CHARACTERISTICS

Age range	1-21 d; ≤ 3-6 mo in TGA/VSD
Male:Female	2:1; 3.3:1 for TGA/IVS
Incidence	7-8% of congenital heart defects
Etiology	Usually no associated syndromes or other noncardiac abnormalities
Associated conditions	ASD; VSD; PDA; LVOTO; pulmonary atresia; coarctation of the aorta

ANESTHETIC CONSIDERATIONS

PREOPERATIVE

Pathophysiology Complete TGA = A-V concordance (RA→RV) and ventriculoarterial discordance (RV→aorta and LV→PA); unlike the normal series circulation, this parallel circulation recirculates deoxygenated systemic venous blood without reaching the lungs and the oxygenated pulmonary venous blood recirculates through the pulmonary circulation. There must be intercirculatory mixing to be compatible with life. Intracardiac mixing occurs through a PFO, ASD, and/or VSD. Extracardiac mixing occurs through a PDA and/or bronchopulmonary collaterals. The amount of mixing is dependent on the size, number and position of communications, as well as ventricular compliance, PVR, SVR and LVOT obstruction (LVOTO).

Respiratory Patients not repaired can quickly develop to PVOD → pulmonary HTN. Hypoxemia is associated with the eventual development of bronchopulmonary collaterals. Some patients are maintained preop on PGE_1, to keep the ductus arteriosus open. PGE_1 can cause apnea; therefore, mechanical ventilation may be required.

Tests: CXR: ✓ enlarged heart and pulmonary edema.

Cardiovascular Patients with VSD have ↑pulmonary blood flow, ↑intercirculatory mixing → CHF. Marked cyanosis is seen in patients with TGA and intact ventricular septum, O_2 saturation depends on degree of mixing (Q_P/Q_S ratio).

Tests: ECG: right axis deviation (RAD) and RVH. ECHO is diagnostic. Cardiac cath defines anatomy, coronary arteries, septal defects, PFO, PDA, bronchopulmonary collaterals, LVOT, pulmonic valve function and pressures, including PVR and LV:RV ratio. Balloon atrial septostomy (Rashkind-Miller) is required to improve mixing in some patients.

Hematologic Polycythemia develops in children with long-term hypoxemia → ↑blood viscosity. Hct > 65 → poor tissue perfusion → thrombosis → end organ infarction. Preop iv hydration is important in these patients.

Laboratory Hct; coags; other tests as indicated from H&P.

Premedication Generally not necessary in children < 9 mo. For older children, midazolam 0.5-0.75 mg/kg po.

Transport to OR Patients are transported from the ICU in a heated transport unit with ECG, SpO_2 and arterial line monitoring. If neonate is intubated, ventilation is assisted with a Jackson Rees circuit. Resuscitative drugs and airway equipment should accompany these patients.

INTRAOPERATIVE

Anesthetic technique: GETA

Induction Infants often arrive in the OR with a PGE_1 infusion and mechanical ventilation in progress. Critically ill infants may present with severe cyanosis, acidosis, ventricular dysfunction and variable ductal

Induction, cont.	patency. IV induction with pancuronium (0.2 mg/kg) and fentanyl (10 μg/kg iv slowly) avoids chest rigidity. An inhalation induction may be tolerated in older, more hemodynamically stable children. Verify ETT placement.	
Maintenance	For patients with ↓intercirculatory mixing and ↓pulmonary blood flow, treatment should include ventilation maneuvers to ↓ PVR (see TOF, Post CPB, p. 906) and improve mixing. Deep GA helps to blunt reactive pulmonary HTN. Avoid ↓HR → ↓CO in infants with limited myocardial reserve.	
Emergence	Extensive vascular suture lines may be responsible for persistent bleeding. Control aortic BP and treat any coagulopathy. ✓ for myocardial ischemia, which can be 2° coronary air emboli or a problem with reimplantation of coronaries. Transport to ICU intubated and ventilated.	
Blood and fluid requirements	IV: 22-24 ga × 1-2 taped securely LR @ TKO Continue iv dextrose in neonates. 5% albumin Fresh, whole blood or PRBCs Blood warmer Humidify gases.	Avoid air bubbles in patients with R→L and L→R shunts.
Monitoring	Standard monitors (see D-1). See TOF for further monitoring, p. 905.	Severely ill infants often present with invasive monitoring and mechanical ventilation. Correct placement of UAC and UVC should be checked preoperatively.
	TEE	TEE helps to evaluate the surgical repair and to ✓ for residual VSD.
CPB	Management of CPB is discussed in Intraoperative Considerations for TOF, p. 906.	A short period of circulatory arrest may be required.
Positioning	✓ and pad pressure points. ✓ and tape eyes.	
Complications	Myocardial ischemia LV dysfunction and failure Persistent bleeding Dysrhythmias Hypothermia Pulmonary HTN Residual structural defects	In patients with TGA and IVS, the LV may be inadequate to support the systemic circulation. The LV becomes "deconditioned" after the PVR drops in early infancy. The LV is then unable to function as the systemic ventricle. Inotropic support (dopamine and epinephrine) and afterload reduction (SNP or amrinone) may be necessary to separate from CPB. ECMO may be required for severe ventricular dysfunction.

POSTOPERATIVE

Complications	Hypothermia Persistent surgical/medical bleeding Pneumothorax/hemothorax Dysrhythmias Cardiac tamponade Myocardial ischemia LV failure Residual structural defects: AI, supravalvular PS or AS	Ischemia 2° coronary artery stenosis, stretching, spasm, compression, etc., can badly damage myocardial tissues. Spasm can be treated with NTG and ↑aortic pressure. If the now-anterior PA dilates (↓PaO_2, ↑$PaCO_2$, ↓temp, ↓pH, excessive or too little PIP, or RV failure), then the coronary arteries may be compressed. Measures to ↓ PA pressure are often essential. Dysrhythmias may require cardioversion or pacing.
Tests	ABGs; electrolytes; coag profile	
	CXR	✓ line, chest tube placement; ✓ for pneumothorax.
	ECHO/TEE	TEE monitoring is an invaluable anatomical and physiological monitor.

References

1. Baue AE, Geha AS, Hammond GL, Laks H, Naunheim KS: *Glenn's Thoracic and Cardiovascular Surgery,* 6th edition. Appleton & Lange, Stamford: 1996.

2. Castaneda AR, Jonas RA, Mayer JE Jr, Hanley FL: D-transposition of the great arteries. In *Cardiac Surgery of the Neonate and Infant.* WB Saunders, Philadelphia: 1994, 409-38.
3. Castaneda AR, Mayer JE: Neonatal repair of transposition of the great arteries. In *Fetal and Neonatal Cardiology.* Long WA, ed. WB Saunders, Philadelphia: 1990.
4. Kambam J: Endocardial cushion defects. In *Cardiac Anesthesia for Infants and Children.* Kambam J, Fish FA, Merrill WH, eds. CV Mosby, St. Louis: 1994, 203-10.
5. Kirklin JW, Barrett-Boyes BG: Complete transposition of the great arteries. In *Cardiac Surgery*, 2nd edition. Churchill-Livingstone, New York: 1993, 1383-1467.
6. Lowe DA, Stayer SA, Rehman MA: Abnormalities of the atrioventricular valves. In *Pediatric Cardiac Anesthesia,* 3rd edition. Lake CL, ed. Appleton & Lange, Stamford, CT: 1998, 407-30.
7. Quaegebeur JM, Auteri JS: Transposition of the great arteries. In *Glenn's Thoracic and Cardiovascular Surgery,* 6th edition. Baue AE, ed. Appleton & Lange, Stamford: 1996, 1393-1407.

SURGERY FOR TRUNCUS ARTERIOSUS

SURGICAL CONSIDERATIONS

Description: Truncus arteriosus is a rare cardiac anomaly in which there is a common aortopulmonary trunk originating from the base of the heart by way of a single, semilunar valve (truncal valve). This single great artery gives rise to the pulmonary, systemic and coronary circulations. A nonrestrictive VSD is almost always found immediately below the truncal valve. An anatomic classification scheme proposed by **Collett** and **Edwards** in 1949 describes four types of truncus. In **type I** truncus (60%), a single arterial trunk gives rise to the aorta and main PA (Fig 12.3-6A). In **type II** truncus (20%), the right and left PAs arise separately from the posterolateral aspect of the truncus. **Type III** truncus (10%) designates cases in which the two PAs also originate from the posterior truncus, but with widely separated orifices. In **type IV** truncus (10%), the PA branches are absent, with pulmonary blood flow derived from bronchial artery collaterals. Pathophysiologically, there is significant L→R shunting at the truncal and ventricular levels, leading to systemic arterial desaturation. Patients become symptomatic in infancy 2° CHF when the PVR ↓ and CO ↑. Untreated, 90% of infants die within 6 mo.

The first total repairs of this congenital anomaly were reported in the early 1960s and included the insertion of **nonvalved artificial conduits** and **aortic allograft and valve conduits.** In the early and mid-1970s, repair was performed at younger ages, with abandonment of palliative banding of the PA branches. Currently, early primary repair is carried out during the first or second mo of life.

Through a median sternotomy, the truncus and PA branches are dissected and cannulation for CPB is performed. The PAs are snared to block pulmonary flow during perfusion. Hypothermia is induced and the aorta is cross-clamped. The PAs are separated from the main truncus, the resultant aortic defect is repaired with a pericardial patch, and a valved homograft (12-14 mm) is prepared. An end-to-end anastomosis of the distal homograft to the PA opening is performed; the VSD is closed through a right ventriculotomy; and the proximal end of the homograft is then anastomosed to the right ventriculotomy (Fig 12.3-6B). The aorta is unclamped, rewarming and resuscitation are performed, and CPB is discontinued.

There are several special considerations associated with this repair which warrant mention. The truncal valve may exhibit insufficiency, necessitating valve replacement using a cryopreserved aortic or pulmonary homograft. In older infants, the PVR may be elevated and pulmonary vasospasm should be anticipated. Finally, the VSD may be small and the ventricular septum oriented in such a way that LVOTO may result if the truncal valve is oriented more toward the RV prior to repair.

Usual preop diagnosis: Truncus arteriosus (types I, II, III, IV)

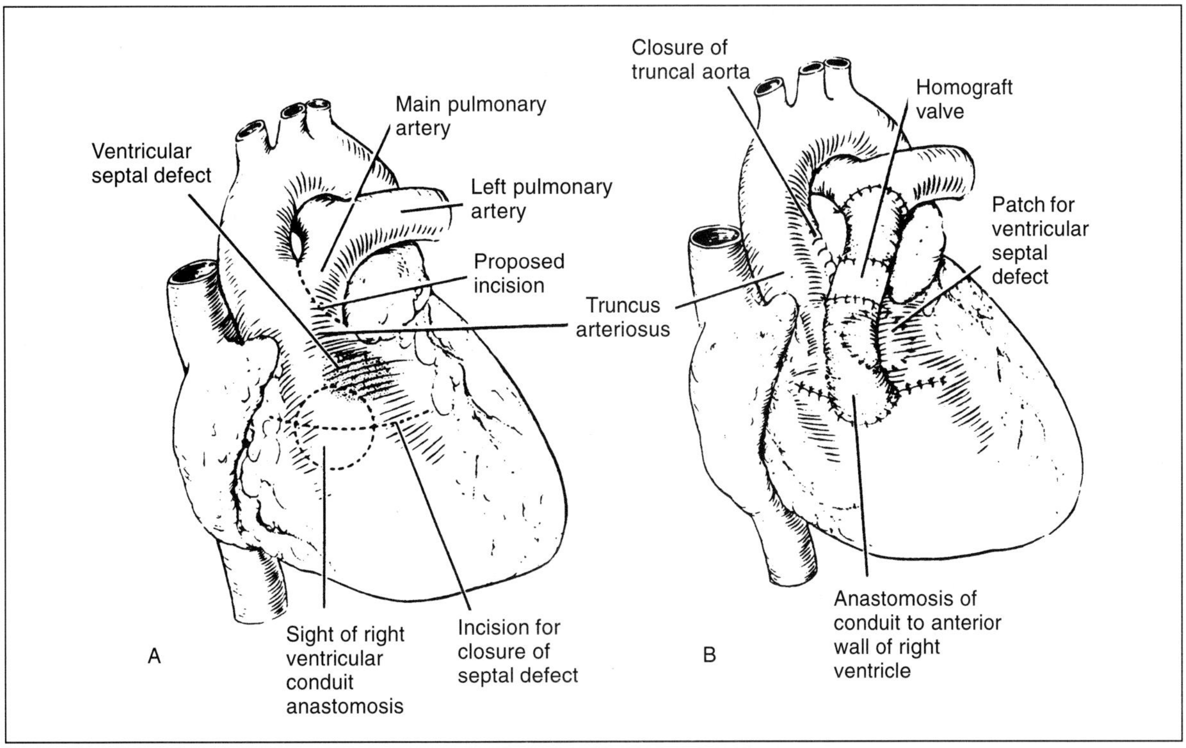

Figure 12.3-6. Truncus arteriosus. (**A**) Cohen-Edwards (Type I). (**B**) Surgical correction involves the separation of the main PA from the truncus, VSD patch closure and insertion of a conduit between the RV and the distal main PA. (Reproduced with permission from Way LW: *Current Surgical Diagnosis and Treatment*, 10th edition. Lange Medical Publications: 1973, 399.)

SUMMARY OF PROCEDURE

Position	Supine
Incision	Standard median sternotomy
Antibiotics	Cefazolin 15-30 mg/kg q 8 h
Surgical time	Aortic cross-clamp: 50-60 min Circulatory arrest: 10-15 min Total: 3 h
Closing considerations	Routine closure with chest tube in the pericardial space; temporary ventricular pacing wire; possible right or left atrial line for monitoring
EBL	Minimal
Postop care	24-48 h of assisted ventilation; pulmonary HTN protocol consisting of hyperventilation and sedation and use of pulmonary vasodilators. Inotropes for adequate CO.
Mortality	10-20%
Morbidity	Hemorrhage Pulmonary vasospasm Truncal valve insufficiency ↓CO
Pain score	8-10

PATIENT POPULATION CHARACTERISTICS

Age range	3 wk–6 mo
Male:Female	1:1
Incidence	1.7-4.6% of congenital heart defects
Etiology	No known etiology; no commonly associated syndromes
Associated conditions	Coexisting interrupted aortic arch or coarctation with PDA (10-20%); right aortic arch (16%); mitral valve anomalies (10%); moderate-size or large ASD (10%); DiGeorge syndrome

ANESTHETIC CONSIDERATIONS

PREOPERATIVE

Pathophysiology Truncus arteriosus is characterized by a single outlet for both ventricles. In type I, the main PA arises from the truncus and is associated with an increase in pulmonary blood flow. In types II and III, the PAs arise separately from posterior and lateral aspects of the truncus and are associated with normal-to-increased pulmonary blood flow. The single arterial trunk allows mixing of systemic and pulmonary blood. The single semilunar valve may be significantly stenotic or regurgitant. In > 1/3 of cases, the coronary artery anatomy is anomalous. This determines the orientation of the infundibulotomy required for VSD closure and RV-to-PA conduit placement. Associated defects are rare. The most frequent surgical anomaly is interrupted aortic arch, found in 12% of cases. DiGeorge syndrome is not uncommon (aplasia or hypoplasia or thymus and parathyroid glands, congenital heart defects, anomalies of the great vessels and facial structures [micrognathia] and esophageal atresia).

As the PVR decreases, untreated truncus → uncontrollable CHF, resulting in significant mortality within 6 mo. The L→R shunt is at the arterial level; therefore, there is augmented pulmonary arterial flow in diastole as well as in systole (compared to a simple VSD). This ↑ the pulmonary shunt, and ↑ the shear forces on the pulmonary endothelium. Thus, an infant who survives the CHF may subsequently develop PVOD and Eisenmenger's syndrome (VSD with pulmonary HTN and cyanosis 2° R→L shunt). These rapid pathologic changes are the rationale for repair shortly after diagnosis, preferably in the neonatal period. ↑PVR and pulmonary HTN may complicate the anesthetic management, especially in older infants.

Airway The facial anomalies (e.g., micrognathia) in DiGeorge syndrome may make intubation difficult.

Respiratory Typically, these infants present with the respiratory Sx of CHF (dyspnea, tachypnea, hypoxemia).
Tests: CXR: ↑pulmonary markings and wide mediastinum.

Cardiovascular The newborn may not manifest overt signs; however, as PVR decreases, CHF develops. Patients become tachypneic, have feeding difficulty and are irritable. A widened pulse pressure and bounding pulses are present.
Tests: ECG: biventricular hypertrophy is common with 1st- or 2nd-degree heart block in 10% of patients. ECHO: Usually diagnostic. Identifies the origin of PA from the common trunk and the presence (subtype A) or absence (subtype B) of a VSD. Evaluates truncal valve competency. Cardiac cath: may be necessary to evaluate PVR and anatomy. A PVR > 8 Wood U/m^2, unresponsive to pulmonary vasodilators (e.g., NO) may indicate inoperability.

Endocrine In DiGeorge syndrome thymic hypoplasia occurs with hypoparathyroidism and symptomatic hypocalcemia.
Tests: ✓ Ca^{++} levels; parathyroid hormone

Premedication Not indicated.

Transport to OR Very sick infants in severe CHF are often intubated, mechanically ventilated and receiving inotropic support. Patients are transported from the ICU in a warmed transport module with ECG, SpO_2 and arterial line monitoring. Maintain the same FiO_2 used in the unit. Resuscitative drugs and airway equipment should accompany the patient.

INTRAOPERATIVE

Anesthetic technique: GETA

Induction Infants often have iv access, UAC and UVC monitoring in place. The correct position of umbilical catheters must be checked preop by x-ray (UAC just above aortic bifurcation; UVC in atrium or IVC). IV induction begins with vecuronium (0.1 mg/kg) or doxacurium (0.05-0.08 mg/kg) to avoid tachycardia → ↓coronary perfusion. Fentanyl 10 μg/kg is administered slowly. It is extremely important in truncus type I (in which pulmonary blood flow is increased) to maintain the delicate balance between PVR and SVR (↓SVR → ↓coronary perfusion → CHF). ↑SVR or ↓PVR → ↑pulmonary blood flow and must be avoided. Just opening the chest can upset the balance, and cardiac arrest may occur. After the chest is open, the surgeon can occlude one of the PAs to improve systemic flow. Other maneuvers to ↑ PVR include the use of PEEP, low inspired FiO_2 (~21%) and mild hypercarbia (~45-50 mmHg). In truncus types II and III, pulmonary blood flow is normal or ↑. The balance between PVR and SVR generally is not as tenuous as in truncus type I.

Maintenance	High-dose narcotic. Fentanyl (100-200 μg/kg). Vecuronium or doxacurium as needed ± midazolam 0.2 mg/kg ± volatile agent. FiO_2 = 0.21. Avoid hyperventilation (↓PVR → ↑ shunt + CHF). PEEP may be useful to maintain PVR. The use of low-flow CPB or DHCA depends on the origin of the PAs and the size of the infant. The surgeon may leave a PFO to serve as a "pop-off" to preserve systemic perfusion when ↑PVR and RV dysfunction occur. A surgical left atrial line is frequently placed for monitoring. Hyperventilation and/or inhaled NO may be necessary for treating ↑PVR and pulmonary HTN. In some cases, the sternum may be left open due to chest-wall and mediastinal edema, and the presence of the anterior RV-PA conduit (Rastelli conduit).	
Emergence	Transport to ICU intubated and ventilated. Maintain narcotic infusion (e.g., fentanyl 1-10 μg/kg/h) for first few d postop to minimize pulmonary hypertensive crises.	
Blood and fluid requirements	See Tetralogy of Fallot (TOF), p. 905.	Continue dextrose infusion in neonates. Only irradiated blood and blood products should be used to prevent graft vs. host disease in patients with DiGeorge syndrome.
Infusions	See TOF, p. 906.	PGE_1 should be continued in patients with interrupted aortic arch.
Monitoring	See TOF, p. 905.	
Positioning	See TOF, p. 907.	
CPB	See TOF, p. 906.	
Complications	Pulmonary HTN Truncal valve insufficiency Coronary artery insufficiency Residual lesion	

POSTOPERATIVE

Complications	A-V block	Generally temporary, injury to conduction system unlikely because it is remote from VSD closure. Occasionally, a pacemaker may be required.
	Pulmonary hypertensive crisis	Frequent in patients > 1 mo old. Rx: NO, sedation, PGE_1, hyperventilation.
	Ventricular dysfunction	May require inotropic support.
	Residual lesions	Residual VSD, severe truncal valve incompetence or obstruction, obstruction of coronary flow, LVOTO.
	Persistent bleeding	
Pain management	Fentanyl infusion	
Tests:	As indicated	

References

1. Baue AE, Geha AS, Hammond GL, Laks H, Naunheim KS: *Glenn's Thoracic and Cardiovascular Surgery,* 6th edition. Appleton & Lange, Stamford: 1996.
2. Bove EL, Beekman RH, Snider AR: Repair of truncus arteriosus in the neonate and young infant. *Ann Thorac Surg* 1989; 47:499-506.
3. Castaneda AR, Jonas RA, Mayer JE Jr, Hanley FL: Truncus arteriosus. In *Cardiac Surgery of the Neonate and Infant.* WB Saunders, Philadelphia: 1994, 281-93.
4. Kambam J: Endocardial cushion defects. In *Cardiac Anesthesia for Infants and Children.* Kambam J, Fish FA, Merrill WH, eds. CV Mosby, St. Louis: 1994, 203-10.
5. Kirklin JW, Barrett-Boyes BG: Truncus arteriosus. In *Cardiac Surgery,* 2nd edition. Churchill-Livingstone, New York: 1993, 1131-51.
6. Lowe DA, Stayer SA, Rehman MA: Abnormalities of the atrioventricular valves. In *Pediatric Cardiac Anesthesia,* 3rd edition. Lake CL, ed. Appleton & Lange, Stamford, CT: 1998, 407-30.
7. Mosca RS, Burke RP: Truncus arteriosus: In *Glenn's Thoracic and Cardiovascular Surgery,* 6th edition. Baue AE, ed. Appleton & Lange, Stamford: 1996, 1211-19.
8. Rosen DA, Rosen KR: Anomalies of the aortic arch and valve. In *Pediatric Cardiac Anesthesia,* 3rd edition. Lake C, ed. Appleton & Lange, Stamford: 1997, 431-69.

SURGERY FOR TRICUSPID ATRESIA

SURGICAL CONSIDERATIONS

Description: In tricuspid atresia, there is a developmental failure of the tricuspid valve, isolating the RA from the RV. There are three types of tricuspid atresia, based on the relationship of the great vessels to the ventricles, otherwise known as **ventriculoarterial concordance.** Type I, the most common type (60-80%), consists of normal ventriculoarterial concordance. Type II (15-25%) consists of *d*-transposition, and Type III (3%) consists of *l*-transposition. In most cases of tricuspid atresia, the RV is hypoplastic, an ASD is present, and pulmonary blood flow is restricted 2° pulmonary stenosis or atresia. Together, these malformations lead to R→L shunting and varying degrees of cyanosis. Those patients with unobstructed pulmonary blood flow develop pulmonary overcirculation and CHF. Consequently, the initial palliative surgical management of this defect depends on the magnitude of pulmonary blood flow; the initial procedure may be either a modified **Blalock-Taussig systemic-to-PA shunt** or a **PA band.** The subsequent definitive surgical management consists of a bidirectional **Glenn shunt** and a modified **Fontan procedure.** Patients may undergo these operations sequentially or, in favorable cases, directly to the definitive Fontan operation.

The systemic-to-PA shunt, developed by Blalock and Taussig in 1944, was the first palliative treatment for this condition. Later, other shunts were introduced by **Potts** (descending aorta-to-left PA) and **Waterston** (ascending aorta-to-right PA). In 1958, Glenn described a shunt from the SVC to the right PA applied specifically to patients with tricuspid atresia. A modification of this shunt to a **bidirectional cavopulmonary anastomosis** was performed clinically by **Azzollina** in 1974 and has since gained widespread acceptance. In 1971, Fontan proposed a surgical repair for tricuspid atresia based upon separation of the right and left circulations. Subsequent modifications to Fontan's original operation were designed to bypass the right ventricle and direct systemic venous return to the pulmonary circulation. The most recent modifications divert vena caval blood directly to the PA, now referred to as a **total cavopulmonary connection** (modified Fontan). In 1988, **Laks** suggested leaving a small fenestration between the right and left circulations, creating a R→L shunt for the purposes of augmenting systemic CO while still maintaining adequate oxygenation.

Bidirectional Glenn shunt: A standard median sternotomy approach is used. If concomitant intracardiac repairs are not anticipated, the bidirectional Glenn shunt may be performed without CPB by placing a temporary shunt between the high SVC and the RA. If the patient has a preexisting Blalock-Taussig shunt on the right, it is divided after instituting CPB. A shunt on the left side may be left open, while the bidirectional Glenn shunt is created on the right. The SVC is divided and the cardiac end is oversewn. The remaining caval end is anastomosed end-to-side to the superior aspect of the right PA.

Fontan procedure: The heart is accessed via a standard median sternotomy. Previously placed systemic-to-PA shunts are dissected and occluded prior to bypass. Bicaval cannulation and CPB with hypothermia are used. The IVC is transected at its PA junction and a Gore-Tex tube graft is interposed end-to-end between the IVC and the inferior surface of the right PA. This operation, in conjunction with the previously performed bidirectional Glenn shunt, establishes a total cavopulmonary connection. After completing the anastomosis, the aortic cross-clamp is removed, the heart is rewarmed and the patient is weaned from CPB. Fenestration of the Fontan circuit may be desirable in high-risk patients, but is generally not required in patients with tricuspid atresia and good ventricular function.

Variant procedure or approaches: A RA→RV connection can be performed in patients with tricuspid atresia without pulmonary obstruction and an adequately functioning RV. This is performed with a direct anastomosis or a valved/ nonvalved conduit (i.e., aortic homograft, Dacron graft).

Usual preop diagnosis: Tricuspid atresia, after Blalock-Taussig shunt or PA banding; univentricular heart or single ventricle after shunt or band; cyanotic congenital heart disease

SUMMARY OF PROCEDURE

	Bidirectional Glenn Shunt	Cavopulmonary Fontan Procedure
Position	Supine	⇐
Incision	Standard median sternotomy	⇐
Unique considerations	Particulate or gaseous emboli from iv lines in the lower extremities can become systemic emboli following a Glenn shunt.	Areas of PA stenosis need to be repaired concomitantly; subaortic obstruction needs to be considered if there is a bulboventricular outlet foramen.
Antibiotics	Cefazolin 15-30 mg/kg q 8 h	⇐

	Bidirectional Glenn Shunt	Cavopulmonary Fontan Procedure
Surgical time	If a simple anastomosis is constructed, the aorta is not cross-clamped; otherwise, aortic cross-clamp: 30-45 min	⇐
	Total: 2-3 h	Total: 3-4 h
Closing considerations	Chest tube in the pericardial space; temporary ventricular pacing wire; possible atrial monitoring line to assess ventricular filling pressures	Chest tube in the pericardial space; possible pleural tubes; temporary ventricular and atrial pacing wires; possible atrial line to correlate with CVP in order to determine the transpulmonary gradient
EBL	Minimal	⇐
Postop care	Cardiac ICU; early extubation to minimize positive intrathoracic pressure	ICU; 24 h ventilation or early extubation; inotropes for ventricular function, including low-dose dopamine, isoproterenol, low-dose epinephrine. Maintain sinus rhythm, A-V pacing, if required.
Mortality	2-4%	4-8%
Morbidity	Bleeding Infection ↑SVC pressure Upper extremity edema (SVC syndrome) ↓CO Cyanosis 2° ↓pulmonary blood flow Pulmonary arteriovenous fistula	Residual R→L shunting through unsuspected systemic venous connections to the atria.
Pain score	8-10	8-10

PATIENT POPULATION CHARACTERISTICS

Age range	6 mo-2 yr	2-5 yr
Male:Female	1:1	⇐
Incidence	1-3% of congenital heart defects	⇐
Etiology	Unknown	⇐
Associated conditions	ASD, TGA	Aortic valve insufficiency requiring repair or replacement; previous palliative shunt or PA banding; residual PA obstruction; dextrocardia; asplenia or polysplenia syndromes

ANESTHETIC CONSIDERATIONS

PREOPERATIVE

Pathophysiology All patients with tricuspid atresia are hypoxemic, since the systemic venous blood must pass from the RA to the LA where it mixes with the pulmonary venous blood. Survival depends on both an interatrial communication (ASD or PFO) to decompress the RA, and a systemic-to-pulmonary shunt (e.g., VSD). Approximately 70% of patients with tricuspid atresia are cyanotic at birth. Most are managed initially (palliative) with a systemic arterial-to-PA shunt (Blalock-Taussig shunt, modified BT shunt or central shunt) to ↑pulmonary blood flow. Approximately 30% of patients with tricuspid atresia have excessive pulmonary blood flow (e.g., large VSD) and CHF without pulmonic stenosis. These patients are managed with PA banding (palliative).

Palliation also can be achieved via the bidirectional Glenn shunt (BDG), which offers the advantage of ↑pulmonary blood flow without LV volume overload. In the Glenn shunt, SVC blood flow is directly shunted into the right PA. The Glenn has been used for interim palliation prior to the Fontan procedure. The infant is generally in the age range of 4-8 mo. Occasionally, an older child not considered a candidate for the Fontan procedure will undergo a palliative Glenn. O_2 sats after BDG are generally 75-85%. Ultimately, treatment of tricuspid atresia requires separation of the systemic and pulmonary circulation using the Fontan procedure. Most patients referred for a Fontan

Pathophysiology, cont. procedure have had a prior Glenn anastomosis or related connection. After completion of the Fontan, the pulmonary and systemic circulations are separated and connected in series. Pulmonary blood flow is then dependent on the pressure gradient between the SVC and the LA. The "external conduit" (modified Fontan) is the preferred and most commonly performed procedure at Stanford, because it obviates the need for circulatory arrest. The approach, however, allows for immediate postop extubation (see TOF Emergence, p. 905). Early spontaneous ventilation has been shown to augment pulmonary blood flow and improve oxygenation in these single-ventricle patients. O_2 sat is approximately 94% following the Fontan operation 2° mixing of coronary sinus blood within the atrium. A baffle fenestration is performed in many patients, permitting shunting into the systemic ventricle to preserve CO in the face of transient ↑PVR. This can result in a further ↓ in O_2 sat.

Respiratory Identify any infectious or asthma-related problems. Optimizing pulmonary function is very important because pulmonary blood flow will be supplied passively from the systemic venous return.

Tests: CXR; O_2 sat

Cardiovascular Patients with ↑↑pulmonary blood flow (e.g., 2° large VSD) → CHF + mild cyanosis. Patients with ↓↓pulmonary blood flow (e.g., 2° small VSD, RVOTO) → marked cyanosis + acidosis. Cardiac cath and ECHO are generally done preop to evaluate PVR, PA anatomy, valvular function, size of the interatrial communication and ventricular function.

Tests: ECG, ECHO, cath

Laboratory Hct (expect ↑Hct 2° chronic hypoxemia); others as indicated by H&P.

Premedication Midazolam 0.5-0.75 mg po 30 min prior to induction in children > 1 yr old

INTRAOPERATIVE

Anesthetic technique: GETA + epidural anesthesia

Induction Children having either the Glenn or Fontan operation generally will tolerate mask induction with halothane or sevoflurane in 50% N_2O and 50% O_2. A smooth induction is essential to avoid exacerbating preexisting hypoxemia. IV access is established and pancuronium (0.1 mg/kg) with remifentanil (1 μg/kg) is given to facilitate ET intubation. Alternatively, the patient may be intubated while deeply anesthetized with sevoflurane or halothane. The epidural anesthetic is then placed (see TOF Epidural analgesia, p. 905). Immediate postop extubation is planned for most children.

Maintenance Sevoflurane/halothane anesthesia in 100% O_2. Bidirectional Glenn: for children who have previously undergone PA banding or who have a contralateral B-T shunt or collateral vessels, a bidirectional Glenn shunt can be performed without CPB. In children in whom a B-T shunt was placed on the right side or who have bilateral SVC, the procedure will require CPB. Fontan: the "external conduit" Fontan requires CPB with moderate hypothermia and a short ischemic interval. The "lateral tunnel" Fontan requires CPB and moderate hypothermia with an ischemic interval, or DHCA. As with the Glenn, adequate pulmonary blood flow and CO must be ensured to wean from CPB.

Emergence Children for whom immediate extubation is planned may be extubated awake or in a deep plane of anesthesia. Factors considered for deep extubation include child's age, activity level and developmental level. Ultimately, clinical experience, judgement and observation are the most important determinants of a smooth extubation and emergence. BP is tightly controlled with vasodilators (e.g., SNP or NTG). Patients extubated in a deep plane of anesthesia rarely require BP control with vasodilators.

Blood and fluid requirements	Blood loss: moderate-to-large IV: 22-24 ga × 1-2 taped securely LR @TKO Blood warmer Humidify gases. PRBC in OR	For patients with Hct > 60%, consider iv LR bolus (5-10 ml/kg) to ↓ viscosity, ↑ CO and ↓ SVR. Expect ↑blood loss in patients with previous cardiac surgery and sternotomies. Blood should be ready for immediate administration.
Infusions	EACA load 150 mg/kg over 30 min	Infusion: 20 mg/kg/h × 5 h, starting at induction
Monitoring	Standard monitors (see p. D-1). Arterial line	Avoid placement of radial arterial line in same side as B-T shunt. An IJ CVP will provide PA pressures postanastomosis.

Monitoring, cont.	CVP Urinary catheter	Some centers avoid upper body central lines because of the risk of thrombosis.
Positioning	✓ and pad pressure points. ✓ and tape eyes.	
CPB	Management of CPB is discussed in Intraoperative Considerations for TOF, p. 906.	Special considerations unique to tricuspid atresia are presented in Post CPB section, below.
Post CPB	PAP - LAP < 10 mmHg PAP < 18 mmHg Maintain CO. S_pO_2 > 70%	Pulmonary blood flow will depend on the transpulmonary pressure gradient (PA pressure–LA pressure). A transpulmonary gradient < 10 mmHg and a PA pressure < 18 mmHg are acceptable in the early postop period. ↓CO is associated with poor perfusion, ↑LA pressure and hypoxemia. Inotropic support with dopamine should be started. If S_pO_2 persistently < 70% following CPB, there should be concern for anastomotic obstruction or ↑PVR. (See TOF for maneuvers for ↑PVR, pp. 906-907).

POSTOPERATIVE

Complications	Persistent bleeding ↑PVR ↓CO Thrombosis of Fontan conduit Cerebral edema Pleural effusions	 Associated with ↑PVR.
Tests	ABG Electrolytes; Hct; coags CXR	

References

1. Baue AE, Gena AS, Hammond GL, Laks H, Naunheim KS: In *Glenn's Thoracic and Cardiovascular Surgery,* 6th edition. Appleton & Lange, Stamford, 1996.
2. Castaneda A, Jonas JA, Mayer JE, Hanley FL: *Cardiac Surgery of the Neonate and Infant.* WB Saunders, Philadelphia: 1994.
3. Cooper JR, Goldstein MT: Septal and endocardial cushion defects and double outlet right ventricle perioperative management. In *Pediatric Cardiac Anesthesia.* 3rd edition. Lake CL, ed. Appleton & Lange, Stamford, CT: 1998, 285-301.
4. Kambam J: Endocardial cushion defects. In *Cardiac Anesthesia for Infants and Children.* Kambam J, Fish FA, Merrill WH, eds. CV Mosby, St. Louis: 1994, 203-10.
5. Kirklin JW, Barrett-Boyes BG: Tricuspid atresia and the Fontan operation. In *Cardiac Surgery,* 2nd edition. Churchill-Livingstone, New York: 1993, 1055-1104.
6. Pearl JM, Permut LC, Laks H: Tricuspid atresia. In *Glenn's Thoracic and Cardiovascular Surgery,* 6th edition. Baue AE, ed. Appleton & Lange, Stamford: 1996, 1431-49.

SURGERY FOR DOUBLE-OUTLET RIGHT VENTRICLE

SURGICAL CONSIDERATIONS

Description: In double-outlet right ventricle (DORV), both of the great arteries arise from the RV. By necessity, there is a VSD which is usually large, but may in some cases be restrictive or, rarely, multiple and muscular. The VSD may be located primarily below the aorta (**DORV/subaortic VSD**) (Fig 12.3-7A) or below the pulmonary valve (**DORV/ subpulmonic VSD** or **Taussig-Bing DORV**) (Fig 12.3-7B). In DORV/subaortic VSD, oxygenated LV blood is directed to the aorta and deoxygenated systemic venous return from the RV is directed to the PA, resulting in minimal-to-no cyanosis. L→R shunting across the VSD, however, leads to pulmonary overcirculation, pulmonary HTN and CHF. In DORV/subpulmonic VSD, oxygenated LV blood is directed to the PA and deoxygenated systemic venous return from the RV is directed to the aorta → pulmonary overcirculation and significant cyanosis. If early PA banding or primary correction is not performed in patients with pulmonary overcirculation, PVOD may result at an early age. In patients with some degree of pulmonary stenosis (usually infundibular), R→L shunting and cyanosis results; the natural history resembles that of patients with tetralogy of Fallot.

The first repairs of DORV were described by **Kirklin** in 1957. The Taussig-Bing DORV was first corrected in 1967. In recent years, management has been simplified for this variant by combining the arterial switch operation with an intraventricular baffle to the pulmonary valve. From a surgical standpoint, the anatomic variations and past attempts at correction may lead to unique intraop challenges. For example, if a previous Blalock-Taussig shunt has been performed, it needs to be controlled prior to initiating CPB. A previous pulmonary band may require removal and PA reconstruction.

DORV/subaortic VSD is generally repaired with an **intraventricular tunnel repair,** in which LV blood from the VSD is channeled through the RV to the aorta. Through a median sternotomy, CPB is instituted and previous shunts are ligated. The aorta is cross-clamped and cardioplegia is administered. After performing a right atriotomy, the interior of the RV is inspected through the tricuspid valve; a right ventriculotomy may be necessary for adequate exposure. A tunnel constructed of Dacron is then placed between the VSD and the subaortic infundibulum. Augmentation of the RVOT, in the form of an outflow patch or extracardiac RV→PA conduit, is often necessary since the outflow tract is commonly obstructed to some degree by the intraventricular tunnel. The heart is then rewarmed and resuscitated, CPB is discontinued, and standard chest closure is commenced.

DORV/subpulmonic VSD (Taussig-Bing DORV) can be corrected with an arterial switch operation and VSD closure under CPB (see Surgery for Complete Transposition of the Great Arteries, p. 911). DORV with significant pulmonary stenosis resembles that for the TOF (see p. 903).

Usual preop diagnosis: DORV ± pulmonary stenosis; s/p PA band or modified Blalock-Taussig shunt; Taussig-Bing type of DORV; CHF

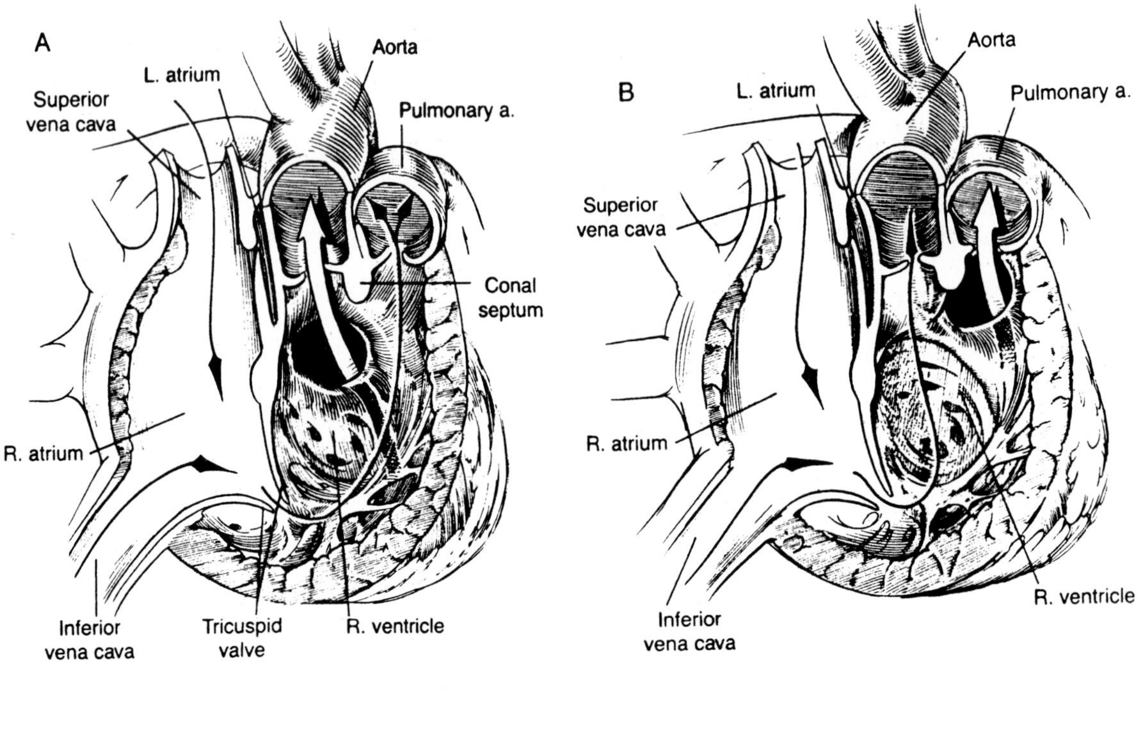

Figure 12.3-7. Double-outlet right ventricle (DORV). (A) DORV with a subaortic VSD. LV flow is directed towards the aorta, resulting in physiology similar to that of tetralogy of Fallot (TOF). (B) DORV with a subpulmonic VSD (Taussig-Bing anomaly). LV flow is directed toward the PA, resulting in physiology similar to that of transposition of the great arteries. (Reproduced with permission from Castaneda AR, et al: *Cardiac Surgery of the Neonate and Infant.* WB Saunders, Philadelphia: 1994, 446.)

SUMMARY OF PROCEDURE

Position	Supine
Incision	Standard median sternotomy
Antibiotics	Cefazolin 15-30 mg/kg q 8 h
Surgical time	Aortic cross-clamp: 50-60 min Total: 3-3.5 h
Closing considerations	Routine closure with chest tube in the pericardial space; temporary ventricular pacing wire; possible LA line for monitoring
EBL	Minimal
Postop care	ICU for 24 h of controlled ventilation; possible pulmonary HTN protocol in cases of unrestricted pulmonary blood flow (see description of management for A-V canal defect, p. 891).
Mortality	5-20%
Morbidity	Hemorrhage ↓CO Intraventricular tunnel obstruction Baffle leakage; residual RVOTO Heart block
Pain score	8-10

PATIENT POPULATION CHARACTERISTICS

Age range	3-24 mo
Male:Female	1:1
Incidence	1-3% of congenital heart defects
Etiology	No specific correlations or associated conditions
Associated conditions	Pulmonary stenosis; complete A-V canal defect; coarctation of the aorta

ANESTHETIC CONSIDERATIONS

PREOPERATIVE

Pathophysiology DORV is a conotruncal abnormality and is almost always associated with a VSD. Other complex abnormalities of venoatrial or atrioventricular connections can coexist with DORV (e.g., pulmonary stenosis, 47%; ASD, 26%; LVOTO, 3-17%). Typically, blood entering the LV must cross through a VSD into the RV, then out the aorta. Systemic venous return follows the usual pathway to the RV. Distribution of RV flow between the pulmonary trunk and aorta depends on several factors, which determine the clinical presentation. If the VSD is just below the aorta ("subaortic") then oxygenated blood from the LV will cross through the VSD and preferentially travel directly out the aorta. The subaortic VSD is frequently associated with infundibular stenosis and obstruction to pulmonary flow. Thus, some deoxygenated blood will enter the aorta. The resulting physiology and clinical picture is similar to that of TOF, and its surgical treatment is analogous, namely, baffle closure of VSD (with aorta to the left side), infundibular muscle resection and possible RVOT patch. On the other hand, if the VSD is just below the pulmonary valve ("subpulmonary"), then oxygenated blood from the LV will cross the VSD and preferentially travel directly out the pulmonary trunk. Because of this, blood from the RA entering the RV will tend to travel out the aorta. The resulting physiology and clinical picture is similar to that of transposition of the great arteries (TGA), and its surgical treatment is usually analogous (i.e., arterial switch with VSD closure, see below). The VSD can have one of two other positions. It may lie under both the aortic and pulmonary valves ("doubly committed"), in which case the repair consists of baffle closure of the VSD. Alternatively, the VSD may lie remote from both valves ("noncommitted"). This anatomy presents the greatest challenge for two-ventricle repair, because a long, intraventricular baffle must be constructed from the VSD to the aortic root. The pathway for this baffle may be too narrow to guarantee lasting, nonobstructed flow from the LV to the aorta. In these cases, a single ventricle repair may be chosen.

Cardiovascular The preop clinical presentation and ECHO findings describe the position of the great vessels and VSD and are the primary determinants of the type of operation chosen for DORV. Young infants

Cardiovascular, cont. with DORV will present with clinical signs of pulmonary overcirculation (with or without mild cyanosis) or pulmonary undercirculation (with mild-to-moderate cyanosis). Diagnosis is made by echocardiography. Catheterization is rarely necessary except in the older infant or young child to determine if there is pulmonary vascular disease. It is important for the anesthesiologist to know precisely which operative approach will be taken for each patient with DORV.

Respiratory Pulmonary overcirculation → CHF + pulmonary edema. Pulmonary HTN may develop.

Laboratory Hct, electrolytes (children on diuretic Rx); others as indicated from H&P.

Premedication Children < 9 mo old rarely need premedication. In older children, effective premedication will help provide for a smooth inhalation induction. It is important to avoid a hyperdynamic cardiovascular response, especially in children with infundibular pulmonary stenosis. (See premedication sections for specific lesions: TOF, VSD, TGA or Glenn shunt).

INTRAOPERATIVE

Intraop management See specific lesion, e.g., TOF, VSD, TGA or Glenn shunt. The management of the infant undergoing palliative operations, such as PA banding, Blalock-Taussig shunt or bidirectional Glenn shunt, is described elsewhere. The corrective surgery follows the general scheme of operations for TOF, TGA or VSD repair. Additional points to consider in the management of infants with DORV follow below.

Pre CPB **DORV/subaortic VSD in infancy:** Patients should be managed similarly to those with TOF. The possibility of a hypercyanotic spell should be considered. Enquire about the use of circulatory arrest or continuous low-flow bypass for the repair, and make appropriate preparations.

DORV/subpulmonary VSD or Taussig-Bing variant: Patients are managed similarly to those with TGA/VSD. Patients with interrupted arch are ductal dependent. Adequate mixing and a relative balance of pulmonary and systemic circulations should be maintained. Anticipate the possibility of a relatively long myocardial ischemic time. Some surgeons will do part of the repair under circulatory arrest.

DORV/noncommitted VSD: Similar to TOF management.

CPB **DORV/subaortic VSD:** Either moderate hypothermia and low flow or deep hypothermia and circulatory arrest will be used. A ventriculotomy may be performed (→ postop ventricular compromise).

DORV/subpulmonary VSD: Repair consists of arterial switch and baffle closure of the VSD. Circulatory arrest may be used for none, part or all of the repair. Upon reperfusion, immediate and careful assessment of coronary perfusion should be made, as in TGA. Pulmonary root reconstruction may be performed while reperfusing and rewarming.

DORV/noncommitted VSD: Intraventricular anatomy will be assessed once the cross-clamp is placed. Be prepared to change the anesthetic plan, depending on the operative findings. If the findings preclude two-ventricle repair, the surgeon may proceed to a Blalock-Taussig or bidirectional Glenn shunt. Otherwise, surgery will proceed with an intraventricular baffle, usually through a right ventriculotomy. Surgical enlargement of the VSD may ↑ risk of damage to the conduction system. RV outflow reconstruction may require a valved homograft. The ischemic and CPB times will be longer than routine TOF repair.

Transition off CPB **DORV/subaortic VSD:** With pulmonary stenosis, the risk of pulmonary HTN is low. RA pressures may be elevated 2° ↓RV compliance. RV/arterial line pressure ratio should be measured post CPB; values > 70-75% suggest inadequacy of RVOT reconstruction. TEE is valuable for assessing completeness of VSD closure and LV function. Patient may require inotropic support (3-5 μg/kg/min of dopamine). SaO_2 = 100% unless there is a PFO and RA pressures are elevated. There is a small incidence of junctional ectopic tachycardia or of surgical damage to the conduction system.

DORV/subpulmonary VSD: Management is similar to that of TGA/VSD postrepair. Response of the LV to weaning must be carefully monitored, considering: (1) the moderate ischemic time, (2) coronary reimplantation, and (3) possibility of residual VSD, coarctation, or semilunar valve insufficiency. These are assessed by arterial line tracing, ABG, ECG, visual appearance of the LV and TEE. Patients may require inotropic support (3-5 μg/kg/min of dopamine and, occasionally, milrinone). SaO_2 should = 100%.

DORV/noncommitted VSD: Patients with intraventricular baffle have the same considerations as for DORV/subaortic VSD, with the possible addition of baffle obstruction to LV outflow. The

Transition off CPB, cont. latter will cause LV failure on attempts to wean from CPB. TEE and direct measurement of LA pressure are useful adjuncts during weaning. Dopamine may be required. If a palliative bidirectional Glenn shunt is performed, PVR should be optimized (adjust ventilation and oxygenation). Direct pressure measurements should be made in the PA and RA (or, more precisely, LA if there is no ASD).

POSTOPERATIVE

Postop management considerations are similar to those of repair for TOF or for TGA/VSD in two-ventricle repairs. Postop care for bidirectional Glenn procedures is discussed elsewhere (p. 921). The mortality associated with DORV repair is greater than that for simple TOF repair or repair of TGA with the usual coronary anatomy and single VSD. This is often caused by problems associated with the intraventricular baffle (e.g., obstruction), anomalies of the coronary origins, residual LVOTO in the Taussig-Bing heart, other associated cardiac anomalies or depression of LV function 2° relatively longer ischemic times in some cases. Careful clinical assessment and ECHO should be performed early in any infant not progressing postop. Cardiac catheterization should not be delayed if a diagnosis of the problem cannot be made with ECHO.

References

1. Baue AE, Geha AS, Hammond GL, Laks H, Naunheim KS: *Glenn's Thoracic and Cardiovascular Surgery,* 6th edition. Appleton & Lange, Stamford: 1996.
2. Castaneda AR, Jonas RA, Mayer JE Jr, Hanley FL: Double-outlet right ventricle. In *Cardiac Surgery of the Neonate and Infant.* WB Saunders, Philadelphia: 1994, 445-59.
3. Kambam J: Endocardial cushion defects. In *Cardiac Anesthesia for Infants and Children.* Kambam J, Fish FA, Merrill WH, eds. CV Mosby, St. Louis: 1994, 203-10.
4. Kirklin JW, Barrett-Boyes BG: Double-outlet right ventricle. In *Cardiac Surgery,* 2nd edition. Churchill-Livingstone, New York: 1993, 1469-1500.
5. Starnes VA, Prendergast TW: Double-outlet right ventricle and double-outlet left ventricle. In *Glenn's Thoracic and Cardiovascular Surgery,* 6th edition. Baue AE, ed. Appleton & Lange, Stamford: 1996, 1417-29.

SURGERY FOR HYPOPLASTIC LEFT HEART SYNDROME

SURGICAL CONSIDERATIONS

Description: Hypoplastic left heart syndrome (HLHS) represents a spectrum of left-sided cardiac malformations centered around a markedly hypoplastic or absent LV, and an atretic aortic valve and ascending aorta; the mitral valve is also usually hypoplastic. Consequently, the RV supports both the pulmonary and systemic circulations. The pulmonary venous return enters the RA via an ASD, and the admixture of systemic and pulmonary venous return is delivered into the RV and main PA. Systemic flow is delivered into the aorta by way of a typically large PDA. Cyanosis, CHF and systemic hypoperfusion result as pulmonary venous return decreases and pulmonary blood flow increases at the expense of systemic blood flow.

Until recently, patients born with this anomaly usually died within the first 2 wk of life, with survival beyond 6 wk being very rare. A palliative surgical treatment was reported by Norwood in 1983. The palliative surgical treatment of HLHS comprises staged operations, with the first stage designated as the **"Norwood operation."** The procedure is directed towards establishing effective CO from the RV to the systemic circulation and to support the pulmonary circulation with a systemic-to-pulmonary arterial shunt. An adequate atrial septal communication is essential.

Norwood Stage I: Through a median sternotomy, a portion of the pericardium is harvested for later use as a patch. The ascending aorta and RA appendage are cannulated and CPB with cooling is instituted. The arch vessels and proximal descending thoracic aorta are dissected. Total circulatory arrest with infusion of cardioplegia is followed by cannulae removal. The ductus arteriosus is then divided and the pulmonary end is oversewn. Next, the main PA is divided and a pericardial patch is placed on the distal PA. An aortotomy is created, extending from the interior aspect of the aortic arch through the lateral aspect of the ascending aorta to the level of the transected pulmonary trunk. The entire aortic arch complex is then augmented, creating a "neoaorta" from the proximal portion of the transected main PA, which is anastomosed to the ascending aorta and arch. A cryopreserved homograft wall is used to facilitate the repair. The RA is opened and the atrial septum is excised to maximize the size of the interatrial communication. The cannulae are then reinserted and CPB with rewarming begins. Finally, a Blalock-Taussig systemic-to-PA shunt is created to provide pulmonary blood flow. The patient is weaned from CPB, a pericardial drainage tube is placed, and the chest is closed in the standard fashion.

Norwood Stage II: As the PVR normally falls in the weeks after the first-stage operation, excessive pulmonary blood flow from the Blalock-Taussig shunt may → RV volume overload and CHF. The second-stage procedure for HLHS is intended to reduce the volume load on the single ventricle while maintaining adequate pulmonary blood flow. Also known as the first stage of the **Fontan procedure** or **"hemi-Fontan,"** this operation consists of a bidirectional cavopulmonary (Glenn) shunt (see Surgery for Tricuspid Atresia, p. 918). This is usually performed in children 6-12 mo old.

Norwood Stage III: The third, and final, stage of the Norwood procedure is usually performed about 6-12 mo after the second stage and consists of the completion of the Fontan procedure (see Surgery for Tricuspid Atresia, p. 918). It is designed to divide the systemic venous return from the pulmonary venous return by establishing continuity from the IVC to the confluence of the PAs and SVC.

Variant procedure or approaches: Successful cardiac transplantation for this condition was performed by **Bailey** in 1985. Cardiac transplantation is associated with a lower operative mortality; however, a significant number of neonates on the waiting lists do not receive donor hearts. Moreover, cardiac transplantation is associated with lifelong immunosuppression and its associated risks.

Usual preop diagnosis: HLHS; mitral and aortic atresia

SUMMARY OF PROCEDURE

Position	Supine
Incision	Standard median sternotomy
Unique considerations	Hypothermia (< 18° C) and circulatory arrest; control of PVR, both preop and postop is extremely important, with the FiO_2 and ventilation being crucial in regulating pulmonary blood flow. For very high pulmonary blood flows and O_2 sats > 85%, consider the addition of N_2 to lower the FiO_2 to < 20%.
Antibiotics	Cefazolin 15-30 mg/kg q 8 h
Surgical time	Aortic cross-clamp: 45-55 min (also circulatory arrest time) Total: 3-3.5 h
Closing considerations	Routine closure with chest tube in the pericardial space; temporary ventricular pacing wire; possible left atrial line for monitoring
EBL	Minimal-to-moderate
Postop care	24-72 h of controlled ventilation; moderate need for inotropic drugs; PGE_1 infusion to ↓PVR
Mortality	15-30%
Morbidity	Hemorrhage Infection ↓CO Inadequate/excessive pulmonary blood flow Tricuspid regurgitation
Pain score	8-10

PATIENT POPULATION CHARACTERISTICS

Age range	5-30 d
Male:Female	2:1
Incidence	3-5% of congenital heart defects
Etiology	Often associated with genetic disorders, but no single associated defect
Associated conditions	CNS defects (29%); microencephaly (25-27%); VSD (5%); TGA

ANESTHETIC CONSIDERATIONS

PREOPERATIVE

Pathophysiology HLHS is characterized by a hypoplastic or atretic aortic valve associated with hypoplasia of the LV, ascending aorta and aortic arch. The mitral valve may be atretic or stenotic. Pulmonary venous

Pathophysiology, cont.	return enters the left atrium and then passes into the RA via an ASD or the PFO. Rarely, pulmonary venous return is via TAPVC to the RA. The systemic circulation is supplied entirely through the ductus arteriosus. Perfusion of the ascending aorta, coronary arteries and transverse arch is retrograde via the ductus. Maintenance of adequate systemic perfusion relies on ductal patency and is achieved with continuous administration of PGE_1. Maintaining a ↑PVR by ↓ the FiO_2 to 0.17-0.20, or by adding CO_2 to breathing gas mixture, also may be necessary. As the ductus closes, the systemic perfusion is compromised, → ischemia, acidosis and eventually death. Hence, survival depends on the patency of the ductus arteriosus; the adequacy of mixing at the atrial level; and maintaining a balance between PVR and SVR to ensure adequate pulmonary and systemic perfusion.	
Respiratory	Evidence of ↑pulmonary blood flow → pulmonary congestion/edema, tachypnea. **Tests:** CXR: enlarged heart; ↑pulmonary vascular markings; ABG	
Cardiovascular	Look for Sx of CHF. These patients are frequently tachycardic and mildly cyanotic. Peripheral pulses may be diminished if systemic perfusion is compromised. Systemic hypoperfusion → ↓renal function, ↓hepatic function. **Tests:** ECG; RAE/RVH; ECHO: assessment of tricuspid or common AV valve regurgitation. Severe TR is a contraindication for 1st stage repair.	
Neurological	Evaluate CNS.	
Laboratory	BUN; creatine; other tests as indicated by H&P.	
Premedication	Not indicated.	
Transport to OR	Patients are transported from the ICU in a warmed transport module with ECG, SpO_2 and arterial line monitoring. Neonates are often intubated because they become apneic from the infusion of PGE_1. During transport to the OR, continue FiO_2 and $FiCO_2$ from ICU. Resuscitative drugs and airway equipment should be readily available during transport.	

INTRAOPERATIVE

Anesthetic technique: GETA

Induction	On arrival in the OR, monitors are applied and ventilation should be adjusted to maintain arterial O_2 sat = 75-85%. Hypoxic gas mixtures with 1-2% CO_2 may be necessary. Avoid hyperventilation (→ ↑pulmonary blood flow). Induction begins with pancuronium (0.2 mg/kg) to avoid opiate-induced chest rigidity. Note: PGE_1 will increase pancuronium dose requirements. Fentanyl (10 μg/kg) is then given. Ventilation needs to be reassessed after muscle relaxation to avoid excessive minute ventilation. A previously placed ETT should be replaced with a new nasotracheal tube to provide an airway free from inspissated secretions. In nonintubated patients, a nasotracheal intubation is appropriate.	
Maintenance	Fentanyl (100-200 μg/kg) in divided doses. Pancuronium prn, midazolam (0.1-0.2 mg/kg) as tolerated. FiO_2 may be increased in the immediate postbypass period → ↓PVR.	
Emergence	Transport to ICU intubated and ventilated.	
Blood and fluid requirements	See Tetralogy of Fallot (TOF), p. 905. 1-2 U PRBC 2 U Plt and 2 U cryo	Continue dextrose infusion in neonates. Blood loss can be due largely to dilutional coagulopathy and multiple suture lines. The use of fresh whole blood, blood products (FFP, cryo and Plt), EACA and modified ultrafiltration (MUF) help to limit hemorrhage and the consequent hemodynamic instability.
Infusions	See TOF, p. 906.	Continue PGE_1 infusion until CPB.
Monitoring	See TOF, p. 905.	
Positioning	See TOF, p. 907.	
CPB	See TOF, p. 906.	Management of CPB is discussed in Intraoperative Considerations for TOF, p. 906. Special considerations unique to HLHS are presented below.
Pre CPB and CPB	See TOF for routine CPB parameters, p. 906.	Maintain the delicate balance between SVR and PVR. Avoid myocardial depression, ↓PVR or ↑SVR, which

		would ↑ pulmonary blood flow at the expense of systemic and coronary blood flows.
Transition off CPB and Post CPB	See TOF, p. 906.	After the Stage I (Norwood) surgical repair, the blood flow continues to be supplied in a parallel fashion from the single ventricle. Optimally, PaO_2 should = 30-40 mmHg with MAP = 45-55 mmHg. In neonates with ↓PaO_2 (20-23 mmHg) the cause can be ↑PVR, inadequate modified B-T shunt or poor myocardial function. The use of NO to ↓ PVR has been controversial in this subset of patients. Most frequently, neonates show Sx of pulmonary overcirculation with PaO_2 > 45 mmHg. Thus, ventilation maneuvers to ↑ PVR should be instituted (↑$PaCO_2$, ↓FiO_2).
Complications	Paradoxical embolism Others, see Postoperative Complications, below	

POSTOPERATIVE

Complications	Pulmonary overcirculation Pulmonary HTN Persistent bleeding Myocardial dysfunction and failure Hypothermia Aortic arch obstruction Renal insufficiency CNS injury	 Aventricular-assist device may be required.
Tests	ABGs Electrolytes; Hct; coags	

References

1. Castaneda AR, Jonas RA, Mayer JE Jr, Hanley FL: Hypoplastic left heart syndrome. In *Cardiac Surgery of the Neonate and Infant.* WB Saunders, Philadelphia: 1994, 363-85.
2. Jacobs ML, Norwood WI: Hyperplastic left heart syndrome. In *Pediatric Cardiac Surgery: Current Issues.* Jacobs ML, Norwood WI, eds. Butterworth-Heinemann, Stoneham, UK: 1992, 182-92.
3. Jacobs ML, Norwood WI: Hypoplastic left heart syndrome. In *Glenn's Thoracic and Cardiovascular Surgery,* 6th edition. Baue AE, ed. Appleton & Lange, Stamford: 1996, 1271-81.
4. Kambam J: Endocardial cushion defects. In *Cardiac Anesthesia for Infants and Children.* Kambam J, Fish FA, Merrill WH, eds. CV Mosby, St. Louis: 1994, 203-10.
5. Kirklin JW, Barrett-Boyes BG: Aortic atresia. In *Cardiac Surgery,* 2nd edition. Churchill-Livingstone, New York: 1993, 1327-42.
6. Nicolson SC, Steven JM, Jobes DR: Hypoplastic left heart syndrome. In *Pediatric Cardiac Anesthesia,* 3rd edition. Lake CL, ed. Appleton & Lange, Stamford: 1998, 337-52.

Surgeon

Gary E. Hartman, MD

12.4 PEDIATRIC GENERAL SURGERY

Anesthesiologists

Alvin Hackel, MD
Gregory B. Hammer, MD

REPAIR OF ESOPHAGEAL ATRESIA/ TRACHEOESOPHAGEAL FISTULA

SURGICAL CONSIDERATIONS

Description: The vast majority (86%) of infants with esophageal atresia (EA) have an associated distal tracheoesophageal fistula (TEF) (Fig 12.4-1). Aspiration of gastric contents or GI distension via the distal fistula generally mandates urgent operative intervention. Many surgeons continue to advocate **gastrostomy**, either as part of the primary repair or as a preliminary procedure in complicated cases. Primary repair with or without gastrostomy is possible in large infants with no associated anomalies or aspiration pneumonitis. **Staged procedures**—initial gastrostomy, followed within days or weeks by **right thoracotomy** for esophageal repair—are used in premature infants with associated anomalies or aspiration, or by surgeons' preference.

Debate continues regarding the choice of retropleural vs transpleural repair. Transpleural repair is faster, but it exposes the pleural space to anastomotic leak and is potentially more disruptive to respiratory physiology. Preop identification of right aortic arch (5%) will allow for consideration of a **left thoracotomy** for the esophageal repair. A **lateral thoracotomy** is used on the side opposite the aortic arch. Initial attention is directed at identification and division of the distal fistula, if present, with the trachea open during the division. The proximal pouch generally requires significant dissection and also may require a circular **myotomy** to gain enough length for a primary anastomosis, which is almost always possible and is done in a single layer.

Variant procedure or approaches: EA without fistula (8%) is treated with initial **gastrostomy**, followed by attempted primary repair, at 6-8 wk, after dilation of the proximal or both pouches. A less desirable alternative is **proximal esophagostomy** with delayed interposition of colon or gastric tube. TEF without atresia (4%) is usually diagnosed later in the first few years of life, due to recurrent aspiration, and is usually approached through a cervical incision.

Usual preop diagnosis: EA; TEF

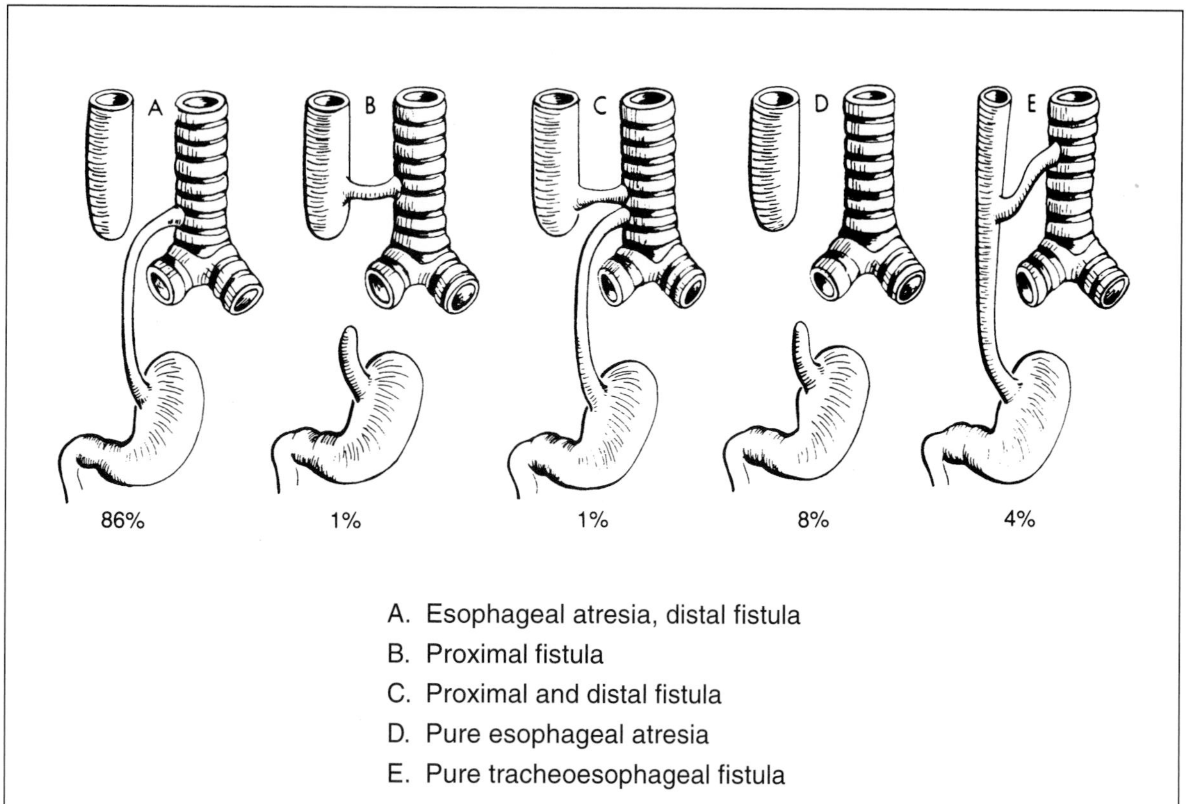

Figure 12.4-1. Types of esophageal atresia. (Reproduced with permission from Ravitch MM, et al, eds: *Pediatric Surgery*, Vol 1, 3rd edition. Year Book Medical Pub: 1979.)

SUMMARY OF PROCEDURE

	Primary Repair	Gastrostomy
Position	Lateral	Supine
Incision	Posterolateral thoracotomy (side opposite aortic arch)	Paramedian, midline
Special instrumentation	Bougie in upper pouch	Whiskey nipple
Unique considerations	Loss of ventilation via fistula	May be done under local anesthesia.
Antibiotics	Preop: ampicillin 25 mg/kg iv + gentamicin 2.5 mg/kg iv	⇐
	Intraop: cephalosporin irrigation (1 g/500 ml NS)	⇐
Surgical time	2-4 h	1 h
Closing considerations	Extubation favored	Local anesthetic; wound infiltration
EBL	10 ml/kg	5 ml/kg
Postop care	NICU; humidified mist; avoid CPAP and neck hyperextension	⇐
Mortality	1-20%, depending on associated anomalies	5%
Morbidity	Stricture: 20-40%	Aspiration
	Leak: 10-20%	
	Aspiration	
	Atelectasis	
	Stridor	
Pain score	7-8	3-4

PATIENT POPULATION CHARACTERISTICS

Age range	Days–weeks
Male:Female	1:1
Incidence	1/4000 births
Etiology	Unknown
Associated conditions	Vertebral, anal, TEF, renal anomalies (VATER association); vertebral, anal, cardiac, TEF, renal, limb anomalies (VACTERL association); trisomy 13, 18; hydrocephalus

ANESTHETIC CONSIDERATIONS

PREOPERATIVE

Esophageal atresia (EA) and tracheoesophageal fistula (TEF) are usually detected in the first day of life, although TEF without atresia may be difficult to diagnose until the patient experiences recurrent pneumonia, cyanosis associated with feeding, or abdominal distention. The fistula is usually at the distal trachea near the carina. Because of the risk of pulmonary aspiration, gastrostomy may be performed within hours of detection. Abnormalities frequently associated with TEF include prematurity (30-40%) and other congenital anomalies, particularly cardiac (20-35%). The VATER association includes the following defects: vertebral anomalies, VSD, anal atresia, TEF with EA and radial (or renal) anomalies. Routine neonatal preop evaluation includes H&P, serum electrolytes, blood sugar and Hct. Evidence of UO is needed before surgery.

Respiratory The upper esophageal pouch is continuously suctioned to minimize aspiration. Premature infants are at risk for RDS. These patients frequently have respiratory insufficiency 2° meconium aspiration or RDS, and may be intubated and on mechanical ventilation with supplemental O_2 prior to surgery.
Tests: CXR; ABG

Cardiovascular Associated cardiac abnormalities include: VSD, PDA, tetralogy of Fallot, ASD and coarctation of the aorta. At risk for pulmonary HTN with R→L shunt (e.g., PFO).
Tests: ECG; ECHO; catheterization, as indicated from H&P in consultation with pediatric cardiologist.

Gastrointestinal Multiple associated GI anomalies may occur (e.g., VATER association, pyloric stenosis, duodenal atresia).

Musculoskeletal Musculoskeletal anomalies are usually of little anesthetic significance, except for cervical spine involvement.
Tests: C-spine flexion, extension

Hematologic For the first 2-3 mo of life, the O_2-carrying capacity of blood is increased because of the presence of fetal Hb with its decreased sensitivity to 2,3-DPG. A shift to the right of the O_2 saturation curve results in ↑O_2-Hb affinity. As a result, tissue oxygenation may be reduced, especially with anemia (Hb < 12 g/dl @ < 2-3 mo). Although TEF repair is not usually associated with significant blood loss, a T&C is indicated.
Tests: Hct; T&C; others as indicated from H&P.

Laboratory Serum electrolytes, UA, ABG, blood glucose, to determine metabolic state.

Premedication Usually none

INTRAOPERATIVE

Anesthetic technique: Combined GETA/epidural, using a pediatric circle or Bain circuit with humidified and warmed gases. Maintain body temperature as close to 37°C as possible. Warm room to 78-80°F. If child is otherwise healthy and extubation is planned at end of the case, consider placing a caudal or lumbar epidural catheter (p. D-5) after airway is secured and the child is anesthetized.

Induction Atropine (0.02 mg/kg iv in children < 6-9 mo) is given before induction to ablate vagal response to laryngoscopy. Advance ETT to right mainstem and withdraw until bilateral breath sounds are present. Have flexible pediatric bronchoscope available to verify placement of ETT and site of TEF. Keep air leak around ETT to a minimum (leak at 10-35 cmH_2O) to minimize alterations in ventilation 2° changes in chest and pulmonary compliance.

Maintenance Avoid high FiO_2; use air/O_2 mixture for ventilation to maintain O_2 sat between 95-100%. Use low PIPs to avoid gastric distention by gasses passing through fistula. Careful adjustment of ventilation will be necessary during surgical retraction of lung. Manual ventilation provides direct monitoring of pulmonary compliance. Air/O_2/opiate (e.g., fentanyl 5-10 μg/kg/h) and low-dose volatile technique preferred because of better hemodynamic stability. Muscle relaxation (pancuronium or vecuronium 0.1 mg/kg iv) is usually necessary. If combined epidural anesthetic is used, GA drug requirements will be reduced. Frequent tracheal suctioning may be needed.

Emergence Extubation in OR is preferable, but not always possible. Supplemental O_2 is necessary to keep PaO_2 = 60-80 mmHg (SpO_2 = 95-100%). Cardiac or pulmonary complications, or any question regarding adequacy of ventilation, mandate continued intubation and ventilation.

Blood and fluid requirements	Blood loss usually minimal IV: 22-24 ga × 2 NS/LR (maintenance) @: 4 ml/kg/h – 0-10 kg 5% albumin	Continue dextrose-containing solution from NICU. Replace 3rd-space losses (6-8 ml/kg/h) with NS/LR. Replace blood loss with 5% albumin ml for ml blood loss; maintain Hct > 35%.
Monitoring	Standard monitors (p. D-1). Left axillary precordial stethoscope Arterial line (e.g., 24 ga)	ABG, Hct and glucose q 60 min
Positioning	✓ and pad pressure points. ✓ eyes. Axillary roll Arms should be positioned to be visible and easily available to anesthesiologist.	The patient is turned to the left lateral decubitus position for a right thoracotomy. Monitor breath sounds in dependent lung.
Complications	Hypothermia Metabolic acidosis Hypo- or hyperventilation Aspiration Pneumothorax Atelectasis	ETT placement may interfere with TEF closure.
	Mucus plug	E.g., in ETT or bronchi

POSTOPERATIVE

Complications	Apnea Pneumothorax Hypoventilation Tracheal leak	Maintenance of normothermia lessens incidence of apnea, hypoventilation and metabolic acidosis.
	Inadequate neuromuscular reversal Recurrent laryngeal nerve injury Pneumonia	Spontaneous hip flexion is the most reliable indication of adequate neuromuscular function.
Pain management	Acetaminophen: 10-20 mg/kg pr q 4 h prn Fentanyl 0.5-1.0 μg/kg iv q 60 min prn Epidural analgesia (p. E-2).	
Tests	ABG; Hct	

References

1. Beasley SW: Esophageal atresia and tracheoesophageal fistula. In *Surgery of Infants and Children.* Oldham KT, Colombani PM, Foglia RP, eds. Lippincott-Raven Publishers, Philadelphia: 1997, 1021-34.
2. Chittmittrapap S, Spitz L, Kiely EM, Brereton RJ: Anastomotic leakage following surgery for esophageal atresia. *J Pediatr Surg* 1992; 27(1):29-32.
3. Goh DW, Brereton RJ: Success and failure with neonatal tracheo-oesophageal anomalies. *Br J Surg* 1991; 78(7):834-37.
4. Gregory GA, ed: *Pediatric Anesthesia*, 3rd edition. Churchill Livingstone, New York: 1994, 430-42.
5. Holzki J: Bronchoscopic findings and treatment in congenital tracheo-oesophageal fistula. *Paediatric Anaesthesia* 1992; 2:297-303.
6. Motoyama EK, Davis PJ, eds: *Smith's Anesthesia for Infants and Children*, 6th edition. Mosby-Year Book, St. Louis: 1996, 464-66.

ABDOMINAL TUMOR: RESECTION OF NEUROBLASTOMA, WILMS' TUMOR, HEPATOBLASTOMA

SURGICAL CONSIDERATIONS

Description: Neuroblastoma and Wilms' tumor (50% of retroperitoneal masses) are the most common abdominal tumors in childhood. Hepatic tumors or malformations (hemangioma) are less common, but challenging lesions. These tumors usually occur in young (< 5 yr) children, and are generally explored with the intent of complete resection. Limited explorations with biopsy only are uncommon. The principles of the operative approach are similar for these tumors and include a generous transperitoneal exposure, followed by careful exploration. If the lesion appears resectable, mobilization of the tumor from the posterior body wall and adjacent viscera usually should precede attempts to control the vascular pedicle. Frequently, the tumor must be divided to preserve major vessels (Fig 12.4-2B). If the tumor is fully mobilized prior to major vessel dissection, then hemorrhage can be controlled by application of vascular clamps and rapid tumor excision. The large size of these tumors often precludes the strategy of early vascular pedicle control, which frequently needs to wait for full mobilization of the mass. Surgeon and anesthesiologist need to be prepared for thoracic extension of the procedure and major vessel control. **Neuroblastoma** arises from sympathetic tissue in the adrenal or other retroperitoneal ganglia. While urinary catecholamine levels are frequently elevated, these tumors rarely produce cardiovascular symptoms. **Wilms' tumor** frequently has direct tumor extension into the IVC or right atrium, particularly with right-side tumors. Preop preparation should include ultrasound imaging and prepping for CPB if major venous extension is suspected. Major **hepatic resections** may be required for tumors or hemangiomas producing CHF or thrombocytopenia not responsive to steroids, hepatic artery embolization or ligation.

Usual preop diagnosis: Neuroblastoma; Wilms' tumor; hepatoblastoma

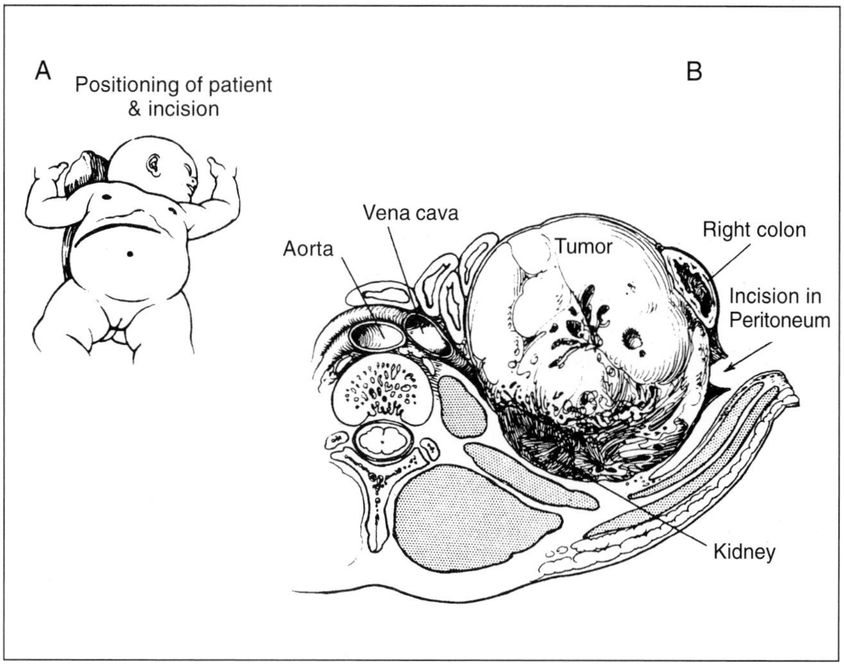

Figure 12.4-2. (A) Patient elevated, with transverse incision that can be extended into the flank. (B) Anatomic relationship of retroperitoneal tumor (Wilms') to major vascular structures. (Reproduced with permission from Ravitch MM, et al, eds: *Pediatric Surgery*. Year Book Medical Pub: 1986.)

SUMMARY OF PROCEDURE

	Neuroblastoma	Wilms' Tumor	Hepatic Resections
Position	Supine, 15° lift (Fig 12.4-2A)	⇐	⇐
Incision	Transverse, possible thoracic extension (Fig 12.4-2A)	⇐	⇐
Special instrumentation	None	Bypass instruments	CUSA; laser
Unique considerations	None	Atrial tumor; IVC may be obstructed → ↓↓CO.	Possible CHF, Plt trapping
Antibiotics	Preop: ampicillin 25 mg/kg iv + gentamicin 2.5 mg/kg iv;	⇐	⇐
	Intraop: cephalosporin irrigation (1 g/500 ml NS)	⇐	⇐
Surgical time	3-6 h	⇐	⇐
Closing considerations	None	None	Hypoglycemia
EBL	20-50 ml/kg	⇐	20-100 ml/kg
Postop care	PICU	⇐	⇐
Mortality	< 5%	⇐	⇐
Morbidity	Intestinal obstruction: 10%	⇐	–
	Postop respiratory atelectasis	⇐	⇐
			Hypoglycemia: 10%
			Bile leak: 5-10%
Pain score	7-8	7-8	7-8

PATIENT POPULATION CHARACTERISTICS

Age range	Few months–school age	⇐	⇐
Male:Female	1:1	⇐	⇐
Incidence	1/10,000	< 1/10,000	⇐
Etiology	Unknown	⇐	⇐
Associated conditions	Beckwith-Wiedemann syndrome; aniridia; hemihypertrophy; HTN (rare)	None	⇐

ANESTHETIC CONSIDERATIONS

PREOPERATIVE

Neuroblastoma, Wilms' tumor (nephroblastoma) and hepatoblastoma commonly present as abdominal masses in infants and children < 4 yr old. Abdominal pain, fever and ↑BP (2° ↑catecholamines or renal ischemia) are often associated findings. These patients may have received chemotherapy or XRT preop, and the timing of surgery may be based on multiple factors.

Respiratory There may be respiratory compromise (as a result of a large abdominal mass pushing up on the diaphragm) which may worsen in the supine position. Wilms' tumor commonly metastasizes to the lungs.
Tests: CXR, if indicated from H&P.

Cardiovascular ↑BP is associated with both Wilms' tumor and neuroblastoma, and volume status should be assessed carefully. Tumor bulk may impede venous return by occluding the IVC. Wilms' tumor may extend through the IVC into the right atrium. These patients may have received doxorubicin, which is associated with cardiomyopathy and CHF (most commonly at doses > 200 mg/m^2). Consultation with a pediatric cardiologist may be appropriate.

Renal Wilms' tumor may present with hematuria and other GU anomalies. Renal function is usually normal.
Tests: BUN; creatinine

Endocrine Neuroblastomas are associated with ↑catecholamine production. Preop adrenergic blockade (as would be required for a pheochromocytoma) is not necessary.
Tests: Urine VMA and HVA

Gastrointestinal Persistent, watery diarrhea (→ hypovolemia, ↓K^+) is associated with neuroblastoma 2° VIP secretion. Intestinal compression from tumor may ↑ risk of gastric aspiration. A surgical bowel prep may cause additional fluid and electrolyte disturbances.
Tests: Electrolytes

Hematologic Severe anemia and thrombocytopenia may be present. Blood should be available because of possible massive intraop blood loss.
Tests: CBC; T&C. ✓ availability of parental/directed donor blood, if requested.

Laboratory Other tests as indicated from H&P.

Premedication In patients at risk for gastric aspiration, prophylaxis with metoclopramide (0.1 mg/kg iv) and ranitidine (0.8 mg/kg iv) should be considered. Patients >12 mo may benefit from midazolam (0.5-0.75 mg/kg po) 30 min before surgery.

INTRAOPERATIVE

Anesthetic technique: Combined epidural/GETA, using a pediatric circle or Bain circuit with humidified and warmed gases. Warm OR to 75°-80°F; use warming pad on OR table. Warming all iv fluids may help to maintain body temperature.

Induction IV catheter insertion prior to induction may be preferable. An upper extremity or EJ site is preferred due to potential for obstruction of IVC during surgery. A modified rapid-sequence induction is recommended in those patients with a large intraabdominal mass compressing the GI tract. Otherwise, standard pediatric induction (p. D-2) is appropriate. Children < 6-9 mo may benefit from a preinduction dose of atropine (0.2 mg/kg iv) to ablate vagal response to laryngoscopy. In children < 6-8 yr of age, an uncuffed ETT commonly is used; however, there is a growing interest in the use of cuffed tubes in infants and children. The appropriate size for the ETT is one that will allow a small leak around the tube when positive pressure is applied (10-35 cmH_2O).

Maintenance Standard maintenance (see p. D-3). Muscle relaxation is appropriate. HTN associated with tumor manipulation can be treated with SNP (0.5-2.0 μg/kg/min) or labetalol (0.1 mg/kg iv) boluses.

Emergence In most instances, patient can be extubated at the end of surgery. Suction NG tube and confirm air leak around ETT before extubation. If there is no air leak, consider laryngeal edema and need for continued intubation.

Blood and fluid requirements Potential for large blood loss/moderate 3rd-space loss

Tumor resection may be associated with massive blood loss, especially with IVC or renal vein involvement. Avoid

Blood and fluid, cont.	IV: 18-20 ga × 1-2 NS/LR @ (maintenance): 4 ml/kg/h – 0-10 kg + 2 ml/kg/h – 11-20 kg + 1 ml/kg/h – > 20 kg (e.g., 25 kg = 65 ml/h)	placement of iv catheter in lower extremities. 5% albumin may be useful to replace 3rd-space losses (8-10 ml/kg/h). Transfuse to maintain Hct > 23. Over 2 mo of age, dextrose-containing solutions are not required.
Monitoring	Standard monitors (p. D-1) Arterial line: (e.g., 22 ga) CVP line: 4 Fr (subclavian or IJ) Urinary catheter	ABG, Hct, blood glucose should be measured hourly. CVP measurement may be useful to evaluate fluid status. UO monitored and kept at 1 ml/kg/h.
Positioning	✓ and pad pressure points. ✓ eyes.	
Complications	Hypotension HTN PE Hypothermia Hypoventilation	↓BP 2° blood loss or IVC obstruction or PE ↑BP 2° tumor or adrenal manipulation 2° tumor embolization usually from IVC → ↓BP. Abdominal retractors and packing will interfere with ventilation.

POSTOPERATIVE

Complications	Atelectasis Hypoventilation	If supplemental O_2 required, pulse oximetry useful for weaning from O_2.
Pain management	Epidural or iv opiates Ketorolac 0.9 mg/kg iv q 6 × 2 d	See p. E-2 for dosing schedule.
Tests	Hct ABG CXR	If CVP placed.

References

1. Charlton GA, Sedgwick J, Sutton DN: Anaesthetic management of renin-secreting nephroblastoma. *Br J Anaesth* 1992; 69(2):206-09.
2. Creagh-Barry P, et al: Neuroblastoma and anaesthesia. *Paed Anaesth* 1992; 2:147-52.
3. Gregory GA, ed: *Pediatric Anesthesia*, 3rd edition. Churchill Livingstone, New York: 1994, 596-97.
4. Kain ZN, Shamberger RS, Holzman RS. Anesthetic management of children with neuroblastoma. *J Clin Anesth* 1993; 5(6):486-91.
5. Motoyama EK, Davis PJ, eds: *Smith's Anesthesia for Infants and Children*, 6th edition. CV Mosby-Year Book, St. Louis: 1996. 579-80.
6. Nagabuchi E, Ziegler MM: Neuroblastoma. In *Surgery of Infants and Children.* Oldham KT, Colombani PM, Foglia RP, eds. Lippincott-Raven Publishers, Philadelphia: 1997, 593-614.
7. Ritchey ML, Andrassy RJ, Kelalis PP: Pediatric Urologic Oncology. In *Adult and Pediatric Urology,* 3rd edition. Gillenwater JY, Grayhack JT, Howards SS, Duckett JW, eds. Mosby-Year Book, Inc, St. Louis: 1996, Vol 3, 2675-93.
8. Shochat SJ: Renal tumors. *Surgery of Infants and Children.* Oldham KT, Colombani PM, Foglia RP, eds. Lippincott-Raven Publishers, Philadelphia: 1997, 581-92.
9. Tagge EP, Tagge DU: Hepatoblastoma and hepatocellular carcinoma. *Surgery of Infants and Children.* Oldham KT, Colombani PM, Foglia RP, eds. Lippincott-Raven Publishers, Philadelphia: 1997, 633-44.

REPAIR OF CONGENITAL DIAPHRAGMATIC HERNIA

SURGICAL CONSIDERATIONS

Description: Congenital diaphragmatic hernia remains a highly lethal anomaly, due to associated pulmonary vascular HTN and pulmonary hypoplasia. Once considered a surgical emergency, it is now common to treat newborns with a period of stabilization or **ECMO support** (see "ECMO," p. 1084) prior to repair of the diaphragmatic defect. Most surgeons prefer an abdominal approach to allow for treatment of associated intestinal anomalies, to close skin only, or to place a Silastic pouch, if replacing the intestine in the abdominal cavity is associated with undue tension. *In utero* diagnosis allows for maternal transport to a tertiary center, preferably one with ECMO capability. **Laparotomy** by subcostal or upper transverse incision is followed by reduction of viscera from thorax. Diaphragm may be repaired by primary suture if adequate tissue remains. Otherwise it is closed with a patch of Silastic or Gortex. Use of a chest tube is optional. If significant adhesions or obstruction related to intestinal malrotation are identified, they are corrected. Replacement of the bowel into the abdomen may be impossible or may produce excessive tension, in which case a Silastic silo may be used or the skin closed without closing the abdominal wall muscles.

Variant procedure or approaches: **Thoracotomy** is preferred by a few surgeons for primary repair, usually of right-sided lesions, and is the approach of choice for recurrent hernias. Hernias initially requiring ECMO support may be repaired prior to or following decannulation. Because the risk of postop hemorrhage is increased if anticoagulation is prolonged, most centers repair the hernia at the completion of the ECMO run. Once the patient has been shown to tolerate weaning from ECMO, the circuit flow is increased to 100 ml/kg/min to allow operating during reduced anticoagulation; patients are then weaned fairly rapidly after repair (12-24 h). **Lateral** or **anterolateral thoracotomy**, using the 6th or 7th interspace, provides adequate exposure for closing the defect in the diaphragm, which is done as from the abdomen. The ability to deal with intestinal abnormalities or abdominal tension, however, is limited by this approach.

Usual preop diagnosis: Diaphragmatic hernia; Bochdalek's hernia (posterolateral diaphragm)

SUMMARY OF PROCEDURE

Position	Supine (lateral for thoracic approach)
Incision	Subcostal (posterolateral for thoracic approach)
Special instrumentation	Pre- and postductal arterial catheters, soft-tissue patch, Gortex
Unique considerations	Reactive pulmonary vasculature
Antibiotics	Preop: ampicillin 25 mg/kg iv + gentamicin 2.5 mg/kg iv Intraop: cephalosporin irrigation (1 g/500 ml NS)
Surgical time	1-2 h
Closing considerations	Assess for changes in ventilation (e.g., PIP, pre- and postductal ABG).
EBL	5-10 ml/kg
Postop care	Paralysis maintained; hyperventilation, fentanyl infusion @ 2-5 μg/kg/min
Mortality	50% without ECMO 25-30% with ECMO
Morbidity	Pulmonary HTN Respiratory failure Sepsis Intestinal obstruction/dysfunction
Pain score	6-7 (7-8 for thoracic approach)

PATIENT POPULATION CHARACTERISTICS

Age range	Newborn–wk or mo
Male:Female	1-2:1
Incidence	1/4000
Etiology	Unknown
Associated conditions	Malrotation (40-100%); congenital heart disease (e.g., PDA) (15%); renal anomalies (rare); esophageal atresia (rare); CNS abnormalities (e.g., myelomeningocele, hydrocephalus) (rare)

ANESTHETIC CONSIDERATIONS

PREOPERATIVE

These infants present with varying degrees of respiratory distress. The majority are already mechanically ventilated, sedated and paralyzed in the NICU prior to anesthesia consultation. The anesthesiologist needs to be aware of the distinction between early and late diaphragmatic hernias. Late events (occurring near or even after delivery) are associated with mature, well developed lungs and minimal problems with ventilation. These babies can often be extubated in the early postop period, facilitated by epidural analgesia. Some infants may be on ECMO (see p. 1084).

Respiratory The lung on affected side is variably hypoplastic and the lung on the contralateral side is compressed and also may be hypoplastic. Pulmonary hypoplasia is most severe in patients with early herniation, and may be minimal in cases of late (even postnatal) herniation. The prognosis is correlated with magnitude of pulmonary hypoplasia and pulmonary muscular abnormalities present on the contralateral side. There is decreased compliance, with resultant risk for hypoventilation. ↑PIP → ↑risk for pneumothorax. Persistent pulmonary HTN and progressive hypoxemia may be present.
Tests: CXR; ABG

Cardiovascular R→L shunting may occur at level of PDA or preductally (e.g., PFO). The degree of R→L shunting may be dramatically increased by ↑pulmonary vasoconstriction (2° ↓PO_2, ↑PCO_2, ↑pH, ↑sympathetic tone) → severe systemic hypoxemia. ↓CO 2° persistent pulmonary HTN and hypoxemia will lead to metabolic acidosis.
Tests: CXR; ECHO; ABG

Neurological Myelomeningocele and/or hydrocephalus may be present. Repeated bouts of hypoxemia predispose to intraventricular hemorrhage (IVH) in preterm infant. These areas of hemorrhage have loss of cerebral autoregulation and BP increases are directly transmitted to the microvasculature, with ↑risk of recurrent hemorrhage and edema.
Tests: Head ultrasound

Hematologic Hct should be maintained at 35%. HbF has ↑affinity for O_2 and ↓sensitivity to 2,3-DPG. This will aggravate cellular hypoxia in the patient with compromised circulatory status. Confirm that vitamin K was administered at birth.
Tests: CBC; T&C; PT; PTT

Metabolic Negligible glycogen stores in neonate; therefore, dextrose hyperalimentation should be initiated early. In patients with CHF, diuretic administration leads to ↓K^+.
Tests: Electrolytes; glucose; BUN; creatinine

Gastrointestinal Constant NG/OG suction. Gastric distention will worsen ventilation.

Laboratory Other tests as indicated from H&P.

Premedication None

INTRAOPERATIVE

Anesthetic technique: GETA, using a pediatric circle or Bain circuit with humidified and warmed gases. Use pressure-limited ventilation (PIP < 30 cmH_2O). Continue NO if administered preop. Maintain body temperature as close to 37°C as possible. Warm room to 75-80°F. Warming blanket on OR table. Consider use of NICU ventilator (e.g., Baby Bird, high frequency oscillator) particularly if high RR (>30/min) is required.

Induction Transported from NICU to OR by anesthesia team. If infant is already intubated, confirm paralysis prior to transport. This is to lessen the risk of patient movement and inadvertent extubation. Transport with full monitoring (ECG, pulse oximetry, arterial pressure tracing). Have airway equipment available (Miller 1 laryngoscope blade, ET 3.0-3.5 with stylets, neonatal mask). Resuscitation drugs (e.g., epinephrine 1 and 10 μg/ml) should be drawn up. Syringe with NS/LR flush. Prior to any further anesthetic administration, reestablish all monitoring in OR. Atropine (0.02 mg/kg iv) given prior to opiates to counteract bradycardia. For nonintubated patients, standard pediatric induction (p. D-2) is appropriate. Avoid N_2O and maintain PIPs as low as possible. For patients with late herniations and healthy lungs, consider caudal/thoracic level epidural instead of iv opioids, and early extubation (OR or NICU); see p. D-5.

Maintenance Opiate-based anesthetic (fentanyl 10-25 μg/kg iv total) with isoflurane supplementation. Ventilate with air/O_2 to maintain O_2 saturation 95-100%, as measured by preductal ABGs/pulse oximetry. Continue neuromuscular blockade with pancuronium, rocuronium or vecuronium.

Emergence	Transport back to NICU with full monitoring, airway equipment and drugs.	
Blood and fluid requirements	Blood loss minimal IV: 22-24 ga × 2 NS/LR @ 4 ml/kg/h maintenance	These infants are fluid-restricted in NICU. Continue dextrose-containing solution from NICU. If umbilical venous line not present, dopamine may be infused via peripheral iv with dextrose solution serving as the carrier fluid. In emergency, NS/LR, albumin 5%, PRBCs (Hct < 50%) may be given via umbilical artery line.
Monitoring	Standard monitors (p. D-1) Right-side precordial stethoscope Arterial line (umbilical artery or radial – 24 ga) ± Umbilical vein line	ABG, Hct, glucose q 30-60 min. Contralateral pneumothorax is detected using a right axillary precordial stethoscope.
	Preductal and postductal pulse oximetry	Changes in pre- and postductal pulse oximetry provide early warning of R→L shunt/pulmonary HTN.
Positioning	✓ and pad pressure points. ✓ eyes.	Arms/iv access sites should be positioned to be visible and easily available.
Complications	Pneumothorax Hypoventilation Hypothermia Metabolic acidosis R→L shunting CHF	With acute deterioration in O_2 saturation, pneumothorax on unaffected side is likely. With removal of abdominal contents from thorax, do not attempt to expand lungs vigorously. Hypoplasia, not atelectasis, is the primary problem. Keep PIP < 30 cmH_2O, if possible.

POSTOPERATIVE

Complications	Same as Intraoperative Complications, above.	Those infants whose oxygenation continues to worsen are possible candidates for ECMO, p. 1084. Discuss with NICU team their criteria for initiation of ECMO.
Pain management	Fentanyl (0.5-2.0 μg/kg/h iv) Epidural analgesia	Tachyphylaxis can develop in 24-48 h.
Tests	CXR; ABG; Hct; glucose; electrolytes	

References

1. Bikhazi GB, Davis PJ: Anesthesia for neonates and premature infants. In *Smith's Anesthesia for Infants and Children*, 6th edition. Motoyama EK, Davis PJ, eds. Mosby-Year Book, St. Louis: 1996, 445-74.
2. Cook DR, Marcy JH, eds: *Neonatal Anesthesia*, 1st edition. Appleton Davies Inc, Pasadena: 1988.
3. Falconer AR, Brown RA, Helms P, Gordon I, Baron JA: Pulmonary sequelae in survivors of congenital diaphragmatic hernia. *Thorax* 1990; 45(2):126-29.
4. Goldsmith JP, Karokin EH, eds: *Assisted Ventilation of the Neonate*, 2nd edition. WB Saunders Co, Philadelphia: 1988.
5. Stehling L, ed: *Common Problems in Pediatric Anesthesia*, 2nd edition. Mosby-Year Book, St. Louis: 1992, 7-11.
6. Wilson JM, Lund DP, Lillehei CW, Vacanti JP: Congenital diaphragmatic hernia: predictors of severity in the ECMO era. *J Pediatr Surg* 1991; 26(9):1028-33.

LAPAROTOMY FOR INTESTINAL PERFORATION, NECROTIZING ENTEROCOLITIS

SURGICAL CONSIDERATIONS

Description: Necrotizing enterocolitis (NEC) is an ischemic/inflammatory condition of the GI tract (1° terminal ileum and splenic flexure of the colon) occurring primarily in stressed premature infants. It may progress to full-thickness necrosis and perforation, which have traditionally been treated by **resection** with **enterostomy** or **primary anastomosis** in selected cases. These infants are usually bacteremic with thrombocytopenia, complex respiratory distress and severe prematurity. Blood loss may be significant. Volume replacement and temperature regulation, therefore, must be precise. Laparotomy via an upper abdominal, transverse incision allows inspection of the entire GI tract for areas of perforation or full-thickness necrosis. Areas of irreversible injury are resected and any questionable areas are retained. Occasionally, primary anastomosis may be suitable, but most often proximal enterostomy and mucous fistula at the lateral margins of the incision are safe and expeditious.

Variant procedure or approaches: In extremely small infants (< 1500 g) a few centers have utilized **peritoneal drainage** under local anesthesia as a temporizing or definitive management. This procedure consists of a small, RLQ incision with evacuation of intestinal contents or purulent material from the peritoneal cavity and placement of Penrose drain(s) through the incision. It is performed in the NICU, with minimal physiologic disturbance.

Usual preop diagnosis: Perforated NEC

SUMMARY OF PROCEDURE

	Resection	Drainage
Position	Supine	⇐
Incision	Transverse	RLQ
Special instrumentation	None	Penrose drains
Unique considerations	Temperature support	⇐
Antibiotics	Ampicillin 50 mg/kg + gentamicin 2.5 mg/kg + clindamycin 10 mg/kg iv preop	⇐
Surgical time	1-2.5 h	0.5 h
EBL	10-100 ml/kg	1-2 ml/kg
Postop care	NICU	⇐
Mortality	20-25%	16-20%
Morbidity	Respiratory failure Sepsis Stricture Intracranial hemorrhage	⇐
Pain score	6-7	3-4

PATIENT POPULATION CHARACTERISTICS

Age range	Newborn–weeks
Male:Female	> 1:1
Incidence	5-8% NICU admissions
Etiology	Multifactorial, including: intestinal ischemia; bacterial colonization; perinatal stress; immaturity; hypoxia; hyperosmolar feeding; splanchnic ischemia
Associated conditions	Prematurity (80-90%); respiratory distress, PDA

ANESTHETIC CONSIDERATIONS

PREOPERATIVE

Most (80-90%) of these patients are premature infants (< 36 wk gestational age) presenting with sepsis and pulmonary insufficiency. In addition to sepsis, significant 3rd-space losses contribute to hypovolemia and metabolic acidosis.

Respiratory	Premature infants are at risk for RDS. These infants are usually on mechanical ventilation with ↑FiO_2 prior to surgery. They also are at increased risk for pneumonia, pneumothorax and pulmonary edema 2° to sepsis and/or CHF. ✓ ventilator settings and recent ABG in preparation for OR mechanical ventilation. **Tests:** CXR; ABG
Cardiovascular	Intrinsically labile BP. Inotropes (e.g., dopamine 5-10 μg/kg/min) may be required to maintain adequate CO. Associated cardiac anomalies (e.g., VSD, PDA) can lead to CHF, further complicating fluid management. Pulmonary overcirculation and intrinsic pulmonary disease contribute to pulmonary HTN. **Tests:** CXR; ABG; ECG; ± ECHO
Neurological	Intraventricular hemorrhage (IVH) may be 2° to prematurity or birth asphyxia. These hemorrhagic regions have impaired autoregulation, and wide variations in BP (20-30 mmHg) can aggravate ischemia/hemorrhage. In addition, these patients may have a seizure disorder. Should this be the case, ✓ medication list for appropriate anticonvulsant therapy. **Tests:** Head ultrasound, if indicated from H&P.
Renal	Presence of PDA and prior Rx with NSAID can lead to impaired renal perfusion and clearance. Aggravating factors are aminoglycoside antibiotics, sepsis and CHF. **Tests:** BUN; creatinine
Metabolic	Metabolic acidosis 2° to sepsis/CHF will further worsen myocardial function. Neonate has minimal glycogen stores and impaired ability to mobilize calcium. **Tests:** ABG; Ca^{++}; glucose; electrolytes
Hematologic	DIC, thrombocytopenia, hemolysis and T-antigen activation on RBCs are present with overwhelming sepsis, particularly clostridial infections. **Tests:** CBC; PT; PTT; fibrinogen; T-antigen; availability of irradiated, washed RBCs and instrumentation (plasma can contain antibody against T-antigen that causes hemolysis)
Laboratory	Others as indicated from H&P.
Premedication	None

INTRAOPERATIVE

Anesthetic technique: GETA, using a pediatric circle, a Mapleson D circuit or Bain circuit, each with warmed, humidified gases. Use air/O_2 mixture for ventilation that maintains SpO_2 between 95-100% to minimize risk of retinopathy. Avoid high concentrations of O_2. Consider use of NICU ventilator (e.g., Baby Bird) if patient requires ↑RR or ↑PIPs. Epidural catheter insertion is not recommended in the presence of sepsis.

Induction	These patients are usually intubated. If not, intubate, with full-stomach precautions (p. B-5). Give atropine 0.02 mg/kg iv (0.1 mg minimum dose) prior to laryngoscopy. Preoxygenate for 2 min. Miller 0/1 blade with O_2 side port, if available. Suction NG. Apply cricoid pressure until airway secured. ETT should have leak at 15-35 cmH_2O pressure.
Maintenance	Narcotic technique (fentanyl 20-30 μg/kg iv total)—avoid myocardial depression from volatile agents. Avoid N_2O (↑bowel size). Muscle relaxation required.
Emergence	Postop ventilation generally is required. Transport to NICU with full monitoring (ECG, arterial line, pulse oximetry). Have laryngoscope and appropriately sized mask and ETT available. Extra volume (albumin 5% in 20 ml syringes) may be needed during transport.

Blood and fluid requirements	Anticipate moderate-to-large blood and fluid losses. IV: 22-24 ga × 2 (or 1 + CVP) Continue dextrose-containing solution from NICU. Warm fluids.	Neonates are usually fluid-restricted in NICU to lessen incidence of PDA. 3rd-space losses are usually significant. Rx: ↓BP with volume before increasing dopamine. Maintain Hct > 35%. Albumin 5% (10 ml/kg iv) boluses as needed. Crystalloid/colloid > 100 ml/kg total not uncommon. Hct, glucose, Ca^{++}, ABG, Plt count, PT/PTT, electrolytes q 30-60 min.
Monitoring	Standard monitors (p. D-1) Arterial line – preferably preductal (RUE)	Central line not as important as arterial line for intraop care, but may be useful for administering inotropic drugs.

Monitoring, cont.	± CVP line (subclavian, IJ, femoral) 3 Fr	
Positioning	✓ and pad pressure points. ✓ eyes.	
Complications	Hypothermia Metabolic acidosis Hypovolemia	Aggressive volume repletion and maintaining normothermia will prevent or ameliorate metabolic acidosis. Bicarbonate replacement = base deficit × wt (kg) × 0.3 → ↓SVR.
	Hemolysis 2° blood products (rare)	Minimized by use of washed PRBCs.
	Pneumothorax	↓O_2 sats, ↑PIPs. ✓ for mucus plugging or mainstem intubation.
	Hypocalcemia	Frequent blood sampling is necessary. Rx: $CaCl_2$ (10 mg/kg iv) via central line or Ca gluconate (30 mg/kg iv) via peripheral line.
	Hypoglycemia	Continue 10% dextrose infusion from NICU.

POSTOPERATIVE

Complications	Retrolental fibroplasia Hypovolemia from continued 3rd-spacing Metabolic acidosis/sepsis Pulmonary edema with fluid remobilization	Maintain PaO_2 < 70 mmHg to lessen incidence of retrolental fibroplasia.
Pain management	Morphine (0.05-0.10 mg/kg iv) q 1-2 h prn or via continuous infusion for initial 24-48 h	
Tests	CBC Electrolytes Ca^{++} Glucose ABG	CXR, if central line placed.

References

1. Ade-Ajayi N, Kiely E, Drake D, Wheeler R, Spitz L: Resection and primary anastomosis in necrotizing enterocolitis. *J R Soc Med* 1996; 89(7):385-88.
2. Diaz JH, ed: *Perinatal Anesthesia and Critical Care*. WB Saunders Co, Philadelphia: 1991.
3. Ein SH, Shandling B, Wesson D, Filler RM: A 13-year experience with peritoneal drainage under local anesthesia for necrotizing enterocolitis perforation. *J Pediatr Surg* 1990; 25(10):1034-37.
4. Grosfeld JL, Molinari F, Chaet M, Engum SA, West KW, Rescorla FJ, Scherer LR III: Gastrointestinal perforation and peritonitis in infants and children: experience with 179 cases over ten years. *Surgery* 1996; 120(4):650-55.
5. Kleigman RM: Neonatal necrotizing enterocolitis: implication for an infectious disease. *Pediatr Clin North Am* 1979; 26:327-42.
6. Kosloske AN: Necrotizing Enterocolitis. In *Surgery of Infants and Children*. Oldham KT, Colombiani PM, Foglia RP, eds. Lippincott-Raven Publishers, Philadelphia: 1997, 1201-14.
7. Luzzatto C, Previtera C, Boscolo R, Katende M, Orzali A, Guglielmi M. Necrotizing enterocolitis: late surgical results after enterostomy without resection. *Eur J Pediatr Surg* 1996; 6(2):92-4.
8. Santulli TV, Schullinger JN, Heird WC, Gongaware RD, Wiggens J, Barlow B, Blanc WA, Berdon WE: Acute necrotizing enterocolitis in infancy: a review of 64 cases. *Pediatrics* 1975; 55(3):376-87.

REPAIR OF PECTUS EXCAVATUM/CARINATUM

SURGICAL CONSIDERATIONS

Description: Pectus excavatum (funnel chest) is a deformity of the sternum and costal cartilages occurring primarily in boys. It is 8-10 times more common than the carinatum (pigeon breast) deformity. While some surgeons believe excavatum deformities are purely cosmetic, recent studies confirm cardiopulmonary deficits in moderate and severe cases. Many children have an antecedent or coincidental respiratory problem, usually in the form of reactive airway disease. The operative procedure consists of **resection** of the costal cartilages of ribs 3-7 bilaterally, **excision** of the xiphoid, and **transverse osteotomy** of the sternum. A transverse incision is used to elevate skin flaps. Pectoralis muscles are elevated from the chest wall and costal cartilages 3-7 are excised, leaving posterior perichondrium intact. The xiphoid is excised and the sternum is fractured at the 2nd interspace. The pectoralis muscles are reattached to the sternum and drains are placed in the mediastinum. If entry into the pleura occurs, the pleura space is evacuated and repaired. In older children and adolescents, the sternum may be reinforced with a metal strut or pin. Operative correction of the excavatum and carinatum deformities is essentially identical, although the timing of operation is frequently different. Excavatum deformities are best repaired at 5-6 yr to allow improved thoracic volume during growth. Carinatum or minor excavatum deformities are usually repaired following the pubertal growth spurt.

Usual preop diagnosis: Pectus excavatum; carinatum

SUMMARY OF PROCEDURE

Position	Supine
Incision	Transverse
Special instrumentation	Air drill; sternal strut; K-wire
Unique considerations	Possible pleural entry
Antibiotics	Preop: ampicillin 25 mg/kg iv + gentamicin 2.5 mg/kg iv Intraop: cephalosporin irrigation (1 g/500 ml NS)
Surgical time	3-5 h
EBL	5-20 ml/kg; greater in older patients
Postop care	PICU (usually); aggressive pulmonary toilet; analgesia (epidural catheter, PCA–p. E-3.)
Mortality	0.2%
Morbidity	Pneumothorax Fluid accumulation
Pain score	7-8

PATIENT POPULATION CHARACTERISTICS

Age range	5 yr–adolescent
Male:Female	5-9:1
Incidence	Uncertain
Etiology	Relationship with reactive airway disease
Associated conditions	Marfan syndrome (5%); mitral valve prolapse (5%)

ANESTHETIC CONSIDERATIONS

PREOPERATIVE

Pectus excavatum (a condition in which there is concave depression of the lower sternum) may be associated with CHD and restrictive lung disease. If the deformity is present without cardiac or pulmonary disease, the patient is asymptomatic and the procedure is cosmetic. Surgery usually occurs between 5-10 years of age. **Pectus carinatum** (a convex lower sternum) is usually repaired for cosmetic reasons only. Surgery usually occurs in the teenage years. Cardiac abnormalities (VSD, PDA, mitral valve anomalies) may be associated with the pectus disorder.

Respiratory Restrictive lung disease 2° chest wall deformity may be present. If a longstanding condition, patient may have chronic hypoxemia, with resultant pulmonary HTN and polycythemia. If patient has exercise limitations, there is a need to differentiate between cardiac and pulmonary components.
Tests: CXR: AP, lateral; PFTs; ABG, if symptomatic

Cardiovascular	In both conditions, CHD should be investigated if present. Pulmonary HTN may be 2° pulmonary overcirculation (e.g., VSD), or chronic hypoxemia. **Tests:** ECG; ECHO	
Laboratory	Hct; T&C; electrolytes	
Premedication	If patient is an asymptomatic child, midazolam (0.75 mg/kg po up to 20 mg) or diazepam (0.1-0.2 mg/kg po up to 5 mg).	

INTRAOPERATIVE

Anesthetic technique: GETA, using a pediatric circle or Bain's circuit with warmed, humidified gases. Heating pad on OR table. Maintain body temperature close to 37°C.

Induction	IV or mask induction. With restrictive lung disease, there is ↓FRC, which will shorten the time to alveolar equilibration for the volatile anesthetics. Hypercarbia will aggravate pulmonary HTN; institute early manual hyperventilation. Tracheal intubation, facilitated by neuromuscular blockade (pancuronium 0.1 mg/kg, rocuronium 1 mg/kg, vecuronium 0.1 mg/kg). Use cuffed ETT for patient > 6-8 yr old. With uncuffed ETT, keep air leak to minimum (10-35 cmH_2O) to avoid alterations in alveolar ventilation with changes in chest and pulmonary compliance.	
Maintenance	Primarily narcotic-based with air/O_2 low-percent volatile agent. Insertion of thoracic lumbar epidural catheter will provide for supplemental anesthesia and treatment of postop pain. Use morphine/hydromorphone-bupivacaine mixture (p. D-3).	
Emergence	Plan for extubation in OR. Ensure adequate reversal of neuromuscular blockade with neostigmine (0.07 mg/kg iv) and glycopyrrolate (0.014 mg/kg iv).	
Blood and fluid requirements	Usually minimal blood and 3rd-space losses IV: 18 or 20 ga × 1 NS/LR @ 3-5 kg/h	With chronic hypoxemia or right-side heart disease, maintain Hct > 30. If otherwise healthy, maintain Hct > 22.
Monitoring	Standard monitors (p. D-1)	Arterial line if pulmonary HTN present.
Positioning	✓ and pad pressure points. ✓ eyes.	Elbow padding to avoid ulnar nerve compression.
Complications	Pneumothorax Atelectasis Subglottic edema	

POSTOPERATIVE

Complications	Respiratory insufficiency 2° splinting, preexisting restrictive pulmonary disease Pneumothorax	
Pain management	Epidural (thoracic or lumbar) or PCA.	Standard epidural infusion (p. E-2) Ketorolac (0.9 mg/kg iv q 6 h × 48 h), in addition to the above measures

References

1. Arn PH, Scherer LR, Haller JA Jr, Pyeritz RE: Outcome of pectus excavatum in patients with Marfan syndrome and in the general population. *J Pediatr* 1989; 115(6):954-58.
2. Chidambaram B, Mehta AV: Currarino-Silverman syndrome (pectus carinatum type 2 deformity) and mitral valve disease. *Chest* 1992; 102(3):780-82.
3. Derveaux L, Ivanoff I, Rochette F, Demedts M: Mechanism of pulmonary function changes after surgical correction for funnel chest. *Eur Respir J* 1988; 1(9):823-25.
4. Gregory GA, ed: *Pediatric Anesthesia*, 3rd edition. Churchill Livingstone, New York: 1994, 445-48.
5. Kandel J, Haller JA: Chest wall and breast. In *Surgery of Infants and Children.* Oldham KT, Colombiani PM, Foglia RP, eds. Lippincott-Raven Publishers, Philadelphia: 1997, 871-82.
6. Motoyama EK, Davis PJ, eds: *Smith's Anesthesia for Infants and Children*, 6th edition. Mosby-Year Book, St. Louis: 1996, 583-84.

PYLOROMYOTOMY

SURGICAL CONSIDERATIONS

Description: Pyloric stenosis due to idiopathic hypertrophy of the muscular layers of the antrum and pylorus occurs in infants, producing projectile vomiting with subsequent dehydration and metabolic alkalosis. Surgical division of the hypertrophied muscle fibers—**pyloromyotomy**—has been the treatment of choice for this condition since the early 20th century. The operative procedure is quite straightforward, with mucosal entry, usually on the duodenal side, being the only significant technical problem. Preop hydration, replacement of electrolytes, and prevention of aspiration are crucial to a successful outcome. The operation is performed through a short, right-upper-quadrant incision. After delivering the antrum and pylorus, a superficial incision through the serosa of the hypertrophied muscle is carried through an avascular region. Blunt division of the muscle fibers can be done with the back of a scalpel handle or the specialized Benson pyloric spreader. Careful inspection for entry into the lumen may be facilitated by injecting air through a NG tube. Mucosal injury is usually at the duodenal end of the myotomy and can be treated either by simple repair or by closing the myotomy and performing another myotomy at an alternate site.

Variant procedure or approaches: **Laparoscopic myotomy** and **balloon dilation** of the pylorus have been done, but cannot match the simplicity, reliability and low complication rate of open myotomy.

Usual preop diagnosis: Pyloric stenosis

SUMMARY OF PROCEDURE

Position	Supine
Incision	Transverse
Special instrumentation	Benson pyloric spreader
Intraop antibiotics	Cephalosporin irrigation (1 g/500 ml NS)
Surgical time	0.5-1 h
EBL	< 5 ml/kg
Postop care	Cardiac/apnea monitoring
Mortality	0.3%
Morbidity	Duodenal perforation Incomplete myotomy Dehiscence
Pain score	4-5

PATIENT POPULATION CHARACTERISTICS

Age range	1-12 wk
Male:Female	4:1
Incidence	3/1000 births
Etiology	Unknown
Associated conditions	Has occurred following repair of other congenital anomalies, such as esophageal atresia, omphalocele.

ANESTHETIC CONSIDERATIONS

PREOPERATIVE

Patients with pyloric stenosis are usually term infants that present in the first month of life with mild-to-moderate dehydration 2° intractable vomiting. Correction of volume deficit and metabolic abnormalities is the first line of treatment. Surgery should proceed only after patients are medically stabilized.

Cardiovascular — Mild-to-moderate dehydration (50-100 ml/kg) is common and this deficit should be replaced with NS over approximately 12 h.
Tests: Urinary Cl > 20 mEq/L or plasma Cl >100 mEq/L, when fluid volume restored.

Metabolic — Protracted vomiting → dehydration with hypochloremic hypokalemic metabolic alkalosis. ↓K^+ should be treated once alkalemia is resolved and UO is confirmed.
Tests: ABGs; electrolytes; Ca^{++}; glucose

Gastrointestinal	Full-stomach precautions	
Laboratory	Hct; other tests as indicated from H&P.	
Premedication	None	

INTRAOPERATIVE

Anesthetic technique: GETA, using a pediatric circle or Bain circuit with warmed, humidified gases. Warm OR to 75-80° F. Use air/O_2 or N_2O/O_2 mixture to maintain O_2 sat @ 95-100%. Maintain body temperature close to 37°C.

Induction An iv catheter will be in place prior to induction for preop fluid management. Decompress stomach with NG or OG tube. Atropine (0.02 mg/kg iv, 0.1 mg minimum) commonly given prior to induction. Preoxygenate 2-3 min. Rapid-sequence induction with cricoid pressure should be performed, using STP (4 mg/kg iv) or propofol (2-3 mg/kg) and succinylcholine (1-2 mg/kg iv) or rocuronium (1 mg/kg). Use awake laryngoscopy if difficulty with intubation is anticipated. Intubate trachea with a 3.5 uncuffed ETT. Should have air leak at 10-35 cmH_2O pressure. Do not wait for return of muscle function before administering vecuronium (0.1 mg/kg iv) or rocuronium (0.6 mg/kg/30 min).

Maintenance Volatile agent (isoflurane) and air/O_2 or N_2O/O_2. Avoid opiates to lessen risk of postop apnea. Maintain muscle relaxation. Surgeon can infiltrate wound site with bupivacaine 0.25% (with epinephrine 1:200,000)—not to exceed 2.5 mg/kg (1.0 ml/kg), for postop pain relief.

Emergence Reverse with neostigmine (70 μg/kg iv) and atropine (0.02 mg/kg iv). Prior to extubation, suction stomach contents via NG/OG tube. Extubate when fully awake.

Blood and fluid requirements	Minimal blood loss IV: 22 ga × 1 NS/LR @ (maintenance): 4 ml/kg/h – 0-10 kg	Minimal 3rd-space loss
Monitoring	Standard monitors (p. D-1)	
Positioning	✓ and pad pressure points. ✓ eyes.	
Complications	Aspiration	ETT in trachea does not prevent aspiration absolutely. Active inspiration and vomiting may permit vomitus to pass around ETT.

POSTOPERATIVE

Complications	Apnea	Pulse oximetry/apnea monitor × 12 h. Differential diagnosis of apnea includes hypoglycemia and hypothermia.
	Hypoglycemia (rare)	Rx of hypoglycemia: dextrose 0.5 g/kg iv
Pain management	Acetaminophen (10-15 mg po/pr q 4 h prn)	
Tests	None routinely indicated.	

References

1. Andropoulos DB, Heard MB, Johnson KL, Clarke JT, Rowe RW: Postanesthetic apnea in full-term infants after pyloromyotomy [see comments]. *Anesthesiology* 1994; 80(1:216-9.
2. Bissonnette B, Sullivan PJ: Pyloric stenosis. *Can J Anaesth* 1991; 38(5):668-76.
3. Eriksen CA, Anders CJ: Audit of results of operations for infantile pyloric stenosis in a district general hospital. *Arch Dis Child* 1991; 66(1):130-33.
4. Goh DW, Hall SK, Gornall P, Buick RG, Green A, Conkery JJ: Plasma chloride and alkalemia in pyloric stenosis. *Br J Surg* 1990; 77(8):922-23.
5. Maher M, Hehir DJ, Horgan A, Stuart RS, O'Donnell JA, Kirwan WO, Brady MP: Infantile hypertrophic pyloric stenosis: long-term audit from a general surgical unit. *Ir J Med Sci* 1996; 165(2):115-17.
6. Oldham KT: Introduction to neonatal intestinal obstruction. In *Surgery of Infants and Children.* Oldham KT, Colombiani PM, Foglia RP, eds. Lippincott-Raven Publishers, Philadelphia: 1997, 1181-82.
7. Scorpio RJ, Tan HL, Hutson JM: Pyloromyotomy: comparison between laparoscopic and open surgical techniques. *J Laparoendosc Surg* 1995; 5(2):81-4.

ESOPHAGEAL REPLACEMENT, COLON INTERPOSITION, WATERSTON PROCEDURE, GASTRIC TUBE PLACEMENT

SURGICAL CONSIDERATIONS

Description: **Esophageal replacement** in children is usually performed for complicated caustic stricture or esophageal atresia (EA). Patients with failed repair of EA usually have a proximal esophagostomy and may have pulmonary dysfunction or other congenital anomalies. Caustic stricture of the esophagus occurs primarily in children 1-3 yr old, and may require esophageal replacement after failed attempts at dilation. The ideal long-term esophageal substitute does not exist, but segments of colon or a tube fashioned from the greater curvature of the stomach are the most suitable. Pulling the stomach up into the bed of the esophagus is also an option. The **proximal anastomosis** is usually performed in the neck at the site of a previous esophagostomy or in the chest, well above the level of stricture. The interposed segment may be brought through the bed of the resected esophagus or transpleural behind the root of the lung. Substernal routes are not favored in children. Depending on the level of the anastomosis, the operation may be accomplished by thoracoabdominal, thoracic or abdominal, or thoracic, abdominal and cervical incisions. Consequently, the operation may be performed in a single position or may require position and drape changes.

Usual preop diagnosis: EA; caustic stricture

SUMMARY OF PROCEDURE

Position	Supine, tilted; or supine, then lateral
Incision	Thoracoabdominal ± cervical; or transverse abdominal, posterolateral thoracic
Special instrumentation	Bougie (upper esophagus)
Antibiotics	Preop: ampicillin 25 mg/kg iv + gentamicin 2.5 mg/kg iv Intraop: cephalosporin irrigation (1 g/500 ml NS)
Surgical time	3-5 h (4-6 h with position change)
EBL	20-40 ml/kg
Postop care	PICU
Mortality	5%
Morbidity	Respiratory failure Anastomotic leak Sepsis Stricture
Pain score	7-8

PATIENT POPULATION CHARACTERISTICS

Age range	1-5 yr
Male:Female	2:1
Incidence	~200/yr in U.S.
Etiology	Caustic ingestion; EA
Associated conditions	Caustic stricture; imperforate anus; VACTERL association

ANESTHETIC CONSIDERATIONS

PREOPERATIVE

These patients usually are children presenting with a Hx of caustic substance ingestion and subsequent development of esophageal stricture. They have undergone multiple esophageal dilations under GA. Previous anesthesia records should be obtained. Preop, these patients are admitted for bowel prep and, consequently, may be hypovolemic.

Gastrointestinal Varying degrees of esophageal reflux may be present. Preop H_2-blocker administration is appropriate (e.g., ranitidine 0.8 mg/kg iv) the night before and morning of surgery. A gastrostomy may be present in some patients.

Tests: Review prior barium swallow studies and upper GI endoscopy reports; electrolytes.

ANESTHETIC CONSIDERATIONS

PREOPERATIVE

Biliary atresia is a postnatal inflammatory disorder of the hepatobiliary tree involving the intrahepatic biliary radicles → obstructive jaundice. The Kasai pocedure is performed when the diagnosis of biliary atresia is made in the first 3-4 mo of life.

Gastrointestinal Hepatic function preserved initially (i.e., normal albumin synthesis). Cholestatic jaundice usually present. There may be impaired elimination of drugs, particularly nondepolarizing muscle relaxants. Glucose homeostasis is usually normal.

Hematologic Anemia 2° hepatic disease. Impaired vitamin K absorption 2° lack of bile salts. Elevated PT will variably correct with vitamin K administration (phytonadione 1 mg im/iv given during the week before surgery). Have FFP available if PT not corrected after vitamin K.
Tests: PT; PTT; CBC; T&C

Laboratory Electrolytes; BUN; creatinine; LFTs; albumin; bilirubin, direct and indirect glucose; others as indicated from H&P. Confirm availability of blood products (PRBCs, FFP). (✓ parental/directed donor blood availability.)

Premedication None

INTRAOPERATIVE

Anesthetic technique: GETA, using a pediatric circle with warmed and humidified gases. Warm OR to 75°-80°F; use warming pad on OR table. (Remember: majority of heat loss is radiant).

Induction Mask induction is appropriate if no iv in place. Nondepolarizing muscle relaxant (e.g., rocuronium 0.6-1 mg/kg) to facilitate tracheal intubation, typically using an uncuffed 3.5-4.0 ETT (with leak at 10-35 cmH_2O).

Maintenance Isoflurane/air/O_2, supplemented with epidural anesthesia if PT/PTT normal. No N_2O, to avoid bowel distension. Continue muscle relaxant to facilitate abdominal closure.

Emergence Patient usually extubated in OR and transported to PACU or, in the case of prolonged surgery and/or significant blood loss, to PICU with O_2 and monitors in place.

Blood and fluid requirements
Moderate blood loss
IV: 22 ga × 1-2
NS/LR @ 10 ml/kg/h
Albumin 5%

Potential for large 3rd-space losses. Plan 10 ml/kg/h of NS/LR for replacement, and be prepared for sudden blood loss. Use albumin 5%, or NS/LR to replace blood loss; transfuse to maintain Hct > 22%. If dextrose infusion required, give 4-6 mg/kg/min.

Monitoring
Standard monitors (p. D-1).
Urinary catheter
NG tube
Arterial line (22-24 ga)
±CVP line

Hct, blood glucose, ±ABG q 1-2 h and prn. Maintain UO @ 1 ml/kg/h. The presence of ↑↑BP variations with respiration is a useful indicator of hypovolemia. CVP may be indicated for blood sampling/intravascular volume monitoring.

Positioning
✓ padding – heels, elbows, occiput.
✓ eyes.

Complications
Hypothermia
Hypovolemia
Hypoventilation
Metabolic acidosis

In upper abdominal surgery, the retractors and abdominal packing may limit diaphragmatic excursion, thus requiring higher PIP to adequately ventilate the patient. ETT leak (PIP) > 20 cmH_2O to insure adequate ventilation.

POSTOPERATIVE

Complications
Hypovolemia
Transfusion-associated disease
Atelectasis
Cholangitis

3rd-space losses continue in the immediate postop period.
Postop mechanical ventilation with TV 10-12 ml/kg and PEEP 3-5 cmH_2O to minimize atelectasis.

Pain management	Fentanyl (1-2 mg/kg/iv q 1 h prn) MS (0.05-0.1 mg/kg iv q 2-4 h prn)	Epidural analgesia if catheter in place (see p. E-2).
Tests	Hct, ABG	

References

1. Engelskirchen R, Holschneider AM, Gharib M, Vente C: Biliary atresia—a 25-year survey. *Eur J Pediatr Surg* 1991; 1(3):154-60.
2. Flake AW: Disorders of the gallbladder and biliary tract. In *Surgery of Infants and Children.* Oldham KT, Colombani PM, Foglia RP, eds. Lippincott-Raven Publishers, Philadelphia: 1997, 1405-1414.
3. Karrer FM, Hall RJ, Stewart BA, Lilly JR: Congenital biliary tract disease. *Surg Clin North Am* 1990; 70(6):1403-18.
4. Karrer FM, Lilly JP: Biliary atresia. In *Surgery of Infants and Children.* Oldham KT, Colombani PM, Foglia RP, eds. Lippincott-Raven Publishers, Philadelphia: 1997, 1395-1404.
5. Kasai M, Suzuki H, Ohashi E, Ohi R, Chiba T, Okamoto A: Technique and results of operative management of biliary atresia. *World J Surg* 1978; 2(5):571-79.
6. Katz J, Steward DJ, eds: *Anesthesia and Uncommon Pediatric Diseases*, 2nd edition. WB Saunders Co, Philadelphia: 1993.

RESECTION OF CYSTIC HYGROMA, BRANCHIAL CLEFT CYST, THYROGLOSSAL DUCT CYST, OR OTHER CERVICAL MASS

SURGICAL CONSIDERATIONS

Description: Lesions requiring extensive dissection in the neck and parotid region that occur during the patient's childhood are generally due to malformations of the lymphatic system (cystic hygroma, lymphangioma), branchial cleft or thyroglossal duct remnants, or infection of the lymph nodes and salivary glands with atypical mycobacteria. Cystic hygromas are usually large lesions centered about the IJ vein. Careful, tedious dissection of the cervical vessels, brachial plexus and the facial, vagus, phrenic, spinal accessory and hypoglossal nerves is common. Extension into the mediastinum occurs in 10-15% of cervical hygromas and should be evaluated preop by x-ray. Branchial cleft anomalies usually require much less extensive dissection. Thyroglossal duct remnants are excised with the central portion of the hyoid bone. Atypical mycobacterial adenitis frequently involves the high jugulodigastric nodes and the submaxillary or parotid gland, with the facial nerve and its marginal mandibular branch being the most vulnerable structures. This midline lesion connects to the pharynx at the foramen cecum and resection must include this tract and the mid portion of the hyoid bone to prevent recurrence. Other lesions in this location are dermoid cysts or ectopic thyroid, which may represent all of the functioning thyroid tissue and, thus, should be preserved.

Usual preop diagnosis: Cystic hygroma; branchial cleft cyst/fistula; thyroglossal duct cyst; atypical mycobacterial adenitis

SUMMARY OF PROCEDURE

	Lateral Lesions/Hygroma/ Branchial Cleft Cysts	Midline Lesions/ Thyroglossal Duct Cysts
Position	Neck extended, head rotated	Neck extended, head midline
Incision	Oblique	Transverse
Special instrumentation	Facial nerve monitor; nerve stimulator	None
Unique considerations	Nerve testing	None
Antibiotics	Preop: ampicillin 25 mg/kg iv + gentamicin 2.5 mg/kg iv Intraop: cephalosporin irrigation (1 g/500 ml NS)	⇐
Surgical time	2-6 h	1 h
EBL	5-20 ml/kg	< 5 ml/kg
Postop care	PICU; airway monitoring	None
Mortality	2-5%	< 1%

	Lateral Lesions/Hygroma/ Branchial Cleft Cysts	Midline Lesions/ Thyroglossal Cysts
Morbidity	Airway compromise	⇐
	Fluid accumulation	⇐
	Infection	⇐
Pain score	3-4	3-4

PATIENT POPULATION CHARACTERISTICS

Age range	Newborn–school age
Male:Female	1:1
Incidence	Common
Etiology	Developmental anomaly; mycobacteria
Associated conditions	Hygroma-mediastinal airway involvement; branchial cleft – 10% (bilateral)

ANESTHETIC CONSIDERATIONS

PREOPERATIVE

These patients generally are otherwise healthy children. A cystic hygroma (cystic lymphangioma), as with other neck masses, may cause airway obstruction and difficult intubation.

Respiratory The size and extent of the neck mass should be defined carefully in an effort to detect the potential for airway compromise and to avoid soft-tissue trauma during intubation, with consequent acute airway obstruction. Inspiratory stridor suggests supraglottic obstruction, while expiratory stridor is associated with subglottic/intrathoracic obstruction. These patients should have had prior CT/MRI imaging; anesthesia records for these studies should be reviewed.
Tests: CXR ± CT/MRI scans

Cardiovascular Cervical masses may be adherent to and/or cause compression of the great vessels.
Tests: CT/MRI scans

Hematologic T&C for cystic hygroma, or if a cervical mass involves great vessels or extends into the mediastinum (~3%).
Tests: Hct

Laboratory Other tests as indicated from H&P.

Premedication If 1-10 yr old and asymptomatic, midazolam (0.5-0.75 mg po) 30 min prior to arrival in OR. Avoid all premedication in patients with potential airway compromise.

INTRAOPERATIVE

Anesthetic technique: GETA with pediatric circle, and warm, humidified gases. OR temperature 75-80°; warming pad on OR table. Use air/O_2 mixture for ventilation. Maintain SpO_2 between 95-100% to minimize retinopathy in premature infants.

Induction Standard pediatric induction (p. D-2) in patients without airway compromise. IV should be secured prior to induction when airway compromise is present or suspected. Mask induction with sevoflurane or halothane in 100% O_2. As plane of anesthesia deepens, gently assist ventilation. (Keep PIP < 20 cmH_2O). Give atropine (0.02 mg/kg iv) if < 9 mo prior to laryngoscopy. If partial airway obstruction exists, maintain spontaneous ventilation and perform laryngoscopy under deep anesthesia (e.g., ~3 MAC of volatile agent). FOB should be available. Have full range of ETT sizes available, since airway narrowing may be present. Once airway is secured, proceed with neuromuscular blockade (e.g., vecuronium 0.1 mg/kg iv or pancuronium 0.1 mg/kg).

Maintenance Standard pediatric maintenance (p. D-3). Surgeon may infiltrate incision with local anesthetic. Limit bupivacaine to 2.5 mg/kg.

Emergence Reverse neuromuscular blockade with neostigmine (0.07 mg/kg iv) and atropine (0.02 mg/kg iv). Confirm air leak around ETT and extubate when fully awake.

Blood and fluid requirements	Minimal blood loss IV: 20-22 ga × 1 Great vessel involvement – IV: 20 ga × 2 NS/LR @ 3 ml/kg/h	Minimal 3rd-space losses. Each ml blood loss can be replaced with 3 ml NS/LR. When great vessels involved, place at least one iv in lower extremity. Blood loss can be quite sudden; have blood available in OR.
Monitoring	Standard monitors (p. D-1) ± Arterial line – 22 ga	An arterial line is used when there is risk of large blood loss or perioperative airway compromise.
Positioning	✓ and pad pressure points. ✓ eyes.	
Complications	ETT dislodged/loss of airway Laryngospasm Bronchospasm Hemorrhage	ETT must be carefully secured. Liberal use of benzoin. Avoid tension on ETT by circuit hoses. Hold ETT during surgeon's intraoral examination.

POSTOPERATIVE

Complications	Subglottic edema Upper airway obstruction from edema related to tumor resection Recurrent laryngeal nerve injury	Dexamethasone (0.5-1 mg/kg iv) and nebulized racemic epinephrine (1.25%) with mist O_2 to treat subglottic edema.
Pain management	Morphine (0.05-0.1 mg/kg iv q 2-4 h) Acetaminophen (10-15 mg/kg po/pr q 4 h)	
Tests	As indicated.	

References

1. Fallat ME: Neck. In *Surgery of Infants and Children.* Oldham KT, Colombani PM, Foglia RP, eds. Lippincott-Raven Publishers, Philadelphia: 1997, 835-56.
2. Gregory GA (ed): *Pediatric Anesthesia*, 2nd ed. Churchill Livingstone, New York: 1989.
3. Motoyama EK, Davis PJ, eds: *Smith's Anesthesia for Infants and Children*, 6th edition. Mosby-Year Book, St. Louis: 1996.

REPAIR OF OMPHALOCELE/GASTROSCHISIS

SURGICAL CONSIDERATIONS

Description: The goals of treatment for the abdominal wall defects (gastroschisis/omphalocele) are the safe return of the herniated viscera to the abdominal cavity and closure of the abdominal wall muscles and skin. Gastroschisis, with no covering membrane and few associated anomalies, generally requires urgent operative treatment. Omphalocele, with an intact membrane, may be managed nonoperatively if associated anomalies require more urgent diagnosis or treatment. While primary closure is ideal, many patients have inadequate abdominal domain, which produces unacceptable respiratory or cardiovascular compromise if primary repair is attempted. Elevation of skin flaps and removal of umbilical cord may require extending the incision in the midline. In omphalocele, the membrane is left intact if possible and the wound closed or Silastic sheeting attached. In gastroschisis, the defect is usually extended and a gastrostomy is placed. If reduction of the viscera is not possible, or if it produces unacceptable respiration or cardiovascular compromise, then a **staged procedure** is performed. This consists of suturing Silastic sheeting to the full-thickness abdominal wall, creating a silo or pouch to contain the abdominal viscera. This pouch is reduced in size day-by-day until the viscera are returned to the abdominal cavity. The reductions may be done in the nursery or the OR and usually will allow definite closure of the abdominal wall in 7-10 d. Omphalocele, under unusual circumstances, can be treated by skin coverage only or by topical application of iodine or mercurochrome to the membrane.

Usual preop diagnosis: Omphalocele; gastroschisis; pentalogy of Cantrell; exstrophy cloaca

SUMMARY OF PROCEDURE

Position	Supine
Incision	Midline
Special instrumentation	None; for staged repair, nylon-reinforced Silastic sheeting
Antibiotics	Preop: ampicillin 25 mg/kg iv + gentamicin 2.5 mg/kg iv Intraop: cephalosporin irrigation (1 g/500 ml NS)
Surgical time	2 h
Closing considerations	Assess respiratory and cardiovascular function after muscle closure by PIP, ABG, MAP. Impaired ventilation and venous return will result from overaggressive attempts at closure.
EBL	5-10 ml/kg
Postop care	Assisted ventilation; volume support (gastroschisis)
Mortality	Omphalocele: 28% Gastroschisis: 15-23%
Morbidity	Respiratory failure Intestinal ischemia/obstruction Infection
Pain score	5-6 (primary); 4-5 (staged repair)

PATIENT POPULATION CHARACTERISTICS

Age range	Newborn
Male:Female	1:1
Incidence	1/3000–1/10,000 live births
Etiology	Unknown
Associated conditions	Gastroschisis – malrotation, intestinal atresia Omphalocele – cardiac, renal anomalies Trisomy 13, 18 Beckwith-Wiedemann syndrome (hypoglycemia, macroglossia) Pentalogy of Cantrell – omphalocele, sternal, diaphragmatic, pericardial, cardiac anomalies Exstrophy cloaca – omphalocele, exstrophy bladder, imperforate anus

ANESTHETIC CONSIDERATIONS

PREOPERATIVE

Newborns with omphalocele/gastroschisis present for urgent surgery. The large exposed surface area of abdominal contents allows substantial evaporative heat and fluid losses. Omphalocele is associated with other congenital anomalies (e.g., VSD, Beckwith-Wiedemann syndrome [infantile gigantism, macroglossia]). The majority of these patients should be medically stabilized in the nursery prior to coming to the OR.

Respiratory	If premature (< 36 wk gestational age), is at increased risk for RDS. Respiratory insufficiency may be present. **Tests:** CXR; ABG
Cardiovascular	With omphalocele, there is a 20% incidence of cardiac anomalies (VSD, PDA). Presence of murmur. **Tests:** ECHO, if indicated
Gastrointestinal	Intestinal atresia may be present. Hypovolemia from evaporative loss also may be present. Use full-stomach precautions. ✓ administration of antibiotics to prevent peritonitis.
Endocrine	Beckwith-Wiedemann associated with hypoglycemia (term infant glucose—normal > 36 mg/dL). **Tests:** Glucose; electrolytes
Laboratory	CBC; T&C; PT; PTT; UA

INTRAOPERATIVE

Anesthetic technique: Epidural anesthesia and GETA, using a pediatric circle or Bain circuit with humidified and warmed gases. Maintain body temperature close to 37°C. Use Bair Hugger and warm room to 78-80°F. (Remember majority of heat loss is radiant.)

Induction Atropine (0.02 mg/kg iv, minimum dose 0.1 mg) is given before induction in patients < 9 mo to ablate vagal response to laryngoscopy. Pass an OG tube to decompress stomach. Assure adequate intravascular volume status (capillary refill < 2 sec; warm, pink extremities). Preoxygenate with 100% O_2 for 2-3 min prior to rapid-sequence intubation. STP (4-6 mg/kg iv) or propofol (2-3 mg/kg) and succinylcholine (1-2 mg/kg iv) or rocuronium (1 mg/kg) administered to facilitate tracheal intubation. 3.5 ETT is most appropriate for this age group. Keep air leak around ETT at 10-35 cmH_2O. Lower pressure air leak may make ventilation difficult if primary closure of abdomen is accompanied by significant rise in intraabdominal pressure. Epidural catheter inserted via the caudal or lumbar route after intubation. If positioning for the epidural catheter insertion is difficult, do not proceed; insert at the end of the case for postop analgesia.

Maintenance Avoid high FiO_2. Use air/O_2 mixture for ventilation to maintain O_2 sat 95-100% and PaO_2 < 100. If no epidural is placed, then use a primarily narcotic-based technique with fentanyl (10-25 μg/kg iv total), low-dose isoflurane as needed. Note initial PIP prior to abdominal closure. Maintain neuromuscular blockade to facilitate abdominal closure. If an epidural catheter is available, dose with local anesthetic and opiate (p. D-5) to supplement inhalation iv agent.

Emergence Remain intubated postop. Transport to NICU on 100% O_2 to increase margin of safety in case of accidental extubation.

Blood and fluid requirements	Marked 3rd-space fluid loss Minimal-moderate blood loss IV: 22-24 ga × 1-2, upper extremities NS/LR @ 4 ml/kg/h	Continue dextrose-containing solution from NICU. Replace 3rd-space losses (10-15+ ml/kg/h). Replace blood loss with albumin 5% and/or blood ml for ml. Maintain Hct > 30%. Lower extremities usually edematous due to abdominal venous and lymphatic compression.
Monitoring	Standard monitors (p. D-1) Arterial line (24-ga radial) ± CVP – 3 Fr subclavian or 4 Fr IJ	ABG pre- and postabdominal closure. Hct, glucose, electrolytes q 60 min. CVP; reserve 1 lumen, for postop TPN. Respiratory variation on arterial waveform is sensitive indicator of hypovolemia.
	± Intragastric catheter Urinary catheter	May be used to measure pressure during abdominal closure.
Positioning	✓ and pad pressure points. ✓ eyes.	Arms positioned to have ready access to arterial line.
Complications	Hypothermia Hypovolemia Respiratory insufficiency/ hypoventilation Atelectasis Volume overload/pulmonary edema	Some institutions monitor intraabdominal pressure during closure. If intragastric pressure is > 20 mmHg and CVP increases by 4 mmHg with initial primary closure, it should be converted to a staged repair. Raised abdominal pressure will cause an acute restrictive ventilatory defect and promote abdominal visceral ischemia.

POSTOPERATIVE

Complications	Respiratory failure Bowel ischemia/necrosis Renal failure Peritonitis Sepsis/metabolic acidosis Pneumothorax RDS Hypothermia	Abdominal 3rd spacing will persist in immediate postop period → ↓intraabdominal pressure → bowel ischemia + ↓renal perfusion. Persistent metabolic and/or respiratory acidosis mandates staged repair.
Pain management	Continuous epidural or iv infusion (p. E-2)	
Tests	ABG; Hct; glucose; electrolytes, Ca^{++} UO maintained at > 0.5 ml/kg/h	

References

1. Gregory GA, ed: *Pediatric Anesthesia*, 3rd edition. Churchill Livingstone, New York: 1994, 557-59.
2. Motoyama EK, Davis PJ, eds: *Smith's Anesthesia for Infants and Children*, 6th edition. Mosby-Year Book, St. Louis: 1996, 455-57.
3. Novotny DA, Klein RL, Boeckman CR: Gastroschisis: an 18-year review. *J Pediatr Surg* 1993; 28(5):650-2.
4. Sauter ER, Falterman KW, Arensman RM: Is primary repair of gastroschisis and omphalocele always the best operation? *Am Surg* 1991; 57(3):142-44.
5. Schier F, Schier C, Stute MP, Wurtenberger H: 193 cases of gastroschisis and omphalocele—postoperative results. *Zentralbl Chir* 1988; 113(4):225-34.
6. Tracy TF Jr: Abdominal wall defects. In *Surgery of Infants and Children.* Oldham KT, Colombani PM, Foglia RP, eds. Lippincott-Raven Publishers, Philadelphia: 1997, 1083-94.
7. Tsakayannis DE, Zurakowski D, Lillehie CW: Respiratory insufficiency at birth: a predictor of mortality for infants with omphalocele. *J Pediatr Surg* 1996; 31(8):1088-90.
8. Yaster M, et al: Hemodynamic effects of primary closure of omphalocele/gastroschisis in human newborns. *Anesthesiology* 1988; 69:84-8.

HERNIA REPAIR

SURGICAL CONSIDERATIONS

Description: Repair of inguinal hernia is the most common operation performed in children. Inguinal hernias in children are almost always indirect type due to failure of the processus vaginalis to obliterate. They are more common and more likely to incarcerate in premature infants. Bilateral hernias are common at < 2 yr of age. Hydroceles are identical to inguinal hernia in origin and treatment. Complications of hernia repair are uncommon and are most commonly related to the effects of GA on an immature CNS and respiratory system. Umbilical hernias are more common in African Americans and will usually undergo spontaneous closure if given enough time; 75-80% will close by 2 yr of age and 95-98% by 5 yr. **Inguinal hernia repair** is performed via an inguinal skin-crease incision. The sac is separated from the spermatic cord structures, dissected to the level of the internal ring, and ligated. The distal sac and floor of the inguinal canal are not disturbed. Bilateral procedures are usually done in children < 2 yr of age. **Umbilical repair** is performed through a transverse incision with excision of the sac after detaching it from the undersurface of the skin. The fascia is repaired transversely and little, if any, intraperitoneal exploration done.

Usual preop diagnosis: Inguinal hernia; hydrocele; umbilical hernia

SUMMARY OF PROCEDURE

	Inguinal	Umbilical
Position	Supine	⇐
Incision	Inguinal, bilateral	Infraumbilical
Unique considerations	Prematurity	Abdominal compression if hernia large
Antibiotics	Intraop: cefazolin irrigation 1 g/500 ml NS	None
Surgical time	1 h	⇐
Closing considerations	Nerve block, caudal	None
EBL	5 ml/kg	⇐
Postop care	Apnea monitor; hospitalization for premature infants	None
Mortality	< 1%	⇐
Morbidity	Apnea Recurrence	None
Pain score	3-5	3-5

PATIENT POPULATION CHARACTERISTICS

	Inguinal	Umbilical
Age range	Premature–adolescent	> 2 yr
Male:Female	5:1	N/A
Incidence	1-2%	1%
Etiology	Patent processus vaginalis	Persistent umbilical defect
Associated conditions	Gonadal dysgenesis	None

ANESTHETIC CONSIDERATIONS

PREOPERATIVE

Hernia repair is most commonly performed in otherwise healthy infants in the first 2 yr of life, often on an outpatient basis. It is also performed on premature infants (< 36 wk gestational age at birth) and other neonates requiring intensive care. Premature infants are particularly prone to inguinal hernias. Postop apnea can occur in infants ≤ 50-60 wk postconceptual age, particularly if the infant was premature, has neurologic disease or required intensive care in the early neonatal period.

Respiratory — Bronchopulmonary dysplasia (BPD), tracheomalacia and subglottic stenosis are consequences of prolonged mechanical ventilation and immature lungs at birth. ✓ prior NICU Hx. ↓FRC and ↑PVR makes infants with this disease more susceptible to hypoxia. They may require supplemental nasal O_2 on a chronic basis.
Tests: CXR

Cardiovascular — Prior PDA ligation is possible. These patients may be on diuretic therapy for intrinsic lung disease (e.g., BPD) with resultant decreased intravascular volume.
Tests: CXR; electrolytes

Neurological — Premature infants may be prone to seizure disorders. Premature infants have immature respiratory centers and may exhibit paradoxical apneic/bradycardic episodes in response to hypoxemia.
Tests: Anticonvulsant levels

Hematologic — Anemia is common at ~ 3 mo of age and increases risk of postop apnea.
Tests: Hct; PT; PTT; Plt, as indicated from H&P.

Laboratory — Other tests as indicated from H&P.

Premedication — If > 1 yr of age, midazolam (0.5-0.75 mg po) 30 min prior to arrival in OR.

INTRAOPERATIVE

Anesthetic technique: Typically, GETA, LMA or mask GA (± caudal or ilioinguinal/iliohypogastric block), using a pediatric circle or Bain circuit with warm, humidified gases. An alternative in ex-preterm infants at high risk for postop apnea is spinal anesthesia without GA or iv sedation (p. D-6). Warm OR to 75°-80° F; use warming pad on OR table.

Induction — Mask induction in children with sevoflurane or halothane/N_2O/O_2. Secure iv. If appropriate, position child for placement of caudal anesthetic: bupivacaine 0.25% ± epinephrine 1:200,000 @ 1 ml/kg. If child otherwise healthy and >1 yr old, can proceed with LMA or mask anesthetic; otherwise, tracheal intubation is preferred. Atropine (0.02 mg/kg iv) given prior to laryngoscopy in patients < 9 mo. Intubation may be facilitated with vecuronium (0.1 mg/kg) or rocuronium (1 mg/kg).

Maintenance — Standard pediatric inhalational anesthetic (p. D-3) is appropriate. With caudal anesthetic or nerve block, decrease amount of volatile anesthetic and avoid or reduce opiates. 2 MAC of inhalational agents at incision is required to avoid laryngospasm in this patient population. Caudal bupivacaine onset time ~15 min.

Emergence — Reverse neuromuscular blockade with neostigmine (0.07 mg/kg iv) and atropine (0.02 mg/kg iv). Extubate only when fully awake.

Blood and fluid requirements — Negligible blood loss
IV: 22-24 ga × 1

Infants receiving diuretics will require 10-20 ml/kg iv of NS/LR to avoid hypotension 2° volatile anesthetics. In

Blood and fluid, cont.	NS/LR @ (maintenance): 4 ml/kg/h – 0-10 kg + 2 ml/kg/h – 11-20 kg	children < 1 mo old, use dextrose-containing iv solution (e.g., D2.5/LR)
Monitoring	Standard monitors (p. D-1)	Premature infants may become hypoglycemic. ✓ blood glucose during surgery.
Positioning	✓ and pad pressure points. ✓ eyes.	With too-large mask, beware ocular compression/corneal abrasion.
Complications	Laryngospasm Bronchospasm Hypothermia Pulmonary hypertensive episode Local anesthetic toxicity Hypoglycemia	Rx bronchospasm: albuterol inhaler. Mist O_2 after extubation. Avoid hyperglycemia → diuresis and dehydration.

POSTOPERATIVE

Complications	Apnea/bradycardia Subglottic edema	Can lessen incidence of apnea/bradycardia by administering caffeine (10 mg/kg iv) intraop or in NICU/PACU.
Pain management	Field block Acetaminophen (10-20 mg po q 4-6 h prn)	If no caudal used, a field block (bupivacaine 0.25% 2-3 ml) at end of surgery reduces pain in the immediate postop period. It is usually performed by the surgeon.
Tests/monitoring	Apnea monitor and pulse oximeter for 12-18 h for premature infants < 60 wk postconception	Caffeine is no substitute for monitoring and attentive parents/nurses.

References

1. Beckerman RC, Brouillette RT, Hunt CE, eds: *Respiratory Control Disorders in Infants and Children.* Williams and Wilkins, Baltimore: 1991, 161-77.
2. Kurth CD, Spitzer AR, Broennle AM, Downes JJ: Postoperative apnea in preterm infants. *Anesthesiology* 1987; 66(4):483-88.
3. Rescorla FJ: Hernias and umbilicus. In *Surgery of Infants and Children.* Oldham KT, Colombani PM, Foglia RP, eds. Lippincott-Raven Publishers, Philadelphia: 1997, 1069-82.
4. Stehling L, ed: *Common Problems in Pediatric Anesthesia*, 2nd edition. Mosby-Year Book, St. Louis: 1992, 69-85.
5. Welborn LG, Hannallah RS, Fink R, Ruttimann VE, Hick JM: High-dose caffeine suppresses postoperative apnea in former preterm infants. *Anesthesiology* 1989; 71(3):347-49.

ESOPHAGOSCOPY FOR FOREIGN BODY REMOVAL, ESOPHAGEAL DILATION

SURGICAL CONSIDERATIONS

Description: Flexible, diagnostic **esophagogastroduodenoscopy**—a common procedure in pediatrics—is usually performed under GA or heavy sedation in an endoscopy suite or special procedure area. **Rigid esophagoscopy** is usually performed for therapeutic indications, such as removal of a foreign body, dilation of an esophageal stricture or injection of varices. The procedure is similar for each diagnosis and generally is performed with ET intubation. Foreign body removal is normally a very short procedure, while dilation and variceal injection can be prolonged and may require multiple insertions/removals of the endoscope. Compression of the trachea, distal to the ETT by the rigid esophagoscope, is a common occurrence.

Usual preop diagnosis: Esophageal foreign body; stricture; esophageal varices

SUMMARY OF PROCEDURE

Position	Supine
Special instrumentation	Rigid esophagoscopes; forceps; dilators
Unique considerations	Esophagoscope may obstruct airway; dilation may perforate esophagus.
Surgical time	5 min-2 h
Closing considerations	Abrupt ending
EBL	< 5 ml/kg
Postop care	Airway support
Mortality	< 5%
Morbidity	Esophageal perforation: 2-5%
Pain score	2-3

PATIENT POPULATION CHARACTERISTICS

Age range	Newborn–school age
Male:Female	1:1
Incidence	1/1000
Etiology	Varices – portal HTN; foreign body – possible stricture
Associated conditions	Esophageal atresia – stricture; portal HTN – varices

ANESTHETIC CONSIDERATIONS

PREOPERATIVE

Esophagoscopy for foreign body removal is usually performed in healthy infants and children, although esophageal lodging of a foreign body can occur in any age group. All of these patients should be treated with full-stomach precautions. Esophageal dilation usually performed in 3 distinct patient populations: (1) those with prior tracheoesophageal fistula (TEF) repair; (2) those with prior ingestion of a caustic substance; and (3) those with skin and connective tissue diseases (e.g., epidermolysis bullosa [EB]).

Respiratory Patients with prior caustic ingestion may have Hx of pulmonary aspiration, with resultant chemical pneumonitis and/or fibrosis. Prolonged intubation after TEF repair may → subglottic stenosis. ✓ any recent anesthesia records for ETT size required. Patients with EB may have limited mouth opening and require special care regarding placing and securing of ETT (see p. 677).
Tests: CXR, if clinically indicated.

Cardiovascular There may be persistent congenital cardiac anomalies in the TEF patient.
Tests: Cardiology consultation, as needed.

Laboratory No routine lab analyses are required if patient has no underlying chronic illnesses.

Premedication For esophageal dilation, patient preference is extremely important since some patients have undergone this procedure several times. For foreign body removal, iv access may be necessary before induction.

INTRAOPERATIVE

Anesthetic technique: GETA, using a pediatric circle or Bain circuit. Room temperature can be maintained at 65-70°F, as long as patient is covered.

Induction If the patient is presenting for dilation alone and has no evidence to suggest reflux, a standard inhalation or iv induction may be performed. Rapid-sequence induction is usually appropriate for foreign-body removal. Atropine (0.02 mg/kg if < 6-9 mo) is administered to attenuate bradycardia from succinylcholine and intubation. Preoxygenate for 2-3 min. Apply cricoid pressure. STP (4-6 mg/kg iv) or propofol (2-3 mg/kg), followed by succinylcholine (1-2 mg/kg). Confirm absence of train-of-four prior to laryngoscopy. Intubate trachea with age-appropriate ETT ([16 + age] ÷ 4). Once airway is secured, administer rocuronium (1 mg/kg) or vecuronium (0.1 mg/kg).

Maintenance Maintain anesthesia with volatile agent/N_2O/O_2 or propofol (100-200 μg/kg/min) + remifentanil (0.05-2 μg/kg/min). Supplement inhalation anesthetic with small doses of fentanyl (e.g., 1-2 μg/kg)

Maintenance, cont.	or morphine (0.05-0.1 μg/kg). Maintain neuromuscular blockade. Movement must be avoided with rigid esophagoscopy.	
Emergence	Extubate when fully awake. Neostigmine (0.07 mg/kg) and atropine (0.02 mg/kg) to reverse neuromuscular blockade. Do not attempt reversal of neuromuscular blockade until first twitch of train-of-four has returned.	
Blood and fluid requirements	IV: 20-22 ga × 1 NS/LR @ 4-6 ml/kg/h	
Monitoring	Standard monitors (p. D-1) Peripheral nerve stimulator	
Positioning	✓ and pad pressure points. ✓ eyes. ✓ radial pulse of dependent arm.	Axillary roll as needed; avoid brachial plexus compression.
Complications	Pneumothorax Aspiration Accidental extubation Stridor 2° subglottic edema	Esophageal perforation, more common with rigid esophagoscopy, will lead to pneumothorax (R > L).

POSTOPERATIVE

Complications	Residual neuromuscular blockade Pneumothorax	
Pain management	Minimal postop pain	If patient reports marked substernal discomfort, suspect esophageal perforation.
Tests	None	

References

1. Gans SL, ed: Esophagoscopy. In *Pediatric Endoscopy*. Grune and Stratton, New York: 1983, 55-66.
2. Rodgers BM, McGahren ED III: Esophagus. In *Surgery of Infants and Children*. Oldham KT, Colombani PM, Foglia RP, eds. Lippincott-Raven Publishers, Philadelphia: 1997, 1005-20.

PULLTHROUGH FOR HIRSCHSPRUNG'S DISEASE; SOAVE, DUHAMEL, SWENSON PULLTHROUGH

SURGICAL CONSIDERATIONS

Description: Congenital aganglionosis (Hirschsprung's disease) produces functional obstruction of the colon with symptoms related to the length of bowel involved. The absence of ganglion cells is continuous in retrograde fashion from the anus with most (75%) cases having the transition to ganglionic bowel in the sigmoid colon. Symptoms range from constipation to complete colonic obstruction, with some patients developing a toxic enterocolitis requiring **emergency colostomy** after initial resuscitation. Most medical centers perform correction of this anomaly in two stages—**initial colostomy** in the transition zone, followed by **definitive pullthrough**. Definitive procedures are generally performed at 10 kg or 12-18 mo of age. Some centers are performing definitive pullthrough in the first mo, without a preliminary colostomy. The abdominal portion of the procedure may be done laparoscopically in selected cases.

The three popular types of pullthrough procedures include resection of most of the aganglionic bowel and delivery of ganglionic bowel to the distal anal canal. They vary in the method of intrapelvic dissection and the type of coloanal anastomosis. All procedures include an initial intraperitoneal dissection, followed by a transanal anastomosis. Some surgeons prefer total lower-body prep, with legs included; others use a modified lithotomy position, with abdominal and perineal prep. After mobilization of the aganglionic colon, the rectum is either transected (**Duhamel**) or dissected to the level of the levator muscle. In the **Swenson procedure** (**abdominal-perineal pullthrough**), the rectal dissection is done on the external surface of the muscular layer, whereas in the **Soave** (**mucosal stripping and pullthrough** of the resulting muscular tunnel) it is done between the submucosal and inner muscular layers. In the **Duhamel** (**double-barrelled pullthrough**), the proximal rectum is closed and the ganglionic bowel is delivered behind the rectum to allow an end-to-side anastomosis just above the levator. The Swenson procedure consists of an end-to-end anastomosis of ganglionic bowel to full-thickness rectal stump. In the Soave procedure, the bowel is delivered within the muscular remnant of rectum and sutured to the remnant of mucosa and submucosa 1 cm above the dentate line.

Some surgeons perform the initial colostomy in the right colon, regardless of the location of the transition zone. In this circumstance, biopsies with frozen sections are required during the definitive pullthrough and a subsequent colostomy closure will follow after adequate healing of the coloanal anastomosis is confirmed.

Usual preop diagnosis: Hirschsprung's disease; congenital aganglionosis; congenital megacolon

SUMMARY OF PROCEDURE

	Preliminary Colostomy	Pullthrough
Position	Supine	Supine → lithotomy
Incision	Left lower-quadrant transverse	Low transverse
Special instrumentation	None	Staplers
Unique considerations	Frozen section to confirm ganglion cells	No monitors or iv lower extremity
Antibiotics	Preop: ampicillin 25 mg/kg iv + gentamicin 2.5 mg/kg iv	⇐
	Intraop: cephalosporin irrigation (1 g/500 ml NS)	⇐
Surgical time	1-1.5 h	4-5 h (Soave) 3-4 h (Duhamel)
Closing considerations	None	Reprep/drape
EBL	< 5 ml/kg	5-10 ml/kg
Postop care	Cardiac/apnea monitor	PICU
Mortality	With enterocolitis: 10% Without enterocolitis: 0-2%	< 5%
Morbidity	Prolapse Stricture Hernia	Anastomotic leak: 5% Wound infection: 4% Pelvic abscess: 3%
Pain score	4	6-7

PATIENT POPULATION CHARACTERISTICS

Age range	Newborn-18 mo (normally)	1 yr
Male:Female	4:1	⇐
Incidence	1/5000	⇐
Etiology	Unknown	⇐
Associated conditions	Trisomy 21: 5% Genitourinary anomalies: < 5% Neurofibromatoses	⇐

ANESTHETIC CONSIDERATIONS

PREOPERATIVE

Infants (~12 mo of age) with Hirschsprung's disease (congenital aganglionosis) have had prior colostomies and now present for colorectal reanastomosis. They may be mildly malnourished, but otherwise healthy.

GI	Diarrhea may be present with associated malabsorption state. **Tests:** Electrolytes
Laboratory	Hct; T&C
Premedication	Midazolam 0.5-0.75 mg/kg po administered 30 min before induction for child >12 mo.

INTRAOPERATIVE

Anesthetic technique: Combined epidural/GETA, using a pediatric circle with humidified and warmed gases. Warm OR to 75-80°F; use warming pad on OR table.

Induction	Mask induction is preferable, unless iv is already in place. Keep air leak around ETT to 10-35 cmH_2O to minimize alterations in ventilation 2° changes in chest and pulmonary compliance. The patient is placed in a lateral decubitus position for lumbar epidural anesthesia (see p. D-5).	
Maintenance	Low-dose volatile agent and air/O_2 with muscle relaxation for majority of cases. During last 30 min, N_2O can be substituted for air. Epidural anesthesia will provide the majority of analgesia, but not the degree of muscle relaxation that will be necessary. Supplemental muscle relaxants (e.g., pancuronium or vecuronium 0.1 mg/kg), therefore, are required.	
Emergence	The goal is to extubate at end of case. Reverse neuromuscular blockade with neostigmine (0.07 mg/kg iv) and atropine (0.02 mg/kg) or glycopyrrolate (0.01 mg/kg).	
Blood and fluid requirements	Mild blood loss IV: 20-22 ga × 1-2 in upper extremities NS/LR @ (maintenance): 4 ml/kg/h – 0-10 kg + 2 ml/kg/h – 11-20 kg + 1 ml/kg/h – > 20 kg (e.g., 25 kg = 65 ml/h)	Potential for large 3rd-space losses; plan 10 ml/kg/h of crystalloid for replacement. Use 5% albumin for rapid volume expansion; transfuse to maintain Hct >23%. As a result of bowel prep, patient may require 10-20 ml/kg iv of NS/LR to offset volume deficit.
Monitoring	Standard monitors (p. D-1) Urinary catheter ± Arterial line (22 ga)	ABG, Hct, blood glucose prn. Maintain UO @ 1 ml/kg/h. Arterial line helpful for monitoring BP, lab draws and presence of respiratory variations as indicator of volume status.
Positioning	✓ padding, particularly over lateral fibular head (common peroneal nerve). ✓ eyes.	
Complications	Hypothermia Hypovolemia	Majority of heat loss is radiant (skin), but potential for large volume shifts mandates warming fluids.

POSTOPERATIVE

Complications	Hypothermia Hypovolemia Respiratory depression 2° opiates	
Pain management	Continuous epidural	Bupivacaine with epinephrine and morphine (as described above) will provide analgesia for 8-16 h (see p. E-5).
Tests	Hct	

References

1. Puri P: Hirschsprung disease. In *Surgery of Infants and Children.* Oldham KT, Colombani PM, Foglia RP, eds. Lippincott-Raven Publishers, Philadelphia: 1997, 1277-1300.
2. Raffensperger JG, ed: *Swenson's Pediatric Surgery*, 5th edition. Appleton & Lange, Norwalk: 1990, 555-78.
3. Swenson O, Sherman JO, Fisher JH, Cohen E: The treatment and postoperative complications of congenital megacolon: A 25-year followup. *Ann Surg* 1975; 182(3):266-73.

PULLTHROUGH FOR IMPERFORATE ANUS, SACROPERINEAL PULLTHROUGH (PERINEAL ANOPLASTY), ABDOMINOSACROPERINEAL PULLTHROUGH

SURGICAL CONSIDERATIONS

Description: Imperforate anus anomalies are classified as high or low, depending on whether the distal end of the rectum ends above or below the levator ani muscle complex. **Low lesions** are repaired from a perineal approach (**perineal anoplasty**), without a preliminary colostomy. Many centers are now doing the anoplasty at 3-6 mo of age. **High lesions** are treated with a preliminary **colostomy**, usually right transverse colon, followed by definitive repair at 10 kg, or 12-18 mo of age. High lesions are initially approached from the sacrum to identify the end of the bowel and deliver it to the perineal location, either through a tunnel created anterior to the levator muscle, or by dividing the levator and external sphincter and reconstructing them around the rectum. If the rectum ends high and cannot be adequately mobilized from behind, the path to the perineum is established and the patient is turned to allow intraperitoneal mobilization of an adequate length of colon. After adequate mobilization, the neoanus is constructed either by passing the colon through the previously identified tunnel or by turning the patient again to perform the perineal anastomosis and reconstruct the muscle complex. The varieties of sacroperineal pullthrough and posterior sagittal anorectoplasty vary in the manner of handling the levator muscle, but the level of the rectal atresia will determine whether the procedure is accomplished entirely from the posterior approach or whether an abdominal procedure will be required.

Usual preop diagnosis: Imperforate anus

SUMMARY OF PROCEDURE

	Low Lesions	High Lesions
Position	Supine, lithotomy	Prone, possible turn to spine or lithotomy
Incision	Midline perineal	Midline sacral, transverse abdominal
Special instrumentation	Muscle stimulator	⇐ + Urethral sound; vaginal pack
Unique considerations	None	Pressure points; prone position
Antibiotics	Preop: ampicillin 25 mg/kg iv + gentamicin 2.5 mg/kg iv	⇐
	Intraop: cephalosporin irrigation (1 g/500 ml NS)	⇐
Surgical time	1-1.5 h	3-6 h
EBL	< 5 ml/kg	5-20 ml/kg
Postop care	Apnea monitor if neonate	PICU
Mortality	≤ 20%, due to associated anomalies	≤ 40%, due to associated anomalies
Morbidity	Anal stenosis: 5-10%	⇐
	Mucosal prolapse: 5%	Intestinal obstruction: 5-10%
		Neurogenic bladder: < 5%
		Urethral stricture: 1-3%
Pain score	3-4	5-6

PATIENT POPULATION CHARACTERISTICS

Age range	Newborn–6 mo	12-18 mo
Male:Female	1.5:1	⇐
Incidence	1/5000	⇐
Etiology	Unknown	⇐
Associated conditions	CHD (common); esophageal atresia (15%); genitourinary anomalies; sacral/spinal cord anomalies; VATER association	⇐

ANESTHETIC CONSIDERATIONS

PREOPERATIVE

Definitive repair is performed via the sacral and/or perineal route at ~12 mo. Children with rectal or anal agenesis without fistula will have had colostomies in newborn period. Other anomalies (e.g., VATER association, VSDs, vertebral anomalies, anal agenesis, tracheoesophageal fistula [TEF]), esophageal atresia (EA), renal or radial bone abnormalities may be present.

Respiratory	If VATER association present, ✓ cervical spine film and neck ROM. Avoid extreme head flexion. If prior TEF repair, concerns as previously noted in Anesthetic Considerations for Repair of Esophageal Atresia/Tracheoesophageal Fistula, p. 932. **Tests:** CXR; cervical spine film
Cardiovascular	Patients with VATER association have a 20% incidence of CHD (e.g., VSD). Prior cardiology consultation.
Gastrointestinal	Colostomy may be present; thus, anesthesia records may be available for review.
Renal	Renal abnormalities may be present. **Tests:** BUN; creatinine; electrolytes
Musculoskeletal	Radial bone deformities may be present. There is no evidence to suggest that VATER patients are at increased risk for malignant hyperthermia (MH).
Laboratory	Hct; T&C (✓ parental/directed donor blood availability.)
Premedication	Midazolam (0.5-0.75 mg/kg po) 30 min prior to arrival in OR. If < 1 yr old, no premedication is given.

INTRAOPERATIVE

Anesthetic technique: Combined epidural/GETA, using a pediatric circle or Bain circuit with humidified and warmed gases. Warm OR to 75°-80°F; heating pad on OR table.

Induction	Awake intubation if airway management problems anticipated; otherwise, standard pediatric induction (see p. D-2). Secure iv access and administer muscle relaxant (e.g., vecuronium or pancuronium [0.1 mg/kg]) to facilitate ET intubation. Maintain air leak at > 10-35 cmH_2O. Lumbar epidural catheter inserted after induction.
Maintenance	Volatile agent/air/O_2 with epdiural analgesia or morphine (0.1-0.25 mg/kg iv total) or fentanyl (5-10 μg/kg iv total). Maintain neuromuscular blockade as surgically indicated.
Emergence	Usually extubated at end of case. Reverse neuromuscular blockade with neostigmine (0.07 mg/kg iv) and atropine (0.02 mg/kg iv). Ability to flex hips is a sign of adequate reversal.

Blood and fluid requirements	Moderate blood/3rd-space losses IV: 20-22 ga × 2 NS/LR @ (maintenance): 4 ml/kg/h – 0-10 kg + 2 ml/kg/h – 10-20 kg	Place iv's in upper extremities, since positioning of legs may impede venous flow. Maintain Hct > 22. This age group does not require dextrose infusions. 3rd-space losses ~5 ml/kg/h.
Monitoring	Standard monitors (p. D-1) Urinary catheter ± 24 ga radial arterial line	Maintain UO @ 0.5-1.0 ml/kg/h. Marked arterial waveform variation with ventilation is a sensitive indicator of hypovolemia. ABG/Hct/glucose prn.
Positioning	✓ and pad pressure points. ✓ eyes.	Patient may be turned during procedure.
Complications	Metabolic acidosis Hypovolemia → ↓BP Hypothermia	Mild metabolic acidosis may occur with significant bleeding, or when 3rd-space losses are replaced with bicarbonate-deficient fluids (NS, albumin 5%, PRBCs).

POSTOPERATIVE

Complications	Subglottic edema Respiratory depression 2° to opiates

Pain management	Continuous epidural analgesia. Fentanyl (1-2 mg/kg iv q 1 h prn) or morphine (0.05-0.10 mg/kg iv q 1-4 h)	See p. E-2. Aggressive pain management warranted.
Tests	Hct, ABG, electrolytes	

References

1. DeVries PA, Pena A: Posterior sagittal anorectoplasty. *J Pediatr Surg* 1982; 17(5):638-45.
2. Paidas C, Pena A: Rectum and anus. In *Surgery of Infants and Children.* Oldham KT, Colombani PM, Foglia RP, eds. Lippincott-Raven Publishers, Philadelphia: 1997, 1323-64.
3. Schecter NL, Berde CB, Yaster M, eds: *Pain in Infants, Children, and Adolescents.* Williams and Wilkins, Baltimore: 1993, 357-83.
4. Smith EI, Tunell WP, Williams GR; A clinical evaluation of the surgical treatment of anorectal malformations (imperforate anus). *Ann Surg* 1978; 187(6):583-92.

MEDIASTINAL MASS—BIOPSY OR RESECTION

SURGICAL CONSIDERATIONS

Description: Mass lesions in the mediastinum may occur at any age, although congenital cystic lesions tend to occur in younger children, with malignant lesions occurring more often in preschool and school-age children. Preop diagnosis is usually quite accurate and is assisted by considering patient age and anatomic location within the mediastinum (anterior, middle or posterior compartments) (Fig 12.4-3). Neurogenic tumors, most often neuroblastoma, and cystic duplications of the esophagus are the common lesions in the posterior compartment. Many of these lesions present with unusual symptoms (e.g., Horner's syndrome, opsoclonus). Minimal extension of neuroblastomas into the neural foramina are common and rarely require direct surgical approach (e.g., **laminectomy**). Although neuroblastomas may reach an impressive size, they are usually resectable. Middle mediastinal masses in older children are commonly lymphoproliferative disorders and may present with respiratory symptoms or SVC compression. They have been associated with cardiorespiratory collapse with GA; hence, obtaining diagnostic tissue safely may be problematic. In younger children (< 2 yr average), middle mediastinal lesions frequently represent hemangioma or lymphangioma, which may extend to other compartments. Anterior mediastinal masses generally represent lesions of the thymus or malignant germ cell tumors or teratomas. The operative approach for most mediastinal tumors is via **posterolateral thoracotomy**, with occasional need for **median sternotomy**. With the availability of current diagnostic techniques, including CT-guided biopsy, the need for exploratory thoracotomy is unusual.

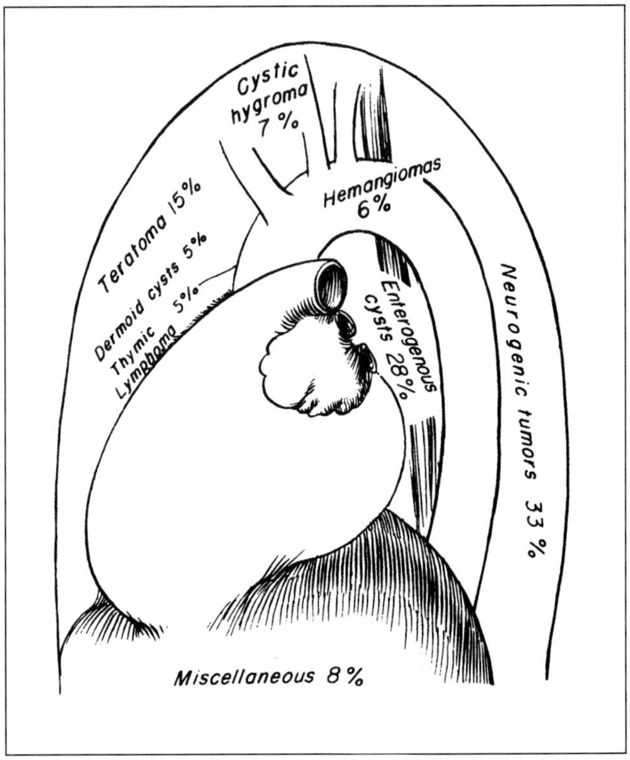

Figure 12.4-3. Distribution of mediastinal cysts and tumor. (Reprinted with permission from Ravitch MM, et al: *Pediatric Surgery.* Year Book Medical Publishers, Chicago: 1986.)

Most lesions can be approached through a right or left posterolateral thoracotomy. Neurogenic tumors are most common and can usually be completely excised, although blood loss may be significant if the chest wall is involved. Extension through a neural foramen usually can be delivered with the tumor. Middle and anterior lesions will require careful dissection around the pulmonary hilum and tracheobronchial tree. Median sternotomy may be required for anterior lesions, including the rare intrapericardial teratoma.

Usual preop diagnosis: Neuroblastoma; teratoma; duplication cyst of foregut; mediastinal mass (lymphoma)

SUMMARY OF PROCEDURE

	Lateral Thoracotomy	Median Sternotomy
Position	Lateral	Supine
Incision	Posterolateral	Median, parasternal
Special instrumentation	None	Bronchoscope; CPB
Unique considerations	Airway or cardiovascular collapse after induction in anterior mediastinal masses	⇐
Antibiotics	Preop: ampicillin 25 mg/kg iv + gentamicin 2.5 mg/kg iv; intraop: cephalosporin irrigation (1 g/500 ml NS)	⇐
Surgical time	2-4 h	1-4 h
Closing considerations	Lung inflation; intercostal block; epidural catheter	⇐
EBL	10-30 ml/kg	10-50 ml/kg
Postop care	Aggressive respiratory therapy; analgesia	⇐
Mortality	< 5%, except symptomatic anterior masses	⇐
Morbidity	Atelectasis/respiratory	⇐
	Cardiovascular collapse with anterior masses	⇐
Pain score	7-8	6-7

PATIENT POPULATION CHARACTERISTICS

Age range	Newborn–teens
Male:Female	1:1
Incidence	1/5000
Etiology	Unknown
Associated conditions	Cervical or axillary cystic hygroma; hemangioma; SVC syndrome

ANESTHETIC CONSIDERATIONS

PREOPERATIVE

The clinical presentation of a mediastinal mass is often nonspecific in an otherwise healthy child. Often, a routine CXR (for some incidental Sx) will show the presence of an anterior mediastinal mass. These patients may suffer acute cardiorespiratory compromise on induction of anesthesia. Hence, a careful preop workup is essential.

Respiratory Respiratory Sx (e.g., dyspnea, cough, stridor, wheezing) are extremely important in guiding additional studies. The ability to lie supine without respiratory embarrassment should be determined. Tracheal and bronchial compression from the tumor may be positional. Preop radiation therapy may ↓ tumor mass and relieve airway obstruction.

Tests: CXR; supine-sitting flow/volume loops (useful for evaluating location and extent of airway obstruction); ABG (or pulse oximetry), if symptomatic; chest CT/MRI

Cardiovascular Sx of a mediastinal mass may include SVC syndrome (e.g., venous engorgement of head and neck, edema of upper body). Other Sx may include syncope and headaches (↑ICP) made worse in the supine position. Papilledema should be sought.

Tests: ECHO; ECG, if symptomatic

Musculoskeletal If thymoma present, ✓ for Sx of myasthenia gravis.

Tests: Presence of acetylcholine-receptor antibodies

Laboratory Electrolytes; CBC; T&C for 2-4 U, depending on body weight and tumor size; other tests as indicated from H&P.

Premedication Avoid premedication in symptomatic patients.

INTRAOPERATIVE

Anesthetic technique: GETA, with warmed and humidified gases, OR temperature 70-75°. Heating pad on OR table.

Induction An iv is mandatory before induction. If SVC syndrome is present, it is important to have iv access in the lower extremity. Atropine (0.02 mg/kg iv) is given to dry secretions and prevent bradycardia from deep inhalation induction and laryngoscopy. An awake FOB and intubation in the sitting position may be necessary. Alternatively, a mask induction with sevoflurane or halothane/O_2 in the semi-Fowler's (reclining) position may be appropriate. Intubation should be performed with preservation of spontaneous ventilation. Have small ETTs available, in light of possible tracheal compression. Fiber optic bronchoscopy is useful to confirm ETT placement and to evaluate trachea/bronchi. Avoid muscle relaxants until the ETT is in place. Surgeon must be present with rigid ★ bronchoscope immediately available in the event of acute airway obstruction on induction. **NB:** A simple positional change (e.g., supine to lateral or sitting) may relieve cardiorespiratory collapse. Following induction, placement of a lumbar or thoracic epidural catheter is beneficial.

Maintenance Spontaneous ventilation/assisted ventilation with volatile agent and 100% O_2 may be appropriate. Supplemental epidural analgesia may be administered (p. D-3). Have surgeon infiltrate wound with bupivacaine 0.25% to reduce volatile anesthetic and opiate requirements.

Emergence Confirm air leak around ETT (with cuff deflated). Have all emergency airway equipment available and surgeon present. Patient should be fully awake before extubation.

Blood and fluid requirements	Usually minimal blood loss. IV: 18-24 ga × 2, depending on age NS/LR @ 10-20 ml/kg iv	If mediastinoscopy is performed, sudden blood loss from torn great vessel may occur. Volume-loading with NS/LR prior to induction may be appropriate because of myocardial depression and venodilation from deep inhalational induction.
Monitoring	Standard monitors (p. D-1) Arterial line	Pulse oximeter on ear lobe detects desaturation sooner than probes on extremities. Esophageal or precordial stethoscope earliest monitor of airway obstruction.
Positioning	✓ and pad pressure points. ✓ eyes.	If obstruction worsens acutely, be prepared to change to lateral decubitus position, which may alleviate tracheal, bronchial compression and cardiovascular collapse.
Complications	Respiratory failure Loss of airway Bronchospasm Laryngospasm Hypotension	Careful attention to ABCs (airway, breathing, circulation). Have all resuscitation drugs (e.g., epinephrine 10 μg/kg iv) drawn up.

POSTOPERATIVE

Complications	Respiratory failure Pneumothorax	Anesthesiologist must be readily available in the PACU to manage acute airway problems.
Pain management	Ketorolac 0.9 mg/kg (up to 30 mg) iv q 6° × 24 h Epidural analgesia PCA (p. E-3)	Cervical biopsy/mediastinoscopy have minimal postop pain and can be effectively treated with NSAID and local anesthetic infiltration.
Tests	Hct, ABG, CXR, as clinically indicated.	

References

1. Ferrari LR, Bedford RF: General anesthesia prior to treatment of anterior mediastinal masses in pediatric cancer patients. *Anesthesiology* 1990; 72(6):991-95.
2. Neuman GB, Weingarten AE, Abramowitz RM, Kushins LG, Abramson AL, Ladner W: The anesthetic management of the patient with an anterior mediastinal mass. *Anesthesiology* 1984; 60(2):144-47.
3. Rodgers BM, McGahren ED III: Mediastinum and pleura. In *Surgery of Infants and Children.* Oldham KT, Colombani PM, Foglia RP, eds. Lippincott-Raven Publishers, Philadelphia: 1997, 915-34.
4. Watcha MF, et al: Comparison of ketorolac and morphine as adjuvants during pediatric surgery. *Anesthesiology* 1991; 76(3):368-72.

Surgeons

Steven P. LaPointe, MD
Linda D. Shortliffe, MD

12.5 PEDIATRIC UROLOGY

Anesthesiologists

Gregory B. Hammer, MD
Cathy R. Lammers, MD

KIDNEY AND UPPER URINARY TRACT OPERATIONS

SURGICAL CONSIDERATIONS

Description: With the increase in perinatal ultrasonographic detection of renal masses and hydronephrosis, the number of pediatric kidney and upper urinary tract surgeries has increased significantly in the past two decades, and children come to surgery at an earlier age to preserve maximal renal function.

Nephrectomy: While the main indications for nephrectomy in the adult population are renal-cell carcinoma or benign renal tumors (e.g., angiomyolipoma, oncocytoma), most nephrectomies in children are performed for congenital anomalies associated with nonfunctioning or infected kidneys. A nonfunctioning kidney can be related to obstruction, or end-stage reflux nephropathy. Multicystic dysplastic kidneys (MCDK) do not require surgery unless they cause symptoms or increase in size. Typically, a nephrectomy is performed using a dorsal lumbotomy approach with the child in the prone position. A transverse skin incision is made parallel to Langers lines (skin crease lines) and a vertical dorsal incision is made parallel to the paraspinous muscles. The retroperitoneum is entered using a muscle-splitting technique with incision of the lumbodorsal fascia. After renal dissection, the vessels are ligated and the kidney is removed. At times a flank incision may be preferred for better exposure of the vessels. The patient is placed in the lateral decubitus position with the affected kidney up, and a transverse incision is made below the 12th rib. The peritoneum is reflected, the upper ureter is dissected to the hilum, and the vessels are ligated. The kidney is excised and the wound is closed. The lumbodorsal approach avoids muscle splitting and is associated with decreased postop pain.

Usual preop diagnosis: MCDK; congenital mesoblastic nephroma; nonfunctioning kidney; dysplastic kidney; ureteropelvic junction (UPJ) obstruction, ureterocele and loss of function

Partial nephrectomy: Partial nephrectomies in children are usually performed for a nonfunctioning upper pole of a duplicated system. Ectopic ureters and ureteroceles are frequently the cause of loss of function. Again, these can be approached from either a dorsal lumbotomy or flank incision. If the upper pole is obstructed and functional, a pyeloureterostomy from the upper pole ureter to the pelvis of the lower pole may be performed in order to salvage as much functioning parenchyma as possible. A partial nephrectomy may be performed for bilateral Wilms' tumor or other renal masses through a chevron or midline incision.

Usual preop diagnosis: Nonfunctioning upper pole of a duplex system; ureterocele; ectopic ureter

Nephroureterectomy: Nephroureterectomy is often performed for the obstructed upper pole of a duplex system 2° a ureterocele or ectopic ureter. After the nephrectomy/partial nephrectomy is performed through a dorsal lumbotomy or flank approach, the ureter is dissected as low as possible (usually to the level of the iliac vessels). The ureteral stump is left open if there is no vesicoureteral reflux and tied off if there is reflux. If indicated, distal ureterectomy can be performed via a second lower abdominal incision.

Usual preop diagnosis: Nonfunctioning upper pole of a duplex system; ureterocele; ectopic ureter

Pyeloplasty: Fetal hydronephrosis is detected in approximately 1/300 pregnancies. Pyeloplasty to correct congenital obstruction of the UPJ is a common infant surgical procedure. The hydronephrotic kidney is usually exposed through either a dorsal lumbotomy (incision parallel to the paraspinous muscle group) or a subcostal flank incision. Gerota's fascia is entered and the kidney is mobilized to expose the upper ureter and renal pelvis. The abnormal UPJ is usually excised, followed by an end-to-end anastomosis (**dismembered pyeloplasty** or **Anderson-Hynes pyeloplasty**). A perirenal Penrose drain is usually placed, and a ureteral stent or nephrostomy tubes may be used.

Usual preop diagnosis: Fetal hydronephrosis 2° UPJ obstruction; hydronephrosis

Transureteroureterostomy (TUU): This procedure, in which a ureter is anastomosed to the contralateral ureter, is used when there is problematic drainage of the distal ureter into the bladder. It is sometimes required to salvage a failed reimplantation or to transform a conduit-type diversion to an orthotopic neobladder or augmented native bladder. This technique also can be used to provide drainage in ureteral trauma. A midline, or Pfannenstiel's, incision is used; and the peritoneum is entered. The ureters are dissected and the affected ureter is retroperitonealized and brought to the contralateral side anterior to the great vessels. It is anastomosed to the contralateral ureter end-to-side with absorbable suture. If required, the recipient ureter is then reimplanted into the neobladder or augmented bladder. (See **urinary diversion**, p. 654).

Usual preop diagnosis: Failed ureteral reimplant; undiversion; distal ureteral trauma

SUMMARY OF PROCEDURE

	Nephrectomy/pyeloplasty	Nephroureterectomy	TUU
Position	Flank/prone	Supine/flank	Supine
Incision	Dorsal lumbotomy; subcostal; flank; midline	Subcostal flank 2nd incision: Pfannenstiel's	Midline or Pfannenstiel's
Antibiotics	Gentamicin 1.7 mg/kg iv	⇐	⇐
Surgical time	2.5 h	3 h	3 h
EBL	Minimal; if partial nephrectomy, 300 ml	Minimal	⇐
Mortality	< 1%	⇐	⇐
Morbidity	Bleeding: < 5%	⇐	⇐
	Infection: < 5%	⇐	⇐
	Ileus: < 5%	⇐	⇐
			Urinary fistula : < 5%
Pain score	Flank: 10 Lumbotomy: 5	10	10

PATIENT POPULATION CHARACTERISTICS

	Ureteroceles	MCDK	UPJ Obstruction	Nephroma
Age range	Pediatric	Neonates	Neonates, children	⇐
Male:Female	1:4	–	M > F	–
Incidence	1:2000	–	1:500 birth	–
Etiology	Congenital	⇐	⇐	⇐
Associated conditions	UPJ; VUR; duplicated collecting system	⇐	VUR; renal insufficiency	–

References

1. Kelalis PP, Maizels M, Das S, Kay R, Williams DI: Kidney Reconstruction. In *Atlas of Pediatric Urologic Surgery.* Hinman F Jr, ed. WB Saunders, Philadelphia: 1994, Part II, 112-17, 123-43.
2. Marshall FF, Massad C, Hensle TW, Parrott TS: Kidney Excision. In *Atlas of Pediatric Urologic Surgery.* Hinman F Jr, ed. WB Saunders, Philadelphia: 1994, Part III, 155-88.
3. Ritchey ML, Andrassy RJ, Kelalis PP: Pediatric urologic oncology. In *Adult and Pediatric Urology,* 3rd edition. Gillenwater JY, Grayhack JT, Howards SS, Duckett JW, eds. Mosby-Year Book: 1996, Vol 3, 2682-93.
4. Snyder HM, D'Angio GJ, Evans AE, Raney RB: Pediatric oncology. In *Campbell's Urology, 6th edition.* Walsh PC, Retik AB, Stamey TA, Vaughn ED Jr. eds. WB Saunders, Philadelphia: 1992, Vol 2, 1967-2014.

ANESTHETIC CONSIDERATIONS

PREOPERATIVE

In infants and children, most upper urinary tract surgical procedures are performed to preserve or restore renal function. Patients may present with renal function that varies from minimally abnormal, requiring little or no modification of anesthetic plan, to end-stage renal failure (ESRD) with its associated abnormalities, including hypoproteinemia, chronic anemia and serum electrolyte disturbances. A careful preop workup is required to determine the presence or absence of abnormal physiologic factors that will affect anesthesia management. For most cases, the workup will have been performed by the patient's physicians before surgery and will provide the rationale for the surgical procedure. Such nonspecific findings as anorexia, headache, nausea, excessive tiredness, as well as alterations in UO and the presence of edema will alert the clinician to the likelihood of renal failure.

Renal abnormalities are often present as one component of a congenital malformation syndrome (e.g., polycystic kidneys, cerebrohepatorenal syndrome). In formulating the anesthetic plan, drugs eliminated by the kidney (e.g., pancuronium, meperidine, etc.) should be avoided.

Respiratory An evaluation of pulmonary function, including auscultation of the lungs, may indicate the presence of pulmonary edema (uremic lung) or a pleural effusion.

Respiratory, cont. **Tests:** ABG; CXR; pulse oximetry

Cardiovascular HTN is commonly seen in these patients, who may be taking antihypertensive medications and diuretics. In the severe cases, CHF or pulmonary edema may be present, necessitating the use of cardioactive drugs and diuretics to optimize the patient's clinical condition before surgery.
Tests: ABG; CXR; digitalis level; electrolytes

Renal In cases requiring unilateral urinary tract surgery, the opposite kidney is usually normal. In the presence of renal insufficiency, a detailed evaluation of renal function is essential. Chronic metabolic acidosis may be present 2° poor kidney function, electrolyte abnormalities (↑K^+, ↓Ca^{++}, ↑ or ↓Na^+), hypovolemia and/or poor tissue perfusion. Children with ESRD will have been dialyzed before surgery. Preop $K^+ < 6$ mEq/L is usually safe. These patients may have an AV fistula which must be protected during surgery (padded, no BP cuff).
Tests: UA; UO; serum electrolytes; BUN; creatinine; total protein; A/G ratio; ABG

Hematologic Anemic, bone marrow depression and coagulopathies are common in patients with poor renal function. An Hct of 15 -18 kg/dL is not uncommon.
Tests: Hb/Hct, PT/PTT; Plt count

Medications Patients with ESRD will be taking many medications, which may influence the anesthetic plan. For example, chronic steroid therapy → Cushing facies, glycosuria; therefore, ✓ blood sugar and ✓ airway (if difficult, mask ventilation). Patients taking digitalis or diuretics → ↓K^+ → arrhythmias. Gentamicin → prolongation of neuromuscular blockade.

Premedication Standard preop medication is administered at 30-50% of the usual dose (see p. D-2.)

INTRAOPERATIVE

Anesthetic technique: GETA ± epidural. Warm OR to 75-80° F; use warming pad on OR table.

Induction Mask induction is preferable, unless iv is already in place. Succinylcholine should not be used if $K^+ > 5.5$ mEq/L. In the presence of renal insufficiency, antibiotics (e.g., gentamicin) may interfere with the metabolism of muscle relaxants and prolong their effect. Tracheal intubation facilitated by a nondepolarizing relaxant (e.g., cisatracurium 0.2-0.3 mg/kg). In appropriate patients (normal coags) epidural anesthesia with bupivacaine (see p. D-5) will reduce inhalation anesthetic ★ requirements and provide postop analgesia (**NB:** local anesthetic clearance may be impaired). Maintain muscle relaxation with cisatracurium or vecuronium.

Maintenance Standard pediatric maintenance (see p. D-3). Moderate hyperventilation may be beneficial (→ ↓K^+ + ↑pH).

Emergence Reverse neuromuscular blockade with neostigmine and atropine or glycopyrrolate.

Blood and fluid requirements	IV × 1 in upper extremities NS @ (maintenance): 4 ml/kg/h (1-10 kg) + 2 ml/kg/h (11-20 kg) + 1 ml/kg/h (over 20 kg)	Usually minimal blood loss; however, renal surgery may be associated with ↑blood loss. Transfuse with whole blood or PRBC as needed to maintain an adequate Hct (25-30%).
Monitoring	Standard monitors (see p. D-1). ± Arterial line	Place arterial line in patients with significant renal failure; ✓ serum electrolytes and ABG frequently.
Positioning	✓ and pad pressure points. ✓ eyes.	✓ eyes frequently if prone or flank positions are used.
Complications	Peripheral nerve injury Eye trauma Hemorrhage	

POSTOPERATIVE

Complications
Hypovolemia
Anemia
Hypothermia
Electrolyte abnormalities
Coagulopathy
Metabolic/respiratory acidosis

Pain management	Acetaminophen (see p. E-1). Narcotics by epidural catheter or PCA (see p. E-3).	In renal failure, reduce analgesic doses by 50% to minimize cumulative effects.
Tests	As indicated.	

References

1. Berry F: Anesthesia for genitourinary surgery. In *Pediatric Anesthesia,* 3rd edition. Gregory GA, ed. Churchill Livingstone, New York: 1994.
2. Davis PJ, Hall S. Deshpande JK, Spear RM: Anesthesia for general, urologic and plastic surgery. In *Smith's Anesthesia for Infants and Children,* 6th edition. Motoyama EK, Davis P, eds. Mosby-Year Book, St. Louis: 1996.

TRANSURETHRAL PROCEDURES

SURGICAL CONSIDERATIONS

Description: Transurethral procedures are not as common in pediatric urology as they are in adult urology; however, the instrumentation, general principles and considerations are similar. The following are the most common pediatric endoscopic procedures: **cystoscopy** and **vaginoscopy,** primarily as a diagnostic procedure; transurethral **posterior urethral valve ablation (PUV)**; transurethral **incision of ureterocele**; **extraction of foreign objects**; **incision and dilatation** of strictures; and **collagen injection** therapy for **vesicoureteral reflux** and **urinary incontinence.**

The positioning and techniques are identical to those in the adult. Patients are placed in the lithotomy position, and a lubricated cystoscope or resectoscope (7-18 Fr) is introduced through the urethra. The patient can remain supine if a flexible cystoscope is used. Cystoscopy is used to identify any pathology, and ureteral catheterization can be performed with a 3-5 Fr ureteral catheter. In infants, posterior urethral valves may be resected using a small cutting electrode, while a resectoscope is used in older children. With the advent of prenatal ultrasonography, posterior urethral valves (→ hydronephrosis and azotemia) may be diagnosed before birth. Unless the infant is premature or medically unstable, posterior urethral valves are often resected in the neonatal period. Foreign bodies or stones are removed using forceps after crushing or pulverization with a lithotrite if necessary.

Usual preop diagnosis: Intravesical foreign body; bladder calculus; bladder outlet obstruction; urethral stricture; ureterocele; hematuria; urethral/vaginal mass; posterior urethral valves

SUMMARY OF PROCEDURE

Position	Lithotomy
Incision	None
Special instrumentation	Cystoscope, resectoscope, catheters, stents, video camera unit, laser (optional)
Unique considerations	Use of cautery, fluoroscopy, PUV (prematurity or azotemia)
Antibiotics	If infected urine preop, gentamicin 1.7 mg/kg iv
Surgical time	Cystoscopy: 10 min Transurethral procedure: 1 h
EBL	Minimal
Postop care	PACU; basic catheter management
Mortality	< 1%
Morbidity	Bleeding Infection
Pain score	2

PATIENT POPULATION CHARACTERISTICS

Age range	0-18 yr
Male:Female	Posterior urethral valves, strictures: male only Ureterocele 1:6 Vesicoureteral reflux 1:4
Incidence	1/1000–1/5000
Etiology	Posterior urethral valves; vesicoureteral reflux; intravesical foreign body; bladder calculus; bladder outlet obstruction; urethral stricture; ureterocele
Associated conditions	Spina bifida; paraplegia/quadriplegia; repeat cystoscopies; strictures; bladder stones; latex allergy

ANESTHETIC CONSIDERATIONS

See Anesthetic Considerations for Transurethral Procedures, Open Bladder Procedures, Penile Surgery, Genital Procedures, p. 981.

Reference

1. Farber GJ, Bloom DA: Pediatric endourology. In *Adult and Pediatric Urology,* 3rd edition. Gillenwater JY, Grayhack JT, Howards SS, Duckett JW, eds. Mosby-Year Book, Inc., St. Louis: 1996, Vol 3, 2739-47.

OPEN BLADDER OPERATIONS

SURGICAL CONSIDERATIONS

Description: Open bladder operations commonly performed on children include **ureteral reimplantation** for correction of vesicoureteral reflux, obstructive megaureters or ureterocele, **vesicostomy (Blocksom)** and **bladder neck operations.**

Ureteral reimplantation: Vesicoureteral reflux (VUR) is one of the most common abnormalities of the urinary tract in children and is present in approximately 25-50% of children who have UTI. While VUR resolves spontaneously in many children, there are a number of indications for correction of VUR. These include: 1) high-grade VUR, 2) progressive VUR and renal scarring, 3) failure to resolve within several years, 4) other bladder surgery, 5) breakthrough UTIs, and 6) poor medical compliance.

Ureteral reimplantations can be performed using different approaches to the bladder (e.g., extravesical, intravesical or a combined approach); however, these different approaches require a similar exposure and abdominal incision. A lower abdominal (Pfannenstiel's) incision is performed, the fascia is opened vertically through the linea alba and the bladder is exposed. The bladder is then opened (intravesical approach) and the ureter(s) is (are) reimplanted, or the bladder is mobilized to expose the posterolateral ureter, which is then reimplanted (extravesical approach). When required, ureteral stents are brought to the abdominal skin through the bladder wall. An initial cystoscopy may be performed to plan a potentially complex reimplantation (e.g., duplex systems, ectopia or periureteral diverticula).

Obstructive megaureters and ureteroceles are other conditions that may require ureteral reimplantation. The abdominal exposure and indications do not differ significantly from ureteral reimplantation for VUR; however, tailoring of the ureter, by reducing its caliber and excising redundant tissue or plicating it, may be necessary. A procedure on the bladder neck also may be required if a ureterocele extends distally through the bladder outlet.

Usual preop diagnosis: VUR; obstructive megaureter; ureterocele

Vesicostomy: Infants and very young children may require bladder drainage until definitive bladder or urethral surgery. A vesicostomy may be performed, allowing the urine to flow continuously from a small lower abdominal vesicocutaneous fistula. A 2 cm transverse incision is made halfway between the umbilicus and the pubis and the bladder is dissected extraperitoneally to expose the dome. The bladder is opened at the dome (urachus) and is anastomosed to abdominal skin with absorbable sutures, creating a small (24 Fr) fistula.

Usual preop diagnosis: Posterior or anterior urethral valves; severe VUR; neurovesical dysfunction; prune-belly syndrome

Bladder neck operations: These procedures are usually required in patients with severe anomalies, such as exstrophy, or severe incontinence due to an incompetent bladder neck. These are more complex procedures, with dissection often difficult. The approach to the bladder is similar to ureteral reimplantation, using a lower abdominal (Pfannenstiel's) incision. The Retzius space is bluntly dissected and the anterior bladder wall and pubic bone exposed. The bladder is opened and the bladder neck dissected and reconstructed. Various techniques to tubularize the anterior bladder wall, elongate the urethra and increase the outlet resistance have been described. Bilateral ureteral reimplantation and bladder neck suspension can be performed at the same time. One special consideration is latex allergy (see Appendix G).

Usual preop diagnosis: Exstrophy/epispadias complex; spina bifida; neurogenic bladder; incontinence; bladder-neck reconstruction

SUMMARY OF PROCEDURE

	Reimplantation	Vesicostomy	Bladder Neck
Position	Supine	⇐	⇐
Incision	Pfannenstiel's or low midline extraperitoneal	⇐	⇐
Unique considerations	None	⇐	Latex allergy (see Appendix G)
Antibiotics	None unless indicated	⇐	Gentamicin 1.7 mg/kg iv slowly
Surgical time	1.5 h	45 min	2 h
EBL	Minimal	⇐	200 ml
Postop care	PACU; urethral catheter ± stents	PACU	Urethral catheter 4-7 d; PACU → ward
Mortality	< 1%	⇐	⇐
Morbidity	Infection: < 3%	⇐	⇐
	Bleeding: < 3%	⇐	< 5%
	Urinary retention:		Urinary retention
	Unilateral: < 5%		
	Bilateral: 8-10%		
	Ureteral obstruction		Ureteral obstruction
	Persistent reflux		
Pain score	7	4	7

PATIENT POPULATION CHARACTERISTICS

Age range	1 mo–teenage	⇐	⇐
Male:Female	1:4	1:1	⇐
Incidence	1%	–	–
Etiology	Unknown	Congenital	⇐
Associated conditions	UTI; renal failure	⇐	⇐

ANESTHETIC CONSIDERATIONS

See Anesthetic Considerations for Transurethral Procedures, Open Bladder Procedures, Penile Surgery, Genital Procedures, p. 981.

References

1. Canning DA, Koo HP, Duckett JW: Anomalies of the bladder and cloaca. In *Adult and Pediatric Urology,* 3rd edition. Gillenwater JY, Grayhack JT, Howards SS, Duckett JW, eds. Mosby-Year Book, Inc., St. Louis: 1996, Vol 3, 2445-88.
2. Dixon Walker R: Vesicoureteral reflux and urinary tract infection in children. In *Adult and Pediatric Urology,* 3rd edition. Gillenwater JY, Grayhack JT, Howards SS, Duckett JW, eds. Mosby-Year Book, Inc., St. Louis: 1996, Vol 3, 2459-95.
3. King LR: Vesicoureteral reflux, megaureter, and ureteral reimplantation. In *Campbell's Urology,* 6th edition. Walsh PC, Retik AB, Stamey TA, Vaughn ED Jr, eds. WB Saunders Co, Philadelphia: 1992, Vol 2, 1689-1742.
4. Smith GHH, Duckett JW: Urethral lesions in infants and children. In *Adult and Pediatric Urology,* 3rd edition. Gillenwater JY, Grayhack JT, Howards SS, Duckett JW, eds. Mosby-Year Book, Inc., St. Louis: 1996, Vol 3, 2411-43.

PENILE SURGERY

SURGICAL CONSIDERATIONS

Description: Pediatric penile operations usually correct congenital urethral abnormalities or involve circumcision. The most common surgical operation performed in the United States, circumcision consists of the excision of the preputial skin to expose the glans. It can be performed for either religious, ethnic, social or medical reasons (e.g., phimosis or recurrent balanitis).

Circumcision: Freehand circumcision involves excising preputial skin using two incisions to remove a sleeve of penile skin to fully expose the glans. At times, various clamps (Gomco, Mogen, etc.) can be used to circumcise.

Hypospadias is the abnormal opening of the urethral meatus resulting from incomplete development of the urethra. The defect can be located anywhere from the corona of the glans to the perineum; accordingly, surgical correction can require minimal dissection, as in the **meatal advancement granuloplasty (MAGPI)** procedure. More proximal defects, however, may require extensive dissection. Preputial or meatal skin flaps are used to reconstruct the defect. Removal of excess preputial skin is usually part of the hypospadias repair. Chordee is a curvature of the penis due to fibrous tissue. If present, it may require additional surgery on the penis, such as a **Nesbitt plication** or **tunica albuginea plication (TAP).** An artificial erection is obtained by infusion of NS through a 25 ga butterfly needle. The curvature is corrected by incising and plicating the tunica albuginea of the penis with absorbable suture. Stenting of the repair is usually reserved for complicated cases. In very complex redo cases, bladder or buccal mucosa may be needed to create a new urethra. Whether a urethral catheter is placed depends on the extent of the repair. Many distal hypospadias repairs do not require a urethral catheter; in any case, postop urethral instrumentation should be avoided because postop catheterization of the newly formed urethra could cause disruption of the repair.

Usual preop diagnosis: Phimosis; circumcision; hypospadias ± chordee; fistula repair; epispadias repair; penile torsion; concealed penis

SUMMARY OF PROCEDURE

	Circumcision	Hypospadias
Position	Supine	⇐
Incision	Circumferential penile	⇐ + ventral penis
Special instrumentation	None	Optical magnification
Unique considerations	1% lidocaine + 1:100,000; epinephrine may be used	⇐
Antibiotics	None	⇐
Surgical time	30 min	1.5-4 h
EBL	Minimal	150 ml
Postop care	Outpatient	Outpatient or ward ± urethral catheter
Mortality	< 1%	⇐

	Circumcision	Hypospadias
Morbidity	Infection: 2%	⇐
	Hematoma: 2%	⇐
		Urethrocutaneous fistula: 5-20%
Pain score	2	5

PATIENT POPULATION CHARACTERISTICS

Age range	Children	> 4 mo
Incidence	61%	1:300
Etiology	Acquired	Congenital
Associated conditions	Infectious	Cryptorchidism; inguinal hernia; bifid scrotum

ANESTHETIC CONSIDERATIONS

See Anesthetic Considerations for Transurethral Procedures, Open Bladder Procedures, Penile Surgery, Genital Procedures, p. 981.

References

1. Cendron M, Elder JS, Duckett JW: Perinatal Urology. In *Adult and Pediatric Urology,* 3rd edition. Gillenwater JY, Grayhack JT, Howards SS, Duckett JW, eds. Mosby-Year Book, Inc., St. Louis: 1996, Vol 3, 2149-52.
2. Duckett JW: Hypospadias. In *Campbell's Urology,* 6th edition. Walsh PC, Retik AB, Stamey TA, Vaughn ED Jr, eds. WB Saunders Co, Philadelphia: 1992, Vol 2, 1893-1919.
3. Duckett JW, Baskins LS: Hypospadias. In *Adult and Pediatric Urology,* 3rd edition. Gillenwater JY, Grayhack JT, Howards SS, Duckett JW, eds. Mosby-Year Book, Inc., St. Louis: 1996, Vol 3, 2549-89.
4. Elder JS: Congenital anomalies of the genitalia. In *Campbell's Urology,* 6th edition. Walsh PC, Retik AB, Stamey TA, Vaughn ED Jr, eds. WB Saunders Co, Philadelphia: 1992, Vol 2, 1920-38.

GENITAL PROCEDURES

(CLITOROPLASTY, VAGINOPLASTY, URETHROPLASTY)

SURGICAL CONSIDERATIONS

Description: Masses of the introitus include urethral prolapse, prolapsed ectopic ureterocele and rhabdomyosarcoma. Genitoplasty is usually performed in female patients with abnormal genitalia, e.g., ambiguous genitalia resulting from abnormal steroidogenesis (congenital adrenal hyperplasia [CAH], danazol exposure) and urogenital sinus or cloacal anomalies.

Urethral prolapse: With the patient in a lithotomy position, a simple circumferential incision is made at the junction between the prolapsed mucosa and the urethral meatus. The prolapsed tissue is excised, and anastomosis is performed with absorbable suture. Introital rhabdomyosarcoma often requires open or transurethral biopsy of the mass, and is usually treated with chemotherapy.

Vaginoplasty/clitoroplasty: These procedures are performed in patients with ambiguous genitalia, and are usually associated with hormonal imbalance (CAH). The initial procedure usually requires reduction of the enlarged clitoris and reconstruction of the labioscrotal folds. With the patient in a lithotomy position, skin incisions are made to allow partial resection of the corporal bodies and glans with nerve sparing. Periclitoral skin flaps are used to reconstruct the clitoris and labial folds. Vaginoplasty is performed through a perineal approach by creating a urethrovaginal septum. The vagina usually can be pulled into its normal position between the urethra and rectum, and anastomosed to perineal skin flaps using absorbable sutures. Vaginoplasty can be performed with clitoroplasty in an infant. If performed later in life (puberty), a vaginoplasty with complex flaps and bowel interposition is necessary. In the latter case, an abdominoperineal approach is required. A loop of sigmoid colon or ileum is isolated, along with its mesentery, and is brought through the perineal incision. It is then anastomosed proximally to the vagina and distally to skin flaps. Also, these procedures may be used for gender reassignment if masculinization of the ambiguous genitalia in a genotypic male is not possible.

Usual preop diagnosis: Ambiguous genitalia; CAH; cloacal exstrophy; urogenital sinus persistence; danazol exposure

SUMMARY OF PROCEDURE

Position	Lithotomy
Incision	Perineal
Special instrumentation	Loupes
Unique considerations	Steroid replacement may be necessary (CAH)
Antibiotics	Gentamicin 1.7 mg/kg iv (children)
Surgical time	2-4 h
EBL	10-15 ml
Postop care	± urethral catheter
Mortality	< 1%
Morbidity	Infection: < 5% Bleeding: < 5% Flap necrosis: < 5%
Pain score	6

PATIENT POPULATION CHARACTERISTICS

Age range	Clitoroplasty: 3-6 mo; vaginoplasty: puberty
Incidence	1:30,000 births (ambiguous genitalia)
Etiology	Congenital
Associated conditions	Hypothalamic-pituitary axis suppression; adrenal hyperplasia; steroid replacement therapy

References

1. Blyth B, Churchill BM: Intersex. In *Adult and Pediatric Urology,* 3rd edition. Gillenwater JY, Grayhack JT, Howards SS, Duckett JW, eds. Mosby-Year Book, Inc., St. Louis: 1996, Vol 3, 2591-2621.
2. Perlmutter AD, Reitelman C: Surgical management of intersexuality. In *Campbell's Urology,* 6th edition. Walsh PC, Retik AB, Stamey TA, Vaughn ED Jr. eds. WB Saunders Co, Philadelphia: 1992, Vol 2, 1951-66.

ANESTHETIC CONSIDERATIONS FOR TRANSURETHRAL PROCEDURES, OPEN BLADDER PROCEDURES, PENILE SURGERY, GENITAL PROCEDURES

PREOPERATIVE

Typically, infants and children presenting for these procedures are otherwise healthy, with some notable exceptions. **Vesicoureteral reflux** may be associated with renal dysplasia and HTN. The **prune-belly (Eagle-Barrett) syndrome** includes dystrophic abdominal musculature, requiring an evaluation of pulmonary function. **Bladder and cloacal exstrophy** may be accompanied by a spinal cord abnormality (e.g., tethered cord, spina bifida).

Pediatric urology patients with lower urinary tract dysfunction and underlying neurologic disorders (e.g., myelomeningocele) and exstrophy are at risk for developing latex allergy as a result of repeated urethral catheterizations or surgical procedures. (See Special Considerations for Latex Allergy, Appendix G.)

Circumcision and hypospadias repair are most commonly performed in the first 2 yr of life in otherwise healthy children.

Respiratory Prune-belly syndrome: pulmonary function may be decreased. These patients are at risk for pulmonary aspiration; therefore, precautions to avoid aspiration of gastric contents should be carried out (e.g., Bicitra, ranitidine, cricoid pressure). ✓ Hx for evidence of recurrent pulmonary disease.
Tests: CXR, others as indicated from H&P.

Renal Renal anomalies may be present as part of a congenital malformation complex.
Tests: As indicated from H&P.

Endocrine Surgery for genital disorders are usually performed to reshape anatomic abnormalities 2° congenital endocrine disorders. Ambiguous genitalia are associated with congenital adrenal abnormalities. They are usually detected in the first month of life and may lead to severe salt-losing crises with ↓Na^+ and ↑K^+. The electrolyte status of these patients must be evaluated in the preop period. Treatment consists of steroid replacement.
Tests: Electrolytes; blood sugar

Premedication Preop medication is usually administered if the child is > 12 mo; midazolam po or iv (see p. D-2).

INTRAOPERATIVE

Anesthetic technique: GA (ETT or LMA) using a pediatric circle with humidified and warmed gases. A combined technique with epidural or caudal anesthesia is often used. For small children, warm OR to 70-75°F. Use warming pad on OR table.

Induction For patients < 10 yr, standard mask induction with sevoflurane or halothane/N_2O/O_2. Older patients may agree to standard iv induction (see p. D-2). For open-bladder and complex genital procedures, an indwelling epidural catheter for intraop and postop pain relief is recommended.

Maintenance Standard pediatric maintenance (see p. D-3). With epidural anesthesia, amount of volatile and/or narcotic anesthetic requirements are diminished.

Emergence Typically, no special considerations. Carefully evaluate patient for adequate ventilation prior to extubation in those with prune-belly syndrome.

Blood and fluid requirements	Minimal blood loss IV: 22 or 24 ga × 1 NS/LR @ (maintenance): 4 ml/kg/h 1-10 kg + 2 ml/kg/h 11-20 kg	Complex cases may be associated with significant blood loss. Transfuse with whole blood or PRBC.
Monitoring	Standard monitors (see p. D-1). ± Arterial line	Place arterial line for measurement of arterial gases, Hct and blood glucose if significant blood loss or long case is anticipated.
Positioning	✓ and pad pressure points. ✓ eyes.	With too-large mask, beware ocular compression/corneal abrasion.
Complications	Nerve damage	In lower extremities, if padding is insufficient with lithotomy position

POSTOPERATIVE

Complications	Prune belly: hypoventilation Adrenogenital syndrome: adrenal insufficiency	Assisted ventilation may be required.
Pain management	Acetaminophen Epidural or PCA analgesia.	See p. E-1.

References

1. Berry F: Anesthesia for genitourinary surgery. In *Pediatric Anesthesia,* 3rd edition. Churchill Livingstone, New York: 1994.
2. Davis PJ, Hall S, Deshpande JK, Spear RM: Anesthesia for general, urologic and plastic surgery. In *Smith's Anesthesia for Infants and Children,* 6th edition. Motoyama EK, Davis PJ, eds. Mosby-Year Book, Inc., St. Louis: 1990.
3. Sheldon CA, Snyder HM III: Principles of urinary tract reconstruction. In *Adult and Pediatric Urology*, 3rd edition. Gillenwater JY, Grayhack JT, Howards SS, Duckett JW, eds. Mosby-Year Book, St. Louis: 1996, Vol 1, 249-50, 2394-95.

INGUINOSCROTAL PROCEDURES

SURGICAL CONSIDERATIONS

Description: Undescended testis (cryptorchidism), hydrocele and inguinal hernia are common in pediatric urology, and surgery is usually performed on an outpatient basis. Testicular torsion is one of the few true pediatric urologic emergencies because testicular infarction will occur within hours of the torsion. Testicular tumors in children, accounting for 1-2% of all pediatric solid tumors, are more frequently benign than those in adults, and represent the main indication for **radical or simple orchiectomy.**

Orchiopexy: Orchiopexy for undescended testis is performed through a small inguinal incision. The external oblique fascia is opened, exposing the inguinal canal. The testis is localized and the cord is dissected to gain adequate length for scrotal fixation, without torsion or tension, to prevent postop ischemia and atrophy. If the testicle is high and adequate inguinal mobilization is not possible, dissection into the retroperitoneum may be required. The scrotal pouch is created by skin incision two-thirds the way down to the scrotum and blunt dissection between the skin and dartos muscle. The testis is fixed with suture material. An initially nonpalpable testis may become palpable with anesthetic relaxation.

Testicular torsion is a pediatric urologic emergency. There is no definitive diagnostic imaging study, although Doppler and isotope scans of the testis can be useful. At times, Sx of testicular torsion may be indistinguishable from epididymitis or torsion of the testicular appendages (embryonic remnants). The testis is delivered through a scrotal incision, examined, detorsed, and viability assessed. If the testis is nonviable, a simple orchiectomy is performed. If the testicle is viable, it is fixed in a scrotal dartos pouch. The contralateral testis is fixed in a similar fashion. A torsion of a testicular appendage is usually treated medically, with pain control and anti-inflammatory agents. If this condition is discovered at surgical exploration, the diseased tissue is excised, the testis is simply reinserted in the scrotum and the wound is closed.

Usual preop diagnosis: Cryptorchidism; nonpalpable testis; testicular torsion; torsion of the testicular appendage

Hydrocelectomy–inguinal hernia repair: This procedure is performed through an inguinal incision and dissection of the inguinal canal. The patent processus vaginalis is carefully dissected from the cord structures; the peritoneal sac is ligated at the level of the internal inguinal ring; and the wound is closed after evacuation of the hydrocele liquid.

Usual preop diagnosis: Hydrocele; inguinal hernia

Radical orchiectomy: While simple orchiectomy is performed through a scrotal incision, radical orchiectomy (used when testicular cancer is suspected) is performed through an inguinal incision. The external oblique fascia is opened, and the spermatic cord is isolated and clamped at the level of the internal ring. The testis is delivered through the incision and examined. If the testis is felt to contain malignancy, the cord is ligated and divided at the level of the internal inguinal ring. If there is uncertainty in the diagnosis, a biopsy can be performed.

Usual preop diagnosis: Testicular mass

SUMMARY OF PROCEDURE

	Hydrocelectomy, Hernia Repair	Orchiopexy, Orchiectomy
Position	Supine	⇐
Incision	Inguinal/scrotal	⇐ + Can be extended to reach retro peritoneum ± laparoscopic exploration.
Antibiotics	None	⇐
Surgical time	1 h	⇐
EBL	Minimal	⇐
Postop care	PACU → home	⇐
Mortality	< 1%	⇐
Morbidity	Infection: 1-2% Recurrence: 1%	Testicular atrophy: 7% Orchiectomy: 5%
Pain score	5	5

PATIENT POPULATION CHARACTERISTICS

Age range	1 yr–puberty	Cryptorchidism: 1-2 yr Torsion: 0-18 yr
Incidence	1-4%	Cryptorchidism: 3% Torsion: 1:4000
Etiology	Congenital	⇐

ANESTHETIC CONSIDERATIONS

PREOPERATIVE

Orchiopexy, orchiectomy, hydrocelectomy and hernia repair are most commonly performed in otherwise healthy children.

Renal	With phimosis, there may be Hx of UTIs. Possible pyelonephritis. Hematuria requires GU workup. **Tests:** UA; renal function (BUN, creatinine), as clinically indicated.	
Laboratory	Hct; others as indicated from H&P.	
Premedication	If > 1 yr of age, consider midazolam (0.5-0.75 mg/kg po) or diazepam (0.1-0.2 mg/kg po up to 10 mg) 1 h before induction. If > 10 yr old: standard premedication (p. D-1).	

INTRAOPERATIVE

Anesthetic technique: GETA or LMA/mask anesthetic, using a pediatric circle with humidified and warmed gases. A combined technique with caudal anesthesia is often used for nonendoscopic procedures. For small children, warm OR to 70-75°F. Use warming pad on OR table.

Induction	In younger patients, mask induction is customary before iv placement. If the surgical procedure will be > 30 min, tracheal intubation or LMA is preferred. Intermediate-acting, nondepolarizing muscle relaxant (e.g., vecuronium 0.01 mg/kg iv) is administered to facilitate tracheal intubation. If appropriate, caudal anesthesia can be obtained using bupivacaine 0.25% with epinephrine 1:200,000, 0.75 ml/kg.	
Maintenance	Standard pediatric maintenance (p. D-3). At least 2 MAC anesthesia is required prior to skin incision to prevent laryngospasm. Caudal anesthesia can be used to provide the majority of analgesia in nonendoscopic procedures.	
Emergence	If neuromuscular blockade is used, reverse with neostigmine (0.07 mg/kg iv) and atropine (0.02 mg/kg iv). Extubate when patient is fully awake.	
Blood and fluid requirements	Negligible blood loss IV: 20-22 ga × 1 NS/LR @ maintenance	Pediatric maintenance: 4 ml/kg/h – 0-10 kg + 2 ml/kg/h – 11-20 kg + 1 ml/kg/h – >20 kg
Monitoring	Standard monitors (p. D-1)	
Positioning	✓ and pad pressure points. ✓ eyes.	Ocular compression/corneal abrasion may occur with oversize mask.
Complications	Laryngospasm	Rx: 100% O_2, jaw thrust, positive pressure. If necessary, administer succinylcholine (1-2 mg/kg iv).
	Intravascular local anesthetic administration	Epinephrine in caudal anesthetic (to detect intravascular administration) does not significantly prolong analgesia.

POSTOPERATIVE

Complications	Bleeding	
Pain management	Caudal or regional block Acetaminophen (10-20 mg po/pr q 6 h prn)	Optimal analgesia and presence of parents in PACU will minimize child's agitation/movement/crying.

References

1. Berry FA: Anesthesia for genitourinary surgery. In *Pediatric Anesthesia,* 3rd edition, Gregory GA, ed. Churchill Livingstone, New York: 1994, 571-606.
2. Motoyama EK, Davis PC, eds: *Smith's Anesthesia for Infants and Children*, 6th edition. Mosby-Year-Book, St. Louis: 1996, 512-13.
3. Rozanski TA, Bloom DA: Male genital tract. In *Surgery of Infants and Children.* Oldham KT, Colombani PM, Foglia RP, eds. Lippincott-Raven Publishers, Philadelphia: 1997, 1543-58.

LAPAROSCOPIC PROCEDURES

SURGICAL CONSIDERATIONS

Description: Laparoscopy is used widely to locate the impalpable testis and for **varicocele ligation. Laparoscopic nephrectomy** (or **heminephrectomy**), **nephroureterectomy** and **pyeloplasty** have been performed.

A pneumoperitoneum is created by insufflating CO_2 (to a pressure of 14-16 mmHg). A trocar is inserted through a small, 1-cm periumbilical incision and positioned in the peritoneal cavity under direct vision (**Hasson technique**). Other trocars (2, 5 or 10 mm) are then inserted, as necessary, under direct laparoscopic vision, avoiding abdominal wall vessels and internal organs.

Impalpable testis: If diagnostic laparoscopy reveals blind ending vessels, confirming the absence of a testis, the procedure is terminated. An inguinal testis remnant usually indicates either antenatal testicular ischemia or torsion. If the vessels are seen to enter the inguinal ring, the laparoscopy is ended and inguinal exploration is performed. If the testis is located intraabdominally, laparoscopic orchiopexy may be performed. Laparoscopic ligation of the spermatic vessels (**Fowler-Stevens orchiopexy**) may be performed if there is adequate cord length. Laparoscopic orchiectomy may be performed for a dysgenetic (streak), nonviable gonad, or for a gonad in which inadequate cord length exists.

Varicocele ligation: The spermatic veins are isolated from the abdominal wall and are ligated with metallic clips, using the same initial laparoscopic approach as for an undescended testis.

Heminephrectomy, nephroureterectomy and pyeloplasty: With the patient in the lateral decubitus position, the initial trocar is inserted extraperitoneally on the anterior axillary line just below the 12th rib. Gas dissection is used to open the retroperitoneal space and kidney dissection is performed. The hilar vessels are ligated with metallic clips. The kidney is then retrieved through the 10 mm port by morcellating it, or the incision can be elongated.

Usual preop diagnosis: Nonpalpable testis; cryptorchidism; varicocele; ambiguous genitalia; UPJ obstruction; infected or nonfunctioning kidney; HTN; multicystic or dysplastic kidney, protein-losing nephropathy in ESRD

SUMMARY OF PROCEDURE

	Undescended Testis/Varicocele	Renal Surgery
Position	Supine; 15° Trendelenburg	Lateral decubitus
Incision	5-10 mm umbilical port + 1 or 2 additional ports	4 ports usually necessary
Special instrumentation	Bladder catheterization, NG tube	⇐
Unique considerations	Secure child firmly to avoid movement with table tilting. Intraabdominal pressure of 14-16 mmHg.	⇐
Antibiotics	None	⇐
Surgical time	1 h	2.5 h
EBL	Minimal	⇐
Postop care	PACU → home	PACU → ward
Mortality	< 1%	⇐
Morbidity	Overall: 0.6-5%	⇐
	Trocar misplacement: bowel perforation	⇐
	Vascular/organ thermal injury from cautery	⇐
	Gas embolus	Bleeding < 5%
	Hypercarbia and acidosis	
	Bowel perforation	⇐
Pain score	2	4

PATIENT POPULATION CHARACTERISTICS

Age range	10 mo-18 yr
Male:Female	Male (cryptorchidism)
Incidence	3% of newborn boys
Etiology	Congenital
Associated conditions	Renal insufficiency

ANESTHETIC CONSIDERATIONS

Creation of a pneumoperitoneum as part of a laparoscopic procedure impairs ventilation and can restrict venous return. The use of Trendelenburg and lithotomy positions can further worsen the respiratory changes that occur. Anesthetic considerations for pediatric patients undergoing laparoscopic procedures are similar to those in adults (see p. 419).

References

1. Farber GJ, Bloom DA: Pediatric endourology. In *Adult and Pediatric Urology,* 3rd edition. Gillenwater JY, Grayhack JT, Howards, SS, Duckett JW, eds. Mosby-Year Book, Inc., St. Louis: 1996, Vol 3, 2739-47.
2. McDougall EM, Gill IS, Clayman RV: Laparoscopic urology. In *Adult and Pediatric Urology,* 3rd edition. Gillenwater JY, Grayhack JT, Howards, SS, Duckett JW, eds. Mosby-Year Book, Inc., St. Louis: 1996, Vol 1, 829-912.

Surgeon

Lawrence A. Rinsky, MD

12.6 PEDIATRIC ORTHOPEDIC SURGERY

Anesthesiologist

Yuan-Chi Lin, MD, MPH

PERCUTANEOUS PINNING OF DISPLACED SUPRACONDYLAR HUMERUS FRACTURE

SURGICAL CONSIDERATIONS

Description: Supracondylar fractures of the humerus are the most common elbow fractures in children, and probably the most common pediatric fracture needing emergent reduction under general anesthesia. They have a justifiable reputation for difficulties because they are often associated with complications, including vascular injuries and compartment syndromes, nerve palsies, malreductions and late deformities. The vast majority of these injuries occur from a fall on an outstretched hand with an extended elbow—a common childhood event. Although an occasional angulated fracture may be stable after reduction with a splint alone, most displaced supracondylar fractures currently are treated by closed reduction and **percutaneous pinning**.

Documentation of the neurovascular examination is mandatory immediately before anesthesia and upon awakening. Reduction is obtained by a combination of traction and manipulation; complete muscular relaxation is essential. Usually two small, smooth, crossed pins are inserted under image intensifier control. Many surgeons use the intensifier screen as a platform, thus requiring the patient to be at the extreme edge of the OR table. Rarely is the fracture irreducible. In that case, the arm is reprepped and a small, lateral incision is made to openly visualize and reduce the fracture. The same type of smooth pin fixation is then carried out. Prolonged skeletal traction has been used extensively in the past for these fractures; however, it is rarely used now in this country.

Usual preop diagnosis: Acute, displaced, supracondylar fracture of the humerus

SUMMARY OF PROCEDURE

	Percutaneous Pinning	Open Reduction
Position	Usually supine, occasionally prone or lateral	⇐
Incision	None	1" lateral
Special instrumentation	Power drill, II	⇐
Unique considerations	Full-stomach compartment syndrome	⇐
Antibiotics	Usually none	Cefazolin 25 mg/kg
Surgical time	30-60 min	30-90 min
Closing considerations	Cast or splint	⇐
EBL	Minimal	⇐
Postop care	PACU → room; close neurovascular monitoring	⇐
Mortality	Rare	⇐
Morbidity	Late angular deformity, especially cubitus varus: 10%	⇐
	Nerve palsy (typically radial nerve) from the fracture itself: 7%	⇐
	Compartment syndrome (Volkmann's contracture): < 0.5% (some degree of vascular spasm or loss of radial pulse much more common)	⇐
	Stiffness, myositis ossificans	⇐
	Ipsilateral fracture	⇐
Pain score	3-5	3-6

PATIENT POPULATION CHARACTERISTICS

Age range	< 10 yr: 84%; most are 5-8 yr
Male:Female	1.6:1
Incidence	Third most common child's fracture (most common: elbow fracture)
Etiology	Trauma
Associated conditions	Usually normal, healthy child

ANESTHETIC CONSIDERATIONS

PREOPERATIVE

The majority of children presenting for repair of upper extremity fractures are otherwise healthy. Most of these patients present for repair of a traumatic injury; thus, the preop workup is routine. Some arm procedures, such as repair of a compound fracture, require immediate attention and necessitate emergency surgery and full-stomach considerations (see p. B-5).

Laboratory Hb/Hct (healthy patients); other tests as indicated from H&P.

Premedication Standard premedication (see p. D-2).

INTRAOPERATIVE

Anesthetic technique: GETA, since small children rarely tolerate regional anesthesia alone. In the older patient, regional anesthesia may be appropriate, and can reduce the risk of aspiration pneumonitis associated with GA in the patient with a full stomach. A combined technique offers the advantages of reduced anesthetic requirements and postop pain relief; however, regional anesthesia is relatively contraindicated in patients with neurovascular damage.

General anesthesia:

Induction Standard induction (see p. D-2) except in acute-trauma patients, where rapid-sequence induction is appropriate (see p. B-5).

Maintenance Standard maintenance (see p. D-3).

Emergence Management of emergence and extubation should be routine, except in difficult airway cases, which require awake extubation. Skin closure is frequently followed by application of a splint; patient should remain anesthetized during splinting procedure.

Regional anesthesia:

Anesthetics and doses
- Lidocaine 2% + crystalline tetracaine 5 mg/10 ml lidocaine ± epinephrine 0.5 ml/kg (for rapid onset of medium duration)
- Bupivacaine 0.5% ± epinephrine 0.5 ml/kg (for long duration).

Interscalene block Phrenic nerve block → hemidiaphragm paralysis is an inevitable consequence of the interscalene block. Major complications (e.g., total spinal or pneumothorax) resulting from interscalene block, are very rare; therefore, this technique is suitable for outpatients. Interscalene block is contraindicated in patients with contralateral recurrent laryngeal nerve or phrenic nerve palsy.

Axillary block The medial aspect of the upper arm is innervated by the intercostobrachial nerve (T2) and requires a separate subcutaneous field block in the axilla, especially when a tourniquet is used. The lateral cutaneous nerve of the forearm, a sensory branch of the musculocutaneous nerve supplying sensation to the lateral forearm, is frequently missed by the axillary approach to the brachial plexus. Thus, a block of this nerve at the elbow is sometimes necessary.

Supplemental sedation Supplemental sedation may be accomplished with use of propofol by continuous infusion (50-150 μg/kg/min).

Blood and fluid requirements
Minimal blood loss
IV: 20 ga × 1
NS/LR @ 1.5-3 ml/kg/h

IV catheter should be placed in the contralateral upper extremity.

Monitoring Standard monitors (see p. D-1).

Positioning
✓ and pad pressure points.
✓ eyes.

Interscalene block complications
Total spinal
Epidural anesthesia
IV injection (seizures/dysrhythmias)
Stellate ganglion block (Horner's syndrome)
Laryngeal nerve block
Phrenic nerve block
Pneumothorax

Resuscitative equipment, including airway management tools, should be immediately available.

Axillary block complications
Inadequate block
Intravascular injection
Peripheral nerve damage
Axillary hematoma

Very minimal doses of local anesthetic can cause CNS toxicity if reverse flow occurs during an intraarterial injection. Axillary thrombosis and pneumothorax are extremely rare.

Axillary block, cont.	Axillary artery thrombosis Pneumothorax	

POSTOPERATIVE

Pain management	PCA (see p. E-3). ± Regional block	Combined regional-GA provides excellent postop pain management.
Tests	None routinely indicated.	

References

1. Salem MR, Klowden AS: Anesthesia for orthopaedic surgery. In *Pediatric Anesthesia*, 3rd edition. Gregory G, ed. Churchill-Livingstone, New York: 1994, 607-56.
2. Wilkins KE: Fractures and dislocations of the elbow region. In *Fractures in Children*. Rockwood CA, Wilkins KE, Beaty JH, eds: Lippincott-Raven Publishers, Philadelphia 1996; 655-669.

POSTERIOR SPINAL INSTRUMENTATION AND FUSION

SURGICAL CONSIDERATIONS

Description: Posterior spinal instrumentation refers to implanted metal rods affixed to the spine to correct and internally splint the deformed spine. Originally designed for scoliosis, posterior spinal instrumentation is commonly performed simultaneously with spinal fusion for a variety of diagnoses including fracture, tumor, degenerative changes and developmental spinal deformity. The original **Harrington rod** is the simplest, and is still considered by many to be "the gold standard."[1,3,4,5,8,10] The spine is approached by an extensive midline posterior incision in which a subperiosteal exposure (typically T2-5 down to L1-4) is used to elevate all the paraspinous muscles as far laterally as the tips of the transverse processes. One hook is placed at each end of the curve on the concave side and anchored by slipping the hook foot into the spinal canal (Fig 12.6-1). A ratcheted single rod is attached to the two hooks and jacked into distraction, thus straightening out the concavity.

Although excellent correction of moderate curves with Harrington instrumentation is possible, the ratchets are a weak point, and the presence of only two fixation points (the hooks) on the spine leaves a risk of hook dislodgement or fracturing of the laminae; thus, a postop body case usually is required. To improve the fixation, many have added sublaminar wire loops[5,9-13] (Fig 12.6-2) at multiple levels (the **"Harri-Luque"**), or switched to two nonratcheted, L-shaped rods with multiple sublaminar wires at each spinal level (**Luque rods**) (Fig 12.6-3). Others, fearful of the neurologic risks[14] caused by the sublaminar wires, have used supplemental wires passed through the base of the spinous processes.[6] This additional fixation eliminates the need for a cast, but a postop brace still is often used. The Luque rod system is most commonly used in scoliosis of neuromuscular etiology.

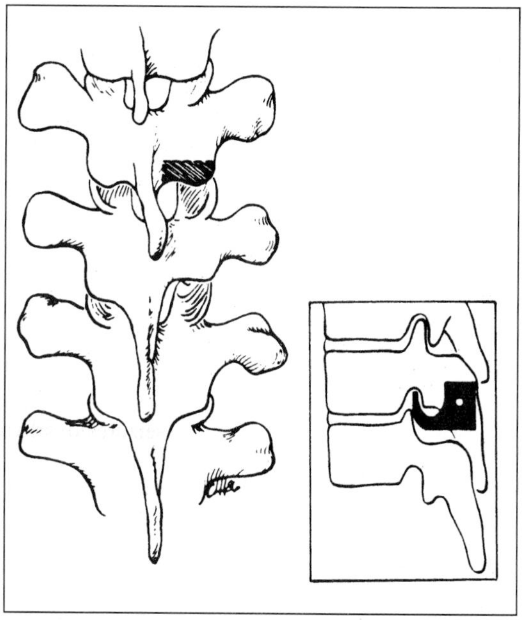

Figure 12.6-1. Placement of Harrington upper hook. (Reproduced with permission from Chapman MW, ed: *Operative Orthopaedics*, 2nd edition. JB Lippincott: 1993.)

Recently, many spinal surgeons have switched to one of several **hook-rod systems** in which multiple hooks are placed along bilateral rods. Hooks in these systems can affix to the pedicles, laminae or transverse processes. Typically, 4-8 hooks are placed

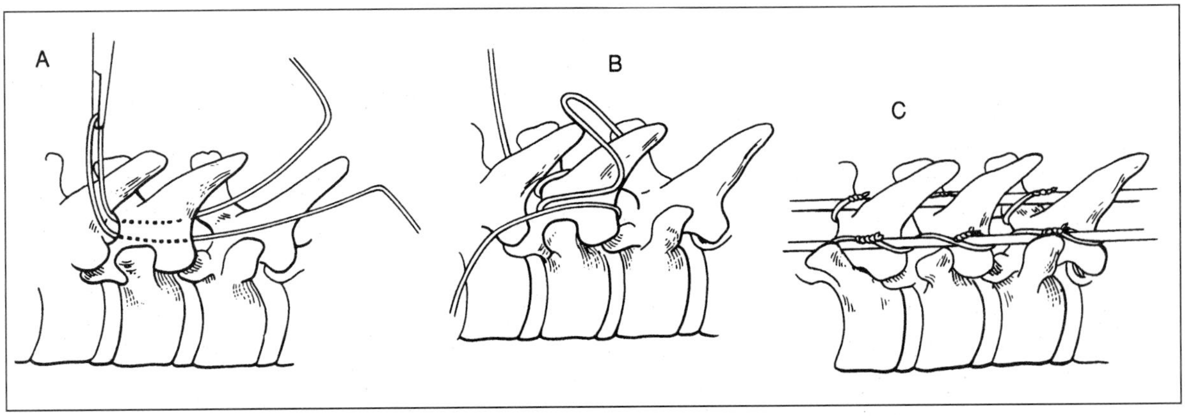

Figure 12.6-2. An example of passing and attaching sublaminar wires. (Reproduced with permission from Chapman MW, ed: *Operative Orthopaedics*, 2nd edition. JB Lippincott: 1993.)

on each rod, with each hook affixed to some posterior element. By compressing along the convex surfaces and distracting along the concave surfaces, some degree of even rotational correction is possible. These systems are by far the most complex, but they offer theoretic advantages in the possibility of a three-dimensional correction. The **Cotrel-Dubousset**[1,2,7] was the first; other popular systems include the Texas Scottish Rite Hospital (**TSRH**) system, Miami Modular Orthopedic Spinal System (**MOSS**) and Universal Spine System (**USS**).

Usual preop diagnosis: Scoliosis (lateral deviation of the spine, usually idiopathic or neuromuscular); kyphosis (increased round back); reconstruction for tumor, trauma and other

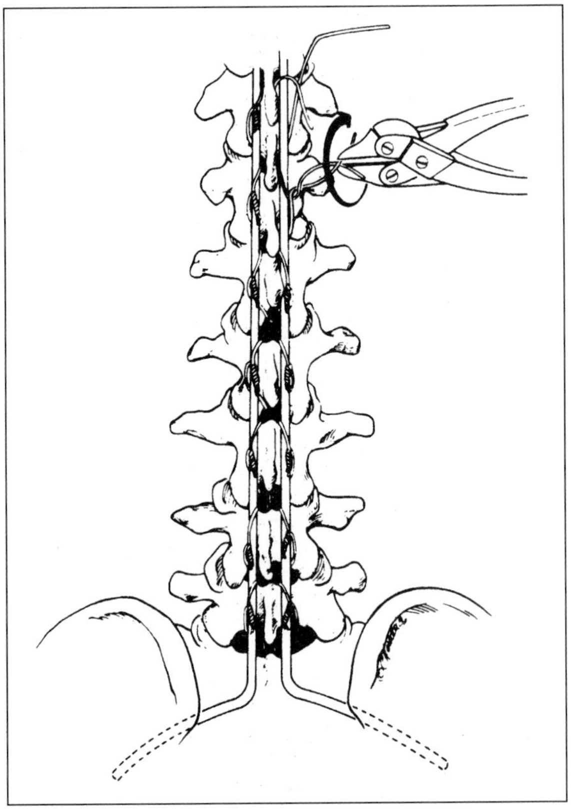

Figure 12.6-3. Positioning rods in pelvis; sublaminar wires being tightened. (Reproduced with permission from Chapman MW, ed: *Operative Orthopaedics*, 2nd edition. JB Lippincott: 1993.)

SUMMARY OF PROCEDURE

	Harrington Rod	Luque Procedure or "Harri-Luque"	Multiple Hook-Rod System
Position	Prone (on spinal frame or bolsters); avoid abdominal compression.	⇐	⇐
Incision	Posterior midline; optional separate iliac crest bone graft	⇐	⇐
Special instrumentation	Rods and hooks	Rods, wires and hooks	Rods, multiple hooks, hook connectors, transverse bars
Unique considerations	"Wake up" test and/or SSEPs; frequently, induced hypotension is requested.	⇐	⇐

	Harrington Rod	Luque Procedure or "Harri-Luque"	Multiple Hook-Rod System
Antibiotics	Cefazolin 1-2 g iv	⇐	⇐
Surgical time	2-6 h	3-7 h	⇐
Closing considerations	Greatest blood loss typically toward the end of procedure. Avoid hypotension after instrumentation is implanted.	⇐	⇐
EBL	800-1500 ml	1200-4000 ml	1200-3000 ml
Postop care	ICU: 1-3 d	⇐	⇐
Mortality[1-6,8]	0-0.5%	⇐	⇐
Morbidity[3-6,8,11-13]	Acute ileus: Very common	⇐	⇐
	Hook dislodgement requiring reoperation: 0-2%	0.01%	1%
	Wound infection: 0-2%	⇐	⇐
	Genitourinary infection: 5-7%	⇐	⇐
	Hematoma, massive bleeding: 1-5%	⇐	⇐
	Pneumothorax, pneumonia, atelectasis, etc: 1-5%	⇐	⇐
	Spinal cord injury: 0.23%	0.86%	0.6%
	Superior mesenteric artery syndrome: 0-1%	⇐	⇐
	Thromboembolism: < 1%	⇐	⇐
	Delayed:		
	Pseudarthrosis: 0-5%	⇐	⇐
	Late rod fracture: 0-5%	⇐	⇐
	Decompensation: 0-2%	< 1%	Coronal decompensation: 0-5%
Pain score	7-9	7-9	7-9

PATIENT POPULATION CHARACTERISTICS

Age range Usually 8-40 yr

Male:Female 1:5

Incidence 1-2/10,000

Etiology Idiopathic (50-75%); neuromuscular (20-30%); associated with syndromes such as osteochondral dystrophies, osteogenesis imperfecta, etc. (5%); congenital scoliosis (2-5%)

Associated conditions

Neuromuscular:
- Freidrich's ataxia (myocarditis and other cardiovascular anomalies; sudden death)
- Myelomeningocele
- Muscular dystrophy (muscle weakness, cardiomyopathy, dysrhythmias, succinylcholine → prolonged muscle contraction, ↑sensitivity to respiratory depressant effect of barbiturates, opiates and benzodiazepines)
- Cerebral palsy
- GE reflux, ↓airway protective reflexes, ↑postop pulmonary complications
- Spina bifida
- Abnormalities of the spinal cord, e.g., tethered spinal cord, syringomyelia

Connective tissue disease:
- Ehlers-Danlos and Marfan syndrome: avoid ↑BP → aortic dissection; ↑risk of pneumothorax.
- Osteogenesis imperfecta: position and intubate with great care.
- Congenital osteochondral dystrophies

Dwarfing syndromes

CHD: 1-4%

Coarctation: 0.5%

Cyanotic CHD: 14%

MVP: 25% (avoid ↑LV emptying; consider antibiotics preop) cerebral palsy

Malignant hyperthermia (MH) risk

ANESTHETIC CONSIDERATIONS

See Anesthetic Considerations for Spinal Reconstruction and Fusion, p. 799.

References

1. Akbarnia BA: Selection of methodology in surgical treatment of adolescent idiopathic scoliosis. *Orthop Clin North Am* 1988; 19(2):319-29.
2. Denis F: Cotrel-Dubousset instrumentation in the treatment of idiopathic scoliosis. *Orthop Clin North Am* 1988; 19(2):291-311.
3. Dickson JH: An eleven-year clinical investigation of Harrington instrumentation. A preliminary report on 578 cases. *Clin Orthop* 1973; 93:113-30.
4. Dickson JH, Harrington PR: The evolution of the Harrington instrumentation technique in scoliosis. *J Bone Joint Surg* [Am] 1973; 55(5):993-1002.
5. Dickson RA, Archer IA: Surgical treatment of late-onset idiopathic thoracic scoliosis. The Leeds procedure. *J Bone Joint Surg* [Br] 1987; 69(5):709-14.
6. Drummond DS, Guadagni J, Keene JS, Breed A, Narechania R: Interspinous process segmental spinal instrumentation. *J Pediatr Orthop* 1984; 4(4):397-404.
7. Lenke LG, Bridwell KH, Baldus C, Blanke K, Schoenecker PL: Cotrel-Dubousset instrumentation for adolescent idiopathic scoliosis. *J Bone Joint Surg* [Am] 1992; 74(7):1056-67.
8. Lovallo JL, Banta JV, Renshaw TS: Adolescent idiopathic scoliosis treated by Harrington-rod distraction and fusion. *J Bone Joint Surg* [Am] 1986; 68(9):1326-30.
9. Luque ER: *Segmental Spinal Instrumentation*. Slack Thorofare, NJ: 1984; 31-165.
10. Morrissy RT: *Atlas of Pediatric Orthopaedic Surgery*. JB Lippincott, Philadelphia: 1992; 1-57.
11. Silverman BJ, Greenberg PE: Idiopathic scoliosis posterior spine fusion with Harrington rod and sublaminar wiring. *Orthop Clin North Am* 1988; 19(2):269-79.
12. Sullivan JA, Conner SB: Comparison of Harrington instrumentation and segmental spinal instrumentation in the management of neuromuscular spine deformity. *Spine* 1982; 7(3):299-301.
13. Wilber RG, Thompson GH, Shaffer JW, Brown RH, Nash CL Jr: Postoperative neurological deficits in segmental spinal instrumentation. A study using spinal cord monitoring. *J Bone Joint Surg* [Am] 1984; 66(8):1178-87.

ANTERIOR SPINAL FUSION FOR SCOLIOSIS, WITH INSTRUMENTATION

SURGICAL CONSIDERATIONS

Description: Anterior spinal fusion is performed through a transthoracic and/or retroperitoneal approach to the vertebral bodies in which the intervertebral discs are removed and a bone graft placed between the vertebral bodies.[1-5, 10-12] The disc removal ("release") loosens the spine and allows greater deformity correction than posterior-only procedures. It is often performed as a first stage to a "front-and-back" fusion but may be performed alone, especially in cases of idiopathic lumbar scoliosis. **Dwyer** originated the technique[2] (1969), using a braided titanium cable through the screw heads that are then crimped onto the cable (Fig 12.6-4). Although the correction is usually dramatic, the cable is not rigid and may decrease normal lumbar lordosis. **Zielke** (1976) exchanged the cable for a threaded rod with nuts holding the rod into slots in the screw head (Fig 12.6-5). The use of nuts allows a gradual controlled correction and a better lordosis control with at least some rigidity from the rod, but a slight increase in the "fiddle factor."[1,11] The procedure also may be performed without anterior instrumentation as a simple anterior release, normally followed by a posterior spinal fusion and instrumentation.[2-4]

The **Zielke procedure** or one of the newer **screw-rod systems** (e.g., Texas Scottish Rite Hospital [TSRH], Miami Modular Orthopedic Spinal System [MOSS]) generally is favored, especially if posterior spinal instrumentation is not otherwise needed. The approach is through a flank incision, then through a rib bed on the convex side (usually the 10th rib). The retroperitoneal plane is entered and developed by blunt dissection behind the transversus abdominis muscle.

The pleural cavity is then entered, and the diaphragm usually must be divided circumferentially near its costal origin and around posteriorly to the spine. The prevertebral areolar plane is then entered and the segmental vessels to each vertebral body are clipped or cauterized in the midline. The psoas muscle is elevated off the lateral aspects of the vertebral bodies. Each disc in the fusion area (usually 3-5 discs) is then excised back to the posterior longitudinal ligament. Next, vertebral screws are inserted transversely across the appropriate bodies and joined at their heads by the Dwyer cable or Zielke rod. Compression is applied through the cable or rod, while the previously flexed OR table is slowly and gradually straightened. It is critical that the anesthesiologist straighten the table with great care to avoid excessive stress on the implants. Prior to closure of the disc spaces, bone graft is placed anteriorly to maintain lordosis.

Usual preop diagnosis: Scoliosis > 45°; idiopathic or neuromuscular

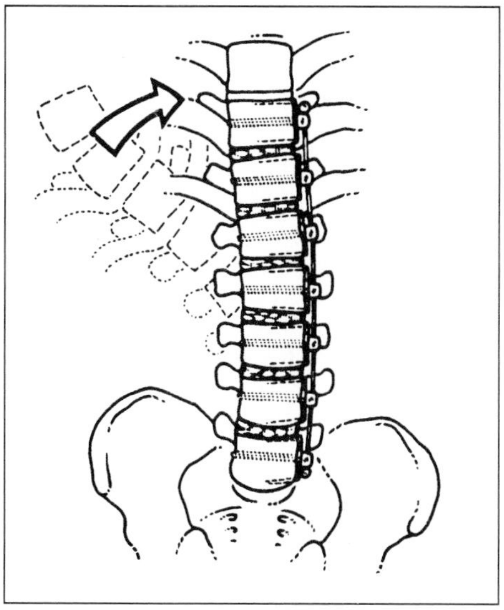

←**Figure 12.6-4.** Dwyer instrumentation used to make spinal correction. (Reproduced with permission from Crenshaw AH, ed: *Campbell's Operative Orthopaedics*, 8th edition. Mosby-Year Book: 1992.)

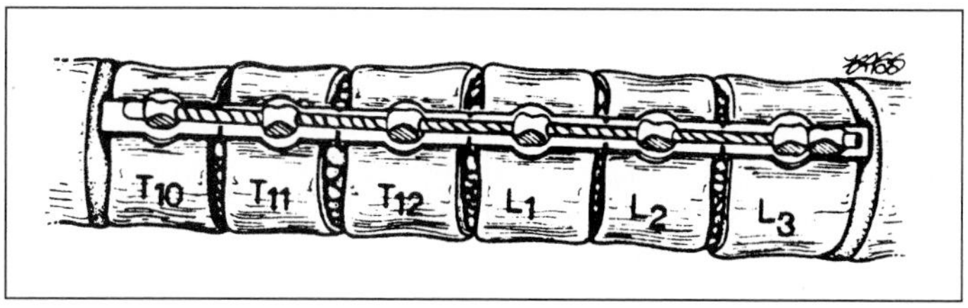

↑**Figure 12.6-5.** Instrumentation from T10-L3 (Zielke). (Reproduced with permission from Chapman MW, ed: *Operative Orthopaedics*, 2nd edition. JB Lippincott: 1993.)

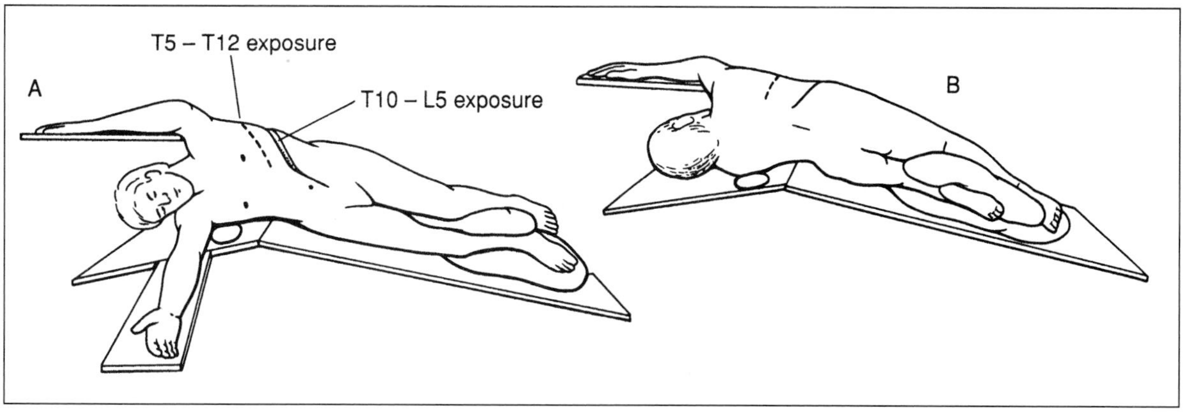

Figure 12.6-6. Lateral decubitus position (diagrammatic) for anterior spinal procedures: (A) anterior view; (B) posterior view. Roll is placed under axilla to minimize axillary artery compression. Skin incision for exposure of T5-T12 is shown with the dotted line. (Reproduced with permission from Chapman MW, ed: *Operative Orthopaedics*, 2nd edition. JB Lippincott: 1993.)

SUMMARY OF PROCEDURE

	Dwyer Procedure	Zielke Procedure, TSRH, MOSS	Release (No Instrumentation)
Position	Full lateral decubitus (Fig 12.6-6)	⇐	⇐
Incision	Flank: over rib at top vertebra in the curve (usually T9-T11)	⇐	⇐
Special instrumentation	Screws, staples, cable, crimper	Screws, staples, rods, nuts	–

	Dwyer Procedure	Zielke Procedure, TSRH, MOSS	Release (No Instrumentation)
Unique considerations	OR table must be "broken" into flexed mode at start, then straightened after discs are removed to aid in reduction. Procedure often followed by posterior spinal fusion, sometimes on same day.[12] Proximity of great vessels, major bleeding a potential problem, although not common.[2,4-5,10-12] Patients with neuromuscular scoliosis often have poor generalized nutrition. Opening and closing sometimes performed by a separate team of general surgeons. Evoked cortical potentials often used to monitor spinal cord function.	⇐	⇐ Uninstrumented release is always followed by posterior spinal fusion and, usually, instrumentation.[2,4]
Antibiotics	Cefazolin 25 mg/kg iv	⇐	⇐
Surgical time	4-7 h	⇐	3 - 6 h
Closing considerations	Chest tube always used; hypotension, if used electively, must be reversed before closure.	⇐	⇐
EBL	500-3000 ml	⇐	250-2000 ml
Postop care	ICU 2-4 d	⇐	⇐
Mortality	0-2%, depending on underlying conditions[4,12]	⇐	⇐
Morbidity	Overall: 30% (significant problem or complication, depending on underlying condition[1-5,10-12]	⇐	20%
	Ileus and atelectasis: ~50%	⇐	⇐
	Urinary tract infection: 10-25% (common in spina bifida)	⇐	⇐
	Minor transient root weakness, or paraesthesia: 10-20%	⇐	1-5%
	Late kyphosis above instrumentation: 5-10%	⇐	⇐
	Nonunion and hardware failure: 5%	⇐	⇐
	Massive blood loss: 2-5%	⇐	⇐
	Respiratory failure: 1-2%	⇐	⇐
	Pneumonia: 1%	⇐	⇐
	Paraplegia (acute anterior spinal artery syndrome): < 1%	⇐	⇐
	Thromboembolism: Rare (< 5% in children)	⇐	⇐
Pain score	5-8	5-8	4-7

PATIENT POPULATION CHARACTERISTICS

Age range	5-35 yr
Male:Female	Idiopathic: 1:10 Neuromuscular: 1:1
Incidence	< 0.1/1000
Etiology	Idiopathic scoliosis; neuromuscular disease (especially cerebral palsy, spina bifida, polio, myopathies, muscular dystrophies); other genetic dysplasias of bone; Marfan syndrome (occasionally)

Associated conditions

Idiopathic: generally healthy
Cerebral palsy patients: often retarded, often with poor general health
Spina bifida: usually with hydrocephalus and chronic urinary tract infection
Myopathy: malignant hyperthermia susceptible
Chronic restrictive lung disease in severe cases
Extremity contractures may make positioning difficult
Muscular dystrophy patients may have cardiomyopathy

ANESTHETIC CONSIDERATIONS

(See Anesthetic Considerations for Spinal Reconstruction and Fusion, p. 799.)

References

1. Brown J, Swank S, Spacht L: Combined anterior and posterior spine fusion in cerebral palsy. *Spine* 1982; 7(6):570-3.
2. Chapman MW: *Operative Orthopaedics*, 2nd edition. JB Lippincott, Philadelphia: 1993, 2899-2913.
3. Dwyer AF, Chafer MF: Anterior approach to scoliosis. Results of treatment in fifty-one cases. *J Bone Joint Surg* [Br] 1974; 56(2):218-24.
4. Ferguson RL, Allen BL Jr: Staged correction of neuromuscular scoliosis. *J Pediatr Orthop* 1983; 3:555-62.
5. Floman Y, Penny JN, Micheli LJ, Riseborough EJ, Hall JE: Combined anterior and posterior fusion in seventy-three spinally deformed patients: indications, results and complications. *Clin Orthop* 1982; 164:110-22.
6. Goldstein LA, Waugh TR: Classification and terminology of scoliosis. *Clin Orthop* 1973; 93:10-22.
7. Goodarzi M, Shier N, Ogden J: Epidural versus patient-controlled analgesia with morphine for postoperative pain after orthopedic procedures in children. *J Pediatr Orthop* 1993; 13:663.
8. Grundy BL: Intraoperative monitoring of sensory-evoked potentials. *Anesthesiology* 1983; 58(1):72-87.
9. Kafer ER: Respiratory and cardiovascular functions in scoliosis and the principles of anesthetic management. *Anesthesiology* 1980; 52(4):339-51.
10. McMaster MJ: Anterior and posterior instrumentation and fusion of thoracolumbar scoliosis due to myelomeningocele. *J Bone Joint Surg* [Br] 1987; 69(1):20-5.
11. Morrissy RT: *Atlas of Pediatric Orthopaedic Surgery*. JB Lippincott, Philadelphia: 1992, 75-97.
12. O'Brien JP, Yau AC, Gertzbein S, Hodgson AR: Combined staged anterior and posterior correction and fusion of the spine in scoliosis following poliomyelitis. *Clin Orthop* 1975; 110:81-9.
13. O'Brien T, Akmakjian J, Ogin G, Eilert R: Comparison of one-stage versus two-stage anterior/posterior spinal fusion for neuromuscular scoliosis. *J Pediatr Orthop* 1992; 12(5):610-15.
14. Phillips WA, Hensinger RN: Control of blood loss during scoliosis surgery. *Clin Orthop* 1988; 229:88-93.
15. Smyth RJ, Chapman KR, Wright TA, Crawford JS, Rebuck AS: Pulmonary function in adolescents with mild idiopathic scoliosis. *Thorax* 1984; 39(12):901-4.
16. Smyth RJ, Chapman KR, Wright TA, Crawford JS, Rebuck AS: Ventilatory patterns during hypoxia, hypercapnia, and exercise in adolescents with mild scoliosis. *Pediatrics* 1986; 77(5):692-97.
17. Sudhir KG, Smith RM, Hall J, Hall JE, Hansen DD: Intraoperative awakening for early recognition of possible neurologic sequelae during Harrington-rod spinal fusion. *Anesth Analg* 1976; 55(4):526-28.

PELVIC OSTEOTOMY

SURGICAL CONSIDERATIONS

Description: Pelvic osteotomy is used to improve hip instability in cases of congenital or developmental hip dysplasia and dislocation by "deepening" the shallow acetabulum.[1,2,5] It is frequently performed in conjunction with open reduction, and occasionally with femoral osteotomy. The surgical approach is made along the iliac crest, always exposing the external (gluteal) surface of the pelvis, and sometimes the internal (iliac) surface. The pelvis is osteotomized closely above the acetabulum, and sometimes through the pubis and ischium as well, depending on the direction of rotation and

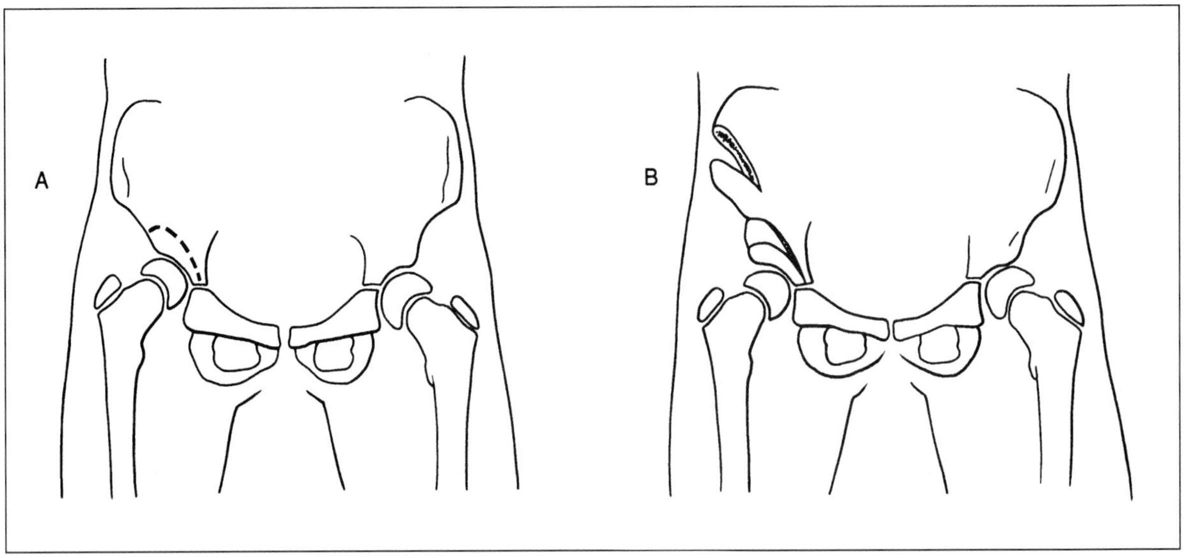

Figure 12.6-7. Pemberton osteotomy: (A) Osteotomy begins slightly superior to iliac spine, curves into triradiate cartilage. (B) Osteotomy completed with acetabular roof in corrected position. Wedge of bone is impacted into osteotomy site. (Reproduced with permission from Crenshaw AH, ed: *Campbell's Operative Orthopaedics*, 8th edition. Mosby-Year Book: 1992.)

reorientation desired. Pelvic osteotomies either reorient an intact acetabular hyaline cartilage surface or are designed as salvage procedures to enlarge the acetabulum by fibrocartilage metaplasia (see Acetabular Augmentation, Chiari, p. 999). **Salter's innominate osteotomy** is the classic reorientation osteotomy, in which a complete cut of the supraacetabular iliac bone allows rotation through the symphysis pubis.[4,7] **Pemberton's operation** is a slightly more difficult incomplete iliac osteotomy, rotating on the triradius cartilage (Fig 12.6-7), which is at the center of the acetabulum in young children.[3] The **Steel**,[6] **"Dial"** or **Eppright osteotomies** are the most difficult reorientation procedures. In each, the acetabulum is freed totally from any bony contact with the remainder of the pelvis and rotated into better position.[5]

Usual preop diagnosis: Acetabular dysplasia due to congenital or developmental hip dislocation

SUMMARY OF PROCEDURE

	Salter	Pemberton	Steel, Dial
Position	Supine	⇐	⇐
Incision	Oblique or longitudinal anterior hip	⇐	⇐
Special instrumentation	Steinmann pins	Special curved, custom osteotomes	Steinmann pins
Unique considerations	Frequently follows previous unsuccessful open-hip surgery.	⇐	⇐ + Additional ischial incision
Antibiotics	Usually, cefazolin 25 mg/kg iv	⇐	⇐
Surgical time	1.5-2 h	2-3 h	2-4 h
Closing considerations	Hip spica	⇐	⇐
EBL	100-300 ml	⇐	200-600 ml
Postop care	PACU → room; care as needed for spica cast	⇐	⇐
Mortality	Minimal	⇐	⇐
Morbidity	Avascular necrosis of the hip: 5-6%	–	–
	Persistent hip subluxation: ~5%	⇐	⇐
	Infection: < 1%	⇐	⇐
	Sciatic or perineal palsy: < 0.1%	–	–

	Salter	Pemberton	Steel, Dial
Morbidity, cont.	Excess bleeding from superior gluteal artery: Rare	⇐	Occasional
	Ileus: Rare	⇐	Occasional
Pain score	2-5	2-5	3-6

PATIENT POPULATION CHARACTERISTICS

	Salter	Pemberton	Steel, Dial
Age range	18 mo-6 yr, if dislocated 18 mo-10 yr, if only subluxated	18 mo-7 yr	> 12 yr
Male:Female	1:2	⇐	⇐
Incidence	0.1/1000	< 0.1/1000	< 0.01/1000
Etiology	Congenital and/or developmental hip dysplasia: 98% Perthes disease: 1%	⇐	⇐
Associated conditions	Torticollis: < 1%	⇐	⇐
	Other joint contractures in cases of neuromuscular dislocation: < 1%	⇐	⇐

ANESTHETIC CONSIDERATIONS

See Anesthetic Considerations for Pediatric Orthopedic Surgery of the Pelvis and Extremities, p. 1020.

References

1. Coleman SS: *Congenital Dysplasia and Dislocation of the Hip*. Mosby Year Book Inc, St. Louis: 1978.
2. MacEwen GD: Treatment of congenital dislocation of the hip in older children. *Clin Orthop* 1987; 225:86-92.
3. Pemberton PA: Pericapsular osteotomy of the ilium for the treatment of congenitally dislocated hips. *Clin Orthop* 1974; 98:41-54.
4. Salter RB, Duboi JP: The first fifteen years' personal experience with innominate osteotomy in the treatment of congenital dislocation and subluxation of the hip. *Clin Orthop* 1974; 98:72-103.
5. Staheli LT: Surgical management of acetabular dysplasia. *Clin Orthop* 1991; 264:111-21.
6. Steel HH: Triple osteotomy of the innominate bone. *J Bone Joint Surg* [Am] 1973; 55(2):343-50.
7. Waters P, Kurica K, Hall J, Micheli LJ: Salter innominate osteotomies in congenital dislocation of the hip. *J Pediatr Orthop* 1988; 8(6):650-55.

ACETABULAR AUGMENTATION (SHELF) & CHIARI OSTEOTOMY

SURGICAL CONSIDERATIONS

Description: Acetabular augmentation is a "salvage" procedure used to deepen the hip socket when a realignment osteotomy of the pelvis and/or femur would not adequately cover the femoral head.[5,8] This is accomplished by securing strips of cortical cancellous bone graft onto the proximal surface of the hip capsule. The surgical approach is anterior to the hip, elevating the gluteal muscles subperiosteally from the outer surface of the ilium. The reflected head of the rectus femoris tendon is elevated, and a domed-shaped slot is created just above the capsular attachment to the ilium. Abundant cortical cancellous strips of bone graft are then harvested from the upper two-thirds of the outer wall of the ilium. These bone grafts have a natural curve and lie on the convexity of the hip capsule. No internal fixation, other than suture repair, is used to hold the bone graft in place. This creates a large bony augmentation (shelf) over the uncovered femoral capsule.

Variant procedure or approaches: The bone graft may be taken as a large, sculpted, solitary, cortical cancellous strut or wedge, or more commonly, as curved "shavings" anchored in a dome-shaped slot just above the hip capsule. In the **Chiari procedure**,[1-4] a complete dome-shaped osteotomy allows lateral displacement of the ilium just above the proximal hip capsule (Fig 12.6-8). The line of the osteotomy corresponds more or less with the slot of the shelf procedure. In either case, the result is abundant bony coverage over the hip capsule, which undergoes metaplasia into fibrocartilage.

Usual preop diagnosis: Acetabular dysplasia (shallow socket) due to congenital hip dislocation or developmental neurologic subluxation

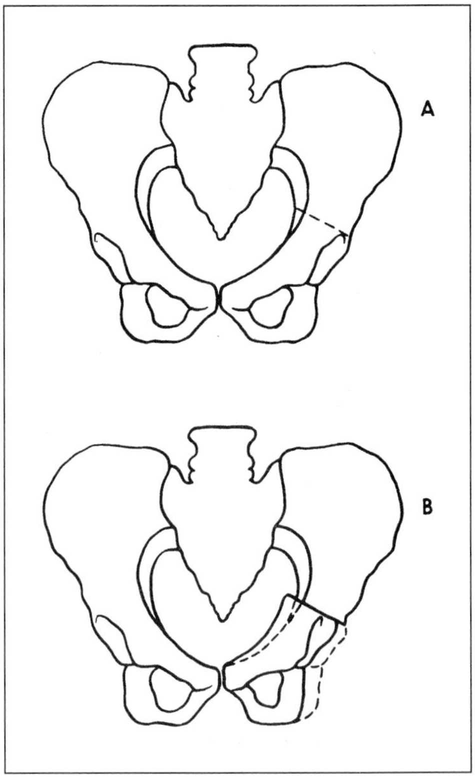

Figure 12.6-8. Chiari osteotomy: (A) Line of osteotomy. (B) Completed osteotomy. (Reproduced with permission from Crenshaw AH, ed: *Campbell's Operative Orthopaedics*, 8th edition. Mosby-Year Book: 1992.)

SUMMARY OF PROCEDURE

	Acetabular Augmentation	Chiari Osteotomy
Position	Supine or slightly tilted up (reverse Trendelenburg)	⇐ or lateral decubitus
Incision	Oblique or longitudinal; anterior hip region	⇐
Special instrumentation	Usually no internal fixation; image intensification or intraop x-ray	Two large screws or pins; image intensification or intraop x-ray
Antibiotics	Cefazolin 25 mg/kg iv	⇐
Surgical time	1.5-3 h	⇐
Closing considerations	Unilateral or 1.5 spica cast mandatory	Spica cast (optional)
EBL	100-500 ml	200-800 ml
Postop care	PACU → room. Care as necessary for cast.	⇐
Mortality	Minimal	⇐
Morbidity	Lateral femoral cutaneous nerve dysfunction: 30-50%[5-8]	Sciatic or peroneal palsy: 2%
	Infection: 1%	Possible need[1-4] for later C-section: Rare
Pain score	4-6	4-6

PATIENT POPULATION CHARACTERISTICS

Age range	6-35 yr
Male:Female	1:1.5
Incidence	< 0.1/1000 in general population; in neuromuscular population (e.g., cerebral palsy, poliomyelitis residuals): ≤ 5-10%
Etiology	Neuromuscular hip subluxation with shallow acetabulum; residual shallow acetabulum (poor coverage from congenitally dislocated hip)
Associated conditions	Cerebral palsy; polio; spina bifida; myopathy; congenital atrophies; Charcot-Marie Tooth disease

ANESTHETIC CONSIDERATIONS

See Anesthetic Considerations for Pediatric Orthopedic Surgery of the Pelvis and Extremities, p. 1020.

References

1. Betz RR, Kumar SJ, Palmer CT, MacEwen GD: Chiari pelvic osteotomy in children and young adults. *J Bone Joint Surg* [Am] 1988; 70(2):182-91.
2. Calvert PT, Augaust AC, Albert JS: The Chiari pelvic osteotomy. A review of the long-term results. *J Bone Joint Surg* [Br] 1987; 69(4):551-55.
3. Chiari K: Medial displacement osteotomy of the pelvis. *Clin Orthop* 1974; 98:55-69.
4. Morrissy RT: *Atlas of Pediatric Orthopaedic Surgery*. JB Lippincott, Philadelphia: 1992, 201-10.
5. Staheli LT: Slotted acetabular augmentation. *J Pediatr Orthop* 1981; 1(3):321-27.
6. Summers BN, Turner A, Wynn-Jones CH: The shelf operation in the management of late presentation of congenital hip dysplasia. *J Bone Joint Surg* [Br] 1988; 70(1):63-8.
7. White RE Jr, Sherman FC: The hip shelf procedure. A long-term evaluation. *J Bone Joint Surg* [Am] 1980; 62(6):928-32.
8. Zuckerman JD, Staheli LT, McLaughlin JF: Acetabular augmentation for progressive hip subluxation in cerebral palsy. *J Pediatr Orthop* 1984; 4(4):436-42.

OBER FASCIOTOMY, YOUNT-OBER RELEASE

SURGICAL CONSIDERATIONS

Description: Ober's fasciotomy is performed to release flexion, abduction and external rotation contracture at the hip.[1-4] This contracture usually occurs as a result of profound flaccid paralysis → prolonged positioning in a so-called "frog" position of 90° flexion, abduction and lateral rotation at the hips. This results in tightening of the iliotibial (IT) band (the greatly thickened lateral aspect of the fascia lata) and related structures. The operation is performed through an anterolateral incision just distal to the iliac crest. All of the fascial investments of the tensor, sartorius and, at times, the rectus femoris and gluteus medias and minimus are divided while preserving any normal-appearing muscle fibers. The limb is stretched into progressively more adduction and extension, until a neutral position can be obtained. The **Yount procedure** is added when the knee is also contracted in a flexed mode due to tightness of the IT band. The Yount procedure consists of further resection of a segment of the IT band and a lateral intermuscular septum through a separate distal mid-lateral longitudinal incision just above the knee. An oblique segment of the IT band and septum are removed and not repaired.

Usual preop diagnosis: Flaccid paralysis and "frog" type contracture due to poliomyelitis, myelomeningocele or myopathy

SUMMARY OF PROCEDURE

	Ober Fasciotomy	Yount-Ober Release
Position	Supine; both legs must be prepped and draped to well above the iliac crest area for intraop stretching.	⇐
Incision	Oblique iliac crest	Mid-lateral longitudinal above knee joint, approximately 10 cm
Unique considerations	Patients with sensory and motor loss have a tendency to get pressure sores.	⇐
Antibiotics	Usually none	⇐
Surgical time	1 h/side	30 min/side
Closing considerations	Bilateral above-knee casts	⇐
EBL	< 150 ml	< 50 ml

	Ober Fasciotomy	Yount-Ober Release
Postop care	PACU → room; extensive physical therapy program of stretching exercises. Myopathic patients will be at risk for postop respiratory compromise.	⇐
Mortality	Minimal	⇐
Morbidity	Hematoma: ~1%	⇐
	Fracture of atrophied bone postop: < 1%	⇐
	Infection: < 1%	⇐
	Pressure sores from positioning or casts: < 1%	⇐
Pain score	3-4	3-4

PATIENT POPULATION CHARACTERISTICS

Age range	2-15 yr
Male:Female	1:1
Incidence	Extremely rare in American-born children; however, polio is seen commonly in southeast Asian and Latin American immigrants.
Etiology	Polio; myelomeningocele; myopathy or dystrophy
Associated conditions	Other contractures; incontinence; pressure sores in myelomeningocele

ANESTHETIC CONSIDERATIONS

See Anesthetic Considerations for Pediatric Orthopedic Surgery of the Pelvis and Extremities, p. 1020.

References

1. Beaty JH: Paralytic disorders. In *Campbell's Operative Orthopaedics*, 8th edition. Crenshaw AH, ed. Mosby Year Book, St. Louis: 1992, 2412-16.
2. Irwin CE: The iliotibial band, its role in producing deformity in poliomyelitis. *J Bone Joint Surg* [Am] 1949; 31:141-52.
3. Ober FR: The role of the iliotibial band and fascia lata as a factor in the causation of low-back disabilities and sciatica. *J Bone Joint Surg* [Am] 1936; 18:105-19.
4. Yount CC: The role of the tensor fasciae femoris in certain deformities of the lower extremities. *J Bone Joint Surg* [Am] 1926; 8:171-82.

HIP, OPEN REDUCTION ± FEMORAL SHORTENING

SURGICAL CONSIDERATIONS

Description: Open reduction of the hip replaces a congenitally or developmentally dislocated femoral head into the anatomic acetabulum, usually after an unsuccessful attempt to reduce the hip by closed means.[1-6] It often is preceded by traction and always followed by spica cast. A developmental dislocation presents with a more normal acetabulum and occurs around birth or later. Teratologic congenital dislocation of the hip occurs early *in utero*; and, as a result, is a high-riding dislocation with a poorly developed acetabulum, presenting much more difficulty in obtaining and maintaining reduction. The most common surgical approach is through an anterior groin incision. The hip capsule is exposed circumferentially, after division and tagging of the origins of the rectus, femoris and sartorius muscles, and retraction of the tensor and gluteal muscles. The capsule is opened in an oblique fashion, the ligamentum teres is excised, and any obstacle to reduction is removed. The iliopsoas tendon is lengthened; then the capsule is repaired in a "vest-over-pants" imbrication, with the hip reduced under direct visualization (Fig 12.6-9). A medial approach through the adductor region can be used in very young children (< 18 mo), but does not allow a capsular repair.[3] If femoral shortening is necessary, the surgical excision is either extended anterolaterally, or a separate lateral incision is made longitudinally over the proximal femur.

Variant procedure or approaches: Most children < 2 yr old can simply have the hip repositioned—closed or open—and subsequently have normal hip development. In older children, especially with a high dislocation, a segment of the femur is removed subtrochanterically to allow reduction without pressure (thus allowing "descent" of the femoral head). If the acetabulum is very shallow, a pelvic osteotomy may be added.

Usual preop diagnosis: Developmental dislocation of hip; teratologic congenital dislocation of hip

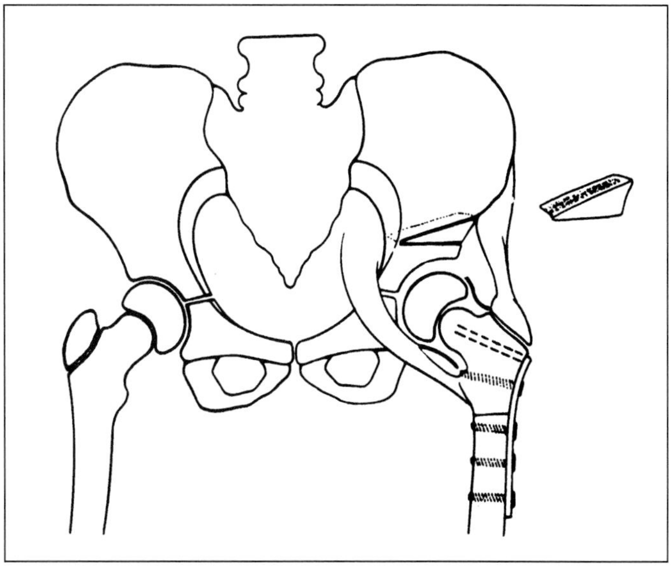

Figure 12.6-9. Open reduction with femoral shortening. (Reproduced with permission from Crenshaw AH, ed: *Campbell's Operative Orthopaedics*, 8th edition. Mosby-Year Book: 1992.)

SUMMARY OF PROCEDURE

	Open Reduction	Open Reduction + Femoral Shortening
Position	Supine	⇐
Incision	Oblique groin ("bikini") or medial longitudinal over joint	⇐ + Anterolateral thigh over joint
Special instrumentation	None	Plates and screws
Unique considerations	Preliminary arthrogram and, often, attempted closed reduction. Image intensifier is used.	⇐
Antibiotics	Usually cefazolin 25 mg/kg iv	⇐
Surgical time	1.5-3 h	2-4 h
Closing considerations	Hip spica cast applied on child's spica frame. ★ **NB**: Do not wake patient until last radiograph is taken in case cast has to be reapplied.	⇐
EBL	< 100 ml	100-400 ml
Postop care	PACU → room; care as necessary for spica cast.	⇐
Mortality	Minimal	⇐
Morbidity	Avascular necrosis of femoral head	⇐
	Stiffness and late arthritis	⇐
	Limb-length discrepancy	⇐
	Marked scrotal or labial swelling: Temporary	⇐
	Redislocation	⇐
	Infection	⇐
Pain score	2-4	3-5

PATIENT POPULATION CHARACTERISTICS

Age range	Closed reduction: 3 mo-3 yr Open reduction: 6 mo-10 yr Open reduction femoral shortening: 2-14 yr
Male:Female	1:5 (approximate)
Incidence	1:10,000
Etiology	Genetic background; breech presentation; first-born girl
Associated conditions	Arthrogryposis; Larsen's disease; myelomeningocele; chromosomal anomalies; congenital torticollis; cerebral palsy

ANESTHETIC CONSIDERATIONS

See Anesthetic Considerations for Pediatric Orthopedic Surgery of the Pelvis and Extremities, p. 1020.

References

1. Chapman MW: *Operative Orthopaedics*, 2nd edition. JB Lippincott, Philadelphia: 1993, 3101-62.
2. Coleman SS: *Congenital Dysplasia and Dislocation of the Hip*. Mosby Year Book Inc, St. Louis: 1978.
3. Galpin RD, Roach JW, Wenger DR, Herring JA, Birch JG: One-stage treatment of congenital dislocation of the hip in older children, including femoral shortening. *J Bone Joint Surg* [Am] 1989; 71(5):734-41.
4. Ferguson AB: Primary open reduction of congenital dislocation of the hip using a median adductor approach. *J Bone Joint Surg* [Am] 1973; 55:67189.
5. Morrissy RT: *Atlas of Pediatric Orthopaedic Surgery*. JB Lippincott, Philadelphia: 1992, 137-54.
6. Schoenecker PL, Strecker WB: Congenital dislocation of the hip in children. Comparison of the effects of femoral shortening and of skeletal traction in treatment. *J Bone Joint Surg* [Am] 1984; 66(1):21-7.

ADDUCTOR RELEASE OR TRANSFER, PSOAS RELEASE

SURGICAL CONSIDERATIONS

Description: The adductor tendon origins and/or the iliopsoas insertion are frequently released in spastic and other neurologic conditions (especially cerebral palsy) which cause crossing of the legs ("scissoring").[1-6] The goal is to allow greater abduction by decreasing the strength of the adductors and flexors. The releases are also performed for other causes of hip contracture due to developmental hip dislocation, juvenile arthritis, etc. The procedure is always performed on a supine patient through a groin incision in which the tendons (usually the adductor longus, brevis and gracilis) are isolated by blunt section and divided by electrocautery. In the classic procedure popularized by **Banks** and **Green**, the anterior branch of the obturator nerve is divided on the surface of the adductor brevis to effect more permanent adductor weakness. **Neurectomy** is now less popular because of the fear that the denervated muscle will fibrose into a worse scar.[6] The iliopsoas tendon may be released at its insertion on the lesser trochanter, in the base of the adductor incision; or, just the tendinous portion of the combined iliopsoas may be released at the pelvic rim, which produces a more modest degree of the flexor lengthening. Some surgeons transfer the adductor longus and gracilis muscles proximally and laterally, suturing them to the ischium to convert the adductors to hip extensors by changing their mechanics.[4,5] Theoretically, this is desirable; but it has not proven to be more effective overall than simple adductor release, and is a more complicated procedure.

Usual preop diagnosis: Adduction and flexion contracture of the hip with subluxation due to cerebral palsy, acquired encephalopathy or progressive neurologic disorder

SUMMARY OF PROCEDURE

	Adductor Release	Adductor Transfer	Psoas Release
Position	Supine	Supine or lithotomy	⇐
Incision	Medial proximal groin, longitudinal or transverse	Transverse medial groin	Anterior groin
Unique considerations	Frequently bilateral; often poor hygiene, especially if severe contracture; proximity to perineum	⇐	⇐
Antibiotics	± Cefazolin 25 mg/kg iv	⇐	⇐
Surgical time	1 h	1.5 h	1 hr
Closing considerations	Bilateral leg casts or double spica cast	⇐	⇐

	Adductor Release	Adductor Transfer	Psoas Release
EBL	< 100 ml	⇐	⇐
Postop care	PACU → room; care as necessary for spica cast.	⇐	⇐
Mortality	Minimal	⇐	⇐
Morbidity	Hematoma, drainage Infection: < 1% Recurrence of adduction deformity	⇐	⇐
Pain score	2-4	2-4	2-4

PATIENT POPULATION CHARACTERISTICS

Age range 2-20 yr

Male:Female 1:1

Incidence 0 in general population; ≤ 30% of cerebral palsy patients (0.6-5.9/1,000)[6]

Etiology Cerebral palsy (90%); slowly progressive degenerative neurologic conditions (8-10%); head injury and drowning (1-2%)

Associated conditions Multiple other contractures; gastroesophageal reflux; poor general nutrition; mental retardation

ANESTHETIC CONSIDERATIONS

See Anesthetic Considerations for Pediatric Orthopedic Surgery of the Pelvis and Extremities, p. 1020.

References

1. Banks HH, Green WT: Adductor myotomy and obturator neurectomy for the correction of adduction contracture of the hip in cerebral palsy. *J Bone Joint Surg* [Am] 1960; 42:111-26.
2. Bleck EE: *Orthopaedic Management in Cerebral Palsy*. JB Lippincott, Philadelphia: 1987, 282-319.
3. Bleck EE: The hip in cerebral palsy. *Orthop Clin North Am* 1980; 11(1):79-104.
4. Reimers J, Poulsen S: Adductor transfer versus tenotomy for stability of the hip in spastic cerebral palsy. *J Pediatr Orthop* 1984; 4(1):52-4.
5. Root L, Spero CR: Hip adductor transfer compared with adductor tenotomy in cerebral palsy. *J Bone Joint Surg* [Am] 1981; 63(5):767-72.
6. Tachdjian MD: *Pediatric Orthopaedics*. WB Saunders, Philadelphia: 1990, 1613-45.

PINNING OF SLIPPED CAPITAL FEMORAL EPIPHYSIS (SCFE)

SURGICAL CONSIDERATIONS

Description: During the rapid growth period of adolescence, the shearing stress of the body weight on the proximal femoral growth plate may cause the femoral head (capital epiphysis) to gradually move relative to the femoral neck physis (growth plate). The displacement occurs over weeks-to-months, with the head appearing to move posteriorly and inferiorly on the neck. ***In situ* pinning** (no reduction) is the most common treatment.[2-7] The goal is to prevent further slipping and subsequent arthritis by causing closure of the growth plate. The procedure must be performed under radiographic control (usually image intensifier), using a variety of threaded pins or screws which are passed through the neck into the femoral head. Currently, the favored technique uses 1 stout cannulated screw, which is passed percutaneously over a guide wire from the anterolateral aspect of the proximal femur. Traditionally, a small lateral incision was used at the base of the trochanter, with 2-4 pins placed; however, screws now in use are strong enough so that 1 is adequate for most chronic slips. More importantly, 1 screw can be placed "dead center" in the femoral head, avoiding the frequent complication of having a pin penetrate the joint.

Variant procedure or approaches: Although most slips are chronic, occasionally following mild trauma, an acute slip will supervene. Following severe trauma, a previous normal hip with an open physis (growth plate) may suffer an acute displacement, but this is rare. In such acute slips, some degree of reduction may be possible, and two pins are usually necessary.[3,7] Because pin-related complications are common, some surgeons prefer to close the growth plate by open drilling and curettement, with bone grafting across the cartilaginous plates.[1,8] This is performed through an anterior incision, opening the hip capsule widely from an oblique groin incision. No pins are used, but an iliac bone graft is placed across the physis. A body spica cast is frequently needed. Once the physis is closed, if there is severe residual deformity, a corrective osteotomy is performed in the trochanteric region (see Proximal Femoral Osteotomy, Southwick procedure, p. 1007).

Usual preop diagnosis: Acute or chronic SCFE

SUMMARY OF PROCEDURE

	Pinning of SCFE	Variant Open Epiphysiodesis
Position	Supine	⇐
Incision	Short, proximal thigh or stab incision	Anterolateral groin
Special instrumentation	Guide wires; cannulated screws; image intensifier; ± fracture table	Image intensifier (recommended)
Unique considerations	Frequently bilateral (≤ 20%); often obese	⇐
Antibiotics	Cefazolin 1 g iv	⇐
Surgical time	0.5-2 h	1-3 h
Closing considerations	None	Frequently needs spica cast
EBL	Negligible	200-500 ml
Postop care	PACU → room	⇐ + Body spica cast, occasionally
Mortality	Minimal	⇐
Morbidity	Unsuspected pin penetration: ≤ 37%[4,7]	⇐
	Avascular necrosis: ≤ 33% (in acute slip cases)	⇐
	Chondrolysis, hip stiffness: 1-28%	⇐
	Fracture after pin removal: < 1%	⇐
	Infection: < 1%	⇐
Pain score	2-3	2-3

PATIENT POPULATION CHARACTERISTICS

Age range	10-16 yr
Male:Female	2-3:1
Incidence	1-3/100,000 (higher in African Americans)
Etiology	Excessive loading of the growth plate (obesity or increased angle of inclination of the physis) Insufficient tensile strength of collagen and proteoglycans around the femoral neck Increased thickness of the physis as from excessive growth hormone, hypogonadism, hypothyroidism, hyperparathyroidism, renal osteodystrophy, almost any other significant endocrinopathy Radiation therapy
Associated conditions	Obesity; endocrinopathies; renal osteodystrophy

ANESTHETIC CONSIDERATIONS

See Anesthetic Considerations for Pediatric Orthopedic Surgery of the Pelvis and Extremities, p. 1020.

References

1. Aadalen RJ, Weiner DS, Hoyt W, Herndon CH: Acute slipped capital femoral epiphysis. *J Bone Joint Surg* [Am] 1974; 56(7):1473-87.

2. Asnis SE: The guided screw system in slipped capital femoral epiphysis. *Contemp Orthop* 1985: 11:27-31.
3. Carlioz H, Vogt J, Barba L, Doursounian L: Treatment of slipped upper femoral epiphysis: 80 cases operated on over 10 years (1968-1978). *J Pediatr Orthop* 1984; 4(2):153-61.
4. Lehman WB, Menche D, Grant A, Norman A, Pugh J: The problem of evaluating *in situ* pinning of slipped capital femoral epiphysis: an experimental model and a review of 63 consecutive cases. *J Pediatr Orthop* 1984; 4(3):297-303.
5. Morrissy RT: *Atlas of Pediatric Orthopaedic Surgery*. JB Lippincott, Philadelphia: 1992, 212-44.
6. O'Brien ET, Fahey JJ: Remodeling of the femoral neck after *in situ* pinning for slipped capital femoral epiphysis. *J Bone Joint Surg* [Am] 1977; 59(1):62-8.
7. Tachdjian MO: *Pediatric Orthopaedics*. WB Saunders, Philadelphia: 1990, 1016-81.
8. Weiner DS, Weiner S, Melby A, Hoyt WA Jr: A 30-year experience with bone graft epiphysiodesis in the treatment of slipped capital femoral epiphysis. *J Pediatr Orthop* 1984; 4(2):145-52.

PROXIMAL FEMORAL OSTEOTOMY

SURGICAL CONSIDERATIONS

Description: Femoral osteotomy is performed in the inter- or subtrochanteric area in order to redirect the proximal femur more superiorly (valgus), or inferiorly (varus), and/or for rotational correction of excessive medial/femoral torsion (anteversion). A plate and screws are commonly used, but an **external fixator** and/or spica cast may be placed instead. The usual surgical approach is directly and laterally over the proximal shaft of the femur, beginning at the greater trochanter. The deep fascia is split and the underlying vastus muscle is elevated subperiosteally to expose the femoral shaft. Normally, a power saw is used to make the osteotomy; and, depending on the correction desired, there are a variety of internal fixation devices which can be used.

Variant procedure or approaches: Different named plates (e.g., AO blade, Coventry screw, Richards screw, Wagner, etc.) may be used to affix the proximal to the distal femoral segments.[1,2,5,6] A 1-4 cm segment of femur may be removed in cases of superior hip dislocation to allow soft-tissue relaxation and descent of the femoral head into the socket.[3] Most proximal femoral osteotomies are performed in the subtrochanteric area, but some are performed in the intertrochanteric or base of the neck (**Kramer compensating**).[4] The **Southwick osteotomy** is a more complicated example of a subtrochanteric osteotomy, which corrects for three directions (varus, lateral rotation and extension).[6]

Usual preop diagnosis: Developmental hip subluxation; excessive hip anteversion; residual deformity from Perthes disease; coxa vara; slipped capital femoral epiphysis (SCFE); residual deformity

SUMMARY OF PROCEDURE

	Varus Derotation Osteotomy with Plate and Screws	External Fixator	Southwick or Kramer
Position	Supine	⇐	⇐
Incision	Lateral thigh or, occasionally, long anterior thigh	⇐	⇐
Special instrumentation	Plate and screws; power drill and saw; image intensifier	External fixator; multiple pins; image intensifier	Plate and screws; power drill and saw; image intensifier
Unique considerations	Fracture or radiolucent table	⇐	⇐
Antibiotics	± Cefazolin 25 mg/kg iv	⇐	⇐
Surgical time	1.5-2.5 h	⇐	2-4 h
Closing considerations	Spica cast, frequently	± Spica cast	Spica cast, occasionally
EBL	250-750 ml	⇐	500-1000 ml
Postop care	PACU → room. Spica cast; nonweight-bearing ~6 wk; no full weight-bearing, 3 mo.	⇐	⇐

	Varus Derotation Osteotomy with Plate and Screws	External Fixator	Southwick or Kramer
Mortality	Minimal	⇐	⇐
Morbidity	Persistent hip dysplasia: 5-20% (depending on etiology)	⇐	⇐
	Excess blood loss from a perforating branch of the profunda femoris: < 1%	⇐	⇐
	Infection: < 1%	⇐	⇐
	Loss of fixation, instrument failure: < 1%	⇐	⇐
	Nonunion: < 1%	⇐	⇐
	Persistent hip stiffness: < 1%	⇐	⇐
	Avascular necrosis: Rare	⇐	⇐
Pain score	6-8	6-8	6-8

PATIENT POPULATION CHARACTERISTICS

Age range	2-21 yr
Male:Female	1:1
Incidence	Depending on diagnosis
Etiology	Coxa varum, coxa valgum due to muscle imbalance; hip dislocation; excessive medial femoral torsion (anteversion); osteochondrodystrophies (dwarfing syndromes); Perthes disease, SCFE
Associated conditions	Cerebral palsy; myelomeningocele, neuromyopathies; congenital hip dislocation; occasionally, hypothyroidism as a cause of SCFE

ANESTHETIC CONSIDERATIONS

See Anesthetic Considerations for Pediatric Orthopedic Surgery of the Pelvis and Extremities, p. 1020.

References

1. Alonso JE, Lovell WW, Lovejoy JF: The Altdorf hip clamp. *J Pediatr Orthop* 1986; 6(4):399-402.
2. Canale ST, Holand RW: Coventry screw fixation of osteotomies about the pediatric hip. *J Pediatr Orthop* 1983; 3(5):592-600.
3. Coleman SS: *Congenital Dysplasia and Dislocation of the Hip*. Mosby, St. Louis: 1978.
4. Kramer WG, Craig WA, Noel S: Compensating osteotomy at the base of the femoral neck for slipped capital femoral epiphysis. *J Bone Joint Surg* [Am] 1976; 58(6):796-800.
5. Morrissy RT: *Atlas of Pediatric Orthopaedic Surgery*. JB Lippincott, Philadelphia: 1992, 264-304.
6. Southwick WO: Osteotomy through the lesser trochanter for slipped capital femoral epiphysis. *J Bone Joint Surg* [Am] 1967; 49(5):807-35.

EPIPHYSIODESIS

SURGICAL CONSIDERATIONS

Description: Epiphysiodesis[1-7] is performed in skeletally immature adolescents to eliminate or retard growth of the longer limb in cases of leg-length discrepancy (anisomelia). The timing of the procedure[1,5,7] is critical, based on the child's bone age and discrepancy, which are plotted on a graph or computer program. The procedure is most commonly performed through small incisions (1") about the knee, centered on the growth plate (physis) of the distal femur or proximal tibia. The original **Phemister technique**[6] is an approach in which a 3/4"-1 1/4" square or rectangular block of bone is removed using a box chisel centered on the physis, visualized directly. The bone block is rotated 90° or 180° and reinserted, causing a bony bridge across the physis. **Blount**[2] subsequently used stout, reinforced staples to bracket the physis and "lock it." This provides theoretical advantage of reversibility (i.e., if staples are removed, growth may resume if the procedure was performed at too early an age). More recently, a **percutaneous technique** of simply drilling directly across the cartilaginous physeal growth plate, causing a bony bridge, has been used. This is accomplished through small stab incisions, under image intensifier control.[3]

Usual preop diagnosis: Limb-length discrepancies of 2-5 cm in adolescents (willing to accept a slight diminution in adult stature)

SUMMARY OF PROCEDURE

	Open Epiphysiodesis	Percutaneous Epiphysiodesis	Epiphyseal Stapling
Position	Supine, with tourniquet	Supine	Supine, with tourniquet
Incision	3-4 cm longitudinal incision, medial and laterally centered incisions over distal femoral and/or proximal tibial epiphysis	1 cm, same area as open epiphysiodesis	4-5 cm, same area as open epiphysiodesis
Special instrumentation	Box chisel	Drill point and sleeve	Heavy, reinforced staples
Unique considerations	Tourniquet used	Image intensifier control mandatory; tourniquet (optional)	⇐
Antibiotics	± Cefazolin 25 mg/kg iv	⇐	⇐
Surgical time	1 h	⇐	⇐
Closing considerations	Cylinder cast or knee immobilizer	⇐	⇐
EBL	< 50 ml	⇐	⇐
Postop care	PACU → room; crutches for comfort	⇐	⇐
Mortality	Minimal	⇐	⇐
Morbidity	Under- or overcorrection with regard to length: 5-10%	⇐	⇐
	Wound problems: < 5%	⇐	⇐
	Asymmetric growth arrest → valgus or varus deformity: 2-5%	⇐	⇐
	Anterior or lateral compartment syndrome: 1%	–	–
	Fracture: 1%	–	–
	Peroneal palsy: < 1%	–	–
Pain score	3-5	2-3	3-5

PATIENT POPULATION CHARACTERISTICS

Age range	9-14 yr (adolescents, usually healthy with limb-length discrepancy 2-6 cm)
Male:Female	1:1
Incidence	< 1/1000
Etiology	Idiopathic hemihypertrophy; neurologic (e.g., polio, hemiplegia); congenital deformities of the lower extremities (e.g., congenitally short femur, fibular hemimelia); osteomyelitis; development of tumorous conditions (e.g., enchondromatosis); traumatic growth plate injuries occurring near puberty; epiphyseal problems related to hip (slipped epiphysis, sequelae of Perthes disease); Klippel-Trenaunay-Weber syndrome
Associated conditions	Other contractures in neurologic conditions (e.g., polio); neurofibromatosis, AV fistulae; Wilms' tumor (rare)

ANESTHETIC CONSIDERATIONS

See Anesthetic Considerations for Pediatric Orthopedic Surgery of the Pelvis and Extremities, p. 1020.

References

1. Blair VP III, Walker SJ, Sheridan JJ, Schoenecker PL: Epiphysiodesis: a problem of timing. *J Pediatr Orthop* 1982; 2(3):281-4.
2. Blount WP, Clarke GR: Control of bone growth by epiphyseal stapling. *J Bone Joint Surg* [Am] 1949; 31:464-78.
3. Liotta FJ, Ambrose TA II, Eilert RE: Fluoroscopic technique vs Phemister technique for epiphysiodesis. *J Pediatr Orthop* 1992; 12(2):248-51.
4. Mayhall WST: Leg length discrepancy treated by epiphysiodesis. *Orthopaedics Rev* 1978; 7:441-4.
5. Moseley CF: A straight line graft for leg length discrepancies. *Clin Orthop* 1978; 136:33-40.
6. Phemister DB: Operative arrestment of longitudinal growth of bones in the treatment of deformities. *J Bone Joint Surg* 1933; [Am] 15:1-15.
7. Stephens DC, Herrick W, MacEwen GD: Epiphysiodesis for limb length inequality: results and indication. *Clin Orthop* 1978; 136:41-8.

SOFIELD PROCEDURE

SURGICAL CONSIDERATIONS

Description: The **Sofield procedure**, or "**fragmentation rodding**," is most commonly performed for deformity of the long bone, and to prevent recurrent fracture, usually a result of osteogenesis imperfecta.[1-3,5,6] The procedure involves exposure of at least one end and a varying amount of the bony shaft. If the deformity is severe, the entire shaft is exposed via a longitudinal incision, usually laterally. The bone is divided (osteotomized) into the minimum number of segments that will allow a straight intramedullary rod to traverse the segments (usually 2-4 osteotomies). The construct is justly referred to as a "shish-ka-bab." It is needed less frequently in the upper extremities.

Variant procedure or approaches: Because a growing bone will elongate beyond the end of a simple intramedullary rod after 1-2 yr, the resulting unsupported portion of the bone will be liable to fracture or new deformity. To obviate this problem, **Bailey** and **Dubow** developed an **elongating rod system**,[1] consisting of an outer tubular rod sleeve (the female portion) and an inner obturator portion (male). Both ends of the telescoping rod are anchored in the ends of the bones. The system elongates much like a car radio antenna and decreases the need for frequent revisions. The surgical technique is, however, identical to any fragmentation rodding, except that both ends of the bone must be exposed.

Usual preop diagnosis: Osteogenesis imperfecta; fibrous dysplasia (occasionally); rickets; congenital pseudarthrosis of the tibia

SUMMARY OF PROCEDURE

Position	Supine
Incision	Lateral for femur; anterolateral for tibia
Special instrumentation	± Image intensifier table
Unique considerations	Tendency to hyperthermia; other bones may fracture in more severe cases, even as a result of a BP cuff. If dentinogenesis imperfecta is present, extreme care should be taken during intubation to prevent tooth trauma. In these patients, neck motion is often limited.
Antibiotics	Cefazolin 25 mg/kg iv
Surgical time	1-1.5 h/tibia; 1.5-2.5 h/femur (often done sequentially on the same day)
Closing considerations	Double spica cast if femur is rodded.
EBL	Depending on age and size, as well as use of a tourniquet for the femur, 50-250 ml; for the tibia, 50-100 ml
Postop care	PACU → room; avoid trauma to teeth, mouth or other bones in PACU.
Mortality	< 1% (usually related to severe restrictive lung disease, in the most severely involved cases[1-3,5])

Morbidity	Intraop hyperthermia: Common Intraop fracture of other bones or teeth Late rod migration: Common Late refracture: Common Nonunion: Rare Exuberant callus simulating osteosarcoma: Rare Infection: < 1% of rodding Radial nerve palsy (in cases of humerus or radius rodding)
Pain score	2-3 (It is surprising how little discomfort these children have, especially the 2nd or 3rd time a bone is rodded.)

PATIENT POPULATION CHARACTERISTICS

Age range	2-25 yr
Male:Female	1:1
Incidence	1/20,000 (osteogenesis imperfecta); other etiologies much less common
Etiology	Congenital (hereditary deficit in collagen synthesis) most commonly as autosomal dominant or spontaneous mutation): All cases
Associated conditions	Dentinogenesis imperfecta; diminished vital capacity due to associated kyphoscoliosis; decreased hearing due to otosclerosis and impingement of the 8th cranial nerve; pelvic distortion causing chronic constipation; basilar impression and other C-spine abnormalities[4] causing brain stem compression or even hydrocephalus (rare)

ANESTHETIC CONSIDERATIONS

See Anesthetic Considerations for Pediatric Orthopedic Surgery of the Pelvis and Extremities, p. 1020.

References

1. Bailey RW, Dubow HI: Evolution of the concept of an extensible nail accommodating to normal longitudinal bone growth: clinical considerations and implications. *Clin Orthop* 1981, 159:157-70.
2. Gamble JG, Strudwick WJ, Rinsky LA, Bleck EE: Complications of intramedullary rods in osteogenesis imperfecta: Bailey-Dubow rods versus non-elongating rods. *J Pediatr Orthop* 1988; 8(6):645-49.
3. Marafioti RL, Westin GW: Elongating intramedullary rods in the treatment of osteogenesis imperfecta. *J Bone Joint Surg* [Am] 1977; 59(4):467-72.
4. Pozo JL, Crockard HA, Ransford AO: Basilar impression in osteogenesis imperfecta. A report of three cases in one family. *J Bone Joint Surg* [Br] 1984; 66(2):233-38.
5. Rodriquez RP, Bailey RW: Internal fixation of the femur in patients with osteogenesis imperfecta. *Clin Orthop* 1988; 159:126-33.
6. Sofield HA, Millar EA: Fragmentation, realignment and intramedullary rod fixation of deformities of the long bones in children. A ten-year appraisal. *J Bone Joint Surg* [Am] 1959; 41:1371-91.

LIMB LENGTHENING

SURGICAL CONSIDERATIONS

Description: Limb lengthening usually is performed in the lower extremity for congenital or acquired leg-length discrepancies of at least 5 cm.[1-8] Lesser discrepancies are dealt with by bone shortening or epiphysiodesis of the long side. The basic principles include: (1) application of an adjustable, external fixator; (2) "low-energy," transverse bone cut (osteotomy without use of a power saw) through a small, longitudinal incision over the involved bone; (3) preservation of the periosteal sleeve; (4) gradual lengthening, usually 1 mm/day in fractional adjustments; and (5) when desired limb length is obtained, either use bone graft and plate acutely, or leave until the bone gap fills in and stabilizes (average 38 d/cm gained).[5]

Limb lengthening dates back to the early 1900s; but it fell into disfavor because of the high rate of major complications.[1-2] **Wagner** improved the technique by introducing a simplified, unilateral, large-pin fixator, but performed the osteotomy in the midshaft and began lengthening immediately[3-7] (Fig 12.6-10). This technique usually requires a bone graft and later plating as a second operation, to obtain healing. **DeBastiani** uses a similar large-pin fixator (**Orthofix**), but performs the osteotomy more toward the end of the bone (metaphysis), and waits a week before beginning the lengthening.[5] Spontaneous healing is usual. **Ilizarov** introduced a more complex, but more adaptable, small-pin transfixation system with a circular fixator.[4] In a similar fashion, the Ilizarov method stretches the healing callus[4] (callostasis). Typically, 4-10 cm/bone are gained with any of the above techniques.

Usual preop diagnosis: Congenital or acquired anisomelia (limb-length discrepancy) due to overgrowth or growth retardation > 5 cm

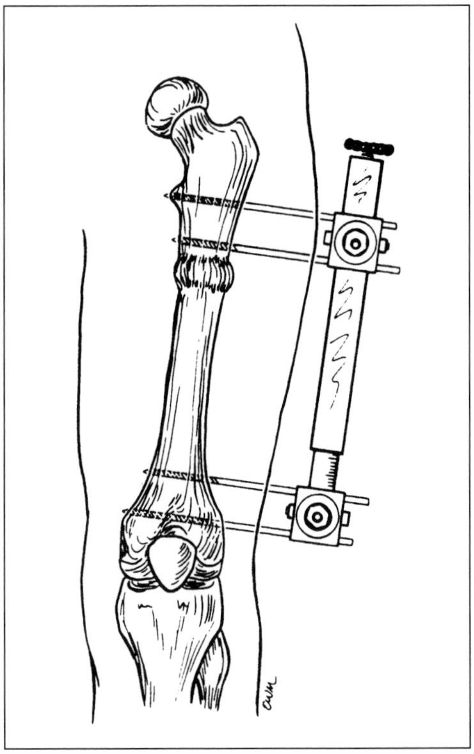

Figure 12.6-10. Wagner apparatus for leg lengthening. (Reproduced with permission from Chapman MW, ed: *Operative Orthopaedics*, 2nd edition. JB Lippincott: 1993.)

SUMMARY OF PROCEDURE

	Wagner	Orthofix	Ilizarov
Position	Supine	⇐	⇐
Incision	Longitudinal midshaft	Longitudinal proximal shaft (metaphyseal)	⇐
Special instrumentation	Image intensifier; Wagner device (Fig 12.6-10); large bone pins	Image intensifier; Orthofix device; large bone pins	Ilizarov frame ("Erector set"); multiple 1.5-1.8 mm small-diameter wires
Unique considerations	Acute lengthening may cause ↑BP.	–	Frame should be prepped prior to surgery because of "fiddle factor."
Antibiotics	Cefazolin 25 mg/kg iv	⇐	⇐
Surgical time	1-2 h	⇐	2-4 h
EBL	< 100 ml	⇐	⇐
Postop care	PACU → room; early initiation of physical therapy and/ or continuous passive motion (CPM) machine	⇐	⇐
Mortality	Minimal	⇐	⇐
Morbidity	While device remains in place, at least one of the following complications is usual; frequently, several occur before healing is complete:[3,6]	⇐	⇐
	Joint stiffness or localized pin infection: Very common - 50% (temporary)	⇐	⇐

	Wagner	Orthofix	Ilizarov
Morbidity, cont.	Edema, swelling, pressure sores: Common	⇐	⇐
	Joint subluxation: Common	⇐	⇐
	Psychological decompensation due to pain: Common	⇐	⇐
	Premature consolidation: Common	⇐	⇐
	Skin necrosis: Common	⇐	⇐
	Wound infection: Common	⇐	⇐
	Localized osteomyelitis: Common	⇐	⇐
	Axial deviation of the bone: Common	⇐	⇐
	Delayed union, nonunion, late fracture: Common	⇐	⇐
	Pin penetration of a vessel or nerve: Rare	⇐	⇐
	Compartment syndrome: Rare	⇐	⇐
	Sudeck's atrophy: Rare	⇐	⇐
Pain score	7-8	7-8	7-8

PATIENT POPULATION CHARACTERISTICS

Age range	10-30 yr
Male:Female	1:1
Incidence	Dependent on underlying diagnosis (common in polio)
Etiology	Congenital deficiencies of the lower extremities (e.g., proximal focal femoral deficiency, congenitally short femur, fibular hemimelia, etc.); osteomyelitis, traumatic growth plate injury, fracture; asymmetric neurologic conditions (e.g., polio or cerebral palsy); congenital hemihypertrophy
Associated conditions	Hip and knee contractures; in cases of polio, other deformities and weaknesses; arteriovenous malformations (AVMs); congenital or developmental hip dislocation

ANESTHETIC CONSIDERATIONS

See Anesthetic Considerations for Pediatric Orthopedic Surgery of the Pelvis and Extremities, p. 1020.

References

1. Abbott LC: The operative lengthening of the tibia and fibula. *J Bone Joint Surg* [Am] 1927; 9:128-52.
2. Anderson WV: Leg lengthening. *J Bone Joint Surg* [Br] 1952; 34:150.
3. Coleman SS, Stevens PM: Tibial lengthening. *Clin Orthop* 1978; 136:92-104.
4. Dal Monte A, Donzelli O: Tibial lengthening according to Ilizarov in congenital hypoplasia of the leg. *J Pediatr Orthop* 1987; 7(2):135-38.
5. DeBastiani G, Aldegheai R, Renzi-Briviol, Trivella G: Limb lengthening by callus distraction (callotasis). *J Pediatr Orthop* 1987; 7(2):129-34.
6. Tachdjian MO: *Pediatric Orthopaedics*. WB Saunders, Philadelphia: 1990, 2895-3012.
7. Wagner H: Operative lengthening of the femur. *Clin Orthop* 1978; 136:125-42.

PATELLAR REALIGNMENT

SURGICAL CONSIDERATIONS

Description: Patellar realignment encompasses over 100 procedures designed to prevent lateral subluxation and dislocation of the patella.[1-10] These disorders include a spectrum of malalignments of the patella, ranging from simple excess lateral tilt, recurrent partial subluxation, and recurrent episodic dislocation, to irreducible chronic dislocation.[9] As such, the surgical procedures also encompass a spectrum of complexities, depending on the degree of instability. Nowadays, an arthroscopic inspection often is performed first. The basic principles of the repair include both proximal and distal realignment.[2-9] **Proximal realignment** includes: (1) lateral release, which is the division of the contracted lateral patellar retinacular joint capsule and other tight lateral tissue—the first step in all surgical repair—(2) medial tightening, including reefing and/or advancement of the medial capsule and vastus medialis muscle insertion; and (3) **distal realignment**, consisting of redirection of the patellar tendon more medially (and sometimes more anteriorly).

Variant procedure or approaches: Arthroscopic or open lateral release is the simplest and first-step procedure. It may be sufficient when there is only subluxation and not true dislocation; and it has the advantage of being an outpatient procedure. For frank dislocation, an open "proximal realignment" also includes the medial tautening. If this is not sufficient to hold the patella centralized, and if the patient has open epiphyses (< 16 yr), the lateral half of the patellar tendon may be released (distal realignment) and reattached medially (**Roux-Goldthwait**); or the patella may be held medially by tenodesing the semitendinosis tendon to it.[1,8] In skeletally mature patients, the bony insertion of the patellar tendon is osteotomized and transferred medially (**Trillat**),[4] or anteriomedially (**Macquet**).[7] The **Hauser procedure** of distal and medial transfer of the tibial tubercle has had a very poor long-term outcome and is seldom performed.

Usual preop diagnosis: Lateral patellar subluxation; recurrent dislocation; congenital or chronic lateral patellar dislocation

SUMMARY OF PROCEDURE

	Proximal Realignment	Trillat	Macquet
Position	Supine, with tourniquet	⇐	⇐
Incision	Anterior transverse or longitudinal or oblique, about the knee or arthroscopic	Anterior longitudinal	Transverse or oblique
Special instrumentation	None	Single bone screw	⇐
Unique considerations	Tourniquet	⇐	May use iliac or bank bone graft.
Antibiotics	Optional, cefazolin 25 mg/kg iv	Usually, cefazolin 25 mg/kg iv	⇐
Surgical time	1.5 h	1-2 h	⇐
Closing considerations	Cylinder cast	⇐	Skin closure may be difficult, depending on elevation of tibial tubercle.
Postop care	PACU → home, if arthroscopic	PACU → room	⇐
EBL	< 100 ml	⇐	⇐
Mortality	Minimal	⇐	⇐
Morbidity	Recurrence: 5-10%	⇐	⇐
	Late stiffness or increased knee pain: 5%	⇐	⇐
	Superficial wound dehiscence or infection: ≤ 5%	> 5%	≤ 5%
	Anterior compartment syndrome of the leg (Hauser procedure): 1-5%	⇐	⇐
	Deep infection: 1-2%	⇐	⇐
	Peroneal palsy: < 1%	⇐	⇐
Pain score	4-6	4-6	4-6

PATIENT POPULATION CHARACTERISTICS

Age range	2-20 yr (most commonly, 13-20 yr)
Male:Female	1:3[2]
Incidence	Subluxation: Very common Recurrent dislocation: Rare Congenital dislocation: Very rare[9]
Etiology	Generalized ligamentous laxity; familial tendency, congenital hypoplasia at a lateral femoral condyle; abnormal attachment or contracture of the IT band; medial femoral torsion or genu valgum; trauma
Associated conditions	Diffuse hyperlaxity syndromes (Ehlers-Danlos, Marfan, etc.); nail patella syndrome (hypoplastic nails and dislocated radial heads, as well as hypoplastic patellae)

ANESTHETIC CONSIDERATIONS

See Anesthetic Considerations for Pediatric Orthopedic Surgery of the Pelvis and Extremities, p. 1020.

References

1. Baker RH, Carroll N, Dewar FP, Hall JE: The Semitendinosus Tenodesis for recurrent dislocation of the patella. *J Bone Joint Surg* [Br] 1972; 54(1):103-9.
2. Bowker JH, Thompson EB: Surgical treatment of recurrent dislocation of the patella. A study of forty-eight cases. *J Bone Joint Surg* [Am] 1964; 46:1451-61.
3. Chrisman OD, Snook GA, Wilson TC: A long-term perspective study of the Hauser and Roux-Goldthwait procedures for recurrent patellar dislocation. *Clin Orthop* 1979; 144:27-30.
4. Cox JS: Evaluation of the Roux-Elmslie-Trillat procedure for knee extensor realignment. *Am J Sports* Med 1982; 10(5):303-10.
5. Fondren FB, Goldner JL, Bassett FH III: Recurrent dislocation of the patella treated by the modified Roux-Goldthwait procedure. A prospective study of forty-seven knees. *J Bone Joint Surg* [Am] 1985; 67(7):993-1005.
6. Hughston J, Walsh WM: Proximal and distal reconstruction of the extensor mechanism for patellar subluxation. *Clin Orthop* 1979; 144:36-42.
7. Maquet P: Mechanics and osteoarthritis of the patellofemoral joint. *Clin Orthop* 1979; 144:70-3.
8. Morrissy RT: *Atlas of Pediatric Orthopaedic Surgery*. JB Lippincott, Philadelphia: 1992, 425-38.
9. Tachdjian MO: *Pediatric Orthopaedics*. WB Saunders, Philadelphia: 1990, 1551-95.
10. Trillat A, DeJour H, Louette A: Diagnostic et traitement des subluxations récidiventes de la rotule. *Rev Chir Orthop* 1964; 50:813-24.
11. Wall JJ: Compartment syndrome as a complication of the Hauser procedure. *J Bone Joint Surg* [Am] 1979; 61(2):185-91.

TENDON TRANSFER, LENGTHENING (POSTERIOR TIBIAL)

SURGICAL CONSIDERATIONS

Description: Extremity tendons may be lengthened (for contracture) or transferred to change the muscle force vector and compensate for paralysis or paresis of other muscle groups.[1,6] Originally used for the treatment of poliomyelitis sequelae, such lengthenings and transfers are now used for a variety of deformities 2° more common neuromuscular disorders such as cerebral palsy, muscular dystrophies, Charcot-Marie-Tooth disease, traumatic nerve palsies, etc. Basic principles are that the muscles to be transferred should be at least grade 4/5 strength, and that the loss of normal function should be well compensated. The posterior tibial muscle (PTM) is a representative example, but many extremity muscles have one or more described lengthenings or transfers. Such procedures frequently are combined with other transfers or fusions.

For moderate spastic ankle varus, the simplest procedure, **PTM lengthening**, is accomplished by an intramuscular myotendinous "slide." This refers to simply cutting the tendinous fibers well within the distal muscle belly and leaving a small gap in the tendon, while the surrounding muscle fibers remain intact.[6] An alternative for spastic varus is the **split posterior tibial transfer** of the PTM.[1,4] Four short, 2 to 3 cm incisions are used to expose and dissect 1/2 of the posterior tibia tendon at its insertion on the navicular. Then, 1/2 of the tendon is passed proximally up its sheath to a second incision just posterior to the distal tibial shaft medially. The freed 1/2 tendon is passed laterally to the peroneal tendon sheath just distal to the lateral malleolus, where, through a final incision, the tendon is anastomosed to the peroneus brevis.

For complete flaccid foot drop (e.g., peroneal nerve palsy), the entire posterior tibial tendon is transferred.[4,5] First, it is detached at its medial insertion, delivered proximally at the distal tibia posteriorly, passed **anteriorly** through a window in the interosseous membrane, and then subcutaneously passed to the mid-dorsal surface of the foot, where it is fixed into the middle cuneiform by a pull-out stitch.

Usual preop diagnosis: Flaccid or spastic developmental deformity such as varus or valgus foot neuromuscular disease

SUMMARY OF PROCEDURE

	Lengthening	Split Transfer	Anterior Transfer
Position	Supine	⇐	⇐
Incision	Longitudinal posteromedial calf	Medial foot; posteromedial calf; lateral ankle; lateral foot	Medial foot; posteromedial calf; anterior ankle; dorsal foot
Special instrumentation	None	Tendon passer	Pull-out suture; buttons
Unique considerations	Underlying neurologic disease. Usually added to other procedures (e.g., Achilles tendon lengthenings.)	⇐	⇐
Antibiotics	Usually none	⇐	⇐
Surgical time	30 min	1 h	⇐
Closing considerations	Below-knee cast	⇐	⇐
EBL	< 20 ml	< 50 ml	⇐
Postop care	PACU or room	⇐	⇐
Mortality	Rare	⇐	⇐
Morbidity	Over- or undercorrection	⇐	⇐
	Hematoma	⇐	⇐
	Drainage: < 1%	⇐	⇐
Pain score	1-3	3-4	3-4

PATIENT POPULATION CHARACTERISTICS

Age range	3-30 yr
Male:Female	1:1
Incidence	Dependent on diagnosis
Etiology	Poliomyelitis; cerebral palsy, spina bifida; traumatic peroneal nerve injury; neuropathies, myopathies (e.g., Charcot-Marie-Tooth disease)
Associated conditions	Multiple other contractures

ANESTHETIC CONSIDERATIONS

See Anesthetic Considerations for Pediatric Orthopedic Surgery of the Pelvis and Extremities, p. 1020.

References

1. Green NE, Griffin PP, Shiavi R: Split posterior tibial-tendon transfers in spastic cerebral palsy. *J Bone Joint Surg* [Am] 1983; 65(6):748-54.
2. Hoffer MD, Barakat G, Koffman M: 10-year follow-up of split anterior tibial tendon transfer in cerebral palsied patients with spastic equinovarus deformity. *J Pediatr Orthop* 1985; 5(4):432-34.

3. Miller G, Hsu JD, Hoffer MM, Rentfro R: Posterior tibial tendon transfer: a review of the literature and analysis of 74 procedures. *J Pediatr Orthop* 1982; 2(4):363-70.
4. Morrissy RT: *Atlas of Pediatric Orthopaedic Surgery*. JB Lippincott, Philadelphia: 1992, 645-68.
5. Richards BM: Interosseous transfer of tibialis posterior for common peroneal nerve palsy. *J Bone Joint Surg* [Br] 1989; 71(5):834-37.
6. Ruda R, Frost HM: Cerebral palsy. Spastic varus and forefoot adductus, treated by intramuscular posterior tibial tendon lengthening. *Clin Orthop* 1971; 79:61-70.

TRIPLE ARTHRODESIS AND GRICE PROCEDURE (EXTRAARTICULAR SUBTALAR ARTHRODESIS)

SURGICAL CONSIDERATIONS

Description: Triple arthrodesis is used to realign the hind foot of skeletally mature patients with significant fixed or flexible deformities of multiple etiologies. The technique involves denuding the cartilaginous surfaces of the talonavicular, talocalcaneal (subtalar) and calcaneocuboid joints and fusing them.[1-5] The approach is always through an oblique lateral sinus tarsi incision and often an additional short medial incision over the talonavicular joint. For supple (passively correctable) deformities, the fusion is performed easily *in situ*. Fixed deformities are more difficult; but, basically, any deformity (valgus, varus, planus, cavus, etc.) can be corrected by resecting appropriate wedges of bone. Fixation is usually internal with pins, screws or staples, in addition to an external cast.

Variant procedure or approaches: Because the triple arthrodesis removes growth cartilage, it is unsuitable in growing children (< 12-14 years). **Grice** developed an **extraarticular subtalar fusion** which can be performed as early as age 3. It is basically a block of autologous bone graft placed between the talus and the calcaneus to stabilize a valgus heel. Tibial, fibular or, preferably, iliac autologous graft is used through the same lateral sinus tarsi incision as for a triple arthrodesis.

Usual preop diagnosis: Varus or cavovarus foot deformities; severe valgus or equinovalgus

SUMMARY OF PROCEDURE

	Triple Arthrodesis	Grice Procedure
Position	Supine, slightly tilted up on the operative side	⇐
Incision	2" oblique over the sinus tarsi; optional medial incision	⇐
Special instrumentation	Pins, screws or rods	Pin or screw
Unique considerations	Intraop x-ray to confirm pin position	Iliac or tibial autologous graft
Antibiotics	Usually, cefazolin 1 g iv	Cefazolin 25 mg/kg iv
Surgical time	1-2 h	1.5 h
Closing considerations	Above-the-knee cast	⇐
EBL	< 100 ml	< 50 ml
Postop care	PACU → room	⇐
Mortality	Rare	⇐
Morbidity	Superficial skin slough	⇐
	Superficial infection	⇐
	Nonunion of at least one arthrodesis site (usually talonavicular)	⇐
	Aseptic necrosis of the talus: Rare	⇐
Pain score	6-8	4-5

PATIENT POPULATION CHARACTERISTICS

	Triple Arthrodesis	Grice Procedure
Age range	> 12 yr	3-10 yr
Male:Female	1:1	⇐
Incidence	< 1% (depends on diagnosis and severity of deformity)	⇐
Etiology	Neuromuscular imbalance: Most cases	⇐
	Congenital malformations (e.g., coalitions, severe pes planus)	⇐
	Incompletely treated or overcorrected clubfoot	⇐
	Postfracture of calcaneus or talus	⇐
Associated conditions	Poliomyelitis	⇐
	Cerebral palsy: ↑GE reflux, ↓airway protective reflexes, ↑postop pulmonary complications	⇐
	Myelomeningocele	⇐
	Charcot-Marie-Tooth disease: ↑sensitivity to muscle relaxants	⇐
	Congenital tarsal coalition	⇐

ANESTHETIC CONSIDERATIONS

See Anesthetic Considerations for Pediatric Orthopedic Surgery of the Pelvis and Extremities, p. 1020.

References

1. Chapman MW: *Operative Orthopaedics*, 2nd edition. JB Lippincott, Philadelphia: 1993, 2272-74.
2. Dennyson WG, Fulford GE: Subtalar arthrodesis by cancellous grafts and metallic internal fixation. *J Bone Joint Surg* [Br] 1976; 58(4):507-10.
3. Duncan JW, Lovell WW: Hoke triple arthrodesis. *J Bone Joint Surg* [Am] 1978; 60(6):795-98.
4. Grice DS: An extra-articular arthrodesis of the subastragalar joint for correction of paralytic flat feet in children. *J Bone Joint Surg* [Am] 1952; 34:927-40.
5. Morrissy RT: *Atlas of Pediatric Orthopaedic Surgery*. JB Lippincott, Philadelphia: 1992, 589-99.

TURCO, SURGICAL CORRECTION OF CLUBFOOT

SURGICAL CONSIDERATIONS

Description: Turco popularized the one-stage surgical correction of resistant (uncorrected by casting) clubfoot in 1971. The orthopedic literature, however, is replete with reports of varying techniques for surgical correction of clubfoot (talipes equinovarus). The three components of the deformity are: (1) hindfoot equinus (back of the heel is up); (2) varus (rolled inwardly); and (3) forefoot adductus (medial deviation). Beyond this, however, there exists considerable disagreement as to the pathologic anatomy, ideal skin incision, position, and which structures to release. Most surgeons vary the degree of release in proportion to the degree of deformity, often performing release of the same deep structures through totally different skin incisions. The most important structures released include: the entire posterior capsule of the ankle and subtalar joint; capsule of the subtalar, talonavicular and calcaneal cuboid joints; tendo-Achilles, posterior tibial tendon, and usually the toe flexors; and origin of the abductor, halluces and the plantar fascia. The navicular is repositioned on the talus and usually held with a small pin.

Variant procedure or approaches: **Turco's procedure**[10,11] is essentially a posteromedial procedure only and is performed through one incision on the medial aspect of the foot. **Crawford**[3] described a much more extensile approach through an incision (**Cincinnati**) that runs from anteromedial, around the back of the tendo-Achilles, and then anterolateral to the calcaneal cuboid joint. This approach is also used by **McKay**[5], **Simons**[7,8] and others for a more complete release. If there is severe equinus deformity, however, the incision is difficult to close posteriorly when the foot is brought up. **Carroll**[2] accomplishes much the same correction using a separate medial and posterolateral incision.

Usual preop diagnosis: Resistant idiopathic clubfoot; secondary clubfoot due to paralysis

SUMMARY OF PROCEDURE

	Turco	Cincinnati/McKay/Simons	Carroll
Position	Supine	Prone or supine	Supine
Incision	Straight medial foot	Transverse from the navicular bone medially-posteriorly across the heel cord, then laterally to the cuboid	Medial zigzag and posterolateral longitudinal
Special instrumentation	Usually loupe magnification; small K wires to hold reduction	⇐	⇐
Unique considerations	Tourniquet mandatory and often bilateral	⇐	⇐
Antibiotics	Cefazolin 25 mg/kg iv	⇐	⇐
Surgical time	1-2 h/foot	⇐	⇐
Closing considerations	Well padded, loose-fitting, above-the-knee cast × 10-14 d	⇐	⇐
EBL	< 30 ml	⇐	⇐
Postop care	PACU → room	⇐	⇐
Mortality	Rare	⇐	⇐
Morbidity[5-11]	Mild, persistent deformity: Very common Hematoma: 2% Superficial infection: 1-2% Avascular necrosis Overcorrection valgus, planus Pressure changes of the navicular Wound dehiscence or necrosis Transection of posterior tibial nerve or artery branch (rare, except in previously multiple-operated patient)	⇐	⇐
Pain score	2-5	2-5	2-5

PATIENT POPULATION CHARACTERISTICS

Age range	3 mo-6 yr
Male:Female	2:1 (idiopathic type)
Incidence	1.2/1000 live births (idiopathic type[9])
Etiology	Genetic, or hereditary effects; neuromuscular defects of the calf muscles; primary defect of formation of the talus and/or other tarsal bones; shortened ligaments and muscles
Associated conditions	Arthrogryposis (difficult intubation; ± VSD, other CHD); Larsen's syndrome (difficult intubation; ± ↑ICP); Freeman-Sheldon syndrome (difficult intubation); osteochondral dystrophies (e.g., diastrophic dwarfism); spinal dysraphism; tethered spinal cord; congenital constricting bands; poliomyelitis

ANESTHETIC CONSIDERATIONS

See Anesthetic Considerations for Pediatric Orthopedic Surgery of the Pelvis and Extremities, below.

References

1. Beat JH: Congenital anomalies of the lower extremity. In *Campbell's Operative Orthopaedics*, 8th edition. Crenshaw AH, ed. Mosby Year Book, St. Louis: 1992, 2075-91.
2. Carroll NC: Congenital clubfoot: pathoanatomy and treatment. *AAOS Instr Course Lect* 1987; 36:117-21.
3. Crawford AH, Marxen JL, Osterfeld DL: The Cincinnati incision: a comprehensive approach for surgical procedures of the foot and ankle in childhood. *J Bone Joint Surg* [Am] 1982; 64(9):1355-58.
4. Lichtblau S: A medial and lateral release operation for clubfoot. *J Bone Joint Surg* [Am] 1973; 55(7):1377-84.
5. McKay DW: New concept of and approach to club foot treatment: Section II – correction of the club foot. *J Pediatr Orthop* 1983; 3(1):10-21.
6. Morrissy RT: *Atlas of Pediatric Orthopaedic Surgery*. JB Lippincott, Philadelphia: 1992, 523-28.
7. Simons GW: Complete subtalar release in clubfeet: Part I – a preliminary report. *J Bone Joint Surg* [Am] 1985 67(7):1044-55.
8. Simons GW: Complete subtalar release in clubfeet: Part II – comparison with less extensive procedures. *J Bone Joint Surg* [Am] 1985; 67(7):1056-65.
9. Tachdjian MO: *Pediatric Orthopaedics*. WB Saunders Co, Philadelphia: 1990, 2428-57.
10. Turco VJ: Resistant congenital club foot - one-stage posteromedial release with internal fixation. A follow-up report of a fifteen-year experience. *J Bone Joint Surg* [Am] 1979; 61(6A):805-14.
11. Turco VJ: Surgical correction of the resistant club foot. One-stage posteromedial release with internal fixation: a preliminary report. *J Bone Joint Surg* [Am] 1971; 53(3):477-97.

ANESTHETIC CONSIDERATIONS FOR PEDIATRIC ORTHOPEDIC SURGERY OF THE PELVIS AND EXTREMITIES

(Procedures covered: pelvic osteotomy; acetabular augmentation & Chiari osteotomy; Ober fasciotomy; Yount Ober release; hip, open reduction; adductor release and/or transfer; psoas release; pinning of SCFE; femoral osteotomy; epiphysiodesis; Sofield procedure; limb lengthening; tendon transfer or lengthening; triple arthrodesis, Grice procedure; Turco procedure)

PREOPERATIVE

Children undergoing orthopedic procedures of the extremities typically fall into two groups: (1) post trauma but otherwise healthy; and (2) those with a variety of chronic medical problems, including cerebral palsy, congenital hip dislocation, limb deformities, osteogenesis imperfecta, juvenile rheumatoid arthritis, epidermolysis bullosa, various myopathies and muscular dystrophies. The anesthesiologist should review the anesthetic implications of these various syndromes or diseases (see Table 12.6-1). Many of these patients will have cardiac, respiratory, endocrine and metabolic derangements, as well as airway abnormalities that may affect anesthetic management. In addition, the surgical procedures may run the gamut from a simple syndactyly repair of the fingers with little blood loss to pelvic osteotomies (in small children) with blood loss approaching patient blood volume.

Respiratory Patient's preop activity level is a good indication for baseline respiratory function. Careful assessment is necessary as associated anomalies may affect airway or lungs. Chronic otitis 2° eustachian tube dysfunction is common. Treat with antibiotics before surgery. Postpone surgery (~2 wk) if Sx of acute URI (e.g., runny nose, fever, sore throat, cough) are present.
Tests: As indicated from H&P.

Cardiovascular Some pediatric patients with congenital musculoskeletal anomalies presenting for orthopedic procedures have coexisting cardiovascular anomalies. Although this is not common, preop review of patient's H&P is essential. Patients should not be accepted for orthopedic surgery and anesthesia until they are in the best possible physical and emotional condition. For children with CHD or who require cardiac medication, it is advisable to consult with a pediatric cardiologist before surgery.
★ **NB:** The consequences of VAE may be disastrous (e.g., cerebral or myocardial embolization) in patients with R→L shunt lesions. All iv lines, injection ports and syringes should be air-free.
Tests: ECG; Hct; baseline O_2 saturation; chest radiograph, as necessary

Neurological For patients with cerebral palsy presenting for orthopedic surgery, preop understanding of their intellectual functional capacity is necessary. Information about patient's behavioral or intellectual

Table 12.6-1. Preop Anesthesia Considerations for Pediatric Orthopedic Diseases

Disease	Anesthesia Considerations
Klippel-Feil syndrome	Limited cervical spine mobility; CHD
Septic arthritis	Systemic infection
Apert's syndrome	Hypoplastic maxilla → difficult airway management, ↑ICP, CHD
Marfan syndrome	Aortic dilation → aortic insufficiency; aortic dissection and aneurysm. Avoid ↑BP. Anticipate difficult intubation 2° narrow palate; lung cysts → pneumothorax.
Osteogenesis imperfecta	Bones fracture easily (e.g., with BP cuff): use extreme care in positioning and intubation. Hypermetabolic fever during anesthesia; Plt dysfunction; CHD; difficult airway.
Achondroplasia	Restrictive lung disease; poor cervical mobility. Anticipate difficult intubation.
Muscular dystrophy	↑sensitivity to muscle relaxant; ↑MH susceptibility. Avoid succinylcholine. May have MVR and cardiac conduction abnormalities. May require postop ventilation. ✓ ECG, ↓gastric emptying and weak laryngeal reflexes.
Myopathies	Avoid all muscle relaxants and respiratory depressants. Postop ventilation may be necessary.
Juvenile rheumatoid arthritis	Poor cervical mobility; TMJ ankylosis; carditis; possibility of difficult intubation
Arthrogryposis	Poor cervical mobility; TMJ ankylosis; CHD; possible airway problems
Cerebral palsy	Gastroesophageal reflux and pulmonary problems; ↑sensitivity to muscle relaxants

Neurological, cont. abilities is usually best obtained from parents or guardian. If patient is on seizure-control medication, it is recommended that the medication be continued until surgery. ✓ levels.

All patients who require Ober fasciotomy or Yount release will have profound weakness of lower extremities, if not of the entire body. Must be careful in choice of muscle relaxant (generally avoid depolarizing agents).

Laboratory Tests as indicated from H&P.

Premedication Premedication for separation anxiety (e.g., midazolam) and facilitating induction. Dosage must be individualized (see p. D-2). Children with valvular disease, prosthetic valves, and/or most forms of CHD, as well as post cardiac-correction patients, should receive antibiotics for bacterial endocarditis prophylaxis preop.[4]

INTRAOPERATIVE

Anesthetic technique: As indicated in the preop considerations, these patient populations cover a vast spectrum, from fit and healthy children to those suffering from a variety of clinical syndromes with airway and cardiorespiratory problems. Hence, anesthesia needs to be tailored to the individual patient. Some older children may benefit from regional anesthesia with sedation. Others may do well with a combined regional/GA technique, while still others with difficult airways may require awake FOL. The following sections address some (not all) of these concerns.

Induction

Normal: standard pediatric (< 12 yr) or adult induction (see p. D-2).

Difficult airway: a mask induction and FOL during spontaneous respiration should be considered. Alternatives include use of an anterior commissure scope, blind oral or nasal intubation, use of FOL or light wand stylet, retrograde wire intubation and tracheostomy.

Muscle abnormalities: these patients may be very sensitive to muscle relaxants, have gastric hypomotility and may be predisposed to MH. Induction should be accomplished by "nontriggering" agents (e.g., thiopental 1-3 mg/kg and atracurium or vecuronium if necessary for intubation). Succinylcholine is usually contraindicated in these patients. Dantrolene must be available, but it need not be administered prophylactically. A study of MH patients showed that 32 out of 89 had preexisting musculoskeletal abnormalities.[1]

Cardiorespiratory compromise: inhalational induction, when administered cautiously, may be used safely in this group of patients. IV (e.g., etomidate 0.1-0.4 mg/kg iv) and intramuscular (e.g.,

Induction, cont. ketamine 4-8 mg/kg im) inductions are usually safe and effective in neonates and infants with severe cardiac disease.

Maintenance

Normal: standard maintenance (see p. D-3).

Muscle abnormalities: maintenance of anesthesia with a nontriggering agent (e.g., N_2O, opiates) and short-acting, nondepolarizing muscle relaxants is prudent. A peripheral nerve stimulator should be used to monitor muscle relaxation as the effects of muscle relaxants may be unexpectedly prolonged.

Cardiorespiratory compromise: the maintenance of anesthesia in this group is most commonly accomplished by use of inhalational agents, additional narcotics or other iv agents, depending on patient tolerance and postop plans for ventilatory management.

Emergence

Normal: if muscle relaxant used, reverse with neostigmine (0.07 mg/kg) and glycopyrrolate (0.01 mg/kg iv) or edrophonium (0.5 mg/kg) and atropine (0.015 mg/kg iv). Make sure patient is awake and able to protect airway. A vital capacity of > 15 ml/kg is considered an adequate sign of recovery of respiratory reserve.[5]

Muscle abnormalities: Anticipate postop respiratory impairment. Suction airway carefully. The response to neostigmine is unpredictable and may precipitate myotonia. Continued postop mechanical ventilation may be required.

Cardiorespiratory compromise: Tourniquet release may cause significant ↓CO and ↓BP, requiring temporary inotropic support. Otherwise, emergence as in normal patients.

Regional anesthesia: Used in patients undergoing lower extremity surgery.

Caudal epidural Use bupivacaine 0.25% or lidocaine 1%, ± epinephrine 1:200,000. Volume = 0.05 ml/kg/dermatome to be blocked.[7]

Continuous epidural infusion Use bupivacaine 0.1-0.125% at rate of 0.1 ml/kg/h in patients < 5 yr; thereafter, patients may require 0.05-0.15 ml/kg/h.

Blood and fluid requirements

IV: 22 ga or greater × 1-2
NS/LR @:
4 ml/kg/h – 0-10 kg
+ 2 ml/kg/h – 11-20 kg
+ 1 ml/kg/h – >20 kg
(e.g., 25 kg = 65 ml/h)
Warm fluids.
Humidify gases.

There may be rapid fluid shifts in pediatric patients undergoing orthopedic procedures. Close monitoring and adequate fluid replacement will ensure hemodynamic stability. In hip or pelvis surgery, blood loss may be substantial, and adequate iv access is important as blood transfusion may be required.

Control of blood loss

Tourniquet – 120-min limit

Use of pneumatic tourniquets has become common practice in peripheral orthopedic procedures. They reduce intraop blood loss; however, they cause pain and, upon removal, release products of anaerobic metabolism.[3]

Monitoring

Standard monitors (see p. D-1).
± Arterial line
± CVP line

Most pediatric patients presenting for extremity surgery do not require invasive monitoring. An arterial or CVP line may be helpful, depending on patient's medical condition, length of surgery and anticipated blood loss.

Positioning

✓ and pad pressure points.
✓ eyes.

Patients with osteogenesis imperfecta or osteoporosis are at risk for fractures and joint dislocations and require special care in positioning.

Complications

MH

Early Sx of MH include: tachycardia, tachypnea, unstable BP, dysrhythmias, cyanotic mottling of skin, rapid rise in temperature (1°/15 min), discolored urine, metabolic acidosis, respiratory acidosis, hyperkalemia, myoglobinuria. Rx: stop surgery and anesthesia immediately; hyperventilate with 100% O_2; administer dantrolene sodium iv (starting dose = 1-2 mg/kg q 5-10 min; maximum cumulative dose = 10 mg/kg) by rapid infusion. Procainamide (15 mg/kg) over 15 min may be required for dys-

Complications, cont.		rhythmias. Initiate cooling, correct acidosis and hyperkalemia. Maintain UO of at least 2 ml/kg/hr. Monitor patient in ICU until danger of subsequent episodes is over (24 h).

POSTOPERATIVE

Complications	MH Respiratory insufficiency	For MH considerations, see above.
Pain management	PCA (see p. E-3). Parenteral opiates Spinal opiates	Caudal epidural morphine (0.05 mg/kg) provides 8-24 h postop analgesia. Epidural fentanyl (0.3-1.0 μg/kg/hr) or hydromorphone (1 μg/kg/hr) may be administered by continuous infusion, ± low doses of bupivacaine. Patients with distal realignment are at risk for compartment syndrome postop and should not have a pain-relieving technique that could mask a compartment syndrome (e.g., epidural, etc.).

References

1. Britt BA, Kalow W: Malignant hyperthermia: a statistical review. *Can Anaesth Soc J* 1970; 17(4):293-315.
2. Brownell AK, Paasuke RT, Elash A, Fowlow SB, Seagram CG, Diewold RJ, Friesen C: Malignant hyperthermia in Duchenne muscular dystrophy. *Anesthesiology* 1983; 58(2):180-82.
3. Brustowicz RM, et al: Metabolic responses to tourniquet release in children. *Anesthesiology* 1987; 67(5):792-94.
4. Prevention of bacterial endocarditis. American Heart Assoc, Committee on Rheumatic Fever, Endocarditis and Kawasaki Disease of the Council on Cardiovascular Disease in the Young of the American Heart Association. *JAMA* 1990; 264(22):2919-22.
5. Shimada Y, Yoshiya I, Tanaka K, Yamazaki T, Kumon K: Crying vital capacity and maximal inspiratory pressure as clinical indicators of readiness for weaning of infants less than a year of age. *Anesthesiology* 1979; 51(5):456-59.
6. Tait AR, Knight PR: The effects of general anesthesia on upper respiratory tract infections in children. *Anesthesiology* 1987; 67(6):930-35.
7. Takasaki M, Dohi S, Kawabata Y, Takahashi T: Dosage of lidocaine for caudal anesthesia in infants and children. *Anesthesiology* 1977; 47(6):527-29.

Surgeon

Stephen A. Schendel, MD, DDS

12.7 REPAIR OF CONGENITAL MALFORMATIONS

Anesthesiologist

Yuan-Chi Lin, MD, MPH

CLEFT LIP REPAIR—UNILATERAL/BILATERAL

SURGICAL CONSIDERATIONS

Description: Cleft lip may be either unilateral or bilateral, associated frequently with clefts of the alveolus and palate. Surgical repair involves the design and execution of geometric flaps on the medial and lateral sides of the cleft. The most common technique is the **rotation advancement flap of Millard** (Fig 12.7-1).

Variant procedure or approaches: Other approaches commonly performed are those of the **Davies-** or **Tennison**-type (Z-plasty) lip repairs (Fig 12.7-2). In large clefts, a lip adhesion may be performed as an initial stage several months prior to the actual definitive correction of the cleft lip. This procedure basically involves creating a wound on either side and suturing the muscles, mucosa and skin together. The procedure itself is very short—approximately one-half h or less of surgical time. Actual cleft lip repair requires 1.5 h.

Usual preop diagnosis: Cleft lip/palate

SUMMARY OF PROCEDURE

Position	Supine; table rotated either 90° or 180° with oral RAE or anode tube.
Incision	Medial and lateral cleft margins into the nose and in the maxillary vestibule on the cleft side
Special instrumentation	★ Plastic surgery throat pack (**NB:** ✓ removal before extubation); oral RAE or anode tube.
Unique considerations	Pediatric patients should wake up in an unagitated state, as undue crying may place excessive tension on repair. Elbow restraints for children.
Antibiotics	Cefazolin 25 mg/kg iv
Surgical time	0.75-1.5 h
Closing considerations	Smooth emergence
EBL	5-10 ml
Postop care	Elbow restraints for 2 wk; PACU → room
Mortality	Minimal
Morbidity	Infection Wound breakdown
Pain score	4

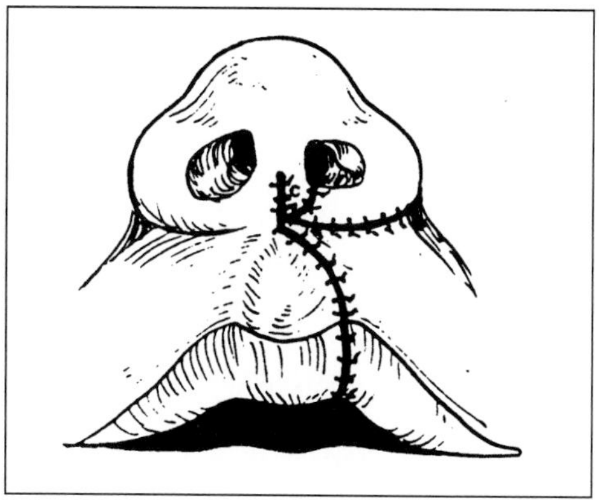

Figure 12.7-1. Completion of the rotation flap of Millard. (Reproduced with permission from McCarthy JG, ed: *Plastic Surgery*. WB Saunders: 1990).

PATIENT POPULATION CHARACTERISTICS

Age range	1 wk-6 mo
Male:Female	2:1 – cleft lip and palate. Isolated cleft palate more common in females.
Incidence	1/750 for Caucasians; more common in Asians; less in Blacks. Left cleft more common than right; both more common than bilateral, in the ratio of 6:3:1.
Etiology	Multifactorial, including both genetic and environmental aspects
Associated conditions	Associated anomalies are seen in approximately 29% of cleft lip cases, and may include major chromosomal deletions and/or duplications, along with possible severe mental retardation and CHD. Pierre Robin syndrome; Klippel-Feil syndrome; Treacher-Collins syndrome; subglottic stenosis

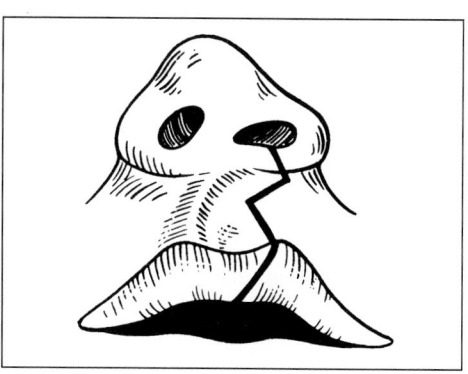

Figure 12.7-2. Z-plasty closure of lip. (Reproduced with permission from McCarthy JG, ed: *Plastic Surgery*. WB Saunders: 1990).

ANESTHETIC CONSIDERATIONS

See Anesthetic Considerations for Lip and Nose Surgery, p. 1033.

Reference

1. Gorlin RJ, Cohen MM, Levin LS: *Syndromes of the Head and Neck*, 3rd edition. Oxford University Press, New York: 1990.

ABBE-ESTLANDER REPAIR/CROSS LIP FLAP

SURGICAL CONSIDERATIONS

Description: Occasionally, the individual born with a cleft lip and palate is severely deficient in tissue of the upper lip. This occurs most frequently in the bilateral condition. Correction involves switching tissue from the midline of the lower lip to the central portion of the upper lip, maintaining a pedicle of soft tissue between the lips, which usually contains the labial artery on one side. This pedicle normally is cut between 7-11 d. The redundant tissue in the mid portion of the upper lip is transferred to the columellar portion of the nose at the same time, which elongates this section (Fig 12.7-3). To avoid disruption of the flap, the older child should be cautioned to avoid wide mouth opening in the postop period.

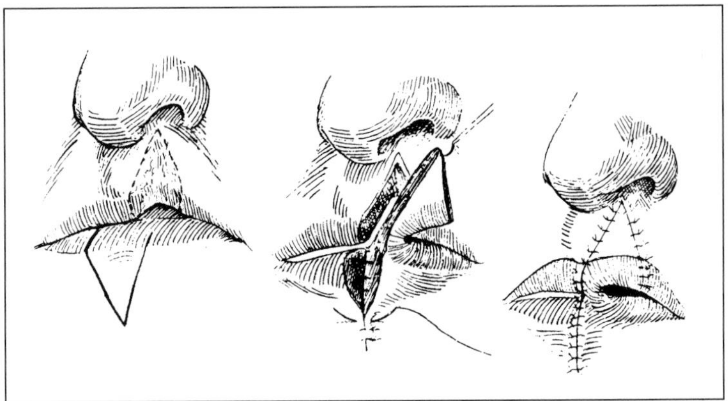

Figure 12.7-3. Abbe-Estlander flap. Note lips sutured together. (Reproduced with permission from Converse JM, ed: *Reconstructive Plastic Surgery*, Vol 3, 2nd edition. WB Saunders Co: 1977.)

Variant procedure or approaches: Only minor technical variants

Usual preop diagnosis: Severely cleft lip/palate

SUMMARY OF PROCEDURE

Position	If nasal RAE tube used, table is either rotated 90° or left in usual position. If oral RAE tube is used, table is rotated either 90° or 180°. The nasal RAE tube has the advantage of easier extubation of a patient with the central portion of his lips essentially sewn together. Nasal intubation, however, somewhat limits the surgeon's ability to visualize and reconstruct the nasal section of the surgery. The oral RAE tube has the opposite advantages and disadvantages.
Incision	Midline upper and lower lips (Fig 12.7-3)
Special instrumentation	Nasal or oral RAE tube (surgeon's preference); plastics setup
Unique considerations	Central portion of lips are attached by a thin, easily damaged soft-tissue pedicle. Patient should wake up unagitated.
Antibiotics	Cefazolin 25 mg/kg iv
Surgical time	1-2 h
Closing considerations	★ **NB:** Remove throat pack.
EBL	25-50 ml
Postop care	Elbow restraints (young child); PACU → room; caution to avoid wide mouth opening
Mortality	Rare
Morbidity	Flap necrosis: < 1%

Morbidity, cont.	Suture line dehiscence: < 1% Bleeding
Pain score	4

PATIENT POPULATION CHARACTERISTICS

Age range	3+ yr
Male:Female	2:1
Incidence	1/750 Caucasians (> Asians; < Blacks)
Etiology	Multifactorial, including both genetic and environmental aspects
Associated conditions	Associated anomalies are seen in approximately 29% of the clefts and may include major chromosomal deletions or duplications, with a possibility of severe mental retardation.[1] CHD; Pierre Robin syndrome; Treacher-Collins syndrome; subglottic stenosis

ANESTHETIC CONSIDERATIONS

See Anesthetic Considerations for Lip and Nose Surgery, p. 1033.

Reference

1. Gorlin RJ, Cohen MM, Levin LS: *Syndromes of the Head and Neck*, 3rd edition. Oxford University Press, New York: 1990.

PALATOPLASTY

SURGICAL CONSIDERATIONS

Description: Cleft palate can be seen as either an isolated condition or in conjunction with clefting of the lip. The mildest form of cleft palate is the submucous, or occult cleft, in which there is no visible cleft but, rather, a nonunion of the soft-palate muscles. This is followed by the incomplete soft-palate cleft and, finally, the complete cleft, which includes soft and hard palates and may extend through the alveolar portion of the maxilla. Repair involves mobilizing the lateral soft tissue and moving it toward the midline to close the cleft and elongate the palate, if necessary. The most important goal of cleft-palate repair is the attainment of normal speech. Children with unrepaired or inadequately repaired clefts develop nasal-sounding speech patterns termed "rhinolalia." Cleft-palate repair, therefore, is usually done when the child is 9-18 mo old, before consequential speech development. In addition to closing the cleft itself, an important goal of palate repair is approximation, in normal alignment, of the levator palati muscles, which are responsible for oronasal valving in speech and swallowing. The cleft palate is closed by loosening the palatal mucoperiosteum from the underlying bone and either approximating it in the midline (**Langenbeck technique**) or using a V-Y type of retrodisplacement and closure (**Wardill-Kilner technique**). In either method, the levator muscles are specifically dissected and the levator sling is reconstructed. A layered closure is usually done, including repositioning of the alveolar muscles.

There are several different approaches to the muscle reconstruction in the soft palate, which can generally be termed **intravelarveloplasties**. One of the newer techniques is a Z-plasty of the soft palate, also called a **Furlow procedure**. The other procedures are basically closures of the muscles and a push-back to lengthen the palate.

Usual preop diagnosis: Cleft palate

SUMMARY OF PROCEDURE

Position	Supine; table rotated 90°-180° with oral RAE tube extending down the midline of the lower jaw and taped to the chin.
Incision	Edges of the cleft palate and possibly the alveolar and pterygomandibular raphe areas
Special instrumentation	Dingmann mouth gag and, usually, a headlight; oropharyngeal pack

Unique considerations	Minimal-to-moderate amount of blood in the oropharynx at end of procedure – should be carefully suctioned. Also, there may be some respiratory difficulties on emergence. Traction with a tongue suture often proves helpful in restoring patient's airway. Usually oral or nasopharyngeal airways should not be placed in children.
Antibiotics	Cefazolin 25 mg/kg q 5-6 h (up to 1 g) × 5 d
Surgical time	1-1.5 h
Closing considerations	Child should not wake up crying and hypertensive. Tongue suture may be placed prior to extubation.
EBL	50 ml
Postop care	Elbow restraints; PACU → room
Mortality	Rare
Morbidity	Recurrent bleeding Hematoma under the palate Dehiscence of the palate
Pain score	4

PATIENT POPULATION CHARACTERISTICS

Age range	6-18 mo
Male:Female	1:3 (isolated cleft palate)
Incidence	1/1,000
Etiology	Failure of fusion of the palatal shelves from anterior to posterior. (Can be due to a persistent high-tongue position *in utero*, increased facial width, reduced facial mesenchyme and/or drugs such as steroids, anticonvulsants and benzodiazepines, or infection.)
Associated conditions	Multiple associated conditions. Most common is the Pierre Robin anomaly, in which cleft palate is found in association with glossoptosis and a micrognathic retruded mandible. These children frequently have airway obstruction and, even at an older age, may have sleep apnea.[1] Other associations include Klippel-Feil syndrome, Treacher-Collins syndrome, CHD, chronic URI and chronic otitis media.

ANESTHETIC CONSIDERATIONS

See Anesthetic Considerations for Lip and Nose Surgery, p. 1033.

Reference

1. Gorlin RJ, Cohen MM, Levin LS: *Syndromes of the Head and Neck*, 3rd edition. Oxford University Press, New York: 1990.

PHARYNGOPLASTY

SURGICAL CONSIDERATIONS

Description: Following the initial repair of palatal clefts, some children or young adults demonstrate continued hypernasal speech patterns, a condition called "velopharyngeal incompetence." This can be 2° a short, soft palate, a large nasopharynx, or a soft palate that has inadequate movement either 2° scarring or due to neurogenic problems. The typical repair would be a superiorly based **pharyngeal flap** to the soft palate.

Variant procedure or approaches: An **Orticochea flap**, using the posterior tonsillar pillars, which are repositioned along with the palatoglossus muscle to the posterior pharynx. A posterior pharyngeal wall implant also may be placed.

Usual preop diagnosis: Velopharyngeal incompetence

SUMMARY OF PROCEDURE

Position	Supine, table rotated 90° or 180°; oral RAE tube exited out the midline and taped in that position.
Incision	Involves incisions in soft and hard palates and in the posterior pharyngeal wall.
Special instrumentation	Dingmann mouth gag; headlight
Unique considerations	Avoid oral or nasopharyngeal airways or nasal suctioning.
Antibiotics	Cefazolin 25 mg/kg q 6-8 h (up to 1 g) × 3 d
Surgical time	1-1.5 h
Closing considerations	Pediatric patients should not become hypertensive (↑bleeding). There will be some nasopharyngeal drainage; thorough oral suctioning is important.
EBL	50-100 ml
Postop care	Avoid postop oral or nasopharyngeal airways or nasal suctioning. Be aware of possible occlusion of nasopharynx with flap and bleeding.
Mortality	Rare
Morbidity	Recurrent bleeding Hematoma under the palate Dehiscence of the palate Nasopharyngeal obstruction Secondary sleep apnea
Pain score	4

PATIENT POPULATION CHARACTERISTICS

Age range	3-11 yr most common
Male:Female	1:1
Incidence	Approximately 15% of children undergoing cleft palate repair will need some type of secondary palatal lengthening procedure after 3 yr.
Etiology	Short and scarred palate; neurogenic palate; palate-to-pharyngeal ratio that is too small
Associated conditions	Sleep apnea; Pierre Robin syndrome, glossoptosis and micrognathia; Treacher-Collins syndrome; microtia with craniofacial malformation; subglottic stenosis; CHD

ANESTHETIC CONSIDERATIONS

See Anesthetic Considerations for Lip and Nose Surgery, p. 1033.

ALVEOLAR CLEFT REPAIR WITH BONE GRAFT

SURGICAL CONSIDERATIONS

Description: Alveolar cleft occurs as both bony and soft-tissue defects in the alveolar portion of the maxilla in the position of the lateral incisor tooth; thus, an oral/nasal fistula exists with this deformity. The size of the cleft is variable; it may be unilateral or bilateral and is associated with cleft lip and palate. The surgical procedure involves raising mucosal gingival flaps, advancing them, and performing a layered closure, starting with the nasal floor and working toward the oral cavity. A bone graft is placed in between these two layers to consolidate the upper arch. Cancellous bone is usually taken from the iliac crest or from the outer table of the skull.

Variant procedure or approaches: In young children, the alveolar cleft procedure may be performed without the use of bone grafts.

Usual preop diagnosis: Congenital alveolar cleft

SUMMARY OF PROCEDURE

Position	Supine; table rotated 90°-180°
Incision	Oral, with the addition of iliac crest incision or scalp incision, either parasagittal or coronal
Special instrumentation	Throat pack; Dingmann mouth gag; headlight. Normally, 2 instrument setups used, with hip instruments kept separate from oral instruments.
Unique considerations	Important to ensure that the hip from which iliac crest bone graft will be procured is on the opposite side from the anesthesiologist if the table is rotated only 90°. Midline oral RAE tube.
Antibiotics	Cefazolin 25 mg/kg (up to 1 g) iv preop
Surgical time	1.5-2.5 h
Closing considerations	★ **NB:** Ensure that throat pack has been removed. Pediatric patients should not wake up in agitated state. Oral mouth gag and gentle oral suctioning permissible; avoid nasal suctioning, especially from the cleft side.
EBL	100-200 ml
Postop care	PACU → ward
Mortality	Rare
Morbidity[2]	Bone graft loss: 2-10% Infection: 2-10% Refistulization: 2-10% Prolonged hip discomfort (bone graft donor site) Bleeding – oral or at bone donor site
Pain score	6

PATIENT POPULATION CHARACTERISTICS

Age range	8-12 yr
Male:Female	2:1
Incidence	Unknown
Etiology	Multifactorial, including both genetic and environmental aspects
Associated conditions	Associated anomalies are seen in approximately 29% of cleft lip cases; and these may include major chromosomal deletions and/or duplications, with the possibility of severe mental retardation.[1] CHD; Pierre Robin syndrome; Treacher-Collins syndrome; subglottic stenosis

ANESTHETIC CONSIDERATIONS

See Anesthetic Considerations for Lip and Nose Surgery, p. 1033.

References

1. Gorlin RJ, Cohen MM, Levin LS: *Syndromes of the Head and Neck*, 3rd edition. Oxford University Press, New York: 1990.
2. Wolfe SA, Price GW, Stuzin JM, Berkowitz SI: Alveolar and anterior palatal clefts. In *Plastic Surgery*, Vol 4. McCarthy JG, ed. WB Saunders Co, Philadelphia: 1990, 2753-70.

LIP/NOSE REVISIONS

SURGICAL CONSIDERATIONS

Description: Secondary deformities of the nose and lip develop following the initial repair of either bilateral or unilateral cleft lip deformities. These subsequent deformities depend on the extent of the initial congenital anomaly, the quality of the surgical repair and resulting oral facial function. Revision can consist of a minimal scar revision, to a complete opening and reconstruction of the lip and nose, with or without ancillary procedures such as **cartilage grafting** to the nose and **septorhinoplasty**.

Usual preop diagnosis: Secondary deformity

SUMMARY OF PROCEDURE

Position	Supine, rotated 90°-180°, with oral RAE tube
Incision	Variable, in lip or nasal areas
Special instrumentation	Throat pack; possibly rhinoplasty instruments; oral RAE tube
Unique considerations	Procurement of a cartilage graft is usually from the nasal septum or ear; thus, the head may need to be turned to one side and this area also prepped. Elbow restraints for children.
Antibiotics	Cefazolin 25 mg/kg (up to 1 g) iv preop
Surgical time	Variable, depending on the extent of revision: 0.5-3 h
EBL	Minimal-75 ml
Postop care	May be obligatory mouth breathing; PACU
Mortality	Rare
Morbidity	Infection Wound breakdown
Pain score	5

PATIENT POPULATION CHARACTERISTICS

Age range	2-50 yr
Male:Female	1:1
Incidence	20-60% of patients with primary clefts
Etiology	Unsatisfactory outcome of previous lip/nose surgery
Associated conditions	Associated anomalies are seen in approximately 29% of the clefts and may include major chromosomal deletions or duplications, with a possibility of severe mental retardation;[1] Pierre Robin syndrome; CHD; Treacher-Collins syndrome; subglottic stenosis.

ANESTHETIC CONSIDERATIONS FOR LIP AND NOSE SURGERY

(Procedures covered: cleft lip repair; Abbe-Estlander repair/cross lip flap; palatoplasty; pharyngoplasty; alveolar cleft repair with bone graft; lip/nose revisions)

PREOPERATIVE

The anesthesiologist should be aware of the parent's feelings about their malformed child.[2] The whole family needs to be treated with sensitivity and compassion. Cleft lip closure may be carried out as early as the first wk of life in the healthy neonate; however, many surgeons and anesthesiologists find the "rule of ten" helpful: the child should have an Hb >10 g, be 10 wk old, and weigh 10 lbs. The hard palate is usually closed between the ages of 1-5 yr; however, the soft palate should be closed prior to speech development (12-15 mo). **Palatoplasty** and **pharyngoplasty** are usually carried out from 1-15 yr. Patients with these midline facial defects are most likely to have other associated anomalies, including CHD, subglottic stenosis and Pierre Robin or Treacher-Collins syndromes.

Respiratory Careful assessment is necessary as associated anomalies may affect airway or lungs. Chronic otitis 2° eustachian tube dysfunction is common. Treat with antibiotics before surgery. Postpone surgery (~2 wk) if Sx of acute URI present (e.g., runny nose, fever, sore throat, cough). Chronic aspiration may be associated with cleft lip/palate.
Tests: as indicated from H&P.

Airway Be aware of other congenital anomalies affecting the airway, such as Apert's, Goldenhar's, Klippel-Feil, Pierre Robin or Treacher-Collins syndromes. Review any previous anesthetic records for insights into airway management. Consider elective tracheostomy under local anesthesia in patients with severe airway abnormalities. Patients with severe subglottic stenosis may require preop tracheostomy.

Cardiovascular CHD is frequently associated with cleft palate.[4] Preop evaluation of a patient with a known or suspected heart defect should include thorough H&P, ECG, Hct, baseline O_2 sat and CXR. For children with Sx of cardiac dysfunction or those requiring cardiac medication, it is advisable to consult with a pediatric cardiologist to optimize the patient's condition prior to surgery.
Tests: Preop ECG indicated for patients with CHD; others as indicated from H&P.

Nutritional Infants with cleft lip/palate may have problems with oral feeding. Assess nutritional status from physical exam and by comparison to expected growth for age.
★ **NB:** NPO after midnight for solids. Patients should continue to have clear liquids up until 2 h preop.

Neurological Delayed development of speech is common in the older child with cleft palate. Some of these children may be hearing impaired. Preop preparation and discussion is important to minimize the impact of these communication problems.

Psychological Many patients with orofacial congenital malformations require multiple procedures; emotional support and psychological assessment of these patients are essential.

Hematologic High incidence of iron deficiency anemia; T&C for 1 U PRBC (cleft palate).
Tests: Hct

Laboratory Other tests as indicated from H&P.

Premedication < 1 yr old rarely needs premedication; > 1 yr old, either oral midazolam (0.75 mg/kg) or oral ketamine (6 mg/kg) ~30 min preop is adequate.

INTRAOPERATIVE

Anesthetic technique: GETA

Induction Typically, an inhalational induction (sevoflurane or halothane ± N_2O/O_2) while patient is breathing spontaneously. Airway obstruction is best treated with an oral airway. Anticipate difficult laryngoscopy if large, prepalatal cleft present. Intubate with oral RAE tube and secure in midline of lower lip. In patients with difficult airways, FOL is the technique of choice. Avoid muscle relaxants for difficult intubations until ETT is placed.

Maintenance Standard pediatric maintenance (see p. D-3) ± muscle relaxant. Airway is shared with the surgeons. The Dingmann mouth gag is used for surgical exposure and may inadvertently compress the ETT or cause an endobronchial intubation. Flexion of the neck may also cause endobronchial intubation. Extension of the neck may cause complete or partial extubation. Adequacy of ventilation should be checked after every position change. Bilateral breath sounds should be equal after final positioning. ETT should be sutured to the alveolar ridge. In palatoplasty the palate is infiltrated with epinephrine (in lidocaine usually) → ↓blood loss + ↑dysrhythmias (halothane > sevoflurane). ↑$PaCO_2$ → ↓dysrhythmias.

Emergence ★ Pharyngeal (throat) packs are usually placed to prevent aspiration of blood. **NB:** Packs must be removed before extubating the trachea. Consider laryngoscopy to inspect airway and remove blood and clots before extubation. A tongue stitch is useful postop following cleft palate surgery. It may be used to pull the tongue forward to relieve postop respiratory obstruction. Extubation in the lateral (tonsillar) position is useful in promoting drainage of blood and secretions.

Blood and fluid requirements IV: 18-20 ga × 1
NS/LR @:
4 ml/kg/h – 0-10 kg
+ 2 ml/kg/h – 11-20 kg
+ 1 ml/kg/h – > 20 kg
(e.g., 25 kg = 65 ml/h)

Blood loss replaced by 3:1 crystalloid or 1:1 colloid (e.g., 5% albumin or 6% hetastarch). Rarely, a blood transfusion may be indicated for hemorrhage.

Monitoring Standard monitors (p. D-1)

Positioning	✓ and pad pressure points. ✓ eyes.	
Complications	Obstructed ETT → ↑PIP	✓ ETT to see that it is not partially or completely obstructed by mouth gag.
	Mucous plugging Hemorrhage	✓ bilateral breath sounds.

POSTOPERATIVE

Complications	Retained throat pack	✓ for retained throat pack if there are Sx of airway obstruction in immediate postop period.
	Airway edema → croup Hemorrhage Obstructive sleep apnea	Rx of postintubation croup consists of cool, humidified, 100% O_2 mask, or nebulization 2.25% racemic epinephrine (0.5 ml in 3 ml NS). Racemic epinephrine is given for its vasoconstrictor, rather than its bronchodilator, effect.
Pain management	Acetaminophen 20 mg/kg (suppository/po) Morphine 0.05-0.1 mg/kg iv q 2-3 h prn	Avoid oversedation in patients with Abbe-Estlander repair 2° airway obstruction.
Tests	Hct, if indicated.	Others as indicated.

References

1. Gorlin RJ, Cohen MM, Levin LS: *Syndromes of the Head and Neck*, 3rd edition. Oxford University Press, New York: 1990.
2. Jones RG: A short history of anaesthesia for hare-lip and cleft palate repair. *Br J Anaesth* 1971; 43(8):796-802.
3. Palmisano BW: Anesthesia for plastic surgery. In: *Pediatric Anesthesia*, 3rd edition, Gregory GA, ed. Churchill-Livingstone, NY: 1994, 699-741.
4. Wallbank WA: Cardiac effects of halothane and adrenaline in hare-lip and cleft-palate surgery. *Br J Anaesth* 1970; 42(6):548-52.

OTOPLASTY

SURGICAL CONSIDERATIONS

Description: There are a number of congenital ear malformations which result in an ear of abnormal shape, frequently with a lack of the antihelical fold. Surgical reconstruction consists of creating an antihelical fold and decreasing the prominence of the ear, as measured by its projection from the mastoid process. This usually involves an elliptical skin incision in the posterior ear area, dissection over the mastoid, and/or cartilage scoring or resection.

Variant procedure or approaches: All procedures are similar, with minor differences in suturing and amount of resection tissue. In addition to the posterior incision, an anterior incision can be used in some approaches. **Microtia reconstruction** is a much larger procedure and, therefore, is staged.

Usual preop diagnosis: Ear malformation; ear trauma

SUMMARY OF PROCEDURE

Position	Supine; table rotated either 90° or 180°; oral intubation
Incision	Posterior ear; occasionally anterior ear
Unique considerations	Head turned from side-to-side during operation.
Antibiotics	Cefazolin 25 mg/kg (up to 1 g) iv preop
Surgical time	2 h
Closing considerations	Ear dressing requires 5-10 min at end of procedure.
EBL	10-20 ml
Postop care	PACU

Mortality	Rare
Morbidity	Hematoma formation: < 1% Infection: < 1% Unsymmetrical ear reduction: < 1%
Pain score	4

PATIENT POPULATION CHARACTERISTICS

Age range	6+ yr
Male:Female	Unknown
Incidence	Unknown
Etiology	Unknown

ANESTHETIC CONSIDERATIONS

See Anesthetic Considerations for Ear Surgery, Chapter 3.0 Otolaryngology, p. 132.

PRIMARY CORRECTION OF CRANIOSYNOSTOSIS, CRANIOFACIAL ANOMALIES

SURGICAL CONSIDERATIONS

Description: Premature closure of cranial sutures causes various abnormal skull shapes, of which the most common are: **scaphocephaly**, involving the sagittal suture; **plagiocephaly**, involving a unilateral coronal suture or lambdoid suture; **bradycephaly,** involving bilateral coronal sutures; and **trigonocephaly**, involving the metopic suture. Surgical correction involves releasing or resecting the affected suture and simultaneously correcting the asymmetric skull by bone flap repositioning or advancement, usually a frontoorbital advancement with supraorbital bar. For example, in plagiocephaly, because of the unilateral coronal synostosis, the frontal bone is retruded on this side. Craniectomy is performed, the forehead removed, the involved coronal suture resected and then the supraorbital bar cut above the orbit and down to the lateral orbital wall across the midline. This bar is then bent, advanced on the involved side—sometimes up to 1.5 cm—and fixed in this position. Additional bone strips are taken from the posterior cranium and split for use as graft material; the other bone pieces are replaced and fixed rigidly with either wires or resorbable plates. Procedures are extradural.

Variant procedure or approaches: In older children (> 2 yr), split cranial bone grafts may be required to correct defects caused by bone-flap advancement. Excision of skull segments is commonly accompanied by rigid fixation.

Usual preop diagnosis: Premature closure of cranial sutures; syndromes such as Apert's and Crouzon's disease; ↑ICP

SUMMARY OF PROCEDURE

Position	Usually supine; prone for correction of lambdoidal suture synostosis
Incision	Usually coronal
Special instrumentation	Horseshoe headrest, usually pediatric; occasionally, Gardiner tongs
Unique considerations	Control of ICP – spinal drain may be placed.
Antibiotics	Pediatric: cefazolin 25 mg/kg q 8 h, or vancomycin 10-15 mg/kg q 6 h, and cefotaxime 25-50 mg/kg q 6 h for oropharyngeal contamination and following dural tears
Surgical time	2-6 h
Closing considerations	Full head-wrap dressing causes head/neck movement → bucking.
EBL	200-800 ml; may be formidable.
Postop care	ICU: 1-2 d
Mortality	0.6-1.6%

Morbidity	Major complications: 14.3% Bone infection: 3-7% CSF leak: 4.5% Air embolus: < 1% Blindness: < 1%[1] Massive bleeding: < 1%
Pain score	4

PATIENT POPULATION CHARACTERISTICS

Age range	2-24 mo (primary correction)
Male:Female	1:1
Incidence	1/10,000 births
Etiology	Idiopathic; however, some are associated with specific genetic conditions (e.g., Crouzon's disease and Apert's syndrome).
Associated conditions	Hydrocephalus; ↑ICP; mental retardation; airway problems; ocular abnormalities; exotropia (20% Crouzon's disease or Apert's syndrome); lagophthalmus; exorbitism

ANESTHETIC CONSIDERATIONS

(Procedures covered: primary correction of craniosynostosis; craniofacial anomalies)

PREOPERATIVE

Patients may have craniofacial anomalies—particularly Apert's syndrome and Crouzon's disease—which are associated with midface hypoplasia and difficult intubation. Hence, detailed preop airway evaluation is necessary. Children with single-suture craniosynostosis are usually healthy. Surgery is often performed between 3-6 mo of age, preferably when the infant weighs > 5 kg.

Respiratory Patients with long-standing upper airway obstruction due to choanal atresia, mandibular and maxillary hypoplasia or other causes, may have chronic hypoventilation and hypoxia, and may experience episodes of apnea. If the patient has Sx of acute URI, delay elective surgery at least 2 wk. The presence of fever, cough and abnormal chest auscultation necessitates radiographic evaluation and pediatric consultation.
Tests: As indicated from H&P.

Airway Be aware of other congenital anomalies affecting the patient's airway, such as Apert's, Klippel-Feil, Goldenhar's, Pierre Robin or Treacher-Collins syndromes or Crouzon's disease. Review any previous anesthetic records for patient to gain insights into appropriate airway management. Consider elective tracheostomy under local anesthesia in patients with severe airway abnormalities.

Cardiovascular Consider the coexistence of congenital cardiopulmonary anomalies, particularly in patients with Apert's syndrome (autosomal dominant trait, craniosynostosis, syndactyly of hands and feet). Preop evaluation of a patient with a known or suspected heart defect should include thorough H&P, ECG, Hct, baseline O_2 sat and CXR. For children with Sx of cardiac dysfunction or those requiring cardiac medication, it is advisable to consult with a pediatric cardiologist to optimize the patient's condition prior to surgery.
Tests: Preop ECG indicated for patients with CHD; others as indicated from H&P.

Neurological If only the sagittal suture is involved, ICP is usually normal. If more than one suture is involved, brain growth will be impaired, the patient will be developmentally retarded, and intracranial HTN may be present.

Hematologic Surgery in early infancy (< 9 mo) is common; thus, allowable blood loss is small; blood transfusion is usually required.
Tests: Hct; PT; PTT; T&C blood.

Laboratory Other tests as indicated from H&P.

Premedication Patients < 12 mo old usually do not require premedication. Antibiotic prophylaxis for CHD (e.g., ampicillin 25 mg/kg + gentamicin 2.5 mg/kg iv).

INTRAOPERATIVE

Anesthetic technique: GETA. Anticipate possible difficult airway. Heat OR to 78-80°.

Induction	Surgery for craniectomies is extradural. Either mask induction with N_2O and inhalational agent or iv induction is suitable for the infant with a normal airway. For a difficult airway, intubation may be facilitated by using a FOL while patient is awake or anesthetized and spontaneously ventilating. In rare situations, tracheostomy, under sedation and local anesthesia, may be necessary. Consider suturing ETT to prevent accidental extubation.	
Maintenance	Maintenance anesthesia with inhalational agent, or balanced anesthesia and long-acting muscle relaxant, should be adequate. Surgery may be prolonged. Control of ICP may be necessary (see below).	
Emergence	Prompt awakening to allow neurological evaluation is an important goal.	
Blood and fluid requirements	Anticipate large blood loss. IV: 18 ga × 1-2 LR @: 4 ml/kg/h – 0-10 kg + 2 ml/kg/h – 11-20 kg + 1 ml/kg/h – > 20 kg (e.g., 25 kg = 65 ml/h) Warm all fluids. Humidify gases.	Have 1-2 U PRBC or whole blood available. Use LR for replacing deficit, maintenance and 3rd-space fluid loss. Replace blood loss with colloid and PRBC ml for ml. Significant blood loss begins with scalp incision; allowable blood loss is small, so that it is important to begin transfusion early before hypovolemia occurs.[1] EBV for an infant in this age group is 75 ml/kg. A good rule is to infuse a volume of blood equal to 10% of EBV prior to incision in the healthy infant. Avoid NS (2° acidosis, bleeding) in children < 5 yr.
Control of ICP	Hyperventilation Osmotic diuretic Loop diuretic	In some cases, it may be desirable to ↓ ICP. This can be accomplished by ↑ ventilation ($PaCO_2$ 25-30 mmHg), diuretics (furosemide 1 mg/kg iv).
Monitoring	Standard monitors (see p. D-1). ± Arterial line ± CVP line ± Precordial Doppler[2] ± Urinary catheter	Arterial cannulation for continuous monitoring of ABG, Hct, electrolytes, etc. ↑K^+ and ↓Ca^{++} is most common following transfusion with whole blood or FFP. VAE has been reported during craniectomies in infants; hence, a precordial Doppler and CVP line will be helpful.
Positioning	✓ and pad pressure points. ✓ eyes.	Positioning depends on surgical approach; most are performed with patient prone; however, use of the head-up position is not uncommon.
Complications	Oculocardiac reflex (OCR) → ↓↓HR and ↓↓BP	Notify surgeons and Rx with atropine 0.02 mg/kg iv.
	VAE	Be prepared to make prompt Dx of VAE (↓$ETCO_2$, change in Doppler sounds, ↑ETN_2 ↓O_2 sat, ↓BP, ↑HR) and Rx: notify surgeons, flood wound, ± head down, aspirate CVP, ± vasopressors.

POSTOPERATIVE

Complications	Hypovolemia with ↓BP Hypothermia	Inadequate volume replacement may result in ↓BP. ✓ Hct to establish need for further fluid or blood therapy.
Pain management	Parenteral narcotics (see p. E-1).	
Tests	Followup Hct postop	Transfuse to keep Hct ≥ 30%.

References

1. Davies DW, Munro IR: The anesthetic management and intraoperative care of patients undergoing major facial osteotomies. *Plast Reconstr Surg* 1975; 55(1):50-5.
2. Harris MM, Yemen TA, Davidson A, Strafford MA, Rowe RW, Sanders SP, Rockoff MA: Venous embolism during craniectomy in supine infants. *Anesthesiology* 1987; 67(5):816-19.
3. Krane EJ, Domino KB: Anesthesia for Neurosurgery. In: *Smith's Anesthesia for Infants and Children*, 6th edition. Motoyama EK, Davis PJ, eds. Mosby-Year Book, St. Louis: 1996, 541-70.
4. McCarthy JG, Thorne CHM, Wood-Smith D: Principles of craniofacial surgery: Orbital hypertelorism. In *Plastic Surgery*, Vol 4. McCarthy JG, ed. WB Saunders Co, Philadelphia: 1990, 2974-3012.
5. Palmisano BW: Anesthesia for plastic surgery. In: *Pediatric Anesthesia*, 3rd edition, Gregory GA, ed. Churchill-Livingstone, NY: 1994, 699-741.

SECONDARY CORRECTION OF CRANIOFACIAL MALFORMATIONS

SURGICAL CONSIDERATIONS

Description: These procedures usually are performed on children 5 yr and older. There are two basic approaches. The first involves advancement of the upper face and frontal bone, frequently described as a **monoblock** or **frontofacial advancement**. The second variation, called **facial bipartition** or **periorbital osteotomies**, is for correction of telorbitism (wide-spaced eyes), usually accomplished by a combined extra- and intracranial approach, using both plastic and neurosurgical teams.

Variant procedure or approaches: Many different variations of the above-named procedures can be performed; but from an anesthetic standpoint, they are not significantly different. The use of cranial bone grafts and rigid fixation have shortened these somewhat lengthy procedures. Other bone grafts, however, from ribs and iliac crest, are occasionally required. These procedures frequently last 6 h or longer and blood loss can be very heavy. Reconstruction of the forehead orbital area following a tumor excision, for example, uses a similar approach, but requires additional bone grafts.

Usual preop diagnosis: Craniofacial malformations, deformities

SUMMARY OF PROCEDURE

	Monoblock or Frontofacial Advancement	Facial Bipartition or Periorbital Osteotomies
Position	Prone	⇐
Incision	Coronal, oral	Coronal, infraorbital
Special instrumentation	Neurosurgical power tools; mini/micro plates	⇐
Unique considerations	↑ICP; may require hyperventilation and spinal drain.	⇐
Antibiotics	Cefazolin (25 mg/kg iv) or vancomycin (10 mg/kg) and cefotaxime (25 mg/kg)	⇐
Surgical time	4-10 h	⇐
Closing considerations	Head and neck movement with application of head-wrap dressing → bucking.	⇐
EBL	400-800 ml	⇐
Postop care	ICU: 1-2 d	⇐
Mortality	0.6-1.6%	⇐
Morbidity	Major complications: 14.3%	⇐
	Bone infection: 3-7%	⇐
	CSF leak: 4.5%	⇐
	Air embolus: < 1%	⇐
	Blindness: < 1%	⇐
	Massive bleeding: < 1%	⇐
Pain score	6	6

PATIENT POPULATION CHARACTERISTICS

Age range	3-20 yr
Male:Female	1:1
Incidence	1/100,000
Etiology	Congenital (80%); occasionally trauma or tumor (20%)
Associated conditions	Depends greatly on the syndrome or disease (e.g., Apert's syndrome, Crouzon's disease, etc.). See Primary Correction of Craniosynostosis, Craniofacial Anomalies, p. 1036.

ANESTHETIC CONSIDERATIONS

PREOPERATIVE

Craniofacial syndromes often are associated with maxillofacial deformities, mandibular abnormalities and challenging airway management.[1]

Respiratory Patients with long-standing upper airway obstruction due to choanal atresia, mandibular and maxillary hypoplasia, etc., may have chronic hypoventilation and hypoxia, and may have apnea episodes. If Sx of acute URI, delay elective surgery at least 2 wk. The presence of fever, cough and abnormal chest auscultation necessitates radiographic evaluation and pediatric consultation.
Tests: As indicated from H&P.

Airway Be aware of other congenital anomalies affecting the airway, such as Apert's, Goldenhar's, Klippel-Feil, Pierre Robin or Treacher-Collins syndromes or Crouzon's disease. Review any previous anesthetic records for insights into airway management. Consider elective tracheostomy under local anesthesia in patients with severe airway abnormalities.

Cardiovascular Frequency of CHD is increased in patients with craniofacial abnormalities. Preop evaluation of patient with known or suspected heart defect should include H&P, ECG, Hct, baseline O_2 sat and CXR. For children with Sx of cardiac dysfunction or those requiring cardiac medication, it is advisable to consult with a pediatric cardiologist to optimize patient's condition prior to surgery.
Tests: Preop ECG indicated for patients with CHD; others as indicated from H&P.

Neurological Neurologic deficits, if any, should be documented preop.

Laboratory Hb/Hct; therapeutic drug levels for patients taking anticonvulsants.

Premedication Premedication is helpful for patients > 1 yr – oral midazolam 0.5-0.75 mg/kg or oral ketamine 6 mg/kg about 30-60 min before induction.

INTRAOPERATIVE

Anesthetic technique: GETA, with special consideration given to associated CHD, pulmonary and airway problems.

Induction In an otherwise healthy patient, inhalational induction with subsequent placement of iv lines is appropriate. Muscle relaxants facilitate intubation but should be used only when adequate mask ventilation can be assured. An oral RAE ETT is useful for this procedure and should be secured carefully in place (often by suturing). Intubation in a patient with airway abnormalities may be facilitated by using a FOL with patient awake or lightly anesthetized and spontaneously ventilating. In rare situations, tracheostomy, under sedation and local anesthesia, may be necessary.[2,3]

Maintenance Standard pediatric maintenance (see p. D-3).

Emergence Extubate trachea when patient is awake and protective airway reflexes have returned. Patients with reactive airway disease may require deep extubation.

Blood and fluid requirements
Anticipate large blood loss.
IV: 18 ga × 1-2
NS/LR @:
4 ml/kg/h – 0-10 kg
+ 2 ml/kg/h – 11-20 kg
+ 1 ml/kg/h – > 20 kg
(e.g., 25 kg = 65 ml/h)
Warm fluids.
Humidify gases.

The goal of intraop fluid therapy is to replace preop deficits, intraop fluid, electrolyte and blood losses, while providing maintenance fluids. Half of the calculated deficit (hours fasting × hourly maintenance fluid requirement) generally is replaced during the 1st h of anesthesia and the balance over the next 1-2 h. Surgical manipulation of tissue will cause 3rd-space fluid loss proportional to the degree of surgical trauma and tissue exposure. It may range from 0-10 ml/kg/h.

Control of blood loss
Deliberate hypotension

Deliberate hypotension can be accomplished by use of SNP, esmolol or potent inhalational agents titrated to effect (MAP 50-60 mmHg).

Monitoring
Standard monitors (see p. D-1).
Arterial line
± CVP line

Arterial line is essential for monitoring BP during deliberate hypotension and for ABGs and blood chemistries.

Control of ICP
Hyperventilation
Mannitol
Loop diuretics
CSF drainage (> 1 yr)

For some procedures, it is essential to reduce intracranial volume to facilitate surgical access. If prolonged brain retraction is required, postop cerebral edema may ensue.

Positioning
✓ and pad pressure points.
✓ eyes.

Positioning head above the heart facilitates venous drainage, but also increases the incidence of VAE. Do not hyperextend or hyperflex the head and neck. Flexion of

Positioning, cont.		the neck will move the ETT downward (mainstem intubation); extension will move the ETT upward (cuff leak).
Complications	Displacement of ETT	Suture ETT to alveolar ridge.
	Oculocardiac reflex (OCR) → ↓↓HR, ↓BP	Notify surgeon. Rx: atropine 0.02 mg/kg.
	VAE Major blood loss	VAE should be suspected if sudden ↑ETN$_2$, ↓ETCO$_2$, ↓O$_2$ sat, ↓BP, ↑HR. Notify surgeon, flood surgical field with NS, support patient hemodynamically and D/C N$_2$O.

POSTOPERATIVE

Complications	↑ADH secretion Diabetes insipidus (DI)	SIADH or DI may follow brain manipulation and may require pharmacologic intervention for Rx.
	Cerebral edema	Cerebral edema may → ↑ICP (headache, N/V, ↓mental status, etc.)
	Pneumothorax Bleeding	Pneumothorax (Sx = ↑respirations, wheezing, ↓BP, ↓CO, ↓O$_2$ sat) may occur 2° rib resection for bone graft. ✓ CXR.
Pain management	PCA (see p. E-3).	
Tests	Hct	

References

1. Christianson L: Anesthesia for major craniofacial operations. *Int Anesthesiol Clin* 1985; 23(4):117-30.
2. MacLennan FM, Robertson GS: Ketamine for induction and intubation in Treacher-Collins syndrome. *Anesthesia* 1981; 36(2):196-98.
3. Rasch DK, Browder F, Barr M, Greer D: Anaesthesia for Treacher-Collins and Pierre Robin syndromes: a report of three cases. *Can Anaesth Soc J* 1986; 33(3P+1):364-70.

13.0 OUT-OF-OPERATING ROOM PROCEDURES

Surgeons

Charles DeBattista, MD (*Electroconvulsive therapy*)
Alexander M. Norbash, MD (*Interventional neuroradiology*)
Robert J. Singer, MD (*Interventional neuroradiology*)
I. Bing Liem, DO (*DC cardioversion; AICD*)
Stephen T. Kee, MD (*TIPS*)
Charles P. Semba, MD (*TIPS*)
Daniel Y. Sze, MD (*Image-guided procedures*)

13.1 OUT-OF-OPERATING ROOM PROCEDURES—ADULT

Anesthesiologists

Richard A. Jaffe, MD, PhD
Stanley I. Samuels, MB, BCh

ANESTHESIA FOR OUT-OF-OPERATING ROOM PROCEDURES

GENERAL COMMENTS

Advances in the fields of radiology, cardiology and neurology have led to an increase in the number of anesthesia procedures performed away from the OR. In line with these changes, the ASA has provided guidelines for the safe delivery of anesthesia at locations remote from the OR environment.

Anesthetic considerations for out-of-OR locations (modified from ASA Guidelines[1]) include:

- Primary and backup O_2 sources (e.g., piped O_2 + 1 full E cylinder)
- Adequate and reliable suction
- Adequate and reliable scavenging system (for inhalational anesthesia)
- Self-inflating hand resuscitator bag with ability to deliver at least 90% O_2
- Adequate anesthetic drug supplies and equipment
- Adequate monitoring equipment to allow adherence to the "Standards of Basic Anesthetic Monitoring"[2]
- Sufficient electrical outlets connected to an emergency power supply
- Wet locations (e.g., cysto, arthroscopy, labor and delivery) should be equipped with either an isolated electrical source or circuits with ground-fault interrupters.
- Adequate illumination for patient observation and monitoring equipment (flashlight backup)
- Sufficient space for expeditious access to patient, machine and support equipment
- Emergency cart with defibrillator immediately available
- Immediate access to skilled anesthesia support personnel

References

1. Guidelines for Non-Operating Room Locations. American Society of Anesthesiologists, Park Ridge, IL: 1997.
2. Standards for Basic Anesthesia Monitoring. American Society of Anesthesiologists, Park Ridge, IL: 1997.

ELECTROCONVULSIVE THERAPY (ECT)

PROCEDURAL CONSIDERATIONS

Description: Electroconvulsive therapy (ECT) is the transcutaneous application of small electrical stimuli to the brain in order to produce generalized seizures for the treatment of selected psychiatric disorders, especially severe depression. There are several important aspects of ECT that are of relevance to the anesthesiologist. The first is the uncontrolled motor activity associated with generalized seizures. Prior to introduction of GA, the most common injuries associated with ECT were compression fractures of the vertebral bodies and broken limbs from violent tonic clonic motor activity. Even with complete paralysis, the masseter muscles are directly stimulated to contract during seizure induction. As a result, the most common malpractice claims in ECT involved dental injuries.

A second consequence of ECT induction is that the electrical stimulus can cause contraction of cranial musculature and, possibly, a brief dilation of sensitive meningeal blood vessels, resulting in postictal headaches in up to 40% of patients. Patients under the age of 50 yr and those with a Hx of migraine headaches appear most at risk for post ECT headaches that may occasionally require aggressive pain management. Finally, ECT may represent a significant hemodynamic stressor. Initially, central parasympathetic centers are activated, resulting in bradydysrhythmias in approximately 30% of patients. Brief sinus pauses are not uncommon. The initial parasympathetic effects are followed by sympathetically mediated increases in HR and BP. Increases of 20-30% above baseline are not uncommon, and MAP may even double. These cardiovascular responses can persist even after the procedure is completed.

The optimal position for ECT is supine. Occasionally, the head is kept slightly raised to help maintain an adequate airway and decrease anxiety. Patients typically come to ECT quite anxious about the procedure. ECT is generally performed in a PACU, or specialized ECT suite. The electrical stimulus is applied through plastic adhesive leads or metal leads prepared with a contact gel. These leads are usually applied to the forehead in a bitemporal or right unilateral placement. Monitoring typically includes a two-lead electroencephalogram (EEG) and frequently an electromyogram (EMG) to measure motor activity. A BP cuff is inflated to act as a tourniquet and prevent neuromuscular blockade in the distal limbs. Thus, an arm or leg can be used to measure motor duration of the seizure. A special ECT device is used to generate the appropriate electrical stimulus. Seizures are typically 30-90 sec in duration and the entire procedure—from the induction of anesthesia to patient awakening—is generally less than 15 min. The recovery period averages 45-90 min and allows for monitoring of vital signs as well as the opportunity for the postictal confusion to clear. Patients can wake up mildly confused to frankly delirious and require close nursing supervision. Treatments are typically performed every other day, and the average number of treatments is 6-12 in the management of major depression.

The most common morbidities associated with ECT include headaches and myalgias. Postictal confusion is the rule and some anterograde and retrograde memory loss occurs in all patients. Memory loss is typically confined to the preop and postop settings; however, there may be a cumulative memory loss with subsequent ECT treatments within a given series. In most patients, memory loss recovers in 1-3 wk following treatment. In rare instances, autobiographical memory loss has been reported for months or years after an ECT series has been completed. Long-term memory loss appears to be more common with bilateral lead placement. ECT-related mortality is estimated at approximately 4/10,000. Cardiac events account for 67% of all ECT-related deaths, with malignant arrhythmias and myocardial infarctions (MIs) accounting for most fatalities. Pulmonary events (obstruction, pulmonary edema or emboli) account for most additional mortality. Cerebrovascular infarctions or hemorrhages have rarely been reported with ECT.

Usual preop diagnosis: Depression; mania; catatonia; refractory psychosis

SUMMARY OF PROCEDURE

Position	Supine
Incision	None
Special instrumentation	Seizure generator & electrodes; EEG/EMG monitors
Unique considerations	Requires complete muscle relaxation to prevent injury. Bite block required to prevent dental injury. Tourniquet (BP cuff) applied before administration of muscle relaxant.
Antibiotics	None
Procedure time	Setup: 5-10 min Treatment: < 10 min (seizure duration 25-280 sec)
Postop care	PACU → room or home
Mortality	4/10,000
Morbidity	Cardiac dysrhythmias: 10-40% (brief asystole common) HA/myalgias: Common Confusion/memory loss: Common MI: Rare Pulmonary edema/pulmonary aspiration CVA: Rare
Pain score	2-3 (headache)

PATIENT POPULATION CHARACTERISTICS

Age range	≥ 18 yr. Some States (e.g., Texas) forbid ECT in minors, and ECT is rarely performed in adolescents; however, patients in their 90s are sometimes candidates for ECT. There is a preponderance of geriatric patients on many ECT services.
Male:Female	1:2
Incidence	The lifetime prevalence of major depression (the primary indication for ECT) is approximately 17%; 26% of women and 12% of men being affected. < 1% of patients with major depression undergo ECT; and approximately 400,000 ECT procedures are performed in North America annually.
Associated conditions	Substance abuse (30% of all depressed patients meet criteria for alcohol or drug abuse); panic attacks (30% of depressed patients); psychotic symptoms (14% of patients); HTN and sinus tachycardia; dehydration; self-inflicted trauma

ANESTHETIC CONSIDERATIONS

PREOPERATIVE

Patients presenting for ECT have often failed to respond to antidepressants; however, most will continue to take psychotherapeutic agents. Many of the older patients will be taking other medications for coexisting medical conditions. Drug interactions are an important consideration for the anesthesiologist (see Drug Interactions, p. F-1). The most commonly used antidepressants are listed in Table 13.1-1.

Table 13.1-1 Commonly Used Antidepressant Medications

Tricyclic	MAOI	SSRI	SNRI and other Antidepressants
amitriptyline (Elavil, others)	isocarboxazid (Marplan)	fluoxetine (Prozac)	venlafaxine (Effexor)
amoxapine (Asendin)	phenelzine (Nardil)	paroxitine (Paxil)	nefazodone (Serzone)
desipramine (Norpramin)	tranylcypromine (Parnate)	sertraline (Zoloft)	sibutramine (Meridia)
doxepin (Sinequan)	St. John's wort	fluvoxamine (Luvox)	mirtazapine (Remeron)
imipramine (Tofranil)		trazodone (Desyrel)	bupropion (Wellbutrin)
maprotiline (Ludiomil)	**Lithium**		
nortriptyline (Pamelor)	(Often used as an adjunctive agent/mood stabilizer in depression)		
protriptyline (Vivactil)			
trimipramine (Surmontil)			

MAOI = monoamine oxidase inhibitor

SSRI = selective serotonin reuptake inhibitor

SNRI = selective norepinephrine/serotonin reuptake inhibitor

Anesthesia for ECT may seem to be a very benign procedure; however, these cases—which seldom take more than 20 min—can prove very challenging, especially in the geriatric population. ECT can place significant stress on the cardiovascular system; therefore, particular care should be taken to evaluate and optimize the patient's pretreatment cardiovascular status. ECT usually takes place in remote locations, so the anesthesiologist must ensure that the location is properly equipped and complies with ASA Guidelines for Out-of-OR Procedures (see p. 1047).

Respiratory These patients will require airway management and positive pressure ventilation. Hence, preop assessment of the airway must focus on the ease of mask ventilation and the potential need for ET intubation (e.g., airway compromise or severe GERD).

Cardiovascular A recent MI (< 3 mo) is a contraindication to ECT. Relative contraindications include aortic aneurysm, angina, CHF and thrombophlebitis. The presence of dysrhythmias, a pacemaker or AICD is not a contraindication for ECT. For the patient with a pacemaker, a means (e.g., a magnet) should be available to convert the pacemaker to an asynchronous mode.
Tests: As indicated from H&P.

Gastrointestinal Patient should be npo. Patients with Sx of GERD should be pretreated with Na citrate (30 ml po), ranitidine (50 mg iv) and metoclopramide (10 mg iv). ET intubation should be considered for all patients at risk for aspiration.

Neurological ECT is relatively contraindicated in the presence of ↑ICP, and recent CVA (< 3 mo), intracranial mass lesions or recent intracranial surgery (< 3 mo).

Endocrine Presence of a pheochromocytoma is a contraindication to ECT. < 1% of hypertensive patients will have a pheochromocytoma, Sx of which may be confused with a psychiatric disorder.

Genetic ✓ for family Hx of pseudocholinesterase deficiency. Mivacurium (0.15 mg/kg) is a suitable alternative to succinylcholine.
Tests: Dibucaine number (normal ≥ 80) and serum cholinesterase level, if indicated from H&P.

Hepatic Hepatotoxicity has been associated with use of MAOI.
Tests: Consider LFTs for patients on chronic MAOI therapy.

Orthopaedic In patients susceptible to bone fracture (e.g., severe osteoporosis, osteoporosis imperfecta), an increased succinylcholine dosage (1.5 mg/kg) is given to ensure profound muscle relaxation. Patients with severe rheumatoid arthritis may have unstable C-spine, and extreme care should be taken during positioning of head and neck.

Ophthalmologic Retinal detachment is a relative contraindication to ECT. Succinylcholine should be avoided in patients with glaucoma treated with cholinesterase-inhibitors (e.g., echothiophate). Mivacurium (0.15 mg/kg) is a suitable alternative.

Pregnancy Pregnancy is not a contraindication for ECT (even in the third trimester). After the fourth mo, the need for full-stomach precautions require rapid-sequence induction and ET intubation (see p. B-5). Left uterine displacement should be maintained during treatment. Monitor fetal heartbeat.

Psychiatric Drugs Patients receiving tricyclic antidepressants (TCAs) may have an exaggerated pressor response to direct-acting sympathomimetic drugs, with the potential for tachycardia, dysrhythmias and hyperthermia. The response to indirect-acting sympathomimetic drugs (e.g., ephedrine) may be attenuated in these patients. TCAs also will increase the effects of anticholinergic drugs (e.g., glycopyrrolate, atropine). Patients receiving MAOIs will exhibit exaggerated responses to indirect-acting sympathomimetic drugs (e.g., ephedrine). Additionally, in these patients succinylcholine metabolism is inhibited (↑NMB), and meperidine is contraindicated (↑↑BP, ↑Sz, ↑↑Temp). It is probably unnecessary to discontinue TCAs or MAOIs prior to ECT, as long as these interactions can be avoided. Lithium should be discontinued for at least 3 d prior to ECT to avoid delayed recovery and subsequent posttreatment agitation and confusion. Lithium also is associated with ↑NMB (succinylcholine and pancuronium). SSRI antidepressants have been associated with prolonged ECT-induced seizure duration, and adverse behavioral/neurological effects following haloperidol administration (use droperidol and metoclopramide with caution). No adverse interactions have been reported between anesthetic agents and SSRIs or SNRIs.

Laboratory Tests as indicated from H&P.

Premedication Although usually not required, some patients may benefit from an antisialagogue (glycopyrrolate 0.2 mg iv). Patients with Hx of postop N/V will benefit from a prophylactic antiemetic (e.g., odansetron 4 mg iv). Patients with postseizure muscle pain and headache may benefit from ketorolac (30 mg iv). Some patients will require 500-1000 mg caffeine iv to decrease seizure threshold. The caffeine effect should be manifest in 5 min. Verapamil (not adenosine, which is blocked by caffeine) should be available to control supraventricular tachycardia (0.07-0.25 mg/kg over 2 min).

INTRAOPERATIVE

Anesthetic technique: A review of previous anesthetic records is very helpful in formulating the anesthetic plan and in anticipating physiological changes unique to each patient. Usually brief iv anesthesia (mask oxygenation and ventilation) with profound muscle relaxation is required to prevent patient injury during seizures. Prior to induction, a tourniquet (BP cuff) is applied to the non-iv arm and inflated to a pressure above systolic. This prevents neuromuscular blockade distal to the cuff and permits direct monitoring of seizure activity. Preop BP control (e.g., labetalol 5-10 mg or esmolol 0.5-1 mg/kg iv in increments) is often necessary.

Induction Preoxygenation should be attempted in all patients. In some patients who are intolerant of a mask, a less intrusive blow-by technique may be tried. Anesthesia is induced with either STP (1.5-3 mg/kg) sodium methohexital (0.5-1 mg/kg) or etomidate (0.1-0.2 mg/kg). Propofol (1-1.5 mg/kg) may be used, but may shorten seizure duration. Remember that TCAs and MAOIs can increase sleep time. Succinylcholine (1 mg/kg) is injected after 3 mg dTC. Hyperventilation is carried out in order to enhance seizure activity. A bite block is placed and then the patient is ready for ECT. In barbiturate-tolerant patients, remifentanil (1-3 μg/kg) has been used as a means of reducing the barbiturate dose, thereby permitting adequate seizure duration. Patients receiving remifentanil need minimal postseizure BP control.

Maintenance Given the brevity of this procedure, maintenance of anesthesia is rarely a concern; however, occasionally a second or third treatment may be necessary if the seizures are of inadequate duration (< 25 sec) and quality. In this case, a subsequent dose (10-30 mg) of succinylcholine may be needed. Assisted ventilation is necessary until spontaneous ventilation resumes. Of major concern during the seizure period is the hypertensive response. Some patients may need to be treated prior to induction of anesthesia with either labetalol (5-20 mg iv) or esmolol (10 mg q 1 min) to control HR/BP. SNP (5-50 μg/bolus iv) is useful to control BP in refractory cases.

Emergence	Patients should be awake within 5-10 min postseizure and may well be disoriented. Small doses of midazolam (e.g., 0.25-0.5 mg iv) may help to control agitation. ASA guidelines for postanesthesia care should be followed (see p. 1047).	
Blood and fluid requirements	No blood loss IV: 20 ga × 1 NS/LR @ TKO	
Monitoring	Standard monitors (p. B-1) Tourniquet EEG EMG	Seizure activity is usually monitored by a psychiatrist observing the tourniqueted limb, and by measuring EMG and EEG activity. (These monitors are usually an integral part of the ECT seizure generator.)
Positioning	Supine	
Complications	Dysrhythmias	Brief periods of asystole and profound bradycardia are not uncommon (usually related to parasympathetic overactivity). Treatment is rarely necessary.
	Tachydysrhythmias	Responds well to esmolol (10-15 mg iv) or lidocaine (1 mg/kg iv) although treatment is usually unnecessary.
	↑BP	↑BP readily responds to esmolol (10-30 mg), or labetalol (5-20 mg). In refractory cases, 10-50 mg of SNP may be necessary.
	Dental damage Pulmonary edema Aspiration	Use of bite block is essential. Dental damage is not prevented by muscle relaxation (direct electrical stimulation of facial and jaw muscles).

POSTOPERATIVE

Complications	Headache, myalgias	Rx: Ketorolac 30 mg iv
	N/V	Rx: Odansetron 4 mg iv
	Disorientation	Rx: Midazolam 0.25-0.5 mg iv
	Memory impairment	
	MI/ischemia	
	Dysrhythmias	
	Pulmonary edema/aspiration	
	↑BP	Prolonged ↑BP is unusual and may suggest the need for further workup.

Reference

1. Martin DE, Kettl P: Anesthesia for electroconvulsive therapy. In *Alternate-Site Anesthesia: Clinical Practice Outside the Operating Room.* Russell GB, ed. Butterworth-Heinemann, Boston: 1997, 243-68.

INTERVENTIONAL NEURORADIOLOGY

PROCEDURAL CONSIDERATIONS

Description: Recent developments in materials technology, surgical techniques and radiotherapy procedures have increased the scope of interventional neuroradiology, with microcatheters now allowing access to previously inaccessible distal circulations. Four broad categories of therapy currently are performed by interventional neuroradiologists: preop or stand-alone hemostasis; treatment of acute and chronic stroke; aneurysm therapy; and embolization of high-flow vascular lesions. There is considerable variability in the duration of these procedures. For example, epistaxis embolizations may be of short duration, whereas more complex procedures, such as multisession, staged embolization of large, high-flow, parenchymal arteriovenous vascular malformations (AVMs), and staged embolizations of Vein of Galen malformations in neonates, may be extremely lengthy. EP monitoring may be used for lesions involving speech, vision, motor centers, basal ganglia and the posterior fossa, thus requiring modification of the anesthetic plan.

Hemostasis: These therapies may take the form of particulate embolization (e.g., epistaxis refractory to traditional nasal packs) or preop embolization of vascular lesions to facilitate surgical resection (e.g., meningiomas, juvenile nasopharyngeal angiofibromas). Shaved gelatin or polymeric particles are used for these embolizations, which are relatively short procedures.

Stroke and ischemia therapy: Stroke therapy encompasses thrombolysis, percutaneous angioplasty and stent placement for a variety of acute and chronic ischemic disorders. For acute events, thrombolysis may be performed in patients presenting within 6 h of a witnessed neurologic event. After 6 h there is an increased risk of converting an otherwise bland stroke into a large and potentially life-threatening hemorrhagic infarct. These procedures are ordinarily preceded by a CT scan to characterize the nature of the infarct, since hemorrhagic stroke is considered by many an absolute contraindication to thrombolysis. Posterior circulation strokes tend to be treated more aggressively, since withholding therapy ordinarily results in death or a vegetative state. Anterior circulation strokes may be treated conservatively, based on the severity of the clinical symptoms.

Aneurysm therapy: The availability of controllable release microcoils has increased the frequency of aneurysm coiling as a substitute for traditional surgical aneurysm clipping in selected cases. These procedures are ordinarily performed with GA, since patient movement during coil placement may interfere with aneurysm visualization. For these procedures, the patient is ordinarily anticoagulated to minimize the risk of accidental thrombosis with downstream embolization. For selected vascular lesions, intraop evoked potential monitoring may be used to minimize complications from therapy. Successful therapy is regarded as complete aneurysm thrombosis. During the procedure, these patients may require elevated perfusion pressures in order to maximize intracerebral perfusion; however, this may risk rerupture in the unprotected aneurysm.

High-flow AVM embolization: High-flow arteriovenous fistulas are primarily supplied by the external carotid artery distribution. These may be treated by transvenous or transarterial routes, and occasionally demand multiple staged treatments. AVMs are groups of microfistulae (nidus) surrounded by parasitized parenchymal branches which involute once the nidus is removed or excluded from the circulation. These lesions have significantly higher morbidity and may be treated with a combination of embolization, cerebrovascular surgery and radiation therapy. Embolization in both types of high-flow lesion may be performed with polymer particles or adhesives, which are chemically related to the superglues. During adhesive embolotherapy, occasionally brief elevations in MAP will assist in placement of specialized "flow-directed" catheters. High-flow embolizations are curative in < 10% of cases and, therefore, these procedures are planned as combined therapy with cerebrovascular surgery and often radiation therapy. Postembolization BP control with SNP and/or esmolol infusions will minimize the risk of intracranial bleeding.

SUMMARY OF PROCEDURE

	Hemostasis	Aneurysm	High-Flow AVM	Stroke/Ischemia
Position	Supine	⇐	⇐	⇐
Incision	Percutaneous femoral artery catheterization	⇐	⇐	⇐
Unique considerations	None	Heparinized; ± EPs	BP control; ± EPs	Variable mental status; anticoagulated BP control
Antibiotics	None	⇐	⇐	⇐
Procedure time	1-3 h	2-4 h	3-8 h	1-4 h
Closing considerations	Femoral artery pressure over catheter site. Minimize leg movement for 15-20 min.	⇐	⇐	⇐
EBL	Minimal	⇐	⇐	⇐
Postop care	Outpatient or ward	ICU: 12-24 h	⇐	⇐
Mortality	Rare	1.5-2%	1-1.6%	~1%
Morbidity	Overall: 0.5% Accidental embolization: < 0.7% Thrombus/embolus: 0.5%	5% Aneurysm rupture: 2% Emboli: 2%	8% Delayed hemorrhage: 4% AVM rupture: 2%	4% Angioplasty rupture: 4% Hemorrhagic stroke conversion: 2%

	Hemostasis	Aneurysm	High-Flow AVM	Stroke/Ischemia
Morbidity, cont.	Blindness: < 1% Cranial neuropathies: < 1% Stroke: < 1% Vessel rupture Postembolization bleeding	Parent vessel occlusion: 1%	Catheter glue-in: 1%	Stent torpedo: 1%
Pain score	1-2	1-2	1-2	1-2

PATIENT POPULATION CHARACTERISTICS

Age range	Varies from neonatal/premature to very elderly
Male:Female	1:1
Etiology	Congenital, degenerative; traumatic
Associated conditions	Elevated ICP; intracranial hemorrhage ± vasospasm; congenital anomalies; HTN/CAD/PVD; anticoagulant therapy

---

ANESTHETIC CONSIDERATIONS

PREOPERATIVE

Patients presenting for diagnostic neuroradiologic procedures frequently may require only local anesthesia and sedation. The newer nontoxic and low osmolality contrast agents have improved patient comfort and tolerance of these procedures while minimizing adverse reactions. Patients presenting for interventional neuroradiological procedures (e.g., embolization or stenting) are likely to experience more discomfort and, therefore, may require GA in order to tolerate the often lengthy procedures. However, the advantages of GA must be balanced against the potential need for intraop neurological monitoring (e.g., speech, vision, and mental status) that requires the patient to be awake and cooperative. In this set of circumstances, close consultation between the neuroradiologist and anesthesiologist is required in formulating the anesthesia plan.

Respiratory — Access to the airway may be limited; therefore, examination should focus on the need for elective ET intubation. Patients with chronic cough may require GA to ensure immobility.
Tests: As indicated from H&P.

Cardiovascular — Patients with recent intracranial hemorrhage may demonstrate ECG abnormalities, which need to be differentiated from new ischemic heart disease (ECHO, cardiac enzymes).
Tests: ECG; other tests as indicated from H&P.

Neurological — Symptoms vary with the location, size and type of lesion. Aneurysms seldom produce neurological symptoms unless they leak or rupture, whereas tumors are commonly associated with symptoms of ↑ICP (HA, N/V, altered mental status, papilledema). Patients with recent cerebral hemorrhages are likely to be medicated with calcium channel blockers (e.g., nimodipine) to ↓arterial vasospasm. Patients with ↑ICP or cranial trauma will usually need GA with mechanical ventilation and intubation.

Premedication — Preop sedation may mask the Sx of ↑ICP or intracranial hemorrhage. Patients at high risk for contrast-media reactions (e.g., patients with previous contrast reaction, allergy to iodine or seafood) should receive prophylactic treatment consisting of prednisone, 50 mg po q 6 h × 3, starting 18 h before the study, and diphenhydramine, 50 mg po/im, 1 h before the procedure.

INTRAOPERATIVE

Anesthetic technique: MAC (p. B-4) may be adequate for patients undergoing diagnostic procedures and necessary for patients requiring neurological assessment during more invasive procedures; otherwise, GETA.

Induction — Standard induction (p. B-2). Patients with ↑ICP should be hyperventilated to an $ETCO_2$ of 30 mmHg. In patients with vascular lesions that may leak or rupture, BP responses to laryngoscopy and intubation should be blunted (e.g., remifentanil 3-5 μg/kg).

Maintenance	Standard maintenance (p. B-3). Muscle relaxation is usually mandatory in order to control ventilation and minimize the chance of movement. Hyperventilation may be necessary to ↓ ICP and may also enhance the quality of the angiogram.	
Emergence	Prompt awakening is important to permit neurologic evaluation. Metoclopramide (10 mg iv) is useful to ↓ postop N/V. Extubate when airway reflexes have returned. Continuous control of BP may be necessary during emergence phase. Patients are typically transported to ICU.	
Blood and fluid requirements	IV: 18 ga × 1-2 NS/LR @ 3-5 ml/kg/h	
Monitoring	Standard monitors (see p. B-1). Arterial line Urinary catheter	BP can be monitored from femoral line placed by radiologist. Place urinary catheter if procedure is lengthy (> 3 h).
	± EPs	Keep inhalation agents < 0.5 MAC to minimize interference with EP monitoring.
Control of BP	Isoflurane (if no EP monitoring) Esmolol (50-200 μg/kg/min) SNP (0.2-2 μg/kg/min) Maintain normovolemia.	BP control may be necessary during intracranial catheter manipulation, embolization and postembolization. Close communication with the radiologist is important. SNP/esmolol may be infused through a second peripheral iv.
Positioning	✓ and pad pressure points. ✓ eyes.	X-ray table may not be well padded → nerve damage.
Contrast-related complications	Common reactions: N/V Itching Urticaria Sensation of warmth Pain Anxiety Rash	These reactions occur in > 5% of patients, and may require no treatment apart from reassurance or a mild anxiolytic. Mild allergic reactions may be treated with diphenhydramine 25-50 mg iv. Monitor patients for progression of Sx, suggesting the need for more aggressive therapy.
	Neurotoxic Sx: Hemiplegia Blindness Aphasia ↓consciousness	These reactions may be related to the hyperosmolarity of the agent. If persistent, procedure should be terminated. Rx may require steroids and vasopressors to improve perfusion. In the anesthetized patient, these Sx will be masked.
	Major allergic reactions: Bronchospasm Hypotension Cardiac arrest Pulmonary edema Laryngeal edema Dysrhythmias	Epinephrine (0.25-0.5 mg iv) should be given immediately. Rx of **anaphylaxis** includes: eliminate antigens (e.g., contrast agent, latex, etc.); secure airway; administer 100% O_2, iv fluids, epinephrine, diphenhydramine. Supplemental Rx may include steroids (e.g., hydrocortisone 5 mg/kg), atropine, $NaHCO_3$ and epinephrine infusion.
Complications, other	Hemorrhage	Aneurysmal rupture or AVM bleeding may require immediate transport to OR for surgical repair.
	Vasospasm	Typically occurs in elderly diabetic or hypertensive patients, especially if the procedure is long and much contrast agent is used. Rx: vasodilators (e.g., NTG) or papaverine delivered by catheter, or balloon angioplasty.
	Occlusion of vessel	2° accidental injection of contrast material into vessel wall. Rx: angioplasty (wire recanalization may be used for thrombotic occlusions).

POSTOPERATIVE

Complications	Neurologic deficits	CT scan for evaluation, as prompt neurosurgical intervention may be required.
	Vasospasm	May require Ca^{++} channel blocker (e.g., nimodipine). Consult with neurosurgeon.

References

1. Bader MK: The complexity of caring for patients with ruptured cerebral aneurysm: case studies. *AACN Clinical Issues* 1997; 8(2):182-95.
2. Cardella JF, Waybill PN: Interventional radiology: diagnostic and interventional vascular applications. In *Alternate-Site Anesthesia: Clinical Practice Outside the Operating Room.* Russell GB, ed. Butterworth-Heinemann, Boston: 1997, 115-32.
3. Clark WM, Barnwell SL: Endovascular treatment for acute and chronic brain ischemia. *Curr Opin Neurol* 1996; 9(1):62-7.
4. Deruty R, Pelissou-Guyotat I, Mottolese C, Bascoulergue Y, Amat D: The combined management of cerebral arteriovenous malformations. Experience with 100 cases and review of the literature. *Acta Neurochirurgica* 1993; 123(3-4):101-12.
5. Gobin YP, Laurent A, Merienne L, Schlienger M, Aymard A, Houdart E, Casasco A, Lefkopoulos D, George B, Merland JJ: Treatment of brain arteriovenous malformations by embolization and radiosurgery. *J Neurosurg* 1996; 85(1):19-28
6. Higashida RT, Halbach VV, Tsai FY, Dowd CF, Hieshima GB: Interventional neurovascular techniques for cerebral revascularization in the treatment of stroke. *Am J Roentgenol* 1994; 163(4):793-800.
7. Kato T, Sato K, Sasaki R, Kakinuma H, Moriyama M: Targeted cancer chemotherapy with arterial microcapsule chemoembolization: review of 1013 patients. *Cancer Chemother Pharmacol* 1996; 37(4):289-96.
8. Nichols DA, Meyer FB, Piepgras D, Smith PL: Endovascular treatment of intracranial aneurysms. *Mayo Clin Proc* 1994; 69(3):272-85.
9. Pollice PA, Yoder MG: Epistaxis: a retrospective review of hospitalized patients. *Otolaryngol Head Neck Surg* 1997; 117(1):49-53.
10. Russell GB: Anesthesia and interventional radiology. In *Alternate-Site Anesthesia: Clinical Practice Outside the Operating Room.* Russell GB, ed. Butterworth-Heinemann, Boston: 1997, 157-70.
11. Spearman MP, Jungreis CA, Wechsler LR. Angioplasty of the occluded internal carotid artery. *Am J Neuroradiol* 1995; 16(9):1791-99
12. Wallace RC, Flom RA, Khayata MH, Dean BL, McKenzie J, Rand JC, Obuchowski NA, Zepp RC, Zabramski JM, Spetzler RF: The safety and effectiveness of brain arteriovenous malformation embolization using acrylic and particles: the experiences of a single institution. *Neurosurgery* 1995; 37(4):606-18.
13. Young WI, Pile-Spellman J: Anaesthetic considerations for interventional neuroradiology. *Anaesthesiology* 1994; 80:427-56.

DIRECT CURRENT CARDIOVERSION

PROCEDURAL CONSIDERATIONS

Description: Direct current (DC) cardioversion is a treatment for cardiac arrhythmias that uses a brief, dosed (50-400 J) discharge of electricity across the heart, depolarizing the entire heart and allowing normal sinus rhythm to resume. The electrical shock is delivered across the chest wall using two external paddles placed in the A-P (preferred) or basilar-apical positions. The pulse is delivered synchronous to the QRS, thus avoiding the vulnerable period. Shock to treat ventricular fibrillation is applied asynchronously and is called "defibrillation." To avoid discomfort, DC cardioversion is performed with the patient under deep sedation or brief GA.

Usual preop diagnosis: Atrial fibrillation; atrial flutter; other supraventricular tachycardia; ventricular tachycardia

SUMMARY OF PROCEDURE

Position	Supine with defibrillator pads positioned A-P or basilar-apical
Unique considerations	Adequate anticoagulation (INR = 2-3) in patients with atrial fibrillation
Antibiotics	None
Procedure time	30 min
Postop care	Monitoring of cardiac rhythm
Mortality	0.1%
Morbidity	Skin burns: ≤ 15% (1st degree), 2% (2nd degree) Embolic event: 2% (↑risk with mitral value disease) Acute pulmonary edema: 1%

Morbidity, cont.	More serious arrhythmia: 1% Myocardial damage: Incidence unknown but estimated to be very low – proportional to delivered energy.
Pain score	2-3

PATIENT POPULATION CHARACTERISTICS

Age range	All ages
Male:Female	3:1
Incidence	100,000/yr in the U.S.
Etiology	Reentry substrates (e.g., atrial flutter, ventricular tachycardia) from hypertensive heart disease, remote MI, cardiomyopathy; idiopathic
Associated conditions	LV dysfunction; CAD; cardiomyopathy; HTN; valvular disease; COPD; obesity; CVA; acute MI; pulmonary edema

ANESTHETIC CONSIDERATIONS

PREOPERATIVE

In general, patients presenting for cardioversion fall into one of two categories: elective or emergent. The presence or absence of hemodynamic instability will define the category. In the emergency patient, full-stomach precautions may be necessary (see p. B-5). Elective cardioversions usually are carried out on patients who have failed drug therapy.

Respiratory Preop evaluation of the airway should focus on the need for elective ET intubation (patients with GERD, difficult mask fit or airway compromise).

Cardiovascular Relative contraindications to elective cardioversion include digitalis toxicity (toxic: > 3 ng/ml), ↓K^+, inadequate anticoagulation, presence of β-blockade, AV block. The presence of significant CHF, CAD or valvular disease may predispose this patient population to ⇊BP in response to anesthetic agents. Consider use of etomidate (0.1-0.2 mg/kg). Patients at ↑risk for embolization include those with: Hx of embolization within 2 yr, mitral stenosis, intraarterial thrombus, CHF or hyperthyroidism. In these patients, ensure adequate anticoagulation (PT 1.5-2 × baseline, INR 2.0-3.0). It has been suggested that NTG patches near the electrodes be removed prior to cardioversion to avoid risk of explosion.
Tests: ECG; TEE (✓ for thrombus and size of atrium); digitalis level (toxic > 3 ng/ml → refractory VF following cardioversion); electrolytes; INR.

Endocrine Hyperthyroidism → atrial fibrillation (AF)

Gastrointestinal Full-stomach precautions (see p. B-5) may be necessary in the emergency patient.

Neurological ✓ Hx for TIAs or CVAs → ↑risk of embolic event. Pre- and postprocedure neurologic exams should be done.

Hematologic ✓ need for anticoagulation (see above).

Laboratory Other tests as indicated from H&P.

Premedication Usually not needed. For the emergency patient, take full-stomach precautions (p. B-5).

INTRAOPERATIVE

Anesthetic technique: Brief GA with mask oxygenation and ventilation

Induction ★ Preoxygenate patient. For hemodynamically fragile patients, etomidate (0.1-0.2 ml/kg iv) is perhaps the agent of choice (**NB**: etomidate-induced clonus → ECG artifact). For the hemodynamically stable patient, use propofol (1.0-1.5 mg/kg iv slowly) until loss of lid reflex. Additional analgesia may be provided by remifentanil (1-2 μg/kg iv), thereby reducing anesthetic requirements.

Maintenance Occasionally necessary to repeat cardioversion. Additional small doses of propofol, etomidate or remifentanil may be required.

Emergence Patients should awaken rapidly with full recovery of airway reflexes. Outpatients are usually discharged to home within 1-2 h.

Blood and fluid requirements	No blood loss IV: 20 ga × 1 NS/LR @ TKO	
Monitoring	Standard monitors (see p. B-1).	Avoid placement of ECG electrodes in precordial area.
Positioning	Hospital bed, supine	Procedure takes place at patient's bedside.
Complications	Loss of airway	Use airway manipulation ± artificial airways; be prepared to intubate.
	VF	Use ACLS protocols.
	↑↑BP/myocardial ischemia	Cardioversion → catecholamine surge → acute MI in susceptible patient population.
	Severe bradycardia	Rx: Atropine (e.g., 0.4 mg iv)
	Thermal injury	Ensure good electrode/skin contact.
	↓CO	2° anesthetic drugs or myocardial stunning from cardioversion. Rx: inotropic support (e.g., ephedrine).

POSTOPERATIVE

Complications	Recall	Especially in hemodynamically fragile patients. Discuss possibility with patient in advance.
	Systemic embolization	Neurological exam should be repeated postcardioversion.
	↓BP/↓CO/CHF	Atrial contraction may not be effective following cardioversion → ↓CO/↓BP.
	New dysrhythmia	
Pain management	Minimal	Myalgias not uncommon; consider ketorolac.
Tests	ECG	Verify NSR.

Reference

1. Stoneham, MD: Anesthesia for cardioversion. *Anaesthesia* 1996; 57:565-70.

IMPLANTATION OF CARDIOVERTER-DEFIBRILLATOR (AICD)

PROCEDURAL CONSIDERATIONS

Description: The automatic implantable cardioverter-defibrillator (AICD) is an effective device for the prevention of premature sudden death from ventricular tachycardia (VT) or ventricular fibrillation (VF). The results of two randomized studies involving survivors of cardiac arrest and those considered at risk for sudden death showed the superiority of AICD therapy over conventional medical therapy in lowering the incidence of sudden death and overall mortality.

The device system consists of a small pulse generator that is capable of producing a 30-40 J shock, and leads that are designed to record ventricular depolarizations and deliver the shock via coils or patches. AICD terminates VT/VF by sensing these rhythms and delivering an appropriate countershock. The most common AICD implantation uses endocardial leads inserted percutaneously (transvenous approach) and, depending on suitability, either a pectoral or abdominal subcutaneous/submuscular pulse generator placement. In the unusual circumstances of difficult endocardial access or high defibrillation threshold (> 25 J), the leads (in the form of patches) are applied epicardially via a thoracotomy approach.

In the transvenous approach, the insertion of leads and pulse generator requires minimal anesthesia; however, during testing of defibrillation efficacy, VF is induced repeatedly. Thus, in addition to continuous monitoring of vital signs and cardiac rhythm, special attention should be directed at the patient's hemodynamic stability prior to VF induction and after the defibrillation. It is customary to allow at least 5 min intervals between VF inductions. In patients with significant LV dysfunction, hypotension should not be treated with excessive fluid administration. If recovery from hypotension is slow, complications such as pneumo/hemothorax or pericardial effusion/tamponade should be considered. In the absence of a PA catheter (which would interfere with AICD lead positioning), accurate assessment of hemodynamic status is impaired. Thus, meticulous attention should be directed at arterial pressure, HR and oxygenation status. Finally, it is not uncommon to encounter acute atrial fibrillation (AF) from induction and conversion of VF. Fortunately, a cardioversion can be easily applied using the AICD or rescue system (external cardioversion).

Usual preop diagnosis: Recurrent ventricular dysrhythmias; poorly tolerated ventricular tachycardia

SUMMARY OF PROCEDURE

Position	Supine with defibrillator pads positioned A-P or basilar-apical
Incision	Left subclavicular (+ abdominal)
Special instrumentation	AICD pulse generator, lead(s) and testing system
Unique considerations	Multiple inductions of VT/VF with associated ↓CO, ↓BP; may require conversion to open thoracotomy approach.
Antibiotics	Cefazolin 1 g iv
Surgical time	1-2 h
Closing considerations	Routine subcutaneous/submuscular pocket closure
EBL	5-20 ml
Postop care	Monitoring of arrhythmia and pocket bleeding
Mortality	0.1% (transvenous); ≤ 5% (thoracotomy)
Morbidity	New-onset arrhythmias: ≤ 5% Pneumothorax: ≤ 5% (transvenous) Pericardial effusion/tamponade: ≤ 1% (transvenous)
Pain score	3 (6-9, thoracotomy)

PATIENT POPULATION CHARACTERISTICS

Age range	6-85 yr
Male:Female	4:1
Incidence	10,000/yr in the U.S.
Etiology	Reentry substrates from remote MI; cardiomyopathy; idiopathic
Associated conditions	LV dysfunction; CAD; cardiomyopathy; HTN; valvular disease; COPD; obesity; atrial fibrillation; CVA; anoxic encephalopathy

ANESTHETIC CONSIDERATIONS

See Anesthetic Considerations for Cardiac Mapping and Ablation Procedures, p. 241.

TRANSJUGULAR INTRAHEPATIC PORTOSYSTEMIC SHUNT (TIPS)

PROCEDURAL CONSIDERATIONS

Description: Portal HTN, most commonly due to hepatic cirrhosis, leads to the development of portosystemic varices and ascites. Portosystemic varices develop in a variety of sites. Gastroesophageal varices, through which portal blood returns to the heart via the azygous system, are a leading cause of massive upper gastrointestinal (GI) hemorrhage. Up to 25% of patients with portal HTN develop variceal hemorrhage within the first yr of diagnosis (incidence increases by 5-10% per yr), with > 50% mortality during the initial episode. Previous treatments have been mainly supportive, including blood replacement therapy and endoscopic sclerotherapy. Surgically created shunts (such as the portocaval shunt), in which a channel is made to direct blood away from the liver, are effective in reducing the risk of hemorrhage; however, they are associated with a high rate of encephalopathy and accelerated liver failure (40-70%).

Rosch created the first transjugular hepatic vein-to-portal vein communication in dogs in 1969. The first percutaneous portosystemic shunts were performed in humans using an angioplasty balloon in 1982. Due to the elastic recoil of the cirrhotic liver tissue, the tract rapidly closed. Palmaz and Richter performed the first successful **transjugular intrahepatic portosystemic shunt** (TIPS) in humans in 1989, using metallic stents to maintain the patency of the tract. Since then, TIPS has gained widespread clinical application, and initial results confirm that it is effective in reducing the frequency of variceal hemorrhage in patients with portal HTN. TIPS also can be used to treat refractory ascites, Budd-Chiari syndrome and hepatorenal syndrome.

TIPS is simply a shunt between the hepatic and portal veins, created in the liver parenchyma and maintained by placing metallic stents across the tract. The aim is to decrease the portal venous pressure, thereby directing blood flow away from the portosystemic varices, and decreasing the formation of ascitic fluid. The procedure can be performed under conscious sedation; however, the balloon dilation of the periportal fibrosis is associated with severe pain, and GA is preferred in many centers.

Via the right IJ, a 10 Fr sheath is placed in the upper IVC. A catheter/guide wire combination normally is used to access the right hepatic vein. A wedged hepatic venogram is performed, using either iodinated contrast, or CO_2, the purpose of which is to reflux contrast through the diseased hepatic sinusoids and demonstrate the location of the portal vein. The catheter is exchanged over a stiff guide wire for a metallic stiffening device, either the Rosch-Uchida or Colapinto transjugular needle (Cook Inc., Bloomington, IN). This device is curved at the tip, and can be steered to puncture the right portal vein (Fig 13.1-1A). The device is rotated anteriorly and medially so that the tip is pointed at the region of the

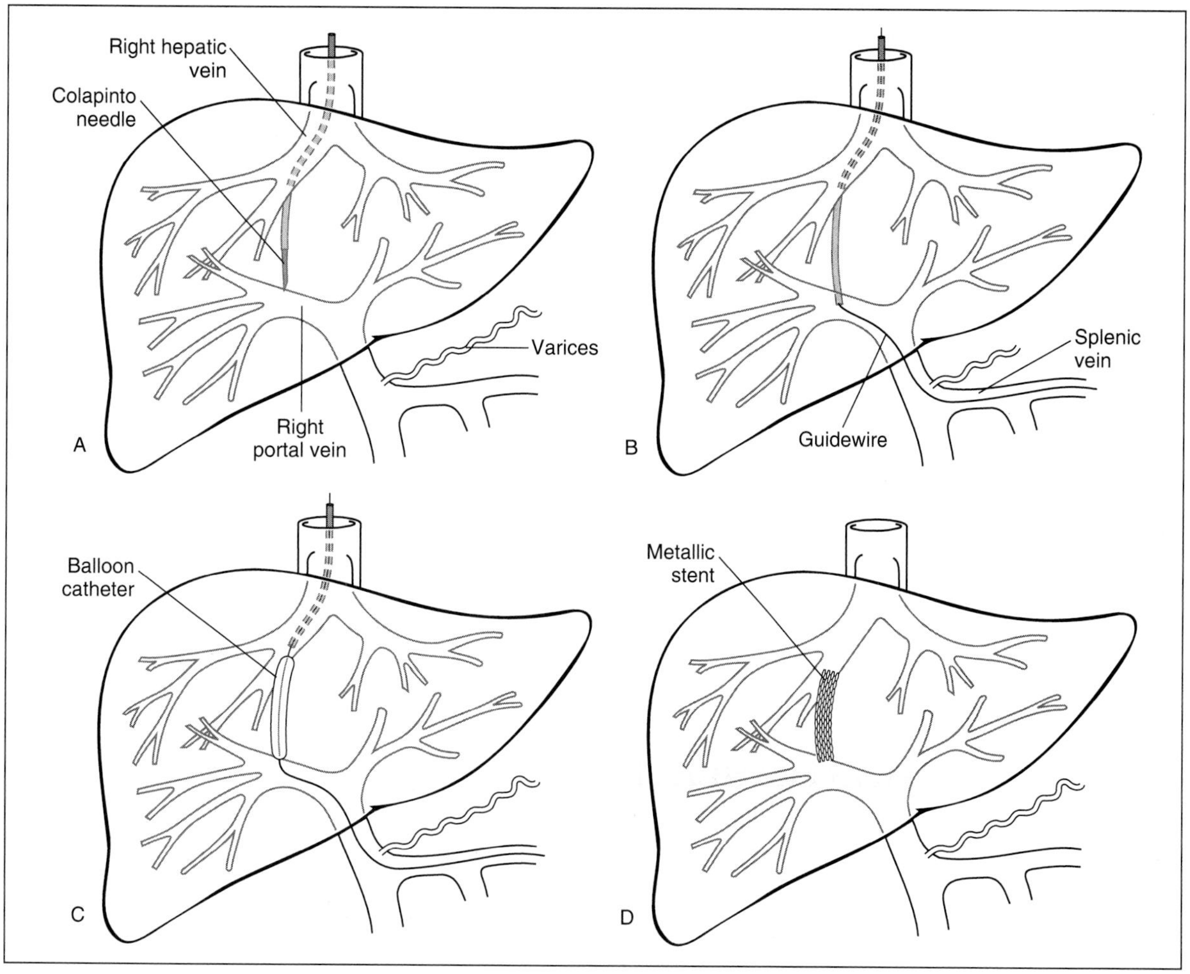

Figure 13.1-1. TIPS placement: (A) Sheathed Colapinto needle is advanced out of hepatic vein into portal vein branch. Varices are present. (B) Guide wire is advanced through the needle sheath into splenic vein. (C) Parenchymal liver tract is dilated using a balloon angioplasty catheter. (D) The metallic stent is deployed within the shunt tract. (Redrawn with permission from Haskal ZJ, Ring F: *Current techniques in interventional radiology.* Cope C, ed. Current Science, Philadelphia: 1994.)

portal vein bifurcation, and the needle advanced 3-4 cm into the hepatic parenchyma towards the hepatic hilum. Suction is applied to the needle as it is slowly withdrawn until blood is aspirated. Contrast is then injected to identify the vascular structure that has been entered. If the portal vein has been successfully punctured, a guide wire is advanced into the splenic vein (Fig 13.1-1B), and the needle exchanged for a 65 cm 5 Fr diagnostic catheter.

Portal venous pressures are measured and the pressure gradient between the portal vein and right atrium determined. Following a portal venogram, the catheter is exchanged for an angioplasty balloon, and the tract dilated (Fig 13.1-1C). A self-expanding stent (Wallstent, Schneider, Minneapolis, MN), is then positioned across the tract and deployed (Fig 13.1-1D). As most TIPS patients are future transplant candidates, care is taken to position the stent within the portal vein-to-hepatic vein tract, without the stent encroaching on either the superior mesenteric vein or the IVC. The stent is then dilated, using an angioplasty balloon, to a diameter 8-12 mm, depending on the pre- and poststent gradients. If necessary, a second stent is deployed to cover any remaining unstented tract. Following stent placement, the portal venogram and pressure gradients are repeated. Ideally the pressure gradient following shunting should be between 6-12 mmHg. If the gradient is too high, there is a risk of rebleeding; if too low, there is overshunting of blood bypassing the entire portal venous system, increasing the risk of encephalopathy.

After successful completion of the shunt, all devices, including the right jugular sheath, are removed, and hemostasis is achieved. Patients are closely monitored in an ICU or step-down unit for 24-48 h.

Usual preop diagnosis: Bleeding esophageal varices (as a result of portal HTN); ascites; Budd-Chiari syndrome

SUMMARY OF PROCEDURE

Position	Supine
Incision	Right IJ access
Special instrumentation	Rosch-Uchida or Colapinto needle set; angioplasty balloons; endovascular stents
Unique considerations	May need FFP.
Antibiotics	Cefazolin 1 g iv
Procedure time	2-6 h
EBL	0-3000 ml
Postop care	Patient → ICU, or step-down unit; careful fluid management
Mortality	Emergency: 50-100% Child's A: 4% } Child's B: 11% } See Table 13.1-2 Child's C: 25% }
Morbidity	Encephalopathy: 18-30% Late liver failure: 10-25% Shunt occlusion: 10%/yr Liver capsule puncture → intraperitoneal hemorrhage (continue procedure to decompress portal venous system → ↓bleeding). Hepatic artery puncture → may require embolization. Allergic reactions (see Contrast-related complications, p. 1054). MI (related to ↑CVP) Renal failure (usually transient)
Pain score	7-8 (first few h only)

Table 13.1-2. Child's Classification

Risk Group	**A**	**B**	**C**
Bilirubin (mg/dL)	< 2.0	2.0-3.0	> 3.0
Serum albumin (g/dL)	> 3.5	3.0-3.6	< 3
Ascites	None	Controlled	Poorly controlled
Encephalopathy	Absent	Minimal	Coma
Nutrition	Excellent	Good	Poor

(Adapted with permission from Child CG: *The Liver and Portal Hypertension.* WB Saunders, 1964.)

ANESTHETIC CONSIDERATIONS

PREOPERATIVE

Patients presenting for TIPS procedures have portal HTN usually 2° end-stage liver disease (ESLD), which will affect the function of a variety of organ systems, as described below.

Respiratory Abdominal distension → atelectasis → ↑pulmonary shunting → hypoxemia (hepatopulmonary syndrome in ESLD).
Encephalopathy → hyperventilation → ↓$PaCO_2$ (respiratory alkalosis with chronic acidosis as compensation). Pulmonary effusion may be present in 5-10% of patients.
Tests: ✓ CXR (for Sx of atelectasis); ABG and PFT, if indicated.

Cardiovascular Cardiomyopathy (ETOH) and CAD (tobacco) occur at higher incidence in this patient population. Diuretic therapy → hypovolemia + ↓K^+ (furosemide) or ↑K^+ (spironolactone). Hyperdynamic circulation 2° to ↓peripheral resistance + ↓cardiac reserve are common findings, and correlate with poor postop outcome.
Tests: ECG; electrolytes; cardiac ECHO, if indicated from H&P.

Neurological Symptoms of hepatic encephalopathy range from mild confusion to coma. These patients may be very sensitive to narcotics and sedatives. A characteristic finding in liver failure is asterixis (liver flap). Hypernatremia and hypoglycemia may mimic hepatic encephalopathy.
Tests: As indicated from H&P.

Hepatic Drug metabolism may be markedly reduced; anticipate prolonged effect with sedative and narcotic drugs. Drugs with particularly prolonged action include midazolam, meperidine, ranitidine and lidocaine. Apparent resistance to pancuronium and all muscle relaxants is most likely due to an increased volume of distribution. Succinylcholine effects may be prolonged in patients with severe end-stage liver disease (ESLD) (2°↓plasma cholinesterase).
Tests: Bilirubin; PT; albumin; LFTs

Gastrointestinal Ascites → ↑intraabdominal pressure → ↑risk of aspiration. Full-stomach precautions and rapid-sequence induction are recommended (see p. B-5). Portal HTN → variceal bleeding. Avoid esophageal instrumentation (e.g., TEE, esophageal stethoscope, etc.). Gastritis and peptic ulceration may be present.

Renal Oliguric renal failure may complicate ESLD (hepatorenal syndrome). This may be reversible if liver failure improves. Differential diagnosis includes prerenal azotemia and acute tubular necrosis.
★ **NB**: bilirubin metabolites interfere with creatinine measurement and may mask ↑creatinine levels.
Tests: BUN; creatinine; electrolytes

Endocrine Hypoglycemia is an infrequent finding (except in presence of severe cirrhosis and CHF). ESLD patients may have decreased response to catecholamines.
Tests: Glucose

Hematologic Patients may be anemic 2° GI bleeding. The majority of patients will exhibit coagulopathy 2° ↓hepatic synthetic function (all factors except VIII and fibrinogen) and ↓Plt. Patients may require vitamin K (if coagulopathy is present and time permits), FFP (if PT > 2 sec above baseline), or Plt transfusion (if Plt < 100 K) before procedure; and these products should be readily available.
Tests: CBC, Plt; PT; others as indicated from H&P.

Premedication Patients with significant ascites will require full-stomach precautions (see p. B-5).
★ **NB:** benzodiazepines should be used with caution in liver failure patients.

INTRAOPERATIVE

Anesthetic technique: In some patients (and at some centers), sedation with local anesthesia may be satisfactory; however, balloon dilation of the intrahepatic tract can be exceedingly painful. Remember, these patients may be very sensitive to narcotics → respiratory arrest. GETA is often necessary to provide adequate analgesia and airway protection.

General anesthesia

Induction Rapid-sequence induction (see p. B-5) is necessary in patients with encephalopathy, abdominal distention and recent variceal bleeds (blood in the stomach).

Maintenance	Standard maintenance (see p. B-3). If muscle relaxation is to be maintained, low-dose vecuronium (0.15 mg/kg) or cisatracurium (3 μg/min infusion) may be used to maintain muscle relaxation.	
Emergence	Extubate when the patient is awake and protective laryngeal reflexes are present. Patient should be transferred to PACU accompanied by anesthesiologist.	
Blood and fluid requirements	Potential for large blood loss IV: 14-16 ga × 1-2 FFP available 2-4 U PRBC available NS/LR (as appropriate)	Glucose-containing solutions may be required for patients with hepatic failure ± CHF. ✓ blood glucose levels frequently. Vasopressor response may be impaired.
Monitoring	Standard monitors (see p. B-1).	Ventricular arrhythmias can be provoked by hepatic vein catheterization.
Positioning	✓ and pad pressure points. ✓ eyes.	Radiology tables usually are not well padded → nerve damage.
Complications	Portal vein rupture Perforation liver capsule Complete heart block CHF	Intraabdominal hemorrhage may be massive and require emergency surgery. Patients with preexisting LBBB may require a pacemaker pre-TIPS (2° risk of RBBB during procedure). Shunt → ↑↑venous return → CHF

POSTOPERATIVE

Complications	Portal vein thrombus ↑encephalopathy Sepsis Bleeding Fluid/electrolyte disturbance	May mimic symptoms of PE or MI. 2° ↓hepatic portal blood flow May require hemodynamic support (e.g., dopamine) Stent insertion → ↑venous return → ↑diuresis → electrolyte/fluid imbalance.
Pain management	IV opiates	

References

1. Cardella JF, Waybill PN: Interventional radiology: diagnostic and interventional vascular applications. In *Alternate-Site Anesthesia: Clinical Practice Outside the Operating Room.* Russell GB, ed. Butterworth-Heinemann, Boston: 1997, 115-32.
2. Cello JP, Ring EJ, Olcott EW, et al: Endoscopic sclerotherapy compared with percutaneous transjugular intrahepatic portosystemic shunt after initial sclerotherapy in patients with acute variceal hemorrhage. A randomized, controlled trial [see comments]. *Ann Intern Med* 1997; 126(11):858-65.
3. Colapinto RF, Stronell RD, Gildiner M, et al: Formation of intrahepatic portosystemic shunts using a balloon dilatation catheter: preliminary clinical experience. *AJR Am J Roentgenol* 1983; 140(4):709-14.
4. Freeman AM, Sanyal AJ, Tisnado J, et al: Complications of transjugular intrahepatic portosystemic shunt: a comprehensive review. *Radiographics* 1993; 13(6):1185-210.
5. Kerlan RK Jr, LaBerge JM, Gordon RL, et al: Inadvertent catheterization of the hepatic artery during placement of transjugular intrahepatic portosystemic shunts. *Radiology* 1994; 193(1):273-76.
6. LaBerge JM, Ring EJ, Gordon RL, et al: Creation of transjugular intrahepatic portosystemic shunts with the Wallstent endoprosthesis: results in 100 patients. *Radiology* 1993; 187(2):413-20.
7. LaBerge JM, Somberg KA, Lake JR, et al: Two-year outcome following transjugular intrahepatic portosystemic shunt for variceal bleeding: results in 90 patients. *Gastroenterology* 1995; 108(4):1143-51.
8. Nazarian GK, Ferral H, Bjarnason H, et al: Effect of transjugular intrahepatic portosystemic shunt on quality of life. *AJR Am J Roentgenol* 1996; 167(4):963-69.
9. Nicoll A, Fitt G, Angus P, et al: Budd-Chiari syndrome: intractable ascites managed by a trans-hepatic portacaval shunt. *Australas Radiol* 1997; 41(2):169-72.
10. Richter GM, Palmaz JC, Noldge G, et al: The transjugular intrahepatic portosystemic stent-shunt. A new nonsurgical percutaneous method. *Radiologe* 1989; 29(8):406-11.
11. Rosch J, Hanafee W, Snow H: Transjugular portal venography and radiologic portacaval shunt: an experimental study. *Radiology* 1969; 92:1112-14.
12. Russell GB: Anesthesia and interventional radiology. In *Alternate-Site Anesthesia: Clinical Practice Outside the Operating Room.* Russell GB, ed. Butterworth-Heinemann, Boston: 1997, 157-71.
13. Semba CP, Saperstein L, Nyman U, et al: Hepatic laceration from wedged venography performed before transjugular intrahepatic portosystemic shunt placement [see comments]. *J Vasc Interv Radiol* 1996; 7(1):143-46.

IMAGING AND IMAGE-GUIDED PROCEDURES

PROCEDURAL CONSIDERATIONS

Description: Cross-sectional imaging includes computed tomography (CT), ultrasound (US) and magnetic resonance imaging (MRI), and has become indispensable in modern diagnosis. In addition, a growing number of invasive procedures are being performed using cross-sectional imaging for guidance, not only for diagnostic purposes but also for therapeutic purposes. Indications include diagnosis of primary or metastatic tumors, tumor staging, diagnosis of benign processes such as infections, drainage of fluid collections and treatment of tumors. Selection of imaging modality reflects ease of identification of the target lesion and resolution of surrounding and intervening structures. Patient compliance is crucial to success, because image resolution and spatial accuracy require the patient to be immobile during image acquisition and the procedure itself. In compliant adults, most of these procedures may be done using conscious sedation. For procedures in the pediatric population, as well as for more invasive procedures in adults, GA is frequently necessary.

Diagnostic imaging: Pediatric: CT scans are performed in a large, ring-shaped gantry, through which the patient is passed on an automated table. US is performed with a handheld transducer attached to a console. Diagnostic MRI scans are performed primarily in a large, circumferential magnet with a cylindrical center bore, also incorporating an automated table. In general, conscious sedation is sufficient to ensure pediatric patient compliance for diagnostic CT, US, or MRI, but occasionally GA is necessary. **Adults:** Almost all CT, US and MRI studies are performed without anesthesia. Approximately 5% of adult patients are too claustrophobic to complete an MRI study. Some of these may benefit from sedation, but use of GA is rare.

Image-guided procedures: Pediatric: Procedures performed on the pediatric patient routinely require GA. For CT- and US-guided biopsies and fluid drainage, initial lesion localization images are obtained after initiation of anesthesia and immobilization of the patient. A skin entry site is then selected and marked, based on coordinates determined from the initial images. Biopsies may require multiple needle passes, either coaxially through a large-bore guiding needle, or separately without such a guide. With CT, confirmation of needle position requires interruption of the procedure to acquire images, while with US, real-time images are obtained. Ideally, adequacy of biopsy sample is determined by an on-site cytopathologist. Fluid drainage may be simple aspiration or, more frequently, will result in placement of an indwelling drainage catheter. **Adults**: CT- and US-guided procedures, such as biopsies, fluid drainage and tissue ablation are routinely performed under conscious sedation.

The developing field of MRI-guided procedures—sometimes referred to as interventional MRI (iMRI) or magnetic resonance-guided therapy (MRT)—reflects the emergence of new magnet geometries, allowing physician access to the patient during imaging. These geometries may be C-arm configurations, parallel discs above and below the patient, or dual rings where the patient is placed either through the apertures of the rings or perpendicularly between the rings. Faster image acquisition pulse sequences are allowing near-real-time feedback. In addition to guiding biopsies and drainage, this technology enables more aggressive procedures, such as craniotomies or percutaneous tumor ablations, to be performed with immediate feedback showing the progress of excision or ablation. Clearly, many of these procedures require GA and, accordingly, require MRI-compatible monitoring and anesthetic equipment. For safety, the anesthesiologist also is subject to the same restrictions that apply to patients, so having a pacemaker, AICD, ferromagnetic aneurysm clips or a metallic foreign body in the orbit precludes that person's suitability to perform these cases.

Usual preop diagnosis: Tumor, primary or metastatic; lymphadenopathy; abscess, effusion, empyema, pseudocyst, or other fluid collection

SUMMARY OF PROCEDURE

	CT	US	MRI/MRT
Position	Supine, prone or lateral decubitus	⇐	⇐ + Sitting
Unique considerations	Metallic objects should be kept out of the imaging field. Exit the procedure room during scanning to avoid radiation exposure.	No ionizing radiation. Room lights are frequently dimmed for better viewing of the screen.	All equipment, including monitors, valves, anesthesia machine, O_2 tanks, laryngoscopes, etc., must be nonferromagnetic. Other metals should be removed from the imaging field to avoid artifact.
Antibiotics	Indicated for open procedures or when draining infected fluid	⇐	⇐

	CT	US	MRI/MRT
Antibiotics, cont.	collections including abscesses, empyemas, obstructed biliary or urinary systems.		
Procedure time	> 1 h	⇐	⇐
EBL	Procedure-dependent; may be internal hemorrhage.	⇐	⇐
Postop care	PACU → room	⇐	⇐
Mortality	Rare	⇐	⇐
Morbidity	Hemorrhage Infection Organ injury/perforation Pneumothorax	⇐	⇐
Pain score	1	1	Procedure-dependent

PATIENT POPULATION CHARACTERISTICS

Age range All
Male:Female 1:1
Incidence Common

Associated conditions **Fluid collections**: Patients may present with fever, sepsis, pain or ileus. Mass effect, such as with empyema or pericardial effusion, may also affect respiratory or cardiovascular function. Instrumentation or relief of mass effect may induce a vasovagal response. Some infections (echinococcus, entamoeba, methicillin-resistant staphylococcus aureus [MRSA], vancomycin-resistant enterococci [VRE]) may require special precautions, such as respiratory isolation.
Solid tumors: Mass effect may result in obstruction of airways, blood vessels, GI/biliary tract or urinary tract, or neural impingement. HTN may be seen with significant renal compression and, occasionally, with neuroendocrine tumors. Hematopoietic, hepatic or renal compromise may result in coagulopathy or Plt dysfunction.

ANESTHETIC CONSIDERATIONS

PREOPERATIVE

The adult patient population requiring anesthesia services for cross-sectioned imaging is medically quite diverse; however, many have in common the inability or unwillingness to lie still during the scanning procedure. Some of these patients are very ill, requiring the services of an anesthesiologist to maintain cardiorespiratory stability. Adult patients should be npo for 6 h preprocedure (elective). In general, US and CT scans present fewer problems for the anesthesiologist than MRI. Regardless of the method of anesthesia chosen, these patients must lie perfectly still, the airway must be protected, and IPPV may be required. Thus, children, mentally retarded, claustrophobic, uncooperative or critically ill patients may all require GA.

Respiratory As a result of limited access to the patient's airway, the preop examination should focus on the need for elective ET intubation in order to protect the airway. ET intubation and mechanical ventilation also may be required in trauma patients, the critically ill or patients with GERD or sleep apnea.

Cardiovascular Presence of a cardiac pacemaker or AICD is a contraindication to MRI, as are PA catheter thermistors or pacing wires.

Neurological Patients with ↑ICP or cranial trauma usually need GA with mechanical ventilation and intubation. The presence of aneurysm clips and/or coils may be a contraindication to MRI (check with surgeon or radiologist). Some of the newer aneurysm clips are nonferromagnetic and are, therefore, MRI compatible.

Musculoskeletal The presence of spinal instrumentation, metal plates, pins, screws, joint replacements or other prostheses is usually not a contraindication to MRI.

Premedication Midazolam 1-5 mg iv (titrated to effect) may be appropriate in the very anxious adult patient; alternatively, lorazepam 1-2 mg po/sl 1 h before procedure.

UNIQUE CONSIDERATIONS FOR MRI/MRT

The MRI/MRT suite poses many challenges to the anesthesiologist. Because of the high magnetic fields involved in MRI, any equipment containing ferromagnetic components—such as ECG monitors, anesthesia machines, etc.—cannot go near the magnet. Thus, MRI-compatible equipment is mandatory in the area of the MRI scanner. The magnetic field will destroy information on credit card/access card magnetic strips, and may damage pagers as well as mechanical devices, including wrist watches and infusion pump motors (a microdrip infusion set is a suitable replacement for an infusion pump).

Noise May be very distressing for some patients and may average 95 dB in a 1.5-T scanner. Exposure to noise levels of this magnitude should not exceed 2 h/d. Ear plugs or earphones with music can be helpful.

Thermal injury Thermal injury is caused by induced currents in metal implants, or in looped conductors in contact with the skin.

Projectile effect The magnet has a strong attraction for ferromagnetic objects that can become lethal missiles; therefore, all objects, such as pens, scissors, iv poles, O_2 cylinders, keys, etc., must be removed prior to entering the scanning room.

Implanted/foreign material There are several reports describing problems that may occur with cardiac pacemakers (failure to pace), aneurysm clips (hemorrhage) and intravascular wires (induced currents). Metal workers may be at special risk for ocular damage 2° imbedded particles.

Contrast agent Currently, gadolinum chelates are the only agents in use and have a higher safety margin than iodinated contrast agents. Adverse reactions, however, occur in ~2% of patients and include: HA, nausea, dizziness, hemodynamic instability and dysrhythmias.

INTRAOPERATIVE

Anesthetic technique: Typically, iv/po sedation, often without the services of an anesthesiologist. Patients unwilling or unable to cooperate will require GA.

IV sedation In patients with a normal airway and no Hx of GERD, sedation can be carried out most easily using a propofol infusion (25-100 μg/kg/min), ± midazolam (0.025-0.10 mg/kg) titrated to effect.

★ **NB:** Infusion pumps may be damaged by the magnet (a microdrip infusion is a useful alternative).

General anesthesia:

Induction Standard induction (p. B-2) on an MRI gantry (typically in the magnet anteroom). The anesthetized patient is then transported into the magnet. Metallic components in the LMA valve assembly may preclude its use in MRI/MRT.

Maintenance Standard maintenance (p. B-3). Most commonly a propofol infusion provides satisfactory sedation for the procedure (see pump considerations, above). Since continuous muscle relaxation is usually not required, spontaneous ventilation may be safest.

Emergence Emergence and extubation are often accomplished after the patient has been moved to the adjacent anteroom, where additional airway and other support equipment are readily available. The patient should be recovered in the PACU, which may be some distance from the MRI suite. Appropriate monitoring and personnel should accompany the patient.

Blood and fluid requirements
No blood loss
IV: 20 ga × 1
NS/LR @ TKO

Monitoring	Standard monitor (see p. B-1).	Monitoring in the MRI/MRT suite presents special problems, discussed below.
Monitoring, MR	ECG	ECG may be distorted by magnetic fields. Use MRI-compatible electrodes. Twist leads together to avoid creating loops (↓artifacts, ↓burns). V5 and V6 are least likely to develop artifacts.
	Pulse oximetry	MRI-compatible oximeters are available. Locate probe outside bore of the magnet (e.g., toe). Avoid burn injury 2° induced current in looped leads.
	BP (NIBP)	Replace all ferrous connections on cuff and tubing with nylon connectors. Use tubing extensions to keep apparatus away from the field.

Monitoring, MR, cont.	± Arterial Line	If an arterial line is medically indicated, keep the transducer close to the patient to avoid recording artifacts. Use MRI-compatible transducers and connectors. Recording equipment should have radiofrequency filters.
	Precordial/esophageal stethoscope	Often unsatisfactory because of magnet noise. An MRI-compatible, infrared, wireless stethoscope is available.
	Temperature	MRI-compatible temp monitors are available, although usually not necessary for adults (short procedure).
	Capnography	MRI-compatible capnographs are available. Long sample lines will distort waveforms, and $ETCO_2$ concentration may not be accurate; however, this is still useful for measuring RR and relative changes in $ETCO_2$.
	PA catheter	PA catheters with thermistors or pacing wires are an absolute contraindication to MRI.
	Urinary catheter	Catheters with temperature probes must be removed to avoid electrical or burn hazards.
	Verbal/visual	The patient and the monitors may be viewed directly (in procedure room) or through a screened window. Contact should be maintained throughout the procedure.
Positioning	✓ and pad pressure points. ✓ eyes.	CT and MRI gantries may be poorly padded → potential nerve injury.
Complications	Contrast-related	Gadolinum → local and systemic reactions (see Contrast-related complications, p. 1054).
	Loss of airway	Patient must be promptly extracted from the magnet bore and moved beyond the range of the magnet to permit use of emergency intubation and resuscitation equipment.
	Psychological	Panic attacks and claustrophobia occur in 5-10% of patients. Use of a blindfold may be helpful in selected patients. Heavy sedation or even GA may be necessary.
	Hearing loss	Temporary hearing loss and tinnitus may be expected in 43% of patients. Prevent by using ear plugs. GA ↑ risk of hearing damage 2° stapedius muscle relaxation.
	Thermal injury	Results from induced current, heating of oximeter probe and looping cables.

POSTOPERATIVE

Complications	Hearing loss Thermal injury	See discussion above. See discussion above.

References

1. Barth KH, Matsumoto AH: Patient care in interventional radiology: A perspective. *Radiology* 1991; 178:11-17.
2. Brown TR, Goldstein B, Little J: Severe burns resulting from magnetic resonance imaging with cardiopulmonary monitoring. Risks and relevant safety precautions. *Am J Phys Med Rehab* 1993; 72:166-67.
3. Charbonneau JW, et al: CT and sonographically guided needle biopsy: Current techniques and new innovations. *Am J Radiol* 1990; 154:1-10.
4. Holshouser BA, Hinshaw DB, Shellock FG: Sedation, anesthesia, and physiological monitoring during magnetic resonance imaging: evaluation of procedures and equipment. *J Magn Reson Imaging* 1993; 3:553-58.
5. Johnson JC, Blackburn TW, Russell GB: Anesthesia for computed tomography. In *Alternate-Site Anesthesia: Clinical Practice Outside the Operating Room.* Russell GB, ed. Butterworth-Heinemann, Boston: 1997, 83-100.
6. Jolesz FA, Kahn T: Interventional MRI: State of the art. *Appl Radiol* 1997; 26:8-13.
7. Jorgensen NH, Messick JM, Gray J, Nugent M, Berquist TH: ASA monitoring standards and magnetic resonance imaging. *Anesth Analg* 1994; 79:1141.
8. Meilstrup JW, Van Slyke MA, Russell GB: Ultrasound-guided interventional diagnosis and therapy. In *Alternate-Site Anesthesia: Clinical Practice Outside the Operating Room.* Russell GB, ed. Butterworth-Heinemann, Boston: 1997, 225-242.
9. Mueller PR, vanSonnenberg E: Interventional radiology in the chest and abdomen. *N Engl J Med* 1990; 322:1364-74.
10. Murphy KJ, Brunberg JA: Adult claustrophobia, anxiety, and sedation in magnetic resonance imaging. *Magn Reson Imaging* 1997; 15:51-4.

11. Russell GB, Taekmann JM, Cronin AJC: Anesthesia and magnetic resonance imaging. In *Alternate-Site Anesthesia: Clinical Practice Outside the Operating Room.* Russell GB, ed. Butterworth-Heinemann, Boston: 1997, 69-82.
12. Shellock FG, Morisoli S, Kanal E: Magnetic resonance procedures and biomedical implants, materials, and devices: 1993 update. *Radiology* 1993; 189:587-99.
13. Smith EH: Complications of percutaneous abdominal fine-needle biopsy. Review. *Radiology* 1991; 178:253-58.
14. Van Slyke MA, Wise SW, Spain JW: Computerized patient imaging. In *Alternate-Site Anesthesia: Clinical Practice Outside the Operating Room.* Russell GB, ed. Butterworth-Heinemann, Boston: 1997, 35-68.
15. Zorab JS: A general anaesthesia service for magnetic resonance imaging. *Eur J Anaesth* 1995; 12:387-95.

Authors

Sarah S. Donaldson, MD, FACR (*Radiation therapy*)
Carol A. Shostak, RN, RTT, CMD (*Radiation therapy*)
Paul T. Pitlick, MD (*Interventional cardiology*)
Gary E. Hartman, MD (*ECMO*)
George F. Van Hare, MD (*Interventional cardiology, EPS*)

13.2 OUT-OF-OPERATING ROOM PROCEDURES—PEDIATRIC

Anesthesiologists

Richard A. Jaffe, MD, PhD (*Radiation therapy*)
Stanley I. Samuels, MB, BCh (*Radiation therapy*)
Cathy R. Lammers, MD (*Interventional cardiology*)
M. Gail Boltz, MD (*Interventional cardiology*)
Gregory B. Hammer, MD (*Oncology, endoscopy, imaging*)

PEDIATRIC RADIATION THERAPY

PROCEDURAL CONSIDERATIONS

Sarah S. Donaldson and Carol A. Shostak

Description: Modern pediatric radiation therapy (XRT) requires that the patient be in a stable and reproducible position for daily treatment. Sharply defined beams with secondary collimation are used to irradiate the tumor volume and to spare normal tissue. Patient movement may undermine techniques for sparing normal tissue and, while movement cannot be completely prevented, it must be minimized. In very young children, it is often impossible to prevent movement and achieve adequate cooperation for radiation treatment. In such cases, daily anesthesia is required. Close cooperation of the radiation oncology and anesthesia teams allows for safe and reproducible daily treatment.[8] In general, children older than 3 or 4 yr can be induced to lie still for radiation therapy. Children from 2.5-4 yr may cooperate during the treatment (which is usually < 15 min), but not for the treatment planning and simulation, in which an immobilization-stabilization device is made (often requiring 1-1.5 h). In most infants and young children (< 2.5 yr), anesthesia is essential.

The optimal position for XRT also must be optimal for the anesthesiologist. Ideally, the area to be treated is determined using 3-dimensional conformal techniques to optimize treatment and to minimize normal tissue exposure. This requires an imaging study (e.g., CT scan), with the patient in the same position as will be used during the radiation treatment. A series of radiographs are taken at the treatment-planning appointment, which typically lasts 1-1.5 h and requires GA. It is essential that there be no patient movement between exposures; if the patient moves, the entire procedure must be repeated. After examining the radiographs, the area to be scanned is determined, and then the patient is transported (anesthetized) to the CT suite for a 3-dimensional treatment-planning CT scan. Thereafter, the specific area can be determined and individual beam-shaping devices made.

One or two d following the initial planning session, the patient has a verification procedure which usually is of shorter duration—often requiring only 30 min of anesthesia time. The verification procedure consists of a series of radiographs using the beam-shaping devices, which simulate the treatment to be given. When this procedure is successfully completed, the anesthetized patient is moved to the treatment room. The child is put in the identical position achieved during the planning/verification procedures, and treatment is administered.

The first day or two, and weekly thereafter, a verification x-ray (called a "port film") is taken to confirm the accuracy of the treatment field. The treatment itself is of only a few min duration for each field; ideally, the entire procedure is completed within 15-30 min. A course of treatment may be only a few d, or may last for 5-6 wk, generally with treatment given 5 times per wk. Occasionally, multiple (2-3) treatments per d are given at 4-8 h (usually 6 h) intervals. At the initial appointment, the patient's optimal position is determined, an immobilization device constructed and measurements taken. The immobilization device is usually a body cradle or cast, and often a head/face mask is made for head and neck or brain treatment. Initially, temporary marks or Band-Aids are used; however, when the final positioning has been determined, a more permanent mark, such as a tattoo, is applied. Often, a head holder with tape or Velcro and/or a belt or mask is applied to ensure the position for XRT.[7]

In managing certain brain tumors (e.g., medulloblastoma, high-grade intratentorial ependymoma, germ cell tumors and CNS leukemia), cranial spinal irradiation (CSI) is used. This procedure requires that the patient be placed in the prone position with the head flexed as much as possible to minimize a cervical lordosis. This positioning, however, creates special difficulties for the anesthesiologist. If the child is intubated for the setup, the radiation stabilization device must allow space for the ETT. If the child is not intubated, there must be adequate access to the airway.

Fractionation: Pediatric protocols are currently testing the efficacy of giving multiple fractions (treatments) of radiation 2-3 times per d, usually at 6-h intervals, to allow higher total radiation doses to be administered with possible less normal-tissue morbidity. These schemes have been, or are being evaluated for children with: brain stem gliomas; supratentorial glial tumors; medulloblastoma and other posterior fossa tumors; soft-tissue sarcomas, including rhabdomyosarcoma; some bone tumors, including Ewing's sarcoma; and total body irradiation in preparation for bone marrow transplantation. Until proven to be of increased efficacy, such schemes should remain part of large protocol studies. The timing of radiotherapy may be at 4, 6, or 8 h intervals 2-3 times per d, depending on the protocol. These studies provide several challenges for anesthesiologists, radiotherapists and parents. Radiotherapy under anesthesia, however, has been successfully administered to infants undergoing multiple fractions per d.[7] Attention must be given to potential malnutrition and/or dehydration from prolonged periods of npo status.

Total body irradiation (TBI): Although most TBI techniques are administered with the patient standing, infants and small children must lie prone and supine for the treatment. This positioning requires sedation and/or anesthesia. Retching and vomiting, sometimes provoked by the radiation, present an additional challenge for proper radiotherapy technique, as well as for anesthetic management. Anesthesia for high-dose TBI has been accomplished with inhalation anesthetics and mechanical ventilation and with ketamine anesthesia.[6]

Radiosurgery: The technique of utilizing stereotactically localized radiosurgery with a highly collimated radiotherapy photon beam, as generated from a linear accelerator, is currently being employed for select patients with small CNS tumors or base-of-skull tumors. There is increasing enthusiasm for this technique for infants and children with recurrent posterior fossa and cerebral tumors, craniopharyngiomas, optic nerve and chiasmal gliomas, and arteriovenous malformations (AVMs). Radiosurgery requires 6-8 h of continuous anesthesia while a patient undergoes application of the metal halo frame, computed tomographic (CT) localization, and multiport radiotherapy treatment. This approach requires close coordination between the anesthesiologist, neurosurgeon and radiotherapist.

Usual preop diagnosis: Leukemia; retinoblastoma; most of the solid tumors of childhood

SUMMARY OF PROCEDURE

	Standard XRT	TBI	Radiosurgery
Position	Supine or prone	Supine and prone	Supine or prone
Unique considerations	If prone: head flexed for maximal straightening of the cervical spine.	May be repeated 2-3 times/d at 4-6 h intervals.	Halo frame placement at CT
Anesthesia time	Planning: 30-120 min Treatment: < 15 min	< 20 min	6-8 h
Postop care	PACU → home	PACU → room	PACU → room or home

PATIENT POPULATION CHARACTERISTICS

Age range	Usually ≤ 4 yr
Male:Female	1:1
Incidence	NA

Associated conditions

Brain tumors: ↑ICP is of concern in these patients. Postradiation edema following the first few treatments may further ↑ICP, with potential for brain stem herniation. Some children with brain stem tumors are particularly difficult to anesthetize, perhaps because of disruption of nerve pathways in those areas of the brain stem which are affected by anesthetics.[8]

Diabetes insipidus (DI): It is often impossible to withhold fluids for 4-6 h prior to radiotherapy in an infant with symptomatic polydipsia from DI.

Neuroblastoma: Neuroblastomas are capable of secreting catecholamines and related substances; hence, there is a potential for paroxysmal HTN during anesthesia induction. In these children, the principles of anesthetic management are similar to those for pheochromocytoma.[3]

Retinoblastoma:[3,5,6,10] It is imperative that the patient be properly immobilized with no movement, as even a mm of change, as occurs with a sigh, may cause unnecessary radiation to the radiosensitive lens and anterior chamber. Optimal anesthesia prevents nystagmus and motion of the head. Even minimal lateral or rotary nystagmus may increase the risk of cataract induction. A course of radiotherapy for retinoblastoma may involve 20-25 GA procedures in 4-5.5 wk.

ANESTHETIC CONSIDERATIONS

Richard A. Jaffe and Stanley I. Samuels

PREPROCEDURE

A detailed preanesthesia visit is essential as this is the prime opportunity to gain the confidence of both child and parents. The importance of npo status needs to be stressed repeatedly to the parents, discussing the potential danger of vomiting during treatment. Breast milk may be given to infants < 6 mo of age, 4-6 h pretreatment. Clear fluids are withheld for 2 h pretreatment, while milk and solids should be withheld 6-8 h pretreatment. Written instructions regarding preop protocol are extremely helpful in this context. In general, these patients are previously healthy children who have developed a life-threatening condition. Some of these children will have Sx of ↑ICP, which must be taken into account when designing an anesthetic plan.

Respiratory Patients with Sx of URI (runny nose, cough, fever) are commonly seen during XRT treatment and may pose problems for the anesthesia team. If the infection is acute, XRT probably should be delayed for a few d or until symptoms abate. Fortunately, most of the children can be managed without the use of an ETT, which might otherwise cause excessive secretions and postop laryngospasm. As always, the benefit of Rx must be balanced against the risks of anesthesia (induction laryngospasm, retained secretions, atelectasis/bronchospasm and postop laryngospasm).
Tests: As indicated from H&P.

Neurological Patients with intracranial tumors may have ↑ICP. Sx include irritability, headache, N/V and papilledema. Suspicion of ↑ICP probably mandates ET intubation and controlled ventilation to induce hypocarbia.

Laboratory Other tests as indicated from H&P.

Premedication Usually unnecessary in this patient group. Reliance on sedation or restraints is ill-advised and will lead to frustration on the part of the child, parents, technologists and physicians. Inappropriate sedation may cause respiratory and cardiovascular depression, and → prolonged period of recovery.

INTRAPROCEDURE

There is increasing enthusiasm for this technique for infants and children with recurrent posterior fossa and cerebral tumors, craniopharyngiomas, optic nerve and chiasmal gliomas and AVMs.

Anesthetic technique: Anesthesia for radiotherapy should be of brief duration, with rapid recovery and minimal cardiopulmonary depression, have good patient acceptance, allow maintenance of nutrition and permit delivery of precise treatment by assuming immobility. Inhalation, iv and intramuscular techniques all have been used successfully in this type of procedure.[9]

Induction **IV:** Propofol (1.5-2 mg/kg) slowly, followed by heparinized saline flush. Intubation is usually unnecessary, except for patients with ↑ICP or patients with potential for airway obstruction.

Inhalation: Mask induction with sevoflurane is appropriate in children without iv access, and may be preferred by some children. Again, intubation is usually unnecessary. The airway may be maintained by extension of the neck and use of a head holder.[1] Alternatively, an LMA may be inserted to maintain airway patency. It is essential that this same degree of head flexion/extension be maintained for each daily treatment. An immobilization device may be molded, with the requirements for anesthesia kept in mind. If extreme neck flexion is required, ET intubation may be necessary.

Maintenance **IV:** Propofol (50-100 μg/kg/min) by continuous infusion. The airway usually can be well maintained by careful positioning and the use of a head strap. Supplemental O_2 should be administered via nasal prongs, mask or LMA.

Inhalation: Maintain anesthesia with sevoflurane in O_2, usually delivered by mask, LMA or insufflation.

Emergence **IV:** Flush iv with heparinized saline to prevent clotting. Patients will awaken rapidly following cessation of propofol infusion or inhaled agents. Extubation should be accomplished when the patient is fully awake, unless there is the possibility of ↑ICP, in which case a deep extubation is appropriate. This is important as there is frequently a long journey between the XRT department and PACU. Antiemetics are usually unnecessary.

Blood and fluid requirements IV: usually permanent access
NS/LR: infusion not usually required

Many children receiving radiotherapy have a central venous access line, placed for long-term administration of chemotherapy.

A planned course of anesthesia for radiotherapy, by itself, is an acceptable indication for placement of a central venous access line, even in the absence of plans for chemotherapy. Alternatively, an indwelling iv catheter with a heparin-lock for repeated iv injections has been effective in outpatient anesthesia for pediatric radiotherapy.

Monitoring	Standard monitors (see p. D-1).	A critical problem is the lack of access to the patient and monitors during XRT. A TV camera can focus on the visual displays of the monitors. Respiration also may be observed by direct visualization through a leaded-glass viewing port or a camera directed at the child. A small marker may be placed on the chest so that the rise and fall of chest motion is easily seen.[8]
Positioning	✓ and pad pressure points. ✓ eyes.	
Complications	Airway obstruction	Respiratory obstruction occasionally occurs; it responds to either nasopharyngeal or oropharyngeal airways. In rare instances, ET intubation may be required for persistent airway obstruction.
	Patient movement	Deepen anesthesia.

POSTPROCEDURE

Complications	Cerebral edema	In patients with ↑ICP, XRT can provoke an acute ↑ICP, with consequent ↑headache, ↑N/V, ↓consciousness → cardiac arrest. These patients should be monitored × 24 h post Rx.
Pain management	Standard approaches	Radiation treatments are not associated with pain, but they may be useful in relieving pain associated with neoplastic disease.

References

1. Browne CH, Boulton TB, Crichton TC: Anaesthesia for radiotherapy. A frame for maintaining the airway. *Anaesthesia* 1969; 24(3):428-30.
2. Casey WF, Price V, Smith HS: Anaesthesia and monitoring for paediatric radiotherapy. *J R Soc Med* 1986; 79(8):454-56.
3. Donaldson SS, Egbert PR: Retinoblastoma. In *Principles and Practice of Pediatric Oncology*. Pizzo PA, Poplack DG, eds, JB Lippincott, Philadelphia: 1989, 555-68.
4. Donaldson SS, Shostak CA, Samuels SI: Technical and practical considerations in the radiotherapy of children. *Front Radiat Ther Oncol* 1987; 21(1):256-69.
5. Harnett AN, Hungerford JL, Lambert GD, Hirst A, Darlison R, Hart BL, Trodd TC, Plowman PN: Improved external beam radiotherapy for the treatment of retinoblastoma. *Br J Radiol* 1987; 60(716):753-60.
6. Lo JN, Buckley JJ, Kim TH, Lopez R: Anesthesia for high-dose total body irradiation in children. *Anesthesiology* 1984; 61(1):101-3.
7. Menache L, Eifel PJ, Kennamer DL, Belli JA: Twice-daily anesthesia in infants receiving hyper-fractionated irradiation. *Int J Radiat Oncol Biol Phys* 1990; 18(3):625-29.
8. Murray WJ: Anesthesia for external beam radiotherapy. In *Pediatric Radiation Oncology,* Halperin EC, Kun LE, Constine LS, Tarbell NJ, eds. Raven Press, New York: 1989, 399-407.
9. Singapuri K, Russell GB: Anesthesia and radiation therapy. In *Alternate-Site Anesthesia: Clinical Practice Outside the Operating Room.* Russell GB, ed. Butterworth-Heinemann, Boston: 1997; 365-80.

INTERVENTIONAL CARDIOLOGY—PEDIATRIC

PROCEDURAL CONSIDERATIONS

Paul T. Pitlick and George F. Van Hare

Description: Vascular access. There are a number of established approaches to the vascular system. The original technique involved a surgical exposure to isolate the desired vessel; however, over the past 20 yr, a percutaneous approach has supplanted this cut-down technique. Some patients, especially after multiple invasive procedures, may have very difficult venous access; for this, a transhepatic approach has recently been described. In all of the approaches, the patient is positioned supine on the catheterization table. The setup of anesthesia equipment (e.g., extension hoses, monitoring lines and iv access) must take into account the final position of the patient and the imaging apparatus, which may be moved during the procedure.

Right femoral artery and vein cannulation: Since most physicians are right-handed, the preferred approach is usually from the right inguinal region, although the left femoral artery and vein are satisfactory alternatives. Both the femoral artery and the vein are readily accessible from this location, unless the patient has had previous procedures, which may have altered the patency of the vessels. This approach usually can be performed using sedation with local anesthesia, unless the procedure is anticipated to be long and/or complex.

Right internal jugular vein: Younger patients may not tolerate this approach without very heavy sedation, and GA is preferred. In patients who have no venous access from either femoral region, this is the preferred approach. Some physicians and older patients also prefer this approach for simpler procedures, such as RV biopsy in transplant patients. In these patients, mild sedation and local anesthesia are usually adequate.

Subclavian vein/axillary artery: This also is an acceptable alternative approach in the patient with thrombosed femoral veins, and it requires patient cooperation and/or GA.

Transseptal approach to the left heart: Normally, the left ventricle and even the left atrium are accessible from a femoral artery. If the patient has a mechanical aortic or mitral valve, attempting to cross the valve with a catheter is contraindicated. For those patients in whom left heart information is important, it is possible to cross the atrial septum with a long needle, threaded from the femoral artery.

Transhepatic: Occasionally, a patient—usually one who has had many previous vascular cannulations—will have completely occluded femoral access, and the SVC also may have thrombosed. An approach via the liver and hepatic veins has been described for this situation.

INTERVENTIONAL PROCEDURES

Balloon dilation: For more than 10 yr, balloon dilation has been performed in the cardiac catheterization laboratory, for a variety of indications. In children, dilation of stenotic pulmonic and aortic valves produces comparable results to conventional surgery. Dilation of coarctations of the aorta, and other vascular structures also compares favorably to surgery, although results with branch PAs are not as uniformly successful.

Coils are used to occlude pulmonary collaterals and AV fistulae, but more commonly are used to occlude a patent ductus arteriosus (PDA).

Stents are used in the pediatric cardiac population to enlarge various vascular structures, such as the PAs in patients with branch pulmonary stenosis after tetralogy of Fallot (TOF) repair, and the SVC after the Mustard procedure.

ASD closure: A device to close intracardiac communications has recently been introduced for clinical testing.

Radiofrequency (RF) ablation is a procedure in which abnormal electrical conducting pathways or automatic electrical foci identified by EPS are destroyed using the application of radiofrequency energy delivered through a deflectable electrode catheter. On some occasions, RF lesions must be placed close to other critical structures in the heart (e.g., AV node). In those cases, in order to prevent the complication of inadvertent AV block, anesthesia care may need to be modified, deepening sedation to provide a motionless patient during application of energy.

DIAGNOSTIC PROCEDURES

Angiography: This is usually performed in conjunction with a hemodynamic evaluation. With injection of contrast agents into appropriate locations, details of cardiac and vascular anatomy are revealed. In the early days of cardiac catheterization, these studies were performed in PA and lateral projections; more recently, they have been enhanced by angling the cameras to the cardiac structures, rather than to the patient's body, which yields better information. This once involved physically moving the patient; however, modern cineangiographic equipment is capable of being moved into a wide range of positions, leaving the patient undisturbed.

CT/MRI: Images are generated in a digital format; each point on an image has x and y coordinates, with the z-axis being obtained from "stacking" the images on each other in the 3rd dimension. With current hardware and software, it is possible to reconstruct the heart and great vessels in 3 dimensions. Patient movement badly distorts the relationship of one slice to the next, however, compromising the image. Quiet respiration is usually tolerated, although breath-holding or GA with controlled ventilation in younger patients works best.

Endomyocardial biopsy: The most common indication for biopsy is for assessing tissue rejection in patients with heart transplants. A RV specimen usually suffices; however, the LV is occasionally biopsied.

Electrophysiologic study (EPS): The heart is a contracting muscle with a well ordered sequence of activation. In patients with arrhythmias (e.g., supraventricular tachycardias), EPS is used to make a diagnosis of the mechanism of arrhythmia, assess the hemodynamic impact of the tachycardia and map the location of abnormal conduction pathways or automatic foci. These procedures may be long, and children may require GA. In some cases, the choice of anesthetic agent may affect the inducibility of the arrhythmia at EPS, making the arrhythmia harder to induce. Furthermore, the arrhythmia itself may complicate anesthetic care, by causing sudden decreases in BP due to excessively rapid rates. The anesthesiologist and cardiologist must carefully plan the approach to each patient to assure both the patient's safety and the optimum data from the EPS.

DIAGNOSTIC INFORMATION

Oxygen saturations: During cardiac catheterization, samples can be taken from all of the chambers of the heart and the associated great vessels. Saturations can be measured, and the location of intracardiac shunting can be detected. In addition, pulmonary blood flow (Q_p) and systematic blood flow (Q_s) can be calculated from this information.

Let VO_2 = Oxygen consumption
PA = Pulmonary arterial oxygen content (ml/L)
PV = Pulmonary venous oxygen content (ml/L)

Then $$Q_p = \frac{VO_2}{(PV - PA)} \quad (1)$$

Let SA = Systemic arterial oxygen content (ml/L)
and MV = Mixed venous oxygen content (ml/L)

Then $$Q_s = \frac{VO_2}{(SA - MV)} \quad (2)$$

In patients with intracardaic shunting—common in children undergoing cardiac catheterization—one must make the distinction between Q_p and Q_s, because these usually will not be equal. For patients without intracardiac shunting, however, SA = PV and MV = PA, and equations (1) and (2) reduce to the same quantity, which is also referred to as cardiac output (CO).

In a patient without intracardiac shunting, the best measure of mixed venous blood is obtained from the pulmonary artery (PA), and it is common in adults to calculate CO by assuming that MV = PA.

Then: $$CO = \frac{VO_2}{(SA - PA)} \quad (3)$$

Note that equation (3) is true *only for patients without intracardiac shunting.*

Intracardiac pressure measurements. Cardiac catheterization allows accurate measurement of pressures in all sites within the right and left sides of the heart, great arteries and major veins.

Calculation of PVR/SVR: Combining the information from outputs and intracardiac pressures, pulmonary vascular resistance (PVR) and systemic vascular resistance (SVR) can be determined:

Let PAP = mean pulmonary arterial pressure (mmHg)
LAP = mean left atrial pessure (mmHg)
SAP = mean systemic arterial pressure (mmHg)
RAP = mean right atrial pressure (mmHg)

Then: $PVR = \frac{PAP - LAP}{Q_p}$ (4)

and $SVR = \frac{SAP - RAP}{Q_s}$ (5)

Calculations of oxygen contents (to derive equations 1-3) in the various sites accessible during cardiac catheterization are as follows.

Let [Hgb] = Hemoglobin concentration (in gm/dl)
sa = Systemic arterial hemoglobin saturation (%)
mv = Mixed venous hemoglobin saturation (%)
pO_2sa = Systemic arterial pO_2 (mmHg)
pO_2mv = Mixed venous pO_2 (mmHg)

Then $SA = 1.34 \times [Hgb] \times sa + 0.003 \times pO_2sa$

and $MV = 1.34 \times [Hgb] \times mv + 0.003 \times pO_2mv$

Let pa = Pulmonary arterial hemoglobin saturation (%)
pv = Pulmonary venous hemoglobin saturation (%)
pO_2pa = Pulmonary arterial pO_2 (mmHg)
pO_2pv = Pulmonary venous pO_2 (mmHg)

Then $PA = 1.34 \times [Hgb] \times pa + 0.003 \times pO_2pa$
$PV = 1.34 \times [Hgb] \times pv + 0.003 \times pO_2pv$

Reference

1. Shim D, Lloyd TR, Cho KJ, Moorehead CP, Beekman RH: Transhepatic cardiac catheterization in children: evaluation of efficacy and safety. *Circulation* 1995;92:1526-30.

ANESTHETIC CONSIDERATIONS

Cathy R. Lammers and M. Gail Boltz

PREOPERATIVE

Pediatric patients presenting for interventional cardiology range from those requiring simple diagnostic procedures to those requiring complex interventional procedures (balloon angioplasty or stenting). These patients can present a challenge, given their abnormal cardiac anatomy and physiology. Many of these patients must undergo repeated catheterizations and will have had multiple anesthetic experiences. All patients must receive a thorough preanesthetic H&P emphasizing cardiorespiratory function and coexisting congenital anomalies that may predict difficult airway management. Children should follow the same npo protocol as they would for surgery (see NPO Guidelines, p. D-1).

Respiratory URIs must be evaluated carefully. If Sx are limited to nasal congestion, the procedure may proceed. Sx of lower respiratory tract involvement—including fever, productive cough or wheezing—warrant postponement for 2-3 wk unless the procedure is urgent.

Cardiovascular Review prior catheterizations, echocardiograms, ECGs and cardiology evaluations. Cardiac transplant recipients can demonstrate HTN 2° cyclosporine use and can develop progressive coronary artery stenosis in their grafts. Antibiotics are given to patients as required for SBE prophylaxis or for those undergoing interventional procedures.

Immunology Cardiac transplant recipients can develop lymphoproliferative disease, which results in redundant lymphoid tissue in the pharynx and epiglottis → possible airway obstruction. Careful evaluation of the airway is required.

Gastrointestinal Chronic steroid use can → significant obesity → difficult airway management.

Renal Cardiac transplant recipients can have renal dysfunction 2° antirejection medications or HTN. Additionally, cyclosporine → $\uparrow K^+$.

Laboratory Tests as indicated from H&P. Most patients will require electrolytes and Hct; however, sometimes these labs can be deferred until after induction and vascular access is acquired. All interventional procedures require a T&C with blood available in the room.

Premedication Usually not needed because parents can accompany child into the catheterization suite and be present during induction. Some children (> 6 mo), however, who have had many prior studies may be anxious and require oral premedication with midazolam 0.5-0.75 mg/kg.

INTRAOPERATIVE

Anesthetic technique: MAC with sedation is preferred for measuring hemodynamic parameters in children because GA will distort these values; however, some patients require GA. Some interventional procedures (e.g., stenting or coiling) require a motionless field or may be too long to tolerate under mild sedation. Patients who require venous access via the IJ vein may not tolerate lying still for long periods of time. Critically ill neonates require intubation and controlled ventilation. Patients with moderate-to-severe pulmonary HTN may be better managed with controlled ventilation in the event of a pulmonary hypertensive crisis. Some older children with studies of shorter duration using groin access may tolerate incremental iv sedation with local anesthesia.

MAC: Sedation can be managed with incremental doses of fentanyl and midazolam or propofol infusion as long as the patient remains normocarbic and normoxic. Hypercapnia or hypocapnia can affect hemodynamic catheterization values.

Induction Standard inhalation or iv induction (see p. D-2). The choice of anesthetic drugs must include careful consideration of their effects on myocardial function and pulmonary resistance.

Maintenance GETA with volatile agents (e.g., sevoflurane) or iv infusion (e.g., propofol, remifentanil). Most catheterizations require the patient to be maintained on room air for accurate O_2 sat and pressure measurements. EPS studies are best managed with iv propofol 50-150 μg/kg/min or midazolam 0.5-0.1 mg/kg load with infusion of 0.001-0.002 mg/kg/min, since these agents have shown the least effect on EPS results. Recent studies, however, demonstrate that halothane, sevoflurane or isoflurane also may be acceptable.

Most cardiologists request heparin 50-100 U/kg for patients with arterial sheaths in place and any interventional procedures. Heparin 50 U/kg is repeated every 90 min. NTG, Ca^{++} channel blockers, or NO may be requested by the cardiologist to evaluate the reversibility of pulmonary HTN.

Emergence Do not allow child to emerge before hemostasis at the access site has been achieved. Use of remifentanil infusion may provide analgesia during the procedure, yet allow for a rapid emergence. Consider remifentanil for patients with pulmonary HTN where a smooth emergence is essential to prevent a hypertensive crisis. Interventional procedures and EPS/ablations require overnight ICU admission for observation. Most other patients can recover in PACU.

Blood and fluid requirements

IV: 20-22 ga × 1
NS/LR @ maintenance:
4 ml/kg/h – 0-10 kg
+2 ml/kg/h – 10-20 kg
PRBCs
Fluid warmer

A second volume iv may be desirable for interventional cases. The cardiologist also will have a venous access line that can be used if necessary. Avoid volume overload. Interventional procedures may result in tearing of vessels and/or myocardium and can cause abrupt hemorrhage; therefore, blood must be available in the room. Neonates can lose significant blood during access and sampling and also may require transfusion. Follow serial Hct.

Monitoring

Standard monitors (see p. D-1).
± Arterial line
± Foley catheter

If arterial access is required, discuss with the cardiologist. Frequently, the femoral artery is cannulated for the catheterization and may be available for use; however, access may be limited at crucial times (e.g., stenting or coiling), so a peripheral arterial line may be desirable. For cases of long duration, consider Foley catheter placement. Monitor temperature and consider a Bair Hugger for maintenance of normothermia.

Positioning

✓ and pad pressure points.
✓ eyes.

Supine, arms flexed above head to allow fluoroscopy of chest. All ECG leads and monitoring wires must be cleared from axilla and chest to allow fluoroscopy.

Complications

Airway obstruction

Rx: Airway support, oral/nasal airway, LMA. Intubate if needed.

Complications, cont.	Arrhythmias	Usually self-limiting; determine etiology (e.g., catheter or wire). Rx: Lidocaine, adenosine or cardioversion, if indicated.
	Hemorrhage	Rx: Fluid resuscitation with crystalloid, 5% albumin and/or blood; vasopressors as needed.
	Hypoxemia	Rx: Airway support; increase FiO_2. Intubate and ventilate as needed.
	Pulmonary hypertensive crisis	Rx: 100% O_2, administer iv opioid, systemic vasopressors. Consider NO and/or nebulized prostacyclin.
	Hypothermia	Rx: Forced air warming device, heat lamp. Increase environmental temperature.
	Contrast reaction/anaphylaxis	Rx: Support airway, 100% FiO_2, intubate if needed: epinephrine, volume resuscitation, steroid, antihistamine.
	Air embolism	Rx: 100% FiO_2; identify and occlude source; Trendelenburg; fluid resuscitation; vasopressor support. Aspirate air from central access if possible.

POSTOPERATIVE

Complications	Hematoma at access site Ischemic limb Emergence delirium	
Pain management	Infiltrate access sites with local anesthetic.	Postop analgesia usually not required.
Tests	CXR If indicated.	

References

1. Hamid RKA: Anesthesia for nonsurgical procedures in children: cardiac catheterization and electrophysiology studies. In *Pediatric Cardiac Anesthesia,* 3rd edition. Appleton-Lange, Norwalk, CT: 1997, 165-80.
2. Lavoie J, Walsh EP, Burrows FA, et al: Effects of propofol or isoflurane anesthesia on cardiac conduction in children undergoing radiofrequency catheter ablation for tachydysrhythmias. *Anesthesiology* 1995; 82:884-87.
3. Yaster MY, Krane EJ, Kaplan RF: Diagnostic evaluation of congenital heart disease. In *Pediatric Pain Management and Sedation Handbook.* Mosby Yearbook, St. Louis: 1997.
4. Zimmerman AA, Ibrahim AE, et al: The effects of halothane and sevoflurane on cardiac electrophysiology in children undergoing radiofrequency catheter ablation. *Anesthesiology* 1997; 87:A1066.

PEDIATRIC ONCOLOGIC PROCEDURES

Cathy R. Lammers and Gregory B. Hammer

Pediatric oncology patients must endure multiple painful procedures, including bone marrow aspirations, biopsies, lumbar punctures and removal of central venous access ports. All of these procedures can be performed in a procedure room with sedation or GA.

PREPROCEDURE

A thorough preanesthetic H&P should be performed in all cases and the usual npo protocol applied (see p. D-1). Prior treatment with chemotherapeutic agents should be identified for evaluation of toxic side effects (see below).

Respiratory Surgeries for patients with Sx of URI (e.g., cough, fever) are usually postponed. Some chemotherapeutic agents have been associated with pulmonary toxicity: bleomycin (2-5%), BNCU (20-50%), busulfan (2.5-11.5%), cyclophosphamide (rare), methotrexate (rare).
Tests: As indicated from H&P.

Cardiovascular Some chemotherapeutic agents have been associated with cardiac toxicity: cyclophosphamide, doxorubicin, Adriamycin, radiation (cardiomyopathy); doxorubicin, m-AMSA (dysrhythmias).
Tests: Consider a functional cardiac study if patient received a chemotherapeutic agent associated with cardiac toxicity (most have already had a study done by this stage of their treatment).

Hematologic Bone marrow suppression with all cytotoxic drugs.
Tests: As indicated.

Laboratory Many patients will have had a recent CBC. In general, no additional labs are required.

Premedication Usually not required because a parent can accompany child into procedure room; however, most children will have venous access and can be given small doses of midazolam if necessary. Consider midazolam 0.5-0.75 mg/kg po (in a few ml of flavored liquid) for the particularly anxious child without iv access in place. For children without venous access, a peripheral iv may be placed (with or without premedication), preferably at least 1 h following application of EMLA cream for topical anesthesia of the skin.

INTRAPROCEDURE

Anesthetic technique: GA (LMA or mask) or MAC in the appropriate patient

Induction Most children have a central venous access line in place for their oncology treatment protocol; thus, induction can proceed with iv propofol 2-3 mg/kg. Infrequently, mask induction is performed.

Maintenance The oncologist infiltrates the area with lidocaine. For Broviac catheter removals, a sufficient bolus of propofol must be given just prior to pulling the catheter. Additional iv usually is not warranted, since the procedure is normally < 10 min. Occasionally, the catheter may break during attempted removal, and the surgeon will have to make a skin incision to allow for removal of the internal fragment. In such cases, a peripheral iv may be inserted quickly to facilitate administration of additional propofol, or mask anesthesia may be given. If the SpO_2 decreases, blow-by O_2 with gentle head and neck positioning are generally sufficient.

Emergence Allow child to awaken in procedure room. Consider ondansetron 0.1 mg/kg for patients receiving intrathecal chemotherapy during their lumbar puncture. Most patients should be recovered in the PACU.

Blood and fluid requirements	No blood loss	IV central line may be *in situ*.
Monitoring	Standard monitors (see p. D-1).	
Positioning	Lateral, fetal position (lumbar punctures) Supine or prone (bone marrow aspiration/biopsy) Supine for Broviac removal	
Complications	Airway obstruction	
	Retained central venous catheter	Rx may require open surgical procedure.
Pain management	Rectal Tylenol	Lumbar punctures are not generally painful afterwards, whereas bone marrow aspirations and biopsies, especially, can be. Rectal Tylenol is usually sufficient for analgesia.

References

1. Cote CJ: Anesthesia outside the operating room. In *A Practice of Anesthesia for Infants and Children.* Cote CJ, Ryan JF, Todres ID, et al, eds. WB Saunders, Philadelphia: 1993.
2. Martin TM, Nicolson SC, Bargas MS: Propofol anesthesia reduces emesis and airway obstruction in pediatric outpatients. *Anesth Analg* 1993; 76(1):144-48.
3. McDowall RH, Scher CS, Barst SM. Total intravenous anesthesia for children undergoing brief diagnostic or therapeutic procedures. *J Clin Anesth* 1995; 7(4):273-80.

UPPER/LOWER GI ENDOSCOPY

Cathy R. Lammers and Gregory B. Hammer

Children presenting for upper and/or lower GI endoscopy may have a wide variety of congenital and acquired abnormalities of the GI tract. Examples include repaired tracheoesophageal fistula (TEF) with residual esophageal dysmotility, presence of a foreign body and various congenital lesions. Patients presenting for gastrostomy tube placement may have encephalopathy 2° cerebral palsy, with associated seizure disorder and muscle contractures. Severe GERD may be present, with the associated risk of pulmonary aspiration following induction of anesthesia. Many GI endoscopy procedures are done without anesthesia. Requests for anesthesia are dependent on the gastroenterologist's preference, as well as the severity of the patient's underlying illnesses. All patients must receive a thorough preanesthesia H&P. Children should follow the same npo protocol used for surgery (see p. D-1).

ANESTHETIC CONSIDERATIONS

Gastroenterology Carefully question the parents for Sx of GERD or esophageal dysfunction resulting in retained food within the esophagus. The stomach and bowel will be insufflated with CO_2 during the procedure, increasing the likelihood of reflux.

Neurologic Patients with seizure disorders that are well controlled do not need to have recent anticonvulsant levels documented. If spasticity 2° cerebral palsy is present, special attention to careful evaluation of the airway is warranted; vascular access may be difficult.

Laboratory As indicated from H&P. Usually none.

Premedication If inhalation induction is planned, premedication may not be required because a parent can accompany the child into the procedure room. Consider midazolam 0.5-0.75 mg/kg po for particularly anxious children and for those in whom iv induction is planned. EMLA cream should be applied at least 1 h in advance for topical anesthesia before iv placement.

INTRAPROCEDURE

Anesthetic technique: Upper endoscopy and gastrostomy tube placement generally require GETA 2° ↑risk of pulmonary aspiration (2° GERD and insufflation of CO_2). In children > 3-4 yr, the indication for tracheal intubation in the absence of Hx of GERD is less clear. Placement of the endoscope in the mouth precludes the ability to use a mask or LMA. Alternatively, an iv sedation technique with propofol (50-100 μg/kg/min), spontaneous respiration, and supplemental O_2 via nasal cannula or blow-by can be used if the risk of aspiration is considered low. For lower GI endoscopy procedures (e.g., colonoscopy), iv sedation may be preferable.

Induction For upper GI endoscopies, if Hx of severe GERD is present, an iv catheter is placed prior to induction of anesthesia. A modified, rapid-sequence intubation is performed with preoxygenation, cricoid pressure, STP (4-6 mg/kg) or propofol (2-3 mg/kg), and rocuronium 1 mg/kg. If the risk of aspiration is relatively low, a standard pediatric iv or mask induction is appropriate (see p. D-2). Alternatively, iv sedation may be performed with propofol (75-150 μg/kg/min), with or without remifentanil (0.05-0.10 μg/kg/min), by continuous infusion.

Maintenance GETA with inhalational agents or iv infusion of propofol ± remifentanil. Alternatively, iv sedation as above. Young children may have tracheal compression caused by passage of the relatively large endoscope into the esophagus.

Emergence Emergence in procedure room. Transport to PACU for recovery.

Blood and fluid requirements No blood loss
IV: 22 or 24 ga × 1
NS/LR @ maintenance

Monitoring Standard monitors (see p. D-1).

Positioning ✓ and pad pressure points.
✓ eyes.
Lateral decubitus for upper and lower endoscopy.
Supine for G-tube placement.

Complications Airway obstruction
Hypoxemia 2° gastric insufflation

Complications, cont.	Pulmonary aspiration GI perforation

POSTPROCEDURE

Pain management	G-tube placements require postop analgesia.	Gastroenterologist infiltrates local anesthetic at the site.
	Rectal acetaminophen (35-40 mg/kg)	Following induction for upper GI endoscopies
	Morphine 0.1-0.2 mg/kg or fentanyl 2-3 μg/kg intraop	Usually provide adequate analgesic in the immediate postop period.

References

1. Balsells F, Wyllie R, Kay M, Steffan R: Use of conscious sedation for lower and upper gastrointestinal endoscopic examinations in children and adults: a twelve-year review. *Gastrointest Endosc* 1997; 45:375-80.
2. Cote CJ: Anesthesia outside the operating room. In *A Practice of Anesthesia for Infants and Children.* Cote CJ, Ryan JF, Todres ID, et al, eds. WB Saunders, Philadelphia: 1993.
3. Haight M. Thomas DW: Pediatric gastrointestinal endoscopy. *Gastroenterologist* 1995; 3:181-86.
4. Squires RH, Morriss F, Schluterman S, et al: Efficacy, safety, and cost of intravenous sedation versus general anesthesia in children undergoing endoscopic procedures. *Gastrointest Endosc* 1995; 41:99-104.

CROSS-SECTIONAL IMAGING (CT, MRI)

Cathy R. Lammers and Gregory B. Hammer

PREPROCEDURE

All patients must receive a thorough preanesthesia H&P. Children should follow the same npo protocol as they would for surgery (see p. D-1). For MRI, thorough questioning regarding metal implants is essential. Any questions regarding appropriateness of specific metal implants should be directed to the radiologist.

Respiratory	URIs must be evaluated carefully. If Sx are limited to nasal congestion, the study may proceed. Sx of lower tract involvement—including fever, productive cough or wheezing—warrant postponement for 2-3 wk unless the study is urgent.
Cardiovascular	Pacemakers are a contraindication for MRI. Prosthetic heart valves may be a contraindication (identify the type of valve present and consult with radiologist).
Neurologic	Head CT or MRI may be performed in patients with primary seizure disorders or brain tumors. Review seizure medications and ✓ serum levels if appropriate. Recent drug levels may not be necessary in children with well controlled or stable seizure disorders. If ↑ICP or ↓intracranial compliance are present (e.g., 2° tumors or hydrocephalus) the anesthesia plan should include tracheal intubation with controlled ventilation. Metal clips or coils are usually contraindications for MRI. For children with head trauma, concurrent injuries involving the cervical spine may be present.
Laboratory	As indicated from H&P. Usually none required.
Premedication	If inhalation induction is planned, premedication may not be required because a parent can accompany child into induction area (either inside CT scan or in outer induction area of MRI). Consider midazolam 0.5-0.75 mg/kg po for particularly anxious children and for those in whom iv induction is planned.

INTRAPROCEDURE

Unique considerations for MRI: See Adult Out-of-OR Procedures, p. 1065.

Anesthetic technique:

CT scans—many children undergo noninvasive CT scans with po sedation without involvement of anesthesia service. For more complex cases requiring the presence of an anesthesiologist, the procedure may be performed with iv sedation or GA. Most commonly, noninvasive CT scans are performed under iv sedation with a continuous infusion of propofol (100-200 μg/kg/min). Alternatively, incremental doses of midazolam (0.025-0.10 mg/kg) may be given. For patients undergoing invasive CT-guided procedures (needle biopsy, placement of drainage tubes, such as thoracostomy tube, etc.), GETA is usually performed. Techniques include spontaneous breathing with inhalational anesthesia and/or propofol infusion or iv anesthesia (propofol with or without remifentanil infusion) and controlled ventilation.

MRI—iv sedation or GA may be performed. A deeper level of anesthesia is needed compared with noninvasive CT because MRI requires the child to be motionless for up to 1-2 h. IV propofol infusion may be administered by gravity via a microdrip device, or inhalational anesthesia may be given with MRI-compatible anesthetic machines. Hypothermia frequently occurs in small children anesthetized for 1-2 h in the MRI scanner. The cooling fan for the magnet can sometimes be turned off to decrease heat loss (discuss with MRI technician). One blanket over patient is usually permissible. The iv, airway circuit and monitors require extensions.

Induction — Standard pediatric iv or mask induction in CT scanner or in MRI induction area (outside MRI scanner). MRI patients transported into scanner after induction.

Maintenance — For iv technique, use propofol infusion pump in CT scanner and microdrip infusion set in MRI (e.g., add 10 ml propofol solution to 90 ml iv fluid to yield propofol concentration of 1 mg/ml [60 drops]; therefore, 1 drop per sec delivers 1 mg/min, or 100 μg/kg/min for a 10-kg child). Typically, these patients do not require muscle relaxants, and spontaneous breathing is appropriate unless controlled ventilation is required to treat ↑ICP.

Emergence — Transport MRI patient back to induction room for emergence (airway equipment available). Patients are usually recovered in PACU. Children having short procedures with propofol anesthesia who are wide awake in the CT or MRI holding area following the study may be recovered there.

Blood and fluid requirements	No blood loss IV if required: 22 or 24 ga × 1 NS/LR @ maintenance	
Monitoring	Standard monitors (see p. D-1 for discussion of monitoring considerations).	For infants, use a child-size NBP cuff on the leg. The length of tubing required significantly alters the values on infant-size cuffs.
Positioning	✓ and pad pressure points. ✓ eyes.	Ear protection for MRI
Complications	Hypothermia Burn injury IV contrast reaction Airway obstruction Hearing loss (MRI)	See adult MRI Complications, p. 1066. From inappropriate placement of pulse oximeter probe or ECG wires in MRI

POSTPROCEDURE

Pain management	Noninvasive procedures are painless.	IV fentanyl or morphine appropriate for invasive procedures.

References

1. Cote CJ: Anesthesia outside the operating room. In *A Practice of Anesthesia for Infants and Children.* Cote CJ, Ryan JF, Todres ID, et al, eds. WB Saunders, Philadelphia: 1993.
2. Jorensen NH, Messick JM, Gray J, Nugent M, Berquist TH: ASA monitoring standards and magnetic resonance imaging. *Anesth Analg* 1994; 79:1141-47.
3. Levati A, Colombo N, Arosio EM, Savoia G, et al: Propofol anesthesia in spontaneously breathing pediatric patients during magnetic resonance imaging. *Acta Anaesth Scand* 1996; 40:561-65.
4. Young AE, Brown PN, Zorab JS: Anesthesia for children and infants undergoing magnetic resonance imaging: a prospective study. *Eur J Anaesthesiol* 1996; 13:400-3.

EXTRACORPOREAL MEMBRANE OXYGENATION (ECMO)

Gary E. Hartman

PROCEDURAL CONSIDERATIONS

Description: **Extracorporeal membrane oxygenation (ECMO)** for prolonged periods (3-21 d) allows cardiopulmonary support for newborns and children with reversible respiratory failure. The most common indications are meconium aspiration and pulmonary HTN associated with congenital diaphragmatic hernia. The procedure is performed in the NICU with OR technique. Patients are given anticoagulants prior to cannulation. Subsequently, repair of the diaphragmatic hernia also is performed in the NICU on ECMO support prior to decannulation. (Fig 13.2-1 shows ECMO schematic.)

The potential detrimental effects of the diaphragmatic repair on respiratory function can be managed with increased circuit flow. ECMO also has been helpful in some newborns with cardiopulmonary failure following correction of congenital cardiac defects. Vascular access is accomplished with one (venovenous) or two (venoarterial) cannulas. The IJ vein is cannulated in both methods with the tip of the cannula in the right atrium. In venoarterial ECMO, the common carotid artery is used with the tip of the cannula at the aortic arch. The wound is closed around the cannulas, which are secured to the infant's scalp.

Usual preop diagnosis: Meconium aspiration; diaphragmatic hernia; Bochdalek's hernia

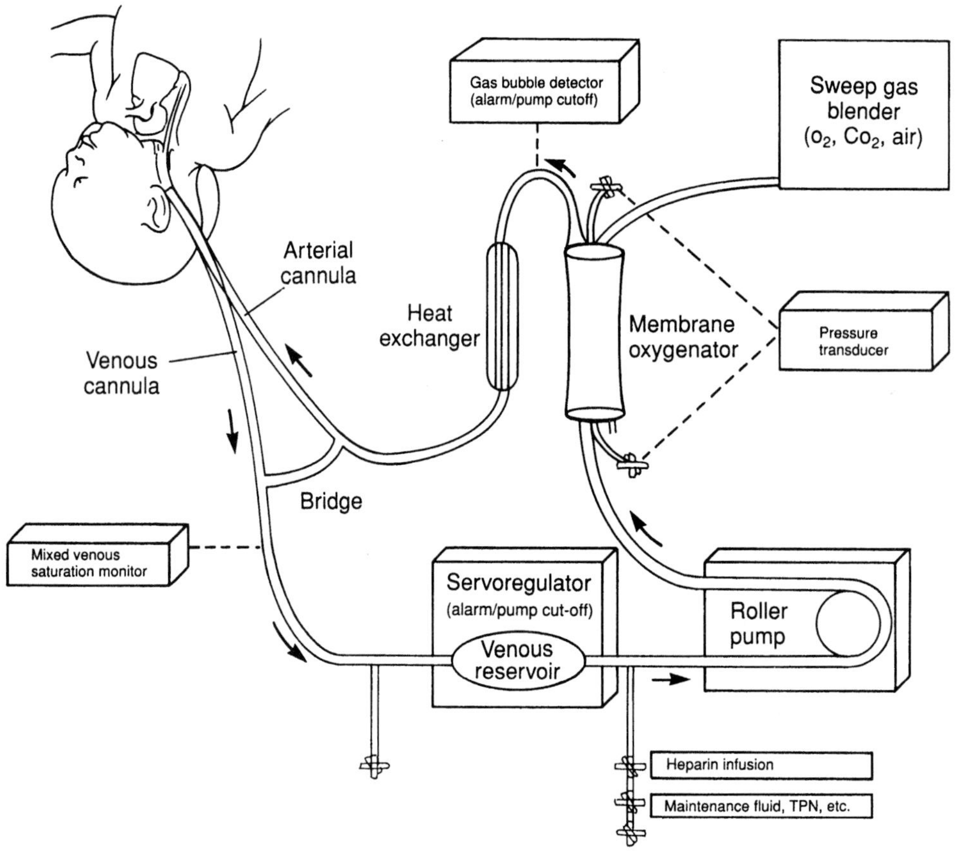

Figure 13.2-1. ECMO circuit. Venous blood is withdrawn by gravity through a servoregulator to prevent pump from actively siphoning venous return. Roller pump delivers blood back to the arterial cannula after it passes through the membrane oxygenator and heat exchanger. Venous return is from the right atrium, arterial infusion is into the aortic arch in double cannula (venoarterial) or right atrium (venovenous) techniques. (Reproduced with permission from Rhine W, Van Meurs K: Extracorporeal membrane and oxygenation. In *Nelson's Textbook of Pediatrics*, Update #8. WB Saunders: 1990.)

SUMMARY OF PROCEDURE

Position	Supine
Incision	Subcostal, right neck incision
Special instrumentation	ECMO circuit (Fig 13.2-1)
Unique considerations	Anticoagulation
Antibiotics	Preop: ampicillin 25 mg/kg iv + gentamicin 2.5 mg/kg iv Intraop: cefazolin irrigation (1 g/500 ml NS)
Surgical time	1-2 h
Closing considerations	Assess for changes in ventilation (e.g., PIP, pre- and postductal ABG).
EBL	> 5-10 ml/kg
Postop care	Paralysis maintained; fentanyl infusion @ 2-4 μg/kg/h
Mortality	25-30%
Morbidity	Respiratory failure Sepsis
Pain score	6-7

PATIENT POPULATION CHARACTERISTICS

Age range	Newborn–weeks or months
Male:Female	1-2:1
Incidence	1/4000
Etiology	Unknown
Associated conditions	For diaphragmatic hernia: malrotation (40-100%); congenital heart disease (15%); renal anomalies; esophageal atresia; CNS abnormalities

References

1. Falconer AR, Brown RA, Helms P, Gordon I, Baron JA: Pulmonary sequelae in survivors of congenital diaphragmatic hernia. *Thorax* 1990; 45(2):126-29.
2. Stolar CJH: Congenital diaphragmatic hernia. In *Surgery of Infants and Children.* Oldham KT, Colombani PM, Foglia RP, eds. Lippincott-Raven Publishers, Philadelphia: 1997, 883-96.
3. Wilson JM, Lund DP, Lillehei CW, Vacanti JP: Congenital diaphragmatic hernia: predictors of severity in the ECMO era. *J Pediatr Surg* 1991; 26(9):1028-33.

Authors

Sandra Leigh Bardas, RPh, BS (*Drug interactions*)
Stephen P. Fischer, MD (*Lab and diagnostic studies*)
Alvin Hackel, MD (*Latex allergy*)
Gregory B. Hammer, MD (*Pediatric anesthetic protocols, pain management*)
Richard A. Jaffe, MD, PhD (*Adult anesthetic protocols*)

APPENDICES

Cathy R. Lammers (*Latex allergy*)
C. Philip Larson, Jr., MD, MS (*Fiber optic intubation*)
Yuan-Chi Lin, MD (*Pediatric pain management*)
Cathy M. Russo, MD (*Adult pain management*)
Stanley I. Samuels, MB, BCh, FFARCS (*Adult anesthetic protocols*)

APPENDIX A: PREOPERATIVE LABORATORY TESTING AND DIAGNOSTIC STUDIES

Stephen P. Fischer

The value and utility of preop diagnostic studies have become central issues in evaluating cost-effective health care in the surgical patient. It is estimated that up to $3 billion is spent in the U.S. annually on preop laboratory and diagnostic studies. Unnecessary testing is inefficient and expensive, and it requires additional technical resources. Inappropriate studies may lead to evaluation of "borderline" or false-positive laboratory abnormalities. This may result in unnecessary OR delays, cancellations and potential patient risk through additional testing and follow-up.

Surgical patients require preop lab and diagnostic studies that are consistent with their medical histories, the proposed operative procedures and the potential for blood loss. Preop lab and diagnostic testing should be ordered for specific clinical indications rather than simply because the patient is about to undergo a certain surgical procedure.

The following preop diagnostic guidelines provide basic recommendations. They are not intended as absolute or standard requirements. Practice guidelines should be modified based on clinical needs and individual practice, to ensure the highest quality of anesthesia and surgical patient care.

SUMMARY OF PREOP STUDIES

Chest x-ray (CXR)

Overview: A preop CXR should be used to assess the presence of acute, progressive or chronic changes in cardiac/pulmonary disease. The decision to obtain a preop CXR should be individualized and based on clinical indications (see Table A-1). CXRs should not be part of a routine preop screening protocol.

Clinical indications: Pneumonia; pulmonary edema; atelectasis; aortic aneurysm; mediastinal or pulmonary masses; tracheal deviation; pulmonary HTN; cardiomegaly; advanced COPD and blebs; dextrocardia; pulmonary embolism

Electrocardiogram (ECG)

Overview: ECGs evaluate cardiac rhythm/conduction disturbances, ischemia, myocardial infarction, hypertrophy and metabolic and electrolyte disorders.

Clinical indications: Patients with suspected or known Hx of CAD; patient age > 50; HTN; chest pain; CHF; diabetes; cerebral vascular disease and PVD; syncope or presyncope; dizziness; SOB; DOE; PND; palpitations; leg/ankle edema; abnormal valvular murmurs

Liver function test (LFT)

Overview: LFTs establish the absence or presence of hepatic injury and the degree of hepatic reserve in disease states. LFTs consist of: AST(SGOT), ALT(SGPT), GGTP, alkaline phosphatase, serum albumin, bilirubin.

Clinical indications: Patients with suspected or known Hx of hepatitis (viral, alcohol, drugs), infiltration (tumor, immunologic); cirrhosis; portal HTN; gallbladder or biliary tract disease; jaundice; intravascular hemolysis

Renal function testing

Overview: Renal function testing measures glomerular filtration and the magnitude of renal tubular dysfunction. These tests include: serum creatinine and BUN.

Clinical indications: Renal function testing is indicated for patients with HTN, increased fluid overload (CHF/peripheral edema/ascites) associated with cardiac, hepatic or renal impairment; dehydration; diabetes; nausea, emesis or anorexia; polyuria; nocturia; oliguria; anuria; high-risk surgery in patients with low CO syndrome; hematuria; CVA pain; renal transplant Hx; renal disease; dialysis.

Hemoglobin (Hb), Hematocrit (Hct), CBC

Overview: The decision to obtain a preop Hb, Hct or CBC should be individualized and based on clinical indications, medical Hx and the proposed surgical procedure. Hb/Hct or CBC should not be part of a routine preop screening protocol.

Clinical indications: Hematological disorder; bleeding/coagulopathy Hx; malignancy; chemotherapy; radiation therapy (CBC); renal disease; anticoagulant and steroid therapy; surgical procedures with high blood loss (> 1500 ml); highly invasive or trauma surgery; malabsorption/poor nutrition status; CNS disease.

Pregnancy testing

Overview: The decision to obtain a preop pregnancy test should be based on clinical Hx and examination. Several assays are available (serum hCG, urine hCG); β-hCG detectable in maternal urine and blood 8-9 d post conception.

Clinical indications: Sexually active; time of last menstrual period; presence or absence of birth control method; patient intuition

Coagulation testing

Overview: Coagulation testing, or clotting function studies, should be obtained in patients with known or suspected coagulopathies as indicated from H&P and drug therapies. Tests include: prothrombin time (PT), partial prothrombin time (PTT), INR, platelet (Plt) count.

Clinical indications: Bleeding disorder Hx; anticoagulants or other drugs affecting coagulation; critical risk surgeries with significant blood loss expected; hepatic disease; malabsorption/poor nutrition

Urine analysis

Overview: Assessment of renal function, infection, intravascular volume status, metabolic disorders

Clinical indications: There are no routine anesthesia preop requirements for a urine analysis.

References

1. Fischer SP: Medical assessment of the surgical patient. In *Fundamentals of Surgery*. Appleton and Lange, Stamford, CT: 1997, 19-30.
2. Fischer SP: Preoperative evaluation of the neurosurgical patient. In *International Anesthesia Clinics*. Little, Brown, Boston: 1996.
3. Friedman LS, Maddrey WC: Surgery in patients with liver disease. *Med Clin North Am* 1987; 71:453.
4. Goldman L, Mangano DT: Preoperative assessment of the patient with known or suspected coronary artery disease. *N Engl J Med* 1995; 333:1750.
5. Kaufman BS, Contereras J: Preanesthetic assessment of the patient with renal disease. *Anesth Analg* 1994; 78:143.
6. MacPherson D: Preoperative laboratory testing: should any tests be "routine" before surgery? *Med Clin North Am* 1993; 77:289.
7. Pasternak LR: Preanesthesia evaluation of the surgical patient. *ASA Refresher Courses in Anesthsiology* 1996; 24:205-19.
8. Roizen MF, Cohn S: Preoperative evaluation for elective surgery—what laboratory tests are needed? In *Advances in Anesthesia*, Vol 10. Stoelting RK, ed. Mosby-Year Book, St. Louis: 1993, 25-47.
9. Schiff RL, Emanuele MA: The surgical patient with diabetes mellitus: guidelines for management. *J Gen Intern Med* 1995; 10:154.

Table A-1. Diagnosis-Based Preop Testing

Preop Diagnosis	ECG	CXR	Hct/Hb	CBC	Lytes	Renal	Glucose	Coag	LFTs	Drug levels	Ca^+
Cardiac disease:											
MI history	X				±						
Stable angina	X				±						
CHF	X	±				±					
HTN	X	±			X[1]	X					
Chronic atrial fib	X									X[2]	
PVD	X										
Valvular heart disease	X	±									
Pulmonary disease:											
Emphysema	X	±								X[3]	
Asthma	(PFT only if symptomatic; otherwise no tests required)										
Chronic bronchitis	X	±		X							
Diabetes	X				±	X	X				
Hepatic disease											
Infectious hepatitis								X	X		
Alcohol/drug-induced								X	X		
Tumor infiltration								X	X		
Renal disease			X		X	X					
Hematological disorders				X							
Coagulopathies				X				X			
CNS disorders:											
Stroke	X			X	X		X			X	
Seizures	X			X	X		X			X	
Tumor	X			X							
Vascular/aneurysms	X		X								
Malignancy				X							
Hyperthyroidism	X		X		X						X
Hypothyroidism	X		X		X						
Cushing's disease				X	X		X				
Addison's disease				X	X		X				
Hyperparathyroidism	X		X		X						X
Hypoparathyroidism	X				X						X
Morbid obesity	X	±					X				
Malabsorption/poor nutrition	X			X	X	X	X	±			
Select drug therapies:											
Digoxin (digitalis)	X				±					X	
Anticoagulants			X					X			
Dilantin										X	
Phenobarbital										X	
Diuretics					X	X					
Steroids				X			X				
Chemotherapy				X							
Aspirin/NSAID	(No tests)										
Theophylline										X	

X = OBTAIN ± = CONSIDER

[1] Patients on diuretics [2] Patients on digoxin [3] Patients on theophylline

APPENDIX B: STANDARD ADULT ANESTHETIC PROTOCOLS

Stanley I. Samuels, Richard A. Jaffe, C. Philip Larson, Jr.

STANDARD MONITORS (NONINVASIVE)

Blood pressure (BP)	
Capnometry/capnography	Measurement of $ETCO_2$/display of wave form
Gas analyzer (e.g., Raman, IR, mass spectometry)	Respired gases and anesthetics
Electrocardiogram (ECG)	5-lead preferred
Esophageal or precordial stethoscope	Breath and heart sounds monitored; dysrhythmias and ↓BP detected
Nerve stimulator	Monitor status of neuromuscular blockade
Oxygen analyzer	Measurement of FiO_2
Pulse oximetry	Measurement of O_2 saturation of hemoglobin
Temperature	Nasal, esophageal, bladder, rectal, tympanic or skin
Visual observation of patient	Skin color, pupils, temperature, edema, sweating, movement
Ventilator function monitors	PIP, TV, disconnect alarm, etc.

STANDARD ANESTHETIC MANAGEMENT (ADULT ASA 1 & 2)

★ **NB:** The following sections are guidelines only (for an otherwise healthy 70 kg adult). Specific drugs and drug dosages should be individualized, based on the physiological and pharmacological status of the patient, including factors such as age, weight, medication and concurrent diseases.

PREMEDICATION

Light	Diazepam 5-10 mg	po 1 h preop
	Lorazepam 1-2 mg	po 1 h preop
	Hydroxyzine 25-100 mg	po 1 h preop
Moderate	Midazolam 1-2 mg iv	Prior to induction (in patient holding area or OR).
	±Fentanyl 25-100 μg iv	Monitor for respiratory depression.
Heavy	Diazepam 10 mg	po 1-2 h preop
	+ Morphine 0.1 mg/kg	im 30-60 min preop
	+ Scopolamine 0.2-0.4 mg	(im 30-60 min preop)

INDUCTION TECHNIQUES

Preinduction

1. ✓ anesthesia machine, suction, airway equipment, drugs.
2. Attach monitors and verify function.
3. Administer 100% O_2 by mask × 1-3 min.
4. Administer supplemental sedation/analgesia (as appropriate).
   e.g.: Fentanyl 1-3 μg/kg iv
   ± Midazolam 0.03-0.1 mg/kg iv

Induction agents

Thiopental	3-5 mg/kg iv
Propofol	1.5-2.5 mg/kg iv (in increments) **NB:** Pain on injection ★
Etomidate	0.2-0.4 mg/kg iv **NB:** Pain on injection; myoclonus ★

Muscle relaxants for intubation

Drugs	Doses	Onset	Duration
Succinylcholine:	1.0 mg/kg	30-60 sec	4-6 min
If given after 3 mg dTC for defasciculation	1.5 mg/kg	30-60 sec	4-6 min
Infusion	1 g/250-500 NS (titrated to effect)	+60 sec	While infusing (phase II block possible)
Vecuronium	0.1 mg/kg	2-3 min	24-30 min
	0.2 mg/kg (rapid onset)	< 2 min	45-90 min
Pancuronium	0.1 mg/kg	3-4 min	40-65 min
Mivacurium	0.1-0.2 mg/kg	1-2 min	6-10 min
Cisatracurium	0.2 mg/kg	90 sec	40-80 min
d-tubocurarine (dTC)	0.5 mg/kg	3-5 min	30 min
Pipecuronium	0.07-0.09 mg/kg	2-3 min	45-120 min
Rocuronium	0.6 mg/kg	60-90 sec	30 min

MAINTENANCE TECHNIQUES

Inhalational anesthesia

30-100% O_2
+ 0-70% N_2O
+ Isoflurane (MAC in 100% O_2 = 1.15%) titrated to effect
Alternatively, for short procedures or for the last hour of long procedures, use sevoflurane (MAC = 1.7%) or desflurane (MAC = 6%)

Balanced anesthesia

30-100% O_2 in N_2O
+ 0-70% N_2O
+ Meperidine 0.5-1.5 mg/kg/3-4 h (intermittent bolus)
or fentanyl 1-10 μg/kg prn response to surgical stimulation
or remifentanil 0.05-2 μg/kg/min prn response to surgical stimulation
+ Isoflurane ~0.5%
or propofol 50-200 μg/kg/min
Alternatively, for short procedures or for the last hour of long procedures, use sevoflurane (MAC = 1.7%) or desflurane (MAC = 6%).

Total intravenous anesthesia

30-100% O_2 in N_2O
0-0% air

+ Remifentanil infusion (infusion off 5 min before end of surgery)	Induction infusion	@ 1 μg/kg/min
	Maintenance	@ 0.25 μg/kg/min
+ Propofol bolus + infusion (infusion off 5 min before end of surgery)	Induction bolus	1 mg/kg
	Maintenance < 30 min	@100 μg/kg/min
	Maintenance > 30 min	@ 80-100 μg/kg/min

★ **NB: No residual analgesia–postop pain management depends on type of surgery and analgesic requirements may be substantial.**

If continued muscle relaxation is required during the above maintenance techniques, several options are available. Always use a nerve stimulator to assess block before redosing.

Short-acting	Mivacurium	0.1 mg/kg/10-20 min or 1-15 μg/kg/min
Intermediate	Vecuronium	0.025 mg/kg/30 min
	Rocuronium	0.6 mg/kg/30 min
	Cisatracurium	0.2 mg/kg/40 min
Long-acting	Pancuronium	0.02 mg/kg/60-90 min
	Pipecuronium	0.015 mg/kg/60-90 min

EMERGENCE

1.	**Reversal of muscle relaxant**	As surgical conditions permit, reverse residual muscle relaxant (when at least 1 twitch is present in train-of-four) with one of the following: Neostigmine 0.05-0.07 (maximum dose) mg/kg iv + glycopyrrolate 0.01 mg/kg iv, or Edrophonium 0.5-1.0 (maximum dose) mg/kg iv + atropine 0.015 mg/kg iv.
2.	**Analgesia**	If remifentanil was used during surgery, supplemental analgesics will be necessary and should be given before emergence.
3.	**Nausea prophylaxis**	Metoclopramide (10 mg iv), or droperidol (0.625 mg iv) or ondansetron (4 mg iv) or dolasetron (12.5 mg iv). Consider OG tube placement and suction to empty stomach.
4.	**O_2**	Discontinue N_2O/volatile agents and administer 100% O_2.
5.	**Suction**	Suction oropharynx thoroughly.
6.	**Extubation**	Extubate after protective airway reflexes have returned, the patient is breathing spontaneously and is able to follow commands.

MONITORED ANESTHESIA CARE (MAC)

1. Standard monitoring with regular verbal contact.
2. Nasal O_2 (qualitative measurement of $ETCO_2$ can be accomplished by attaching a sampling catheter to the nasal cannula).
3. If the initial local anesthetic injection will be painful (e.g., retrobulbar block), then a brief period of analgesia, sedation and amnesia can be induced with:

		Advantages:	Disadvantages:
A.	Midazolam (0.5-2 mg) 3-5 min before injection + Ketamine (10-20 mg) 3 min before injection + alfentanil 3-7 μg/kg 2 min before injection or remifentanil 0.5 μg/kg 2 min before injection or	Profound amnesia Excellent analgesia Usually no apnea Airway reflexes maintained Patient cooperation	Patient not "asleep" Timing important Possible ↑BP and HR
B.	STP (1-3 mg/kg) ± fentanyl (25-50 μg/)	Patient "asleep"	Possible apnea Possible loss of airway ↓BP Patient unresponsive

4. Light-to-moderate levels of sedation (± analgesia) can be maintained using a **propofol infusion** (25-100 μg/kg/min), or with intermittent bolus injections of midazolam (0.25-1mg) ± fentanyl (10-25 μg) or with a remifentanil infusion (0.025-0.05 μg/kg/min), titrated to effect. Monitor closely for respiratory depression.

RAPID-SEQUENCE INDUCTION OF ANESTHESIA (FULL-STOMACH PRECAUTIONS)

1. ↓ gastric volume/acidity	Ranitidine 50 mg iv at least 30-60 min before induction Metoclopramide 5-10 mg iv 30-60 min before induction 0.3 M sodium citrate 30 ml po immediately before induction
2. Induction	Preoxygenation > 3 min Defasciculate: dTC 3 mg 3-5 min before succinylcholine Cricoid pressure (Sellick maneuver) by assistant Etomidate 0.1-0.4 mg/kg or STP 3-5 mg/kg or ketamine 1 mg/kg iv or propofol 1.5-2.5 mg/kg + Succinylcholine 1.5 mg/kg for intubation (stylet ETT). If succinylcholine contraindicated, consider rocuronium (1.2 mg/kg).
3. Intubation	Intubate when patient is fully relaxed. Watch chest movement and auscultate for equal BBS. ✓ expired CO_2 on monitor. Listen over stomach. Secure ETT and release cricoid pressure. Pass NG tube and suction stomach contents.
4. Failed intubation protocol	See Anesthetic Considerations for Cesarean Section, Obstetric Surgery, p. 602.
5. Maintenance	As indicated by patient's condition and type of surgery.
6. Extubation	Extubate when patient is awake and with active laryngeal protective reflexes. Remember, some may require postop ICU care until safe extubation can be assured.

SPECIAL PEDIATRIC CONSIDERATIONS

1. The same principles apply in children requiring surgery, and in those who may have full stomachs. Consider emptying the stomach with an OG tube prior to induction. If iv is placed, continue as indicated above. If iv access is difficult, O_2/halothane or O_2/sevoflurane induction with cricoid pressure, succinylcholine (2-4 mg/kg im) will permit intubation and minimize risks of gastric aspiration.
2. Awake intubation in neonates and sick infants may be the safest method.

AWAKE FIBER OPTIC INTUBATION PROTOCOL

C. Philip Larson, Jr.

Premedication If not contraindicated, patients should receive mild-to- moderate sedation with meperidine 0.5 mg/kg and midazolam 1-2 mg iv.

Topical anesthesia When premedication has been established, the oropharynx is sprayed vigorously ~6 times over a span of 10 min, using lidocaine 10% solution. Initially, the spray is directed at the front of the tongue; gradually, it is directed further back in the throat, until the entire oropharynx is numb. In reality, the lateral recesses of the oropharynx need not be anesthetized topically because both fiber optic laryngoscope and ETT are confined to the midline of the mouth.

Tracheal anesthesia Next, a transtracheal injection of cocaine or lidocaine 4% (2 ml) is made through the cricothyroid membrane, using a 3-ml syringe and a 23 ga, 3/4 inch needle. So that this injection can be made as rapidly as possible, it is important to use a small syringe, making certain that the connection between syringe and needle is tight. The patient is instructed not to cough until the injection is complete. Since this may be impossible for some patients, it is important that the operator's hand be fixed firmly against the patient's upper chest to assure that needle movement is minimized and that the full injection is made into the trachea. When the injection is complete, the patient is urged to cough vigorously.

Laryngoscopy Once the mouth and trachea are anesthetized with local anesthetic, an oral airway with a central orifice (e.g., Tudor-Williams airway) is placed in the midline of the mouth. A 7 mm orotracheal tube, without connector attached, is placed over a fiber optic laryngoscope. With the operator at the patient's side near the waist, the fiber optic laryngoscope is introduced through the hole in the airway and advanced to end of airway. At this point, the epiglottis should be visible. The tip of the fiber optic scope is flexed toward the operator about 15-20°, which should bring arytenoid cartilages and laryngeal opening into view. The scope is advanced into the larynx so that tracheal rings can be visualized. Often, the carina also can be visualized. The laryngoscopist also can place the scope in the airway by darkening the room and using the scope as a light wand, directing the light externally to the sternal notch and advancing it down the trachea.

Intubation The scope is placed on the patient's chest and, holding it so that it is not advanced further, the orotracheal tube is gently advanced into the trachea. To facilitate passage of the orotracheal tube past the arytenoid cartilages and into the larynx, it is often necessary to rotate the tube counterclockwise 90°, or even as much as 180°, several times as it is being advanced. Using this rotational movement, the operator should never need to push hard on the tube to position it in the larynx. Once the tube is in place, the fiber optic laryngoscope and oral airway are removed, and the 15-mm connector is reattached to the tube. To verify that the tube is properly positioned, a device can be attached to the connector that will make a distinct whistle as the patient exhales. Alternatively, $ETCO_2$ confirms proper placement. The orotracheal tube is then firmly taped in place at one side of the mouth.

APPENDIX C: STANDARD ADULT POSTOPERATIVE PAIN MANAGEMENT

Cathy M. Russo

STANDARD ADULT POSTOP ANALGESICS AND ANTIEMETICS

Analgesics	Morphine	1-2 mg/10 min, up to 10 mg iv
	Meperidine	10 mg/10 min, up to 50-70 mg iv
	Hydromorphone	0.5-1 mg/10-20 min, up to 6 mg
	Fentanyl	12.5-25 μg/5 min, up to 100 μg iv
	Ketorolac	30 mg iv slowly; then 15 mg q 6 h × 3 d max
Antiemetics	Metoclopramide	5-10 mg iv
	Ondansetron	4 mg iv – repeat if necessary after 30 min.
	Dolasetron	12.5 mg iv
	Droperidol	0.625 mg iv

EPIDURAL ANALGESIA

	Lumbar Epidural		Thoracic Epidural	
Loading dose	**Morphine**	**Hydromorphone**	**Morphine**	**Hydromorphone**
Lower extremities	2-3 mg	0.4-0.6 mg	1-2 mg	0.13-0.3 mg
Pelvis	3-4 mg	0.5-0.8 mg	1-3 mg	0.15-0.4 mg
Abdomen	5-7 mg	0.5-1 mg	2-3.5 mg	0.2-0.6 mg
Thorax	7-8 mg	0.5-1 mg	2-3.5 mg	0.4-0.8 mg
Infusion	**Morphine**	**Hydromorphone**	**Morphine**	**Hydromorphone**
Lower extremities	0.3-0.5 mg/h	0.1-0.2 mg/h	0.1-0.3 mg/h	0.05-0.1 mg/h
Pelvis	0.3-0.5 mg/h	0.1-0.2 mg/h	0.1-0.3 mg/h	0.1-0.15 mg/h
Abdomen	0.4-0.7 mg/h	0.2-0.3 mg/h	0.2-0.5 mg/h	0.1-0.2 mg/h
Thorax	0.5-1.0 mg/h	0.2-0.3 mg/h	0.2-0.6 mg/h	0.15-0.2 mg/h

Special considerations:

1. Concentrations of opioids used for epidural infusions (in preservative-free solution):
   - Morphine, 0.15 mg/ml
   - Hydromorphone, 0.05 mg/ml
2. Ketorolac may impair hemostasis. Use for breakthrough pain following consultation with the surgical team.

EPIDURAL ANESTHESIA/POSTOP ANALGESIA

Surgical Site	Epidural Catheter Location	Initial Bolus of 0.5% Bupivacaine	Infusion Rate of 0.125% Bupivacaine
Thoracic or upper abdomen	T6-T8*	4-6 ml	5-10 ml/h
Lower abdomen	T10*	10 ml	15 ml/h
Hip or knee	L2-3	8 ml	10 ml/h

*Catheter insertion at L3-4 is a satisfactory alternative for most patients, although the dose will need adjustment.

Special considerations:

1. Give initial bolus dose prior to incision. Then, if hemodynamically stable, give 1/2 bolus dose 30 min before end of surgery.
2. In recovery room, check sensory level. If no sensory block, ✓ whether catheter is functioning with 8 ml 2% lidocaine bolus. (✓ vital signs.)
3. Start infusions: If catheter is functional, as evidenced by loss of sensation, start: local anesthetic + opioid infusions (see table, p. C-1).
4. Best results: Local anesthetics and opioids are mixed in line using two separate infusion pumps. Thus, if either causes side effects, one can be stopped without the other. If the goal is to have patient ambulate POD 1, stop bupivacaine at 5 a.m. on POD 1.

PATIENT-CONTROLLED ANALGESIA (PCA) FOR INTRAVENOUS ADMINISTRATION

Loading dose	Morphine	Titrate to comfort
	Hydromorphone	Titrate to comfort
	Fentanyl	Titrate to comfort
Basal rate	Morphine	0.5-1 mg/h
	Hydromorphone	0.1-0.2 mg/h
	Fentanyl	5-10 μg/h
PCA lock-out dose and time	Morphine	1-2 mg q 10-15 min
	Hydromorphone	0.1-0.2 mg q 10-15 min
	Fentanyl	5-10 μg q 10-15 min

Typical orders:

1. Call anesthesiologist with any questions about PCA.
2. Check respiratory rate q 1 h while PCA in use.
3. Call anesthesiologist if respiratory rate < 10/min. If rate < 8/min, treat with naloxone 0.4 mg iv, push and assist ventilation while waiting for anesthesiologist.
4. Encourage patient to ambulate 4-6 h after surgery (unless contraindicated).
5. After PCA D/C'd, start po pain medications (per surgeon).
6. If patient required a large loading dose, the PCA lockout dose may need to be increased. Expect patient to need about 1/3 loading dose q h. Change PCA dose or lockout time to permit this dosing.

PATIENT-CONTROLLED EPIDURAL ANALGESIA (PCEA) FOR LUMBAR EPIDURAL ADMINISTRATION

Loading dose	Morphine	2-3 mg
	Hydromorphone	0.5-1.0 mg
	Fentanyl	50-75 μg
Basal rate	Morphine	0.2-0.5 mg/h
	Hydromorphone	0.08-.12 mg/h
	Fentanyl	5-10 μg/h
PCA lock-out dose and time	Morphine	0.1-0.2 mg q 10-15 min
	Hydromorphone	0.02-0.03 mg q 10-15 min
	Fentanyl	5-10 μg q 10-15 min

Special considerations:

1. For thoracic epidural, decrease all doses by one-third (1/3).
2. Concentrations of opioids for epidural infusion (in preservative-free solution).
   - Morphine 0.15 mg/ml
   - Hydromorphone 0.05 mg/ml
   - Fentanyl 10 μg/ml
3. Bupivacaine (0.125% @ 5-8 ml/h) may be added to the above regime for supplemental analgesia. Typically, the bupivacaine infusion is stopped on POD 1 to facilitate early ambulation.

TYPICAL ORDERS FOR POSTOP EPIDURAL/SPINAL ANALGESIA

I. EPIDURAL MEDICATIONS

____ 1. **Epidural Infusion – Opiate**

☐ Hydromorphone (Dilaudid) 0.05 mg/ml concentration @ ______ mg/h = ______ ml/h
☐ Morphine sulfate 0.15 mg/ml concentration @ ______ mg/h = ______ ml/h
☐ Fentanyl (Sublimaze) 10 μg/ml concentration @ ______ μg/h = ______ ml/h
☐ Range: May vary infusion between ______ /h to ______ /h prn pain.

____ 2. **Epidural Infusion – Anesthetic**

☐ Bupivacaine 0.125% concentration @ ______ ml/h
☐ Bupivacaine 0.25% concentration @ ______ ml/h
☐ Turn off bupivacaine on POD #1 @ 5 am.

____ 3 **Epidural Bolus – Opiate**

☐ Hydromorphone (Dilaudid) ______ mg q ______ h in 10 ml preservative-free NS (PFNS)
☐ Morphine sulfate ______ mg q ______ h in 10 ml PFNS

____ 4. **Breakthrough Pain**

☐ Fentanyl [*50-100*] μg via epidural q [*1*] h prn pain in 10 ml PFNS
☐ Call MD if ≥ 2 doses in [*2*] h.
☐ Ketorolac (Toradol) [*15*] mg iv q 6 h × [*3*] d (for a maximum of 12 doses)

II. NURSING CARE

____ 1. **Vital Signs**

☐ For opiates: T, P, BP q 4 h; RR q 2 h; then q 8 h, if stable.
Continuous O_2 sats × 24 h; then D/C if O_2 sats > 90% on room air.
☐ For anesthetics: BP & P q 2 h; then q 4 h, if stable.
Orthostatic BP before ambulation × 24 h.

____ 2. Label tubing, pump, infusion as "epidural." Place sign over bed; cover "Y" ports on tubing.
____ 3. Place naloxone (Narcan) and syringe at bedside.
____ 4. Administration of any additional opiates, sedative or antiemetics must be approved by anesthesiologist.
____ 5. Assess patient's pain (0-10 scale – 0 = no pain; 10 = worst pain imaginable) and level of sedation (awake, drowsy, asleep, unresponsive), along with vital signs.
____ 6. D/C Epidural Protocol when epidural D/C'd.

III. SIDE EFFECTS MANAGEMENT

____ 1. **Respiratory depression:** For RR < 6 or O_2 sat < 86% (on 2 separate occasions < 5 min apart): Administer naloxone (Narcan) 0.1 mg-0.2 mg iv STAT; may repeat, to total of 0.6 mg. Administer O_2 10 L/min via nonrebreathing mask. TURN OFF INFUSION. CALL ON-CALL MD STAT.

____ 2. **Excessive somnolence/sedation:**
Administer naloxone (Narcan) 0.1 mg-0.2 mg iv STAT; may repeat, to total of 0.6 mg. Administer O_2 10 L/min via nonrebreathing mask. TURN OFF INFUSION. CALL ON-CALL MD STAT.

____ 3. **Nausea/Vomiting:**

☐ Metoclopramide (Reglan) [*10 mg*] iv q 4-6 h prn
☐ Ondansetron [*4 mg*] q 6 h prn
☐ Nalbuphine (Nubain) [*2.5-5.0 mg*] iv q 4 h prn

____ 4. **Pruritus:**

☐ Nalbuphine (Nubain) [*2.5-5.0 mg*] iv q 2-4 h prn
☐ Diphenhydramine (Benadryl) [*10-25 mg*] iv q 4 h prn

[ ] indicates suggested dosage

APPENDIX D: STANDARD PEDIATRIC ANESTHETIC PROTOCOLS

Gregory B. Hammer

STANDARD MONITORS (NONINVASIVE)

Blood pressure (BP)	
Capnometry/capnography	Measurement of $ETCO_2$/display of wave form
Gas analyzer (e.g., Raman, IR or mass spectroscopy)	Respired gases and anesthetics
Electrocardiogram (ECG)	5-lead preferred
Esophageal or precordial stethoscope	Breath and heart sounds monitored; dysrhythmias and ↓BP detected
Nerve stimulator	Monitor status of neuromuscular blockade
Oxygen analyzer	Measurement of FiO_2
Pulse oximetry	Measurement of O_2 saturation
Temperature	Nasal, esophageal, rectal or skin
Visual observation of patient	Skin color, pupils, temperature, edema, sweating, movement
Ventilator function monitors	PIP, TV, disconnect alarm, etc.

STANDARD PREOP FASTING (NPO) GUIDELINES

- All solid foods and nonclear liquids (e.g., milk, infant formula, orange juice) should be withheld after midnight prior to scheduled surgery.
- All clear liquids (and breast milk) should be given up to 3 h before scheduled surgery. Because breast milk has a relatively short transit time through the stomach, and to simplify (and, therefore, increase compliance with) these guidelines, breast milk is considered a clear liquid.
- In practice, nonemergency cases may proceed 6 h after solids and nonclear liquids and 2 h after clear liquids and breast milk have been ingested.

STANDARD ANESTHETIC MANAGEMENT

★ **NB:** The following sections are guidelines only. Specific drugs and drug dosages should be individualized, based on the physiological and pharmacological status of the patient, including factors such as age, weight, medication and concurrent diseases.

PREMEDICATION

- In general, patients < 9 mo of age do not need premedication—only atropine 0.01 mg/kg iv or im prior to intubation.
- Older children (9 mo-10 yr) can be premedicated successfully by using oral midazolam (0.5-0.75 mg) in apple juice, grape Kool-Aid or cherry-flavored Tylenol elixir (10-15 mg/kg) 20-30 min prior to surgery.
- For patients > 35-40 kg, oral lorazepam (0.03-0.05 mg/kg) or diazepam (0.1-0.15 mg/kg) may be given 60 min prior to surgery with a sip of water.

INDUCTION TECHNIQUES

Preinduction

1. ✓ anesthesia machine, suction, airway equipment, drugs.
2. Attach monitors and verify function.
3. Premedication: < 6-9 mo – consider atropine 0.01 mg/kg iv prior to laryngoscopy to prevent vagally mediated bradycardia.

Induction

Routes of administration:

1. Rectal – methohexital (5%) 30 mg/kg
2. Intramuscular – ketamine hydrochloride 3-5 mg/kg (with atropine 0.02 mg/kg)
3. IV – STP 4-7 mg/kg
   – methohexital 0.5-1 mg/kg
   – propofol 2-3 mg/kg
4. Inhalational-halothane (MAC = 0.87% [neonates], 1-2% [infants], and 0.75% [adults]) or sevoflurane (MAC = 3.3% [neonates and younger infants], 2.5% [older infants and children], 1.7-2.0% [adults]) in N_2O (up to 70%)/O_2. Increase the inspired concentration of halothane incrementally every 3 breaths up to 4%, sevoflurane up to 7%. Monitor BP and HR closely.

Muscle relaxation

1. Succinylcholine (controversial*): 1-2 mg/kg iv or 2-4 mg/kg im
2. Vecuronium or pancuronium: 0.1 mg/kg iv
3. Rocuronium 0.6-1 mg/kg iv
4. Atracurium: 0.3-0.5 mg/kg
5. Cisatracurium 0.1 mg/kg iv
6. Deep halothane or sevoflurane and anesthesia

Laryngoscope

Blade	Age
Miller 0	Neonate
Miller 1	6-9 mo
Wis-Hipple 1.5	9 mo-3 yr
Macintosh 2	1-4 yr
Macintosh 3 or Miller 2	> 4 yr

*Succinylcholine may trigger MH in susceptible patients or cause cardiac arrest in myopathic patients; therefore, many pediatric anesthesiologists avoid the use of succinylcholine.

TYPICAL ETT SIZE AT DIFFERENT AGES

Age	Wt	ETT Size
Newborn	3-4 kg	3.0
≤ 6-8 mo	6-8 kg	3.5
≤ 8-16 mo	10-12 kg	4.0
2-3 yr	13-15 kg	Thereafter use formula:
6 yr	20 kg	4+ (age/4) = ETT size (to allow for a slight
9 yr	30 kg	leak when positive pressure is applied).
12 yr	40 kg	

★ **NB:** This is a guide only; prepare an ETT one size larger and one size smaller than the ETT size selected. ✓✓ ET placement of tube by auscultation of breath sounds bilaterally. ✓ depth of carina by auscultation over left axilla as ETT is slowly advanced. Withdraw and secure ETT 2 cm from position where diminution of breath sounds was first noted. Positive pressure leak between 30-40 cmH_2O is desirable. Leaks < 30 cm result in volume loss and difficulty in providing appropriate ventilation during critical phases intraop or postop. Conversely, leaks > 40 cmH_2O carry a higher risk of subglottic edema and/or stenosis.

MAINTENANCE TECHNIQUES

Inhalational anesthesia

30-100% O_2
+ 0-70% N_2O. In preemies and for cases where N_2O is contraindicated, air may be used to lower FiO_2.
+ Isoflurane, halothane or sevoflurane, titrated to effect

★ **NB**: Warm and humidify all gases. Warm room to 75-80° F for infants, 70-75° F for children.

Balanced anesthesia

30-100% O_2
+ 0-70% N_2O
+ ~0.5% isoflurane
or propofol (50-200 μg/kg/min)

+ Morphine (0.05 mg/kg/h) or fentanyl (1-3 μg/kg/h)

If continued muscle relaxation is required during the above maintenance techniques, several options are available. Always use a nerve stimulator to assess block before redosing.

Short-acting	Mivacurium	0.1 mg/kg → 6-10 min
Intermediate	Vecuronium	0.01 mg/kg → 25-30 min
	Rocuronium	0.6 mg/kg/30 min
	Atracurium	0.4 mg/kg/30 min
	Cisatracurium	0.1 mg/kg/30 min
Long-acting	Pancuronium	0.1 mg/kg → 40-65 min

EMERGENCE	
1. Reversal of muscle relaxant	As surgical conditions permit, reverse residual muscle relaxant (when at least 1 twitch is present in train-of-four) with one of the following: • Neostigmine 0.05-0.07 (maximum dose) mg/kg iv + glycopyrrolate 0.01 mg/kg iv, or • Edrophonium 0.5-1.0 (maximum dose) mg/kg iv + atropine 0.01 mg/kg iv.
2. Nausea prophylaxis	Metoclopramide 0.1 mg/kg iv (~1 h before emergence) or Droperidol 0.025-0.05 mg/kg (single dose only) or Ondansetron 0.1 mg/kg
3. O_2	Discontinue N_2O/volatile agents and administer 100% O_2.
4. Suction	Suction oropharynx thoroughly.
5. Extubation	Laryngeal spasm is common in children. It is, therefore, usual to extubate children when they are awake, moving all limbs and breathing adequately. Infants and children with full stomachs or difficult airways must be extubated when they are fully awake. The pharynx should be suctioned thoroughly prior to extubation. Should laryngeal spasm occur, Rx with 100% O_2 and CPAP or PPV. If spasm fails to resolve and hypoxemia occurs, give succinylcholine 0.1-0.5 mg/kg and administer PPV. Consider reintubation if hypoxemia fails to resolve quickly.

PEDIATRIC EPIDURAL ANESTHESIA

Epidural anesthesia may be combined with GA for infants and children undergoing surgery involving the lower extremities, abdomen, chest or spine. Single-dose ("single-shot") techniques may be used, or epidural catheters may be placed for longer procedures and to facilitate postop epidural analgesia (see below). Bupivacaine 0.25% with or without epinephrine 1:200K is most commonly used. For patients admitted following surgery, opioids (morphine and hydromorphone [Dilaudid]) are generally added. Avoid air-filled syringe for loss-of-resistance technique (→ VAE).

TECHNIQUES AND DOSAGES

1. **Caudal**
   - Single-shot – 22 ga iv catheter (< 5 yr), 20 ga iv catheter (> 5 yr), or 21 to 23 ga short bevel needle may be inserted via sacrococcygeal membrane.
     - Initial dose:
     - 0.5 ml/kg for lower extremity/perineal/genital procedures
     - 1.0 ml/kg for abdominal procedures
   - Catheter technique – in patients < 10 kg, 20 ga epidural catheter may be inserted through 18 ga Critikon iv catheter and advanced so that tip is located near level of incision (e.g., approximately 17 cm from skin to T4 in infant). If resistance is met, try reinserting epidural catheter or securing at level where resistance encountered.
     - Initial dose: 0.5 ml/kg
2. **Lumbar**
   - 17 or 18 ga epidural needle inserted via L3-4 or L4-5 interspace for single-shot injection or placement of 20 ga epidural catheter.
   - Use loss-of-resistance technique with fluid-filled syringe (air may cause VAE).
   - Catheter should be threaded approximately 4 cm (maximum) beyond tip of needle.
   - A test dose with 0.1-0.2 ml/kg bupivacaine with epinephrine 1:100K or 1:200K is given.
   - Initial dose:
     - 0.5 ml/kg for lower abdominal procedures
     - 1.0 ml/kg for upper abdominal and thoracic procedures
3. **Thoracic**
   - The technique described for lumbar epidural catheter placement may be used between T6 and T12 in children.
   - Initial dose: 0.5 ml/kg
   - Local anesthetic dosing guidelines same as above (note that volume will be ~$^1/_3$ less than with caudal approach.

For indwelling catheter techniques, hourly maintenance doses of $^1/_3$-$^1/_2$ the initial dose may be given.

PEDIATRIC SPINAL ANESTHESIA AND ANALGESIA

Spinal anesthesia is used primarily for procedures such as inguinal herniorrhaphy in former preterm infants at risk for postop apnea following GA. By avoiding GA, the incidence of postop apnea is reduced, but not eliminated. In most patients arriving in the OR without iv access, an iv may be inserted in a lower extremity immediately following placement of the spinal anesthetic, as little change in BP or HR occurs in infants < 6 mo of age.

After standard monitors are applied, the infant is placed in a supine or lateral decubitus position. Care is taken to avoid neck flexion, which may cause airway obstruction. The skin is infiltrated with 1% lidocaine using a 27 or 30 ga needle. Lumbar puncture is performed with a 22 ga 1.5" spinal needle to an average depth of 1.5 cm from skin. The most commonly used local anesthetic for spinal anesthesia in infants is tetracaine 1.0%, mixed with an equal volume of 10% dextrose in a dose of 0.8-1.0 mg/kg. Epinephrine 1:1000 0.01 ml/kg is added. This dose usually provides adequate anesthesia for 90-120 min for inguinal herniorrhaphy.

Complications include high spinal anesthesia requiring tracheal intubation. PDPH is very uncommon in children < 12 yr of age, and probably rare in infants.

References:

1. Alifimoff JK, Cote CJ: Regional anesthesia. In *A Practice of Anesthesia for Infants and Children.* Cote CJ, Ryan JF, Todres ID, Goudsouzian NG, eds. WB Suanders Co, Philadelphia: 1993, 429-49.
2. Yaster M, Krane E, Kaplan R, Cote C, Lappe D: *The Pediatric Pain and Sedation Handbook.* Mosby-Yearbook, Inc., St. Louis: 1997.

APPENDIX E: STANDARD PEDIATRIC POSTOPERATIVE PAIN MANAGEMENT

Yuan-Chi Lin and Gregory B. Hammer

STANDARD PEDIATRIC POSTOP ANALGESICS AND ANTIEMETICS

Analgesics	Acetaminophen	10-15 mg/kg po prn q 4 h 30-40 mg/kg pr 1st dose, then 25-35 mg/kg pr q 4 h prn
	Morphine	0.02 mg/kg iv q 5-10 min prn; may repeat up to 0.2 mg/kg total dose
	Fentanyl	0.3-0.5 μg/kg iv q 5-10 min prn, up to 3 μg/kg
Antiemetics	Droperidol*	0.02 mg/kg iv
	Metoclopramide*	0.1 mg/kg, may repeat × 1 iv
	Ondansetron	0.1 mg/kg iv

*NB: Increased incidence of extrapyramidal reactions with both agents.

PATIENT-CONTROLLED IV ANALGESIA (PCA)

PCA is the most commonly utilized technique for postop pain management in patients ≥ 5 yr. Typically, PCA combined with a continuous infusion is the preferred mode for pediatric patients. Loading doses are necessary to establish analgesia in some patients. The lockout time can be as short as 5 min. Common PCA medications are listed below.

Common PCA Medications

Medication	**Loading dose**	**Basal Rate**	**Patient-controlled bolus**
Morphine (1 or 5 mg/ml)	0.03 mg/kg	0.01 mg/kg/h	0.02-0.03 mg/kg
Hydromorphone (100 μg/ml)	5 μg/kg	1 μg/kg/h	2 μg/kg
Fentanyl (50 μg/ml)	0.3 μg/kg	0.1 μg/kg/h	0.2-0.3 μg/kg

Continuous iv infusion: When PCA is not practical (e.g., in uncooperative children), continuous iv infusion of opiates may be used. Morphine infusion of 10-30 μg/kg/h results in serum concentrations of 10-22 ng/ml and provides adequate analgesia. A common technique is to initiate iv morphine infusion with 1 mg/kg of morphine in 100 ml of D5W at 1 ml/h (the effective infusion rate is 10 μg/kg/h); the infusion rate is slowly increased to provide adequate pain relief.

Typical Orders for IV PCA are on p. E-2.

TYPICAL ORDERS FOR PATIENT-CONTROLLED IV ANALGESIA (PCA)

1. Program PCA pump as follows: (Check one order in each area.) WT ________
   a) DRUG: ______ Morphine 1 mg/ml
      ______ Morphine 5 mg/ml
      ______ Hydromorphone 100 μg/ml
      ______ Fentanyl 50 μg/ml
      ______ Other: ________________________________
   b) LOADING DOSE: prn severe pain at beginning of infusion (may repeat × 1 after 15 min)
      ______ Morphine ______ mg (0.03 mg/kg)
      ______ Hydromorphone ______ μg (5 μg/kg)
      ______ Fentanyl ______ (0.3 μg/kg)
   c) MODE: ______ PCA only
      ______ Continuous only
      ______ PCA + continuous
   d) BASAL RATE:
      ______ Morphine ______ mg/h (Start at 0.01 mg/kg/h.)
      ______ Hydromorphone ______ μg/h (Start at 1 μg/kg/h.)
      ______ Fentanyl ______ μg/h (Start at 0.1 μg/kg/h.)
   e) PCA DOSE:
      ______ Morphine ______ mg (0.02-0.03 mg/kg)
      ______ Hydromorphone ______ μg (2 μg/kg)
      ______ Fentanyl ______ μg (0.2-0.3 μg/kg)
   f) LOCKOUT INTERVAL: ______ min (usual range 6-10 min)
2. Do not administer any other opioids, benzodiazepines, sedatives or antiemetics, unless approved by
   ________________________ MD(s) ______________ PAGER(s).
3. O_2 sat monitor continuous for the 1st 24 h or for 24 h after rate increase.
4. For SaO_2 < 94%, administer O_2 per nasal cannula to maintain SaO_2 at or above 94%.
5 Assess HR, RR, BP, and level of pain using appropriate tool (0-10 Scale, Wong-Baker Faces Scale, or Infant/Nonverbal Pain Scale) at least q 4 h, and record.
6. SIDE EFFECTS:
   a) If unable to arouse or SaO_2 < 85%, turn off PCA pump, administer O_2 and/or ambu-bag, stimulate patient, administer naloxone ______ mg (0.005 mg/kg of 0.4 mg/ml) q 1-2 min as needed to restore level of consciousness, and STAT page physician.
   b) Nausea/vomiting: (Check one)
      ______ Metoclopramide (Reglan) ______ mg iv q 6 prn (0.1 mg/kg)
      ______ Ondansetron (Zofran) ______ mg iv q 8 h prn (0.1 mg/kg)
      ______ Other: ________________________________
   c) Pruritus: (Check one)
      ______ Diphenhydramine (Benadryl) ______ mg iv q 6 h prn (0.5 mg/kg)
      ______ Nalbuphine (Nubain) ______ mg iv q 4 h prn (0.05 mg/kg)
   d) Urinary retention: Assess for bladder distention. If no void for ______ h (since surgery or last void) may straight cath prn × 2.

DATE ________ SIGNATURE ____________________ PAGER # ________

POSTOPERATIVE EPIDURAL ANALGESIA

Patients with indwelling epidural catheters may receive postop analgesia with either continuous infusion alone or continuous infusion with intermittent bolus dosing (patient-controlled epidural analgesia, or PCEA). The infusate may be either local anesthetic with an opioid, local anesthetic alone or opioid alone. At Stanford, the most commonly used epidural infusate for continuous infusion is bupivacaine 0.1% with hydromorphone 3 μg/ml. In patients receiving PCEA, bupivacaine 0.1% with hydromorphone 25 μg/ml is often used (see Typical Orders for Continuous Epidural Analgesia and Epidural PCA, pp. E-4, E-5).

At Stanford, patients receiving epidural analgesia are managed by the Pediatric Pain Service.

Opioids:

1. **Hydromorphone** (Dilaudid): The usual bolus dose is 10 μg/kg, although a reduced dose may be given when the epidural catheter tip is near the level of the incision. The duration of action is 6-12 h.

   When opioid epidural analgesia is indicated, hydromorphone is most commonly used because:

   (a) It causes less itching and nausea compared with morphine.

   (b) It is more water soluble than fentanyl (therefore, ↑ spread, ↓ systemic absorption).

   (c) It is less water soluble than morphine (thereby minimizing late respiratory depression).

2. **Preservative-free morphine**: The usual bolus dose is 30-60 μg/kg.

   Morphine is used by some practitioners because of its greater familiarity and because the duration of action may be longer (8-16 h) than hydromorphone.

References

1. Alfimoff JK, Cote CJ: Pediatric regional anesthesia. In *A Practice of Anesthesia for Infants and Children.* Cote CJ, Ryan JF, Todres ID, Goudsouzian NG, eds. WB Saunders, Philadelphia: 1993, 429-49.
2. Yaster M, Krane E, Kaplan R, Cote CJ, Lappe D: *The Pediatric Pain and Sedation Handbook.* Mosby-Year Book, St. Louis: 1997.

TYPICAL ORDERS FOR CONTINUOUS EPIDURAL ANALGESIA

1. Epidural solution in preservative-free normal saline: WT ________
   ________ Bupivacaine 0.1%
   ________ Hydromorphone 3 μg/ml with bupivacaine 0.1%
   ________ Morphine 10 μg/ml with bupivacaine 0.1%
   ________ Other ________
2. Epidural infusion rate: ________ ml/h (0.1-0.5 ml/kg/h)
3. Notify Pain Management Service when patient arrives on unit.
4. No opioids, antiemetics, benzodiazepines or sedatives unless FIRST approved by Pain Management Service.
5. Maintain iv access until epidural catheter D/C'd.
6. Assess HR, BP, RR, level of pain q 4 h until end of infusion. ✓ orthostatic BP before ambulating.
7. Assess level of pain using age-appropriate tool (0-10 Scale, Wong-Baker Faces Scale, or Infant/Nonverbal Pain Scale) at least q 4 h, and record.
8. O_2 sat monitor × 24 h after beginning of infusion or after rate increase.
9. For SaO_2 < 94%, administer O_2 per nasal cannula to maintain SaO_2 at or above 94%.
10. Keep naloxone, syringe, needle and med label with calculated patient-appropriate dose at patient's bedside. To be given IV ONLY.
11. If unable to arouse or SaO_2 < 85%, D/C infusion, STAT page Pain Management Service and primary service, administer O_2 and/or ambu-bag, stimulate patient, administer naloxone ________ mg (0.005 mg/kg of 0.4 mg/ml naloxone) q 1-2 min to restore level of consciousness.
12. a) Urinary retention: Assess for bladder distention. If no void for ________ h (since surgery or last void), may straight cath prn × 2.
    b) Nausea/vomiting:
       ________ Naloxone (Narcan) infusion ________ mg in 100 ml D5W @ ________ ml/h
       (0.1 mg/kg in 100 ml @ 1-2 ml/h)
       ________ Ondansetron ________ mg iv q 6 h prn (0.1 mg/kg)
       ________ Metoclopramide (Reglan) ________ mg iv q 6 prn (0.1 mg/kg)
    c) Pruritus:
       ________ Naloxone infusion ________ mg in 100 ml D5W @ ________ ml/h
       (0.1 mg/kg in 100 ml @ 1-2 ml/h)
       ________ Nalbuphine (Nubain) ________ mg iv q 4 h prn (0.05 mg/kg)
       ________ Diphenhydramine ________ mg iv q 6 h prn (0.5 mg/kg)
13. For any pain management-related issues, notify Pain Management Service.

TYPICAL ORDERS FOR PATIENT-CONTROLLED EPIDURAL ANALGESIA (PCEA)

1. Program PCEA pump as follows: (Check one order in each area.) WT ________
   a) DRUG: ________ Hydromorphone 25 μg/ml
   ________ Hydromorphone 25 μg/ml + bupivacaine 0.1%
   b) LOADING DOSE: prn severe pain at beginning of infusion ________ ml × 1
   c) MODE: PCEA + continuous
   d) BASAL RATE: ________ ml/h (4 ml/h for patients 35-70 kg)
   e) PCEA DOSE: ________ ml (1 ml for patients 35-70 kg)
   f) LOCKOUT INTERVAL: ________ min (usual: 30 min)
2. Do not administer any other opioids, benzodiazepines, sedatives, or antiemetics, unless approved by
   ________________ MD(s) ________________ PAGER(s).
3. O_2 sat monitor continuous for the 1st 24 h or for 24 h after rate increase.
4. For $SaO_2 < 94\%$, administer O_2 per nasal cannula to maintain SaO_2 at or above 94%.
5 Assess HR, RR, BP, and level of pain using appropriate tool (0-10 Scale, Wong-Baker Faces Scale, or Infant/Nonverbal Pain Scale) at least q 4 h, and record.
6. SIDE EFFECTS:
   a) If unable to arouse or $SaO_2 < 85\%$, turn off PCA pump, administer O_2 and/or ambu-bag, stimulate patient, administer naloxone ________ mg (0.005 mg/kg of 0.4 mg/ml) q 1-2 min as needed to restore level of consciousness, and STAT page physician in #2.
   b) Nausea/vomiting: (Check one)
   ________ Metoclopramide (Reglan) ________ mg iv q 6 prn (0.1 mg/kg/dose)
   ________ Ondansetron (Zofran) ________ mg iv q 8 h prn (0.1 mg/kg)
   ________ Naloxone (Narcan) infusion ________ mg in 100 ml D5W @ ________ ml/h
   (0.1 mg/kg in 100 ml @ 1-2 ml/h)
   c) Pruritus: (Check one)
   ________ Diphenhydramine (Benadryl) ________ mg iv q 6 h prn (0.5 mg/kg/dose)
   ________ Nalbuphine (Nubain) ________ mg iv q 4 h prn (0.05 mg/kg)
   ________ Naloxone (Narcan) infusion ________ mg in 100 ml D5W @ ________ ml/h
   (0.1 mg/kg in 100 ml @ 1-2 ml/h)
   d) Urinary retention: Assess for bladder distention. If no void for ________ h (since surgery or last void) may straight cath prn × 2.

APPENDIX F: TABLE OF DRUG INTERACTIONS

Sandra Leigh Bardas

This table is intended only as an advisory overview of potential drug interactions between various drug classes that patients may be taking preoperatively with drugs used in anesthesia practice. In view of the constant flow of new drug information, the reader is strongly urged to check the primary literature of each drug and tailor drug usage to the specific clinical situation.

Preop Drug Or Drug Class	Anesthetic Drug Or Drug Class	Interaction	Clinical Management
Amiodarone	fentanyl	↓↓HR, ↓BP, sinus arrest	Monitor hemodynamic function. Administer inotropic, chronotropic and pressor agents as indicated. Large doses of vasopressors may be required. Bradycardia is usually not responsive to atropine.
Aminoglycosides	enflurane	↑potential for nephrotoxicity 2° fluoride	Monitor renal function postop.
	nondepolarizing muscle relaxants (NMR)	↑block; possible protracted respiratory depression	Administer combination only when necessary. Titrate NMR dose. Antidotal use of Ca salts and anticholinesterases is unreliable. Support respiration.
	succinylcholine	↑depolarizing block	Delay administration of aminoglycosides as long as possible after recovery from block. Support respiration.
Amphetamines	narcotic analgesics	↑analgesia	Titrate dosage of narcotic.
Antacids	oral medication	Delayed drug absorption 2° delayed gastric emptying	Avoid administration within 2 h of each other.
Antibiotics, polypeptide (bacitracin, colistmethate, polymyxin B	NMR	↑block	Monitor neuromuscular blockade. Titrate dosage of NMR. Support respiration.
Anticholinesterases (including ophthalmics)	NMR	↓block	Titrate dosage of NMR to therapeutic effectiveness.
Anticholinesterases	succinylcholine	Blockade may be prolonged or antagonized.	Monitor neuromuscular blockade.
Aprotinin	succinylcholine	Prolonged or recurring apnea	Monitor respiratory status.

Preop Drug Or Drug Class	Anesthetic Drug Or Drug Class	Interaction	Clinical Management
Asparaginase	physostigmine	Possible Parkinsonian effects	**Avoid combination.**
	droperidol	Possible Parkinsonian effects	**Avoid combination.**
Azathioprine	NMR	May ↓ or reverse block.	Titrate NMR dosage.
Barbiturates	inhalation anesthetics, ketamine, narcotic analgesics	↑respiratory depression	Monitor and support respiration.
Benzodiazepines	narcotic analgesics	↓BP	Monitor and support BP.
	NMR	May prolong or antagonize blockade.	Monitor and support respiration.
	barbiturates	Drug actions may be additive.	Titrate dosage of barbiturate.
	bupivacaine	Reduces potential for CNS toxicity, but not for cardiovascular toxicity.	Seizure threshold raised; monitor and support cardiovascular status.
Benztropine	ketamine	↑HR	Use β-blocker if necessary.
β-adrenergic agonists	inhalation anesthetics	Potentiation of cardiovascular effects	Monitor BP, HR and rhythm.
β-blockers	NMR	May prolong or antagonize blockade.	Monitor and support respiration.
	bupivacaine, lidocaine	↓clearance of bupivacaine, lidocaine	Infuse slowly to prevent high peak levels.
	droperidol	↓BP	Monitor and support BP.
	neostigmine	↓HR + ↓BP	Monitor and support cardiovascular status. Use atropine.
	inhalation anesthetics	↓HR, ↓BP; asystole	Monitor and support cardiovascular status.
β-blockers, nonselective	epinephrine	↑BP + ↓HR	**Avoid combination.** Consider discontinuation of nonselective β-blocker 3 d preop.

Preop Drug Or Drug Class	Anesthetic Drug Or Drug Class	Interaction	Clinical Management
Bretylium	inhalation anesthetics	Increased potential for ↓BP due to blunting of compensatory cardiovascular reflexes	Monitor and support cardiovascular status.
	d-tubocurarine	↑block	Monitor and support neuromuscular blockade. Monitor and support respiration.
Calcium channel blockers	NMR or succinylcholine	↑block	Monitor neuromuscular blockade.
	inhalation anesthetics	Increased potential for cardiovascular depression, resulting in ↓BP, ↓HR, asystole	Monitor and support cardiovascular status.
Carbamazepine	NMR	↓block	Monitor neuromuscular blockade. Titrate dosage.
	diltiazem; verapamil	↑carbamazepine levels → CNS toxicity	Monitor for neuromuscular disorders.
Chlorpropamide	barbiturates	↑barbiturate activity	Monitor for CNS depression.
Cimetidine	lidocaine	↑lidocaine toxicity	Monitor for lidocaine toxicity.
	narcotic analgesics	↑CNS depression	Consider naloxone.
	succinylcholine	↑block	Monitor neuromuscular blockade. Titrate succinylcholine.
Clindamycin and lincomycin	NMR or succinylcholine	↑↑block	**Avoid combination, if possible.** Monitor and support respiration. Anticholinesterases or Ca^{++} may be of benefit.
Clonidine	inhalation anesthetics	↓inhalation anesthetic requirements	Titrate inhalation anesthetic.
Clonidine (epidural)	local anesthetics	Prolonged sensory and motor blockade	Titrate dose of local anesthetics.
Corticosteroids	NMR	Altered effectiveness of block	Titrate and monitor NMR. May require higher dosage.
Cyclophosphamide	succinylcholine	↓ metabolism → ↑block duration	↓ succinylcholine dosage.

Preop Drug Or Drug Class	Anesthetic Drug Or Drug Class	Interaction	Clinical Management
Cyclosporine	NMR or succinylcholine	↑block	Monitor neuromuscular blockade and titrate dose. Support respiration.
Dantrolene	calcium channel blockers	Can precipitate hyperkalemia and cardiovascular collapse.	**Avoid combination.**
Digoxin	esmolol	↑digoxin activity	Monitor for signs of digoxin toxicity.
	pancuronium	Precipitate new dysrhythmias or potentiate existing rhythm disturbances.	Monitor cardiac status.
	succinylcholine	Possible precipitation of new dysrhythmias or potentiation of existing rhythm disturbances	Monitor cardiac status.
Disopyramide	NMR	↑block	Monitor neuromuscular blockade. Consider use of a shorter-acting NMR.
Disulfiram	barbiturates	↑barbiturate activity	Monitor for CNS depression. Titrate dose of barbiturates.
Dobutamine	inhalation anesthetics	Ventricular arrhythmias	Monitor HR and rhythm.
Donepezil	succinylcholine	Enhanced blockade	Note ↑ effects of cholinesterase inhibitors and cholinergic agents. Monitor neuromuscular blockade.
Echothiophate, ophthalmic	succinylcholine	Systemic absorption → ↑↑block	**Use with extreme caution.** Titrate NMR dose.
Edetate (disodium EDTA)	barbiturates; inhalation anesthetics	Possible potentiation of cardiodepressant effects	Rx: ↓ BP with $CaCl_2$.
	NMR or succinylcholine	Potentiation of neuromuscular blockade; ↑block; ↑depolarizing block	Titrate dose. Support respiration.
Epoprostenol	vasodilators	↓BP	Titrate vasodilator.
Ergotamine	β-blocker	Severe peripheral vasospasm	**Avoid combination in patients with PVD.**

Preop Drug Or Drug Class	Anesthetic Drug Or Drug Class	Interaction	Clinical Management
Erythromycin	alfentanil	↑effect of alfentanil	Consider ↓dose of alfentanil. Monitor and support respiration.
	midazolam	↑CNS depression	Titrate dose of midazolam.
Esmolol	succinylcholine	↑block	Monitor neuromuscular blockade. Consider ↓dosage of esmolol.
	morphine	↑β-blockade	Monitor cardiovascular function. Consider ↓dose of esmolol.
Estrogens	succinylcholine	↑block	Monitor neuromuscular blockade. Titrate succinylcholine.
Ethanol	alfentanil	Chronic alcohol consumption → pharmacodynamic tolerance to alfentanil.	May need to increase dose of alfentanil.
	barbiturates	Acute ingestion → CNS depression; chronic ingestion → tolerance	**Avoid combination** as tolerance is unpredictable.
	benzodiazepines	Acute ingestion → CNS depression; chronic ingestion → tolerance	Titrate dose of benzodiazepines.
Fludrocortisone	anticholinesterases	Possible antagonism of reversal agents	Monitor neuromuscular blockade.
Furazolidone	sympathomimetics	↑pressor sensitivity due to MAOI activity of furazolidone	**Avoid combination.** In hypertensive crisis, consider phentolamine.
	meperidine	Risk of MAOI/ meperidine interaction toxicity	**Avoid combination.**
Furosemide	NMR	↑block	Monitor neuromuscular blockade.
Glycopyrrolate	ketamine	↑HR	Monitor HR.
	NMR	High doses may ↑block.	Monitor neuromuscular blockade.
Guanethidine	sympathomimetics	↑direct-acting sympathomimetics (epinephrine, phenylephrine). ↓indirect-acting sympathomimetics (ephedrine, dopamine).	Use combination with caution. Titrate dosages. Monitor BP.

Preop Drug Or Drug Class	Anesthetic Drug Or Drug Class	Interaction	Clinical Management
Halothane	doxapram	↑dysrhythmogenicity of halogenated hydrocarbons	Delay administration of doxapram for at least 10 min after discontinuing halothane.
Inhalation anesthetics	NMR or succinylcholine	↑block	Titrate dose of both agents.
Isoniazid (INH)	halothane	↑hepatotoxicity	Avoid giving rifampin-isoniazid after halothane anesthesia.
	meperidine	↓BP; ↑CNS depression	**Use combination with caution.** Monitor BP
	enflurane	Fast acetylators of INH facilitate defluorination of enflurane → high-output renal failure.	Monitor renal function postop.
Ketamine	halothane	↓BP + ↓CO	**Use combination with caution.** Monitor BP.
	succinylcholine	↑block	Monitor neuromuscular blockade. Titrate dosage of succinylcholine.
Labetalol	inhalation anesthetics	↓↓BP	**Use combination** (especially halothane) **with caution.** Monitor BP.
Levodopa	benzodiazepines	Possible antagonism of levodopa	**Avoid combination, if possible.**
	droperidol	Dopamine antagonist	**Avoid combination, if possible.**
Lidocaine and other local anesthetics	NMR or succinylcholine	Possible ↑block	Monitor neuromuscular blockade. Titrate dosage of NMR.
Lithium	NMR	↑↑block	Titrate dosage of NMR. Monitor neuromuscular blockade. Support respiration.
	succinylcholine	↑block	Monitor neuromuscular blockade.
Loop diuretics	NMR	Blockade may be prolonged or antagonized; possibly dosage-dependent; ↓K^+ → ↑block.	Monitor neuromuscular blockade. Titrate dose of NMR. Support respiration.
Magnesium salts, parenteral	NMR	↑block	Monitor neuromuscular blockade. Titrate dosage of NMR.

Preop Drug Or Drug Class	Anesthetic Drug Or Drug Class	Interaction	Clinical Management
Mercaptopurine	NMR	May ↓ or reverse blockade.	Monitor neuromuscular blockade. Titrate dose of NMR.
Methocarbamol	anticholinesterases	Possible severe muscle weakness	Monitor neuromuscular blockade. Titrate dosage of anticholinesterase.
Methyldopa	naloxone	Naloxone may precipitate a mild ↑BP.	Monitor BP.
	ephedrine	↓ephedrine effect	Use alternative pressor agents.
Metoclopramide	sympathomimetics	↑BP	Monitor BP. D/C sympathomimetics.
	succinylcholine	↑block	Monitor neuromuscular blockade. Titrate dosage of succinylcholine.
Monoamine oxidase inhibitors (MAOI)	meperidine	Agitation, seizures, diaphoresis, fever, coma, apnea	**Avoid combination.**
	sympathomimetics (including local anesthetic/ epinephrine combinations)	Indirect- or mixed-acting sympatho-mimetic may cause severe headache, hyperpyrexia, or hypertensive crisis. (Direct-acting sympathomimetics appear to interact minimally.)	**Avoid combination.** Rx: ↑ BP with phentolamine.
Narcotic analgesics	barbiturate anesthetics	Drug actions may be additive.	Monitor for CNS depression.
	NMR or succinylcholine	↑narcotic toxicity	Titrate dose of narcotic.
	propofol	↓BP	Titrate dosage of propofol.
Nifedipine	fentanyl	↓BP with high doses of fentanyl	Monitor BP. Titrate fentanyl dosage.
Nitroglycerin (NTG)	pancuronium	↑block	Monitor and support respiration.
Nondepolarizing muscle relaxants (NMR)	inhalation anesthetics	↑block	Titrate dose of NMR. Monitor neuromuscular blockade.
	ketamine	↑block	Titrate dose of NMR. Monitor neuromuscular blockade.
Oral contraceptives	succinylcholine	↑block	Monitor neuromuscular blockade.

Preop Drug Or Drug Class	Anesthetic Drug Or Drug Class	Interaction	Clinical Management
Oxytocic drugs (oxytocin, ergotamine, methylergonovine)	sympathomimetics	↑BP 2° synergistic and additive vasoconstrictive effect	Monitor BP. Titrate dosage.
Papaverine	droperidol, physostigmine	Possible development of Parkinsonian syndrome	**Avoid combination.**
Phenothiazines	narcotic analgesics	↓analgesic effects	Titrate narcotic to analgesic effect.
	phenylephrine	↓α-adrenergic effects	Use an alternative pressor agent.
Phenoxybenzamine	local anesthetics	↑absorption of local anesthetics	Add epinephrine or other vasoconstrictor to local anesthetic.
Phenytoin	dopamine	↓↓BP; cardiac arrest	**Use combination with extreme caution.** Discontinue phenytoin infusion if ↓BP develops.
	inhalation anesthetics	Potentiation of inhalation anesthetics	Titrate dosage of inhalation anesthetics.
	NMR	Reduced duration of blockade; atracurium not affected by phenytoin.	Increased dosage of NMR may be required. Monitor neuromuscular function.
Piperacillin	NMR	↑block	Monitor neuromuscular blockade.
Probenecid	thiopental	↑CNS depression	Titrate dosage of thiopental.
Procaine, procainamide	succinylcholine	↑neuromuscular blockade 2° competition for pseudo-cholinesterases	Monitor neuromuscular blockade.
	NMR	↑block	Monitor neuromuscular blockade.
Propofol	sedative/hypnotics inhalation anesthetics	↑block	Titrate dose of NMR. Monitor neuromuscular blockade.
	succinylcholine	↓↓HR	Monitor cardiac function. Consider atropine premed when propofol precedes succinylcholine.
	atracurium	Bronchospasm	Anaphylactoid-type reaction
	vecuronium	↑block	Monitor neuromuscular blockade.

Preop Drug Or Drug Class	Anesthetic Drug Or Drug Class	Interaction	Clinical Management
Quinine, quinidine	NMR	↑block	Titrate dosage of NMR. Monitor neuromuscular blockade.
	succinylcholine	↑neuromuscular blockade 2° metabolism of succinylcholine	**Use this combination with caution.**
Ranitidine	NMR	Possible resistance to NMR	↑dosage of NMR; if unsuccessful, use different NMR.
Rauwolfia alkaloids	sympathomimetics	↑direct-acting sympathomimetics; ↓indirect-acting agents	Monitor BP. Titrate dosage.
	inhalation anesthetics	↓inhalation anesthetic requirements; ↑CNS depressant effects; ↓BP.	Monitor CNS status. Monitor cardiovascular status.
Rifampin	halothane	↑hepatotoxicity	Avoid giving rifampin-isoniazid after halothane anesthesia.
Scopolamine	NMR	High doses of scopolamine may ↑block.	Monitor neuromuscular blockade.
	ketamine	↑HR	Monitor HR.
Sildenafil (Viagra)	nitrates	Severe hypotension	Half-life of 4 h may be prolonged by drug interactions, renal or hepatic impairment; **avoid combination in the elderly.**
Succinylcholine	anticholinesterases	↑block	**Use combination with caution.** Monitor neuromuscular blockade.
	thiopental	Possible disseminated intravascular coagulation	Use large veins. Flush tubing with saline. Wait 2-3 min between administration.
Sympathomimetic amines	doxapram	Potentiation of sympathomimetic amines	Monitor cardiovascular and CNS status.
Tacrine	succinylcholine	Enhanced blockade	Monitor neuromuscular blockade.
Terbutaline	succinylcholine	Enhanced blockade	Monitor neuromuscular blockade.
Tetracycline	NMR or succinylcholine	↑block	Monitor neuromuscular blockade.

Preop Drug Or Drug Class	Anesthetic Drug Or Drug Class	Interaction	Clinical Management
Theophylline	halothane	↑catecholamine-induced dysrhythmias	Use an alternative inhalation agent.
	ketamine	Seizures	**Use combination with caution.**
	NMR	Resistance to blockade	May need ↑dosage of NMR.
	narcotic analgesic	↑narcotic effects	Titrate narcotic.
	midazolam	↓midazolam effectiveness	Titrate dose of midazolam.
	propofol	Antagonize sedation	Titrate dose of propofol.
Thiazide diuretics	NMR	↑block (may be 2° ↓K^+)	Correct hypokalemia. Titrate NMR.
Thiotepa	NMR	↑block	Monitor neuromuscular block.
Tricyclic antidepressants (TCA)	sympathomimetics	↑direct-acting sympathomimetics; ↓indirect-acting agents	Monitor for ↑BP and dysrhythmias. Titrate dosage.
	anticholinesterases	Anticholinergic effects of TCA may ↓anticholinesterase effect.	Titrate dose of anticholinesterase.
	halothane, pancuronium	↑dysrhythmia	Monitor cardiac status.
Trimethaphan	NMR or succinylcholine	↑block	Monitor neuromuscular blockade. Titrate dosage of NMR.
	succinylcholine	↑block	**Avoid combination.** Use NTP instead.
Vancomycin	NMR	↑block	Monitor neuromuscular blockade. Titrate dose of NMR.
	succinylcholine	↑block	Avoid administering vancomycin in the postanesthesia period.
Verapamil	etomidate	↑respiratory depression; apnea	Monitor and support respiratory function.
	midazolam	Deep and prolonged sedation	Monitor CNS and respiratory status.
	NMR	↑block	Titrate dose of NMR.

HERBAL AGENTS	
Plant	**Precautions for Anesthesia and Surgery**
Chaste treeberry	May interfere with dopamine receptor agonists.
Feverfew	May interact with anticoagulants to increase bleeding.
Garlic	May inhibit Plt aggregation. May interact with anticoagulants.
Ginger	May result in a prolonged bleeding time.
Ginkgo	Inhibits Plt aggregation. May cause vasodilation.
Guarana	May cause HTN. May inhibit Plt aggregation.
Hawthorn	High doses may cause hypotension and CNS depression.
Kava Kava	High doses may cause muscle weakness. Potentiates CNS depressants. Analgesic effects not reversed by naloxone.
Ma huang	Contains alkaloids of ephedrine and pseudoephedrine → ↑BP.
Passion flower	May have some MAOI activity.
Pau d'arco	May have anticoagulant effects.
St. John's wort	May have some MAOI activity.
Valerian	Potentially synergistic with opiates and CNS depressants, including thiopental.
Yerba mate	May cause HTN.
Yohimbine	May cause CNS stimulation. May have cardiovascular effects. May have MAOI activity.

APPENDIX G: SPECIAL CONSIDERATIONS FOR LATEX ALLERGY

Cathy R. Lammers and Alvin Hackel

In the last decade, it has been observed that sensitization and subsequent exposure to latex can occur in patients following multiple surgical procedures. Repeated exposure to latex leads to increased risk for IgE-mediated latex allergic reactions and life-threatening anaphylaxis. Patients at risk for latex allergy include those with spina bifida (repeated bladder catheterizations) and those who have had multiple neurologic, orthopedic and urologic procedures. Patients with food allergies to kiwi, banana, avocado and chestnuts have been shown to have cross-reactivity with latex. In these high-risk patients, latex-avoidance protocols are recommended, as this may decrease the incidence of subsequent intraop allergic reactions. Skin-prick tests are available to identify patients with a high titer of IgE to latex, but this is not predictive for the development of an allergic reaction.

The latex content of commonly used materials must be identified from package inserts, external labeling or directly from the manufacturers. Even minimal latex exposure (e.g., a tourniquet, injection of drug through a latex port of iv tubing or opening a package of latex gloves) has resulted in anaphylaxis.

Prophylaxis for latex-sensitive patients:

- Prophylaxis consists of diphenhydramine (0.5 mg/kg), ranitidine (0.5 mg/kg iv), hydrocortisone (1-2 mg/kg iv) q 8 h × 24 h before surgery and 24 h after surgery.
- Consider continuing prophylaxis through the patient's entire hospital admission.
- Prophylaxis is recommended by some authors; however, other studies have demonstrated no difference in incidence of anaphylaxis following prophylactic treatment. Most authors agree that prophylaxis is not indicated in patients who are latex-allergy susceptible but have not yet demonstrated a sensitivity.

To prepare a latex-safe environment:

- Notify OR nurses, anesthesia technicians and surgical staff of the need for a latex-free room.
- Place a sign on the door stating: "LATEX-FREE ROOM."
- Schedule the latex-allergic patient as the first case of the day to minimize the presence of airborne latex particles.
- Set up the room with latex-free materials (e.g., bag, bellows, ECG electrodes, pulse oximeter clip, iv tubing without latex ports, vinyl gloves, vinyl BP cuffs, clear micropore tape).
- Avoid bouffant surgical hair caps and shoe covers that contain latex bands.
- Wrap latex tubing on stethoscope, BP cuff or tourniquet with Webril or cotton gauze.
- Remove rubber stoppers from drug vials (do not withdraw drugs through rubber stoppers).

Diagnosis of anaphylaxis or latex allergy:

- Skin: urticaria at site of contact with latex product or generalized urticaria.
- Respiratory: bronchospasm, wheezing, ↑PIP, ↓O_2 SAT, ↓$ETCO_2$.
- Cardiac: ↓BP, ↑HR, cardiac arrest.

Treatment of anaphylaxis:

- 100% O_2 and manually ventilate if needed.
- Epinephrine 1-3 μg/kg iv and escalate dose as needed to support BP.
- Administer iv fluid to ↑ preload and support BP; may require an epinephrine infusion (0.05-0.1 μg/kg/min).
- Consider isoproterenol infusion if resistant to epinephrine.
- Stop administration of any suspected medications and remove latex products. (Instruct surgical staff to change to nonlatex gloves and remove any latex products from surgical field).
- Administer steroids (hydrocortisone 100 mg iv for adults or 2 mg/kg for pediatric patient) and antihistamine (diphenhydramine 50 mg or 0.5 mg/kg iv).
- Continue steroids and diphenhydramine for 24-48 h or until symptoms resolve.
- Consider drawing blood during reaction to send for tryptase level (mediator released from mast cells during degranulation).
- Refer patient to allergist to follow up on diagnosis. Skin prick test or RAST can be performed (after the acute reaction resolves) to specifically test for latex allergy. Neither test is 100% sensitive.

References

1. Hamann CP, Kick SA: What the practicing urologist should know about latex allergies. *AUA Update Series* 1994; 13:110-15.
2. Hirshman CA: Latex anaphylaxis. *Anesthesiology* 1992; 77:223-24.
3. Holtzman RS: Clinical management of latex-allergic children. *Anesth Analg* 1997; 85(3):529-33.
4. Holtzman RS: Latex allergy: an emerging operating room problem. *Anesth Analg* 1993; 76:635-41.
5. Michael T, Niggemann B, Moers A, Seidel U, Wahn U, Scheffner D: Risk factors for latex allergy in patients with spina bifida. *Clin Exp Allergy* 1996; 26(8):934-39.
6. Pollard RJ, et al: Latex allergy in the operating room: case report and a brief review of the literature. *J Clin Anesth* 1996; 8(2): 161-67.
7. Porri F, Pradal M, Lemiere C, Birnbaum J, Mege JL, Lanteaume A, Charpin D, Vervloet D, Camboulives J: Association between latex sensitization and repeated latex exposure in children. *Anesthesiology* 1997; 86(3):599-602.
8. Rao AM et al: Syringes and latex allergy. *Anaesthesia* 1997; 52(5):506.
9. Spears FD, et al: Anaesthesia for the patient with allergy to latex. *Anasth Intensive Care* 1995; 23(5):623-25.
10. Vassallo SA, et al: Allergic reaction to latex from stopper of a medication vial. *Anesth Analg* 1995; 80(5):1057-58.

APPENDIX H: ACRONYMS AND ABBREVIATIONS

2°: secondary to
A-a: alveolar-arterial
AAA: abdominal aortic aneurysm
ABC: argon beam coagulator
ABG: arterial blood gas
abx: antibiotics
ACE: angiotensin converting enzyme
ACL: anterior cruciate ligament
ACLS: advanced cardiopulmonary life support
ACT: activated clotting time
ACTH: adrenocorticotropic hormone
ADH: antidiuretic hormone (vasopressin)
AF: atrial fibrillation
AH: autonomic hyperreflexia
AI: aortic insufficiency
A-I: anterior-inferior
AICD: automatic implantable cardiac defibrillator
ALCAPA: anomalous left coronary artery from pulmonary artery
ALT: alanine amino transferase (SGPT)
AoE: aortic enlargement
AOVM: angiographically occult vascular malformations
A-P: anterior-posterior
AR: aortic regurgitation
ARDS: adult respiratory distress syndrome
AS: aortic stenosis
ASA: American Society of Anesthesiologists
ASD: atrial septal defect
AST: aspartate amino transferase (SGOT)
ATLS: Advanced Trauma Life-Support System
A-V: atrioventricular
AVM: arteriovenous malformation
AVR: aortic valve replacement
BAEP: brainstem auditory evoked potential
BAER: brainstem auditory evoked response
BB: bronchial blocker
BBS: bilateral breath sounds
BDG: bidirectional Glenn shunt
β-HCG: β-human chorionic gonadotrophin
BMR: basal metabolic rate
BNCU: chemotherapy agent
BOR: branchio-oto-renal syndrome
BP: blood pressure
BPD: bronchopulmonary dysplasia
BPF: bronchopleural fistula
bpm: beats per minute
BRCA: breast cancer gene
BSA: body surface area
BSO: bilateral salpingo-oophorectomy
BT: Blalock-Taussig (operation)
BUN: blood urea nitrogen
BVH: biventricular hyperplasia
Bx: biopsy
C-section: cesarean section
Ca^{++}: calcium
CABG: coronary artery bypass graft(ing)
CAD: coronary artery disease
CAH: congenital adrenal hyperplasia
CAJ: cricoarytenoid joint
CBC: complete blood count
CBF: cerebral blood flow
CCU: coronary care unit
CDDP: combination of chemotherapy
CEA: carotid endarterectomy
CHD: congestive heart disease
CHF: congestive heart failure
CI: cardiac index
CMC: carpometacarpal (joint)
cmH_2O: centimeters of water
$CMRO_2$: cerebral O_2 consumption
CNS: central nervous system
CO: cardiac output
CO_2: carbon dioxide
CoA: coarctation of aorta
COPD: chronic obstructive pulmonary disease
CP: cerebral palsy
CPAP: continuous positive airway pressure
CPB: cardiopulmonary bypass
CPD: citrate-phosphate-dextrose
CPK: creatinine phosphokinase
CPM: continuous passive motion
CPP: cerebral perfusion pressure
CPR: cardiopulmonary resuscitation
CSF: cerebrospinal fluid
CSI: cranial spinal irradiation
CT: computed tomography
CTR: carpal tunnel release
CTS: carpal tunnel syndrome
CUSA: Cavitron ultrasonic aspirator
CVA: cerebrovascular accident
CVP: central venous pressure
CXR: chest x-ray
d: day(s)
D5W: dextrose 5% in water
D&C: dilation & curettage
DBP: diastolic blood pressure
D/C: discontinue
DCR: dacryocystorhinostomy
DDAVP: desmopressin acetate
DHCA: deep hypothermic cardiac arrest
DI: diabetes insipidus
DIC: disseminated intravascular coagulation
DIP: distal interphalangeal (joint)
DJD: degenerative joint disease
dL: deciliter(s)
DL: direct laryngoscopy
DLT: double lumen tube
DM: diabetes mellitus
DOE: dyspnea on exertion
DORV: double outlet right ventricle
DP: dorsalis pedis
DPG: diphosphoglycerate
DSA: digital subtraction angiography
dTC: d-tubocurarine
DVT: deep venous thrombosis
Dx: diagnosis
EA: esophageal atresia
EAC: endoaortic clamp catheter
EACA: epsilon aminocaproic acid
EARC: endoaortic return cannula
EB: epidermolysis bullosa
EBL: estimated blood loss
EBV: estimated blood volume
EC-IC: extracranial-intracranial
ECG: electrocardiogram
ECHO: echocardiogram
ECMO: extracorporeal membrane oxygenation
ECT: electroconvulsive therapy
EDAS: encephaloduro-arteriosynangiosis
EEA: end-to-end anastomosis
EF: ejection fraction
EJ: external jugular
EMG: electromyogram
EMLA: eutectic mixture of local anesthetic
ENT: ear-nose-throat
EP: evoked potentials
EPS: electrophysiologic studies
EPV: endopulmonary vent
ER: emergency room
ERCP: endoscopic retrograde colangiopancreatography
ERV: expiratory reserve volume
ESC: endocoronary sinus catheter
ESLD: end-stage liver disease

ESRD: end-stage renal disease
ET: endotracheal
$ETCO_2$: end tidal CO_2
ETN_2: end tidal N_2
ETOH: alcohol
ETT: endotracheal tube
EVD: endovascular drain (extraventricular catheter)
FAP: familial adenomatous polyposis
FB: foreign bodies
FDP: flexor digitorum profundus (tendon)
FDS: flexor digitorum superficialis (tendon)
FDT: forced duction test
FEV_1: forced expiratory volume (in 1 sec)
FFP: fresh-frozen plasma
FHR: fetal heart rate
FIGO: International Federation of Gynecologists & Obstetricians
FiO_2: fraction of inspired oxygen
FOB: fiber optic bronchoscopy
FOL: fiber optic laryngoscopy
Fr: French (size)
FRC: functional residual capacity
FSP: fibrin-split products
FTSG: full-thickness skin graft
FTT: failure to thrive
FVC: forced vital capacity
g: gram(s)
ga: gauge
GA: general anesthesia
GCS: Glasgow coma scale
GERD: gastroesophageal reflux disease
GETA: general endotracheal anesthesia
GFR: glomerular filtration rate
GGTP: liver enzyme
GH: growth hormone
GI: gastrointestinal
GIA: gastrointestinal anastomosis
GnRH: gonadotropin-releasing hormone
GU: genitourinary
h: hour(s)
H&P: history and physical examination
Hb: hemoglobin
Hb/Hct: hemoglobin/hematocrit
HbA: adult hemoglobin
HbF: fetal hemoglobin
HCG: human chorionic gonadotropin
HCO_3: bicarbonate
Hct: hematocrit
HELLP: hemolysis, elevated liver enzymes, and low-platelet count
HFV: high-frequency ventilation
Hg: mercury
HIV: human immune deficiency virus
HLHS: hypoplastic left heart syndrome
HM: hyoid myotomy
Ho:YAG: holmium-yag laser
HPV: hypoxic pulmonary vasoconstrictive (reflex)
HR: heart rate
HSV: highly selective vagotomy
HTN: hypertension
HVA: homovanillic acid
Hx: history
IABP: intraaortic balloon pump
IBD: inflammatory bowel disease
IC: inspiratory capacity
ICP: intracranial pressure
ICU: intensive care unit
IgE: immunoglobin E
IHSS: idiopathic hypertrophic subaortic stenosis
IJ: internal jugular (vein)
im: intramuscular
IMA: internal mammary artery
IMF: intermaxillary fixation
INH: isonicotinic acid (isoniazid)
INR: International Normalized Ratio
IOP: intraocular pressure
IORT: intraoperative radiation therapy
IPPV: intermittent positive pressure ventilation
IRDS: infant respiratory distress syndrome
ISS: injury severity score
IT: iliotibial
ITP: idiopathic thrombocytopenic purpura
iv or IV: intravenous
IVC: inferior vena cava
IVF: *in vitro* fertilization
IVH: intraventricular hemorrhage
IVP: intravenous pyelogram
IVS: intact ventricular septum
J: Joule
JVD: jugular venous distention
K^+: potassium
KCl: potassium chloride
kg: kilogram(s)
LA: left atrium
LAD: left anterior descending
LAE: left atrial enlargement
LAVH: laparoscopy-assisted vaginal hysterectomy
LE: lower extremity
LEEP: loop electrosurgical excision procedure
LFT: liver function test
LGL: Lowen-Ganong-Levine (syndrome)
LH-RH: luteinizing hormone-releasing hormone
LHSV: laparoscopic highly selective vagotomy
LIMA: left internal mammary artery
LINAC: linear accelerator
LMA: laryngeal mask airway
LMG: laser midline glossectomy
LMP: last menstrual period
LP: lingualplasty
LR: lactated Ringer's (solution)
LRD: living related donor
LTA: lidocaine trachial anesthesia
LV: left ventricle/ventricular
LVAD: left ventricular assist device
LVEDP: left ventricular end-diastolic pressure
LVH: left ventricular hypertrophy
LVOT: left ventricular outflow tract
LVOTO: left ventricular outflow tract obstruction
m: meter(s)
M: molar
MAC: monitored anesthesia care
MAGPI: meatal advancement granuloplasty
MAO-B: monoamine oxidase-B
MAOI: monoamine oxidase inhibitor (antidepressant)
MAP: mean arterial pressure
MCA: middle cerebral artery
MCKD: multicystic kidney dysplasia
MEA: multiple endocrine adenopathy
MEP: motor-evoked potential
mEq: milliequivalent
mg: milligram(s)
Mg^{++}: magnesium
$MgSO_4$: magnesium sulfate
MH: malignant hyperthermia
MI: myocardial infarction
μg: microgram(s)
MIF: maximum inspiratory force
min: minute(s)
ml: milliliter(s)
mm: millimeter(s)
$MMEF_{25-75}$: maximum mid-expiratory force
mmHg: millimeters of mercury
mo: month(s)
MOGA: mandibular osteotomy and genioglossal advancement
MR: mitral regurgitation
MS: morphine sulfate
MSRA: methicillin-resistant staphylococcus aureus
MUF: modified ultrafiltration

MUGA: multi-unit gated acquisition (scan)
MUPIT: Martinez Universal Perineal Interstitial Template
MV: minute ventilation
MVA: motor vehicle accident
MVD: microvascular decompression
MVO_2: mixed venous oxygen content
MVP: mitral valve prolapse
N/V: nausea & vomiting
Na^+: sodium
$NaHCO_3$: sodium bicarbonate
NB: nota bene (note well)
Nd:YAG: neodymium-yag laser
NEC: necrotizing enterocolitis
ng: nanogram(s)
NG: nasogastric (tube)
NIBP: noninvasive blood pressure
NICU: neonatal intensive care unit
NLD: nasolacrimal duct
NMB: neuromuscular blocker
NMR: nondepolarizing muscle relaxant
NO: nitric oxide
NPH: neutral protamine Hagedorn (insulin)
npo: nothing per mouth
NS: normal saline (solution)
NSAID: nonsteroid anti-inflammatory drug
NS/LR: normal saline/lactated Ringer's (solution)
NSR: normal sinus rhythm
NTG: nitroglycerin
NTP: nitroprusside
N_2O: nitrous oxide
OA: osteoarthritis
OCR: oculocardiac reflex
OG: orogastric (tube)
OLT: orthotopic liver transplant
OLV: one-lung ventilation
OPLL: ossification of the posterior longitudinal ligament
OR: operating room
ORIF: open reduction and internal fixation
OSA: obstructive sleep apnea
O_2: oxygen
O_2sat: oxygen saturation
PA: pulmonary artery
PACU: post anesthesia care unit
$PaCO_2$: partial pressure of CO_2 (arterial)
PAD: pulmonary artery diastolic
PADP: pulmonary artery diastolic pressure
PaO_2: partial pressure of oxygen (arterial)
PAP: pulmonary artery pressure
PAR: postanesthesia room
PAWP: pulmonary artery wedge pressure
PCA: patient-controlled analgesia
PCEA: patient-controlled epidural analgesia
PCL: posterior cruciate ligament
PCO_2: partial pressure of carbon dioxide
PCV: parietal cell vagotomy
PCWP: pulmonary capillary wedge pressure
PDA: patent ductus arteriosus
PDPH: postdural puncture headache
PE: pulmonary embolus
PEEP: positive end-expiratory pressure breathing
$PetCO_2$: end-tidal CO_2 partial pressure
PFO: patent foramen ovale
PFT: pulmonary function test
PGE: prostaglandin E
PICU: pediatric intensive care unit
PID: pelvic inflammatory disease
PIH: pregnancy-induced hypertension
PIP: peak inspiratory pressure
Plt: platelet
PND: paroxysmal nocturnal dyspnea
po: per mouth
PO_2: partial pressure of oxygen
POC: product of conception
POD: postoperative day
ppm: parts per million
PPV: positive pressure ventilation
pr: per rectum
PRBC: packed red blood cell
prn: as needed
PT: prothrombin time
PTCA: percutaneous transluminal coronary angioplasty
PTT: partial thromboplastin time
PUV: posterior valve ablation
PVC: premature ventricular contraction
PVD: peripheral vascular disease
PVOD: pulmonary vascular occlusive disease
PVR: pulmonary vascular resistance
q: every
qd: every day
Q_P/Q_S: pulmonary-to-systemic flow ratio
QRS: QRS complex of ECG
qs: quantum satis (sufficient quantity)
RA: radial artery
RAD: right axis deviation
RAE: right atrial enlargement
RAST: radioallergosorbent test
RBBB: right bundle branch block
RBC: red blood cell
RCA: right coronary artery
RDS: respiratory distress syndrome
RF: regurgitant factor
RFT: renal function test
RIND: reversible ischemic neurological deficit
RLQ: right lower quadrant
r/o: rule out
ROM: range of motion
ROP: retinopathy of prematurity
RR: respiratory rate
RSD: reflex sympathetic dystrophy
RUE: right upper extremity
RUQ: right upper quadrant
RV: right ventricle
RVE: right ventricular enlargement
RVEDP: right ventricular end-diastolic pressure
RVESV: right ventricular end-systolic volume
RVH: right ventricular hypertrophy
RVOT: right ventricular outflow tract
RVOTO: right ventricular outflow tract obstruction
Rx: treatment
SA: sinoatrial (node)
SAB: subarachnoid block
SBE: subacute bacterial endocarditis
SBO: small-bowel obstruction
SBP: systolic blood pressure
sc: subcutaneous
SCD: sequential compression device
SCFE: slipped capital femoral epiphysis
sec: second(s)
SGOT: serum glutamic-oxaloacetic transaminase
SGPT: serum glutamate pyruvate transaminase
SI: sacroiliac
SIADH: syndrome of inappropriate antidiuretic hormone
SICU: surgical intensive care unit
SLT: single-lumen tube
SMV: superior mesenteric vein
SNP: sodium nitroprusside
SOB: short(ness) of breath
S/P: status post
SpO_2: oxygen saturation measured by pulse oximetry
SSEP: somatosensory evoked potential
SSRI: selective serotonin reuptake inhibitor
SSS: sick sinus syndrome

ST-T: ST-T wave of ECG
STA: superficial temporal artery
STP: sodium thiopental
STSG: split-thickness skin graft
SVC: superior vena cava
S_vO_2: venous O_2 saturation
SVR: systemic vascular resistance
SVT: supraventricular tachycardia
Sx: signs and symptoms
T&C: type and cross-match
T&S: type and screen
T/A: tonsillectomy/adenoidectomy
TAAA: thoracoabdominal aortic aneurysm
TAH: total abdominal hysterectomy
TAPVC: total anomalous pulmonary venous connection
TB: tuberculosis
TBI: total body irradiation
TBSA: total body surface area
TCA: tricyclic antidepressant
TCD: transcranial Doppler
TE: tangential excision
TEA: thromboendarterectomy
TEE: transesophageal echocardiogram(graphy)
TEF: tracheoesophageal fistula
TEG: thromboelectrograph
TGA: transposition of great arteries
TGV: transposition of the great veins
TIA: transient ischemic attack
TID: 3 times per day
TIPS: transjugular intrahepatic portosystemic shunt
TIVA: total intravenous anesthesia
TKO: to keep open
TMJ: temporomandibular joint
TMJD: temporomandibular joint dysfunction
TOF: tetralogy of Fallot, train of force
TPN: total parenteral nutrition
TR: tricuspid regurgitation
TRAM: transverse rectus abdominus muscle (flap)
TSH: thyroid-stimulating hormone
TTP: thrombotic thrombocytopenic purpura
TUMT: transurethral microwave thermotherapy
TUNA: transurethral needle ablation
TUR: transurethral resection
TURP: transurethral resection of the prostate
TUVP: transurethral vaporization of the prostate
TV: tidal volume
TW airway: Tudor-Williams airway
Tx: transplant
U: unit(s)
UA: urinalysis
UAC: umbilical artery catheter
UE: upper extremity
U/O: urine output
UVC: umbilical vein catheter
UPJ: ureteropelvic junction
UPPP: uvulopalatopharyngoplasty
URI: upper respiratory infection
UTI: urinary tract infection
V&A: vagotomy and antrectomy
V&P: vagotomy and pyloroplasty
VA: ventriculoatrial
VAE: venous air embolism
VAT: video-assisted thoracoscopy
VC: vital capacity
Vd: volume of distribution
VF: ventricular fibrillation
VLAP: visual laser ablation of the prostate
VMA: vanillylmandelic acid
VO_2: oxygen consumption
VP: ventriculoperitoneal
V/Q: ventilation-perfusion ratio
VRE: vancomycin-resistant enterococci
VSD: ventricular septal defect
VT: ventricular tachycardia
VUR: vesicoureteral reflux
WBC: white blood cell
WPW: Wolff-Parkinson-White (syndrome)
W/U: work-up
XRT: x-ray therapy
yr: year(s)

SUBJECT INDEX

Note: Page numbers appearing in bold refer to figures.

A

C

D

E

F

G

H

I

J

M

N

O

Q

U